SMALL ANIMAL
Clinical Pharmacology

For Elsevier:
Commissioning Editor: Joyce Rodenhuis
Development Editor: Rita Demetriou-Swanwick
Project Manager: Kerrie-Anne Jarvis
Designer: George Ajayi
Illustrator: David Gardner
Illustrations Manager: Gillian Richards

SMALL ANIMAL Clinical Pharmacology

SECOND EDITION

Edited by

JILL E MADDISON BVSc DipVetClinStud PhD FACVSc MRCVS

Department of Veterinary Clinical Sciences, The Royal Veterinary College, North Mymms, Hertfordshire, UK

STEPHEN W PAGE BSc(Vet) BVSc MVetClinStud MAppSci MACVSc

Advanced Veterinary Therapeutics, Berry, New South Wales, Australia

DAVID B CHURCH BVSc PhD MACVSc ILTM MRCVS

Department of Veterinary Clinical Sciences, The Royal Veterinary College, North Mymms, Hertfordshire, UK

SAUNDERS

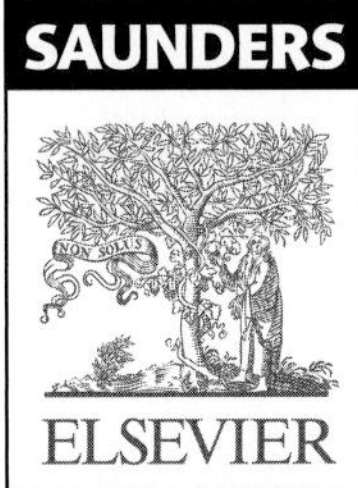

EDINBURGH LONDON NEW YORK OXFORD PHILADELPHIA ST LOUIS SYDNEY TORONTO 2008

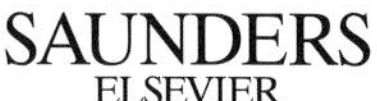

An imprint of Elsevier Limited

First published 2002
Second edition 2008

ISBN: 978 0 7020 2858 8

British Library Cataloguing in Publication Data
A catalogue record for this book is available from the British Library

Library of Congress Cataloging in Publication Data
A catalog record for this book is available from the Library of Congress

Notice

Knowledge and best practice in this field are constantly changing. As new research and experience broaden our knowledge, changes in practice, treatment and drug therapy may become necessary or appropriate. Readers are advised to check the most current information provided (i) on procedures featured or (ii) by the manufacturer of each product to be administered, to verify the recommended dose or formula, the method and duration of administration, and contraindications. It is the responsibility of the practitioner, relying on their own experience and knowledge of the patient, to make diagnoses, to determine dosages and the best treatment for each individual patient, and to take all appropriate safety precautions. To the fullest extent of the law, neither the Publisher nor the Authors assume any liability for any injury and/or damage to persons or property arising out of or related to any use of the material contained in this book.

The Publisher

Printed in China

Contents

Contributors vi
Preface viii
Dedication ix

1 Principles of clinical pharmacology 1
Stephen W Page and Jill E Maddison

2 Clinical pharmacokinetics 27
Jill E Maddison, Stephen W Page and Timothy M Dyke

3 Adverse drug reactions 41
Jill E Maddison and Stephen W Page

4 The pharmacology of the autonomic nervous system 59
Matthias J Kleinz and Ian Spence

5 Anesthetic agents 83
Patricia Pawson and Sandra Forsyth

6 Sedatives 113
Patricia Pawson

7 Behavior-modifying drugs 126
Kersti Seksel

8 Antibacterial drugs 148
Jill E Maddison, A David J Watson and Jonathan Elliott

9 Systemic antifungal therapy 186
Joseph Taboada and Amy M Grooters

10 Antiparasitic drugs 198
Stephen W Page

11 Glucocorticosteroids and antihistamines 261
Michael J Day

12 Immunomodulatory therapy 270
Michael J Day

13 Nonsteroidal anti-inflammatory drugs and chondroprotective agents 287
Peter D Hanson and Jill E Maddison

14 Opioid analgesics 309
Richard Hammond, Macdonald Christie and Anthony Nicholson

15 Cancer chemotherapy 330
Jane M Dobson, Ann E Hohenhaus and Anne E Peaston

16 Anticonvulsant drugs 367
Karen M Vernau and Richard A LeCouteur

17 Drugs used in the management of heart disease and cardiac arrhythmias 380
Sonya G Gordon and Mark D Kittleson

18 Drugs used in the management of respiratory diseases 458
Philip Padrid and David B Church

19 Gastrointestinal drugs 469
Alexander J German, Jill E Maddison and Grant Guilford

20 Drugs used in the management of thyroid and parathyroid disease 498
Boyd Jones and Carmel T Mooney

21 Drugs used in the treatment of disorders of pancreatic function 509
David B Church

22 Drugs used in the treatment of adrenal dysfunction 517
David B Church

23 Drugs and reproduction 528
Philip G A Thomas and Alain Fontbonne

24 Topical dermatological therapy 546
Ralf S Mueller

25 Ocular clinical pharmacology 557
Robin G Stanley

Index 574

Contributors

Macdonald Christie
Royal North Shore Hospital
The University of Sydney
Sydney, NSW, Australia

David B Church
Department of Veterinary Clinical Sciences
The Royal Veterinary College
North Mymms, Hertfordshire, UK

Michael J Day
School of Clinical Veterinary Science
University of Bristol
Langford, Bristol, UK

Jane M Dobson
Department of Veterinary Medicine
University of Cambridge
Cambridge, UK

Timothy M Dyke
Australian Pesticides and Veterinary Medicines Authority
Kingston, ACT, Australia

Jonathan Elliott
The Royal Veterinary College
London, UK

Alain Fontbonne
Ecole Nationale Vétérinaire d'Alfort
Maisons-Alfort, Paris, France

Sandra Forsyth
Institute of Veterinary, Animal and Biomedical Sciences
Massey University
Palmerston North, New Zealand

Alexander J German
Department of Veterinary Clinical Sciences
University of Liverpool Small Animal Hospital
Liverpool, UK

Sonya G Gordon
Department of Small Animal Clinical Science
College of Veterinary Medicine and Biomedical Science
Texas A&M University
College Station, Texas, USA

Amy M Grooters
Department of Veterinary Clinical Sciences
School of Veterinary Medicine
Louisiana State University
Baton Rouge, Louisiana, USA

Grant Guilford
Institute of Veterinary, Animal and Biomedical Sciences
Massey University
Palmerston North, New Zealand

Richard Hammond
Associate Professor of Pharmacology and Anaesthesia
Head of the Division of Surgery
School of Veterinary Medicine and Science
University of Nottingham, Sutton Bonington, Leicestershire, UK

Peter D Hanson
Merial Limited
Duluth, Georgia, USA

Ann E Hohenhaus
The Animal Medical Center
New York, USA

Boyd Jones
Veterinary Sciences Centre
School of Agriculture, Food Science and Veterinary Medicine
University College Dublin
Belfield, Dublin, Ireland

Mark D Kittleson
Department of Medicine and Epidemiology
School of Veterinary Medicine
University of California, Davis
Davis, California, USA

Matthias J Kleinz
Department of Veterinary Basic Sciences
The Royal Veterinary College
London, UK

Richard A LeCouteur
Department of Surgical and Radiological Sciences
School of Veterinary Medicine
University of California, Davis
Davis, California, USA

Jill E Maddison
Department of Veterinary Clinical Sciences
The Royal Veterinary College
North Mymms, Hertfordshire, UK

Carmel T Mooney
University Veterinary Hospital
School of Agriculture, Food Science and Veterinary Medicine
University College Dublin
Belfield, Dublin, Ireland

Ralf S Mueller
Medizinische Kleintierklinik
Ludwig-Maximilians-University
Munich, Germany

Anthony Nicholson
The Jackson Laboratory
Bar Harbor, Maine, USA

Philip Padrid
Chicago, Illinois, USA

Stephen W Page
Advanced Veterinary Therapeutics
Berry, NSW, Australia

Patricia Pawson
Veterinary Clinical Services Unit
Faculty of Veterinary Medicine
University of Glasgow
Glasgow, Scotland, UK

Anne E Peaston
The Jackson Laboratory
Bar Harbor, Maine, USA

Kersti Seksel
Seaforth Veterinary Hospital
Seaforth, NSW, Australia

Ian Spence
Discipline of Pharmacology
School of Medical Sciences
The University of Sydney
Sydney, NSW, Australia

Robin G Stanley
Animal Eye Care
Malvern East, Victoria, Australia

Joseph Taboada
Department of Veterinary Clinical Sciences
School of Veterinary Medicine
Louisiana State University
Baton Rouge, Louisiana, USA

Philip G A Thomas
Queensland Veterinary Specialists
Stafford Heights, Queensland, Australia

Karen M Vernau
Department of Surgical and Radiological Sciences
School of Veterinary Medicine
University of California, Davis
Davis, California, USA

A David J Watson
Glebe, NSW, Australia

Preface

The philosophy and rationale behind the first edition of *Small Animal Clinical Pharmacology* developed out of my experience, as a small animal internal medicine clinician, of teaching pharmacology to undergraduates and subsequently to practitioners. It became clear as I strove to develop a course that would encourage understanding, facilitate deep learning and above all foster student interest and enthusiasm, that pharmacology cannot be taught in isolation from physiology, pathology or clinical medicine otherwise it becomes just a bewildering blur of drug names and doses. The same philosophy and rationale has informed the second edition.

A fundamental understanding of clinical pharmacology is essential for good clinicians. Certainly our clinical mentors impressed upon us the importance of understanding the clinical application, mechanism of action and potential side effects of any drug we prescribed. Similarly, knowledge of the pharmacological action of drugs is meaningless unless one also has a basic understanding of the relevant physiology and pathophysiology of the system or tissue adversely affecting the health or welfare of the patient. Hence our undergraduate and continuing education courses in clinical pharmacology evolved over many years to meet these needs culminating in the particular and perhaps unique approach and format of *Small Animal Clinical Pharmacology*.

The aim of the 2nd edition expands that of the 1st – to provide up to date drug information that is practical and relevant to students and practitioners, and sufficiently comprehensive to increase the reader's understanding of clinical pharmacology without being prescriptive. It is not intended to be a therapeutics or "how to treat" textbook – the drugs, not diseases, are the "stars". Nor is it intended to be a complete pharmacological reference book. The authors of the chapters are all recognized specialists in their field. They have an intimate understanding of how and why drugs are used in their area of clinical specialty and the clinical pharmacological features of the drugs that are relevant to the practicing clinician.

I am indebted to my co-editors, Stephen Page and David Church, who have brought skills to the editing process that have immeasurably enhanced the depth, breadth and quality of *Small Animal Clinical Pharmacology*. They both have expertise that far exceeds my own in many areas of basic and clinical pharmacology even if their interpretation of the meaning of the word "deadline" is somewhat looser than mine and our publishers.

The support and patience of the staff at Elsevier, in particular Joyce Rodenhuis, Rita Demetriou-Swanwick, and Kerrie-Anne Jarvis, have been superb and we extend to them our deepest thanks and appreciation.

I hope that practitioners and veterinary students find the second edition of *Small Animal Clinical Pharmacology* an invaluable addition to the resources they access to increase and deepen their knowledge and understanding of drugs used in veterinary practice.

Jill Maddison
Senior Editor
London, 2007

Dedication

To Tom, Rosalind and Jimmy, who are working on the music for the feature film.

Principles of clinical pharmacology

Stephen W Page and Jill E Maddison

INTRODUCTION

Clinical pharmacology in the veterinary setting is the clinical discipline devoted to the optimal use of drugs in veterinary patients, maximizing their prophylactic or therapeutic benefits while ensuring that the adverse consequences of drug use are minimized. The first principle of clinical pharmacology was recognized and enunciated by the famous Greek physician Hippocrates (460–377 BC), traditionally regarded as the father of medicine: *primum non nocere*, 'above all, do no harm'. Later, Aureolus Paracelsus (1493–1541), a German-Swiss physician and the grandfather of modern pharmacology, stated that 'all things are poisons, for there is nothing without poisonous qualities. It is only the dose that makes a thing a poison.' These seminal observations have been reinforced by the accumulation of centuries of experience, remaining as pertinent and germane today. At the extremes the use of medicines can be either life saving or lethal. Patient outcome can be biased towards benefit by the appropriate application of the principles of clinical pharmacology. It is salutary to recall the words of Arthur Bloomfield, an eminent physician at Stanford University during the first half of the 20th century, that 'there are some patients whom we cannot help; there are none whom we cannot harm.'

Clinical pharmacology, then, is concerned with ensuring that patients receive the right drug at the appropriate dose for the correct duration, with appropriate supervision and surveillance of the response, guiding modification and refinement of the dose regimen as indicated. Figure 1.1 illustrates these important decisions. Both Hippocrates and Paracelsus recognized that the body has an extraordinary ability to heal itself, if given the opportunity. Thus, while drugs can be powerful and effective tools, underlying every decision to treat must be a thorough and accurate diagnosis and the development of a therapeutic plan. The decision to avoid interventions with drug treatment may frequently be as valid and scientifically and clinically sound as the decision to administer drugs. The judgment remains with the clinician in consultation with the client.

The outcome of successful drug treatment may be alleviation of signs or cure of disease. By contrast, the inappropriate use of a drug may result in delay in diagnosis, lack of effective intervention for a life-threatening though curable disease, induction of toxicity, prolongation of disease, development of a disorder that would otherwise not be present, selection for antibiotic resistance, false rejection of a drug wrongfully used and increased cost.

The response of each patient to treatment is an individual event, with the possibility of a high degree of interpatient variability. In determining the correct dosage regimen for an individual patient, it may often be appropriate to use a fixed and predetermined dosage schedule. However, in other cases, particularly in the presence of serious disease, the dosage regimen may need to be individualized to provide an improved balance of benefits and risks. The process of defining the nature of the appropriate individualization is an important function of clinical pharmacology and relies on a thorough knowledge of those characteristics of the patient, the disease and the drug and its dosage form that may lead to variation in clinical response. This chapter introduces key concepts and definitions that underpin the discipline of clinical pharmacology, highlighting major sources of clinical variability and summarizing the principal responsibilities of veterinarians in prescribing and dispensing drugs.

DEFINITIONS

- **Pharmacology** is the study of the properties of drugs and all aspects of their interaction with living organisms. Drugs include any chemical agent (other than food) used in the treatment, cure, prevention or diagnosis of disease or the control of physiological processes. The science of pharmacology draws on the knowledge and methods of many allied clinical and nonclinical disciplines, including chemistry, biochemistry, biology, physiology, pathology and medicine.
- **Clinical pharmacology** is a subset of the broad study of pharmacology and is devoted to the study of the clinical effects of drugs on patients with a goal of optimizing therapeutic dosage regimens. Knowledge of the pharmacokinetic and pharmacodynamic properties of drugs and their toxic effects is inherent in this discipline.

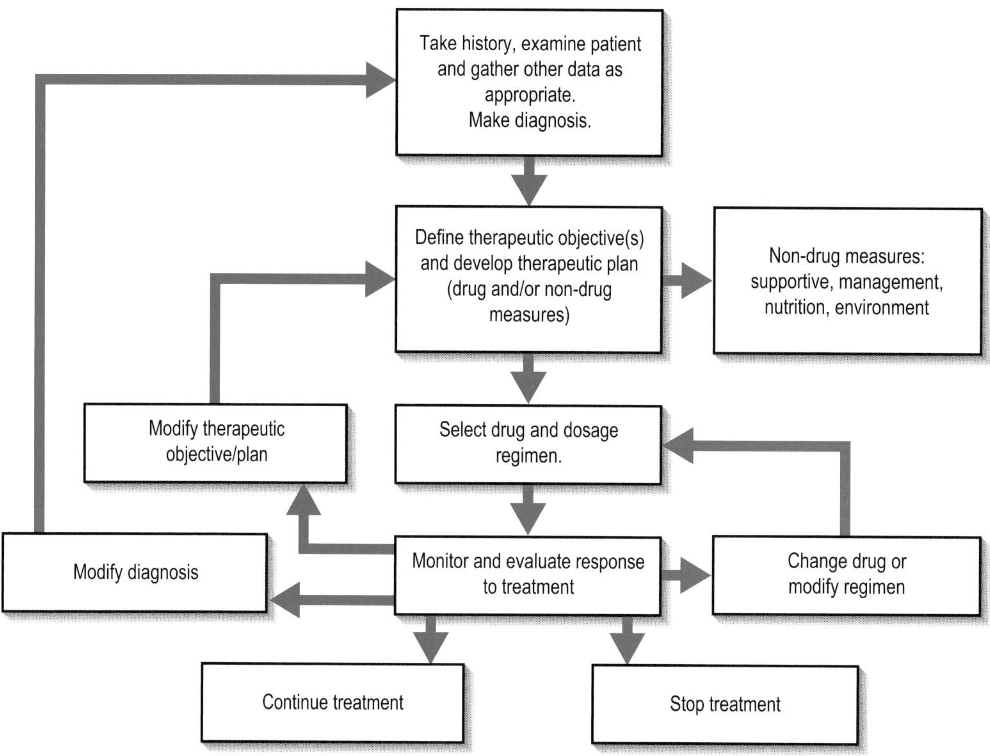

Fig. 1.1 **Steps in the initiation, management and reassessment of drug therapy.**

- **Pharmacokinetics** is the study of the characteristics of the time course and extent of drug exposure in individuals and populations and deals with the absorption, distribution, metabolism and excretion (ADME) of drugs. Pharmacokinetics has been described as 'what the body does to the drug'. Important pharmacokinetic terms are briefly described below and are discussed more comprehensively in Chapter 2.
  - *Volume of distribution* (V) is the constant that relates the amount of drug in the body (A) to the plasma drug concentration (C) (i.e. $V = A/C$), but does not necessarily correspond to any actual anatomic volume or compartment. V is a characteristic of a drug rather than of the biological system, although it may change in the presence of disease, pregnancy, obesity and other states. By knowing the value of V, it is possible to calculate the dose necessary to obtain a target plasma concentration (i.e. $A = V \cdot C$), which corresponds to the loading dose. The greater the volume of distribution of a drug, the higher the dose necessary to achieve a desired concentration. Amongst the antibibacterial drugs, β-lactams are ionized at physiological pH and generally have a low V, while macrolides are concentrated in cells and have a high V.
  - *Clearance* (Cl) describes the efficiency of irreversible elimination of a drug from the body (principally by the major organs of biotransformation and elimination, the liver and kidney) and is defined as the volume of blood cleared of drug per unit time. Clearance determines the maintenance dose rate required to achieve a target plasma concentration at steady state, as at steady state there is an equilibrium whereby the rate of drug elimination is matched by the rate and extent of drug absorption.
  - *First-pass effect* is a type of drug clearance and defined as the extent to which an enterally administered drug is removed prior to reaching the systemic circulation by prehepatic and hepatic metabolism. First-pass effects are important as a possible source of variability in clinical response to a drug and in explaining a component of the difference in response between parenteral and enteral administration of the same drug.
  - *Half-life* ($t_{1/2}$): is the time taken for the amount of drug in the body (or the plasma concentration) to fall by half. In most cases it is the *elimination*

half-life that is referred to, to distinguish it from the *absorption half-life*, a parameter that describes the rate of drug absorption and increase in plasma concentration. Half-life is a function of *V* and *Cl* ($t_{1/2} = 0.693\ V/Cl$) and frequently determines the duration of action after a single dose of a drug, the time taken to reach steady state with repeated dosing (generally 3–5 half-lives) and the dosing frequency required to avoid large fluctuations in peak and trough plasma concentration during the dosing interval (dosing at intervals of one half-life will lead to plasma concentrations covering a twofold range).

- T_{max} represents the time after dosing at which the maximum plasma concentration is observed and indicates the time at which the rate of absorption equals the rate of dissipation (distribution and elimination).
- C_{max} represents the maximum concentration of the drug observed (or calculated) in plasma after administration and occurs at T_{max}.
- *Area under the curve* (AUC) is the area integrated below the plasma concentration versus time curve and is a measure of the extent of drug absorption.
- *Bioavailability* (*F*) is defined as the rate and extent to which the active constituent or active moiety of a drug is absorbed from a drug product and reaches the circulation. For systemically active drugs, absolute (100%) bioavailability is assigned to intravenously administered drug (unless the drug is likely to precipitate in blood). The bioavailability of alternative formulations of the same drug administered by other routes is compared to that of the IV route. In this case relative bioavailability is assessed by determining the AUC and comparing it to the AUC following IV administration. For nonsystemically active drugs, bioavailability is frequently determined by non-pharmacokinetic means, often by comparing the time course and degree of clinical response or effect of a test drug with a standard (or reference) drug preparation.
- *Bioequivalence* is a clinical term referring to formulations of a drug with rates and extents of absorption that are sufficiently similar that there are not likely to be any clinically important differences with respect to either efficacy or safety. In order to demonstrate bioequivalence for systemically active drugs, a comparative pharmacokinetic study is generally undertaken and the similarity (defined by statistical and biological criteria) of C_{max} and AUC of the formulations is assessed. For drugs not acting systemically, comparisons of clinical or other pharmacological endpoints may be necessary.

- **Pharmacodynamics** is the study of the biochemical and physiological effects of drugs, their modes of action and the relationship between drug concentration and effect. Pharmacodynamics has been described as 'what the drug does to the body'. An understanding of pharmacodynamics forms the foundation of rational therapeutic drug use and provides insights into improved dosage regimens and possible drug interactions as well as the design of new drugs.

HOW DRUGS WORK

Drug action = initial consequence of drug–receptor combination
Drug effect = biochemical and physiological changes that occur as a consequence of drug action

Structure-dependent drug action

The actions of the majority of drugs are intimately related to their three-dimensional chemical structure. Seemingly minor alterations to a drug molecule can result in major changes in pharmacological properties. This can be exploited to develop drugs with a more favorable therapeutic index, fewer side effects or a shorter or longer duration of action. As an example, chemical modification of the penicillins and cefalosporins has led to the availability of many new groups or generations of antibacterial agents with differing pharmacokinetic (orally active, broader distribution, longer acting) and microbiological (broader spectrum, β-lactamase resistant) characteristics, overcoming many of the limitations of the originally isolated substances.

The actions of drugs on receptors that lead to responses are governed by the same factors that influence the rate and direction of chemical or biochemical reactions, i.e.:

- temperature (although this is usually kept within tight limits in homeotherms but may be modified during episodes of fever or hypothermia)
- the concentration of each reactant (including cofactors)
- catalysts (enzymes that activate drug precursors).

In addition, there are biological processes that tend to reduce the concentration of a drug at the site of action, including concentration gradients affected by local blood flow, degradative enzymes, cell uptake mechanisms and changes in the characteristics of the receptors (allosteric changes, for example).

Structural nonspecificity

A few drugs share the ability to accumulate in certain cells because of a shared physicochemical property rather than a specific chemical structure. For example, one of the theories of the mode of action of volatile anesthetics relates to the oil–water partition coefficients: the more lipid soluble a gas, the more potent. Also, anesthetic compounds have diverse structures, suggesting that biophysical rather than specific receptor-mediated mechanisms of action may be important.

Other examples of physicochemical actions include:

- adsorbents bind toxins or poisons nonspecifically in gut, rendering them biologically unavailable, e.g. activated charcoal
- oily laxatives work partly because of their lubricant properties
- osmotic diuretics, e.g. mannitol.

Noncellular mechanisms of drug action

Drug reactions may occur extracellularly and involve noncellular constituents.

- **Physical effects**, e.g. protective, adsorbent and lubricant properties of agents applied to the skin.
- **Chemical reactions**, e.g. neutralization of gastric HCl by antacids.
- **Physicochemical mechanisms** may alter the biophysical properties of specific fluids, e.g. surfactants, detergents, antifoaming agents.
- **Modification of the composition of body fluids**. Substances may exert osmotic influence across cellular membranes, e.g. mannitol, poultices, electrolyte solutions, acidifying and alkalinizing salts to alter urine pH.

Cellular mechanisms of drug action

Most responses elicited by drugs occur at the cellular level and involve either functional constituents of the cell or, more commonly, specific biochemical reactions.

- **Physicochemical and biophysical mechanisms**. Some drugs can alter the physicochemical or biophysical characteristics of specific components of the cell, e.g. inhalant anesthetics may affect the lipid matrix of the cell membrane and polymyxins are cationic surface active agents that disrupt membrane phospholipids.
- **Modification of cell membrane structure and function**. Various drugs may influence the structure or function of specific functional components of the cell membrane. Their action may also involve enzyme systems or receptor-mediated reactions. For example:
  - local anesthetics bind to sodium channels in excitable membranes and prevent depolarization
  - calcium channel blockers inhibit entry of calcium into cells
  - insulin facilitates transportation of glucose into cells
  - neurotransmitters increase or decrease sodium ion permeability of excitable membranes.
- **Enzyme inhibition**. Certain drugs exert their effects by inhibiting the activity of specific enzyme systems, either in the host animal or in invading pathogens. This inhibition may be competitive or noncompetitive, reversible or irreversible.
- **Receptor-mediated effects**. Many drugs interact with specific cellular proteins known as receptors. As a result of this interaction, activation or inhibition of a sequence of biochemical events is usually initiated. Receptors may be located on the cell membrane, in the cytosol or in the nucleus. There is usually a close correlation between drug structure and drug activity (see Table 1.1).

DRUG RECEPTORS

Drug–receptor interactions are similar in concept to enzyme reactions. The simplest concept is the analogy of a lock and key (receptor and drug), although receptor and drug structure are not necessarily rigid and may be relatively plastic. The most potent drug at a receptor will 'fit perfectly' and other drugs with similar but nonidentical structure may fit less effectively and therefore be less potent and have no effect, a partial effect or indeed inhibit (antagonize) the interaction of the reference drug.

Within a class of drugs one or more parts of the molecule will be the key in the receptor interaction. Paul Ehrlich, a pioneer of pharmacology, described the essential molecular characteristics responsible for drug–receptor interaction as the pharmacophore. To convey some specificity, receptor pharmacophores generally have multiple spatial and chemical requirements for full effect. Different drugs in that class will have the same key structure but the rest of the structure will be different. This often results in different pharmacological properties such as potency, duration of action, absorption, protein binding, metabolism and adverse effects.

Drug response may be graded (continuous) or quantal (present or absent). Examples of quantal drug responses include prevention of seizures, prevention of death, induction of parturition. They require a group of animals for study. Graded responses, e.g. changes in blood pressure, changes in hormone concentrations after therapy, can be studied in an individual though to detect interindividual differences, groups of patients will need investigation.

Drug–receptor binding

Drug–receptor interactions involve all known types of bond: ionic, hydrogen, van der Waals, covalent. Drugs with short duration of action generally have weaker bonds; long-duration or irreversible drug–receptor interactions may have stronger bonds such as covalent. The drug–receptor interaction can be described as follows.

$$\text{Drug } (D) + \text{receptor } (R)\ k_1 \leftrightarrow k_2\ DR \rightarrow \text{effect}$$

k_1 = rate of association

k_2 = rate of dissociation

$$\text{Effect} = \frac{(\text{maximal effect} \times [D])}{(K_\text{d} + [D])}$$

K_d = dissociation constant

= affinity of the drug for the receptor

= k_2/k_1

Effect is half maximal when $[D] = K_\text{d}$.

Describing the drug–receptor interaction

A measurable drug response can be illustrated in a number of ways.

- Dose–response curve (Fig. 1.2)
- Log dose–response curve (Fig. 1.3)
- Lineweaver–Burk plot (linear), which is described by the equation (Fig. 1.4):

$$1/\text{effect} = K_\text{d}/\text{max effect } [\text{D}] + 1/\text{max effect}$$

Several terms are useful when evaluating a drug dose–response curve.

- **Potency** is a measure of the drug concentration required to elicit a particular effect and is related to the distance between the response (y) axis and the ED_{50}. Therefore, a shift to the right means a decrease in potency, a shift to the left an increase in potency (Fig. 1.5).
- The **slope** of the linear part of the dose–response curve indicates the degree to which a change in dose results in a change in effect. The steeper the slope, the greater the change in effect with small increments of dose.
- **Maximum effect** is where the dose–response curve reaches a plateau.

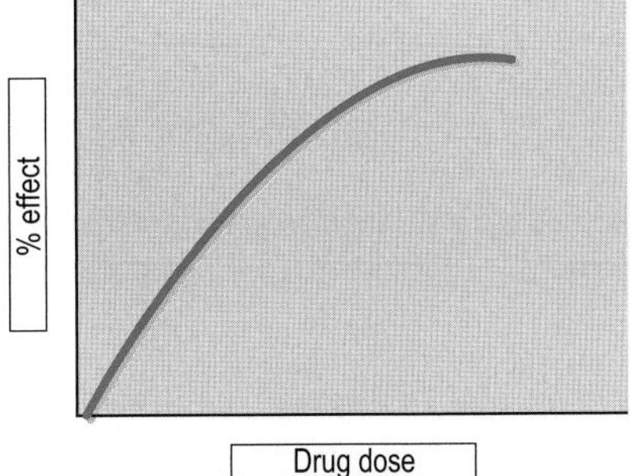

Fig. 1.2 **Dose–response curve.**

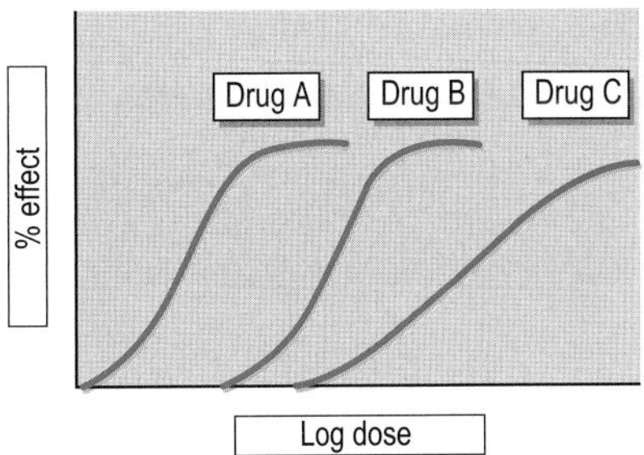

Fig. 1.3 **Log dose–response curve. Drug A is more potent than drug B or drug C. The curves for drugs A and B have the same shape, indicating that they probably interact with the same receptor to achieve the drug effect. Drug A and drug C have different-shaped curves indicating that, although the drugs cause the same effect, they most probably do so through interacting with different receptors.**

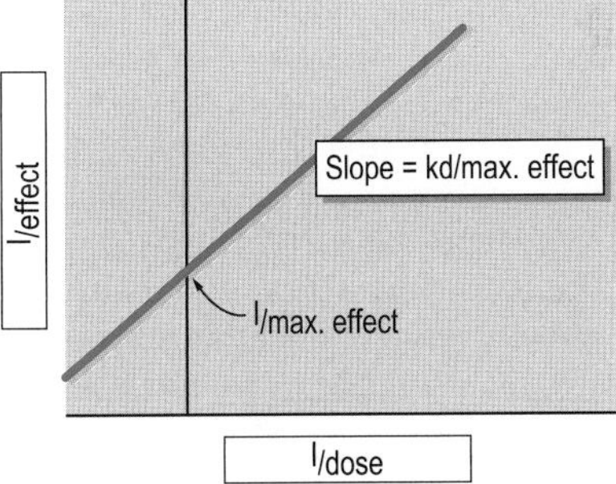

Fig. 1.4 **Lineweaver–Burk plot.**

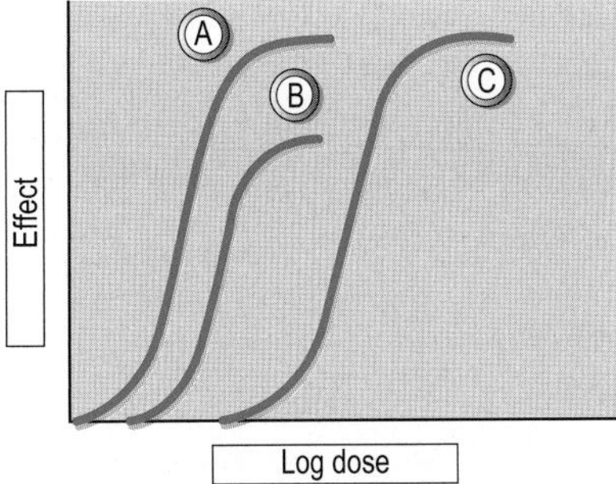

Fig. 1.5 **Log dose–response curves. (A) Log dose–response curve of an agonist (drug X). (B) Log dose–response curve of the agonist, drug X, in the presence of a noncompetitive antagonist or log dose–response curve of a partial agonist (drug Y). (C) Log dose–response curve of the agonist, drug X, in the presence of a competitive antagonist or log dose–response curve of a less potent agonist (drug Z).**

- ED_{50} (50% effective dose) is the dose of drug that produces an effect in 50% of the population (quantal) or causes 50% of maximal effect (graded).
- LD_{50} is the dose that kills 50% of an exposed population.
- The **therapeutic index** is a measure of a drug's safety and is equal to LD_{50}/ED_{50}.
  - The higher the value, the safer the drug.
  - Only valid if ED_{50} and LD_{50} curves (concentration versus effect) are parallel.
  - If the ED_{50} and LD_{50} curves have different shapes, the flatter the LD_{50} curve the safer the drug, as it indicates that, for a given change in concentration, the increase in toxicity is lower than for a steeper curve.
- Indices that consider the steepness of the dose–response curve, for example LD_{25}/ED_{75}, are more useful but are seldom used. One example of use is in defining the selectivity of nonsteroidal anti-inflammatory drugs for COX-2 effects (see Chapter 13).

Agonists and antagonists

- An **agonist** is defined as a drug that combines with a receptor and initiates a sequence of events that lead to a response.
- An **antagonist** interacts with a receptor to inhibit the action of an agonist without initiating any effect itself. Antagonists may be competitive or noncompetitive.
  - The effects of a competitive antagonist can be overcome by increasing the dose of drug; thus the antagonist is acting reversibly at the receptor site.
  - The effect of a noncompetitive antagonist cannot be completely overcome regardless of dose, because of either irreversible binding of antagonist at the receptor or interaction of the antagonist at a site away from the receptor (but to which the agonist doesn't bind) that prevents initiation of effect.
- A **partial agonist** acts at a receptor but produces less than maximal effect. If a partial agonist occupies a significant fraction of the available receptor population, it antagonizes the action of the agonist.

The comparative log dose–response curves for an agonist, the agonist in the presence of an antagonist (competitive and noncompetitive) and a partial agonist are diagrammatically represented in Figure 1.5.

Effect of the drug–receptor interaction

Selectivity and specificity

The selectivity and specificity of the effect of a drug relate to the receptors it interacts with and the distribution of those receptors. A drug may have a widespread effect throughout the body or may have a very localized or specific effect.

Widespread effects occur as a result of several mechanisms.

- A relatively nonspecialized receptor serves a function common to most cells. Therefore, a drug interacting with this type of receptor will have a widespread effect. If this is a vital function, drug exposure is potentially dangerous. For example, cardiac glycosides (digoxin) are potent inhibitors of a fundamental and vital ion transport process common to most cells. Thus cardiac glycosides affect many organs in addition to the target organ (heart) and the therapeutic index is consequently small.
- Even if all effects of a drug are due to a single mechanism of action and the drug is described as selective, it may produce multiple pharmacological effects because of the location of receptors in various organs. For example, atropine affects gut motility, heart rate and salivation, all as a result of the location of muscarinic receptors within these organs.
- Most drugs produce multiple effects, although they are usually described on the basis of their most prominent effect. For example, morphine is described as an opioid analgesic but it also causes respiratory depression, release of antidiuretic hormone and constipation. All these responses are mediated by actions on opiate receptors.
- The effects of nonselective drugs may also result from the drug having several mechanisms of action. For example, phenothiazine tranquilizers produce sedation (increased rate of dopamine turnover in brain), prevent vomiting (depress activation of vomiting center and chemoreceptor trigger zone), prevent morphine-induced excitement in cats (blockade of central dopaminergic receptors), reduce blood pressure (α-adrenergic receptor blockade), have an antispasmodic effect on gut (anticholinergic action) and induce hypothermia (interference with hypothalamic control of temperature regulation).

Selective and specific drug effects may occur through several mechanisms.

- Specialized receptors are unique to specific types of cell. Therefore, the effects of the drug interacting with this type of receptor are more specific. Adverse effects are minimized although toxicity may not be precluded.
- Other drugs are selective by virtue of the route of administration. For example, atropine given by injection has a wide range of effects on gut and other organs. However, if it is administered as an ophthalmic preparation its effect is confined to the eye. Some

antibiotics are poorly absorbed if given by mouth, e.g. neomycin; thus they will have a selective effect on gut bacteria. However, if neomycin is administered parenterally it will gain access to bacterial infections in other tissues, as well as potentially causing systemic toxicity. Intra-articular administration of corticosteroids reduces the systemic effects of the drug while achieving a local effect.

Increasingly, as more is understood about the nature of receptors, it is clear that there are different subtypes of receptor within a given class, each mediating a different response. For example, there are a number of different dopamine receptors, some confined to the central nervous system, others to the cardiovascular system. While dopamine may be the endogenous agonist, through selective structural modifications, drugs have been synthesized that act selectively either as agonists or antagonists at each of the receptor subtypes. A similar approach has been applied to histaminergic, opioid and serotonergic drugs. GABA receptors have several subunits (α, β and γ). GABA receptors throughout the CNS are composed of different combinations of subunits, which affects their function and interaction with different drugs. It is important to recognize the complexity of physiological pathways and their interactions and interdependence. Specificity of drug–receptor interactions may be evident at the molecular level, but loss of apparent specificity of action may be evident as effects at the cellular, tissue and whole organism level are investigated and homeostatic compensatory processes are recruited.

Receptor occupancy

In the classic theory of receptor occupancy, drug effect is proportional to the number of receptors occupied by drug. Maximal effect occurs when all receptors are occupied. There are, however, many exceptions to this where maximal effect can be achieved when only a critical proportion of receptors is occupied, indicating that spare receptors exist.

Other receptors may have multiple drug binding sites (allosteric sites), which may not act independently. Drug attachment at one point may alter the characteristics of agonist– or antagonist–receptor interactions at other locations.

Regulation of receptors

Receptor density and sometimes affinity for agonists and antagonists are dynamic and often influenced by receptor–drug interactions.

- **Downregulation.** Continual stimulation of cells by an agonist may result in a state of desensitization, whereby the concentration of agonist required to produce a certain effect is increased. This may occur, for example, with benzodiazepine therapy. Downregulation of myocardial β-receptors occurs in cardiac failure as a result of increased sympathetic stimulation.
- **Upregulation.** Additional receptors can be synthesized in response to chronic receptor antagonism. When the cell is subsequently exposed to the agonist, more receptors are available, causing a hyperreactive response or supersensitivity.

Signaling mechanisms and drug action

When a drug binds to a receptor it initiates a sequence of events that culminates in the drug effect. How does the message get from a membrane-bound receptor to the site of action within the cell? Several mechanisms have been identified.

- **Induction of synthesis of specific proteins by intracellular receptors that regulate gene expression.** For example, lipid-soluble hormones such as corticosteroids, sex steroids, vitamin D and thyroid hormones are sufficiently lipid soluble to cross plasma membranes. Interactions with intracellular receptors (notably members of the superfamily of nuclear receptors) stimulate transcription of genes by binding to specific DNA sequences. In some cases (e.g. glucocorticoids), once the hormone has bound to the receptor in the cytoplasm, the receptor–ligand complex moves to the nucleus. In other cases (e.g. estrogen and thyroid hormone), the receptor is principally located in the nucleus. As a result of this mechanism these hormones produce their effects after a lag period (30 min to several hours) as their effects depend on regulation of gene expression and protein synthesis. The effects of these agents can persist for hours or days after the agonist concentration has been reduced below the level of detection because new enzymes and proteins that have been synthesized remain active until degraded by normal mechanisms.
- **Regulation of gated ion channels in the plasma membrane.** Drugs may mimic or block actions of endogenous ligands that regulate the flow of ions through transmembrane ion channels. Natural ligands include glutamate, γ-amino butyric acid (GABA) and acetylcholine. For example, barbiturates and benzodiazepines influence chloride ion channel function; local anesthetic agents influence sodium channel function.
- **Regulation of plasma membrane enzymes.** Numerous receptors activate or inhibit plasma membrane enzymes. The primary enzyme affected is adenyl cyclase, which is the enzyme responsible for intracel-

lular production of cyclic adenosine monophosphate (cAMP). cAMP in turn acts within the cytoplasm to stimulate cAMP-dependent protein kinases, which catalyze the phosphorylation of serine hydroxyl groups present within numerous enzymes and other proteins. Guanyl cyclase is activated by specific receptor interactions to synthesize the second messenger, cyclic guanosine monophosphate (cGMP). cGMP is a 'specialist' messenger with established signaling pathways in many cell types, e.g. intestinal mucosa, vascular smooth muscle.

- **Calcium entry into the cell.** Many hormones and neurotransmitters exert their effects by increasing calcium concentration in the cytosol of their target cells. Calcium ions enter across the cell membrane or are released from intracellular storage sites. Calcium enters cells either through selective membrane channels that are membrane potential dependent, membrane potential independent or via sodium/calcium ion exchange.
- **Accumulation of multiple intracellular second messengers.** Receptors for many hormones and neurotransmitters cause accumulation of multiple second messengers. A fundamental event in some of these systems appears to be the receptor-stimulated formation of inositol-1,4,5,-triphosphate (IP3) and diacylglycerol (DAG).
- **Stimulation of plasma membrane-bound protein kinases.** Physiological substrates for these kinases have not all been identified but their phosphorylation is distinctive (from cAMP-mediated phosphorylation) in that it is confined to tyrosine rather than serine.

All these mechanisms are targeted in drug development. Increased understanding of the cellular mechanisms by which drugs work enhances the development of specifically targeted and rational drug treatment. A survey of a number of important receptors and their ligands is presented in Table 1.1.

DRUG NOMENCLATURE

In order to avoid mistaken identification and potential adverse consequences, it is critical that drugs and drug products are uniquely, clearly and unambiguously named. In addition, unique names are important to ensure that in international correspondence it is clear which drug or drug product is studied, described or recommended.

- The **chemical name** describes the precise atomic arrangement of the molecule. The chemical name may be derived from the rules of the International Union of Pure and Applied Chemistry (IUPAC) or the Chemical Abstracts Service (CA).
- The **Chemical Abstracts Registry number (CAS RN)** is a unique reference number, specific for each chemical moiety, with distinct numbers for each salt, hydrate, isomer and racemic form.
- The **nonproprietary** (**common** or **generic**) **name** is assigned at the request of a manufacturer. While an internationally accepted common name is preferred, e.g. the international nonproprietary name (INN), there are a number of bodies that issue such names. Therefore, there can be a United States adopted name (USAN), an Australian approved name, a British adopted name (BAN) and an International Standards Organization name (which may be different in English and in French). The nonproprietary name is usually adopted by and incorporated into the various official drug compendia (e.g. the *United States Pharmacopeia*, USP; the *British Pharmacopoeia*, BP; and the *European Pharmacopoeia*, EP).

Table 1.1 Receptors and ligands

Receptor type	Examples of ligands
G protein-coupled receptors (all members of the GCPR superfamily consist of seven transmembrane α-helices, an extracellular ligand binding site which when activated triggers conformation changes in the associated G protein on the cytoplasmic side of the membrane leading to decreased affinity for its bound guanosine diphosphate [GDP] and replacement with GTP, in turn activating associated effector mechanisms, usually an enzyme or ion channel)	Adenosine receptors (adenosine [agonist], theophylline [antagonist]) Adrenoceptors (adrenaline, noradrenaline, isoprenaline [agonists], phenoxybenzamine, salbutamol [antagonists]) Dopamine receptors (dopamine, apomorphine [agonist], metoclopramide [antagonist]) Histamine receptors (cimetidine [antagonist]) Muscarinic acetylcholine receptors (pilocarpine [agonist]; atropine [antagonist]) Opioid receptors (morphine, buprenorphine [agonists], naltrexone [antagonist]) Prostanoid receptors (misoprostol [agonist]) Serotonin (5-hydroxytryptamine or 5-HT) receptors (ergotamine [agonist], granisetron [5-HT3 antagonist])

Table 1.1 Receptors and ligands (*continued*)

Receptor type	Examples of ligands
Ligand-gated ion channel receptors	GABA receptor (pentobarbitone, diazepam [agonists], flumazenil [antagonist]) Glutamate receptor (ketamine [NMDA subtype antagonist]) Nicotinic receptor (suxamethonium [antagonist])
Tyrosine kinase-associated receptors	Insulin receptor (insulin [agonist], biguanides [sensitizer])
Nuclear receptors	Androgen receptor, glucocorticoid receptor, mineralocorticoid receptor (aldosterone [agonist], spironolactone [antagonist]), estrogen receptor, progesterone receptor, retinoic acid receptor (isotretinoin [RARα agonist]), thyroid hormone receptor, vitamin D receptor
Enzymes	
Oxidoreductases (enzymes catalyzing the transfer of electrons from one molecule [oxidant, hydrogen donor or electron acceptor] to another [reductant, hydrogen acceptor or electron donor])	Cyclo-oxygenase (acetylsalicylic acid [COX-1 inhibitor], meloxicam [COX-2 inhibitor]) Dihydrofolate reductase (methotrexate [inhibitor]) Iodothyronine-5′ deiodinase (propylthiouracil [inhibitor]) Lanosterol demethylase (azole antifungals [inhibitor]) Lipoxygenase (tepoxalin [inhibitor]) Monoamine oxidase (MAO) (selegiline [inhibitor]) Xanthine oxidase (allopurinol [inhibitor])
Transferases (enzymes catalyzing the transfer of a function group [for example, methyl, phosphate] from one molecule [donor] to another [acceptor])	DNA polymerase (aciclovir [inhibitor]) GABA transaminase (valproic acid [inhibitor]) Peptidyl transferase (bacterial) (chloramphenicol [inhibitor]) Reverse transcriptase (zidovudine [inhibitor]) Tyrosine kinase
Hydrolases (enzymes catalyzing the hydrolysis of a chemical bond)	Angiotensin-converting enzyme (captopril [ACE inhibitor]) β-Lactamase (bacterial) (clavulanic acid [inhibitor]) Esterase (acetylcholine esterase) (organophosphates [inhibitors]) Phosphodiesterase (caffeine [inhibitor])
Lyases (enzymes catalyzing the breaking of chemical bonds by processes other than hydrolysis and oxidation)	Carbonic anhydrase (acetazolamide [inhibitor]) Ornithine decarboxylase (eflornithine [inhibitor])
Isomerases (enzymes catalyzing the interconversion of isomers)	DNA gyrase (bacterial) (fluoroquinolones [inhibitor]) Topoisomerase II (etoposide [inhibitor]) Δ8,7 isomerase (fungal) (amorolfin [inhibitor])
Ligases (enzymes catalyzing formation of new molecule from two separate molecules)	Thymidylate synthase (fungal and mammal) (fluorouracil [inhibitor]) Phosphofructokinase (protozoal) (meglumine antimonate [inhibitor]) 1,3-β-d-glucan synthase (fungi) (caspofungin [inhibitor])
Ion channels	
Calcium (Ca^{2+}) channels	L-type channels (diltiazem, verapamil [inhibitors])
Sodium (Na^{+}) channels	Epithelial Na^{+} channels (bupivacaine, lidocaine [inhibitors]) Voltage-gated Na^{+} channels (carbamazepine, phenytoin [inhibitors])
Potassium (K^{+}) channels	Epithelial K^{+} channel (minoxidil [opener], sulfonylureas [inhibitor])
Chloride (Cl^{-}) channels	Mast cell Cl^{-} channel (cromolyn sodium [inhibitor])
Transport proteins	
Cation-chloride cotransporter (CCC) family	Thiazide-sensitive NaCl symporter (thiazide diuretics [inhibitor]) Bumetanide-sensitive NaCl/KCl symporters (furosemide [inhibitor])
Proton pumps	Omeprazole [inhibitor]
H^{+}/K^{+}-ATPase	Cardiac glycosides [inhibitors]
Neurotransmitter/Na^{+} symporter (NSS) family	Serotonin/Na^{+} symporter, dopamine/Na^{+} symporter (tricyclic antidepressants [inhibitors])
Nucleic acids	DNA and RNA alkylation (chlorambucil, cyclophosphamide) DNA intra-strand stabilization (cis-platin)
Ribosomes	30S subunit (bacterial) (aminoglycosides, doxycycline [inhibitors]) 50S subunit (bacterial) (chloramphenicol, clindamycin, macrolides [inhibitors])

- **Proprietary** or **trade names** are usually specific to a particular manufacturer and protected as trademarks. They more frequently apply to a drug product. One particular drug may be incorporated into a number of different drug products that have a multitude of trade names. As set out below in sections describing intraspecies sources of variability, dosage forms that are not identical can not uncommonly be significant sources of variation in pharmacological and clinical response.

EXAMPLE

Proprietary name:	Rapifen®, Alfenta®
Common name:	Alfentanil hydrochloride
Chemical name:	N-(1-(2-(4-ethyl-4,5-dihydro-5-oxo-1H-tetrazol-1-yl)ethyl)-4-(methoxymethyl)-4-piperidinyl)-N-phenylpropanamide hydrochloride
CAS RN:	70879-28-6

CLASSIFICATION OF DRUGS

Humans are predisposed to taxonomy and consequently there is no single and unified system of drug classification. Depending on the context, the following classifications may prove useful.

- Chemical structure, e.g. steroids, barbiturates, benzodiazepines, glycosides
- Principal pharmacological effect, e.g. bacteriostatic, diuretic, sedative, anesthetic, analgesic, purgative, antiemetic, anthelmintic, etc.
- Physiological effect, e.g. parasympathomimetic, adrenergic, β-blocker, neuromuscular blocker
- Diagnostic use, e.g. radio-opaque dyes for contrast radiography
- Prophylactic drugs, e.g. diethylcarbamazine for heartworm prophylaxis
- Placebo (Latin: 'I shall please') – pharmacologically inert but psychologically active
- Poisons – recall that Paracelsus stated that 'all drugs are poisons. It is only the dose that makes a drug a poison'

Clearly, one drug may be classed a number of different ways.

SOURCES OF INFORMATION

The field of clinical pharmacology is rapidly expanding and it is important to keep abreast of significant new findings and high-quality objective evidence that may allow refinements of therapeutic regimens. Continuing education is frequently best if a variety of sources of information are sought, particularly a mix of conferences, symposia, meetings, discussions and journal subscriptions. Some of the key written and electronic sources are listed below. However, this list is far from complete and clinicians are strongly encouraged to critically appraise as broad a base of peer-reviewed information as possible that is pertinent to each individual's field of practice.

Journals

There are a large number of journals available to veterinarians. Those that have a particular and regular focus on rational veterinary therapeutics and provide reviews pertinent to clinical pharmacology include:

- Acta Veterinaria Scandinavica
- Annales de Recherche Veterinaire
- Compendium of Continuing Education for the Practicing Veterinarian
- Journal of the American Veterinary Medical Association
- Journal of Veterinary Internal Medicine
- Journal of Veterinary Pharmacology and Therapeutics
- Veterinary Clinics of North America: Small Animal Practice
- Veterinary Medicine
- Veterinary Record.

Valuable background information from the human medical arena is frequently found in the following medical journals:

- British Medical Journal
- Clinical Pharmacokinetics
- Drug Information Journal.
- Journal of Clinical Pharmacology
- New England Journal of Medicine
- The Lancet.

Texts

- Adams HR (ed) 2001 Veterinary pharmacology and therapeutics, 8th edn. Iowa State University Press, Ames, IA.
- Bonagura J, Kirk R (ed) 1992/1995/2000 Kirk's current veterinary therapy, XI, XII and XIII. WB Saunders, Philadelphia, PA.
- Brunton LL, Lazo JS, Parker KL (eds) 2005 Goodman and Gilman's the pharmacological basis of therapeutics, 11th edn. McGraw-Hill, New York.
- Gibaldi M (ed) 1991 Biopharmaceutics and clinical pharmacokinetics, 4th edn. Lea and Febiger, Philadelphia, PA.

- Hardee GE, Baggot JD (eds) 1998 Development and formulation of veterinary dosage forms, 2nd edn. Marcel Dekker, New York.
- Katzung BG (ed) 2007 Basic and clinical pharmacology, 10th edn. Lange Medical Books/McGraw-Hill, New York.

Drug compendia

- Bishop Y (ed) The veterinary formulary, 6th edn. Pharmaceutical Press, London.
- British pharmacopoeia (BP) and supplements. Stationery Office, London.
- Compendium of data sheets for animal medicines. Data sheets on products available in the UK, updated annually and available from the National Office of Animal Health at noah@noah.co.uk and online at www.noah.co.uk/.
- Compendium of veterinary products (CVP), 6th edn. North American Compendiums, Port Huron, MI, 2001.
- Index of veterinary specialities (IVS). Updated annually and available in Australian, New Zealand and South African editions from MIMS at www.mims.com.au.
- Sweetman SC (ed) 2006 Martindale. The complete drug reference, 35th edn. Pharmaceutical Press, London.
- National formulary (NF).
- Plumb DC 2005 Veterinary drug handbook, 5th edn. Blackwell Publishing Professional, Ames, IA.
- United States pharmacopeia (USP).

Websites

Online journals

Many veterinary and medical journals are available online, but usually only to subscribers. Access is frequently available to students via university library electronic catalogs.

Medical and veterinary databases

- PubMed: database of the US National Library of Medicine – free search service that provides access to more than 16 million citations in MEDLINE, PreMEDLINE and other related databases, with links to participating online journals. www.ncbi.nlm.nih.gov/entrez/query.fcgi
- CAB Abstracts: subscription-only database that provides access to more than 150 veterinary journals, as well as many medical publications.

Regulatory sites

The websites set out in Table 1.2 focus principally on guidelines for establishing the efficacy and safety of veterinary drugs as well as postmarketing pharmacovigilance and other regulatory information. At some of the sites (CVM, EMEA, ACVM and APVMA), summaries of product approvals are available, which contain useful information on the results of clinical studies. At the APVMA and CVM sites there are summaries of reported suspected adverse drug events.

FACTORS THAT MODIFY DRUG EFFECTS AND DOSAGE

There are many factors that can affect the pharmacological response to the administration of a particular intended dose of drug. The most important of these factors are summarized in Figure 1.6. Recognition of these sources of variation allows the prescriber to intervene and ensure that the source of variation is minimized (e.g. compliance can be improved), controlled (e.g. a standard dosage form can be used) or eliminated (e.g. concomitant drug administration can be stopped). For those sources of variation that cannot be controlled by the clinician (e.g. presence of organ dysfunction due to disease or a patient with a genotype with a metabolic

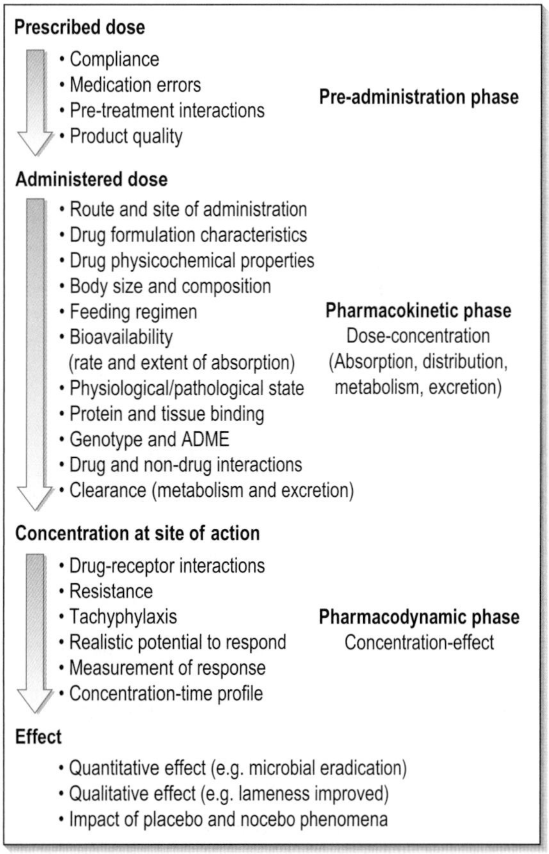

Prescribed dose

- Compliance
- Medication errors
- Pre-treatment interactions
- Product quality

Pre-administration phase

Administered dose

- Route and site of administration
- Drug formulation characteristics
- Drug physicochemical properties
- Body size and composition
- Feeding regimen
- Bioavailability (rate and extent of absorption)
- Physiological/pathological state
- Protein and tissue binding
- Genotype and ADME
- Drug and non-drug interactions
- Clearance (metabolism and excretion)

Pharmacokinetic phase
Dose-concentration
(Absorption, distribution, metabolism, excretion)

Concentration at site of action

- Drug-receptor interactions
- Resistance
- Tachyphylaxis
- Realistic potential to respond
- Measurement of response
- Concentration-time profile

Pharmacodynamic phase
Concentration-effect

Effect

- Quantitative effect (e.g. microbial eradication)
- Qualitative effect (e.g. lameness improved)
- Impact of placebo and nocebo phenomena

Fig. 1.6 **Factors influencing the relationship between dose and effect.**

Table 1.2 Regulatory websites

Country / region	Website address	Description
Australia	www.apvma.gov.au/	Veterinary medicines must be approved by the Australian Pesticides and Veterinary Medicines Authority. This website contains information on all approved small animal products and their labels as well as summaries of ADRs
Canada	www.hc-sc.gc.ca/dhp-mps/vet/index_e.html	Veterinary Drugs Directorate (VDD) site includes information on regulations and adverse drug reactions and antimicrobial resistance
Europe	www.emea.europa.en/index/indexv1.htm	European Medicines Evaluation Agency (EMEA). Information on veterinary medicines, guidelines, European Public Assessment Reports (EPARs) and pharmacovigilance
International	http://vichsec.org/	VICH International Co-operation on Harmonization of Technical Requirements for Registration of Veterinary Medicinal Products. This website provides efficacy and pharmacovigilance guidelines
New Zealand	www.nzfsa.govt.nz/acvm/	The Agricultural Compounds and Veterinary Medicines (ACVM) Group is responsible for registration of veterinary medicines. The site contains information on all approved products and copies of many labels
South Africa	www.nda.agric.za/act36/main.htm	Act 36 (Fertilizers, Farm Feeds, Agricultural Remedies and Stock Remedies Act, 1947) applies to over-the-counter products. This site contains information on the reporting of adverse drug reactions
South Africa	www.mccza.com	Act 101 applies to veterinary prescription medicines and is administered by the Medicines Control Council
United Kingdom	www.vmd.gov.uk	The Veterinary Medicines Directorate is an Executive Agency of the Department for Environment, Food and Rural Affairs (DEFRA). This site contains information on legislation, ADRs, Veterinary Medicines Regulations 2005, and many useful links
United Kingdom	www.noah.co.uk/	National Office of Animal Health (NOAH). The site contains access to an online compendium of approved products
United Kingdom	www.rcvs.org.uk	Royal College of Veterinary Surgeons. Guide to Professional Conduct, including 'The Use of Veterinary Medicinal Products'
USA	www.fda.gov/cvm	The Center for Veterinary Medicine (CVM) regulates the manufacture and distribution of drugs that will be given to animals. This site contains a database of all approved products (Green Book), information on ADRs as well as FOI summaries
USA	www.aphis.usda.gov/	The US Department of Agriculture regulates animal vaccines and bacterins
USA	www.epa.gov/pesticides/	The US Environmental Protection Agency regulates topically applied external parasiticides

idiosyncrasy) the dose regimen can be modified in an attempt to accommodate the particular patient characteristics. The following paragraphs provide further information on the many important sources of variation that can exist both between and within patients.

Drug and dosage form

In the development of dosage forms there are many factors that must be standardized in order to ensure that the biological availability of the active constituent is both predictable and reproducible. The following physicochemical and formulation-induced factors have been described as sources of potential bio-inequivalence between products.

- **Amorphous state.** Drugs that exist in a random solid structure (i.e. they are amorphous) generally have increased solubility compared with their crystalline counterparts and are associated with increased bioavailability. Drugs that can be present in either form include chloramphenicol, fluprednisolone and zinc insulin.
- **Polymorphous state.** Some drugs can exist in more than one crystalline state, each having different solubility and bioavailability. Examples include mebendazole and methylprednisolone. It is of particular importance that the drug does not change from one state to another during storage, as this will result in an unpredictable and significant variation in bioavailability.

- **Solvated state.** Crystal solvates are substances that contain a solvent as a defined part of their lattice network structure. Crystal hydrates include the most commonly encountered examples. There are significant differences in stability, solubility and bioavailability between solvated and solvent-free crystals. Drugs that can exist in either state are numerous and include ampicillin, amoxicillin, phenobarbital, theophylline, prednisolone and morphine.
- **Particle size.** Both particle size and particle size distribution can influence solubility and bioavailability, principally by changes in surface area of the drug. Clinically important examples of active constituents in solid or aqueous dosage forms include mebendazole, digoxin and nitroscanate, the bioavailability of all being increased as particle size is reduced. Penicillin and erythromycin suffer reduced oral bioavailability with reduced particle size as a greater surface area is exposed to acid degradation in the stomach. It should be noted that, for parenterally administered oily suspensions, the converse is observed: the smaller the particle size, the slower the absorption.
- **Salt form.** Salt forms of drugs generally exhibit a higher dissolution rate than the corresponding acid or base and if the rate of absorption is dissolution limited, then salts will provide improved bioavailability. While different salts frequently have similar pharmaceutical characteristics, this is not always the case. The relative order of dissolution rates and plasma C_{max} for penicillin V was potassium salt > calcium salt > free acid > benzathine salt. It should be noted, however, that the stability of different salt forms may vary. For example, the thermal stability of the sodium and potassium salts of penicillin G is superior to that of the procaine salt. The calcium salt of penicillin V is less hygroscopic than the sodium salt.
- **Excipients.** Excipients are the pharmaceutically important but (generally) pharmacologically inactive components of a formulation that in great part determine the physical form, release characteristics and stability of the dosage form. In solid dosage forms excipients function to control the rate of disintegration and dissolution, which may also be influenced by both the compression characteristics of tablets and any special coatings that may be applied (e.g. pH-sensitive enteric coatings). Excipients act as binders (sucrose, methylcellulose), disintegrants, lubricants (magnesium stearate), glidants (talc), wetting agents, adsorbents, buffers, surfactants, micellization agents, solvents, cosolvents, emulsifiers, suspending agents, viscosity enhancers, desiccants, flavor enhancers, coloring agents, antioxidants, preservatives and fillers. While the relative proportions may be constant and controlled within any one defined dosage form, there may be subtle or extreme differences between products, all potentially influencing bioavailability either positively or negatively.
- **Physiological effects.** Depending on both the active constituent and the formulation, there may be significant physiological effects on the recipient of the dosage form. These include pain and tissue damage from injections (intravenous, intra-articular, intramuscular and subcutaneous), skin damage from topical preparations, increased tear production from ophthalmic products, emesis and mucosal irritation from oral dosage forms. All of these physiological effects can impair the bioavailability of the drug and lead to variation in clinical response between and within individuals.

Compliance

There is little published data on patient (client) compliance in veterinary medicine but some guidelines exist from human studies and unpublished work. Studies have shown that a substantial proportion of human patients comply poorly with drug therapies prescribed by physicians. Limited observations suggest that non-compliance is also important in veterinary medicine. In two canine studies, only 27% of owners gave the prescribed number of doses each day during short-term antibiotic treatment. Other reported examples of poor compliance apply to long-term prophylaxis of heartworm with daily or monthly preparations, insulin administration in diabetic patients and chronic administration of behavior-modifying drugs. In one additional case of compliance failure, veterinary support staff withheld postoperative opioid treatment or substituted another analgesic agent in dogs displaying pain because of concern about possible adverse effects.

Errors of compliance include the following.

- **Omission of treatment**, including 'drug holidays'.
- **Incorrect treatment administration**, e.g. oral products given with food when fasting was required or, in dermatological therapy, dipping technique may be inadequate to penetrate the hair or the preparation may be rinsed out of the hair coat instead of being left to dry; dips for scabies may miss the ears and face; shampoos may not be left on long enough.
- **Dosage**: under- or overdosing.
- **Timing or sequence**: for example, a recommendation for morning treatment may not be observed; dosing may be after feeding instead of before feeding.
- **Addition** of medications that were not prescribed.

- **Premature termination** because of apparent control of the disease or the presence of adverse effects.

Factors influencing the thoroughness of compliance include the following.

- **Disease being treated**
  - Seriousness and chronicity
  - Natural history and susceptibility to treatment
  - Rapidity of relapse once medication is stopped
- **Client**
  - Degree of commitment to the wellbeing of the companion animal
  - Language skills and ability to understand the importance of compliance
  - Complexity of daily schedule
  - Respect for and trust in the veterinarian
- **Patient (dog or cat)**
  - Acceptance or rejection of medications; brachycephalic breeds and cats may pose particular challenges to oral medication. Palatable dosage forms may improve compliance
- **Veterinarian**
  - Strength of relationship with client
  - Ability to communicate with, motivate and provide encouragement of client
- **Medication**
  - Physical form (taste, odor, size) and ease of administration
  - Frequency of administration
  - Propensity for side effects
  - Influence on the disease being treated, whether specific, supportive, symptomatic or palliative
  - Rapidity of onset of improvement

Compliance can be positively influenced by the following factors.

- **Clinician/client communication.** Clinicians should tailor their style of communication to the client and ensure full understanding of the disease being treated, the prognosis, the expected response to treatment and the nature of any expected side effects, as well as the circumstances that warrant reassessment. Interactive development of a mutually agreeable therapeutic plan with achievable expectations is most likely to succeed. The clinician should provide an environment in which the client feels comfortable about raising any concerns or objections.
- **Written instructions.** Provide precise, simple but thorough and legible instructions, which may include a treatment calendar.
- **Medication.** Select a medication with physical characteristics suitable to the skills of the client and acceptable to the patient. Demonstration of administration technique and observation of the competence of the client in administration will allow appropriate training or adjustment of the plan to be instituted.
- **Dosage regimen.** Frequency of dosage and duration of therapy should be as simple as efficacy, safety and cost considerations permit. The most sophisticated treatment regimen is destined to fail if it cannot be translated into a plan that can be implemented by the client.
- **Follow-up.** At the appropriate time, it can be important to contact the client and assess whether the therapeutic plan is operating as expected.

Undesirable consequences of poor compliance include:

- inadequate response to treatment, depriving the patient and client of potential benefits
- recurrence or relapse of the poorly treated condition
- increased costs caused by continuing need for reassessment and further treatment
- creation of doubt in the mind of the client and the clinician about the effectiveness of the drug
- possible use of an elevated dose rate that increases the likelihood of an adverse effect if compliance is restored
- underdosing which, in addition to being ineffective, may be a strong selection force for antibiotic, arthropod or helminth resistance.

Whenever there is unexpected lack of efficacy or an adverse response, the investigation should include an examination of the likelihood of deficient compliance. A number of studies have shown that owner compliance cannot be readily predicted by the prescribing veterinarian.

Medical and medication errors

It has been estimated that the human toll due to medical management errors exceeds the combined number of deaths and injuries from motor vehicle and air crashes, suicides, falls, poisoning and drowning. While there are a number of important differences between medical and veterinary practice, it should be expected that errors are not uncommon in the veterinary arena. Though half the errors in two large medical studies were related to surgical procedures, complications arising from drug administration were the next largest category.

The psychology of human error has been a fruitful field for psychologists, who have described a combination of active failures and latent conditions frequently associated with breaches in safeguards leading to adverse events.

Active failures can be divided into mistakes, slips and lapses. Mistakes can result from cognitive errors (e.g. failing to verify the existence of a sign of disease) or rule-based errors, incorrectly applying a good rule (oral administration of aspirin on an empty stomach instead of with food or injecting melarsomine into the caudolateral thigh rather than the epaxial musculature) or applying a bad rule. Slips and lapses are defects in unconscious processes and can result from slips of action (illegibly writing amoxicillin, which is then misread as digoxin) or lapses of memory (administering penicillin and forgetting that you have already been advised that the patient is allergic).

Latent conditions are the inevitable consequences of the systems operating to define the work environment. The most notable example is the error-provoking conditions induced by time pressure, understating, fatigue, inadequate equipment and inexperience. Clearly, the combination of latent conditions and active failures is an excellent recipe for error.

While all clinicians will have experienced and recognized errors, it is unfortunate that systematic reporting and analysis is rare to nonexistent. Encouragement of nonpunitive, protected, voluntary incident reporting combined with case review and auditing of diagnoses would help to identify errors and limit their relentless reproduction.

With respect to variability in clinical response to treatment, medical errors should be actively sought and corrected before adjusting therapeutic plans.

Feeding

There are many potential interactions of food and drugs in companion animals; however, the clinical significance of many of these effects is still under investigation. While it is of some importance with short-term dosing, when administering drugs chronically it is a therapeutic goal that the pharmacokinetics (and bioavailability) of the drug remain constant, predictable and reproducible, as this will be reflected in the response of the patient. Differences in feeding regimens may be one source of variation in drug behavior. The degree of variation that is clinically acceptable will depend on:

- the need to exceed a minimum plasma concentration for as long as possible or to attain a maximum plasma concentration (particularly important for antibiotics)
- the therapeutic index of the drug being administered (e.g. the digitalis glycosides, mitotane and many antineoplastic agents have a low therapeutic index and the likelihood of adverse effects can only be reduced by minimizing pharmacokinetic variability)
- the seriousness of the condition being treated.

The interaction of food and drugs is principally manifested as effects on drug absorption, the rate and extent of which can be decreased, delayed, less commonly increased or be unaffected. There are also possible effects of food on drug metabolism. Advantage can be taken of the interaction of food and drugs in minimizing tissue irritation (useful with a number of acidic drugs such as ibuprofen and aspirin) and in reducing the likelihood of toxicity by delaying absorption to produce a reduced C_{max} (e.g. digoxin).

The mechanisms by which food can interact with a drug include effects on the following.

- **Gastric emptying.** Most absorption of orally administered drugs takes place in the small intestine. The rate at which drugs reach the small intestine is dependent on the rate of gastric emptying, which in turn is dependent on the presence or absence of food, meal size, energy content, form of meal (solid or liquid) and particle size distribution. In the fasting state, drugs usually leave the stomach rapidly but exit is dependent on the time of administration in relation to the gastroileal contractile waves of the interdigestive migrating motor complex. Intestinal transit time is relatively constant and little influenced by feeding, but may be affected by disease.
- **Dissolution of dosage forms.** Changes in gastric emptying rate combined with changes in gastric pH induced by food can significantly impact the rate and extent of dosage form disintegration and drug dissolution. Gastric acid promotes the dissolution and absorption of basic drugs and accelerates the degradation of acid-labile compounds. Increased gastric dissolution of carbamazepine and phenytoin will increase the drug available for absorption by the small intestine. By contrast, some drugs (e.g. penicillin G) are susceptible to degradation in low pH environments and, if dosage forms disintegrate and release their drug content, less drug will be available for absorption.
- **Bile acid activity.** The absorption of some insoluble (fenbendazole) or lipid-soluble (griseofulvin and mitotane) drugs can be enhanced by coadministration of a high-fat meal, which increases the biliary output of bile acids. However, with some drugs (e.g. kanamycin and polymyxin) bile salts may form stable complexes, reducing their bioavailability.
- **Pancreatic and intestinal mucosal enzyme activity.** The presystemic metabolism of drugs susceptible to enzymatic biotransformation by pancreatic proteases, lipases and other enzymes can be affected. While prodrugs may be activated and bioavailability increased (particularly with esters of active drugs), many peptide drugs will be inactivated.
- **Splanchnic blood flow.** Splanchnic blood flow increases in response to feeding and a greater proportion of blood flow bypasses the liver, thus allowing drugs subject to first-pass hepatic metabolism (e.g. clomipramine) to avoid this process, with an apparent increase in systemic bioavailability.

- **Barrier to absorptive surfaces.** Food may impose a physical barrier to the dissemination of drugs to mucosal absorptive surfaces. In addition, some food constituents (particularly fiber) can be a site of drug adsorption, effectively reducing the quantity of drug available for absorption.
- **Pharmacologically active food constituents.** While not a usual component of the diet of dogs and cats, in humans the ingestion of Seville oranges, limes or grapefruit juice (which all contain biologically active polyphenolic furanocoumarins) has been reported to inhibit certain cytochrome P450 isoenzymes (particularly CYP3A), leading to increased bioavailability of a number of drugs that otherwise would have been metabolized. Inhibition of CYP has also been reported in humans consuming garlic extracts or St John's wort.

The magnitude of a food–drug interaction is dependent on the following factors.

- **The physicochemical properties of the drug**
  - The main considerations include the pKa and chemical lability of the drug.
  - Nonionized forms of drugs are most readily absorbed and the pH of the milieu in which the drug is absorbed will determine the relative concentrations of ionized and nonionized drug.
  - Acid-labile drugs may benefit (though unpredictably) from coadministration with food, as gastric pH is buffered and elevated to a variable extent.
- **Formulation**
  - Egress from the stomach is quickest for solutions, followed by suspensions, pastes, tablets and capsules.
  - It has been observed that particles of diameter up to 1.6 mm empty more rapidly than the meal, while particles larger than 2.4 mm empty more slowly.
  - The protective barriers provided by enteric-coated tablets may be breached and protection from gastric acid reduced if the dosage form resides for protracted periods in the stomach.
  - Formulations with a density less than unity may have increased residence in the stomach due to buoyancy effects. Experimentally, advantage has been taken of this phenomenon in the design of sustained-release formulations.
- **Type and size of meal**
  - Liquid and low-viscosity meals are associated with rapid gastric emptying and may lead to increased or decreased bioavailability of co-administered drugs, depending on the time necessary for disintegration and dissolution of dosage forms.
  - High-fat meals are followed by increased concentrations of circulating free fatty acids, which bind to albumin and limit the number of binding sites available for acidic drugs. This can lead to increased free drug and more rapid clearance. Notably, fasting is also associated with increased concentrations of free fatty acids from the mobilization of endogenous depots and can lead to the same effect on drugs.
  - In humans, diets high in protein and low in carbohydrate have been associated with increased hepatic mixed function oxidase activity, which led to more rapid clearance of theophylline and propranolol.
  - The bioavailability of a number of drugs (especially the fluoroquinolones and tetracyclines; doxycycline is an exception) is adversely affected by the presence of divalent and trivalent cations, as may be present in dairy products (Ca^{2+}) and antacids (Mg^{2+} and Al^{3+}). Insoluble complexes are formed, resulting in reduced absorption. Dietary milk can elevate gastric pH and accelerate the dissolution of enteric-coated tablets, leading to drug release and possible gastric irritation or drug degradation.
  - A number of studies in dogs have demonstrated a more marked effect on drug availability of dry food than semi-moist canned food, presumably because of a more delayed gastric emptying.
- **Time interval and sequence between eating and drug administration**
  - While the optimum fasting period will depend on the animal, the drug and the meal, for those drugs that may be adversely affected by feeding it is generally recommended that 1–2 hours should elapse between feeding (either before or after) and drug administration.
  - A possible exception is that a greater period may be necessary after feeding when a dry ration is consumed.

Drug interactions

A drug interaction occurs when the effect of one drug is changed by the presence of another drug. The interaction can have positive (e.g. the synergism of co-administered amoxicillin and clavulanic acid) or harmful consequences (as may be associated with the interaction of potassium-depleting diuretics and digoxin). Many possible interactions have been described in both medical and veterinary practice, but a caution has been issued that the data are widely variable in quality and reliability. While some interactions have been critically evaluated under controlled conditions, others 'are no more than speculative and theoretical scaremongering guesswork, hallowed by repeated quotation'.

When studied, the incidence of drug interactions has been found to be much lower than would be anticipated on the basis of the frequency of use of multiple drugs. However, clinicians should always be conscious of the possibility of drug interactions whenever more than one drug is administered, considering both prescribed treatment and concurrent owner-initiated medications. Interactions can be serious, but a critical, objective and investigative mind should be retained, as it is important always to endeavor to determine the cause of any unintended clinical outcomes in order that future prescribing decisions can be modified appropriately.

Interactions may be:

- physicochemical or pharmaceutical, generally interacting prior to administration
- pharmacokinetic, leading to alterations in the absorption, distribution, metabolism or elimination of one drug by another
- pharmacodynamic, whereby one drug affects the action of another drug.

The net outcome of the interaction may be:

- enhancement of the effects of one or other drug
- development of totally new effects not seen when either drug is used alone
- inhibition of effect of one drug by another
- no change in net result despite the pharmacokinetics of one or both drugs being substantially altered.

Mechanisms of interactions

- Direct **chemical** or **physical** interactions, e.g. inactivation and precipitation of penicillin when mixed in the same syringe or infusion set with phenytoin or B complex vitamins. Similarly with carbenicillin and gentamicin.
- Interactions in **gastrointestinal tract** (GIT) **absorption:**
  - physical interactions (tetracyclines or fluoroquinolones given with milk (calcium) or iron; levothyroxine (thyroxine) complexed to coadministered colestyramine)
  - altered GIT motility by one drug (metoclopramide can decrease and propantheline can increase the absorption of digoxin)
  - change in pH by one drug (reduced ketoconazole absorption due to reduced dissolution when administered with antacids or H_2 blockers)
  - alteration in bacterial flora can cause dysbiosis and altered GIT motility; in addition, antimicrobial drugs can eliminate the flora that may be necessary to activate (e.g. sulfasalazine) or inactivate (e.g. digoxin) a drug, leading to decreased and increased bioavailability respectively.
- **Protein binding.** Many drugs bind to plasma proteins. Acidic drugs bind to albumin while basic drugs bind to α_1-acid glycoprotein. Competition between drugs for binding sites depends on the affinity of each drug for the binding sites and drug concentration. Usually only the free (nonbound) portion of the drug is able to exert a pharmacological effect. If the drug is highly protein bound (>95%), even a minor percentage change in the extent of binding will lead to a large change in the concentration of free drug. The free drug is immediately available for distribution and elimination and a new equilibrium of free and bound drug is established, rendering this type of interaction more hypothetical and perceived than real and of clinical importance.
- Interactions at **receptor sites** by:
  - agonist and antagonist will negate an effect, which may be beneficial (organophosphate and pralidoxime, naloxone and morphine, vitamin K and coumarin anticoagulant) or harmful (α_2-adrenoceptor agonist and α_2-adrenoceptor blocker)
  - multiple agonists or antagonists may lead to increased effect (increased likelihood of ototoxicity with concurrent use of aminoglycosides and furosemide (frusemide), potentiation of effects of nondepolarizing muscle relaxants with concurrent use of aminoglycosides).
- Interaction due to **accelerated metabolism** after induction of drug-metabolizing enzymes, especially hepatic (e.g. phenobarbital significantly decreases the half-life of quinidine and digoxin; other enzyme inducers include phenytoin, griseofulvin and carbamazepine).
- **Inhibition of metabolism** by chloramphenicol, phenylbutazone, azole antifungal agents, cimetidine and verapamil can be associated with prolonged action, accumulation and toxicity of concurrent medications that would normally be cleared by hepatic biotransformation.
- Alteration of **renal excretion.** Increased digoxin concentrations have been associated with use of aminoglycosides and consequent renal impairment. Probenecid reduces the renal clearance of penicillin by competitively inhibiting renal tubular secretion.
- Alteration of **urine pH** by alkalinizing agents (sodium bicarbonate and acetazolamide and other carbonic anhydrase inhibitors) or acidifying agents (ascorbic acid or ammonium chloride) can hasten or delay the excretion of drugs. Renal clearance of basic drugs (e.g. amfetamine) is increased in acid urine while clearance of acidic drugs (e.g. aspirin and barbiturates) is enhanced in alkaline urine.

Inter- and intraspecies differences

Between-species differences

It is perhaps surprising that, although dogs and cats have evolved independently, when drug dose rates are scaled according to bodyweight the majority of drugs behave similarly in both species. However, there are a number of notable differences and it is prudent therefore to consider that, in the absence of information to the contrary, each species should be treated as unique.

The principal pharmacological differences between dogs and cats can be classified as pharmacokinetic, pharmacodynamic and behavioral.

Pharmacokinetic differences

While there are differences in enteric and dermal absorption, distribution and elimination, the most notable pharmacological differences are in metabolism. Cats have a slow rate of hepatic phase II glucuronidation, resulting in decreased clearance of drugs that depend on this means of biotransformation prior to elimination. Important clinical examples include the metabolism of acetylsalicylic acid (aspirin) and morphine. While the dose rate of aspirin is the same in the dog and cat (10 mg/kg) as the drug has similar volumes of distribution, the dosage interval to allow maintenance of a therapeutic concentration is 12 hours in the dog and 48 hours in the cat. This reflects the significant differences in half-life of elimination (8.6 hours in the dog and 37.6 hours in the cat) as a result of the reduced clearance and rate of metabolism in the cat.

In contrast to cats, dogs are deficient in hepatic phase II acetylation, reducing the dog's ability to metabolize aromatic amines. This can be beneficial to the dog when treated with sulfonamides, as acetylated metabolites produced in species with active acetylation pathways are less soluble than the parent compound and more likely to precipitate and cause damage in the renal tubules. Alternative metabolic pathways for aromatic amines include glucuronidation and hydroxylation.

Other drugs displaying pharmacokinetic differences include succinylcholine, which is metabolized more slowly in the cat than in the dog, presumably because of reduced blood pseudocholinesterase activity.

Pharmacodynamic differences

Differences between dogs and cats with respect to drug receptor distribution and affinity have been described, with morphine representing the archetypal example. In addition to a slower rate of biotransformation because of the deficiency of glucuronidation in the cat, morphine is associated with CNS stimulation (CNS depression in the dog), centrally mediated emesis at much reduced sensitivity compared to the dog (dog requires dose 1/740 that of cat) and pupillary dilation (miosis in the dog). However, at a dose rate of 0.1 mg/kg subcutaneously (compared with 0.1–2 mg/kg in the dog), morphine provides effective analgesia in the cat.

Other examples of drugs subject to pharmacodynamic differences include xylazine and febantel (which induce emesis much more readily in cats than dogs), digitalis glycosides (the cat is less tolerant than the dog, presumably because of increased sensitivity of feline cardiac Na^+,K^+-ATPase to inhibition) and drugs affecting oxidative processes such as some of the sulfonamides, nitrofurans and sulfones (cat erythrocytes more sensitive to oxidative challenge than those of dogs). The increased sensitivity of cats to the toxic effects of permethrin and chlorpyrifos may also be due to pharmacodynamic differences between cats and dogs.

Behavioral differences

The grooming behavior of cats increases the likelihood that topically applied medications will be ingested. Advantage can be taken of this behavior by applying medications intended for ingestion to accessible parts of the cat's body (e.g. anthelmintic or antibiotic paste preparations). However, cats are at greater risk of exposure to purposefully or adventitiously applied topical toxicants such as disinfectants (particularly phenolics, which are principally candidates for glucuronidation) or pesticides. Indeed, concentrated preparations of permethrin applied topically to cats can be lethal when ingested.

Within-species differences

There are many real and potential factors that influence the clinical pharmacology of a drug within an individual (see Table 1.3).

- **Age**, bounded by the extremes of the pediatric and geriatric patient. In many cases metabolic enzymes have not reached full activity in neonatal animals. The aged frequently have increased pharmacodynamic sensitivity of the cardiovascular and central nervous systems.
- **Sex.** With the exception of the reproductive hormones, surprising little impact of sex has been described to account for within-species differences in drug pharmacology.
- **Disease.** Febrile state; dysfunction of organs of metabolism and excretion; cardiovascular and renal dysfunction affecting water balance and drug distribution; and gastrointestinal disorders affecting drug absorption can all account for significant within-species differences. Adjustment of dosage regimens or avoidance of use of particular drugs may be necessary in patients with particular disease states.
- **Physical state.** Pregnancy, obesity and lean or malnourished states can all have effects on drug distribu-

Table 1.3 Pharmacokinetic variation due to physiology and pathology

Pharma-cokinetic stage	Physiological or pathological condition		
	Neonate	*Pregnancy*	*Pyrexia*
Absorption	Near neutral stomach pH Decreased gastric emptying Increased gut permeability	Increased gastric emptying Decreased intestinal transit time Increased skin perfusion	Decreased feed and water intake Decreased gut motility Fluid diarrhea Blood flow redistribution (from skin and GIT to shivering muscle)
Distribution	Increased total body water Decreased body fat Decreased plasma albumin Decreased blood–brain barrier	Increased plasma volume Increased total body water Increased body fat Decreased plasma albumin	Increased cell permeability Increased α_1 acid glycoprotein Decreased plasma albumin Increased free fatty acids
Metabolism	Decreased gut wall metabolism Decreased hepatic phase I and II activity	Increased hepatic phase I and II activity	Decreased hepatic phase I and II activity
Excretion	Decreased GFR & RPF Decreased tubular secretion Higher urine pH Reduced bile flow	Increased GFR Increased RPF	Decreased GFR Decreased tubular secretion Decreased urine pH

Most observations from dogs. Cat assumed to have similar trend in parameters.

tion. The volume of distribution of highly lipophilic drugs may be dependent on the fat content of the individual treated and higher dose rates may be necessary in the obese. By contrast, dose rates of poorly lipophilic drugs administered to the obese may be better based on estimated lean weight rather than on actual total weight.

- **Mobility.** Sedentary and athletic individuals may experience differences in drug absorption from parenteral sites.
- **Diet.** See discussion above on effects of food on drug absorption.
- **Genetics.** The discipline of pharmacogenetics explores differences between individuals in their response to drugs, including study of the polymorphic nature of metabolic enzyme systems. This is more thoroughly described in the human than in companion animals. Breed effects include:
  - the sensitivity of collies and other related breeds to the CNS toxicity of the avermectins (related to mutations in the genes coding for P-glycoprotein, an important transport protein in brain capillary endothelium)
  - the sensitivity of greyhounds and similar breeds to the actions of many parenteral anesthetics (e.g. the thiobarbiturates and propofol)
  - the apparent predisposition of some Doberman pinschers to adverse effects of the sulfonamides (possibly associated with decreased ability to detoxify hydroxylamine metabolites)
  - breed differences in elimination of naproxen by dogs (elimination half-life of 35 hours in beagles compared with 74 hours in mongrels).
- **Circadian rhythms.** The time of day may influence the effect of drug administration. Diurnal variations in efficacy or toxicity have been reported for the adrenocorticosteroids, methylxanthines and cisplatinum.

PLACEBO EFFECTS

The act of administering a medication may itself elicit a response (beneficial or adverse) that is unrelated to the pharmacodynamics of the drug in question but may be more related to psychologically induced effects. These effects are well described in humans, less so in veterinary practice and can be evaluated by the use of an inert placebo or dummy medication. However, the placebo effect can also be an important and additive component of the response to actual drug administration.

In humans, the placebo effect is thought to result from the motivation for a successful outcome induced by a strong relationship between the doctor and the patient. By contrast, overemphasis of warnings and precautions may encourage a propensity to observe adverse effects, a manifestation of the nocebo effect. Positive motivation may be important when owners evaluate the response of their companion animal to a treatment. However, for reasons that are far from clear, a placebo effect may also be encountered when an objective assessment of clinical improvement is made in dogs or cats receiving a dummy medication.

Placebo effects are unpredictable and can vary significantly between patients and within a patient at different times. It is important that this effect is controlled when undertaking a clinical study to evaluate the efficacy of a treatment in order that one can clearly separate pharmacodynamic and placebo effects. Recognizing the existence and possible benefits of placebo effects, it is good practice to maximize use of the placebo effect to supplement the pharmacological response to treatment, although the effect may not be sustained and may be a source of variability in response with time.

DEVELOPMENT OF NEW ANIMAL DRUGS

In approving new animal drugs, regulatory agencies must first be satisfied with the efficacy, safety and quality of the proposed new product. While each regulatory agency has a unique set of requirements that must be satisfied, common to all is the high quality and integrity of information that is currently demanded and supplied. The development of a new animal drug product is a costly, time-consuming and high-risk exercise. It is estimated that from discovery to marketing of a new chemical entity for a companion animal can take 6–8 years, cost in the order of US$100m and result from the selection of one candidate from thousands originally screened for biological activity.

Clearly, the development of new animal drugs can only be undertaken by large companies with the appropriate competencies, skills and commitment. To lessen the risks associated with investment in drug candidates that will not ultimately meet the stringent requirements of the regulatory agencies or the marketplace, it is critical that developers can clearly identify as early as possible in the development process the limitations of candidate molecules. Successful new animal drugs must satisfy a clinical need and be effective, safe and economically acceptable. Decisions concerning the therapeutic areas to which to devote development resources will consequently require a blend of scientific and commercial considerations. Because of the high costs and the inherent need to achieve a financial return on the investment, many minor therapeutic needs will be left without approved animal drugs for treatment and require the use of alternative remedies, e.g. human drugs.

Much of the high cost of bringing a new animal drug to market is associated with the manufacturing and preclinical (especially toxicity testing) requirements. In many cases this cost can be reduced by selecting for development those compounds already under development or approved for human or agricultural use. Examples of development cost reduction include the development of enrofloxacin (the *N*-ethyl analog of ciprofloxacin) for animals, having previously developed ciprofloxacin for humans; the application of enalapril in dogs, having established its use in humans; the development of imidacloprid and fipronil for dogs and cats, having initially developed these actives for agricultural pest control.

Complete details of the requirements of individual agencies for the approval of new animal drugs can be obtained by consulting the appropriate web addresses provided earlier. A summary of the process from discovery to marketing and beyond is presented below.

Discovery

While new indications for an existing drug may arise from astute observations during treatment of patients for approved indications (e.g. unexpected control of erythema nodosum leprosum noted when thalidomide is used as a soporific in lepers; botulinum toxin type A originally approved for treatment of strabismus and blepharospasm associated with dystonia and found useful for temporary improvement in the appearance of moderate-to-severe glabellar lines associated with corrugator and procerus muscle activity; sildenafil for diabetic gastroparesis arose from astute observations during treatment of patients for erectile dysfunction), the most fruitful area of discovery is the biological screening of new chemical entities (NCEs). NCEs may be derived by chemical synthesis (e.g. fluoroquinolones), by screening of secondary metabolites elicited by fermentation of micro-organisms (cyclosporin, penicillin and ivermectin) or from extracts of plants or animals (digitalis glycosides from foxglove, morphine from poppies, salicylic acid from willow bark, insulin from pancreas).

Recently there has been renewed interest in evaluating the traditional remedies of various indigenous peoples. Compounds such as digoxin, quinine, aspirin and morphine were discovered historically in this way and more recently a number of antimalarial and antineoplastic compounds have been identified in ethnobotanical investigations. Other natural sources of NCEs include the toxins of snakes, spiders and marine organisms, bacterial and fungal metabolic products (including antibiotics, anticoccidials and other pesticides) as well as antibiotic products from insects and amphibians.

Chemical synthesis is often directed by planned three-dimensional structure–activity analysis of known interactions with isolated receptors. The most recent source of NCEs has emerged from the genomic, proteomic, transcriptomic and metabolomic revolutions. By isolating and identifying genes and proteins involved in disease processes (either in the mammalian host or a pathogen) it is possible (in theory) to identify receptors and pharmacophores and use them to guide development of novel agonists or antagonists that may serve important therapeutic roles.

In vitro broad-spectrum high-throughput screens have been developed to quickly characterize the biological activity of NCEs, identifying propensity for tissue toxicity as well as therapeutic activity. Any compound with interesting biological activity (satisfactory selectivity arising from low toxicity combined with therapeutic activity at low dose rate) may be targeted for further study.

Research

Promising candidates will be subject to additional studies to more completely characterize their safety, efficacy and pharmacology, generally in laboratory animals (mice, rats and dogs). In addition, assessments are made of the routes and costs of synthesis (or fermentation if appropriate) and early formulation studies are undertaken. Those candidates that continue to show therapeutic and financial promise may be patented and move to the next stage.

Development

Formal development plans are designed to satisfy all regulatory requirements prevailing in those countries in which it is intended to market the drug. The methods of designing, conducting, analyzing and reporting studies together with the responsibilities of those involved have been described in codes of Good Clinical Practice (GCP), Good Laboratory Practice (GLP) and Good Manufacturing Practice (GMP). Specific details of these codes can be accessed via the regulatory web addresses provided earlier. The areas of particular interest in the development of a new animal drug include the following.

- **Efficacy.** Studies are undertaken in the target species to determine the effective dose rate or range and regimen to achieve acceptable efficacy for the selected indication(s). The dose regimen may be first selected on the basis of pharmacokinetic study, the integration of pharmacokinetic and pharmacodynamic characteristics (increasingly useful for antimicrobial agents and nonsteroidal anti-inflammatory drugs) or from a disease model. However, a series of confirmatory clinical studies (using the final proposed drug product) are also undertaken, usually in compliance with the principles of Good Clinical Practice (GCP).
- **Target animal safety.** Elevated-dose and protracted-use studies are generally instigated to define and confirm the margin of safety. Studies must normally conform to the requirements of Good Laboratory Practices (GLP). Special studies in neonates, breeding animals (male and female), pregnant animals and other potentially at-risk groups may also be undertaken if use in these groups is required.
- **Chemical characterization.** Each NCE requires comprehensive and unique characterization, including structural description, impurity profile, stability and analytical methods.
- **Manufacturing process.** New animal drugs must generally meet the requirements of codes of GMP in order that quality, potency and purity can be assured. Finished product stability and shelf-life must be investigated and storage conditions defined.
- **Human safety.** The composition of the human safety package is determined in part by the degree of reasonably expected human exposure during manufacture, transport, distribution and use. The human safety needs of a product intended exclusively for companion animals are less comprehensive than products for food animal use, where potential human exposure to tissue residues is a major consideration. Generally, toxicity studies (conducted according to GLP guidelines) in laboratory animal species will address toxicokinetics, acute toxicity of the active constituent and drug product (lethality – LD_{50} – or lowest toxic dose, skin and eye irritancy, skin sensitization and corrosiveness), repeat dose studies (short term 7–28 days, subchronic up to 90 days and chronic 18–24 months), reproductive toxicity (teratogenicity, fertility, perinatal toxicity) and genotoxicity. Carcinogenicity and special studies (e.g. specific organ toxicity, neurotoxicity, immunotoxicity, toxicity of metabolites and impurities or toxicity of mixtures) may be necessary on a case-by-case basis. For antimicrobial products it is possible that a risk assessment of the likelihood of microbial resistance selection and transfer to humans may also be required.
- **Environmental fate and toxicity.** The likelihood of adverse environmental effects arising from either direct accidental exposure to the drug product or indirect exposure via the excretion of drug or metabolites from treated animals may need to be addressed. Appropriate studies may be derived from an understanding of the physicochemical and pharmacokinetic properties and quantitative description of excretion products combined with study of environmental fate and toxicity to a variety of environmental organisms (typically aquatic invertebrates, fish, terrestrial plants and earthworms).
- **Occupational health and safety.** On the basis of the manufacturing process and the toxicity profile of the developed drug and its formulation, particular measures may need to be instituted to minimize occupational exposure. Other possible sources of occupational exposure may be encountered during the storage and transport of the finished product. Again, depending on the degree and consequences of likely exposure, safeguards (e.g. protective clothing or special packaging) may need to be implemented.

Regulatory review

Regulatory evaluation of submissions in support of a new animal drug is a multidisciplinary activity, involving chemists, toxicologists, environmental scientists, clinically trained veterinarians and sometimes epidemiologists and other skills. The review may take 1–2 years or longer, depending on the novelty of the product and completeness or complexity of the data evaluated.

Among the critical elements of the review is the generation of the labeling of the product (described below) and a decision as to the availability of the drug, particularly if the product should be available only from veterinarians or be obtained from pharmacists or more readily available without restriction over-the-counter (OTC). This important decision involves a balancing of risks and benefits and comprises a number of criteria that vary from country to country but generally include the following considerations:

- the ability to prepare adequate labeling instructions for nonprofessional use
- the potential for abuse, particularly for drugs of addiction
- the potential for misuse, e.g. anabolic steroids, which may have illicit uses in humans
- the safety of the drug in the target species
- the safety of the drug in humans
- the seriousness of side effects
- the need for further information and evaluation of safety and efficacy
- the nature of the indications (disease being treated) and the need for professional diagnosis and monitoring
- the route and complexity of administration (e.g. is special or sophisticated equipment or skill necessary)?
- other public health considerations, e.g. impact of use of a new antimicrobial agent on microbial resistance and its transfer to human pathogens.

Once all issues are resolved and the regulatory agency is satisfied with the safety, efficacy, quality and labeling of the proposed product, the application is approved and marketing can commence.

Pharmacovigilance/postmarketing experiences

For those few new products that are commercialized, study, data collection and analysis continue in order to ensure that important new information on safety and efficacy is not overlooked. During the development of new animal drugs only small numbers of treated animals (generally fewer than 2000) are closely monitored. Consequently, unusual or rare manifestations of toxicity may not be encountered. Only after marketing, when large numbers of animals receive the treatment, is there an opportunity to seek this information. On the basis of postmarketing surveillance, high-risk groups may be identified and product label details amended accordingly to ensure continued safe use.

LABELING OF DRUGS

The labeling of a drug product is a legal document and provides critical information permitting proper use of the product. It includes all the information presented on the immediate label, outer packaging and any package inserts and consumer information leaflets. Label information is based on the findings of the multitude of studies undertaken during the development of the drug and any additional experience gained after approval.

The importance of familiarity and understanding of the content of labeling information is underscored by a recognition that it is frequently illegal (in some cases even for veterinarians) to use a product in a way that is inconsistent with the directions presented on the label. Apart from the importance of legal responsibilities, the information on the label should be sufficient to allow the effective and safe use of the product for the approved indications.

Labels contain a large amount of information that is frequently presented poorly, both with respect to font size and clarity of layout and expression. There is no standard label presentation and data requirements for inclusion on labels vary widely both within a country (e.g. there are differences between pesticide labels, OTC labels and veterinarian-only labels) and between countries. Nevertheless, it is an important responsibility of the prescriber and user to be completely familiar with the labeling details before use of a product.

Information that typically is presented on a label includes the following. However, veterinarians should be familiar with the labeling requirements of their own jurisdictions. Many of the label requirements as well as copies of labeling information can be accessed via the regulatory web addresses previously presented.

- **Signal heading.** A prominent statement that indicates if the product is scheduled or controlled or available only by prescription. Examples of signal headings include 'PRESCRIPTION ANIMAL REMEDY' or 'Caution. Federal law restricts this drug to use by or on the order of a licensed veterinarian'. Other components of the heading may be related to the safety of the product (CAUTION, POISON, DANGEROUS POISON, CONTROLLED DRUG) and exposure of children (KEEP OUT OF REACH OF CHILDREN).

- When there are particular **safety instructions** that are required, there may be a statement 'READ SAFETY DIRECTIONS BEFORE OPENING OR USING'.
- 'FOR ANIMAL TREATMENT ONLY'. A **cautionary statement** required in most countries.
- **Distinguishing name.** Usually the proprietary and/or nonproprietary names are provided. To limit errors, a unique name that cannot be confused with the name of another product should be selected. Often the name will describe the product type, route of administration and intended species and use.
- **Active constituents.** The approved nonproprietary name of the active constituent expressed qualitatively and quantitatively. Some labels may also contain details of particular preservatives (particularly with parenteral or ophthalmic preparations) and, for pesticides, either the solvent or all excipients.
- **Statement of claims.** An accurate description of the approved indications or claims.
- **Contents.** A statement of the net weight or volume and quantity of the product.
- **Dosing directions.** Includes essential product information needed for proper administration. This includes species of animal for which the product is intended, the route of administration, mixing directions if relevant (e.g. 'Shake well before use'), dose rate (for systemic products: usually, but not always, mg/kg bodyweight), the dosing frequency, the duration of dosing and any special instructions relating to dosage or administration (For topically applied products, this may include a statement such as 'For external use only' or 'Not to be taken internally'.).
- **Pharmacology.** Information may be provided concerning the pharmacokinetic and pharmacodynamic (including microbiology if appropriate) characteristics of the drug.
- **Restraints.** Absolute limitations or restrictions on use.
- **Contraindications.** Conditions that may cause use of the product to be inadvisable.
- **Adverse reactions.** Clinical signs of adverse reactions that have been observed and may be encountered.
- **Precautions.** Situations that may require special care for safe and effective product use. This section may include information regarding product use in the very young, the aged, breeding animals or during pregnancy. In addition, information on drug interactions may be provided.
- **Safety directions.** Advice to the user concerning special protective clothing, washing of hands, ventilation, etc. which enable safe use.
- **First aid statement.** Advice to the user in case of human exposure and anticipated or actual signs of intoxication.
- **MSDS reference.** A Material Safety Data Sheet contains information about the toxicity of the drug and details about safe transport and handling. When appropriate, reference may be made allowing access to this document.
- **Precautionary environmental statement.** Advice to ensure the protection of the environment during use of the product.
- **Emergency and transport advice.** Advice on steps to be taken in case of leakage, spillage or fire. Often only needed for products classified as dangerous goods.
- **Company name.** Name, business address and preferably the contact phone number of a suitably qualified person.
- **Disposal statement.** Disposal instructions designed to ensure the protection of humans and the environment. This may relate to excess product as well as packaging, needles or other sharps.
- **Storage instructions.** The stability of most products is dependent on the conditions of storage. Details of temperature, humidity, protection from light and other special requirements will be provided.
- **Regulatory agency approval number.** Generally a unique number designated by the prevailing authority.
- **Expiry date.** This indicates the date (often month and year) after which the drug should not (sometimes must not) be used. The date is dependent on compliance with the storage conditions. Multiple-use products (particularly injections) may have a different expiry date once the product has been opened or seals have been breached.
- **Batch number.** The number, letters or combination applied by a manufacturer that uniquely identifies a production batch and allows the tracing of each batch from manufacturer to end-user.

PRINCIPLES OF GOOD PRESCRIBING PRACTICE/RESPONSIBILITIES OF COMPANION ANIMAL CLINICIANS

Veterinarians have been entrusted with the responsibility to prescribe and dispense those drugs that are considered incapable of being effectively or safely used by lay people or may have particular public health considerations rendering them unsuitable for unrestricted availability. Veterinarians are considered suitable prescribers of such products by virtue of their training and experience in the practice of veterinary medicine and clinical pharmacology. These responsibilities must be viewed seriously – they are indeed responsibilities and not rights.

Veterinarians must be aware of, understand and observe their various legal obligations under relevant national/federal, state and local acts and regulations.

These obligations will encompass a broad range of activities from authorization to practice veterinary medicine, to hospital registration, to supply, use, storage, prescription and disposal of drugs or veterinary medicines. While recognizing the diversity of rules and regulations that specify actual requirements in each jurisdiction, general principles of good prescribing practice are set out below and an example of the application of these principles to the appropriate use of antimicrobial agents is set out in Table 1.4.

- **Veterinary medicines must be used only by or under the supervision of a licensed veterinarian.**
- **Veterinarian–client–patient relationship (VCPR):** veterinary medicines must only be used in the context of a valid VCPR, which exists if:
  - the veterinarian has assumed the responsibility for making clinical judgments regarding the health of the patient and the need for medical treatment and the client has agreed to follow the veterinarian's instructions
  - there is sufficient knowledge of the animal by the veterinarian to initiate at least a general or preliminary diagnosis of the medical condition of the animal

Table 1.4 Principles of appropriate drug use

Parameter	Example: antimicrobial therapy
Professional intervention	Establish a veterinarian–client–patient relationship
Diagnosis	Clinical diagnosis History, physical examination, other assessments Microbiological diagnosis Sampling of appropriate fluids or tissues Likely etiological agent identified (i.e. not normal flora) Culture and susceptibility testing
Therapeutic objective	Options include: Eradication of infecting organism Clinical improvement
Therapeutic plan	Therapeutic choices (drug and non-drug therapy) Supportive therapy (drainage, debridement, nutrition, management, etc.) Host factors (concurrent illness, age, immunocompetence, pregnancy, lactation)
Drug treatment	Selection of appropriate drug; considerations include: Activity against infectious agent Activity against nontarget agents Factors influencing effective concentration at site of infection Availability of approved product Acceptable dosage form Target animal and environmental safety Public health implications (e.g. antimicrobial resistance transmission) Cost Dosage regimen: PK-PD factors Dose rate Route of administration Site of administration Dosage interval Duration
Monitoring	Institute plan to monitor response to treatment to enable ongoing reassessment of the objectives and plan and identification of any significant adverse events
Record keeping	Date of examination Diagnosis Animal identification Drugs used Dosage regimen (including dose rate, route and duration) Date(s) administered Other treatment advice and measures implemented
Disease prevention	Prevention plan (health program, including consideration of vaccination, hygiene, nutrition, environment, routine monitoring)

  - the veterinarian is readily available for follow-up evaluation in the event of adverse reactions or failure of the treatment regimen.

This description of the VCPR is taken from the US FDA (Extralabel Drug Use in Animals, 21 CFR Part 530, 9 December 1996) and, while directly applicable in the USA, provides general guidance elsewhere.

- **Diagnosis.** An accurate diagnosis underpins each decision to treat.
- **Therapeutic plan.** A plan including clear objectives of treatment should be developed. It is useful to consider each therapeutic intervention as an experiment to be conducted judiciously but thoroughly.
- **Drug knowledge**
  - The label of all drugs used should be fully understood and the use of the drug should be consistent with the labeled directions, unless compelling reasons direct alternative use. In addition, veterinarians should familiarize themselves with any further relevant information that may allow the drug to be used more effectively or with greater safety.
  - For example, if there is a precaution concerning use in neonatal animals, inquiry may establish that the drug has been universally used safely by other practitioners in this category of animal.
  - Similarly, inquiry of the literature or other practitioners may enable dose adjustments as necessary in the presence of specific organ dysfunctions. Whenever collecting additional information, it is incumbent on the inquirer to evaluate the relevance, quality and strength of the evidence obtained before incorporating it into a therapeutic plan.
- **Client communication.** The client should be involved in the development of the plan, both to ensure that s/he concurs with the decision to treat and the objectives of treatment, as well as to ensure that compliance with the dosage regimen is assured. The risks and benefits of the plan should be discussed.
- **Client consent.** Particularly when using an untested approach or extra-label program, the informed consent of the client should be obtained.
- **Client instructions**
  - Clear and comprehensible written instructions should be provided to the client, outlining the method of administration, dose rate, frequency and duration.
  - Details of product storage and disposal should be provided.
  - Other instructions should describe the expected response to treatment, identifying any expected side effects and encouraging the client to contact the prescribing veterinarian if any concerns arise.
- **Follow-up.** As considered appropriate, plans for either passive (allowing the client to call if concerned) or active (scheduled by veterinarian) follow-up should be considered in order to determine if the therapeutic plan is working as expected.
- **Reassessment.** The success of the therapeutic plan should be always open to objective reassessment. As discussed earlier in this chapter, there are a multitude of factors that can lead to variation in clinical response to treatment. These factors (including reassessment of the diagnosis, compliance, medication errors and comorbidities) should be systematically evaluated if either lack of efficacy or untoward effects are encountered.
- **Adverse events.** Suspected adverse events, including drug interactions, should be thoroughly investigated and the manufacturer and regulatory agency informed.
- **Prescriptions.** Veterinarians must be familiar with requirements for prescription writing, particularly the minimum labeling needs (see further information below). In addition, the quantity of medication prescribed should be commensurate with the needs of the patient, the disease, the expiry date and the potential for misuse.
- **Special requirements.** When prescribing drugs for companion animals, veterinarians should be aware of any rules and regulations of breed societies, sporting bodies or other parties that may be applicable.
- **Containers.** Products should preferably be dispensed in their original labeled container. If this cannot be done, then the product should preferably be dispensed in a childproof container labeled with the appropriate information, as for example described below under Prescriptions.
- **Record keeping.** Thorough records of each case, including the dates of consultations and treatment, details of drug dosage regimens and identification of the animal treated, should be maintained in a readily retrievable system for the necessary time. For certain scheduled or controlled drugs (particularly drugs of addiction) there may be additional record-keeping requirements.
- **Storage of medicines.** Medicines should be stored according to appropriate legislation, but generally this will include storage in a secure site, away from the public. The storage conditions of each drug should be observed and expired product removed. The flammability of stored products should be determined and appropriate precautionary measures implemented. In addition to segregation of flammable and nonflammable products, it may be necessary to have a bonded storage area and specific fire extinguishers.

- **Disposal of medicines.** Knowledge of prevailing legislation is essential and must be observed during disposal.
- **First aid and antidotes.** It is prudent to be familiar with the adverse consequences of either human or animal exposure to drugs stored on site and to have the appropriate first aid materials and antidotes readily available.
- **Extra-label (off-label) use of drugs**
  - This refers to use of a drug in an animal that is not in accordance with the approved labeling. This includes use in species not listed in the labeling, use for indications not listed in the labeling, use at dosage levels, frequencies or routes of administration not listed in the labeling. Extra-label use may arise from use of an animal drug, a drug approved for use in humans or extemporaneous preparations.
  - Generally, extra-label use is limited to situations when the health of an animal is threatened or suffering or death may result from failure to treat and no approved animal drug is available that is considered likely to be effective.

The collection of responsibilities described above is especially relevant to extra-label drug use, in particular the need for a minimum base of drug knowledge, a reasonable expectation that the selected drug may be effective in the prevailing circumstances, combined with client consent.

Veterinary prescriptions

To preclude errors and avoid ambiguity, prescriptions should be written legibly and indelibly. The form and content of a prescription are usually subject to rules and regulations prevailing in the prescriber's jurisdiction and must be observed. However, the content of the prescription usually includes:

- name, address and telephone number of the prescriber
- date of prescription issue
- name and address of client
- identification (name and species) of the animal(s) to be treated
- name and strength of the drug(s) to be dispensed (e.g. amoxicillin 100 mg): the name may be the proprietary name if a specific product is required or the nonproprietary name if a choice of available products can be made by the pharmacist who dispenses the prescription – for extemporaneous products, full details of preparation should be provided
- dosage form and total amount to be dispensed (e.g. 25 tablets)
- information for the package label: this usually includes directions for use (route, amount and frequency of administration), special instructions (e.g. 'give with food') and warnings; in addition, some jurisdictions require the statements 'For Animal Treatment Only' and 'Keep Out of the Reach of Children', unless already on the printed label of the product being dispensed
- signature and qualifications of the prescriber.

CONCLUSION

Veterinarians are in a unique position to improve the health and wellbeing of their companion animal patients. A number of responsibilities accompany the practice of veterinary medicine, particularly relating to the use of drugs. Of high importance is the application of clinical pharmacology to the judicious development of individualized therapeutic plans. There are many factors that lead to variations in the expected clinical outcome of treatment. An accurate diagnosis and thorough understanding of the patient's disease or disorder, age and physiological state, combined with knowledge of the pharmacology, efficacy and safety of the selected drug, permit a therapeutic plan to be prepared. Implementation of the plan and measures to increase compliance while minimizing errors, combined with subsequent reassessment and plan refinements if necessary, provide the best opportunity for a successful outcome.

FURTHER READING

Barach P, Small D 2000 Reporting and preventing medical mistakes: lessons from non-medical near miss reporting systems. Br Med J 320:759-763

Baxter K (ed) 2006 Stockley's drug interactions: a source book of interactions, their mechanisms, clinical importance and management, 7th edn. Pharmaceutical Press, London

Brunton LL (ed) 2005 Goodman and Gilman's the pharmacological basis of therapeutics, 11th edn. McGraw-Hill, New York

Dean B, Schachter M, Vincent C, Barber N 2002 Causes of prescribing errors in hospital inpatients: a prospective study. Lancet 359:1373-1378

Gibaldi M (ed) 1991 Biopharmaceutics and clinical pharmacokinetics, 4th edn. Lea and Febiger, Philadelphia, PA

Hardee GE, Baggot JD (eds) 1998 Development and formulation of veterinary dosage forms, 2nd edn. Marcel Dekker, New York

Weingart SN, Wilson RML, Gibberd RW, Harrison B 2000 Epidemiology of medical error. Br Med J 320:774-777

Clinical pharmacokinetics

Jill E Maddison, Stephen W Page and Timothy M Dyke

INTRODUCTION

More often than not, veterinarians calculate drug doses on the basis of a fixed dose recommended on a product label or in a textbook, expecting that the recommended dose will give a described drug response. It is expected that the 'average' dose of drug will achieve 'average' blood concentrations and 'average' responses in 'average' patients. However, a recommended dose may give a response that differs markedly from that which is expected: either little response is seen or side effects or toxicity result.

Variability in the handling of the drug by the body affects the concentration of the drug at its site of action and consequently responses to drugs. This variability occurs between individual patients of the same species, between species and, not infrequently, within the individual patient at different times. Some diseases impact the extent and direction of this variance from 'average'. These sources of variability need to be considered when predicting or assessing an individual animal's response to therapy, especially when the response is unexpected.

Knowledge of pharmacokinetics, the study of the rate and extent of movement of drug through the animal body, can be used to maximize the likelihood of success with drug therapy in small animal patients. We 'individualize' drug doses to optimize the effectiveness and safety of a drug in an individual patient. This chapter addresses basic pharmacokinetic principles that will benefit veterinary practitioners attempting to 'individualize' drug therapy. The chapter should be used in conjunction with specific pharmacokinetic information found in other chapters of this text dealing with specific drugs.

Pharmacokinetics is perhaps most easily thought of as 'what the body does to the drug', as distinct from pharmacodynamics which is 'what the drug does to the body'. Clinical pharmacokinetics can be defined as the use of pharmacokinetic information to select and define rational drug therapy in clinical patients. Pharmacokinetics can be categorized into several sequential and often overlapping phases: product dissolution, absorption, distribution, metabolism and excretion.

After the drug formulation has disintegrated and allowed its active constituents to dissolve in enteric or intercellular fluid at the site of administration, molecules of the 'parent' drug are absorbed into the bloodstream (or rarely lymphatics), wherein they are distributed throughout the body. They may be metabolized and excreted or they may be excreted as unchanged parent molecules.

For systemically active drugs the circulatory system is 'central' to the movement of drug throughout the body and it is from this central compartment that drug is distributed to the peripheral tissues. The effect of most drugs occurs in a peripheral tissue. Usually, but not always, the drug must be returned to the blood in order to be eliminated from the body. However, the concentration of drug present in peripheral tissues is often extrapolated from the plasma concentration of drug. Serum, rather than plasma, is also sometimes used for drug concentration analyses. Plasma is relatively easy to collect and analyze and, because plasma concentration usually reflects blood concentration, which often bears some relationship to concentration at the site of action, pharmacokinetic information is often developed from the study of changes in plasma drug concentrations over time.

THE PHYSIOLOGICAL BASIS OF PHARMACOKINETICS

For a drug to exert an effect on the body, it must be absorbed and distributed to the site of action. Having exerted its effect, it then must be metabolized and/or eliminated from the body. Therefore, an understanding of absorption, distribution, metabolism and excretion (or ADME) of drugs is critical to maximizing the likelihood of successful drug therapy in small animals.

Transport across membranes

The movement of drug molecules across membranes is an important aspect of the absorption, distribution and elimination of drugs. Biological membranes can be viewed as trilaminar sheets, an outer and inner layer formed by the hydrophilic ends of phospholipids sandwiching an intermediate hydrophobic lipid matrix. Proteins embedded in the membrane, traversing it in places, serve as receptors, ion channels and drug transporters.

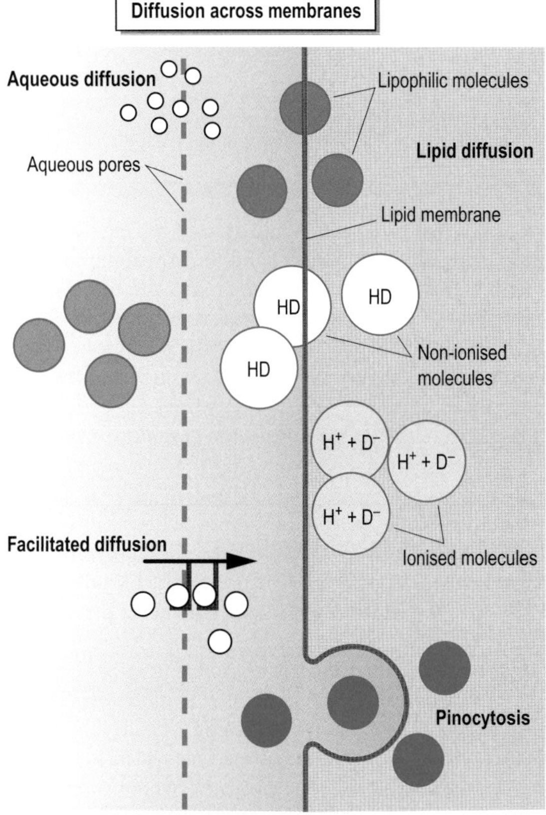

Fig. 2.1 **Different ways in which drug molecules may passively cross membranes. H, hydrogen; D, drug.**

Drugs may cross membrane barriers by one of five major mechanisms (Fig. 2.1):

- passive aqueous diffusion (especially via aquaporins)
- passive lipid diffusion
- facilitated diffusion (including transport proteins such as P-glycoprotein)
- pinocytosis
- active (energy-expending) transport.

The rate of transfer of a drug across a biological membrane by passive diffusion (J) can be described by Fick's law of diffusion:

$$J = k(C_1 - C_2) \textit{ where}$$
$$k = D \times A \times P/T$$

C_1 and C_2 denote the drug concentrations on each side of the membrane and k is a proportionality constant that incorporates the diffusion coefficient of the drug (D), the thickness (T) and surface area (A) of the exposed membrane and the partition coefficient (P) of the drug product.

- *D*: the **diffusion coefficient** of the drug. Nonpolar (nonionized) drugs are expected to diffuse quickly through lipid and aqueous membranes.
- *A*: The **surface area of the tissue exposed to the drug.** Transfer across membranes is usually faster in tissues with a very large surface area (e.g. lung alveoli, small intestinal villi) than across the membranes of organs with a smaller surface area (e.g. stomach).
- *T*: The **thickness** of the membrane through which drug transfer is occurring. The thicker the barrier, the slower will be the rate of transfer.
- *P*: the **partition coefficient** describing the movement of drug from the drug product into the biological membrane.
- ΔC (*i.e.* $C_1 - C_2$): The **concentration gradient** is the difference between the concentration of the drug on either side of a membrane. This gradient is dependent upon processes on both sides of the membrane, e.g. the amount of drug administered (gradient source) and the rate of removal from the contralateral side of the membrane (gradient sink). If the drug is removed very rapidly from the contralateral side (e.g. because of high blood flow or rapid ionization due to a different pH), the concentration gradient will remain high and the rate of diffusion is expected to be high.

While Fick's law holds true for monolayers and can be predictive for complex multilayer biological membranes, transfer across biological membranes is highly complex and deviations from Fick's law point to the presence of unaccounted factors influencing transmembrane permeation.

Aqueous diffusion

Membranes have aqueous pores (protein channels termed aquaporins) through which water and some drugs can diffuse. However, the number and size of the pores vary greatly between different membranes and the membrane may have limited capacity to allow aqueous diffusion. Aqueous diffusion can also be paracellular via intercellular gaps. The epithelial cells lining the surface of the body (e.g. gut, cornea and bladder) are connected by tight junctions and only very small molecules can pass through. In contrast, most capillaries have very large pores and much larger molecules can pass along hydrostatic and concentration gradients. An exception to this is the capillaries of protected parts of the body such as the choroid plexus and the blood–brain barrier.

Lipid diffusion

One of the most important methods of drug permeation is movement of molecules across cell membranes by dissolution in the lipids of the membrane. The movement is passive and driven by the concentration gradient. A high degree of lipid solubility relative to aqueous solubility will favor this mode of transportation. But note that drugs must be in the aqueous solution (i.e. plasma) to gain access to the lipid membrane; thus a degree of both lipid and aqueous solubility is a useful characteristic.

Facilitated diffusion

Solutes are transported according to the concentration gradient but at an accelerated rate. Some drugs are transported by special transmembrane carriers in the membranes of cells, e.g. thiamine transport across the blood–brain barrier. There are also an increasingly recognized number of cation and anion transport proteins that regulate influx and efflux of drugs and endogenous compounds. These transport proteins often act vectorially by virtue of their cellular distribution to ensure drugs are either excreted from the body (for example, into bile, urine or gut lumen) or from certain tissues (for example, drug efflux from the brain into the blood via P-glycoprotein, a most notable example being the efflux of ivermectin from endothelial cells lining the brain vasculature) or absorption into blood is enhanced (for example, certain amino acids and other key nutrients).

Active transport

Drugs can also be transported actively against a concentration gradient, e.g. penicillamine, 5-fluorouracil.

Pinocytosis (receptor-mediated endocytosis)

Very large molecules (mol. wt > 1000) can pass through cells by pinocytosis, the process of engulfing extracellular material within membrane vesicles and retaining such material within the cell or expelling it on a contralateral side of the cell.

Absorption

General principles of drug absorption

- Drug molecules are small (mol. wt less than 1000).
- Drug molecules are usually either weak acids or weak bases.
- The extent of ionization of drug molecules is determined by both the inherent pKa of the drug and the pH of surrounding fluid.
- Drug molecules tend to be ionized when in a pH-opposite fluid (e.g. basic drugs are ionized and retained in acidic fluid).
- Nonionized drug molecules move across biological membranes by passive diffusion.
- Ionized drug molecules cannot move across biological membranes by passive diffusion and can only cross by specific, selective active transport mechanisms, facilitated diffusion or pinocytosis.
- The degree of ionization is especially important in those body compartments in which pH may change, e.g. gastric fluid, urine.
- Bioavailability is defined as the fraction of unchanged drug reaching the systemic circulation following administration by any route and can be estimated experimentally. For an intravenous drug, the bioavailability is usually regarded as complete (i.e. 100%).
- In most cases, a drug must enter the blood to be transported to its site of action.
- Some drugs used topically for local effect on the skin or mucous membranes and drugs that are orally administered and then act within the intestinal lumen do not need to be absorbed into the blood as they are already at their site of action.
- Absorption into the blood is significantly influenced by the route of administration and the formulation of the drug: factors such as particle size, rate of dissolution of a tablet, volume of injection, vehicle characteristics, controlled release formulations, etc. can affect the release and absorption of drugs into the blood.

Routes of administration

The different routes by which a drug may be administered include the following.

- Parenteral (intravenous, intramuscular, subcutaneous, intra-arterial)
- Enteral (oral, sublingual, rectal)
- Topical (intra-aural, dermal, transdermal, topical, ocular)
- Inhalational
- Intrathecal
- Intramammary
- Intravaginal
- Intrauterine

Oral

Oral administration is convenient and many drugs are absorbed efficiently from the gastrointestinal tract (GIT). However, some drugs are destroyed or altered by gastric acid or intestinal flora. Many drugs are absorbed from the gastrointestinal tract by lipid diffusion, as tight epithelial junctions limit aqueous diffusion. Thus lipid-soluble drugs are more readily absorbed. However, aquaporins and transport proteins are abundant along the GIT and serve to regulate and control drug absorption. Drugs given orally may be in a variety of pharmaceutical formulations including solids (tablets, capsules), semisolids (pastes, gels) or liquids (aqueous and nonaqueous). Absorption is principally from the small intestine because of the large surface area associated with three levels of magnification: tissue folding, villous formation and the presence of microvilli. Rate of gastric emptying is therefore an important determinant of the rate of absorption of drugs from the small intestine.

Drugs susceptible to destruction in the acidic gastric environment can be coated to resist dissolution in the stomach but allow dissolution by the higher pH in the small intestine.

Once absorbed from the gastrointestinal tract, drugs enter the portal vein and are conveyed to the liver. Here they are exposed to metabolizing hepatic enzymes. Some drugs are extensively metabolized to inactive metabolites and do not reach the systemic circulation, while other drugs are excreted into bile and do not reach the systemic circulation. The removal of recently absorbed drug by hepatic metabolism and/or biliary excretion is called the first-pass effect. Some drugs undergo enterohepatic circulation, where they are absorbed, conjugated in the liver, excreted in bile into the small intestine, deconjugated by intestinal flora and then reabsorbed, increasing the persistence of the drug, for as long as recycling takes place.

Intravenous

Intravenous administration bypasses absorption barriers. It is potentially the most hazardous route of administration as a high concentration of drug is delivered to organs as rapidly as the rate of injection, which may elicit toxic effects. Intravenous administration is used primarily where a rapid onset of action is required (e.g. anesthesia, emergency medicine) or where a drug cannot be given orally either because of its inherent physicochemical properties or because of patient factors (e.g. the patient is persistently vomiting, is unconscious or is too young to safely swallow solid forms of medication). Drugs in the form of suspensions or oily solutions cannot generally be given intravenously.

In common with all parenteral injections, products should be sterile, free of pyrogens, buffered to physiological pH and isotonic.

Intramuscular

The intramuscular route is used where effects are desired over a longer period of time than can be expected after intravenous injection, for drugs that are too irritant to be given subcutaneously, or for oily solutions, which cannot be given intravenously. Drugs in aqueous solution are often absorbed rapidly from intramuscular sites. Drugs dissolved in oil ('depot' injections) are absorbed more slowly and absorption can continue for weeks after injection. Some drugs (e.g. thiacetarsamide) should not be given intramuscularly due to pain and tissue damage at the injection site. Choice of injection site should include consideration of the volume to be injected, the presence of fascial planes, important anatomical features (e.g. vessels and nerves) and the consequences of any tissue reaction.

Subcutaneous

Subcutaneous injections are convenient and usually less painful than intramuscular injections for low-volume drugs, e.g. vaccines. In normovolemic patients, drugs may be absorbed from subcutaneous sites at rates similar to adjacent intramuscular sites. Subcutaneous injections are only suitable for drugs that are nonirritant. The site of subcutaneous administration has a significant bearing on the rate of absorption, as do factors that affect local circulation such as warmth and exercise, dehydration and hypovolemic shock.

Inhalational

Pharmacological agents that can be vaporized or dispersed in an aerosol of fine aqueous droplets can be administered by the inhalational route (e.g. anesthetic gases, asthma therapy, antibiotics and mucolytics administered for treatment of respiratory disease).

Topical and transdermal

Topical administration is used to achieve a local effect to areas such as the skin, nose, eye, throat and vagina.

Transdermal administration allows application of drugs to the skin for systemic effect (e.g. nasal spray for hormonal treatment, nitroglycerin for angina, fentanyl patches and a variety of antiparasitic topical preparations), either the formulation or the stratum corneum usually acting as the rate-limiting barrier to absorption.

Buccal or sublingual

Buccal or sublingual administration is useful for drugs that are extensively cleared by the liver (first-pass effect) if given orally. Drug is absorbed across buccal mucosa and venous drainage directly into systemic veins, avoiding the portal circulation.

Rectal

Rectal administration may be used for local effect in the rectum or for systemic effects instead of oral administration, e.g. use of antiemetic pessaries for patients with severe vomiting. The first-pass effect may also be avoided by rectal administration, provided the drug remains in the terminal rectum and does not drift towards the colon, an area drained by the portal circulation.

Intrathecal

Intrathecal administration is where drug is injected into the cerebrospinal fluid (e.g. epidural anesthetics, administration of some cytotoxic drugs to treat brain tumors).

Intra-arterial

Intra-arterial administration is intended to provide high concentrations of drug at a specific site, e.g. tumor or infection. Intra-arterial injection tends to reduce systemic effects as administration is more direct.

Distribution

General principles of drug distribution

1. Drug molecules can bind to plasma protein and tissue protein.
   - Acidic drugs bind to albumin.
   - Basic drugs bind to α_1-acid glycoprotein.
2. Drugs diffuse into peripheral tissues by capillary filtration.
   - Drug–protein complexes do not cross normal biological membranes.
   - Drug bound to protein complexes is not active.
   - The amount of active drug available is represented by the concentration of 'free' unbound drug.
3. Lipophilicity of nonionized drug molecules affects diffusion; more lipophilic drugs diffuse faster and are retained for longer in fat-containing tissues.
4. Depending on a drug's potential for ionization, protein binding and lipophilicity, drugs distribute into various anatomical/physiological spaces.
   - Drugs may distribute predominantly within the plasma space and have a 'volume of distribution' similar to plasma volume (e.g. if extensively bound to plasma protein).
   - Some drugs distribute within body spaces occupied by water and have a 'volume of distribution' similar to total body water.
   - Some drugs become extensively bound to peripheral tissue sites and have a 'volume of distribution' that is many times body volume.
   - Unless shown otherwise, assume that all drugs cross the placenta and enter milk during lactation.

Once a drug has been absorbed into blood it will be distributed to various parts of the body. Within each part of the body, diffusion into specific organs and tissues may or may not occur, depending upon the physicochemical characteristics of the drug, as well as circulatory and tissue factors. The apparent **volume of distribution** (V_d) of a drug relates the amount of drug in the body to the concentration of drug in blood or plasma.

$$V_d = \frac{A(\text{amount of drug in body})}{C(\text{drug concentration in plasma})}$$

Knowledge of V_d allows calculation of the loading dose (in this case, loading dose = A) necessary to obtain a target plasma concentration (in this case C).

In this context, the body is thought of as a group of compartments including total body water (plasma plus intracellular water plus extracellular water), fat and bone.

The distribution of some drugs is limited to the plasma (e.g. nonsteroidal anti-inflammatory drugs); other drugs may enter the extracellular fluid (e.g. phenobarbital) while others may be distributed throughout the total body water (theophylline). Some drugs are highly lipid soluble and accumulate in fat (halothane) while others, e.g. heavy metals and fluoride, are slowly sequestered in bone.

Table 2.1 Volumes of body fluids in dogs

Body fluid	Volume (mL/kg)
Total body water	600–650
Extracellular fluid	200–250
Intracellular fluid	300–350
Circulating blood volume	85–90
Plasma volume	49–50

Drugs can bind to cell surfaces and intercellular macromolecules; therefore the apparent volume of distribution of a drug is often much larger than the actual volumes that physically exist. There does not need to be any correlation between physiological volumes of body fluids (Table 2.1) and apparent volumes of distribution.

The most important factors determining drug distribution are:

- protein binding
- tissue binding
- organ blood flow
- membrane permeability
- drug solubility.

Protein binding

In blood drugs may bind (usually reversibly) to albumin, α_1-acid glycoprotein and several other plasma transport proteins. The binding sites are referred to as inert or nonreceptor binding sites, as no specific pharmacological response is elicited as a result of the binding. Drug molecules bound to inert binding sites are not immediately available for diffusion or interaction with receptors. They are in equilibrium with free drug so alterations in the concentration of free drug will alter the amount (but not the percentage) bound. Nonreceptor binding sites are not very specific and different drugs can compete for the same binding sites. This can have important consequences; for example, if drug A is highly protein bound (i.e. only a small percentage is free and therefore 'active'), the addition of drug B, which competes with higher affinity for the same binding site, might displace drug A from the protein-binding sites, causing a significant increase in free drug concentration. Toxicity associated with displacement is unusual as the displaced drug is instantly available for distribution, metabolism and excretion and a new equilibrium is rapidly attained.

Tissue binding

Unlike protein binding which retains drug in the blood and keeps V_d close to blood volume, tissue binding, which can be specific or nonspecific, can cause extravascular accumulation of drug and very high V_d. Examples include digoxin, which binds to receptors widely distributed in muscle, and macrolide antibiotics that are concentrated in subcellular organelles.

Organ blood flow

Initially the distribution of a drug depends on blood flow and organs with high blood flow (brain, heart, liver, kidney) receive the greater proportion of the drug. Delivery of drug to less well-perfused organs (e.g. resting muscle, skin) is slower. Fat and bone are particularly poorly perfused and it may take some hours before drug reaches equilibrium in poorly perfused tissues.

Membrane permeability

Transport across membranes has already been discussed. Note that distribution across the placenta is most likely for drugs that are lipid soluble and may have pharmacological effects on the fetus and interfere with fetal development.

Drug solubility

Drugs that are highly lipid soluble can accumulate in fat. Other organs may specifically accumulate certain substrates because of specific uptake mechanisms, e.g. copper in liver.

Metabolism

General principles of drug metabolism

- Most drugs are metabolized and mostly by the liver.
- Metabolism often involves the addition of or exposure of a polar group, particularly by oxidative, hydrolytic or less commonly reductive reactions (phase I metabolism) followed by the addition of a large chemical group (conjugative phase II metabolism) to increase water solubility and excretion from the body.
- Hepatic phase I drug metabolism involves primarily cytochrome P450 enzyme reactions.
- Drugs are often metabolized by specific cytochrome P450 enzyme pathways.
- Drug-metabolizing enzymes can be inhibited or induced.
- For most therapeutic drugs, the rate of drug metabolism is proportional to the concentration of the drug (first-order reaction), i.e. more drug is removed when there is more drug present.
- Some drugs are activated by metabolism (e.g. morphine, ceftiofur).
- Some drugs are metabolized to toxic metabolites (e.g. acetaminophen).

Termination of the effect of a drug is sometimes dependent on excretion from the body but more commonly is the result of biotransformation of the drug to inactive products that are then excreted. In some cases the products of biotransformation may have activity (e.g. enrofloxacin) and in a few cases the drug itself may be administered as an inactive prodrug that requires biotransformation to become active (e.g. enalapril, febantel).

Many pharmacologically active molecules tend to be lipophilic and are often strongly bound to proteins. Such substances are not readily filtered by the kidney. The kidney excretes polar (water-soluble) compounds most efficiently; thus lipid-soluble drugs must be metabolized to more water-soluble substances prior to renal excretion.

Although almost every tissue has some ability to metabolize drugs, metabolism primarily occurs in the liver. The gut, skin, kidney and lungs also have some activity. Metabolism can essentially be divided into two categories: phase I and phase II reactions. The enzymes involved in phase I drug metabolism (microsomal enzymes) are associated with the endoplasmic reticulum of hepatocytes and those involved with phase II can be in the cytosol (methylation, acetylation), endoplasmic reticulum (microsomes; glucuronidation) or mitochondria (glycine conjugation).

Phase I reactions usually convert the parent drug to a more polar metabolite. The reaction usually involves oxidation (requiring mixed function oxidases, including cytochrome P450), reduction or hydrolysis. Often the metabolites are inactive, although occasionally activity may be modified, not terminated. If phase I metabolites are sufficiently polar they may be readily excreted by the kidney. However, often further reaction is required to form a sufficiently polar compound.

Phase II reactions involve conjugation of the products of phase I reactions with natural substrates. The process requires input of energy and results in the formation of a compound with increased polarity, which can be readily excreted by the kidney or biliary system. Glucuronic acid and glutathione are two of the most common conjugates; others include acetylation, methylation or conjugation with sulfate or glycine groups. Dogs cannot effectively metabolize drugs via acetylation while cats are deficient in glucuronidation. Phase II reactions involve specific transfer enzymes (transferases), which may be located in the microsome or the cytoplasm. Although, in general, drug conjugation is a true detoxification process, in some cases certain conjugation reactions may lead to the formation of reactive species responsible for the hepatotoxicity of the drug.

Enzyme induction can occur with repeated administration of a drug (e.g. phenobarbital, phenytoin) and usually involves increased gene expression leading to increased enzyme synthesis or, less commonly, involves decreased enzyme degradation. When new enzyme synthesis is involved, enzyme induction evolves over a prolonged period. In most cases induction results in an acceleration of metabolism and a decrease in the activity of drugs that are metabolized by induced enzymes. Such changes may account for the patient developing apparent tolerance to the drug. However, in some instances where drugs are biotransformed to active metabolites or reactive intermediates, enzyme induction may exacerbate drug-mediated toxicity. Enzyme activity can also be inhibited by certain drugs (e.g. chloramphenicol, metronidazole, cimetidine, verapamil, fluoroquinolones) leading to persistence of drug and possibly toxicity.

Other factors that can alter enzyme activity and hence the drug-metabolizing capacity of the patient are diseases, hormonal status, age, genetics, environmental factors, drug–drug interactions during metabolism, interactions between drugs and endogenous compounds and nutritional status.

Excretion

General principles of drug excretion

- Most drugs (or metabolites) are excreted by the kidneys.
- Three process can occur in renal excretion: glomerular filtration, tubular secretion and passive reabsorption.
- Some drugs are eliminated by the liver in the bile and excreted in feces.
- Enterohepatic circulation can occur (drug excreted in bile is absorbed by the gut and re-excreted by the liver in bile).
- Many of the concepts summarized under Absorption apply to excretion.

Renal excretion is the most common route of drug elimination. However, many drugs are excreted into bile via the liver and some volatile substances (primarily gaseous anesthetics) can be excreted via the lungs. Saliva often contains very small quantities of drug and this may be regarded as a mechanism of excretion although the amount is inconsequential in companion animal species. The gastrointestinal tract can also be involved in elimination of some drugs. The excretion of drugs into milk is a minor excretion pathway but may cause a nursing neonate to receive a significant dose.

Kidney

Drugs may be excreted by the kidney by glomerular filtration (passive) or by tubular secretion (active). They may also be reabsorbed from the filtrate across the renal tubular epithelial lining, usually by passive diffusion. Glomerular filtration is a passive process that removes small molecules (less than the size of albumin). Therefore drugs that are highly protein bound are not filtered and small molecule drugs that are not protein bound are cleared rapidly. The pH of the ultrafiltrate, which determines the degree of ionization of the drug, significantly influences the rate of excretion of acidic and basic drugs by ion trapping and reduced passive resorption. This can be exploited by altering urine pH to enhance excretion of a drug or increase reabsorption to increase drug persistence.

For example, if a weakly acidic drug is excreted into an alkaline urine, the drug is highly ionized and therefore not lipid soluble. It therefore will not be reabsorbed across the renal epithelial membrane and excretion will be enhanced. Excretion can also be enhanced by increased urine flow following osmotic diuresis.

Some drugs are actively secreted by special mechanisms located in the renal tubules (e.g. furosemide (frusemide)). Active secretion is a saturable process and requires the expenditure of energy.

Changes in renal blood flow may alter the rate of drug excretion and the dose of a drug may have to be altered accordingly in a patient suspected of having reduced renal blood flow.

Liver

A few drugs are actively secreted into the bile (e.g. carprofen). Some drugs undergo enterohepatic recycling, by which the drug is excreted into the bile (often as a glucuronide) and reabsorbed from the gut after deglucuronidation by gut microflora, which may be followed by renal or further biliary excretion. In the latter case continued resorption of the drug can greatly extend its duration of action.

PHARMACOKINETICS AND THE VETERINARY CLINICIAN

There are several pharmacokinetic definitions that the clinician should be aware of and understand as they are important in determining drug individualization.

Processes such as absorption, metabolism and elimination can be described by equations that are either zero or first order. The curious reader is referred elsewhere for the mathematics involved in the derivation of these equations.

Zero-order processes are those in which the change of drug concentration in a body fluid such as plasma or urine occurs at a constant rate, irrespective of the concentration of the drug present in that body fluid. $\delta C/\delta t = kC^0 = k$ (i.e. the rate of change of concentration (C) over time (t) equals a constant). The exponent of C is zero, leading to the description, zero order.

Examples where absorption is a zero-order process include many drugs that are prepared as sustained-release formulations, many drugs when administered by constant intravenous infusion and many drugs administered by transdermal patches.

Some drugs that are eliminated by zero-order processes in some species include ethanol, salicylate, phenytoin (in humans but not in dogs), propranolol in some species, phenylbutazone in the horse at some dose rates and paracetamol (acetaminophen) in the cat. Zero-order elimination is usually due to saturation of metabolism or excretion processes.

In summary, zero-order rates remain constant irrespective of the concentration of drug present.

In contrast, a **first-order process** is one where the change in concentration of drug in the body fluid is proportional to the concentration of the drug in that fluid at that time. $\delta C/\delta t = kC$ (i.e. the rate of change of C over time equals a constant proportion of C). The exponent of C is one, leading to the description, first order.

The vast majority of drugs used at therapeutic doses in veterinary clinical practice conform to first-order pharmacokinetics with respect to their elimination from the body, but there are some drugs that are absorbed and eliminated by zero-order processes.

In order to discuss manipulation of drug dose and dosing frequency, some pharmacokinetic characteristics must be introduced and described mathematically. The most useful clinically (and referred to later in this chapter) are as follows.

- *F* (the fraction absorbed): the extent of a drug's systemic availability (bioavailability) after administration, usually considered as the percentage of unchanged drug absorbed that reaches the systemic circulation, e.g. $F = 80\%$ means that 80% of the administered drug reaches the blood in comparison with intravenous bioavailability which is usually accepted as being 100%.
- *Cl*, the plasma clearance, is the volume of plasma cleared of drug per unit time. Clearance is a measure of the efficiency of removal of drug from the blood by all means, though principally hepatic and renal processes. Plasma clearance is expressed in units of flow (e.g. mL/min). Clearance determines the maintenance dose rate required to achieve a target plasma concentration at steady state. Maintenance rate (mg/min) = *Cl* (mL/min) × [target concentration (mg/mL)].
- V_d: the apparent volume of distribution of a drug. V_d is expressed in units of volume (e.g. mL). It does not have physiological meaning but is useful in predicting the loading dose.
- **Elimination half-life** ($t_{1/2}$): the time taken for the plasma concentration to halve, e.g. if the plasma concentration of a drug decreases from 8 μg/mL to 4 μg/mL in 4 hours, the half-life of the drug is 4 hours. Half-life is a hybrid term, being a function of both *Cl* and V_d.
  - $t_{1/2} = kV/Cl$ ($k = 0.693$). As V increases, $t_{1/2}$ increases. As *Cl* increases, $t_{1/2}$ decreases. If both parameters vary together, $t_{1/2}$ can remain unchanged.
  - Half-life determines duration of action after a single dose, time needed to reach steady state with repeated dosing and dosing frequency required to avoid large fluctuations in plasma concentration during the dosing interval. As a general rule, when the effect is related to drug concentration, doubling the dose adds one half-life to the duration of effect.

In summary, the volume of distribution and bioavailability are important for determining the first drug dose, clearance is important for the maintenance dose and half-life is important for determining the time needed to reach steady state and the dosing interval. These concepts are explored further in the Appendix to this chapter (p. 38).

Individualization of dosage regimens

When a veterinarian is considering drug therapy in an animal patient, critical questions include:

- What drug?
- What dose?
- What dosing interval and frequency?

Within each animal species, each drug is expected to have a predictable absorption, distribution, metabolism and excretion in normal animals and dosing regimens suggested in textbooks reflect this 'predictability'. However, there can be substantial individual variation in drug kinetics in individual dog and cat patients to which additional variability may be presented by pharmacodynamic processes. In addition, certain diseases may alter the pharmacokinetics of a drug. This variability is greater for some drugs than for others and has clinical importance when concentrations that are associated with toxicity are similar to therapeutic concentrations (e.g. drugs with low therapeutic margin such as digoxin, many cytotoxic drugs).

The variability in how the body 'deals' with the drug can be very difficult to predict. While approaches to alter the inherent pharmacokinetic nature of a drug in an individual animal are limited, veterinarians can manipulate the dose and dosing frequency of a drug to compensate for expected pharmacokinetic changes. Such manipulations can be made on a trial-and-error basis where the effects of the drug are closely monitored. Unfortunately, for many drugs used in small animal practice, drug effects cannot readily be measured, so monitoring the effectiveness of a dosing regimen manipulation can be difficult. Since it takes approximately 3–5 half-lives for drug concentrations to reach steady state, monitoring the impact of a change requires at least this time to elapse.

Some patients may benefit from drug concentrations that exceed the accepted therapeutic concentrations while others may suffer significant toxicity at doses that achieve therapeutic concentrations. An example of this is phenobarbital therapy for epilepsy, where some patients require much higher plasma concentrations and do not experience toxicity at doses that substantially exceed the standard therapeutic range for the drug.

What drug?

When choosing a drug, clinicians should be aware of the inherent pharmacokinetic characteristics of a particular drug.

- Is the drug well absorbed from the gastrointestinal tract? Is the drug subject to first-pass liver metabolism? Drugs that are poorly absorbed from the gut may not be in a suitable oral form for client use.
- Is gut absorption affected by food? Drugs may need to be given with food or, conversely, at times when food is not expected to be present in the upper gut.
- Does the drug distribute to particular body tissues? Drugs within a certain class may be chosen for particular pharmacokinetic characteristics, e.g. an antibiotic may be chosen because it is known to distribute to the prostate gland, whereas other antibiotics do not.
- How is the drug excreted (e.g. liver and/or kidney)? Drugs may be chosen for particular characteristics when a particular disease is present; for example, one may choose to avoid drugs that are predominantly cleared by the kidney when an animal presents with renal failure.

What dose?

Drug doses recommended on product labels are usually derived from dose determination studies, in which the clinical effects of various doses are examined. In such studies it may be determined that a 10 mg/kg bodyweight (bw) dose is ineffective, 20 mg/kg bw and 30 mg/kg bw doses are effective but a 100 mg/kg bw dose is toxic; 20 mg/kg would then be considered the minimally effective dose and would be the lowest dose (possibly of a range) recommended on product labels.

Veterinary drugs can be split into two types: those given once for an immediate effect (e.g. sedation, intravenous anesthesia) and those given repeatedly for a prolonged effect (e.g. antibiotics, nonsteroidal anti-inflammatory drugs, anticonvulsants). Where drugs are given once for an effect, the potential effects of disease on the pharmacokinetics of a drug in an individual animal patient are minimal. The reasons for this are discussed below.

The concentration of a drug in the body is determined by the amount of drug administered (e.g. the dose), bioavailability and the volume in which the drug is distributed. This relationship is:

$$\text{Concentration} = \text{amount absorbed/volume}.$$

To achieve a certain (therapeutic) plasma concentration of a drug when a clinician suspects that the volume of distribution of a drug may be altered because of a particular disease process, the amount of drug (dose) must be altered to allow for the suspected change in the volume of distribution of the drug. The most common reason for V_d of water-soluble drugs to change is dehydration. Since dehydration will only alter total body water by approximately 10%, changes in V_d do not often lead to changes in administered dose. V_d can be increased as a result of disease (for example, with hypoproteinemia leading to decreased protein binding, ascites leading to increased body water), pregnancy, obesity and age.

Note that clearance has little influence on this 'once-only' dose and therefore diseases that affect clearance do not usually require dose adjustments.

If therapy involves multiple drug administrations, then the frequency and interval of drug administration should be determined (see below).

Loading dose

The above points are relevant to the first dose given in a multiple drug administration protocol. This first dose is often called a 'loading dose', because it 'loads' the volume of distribution of the drug (even though this is not strictly correct) and allows steady-state concentrations to be approached more rapidly. Note that the loading dose is usually much higher than the maintenance doses given in subsequent drug administrations. As an example, a drug that is initially given as a dose of 2 mg/kg may then be given as maintenance doses of 1 mg/kg q.half life. The magnitude of the first 'loading' dose is predominantly related to the volume of distribution of the drug, whereas subsequent doses are related to the clearance of the drug (see below).

A loading dose may be desirable if the time required to attain steady state by the administration of the drug at a constant rate (3–5 elimination half-lives) is long relative to the temporal demands of the condition being treated. Potential disadvantages of using a loading dose include increased risk of toxicity and prolonged time for the concentration to fall if the drug has a long half-life.

What dosing frequency?

Dosing frequency is critical to the successful treatment of many diseases. When a drug has to be given repeatedly, the usual aim of therapy is to maintain a (relatively) constant drug concentration at the site of effect.

This 'steady-state' concentration (C_{ss}) is determined by the dose (D), the bioavailability (F), the dosing frequency (T) and the clearance of the drug (Cl). Mathematically this is defined as:

$$C_{ss} = F \times D/T/Cl$$

Using the equation:

- when the dose (D) is increased, concentration at steady state (C_{ss}) is increased
- when the dosing frequency (T) is decreased (e.g. every 12 h rather than every 8 h), C_{ss} decreases
- when clearance (Cl) decreases, C_{ss} increases
- a decrease in clearance (Cl) will need to be balanced by a decrease in dose/frequency (D/T) to keep C_{ss} constant
- either a decrease in dose (D) or an increase in dosing frequency (T) or both will lead to a decrease in D/T
- decreases in drug clearance may occur frequently as a result of renal and liver diseases
- significant increases in drug clearance are uncommon in small animal practice.

Example

If a D/T of 100 mg/h is required, this could be achieved by:

- a dose of 1000 mg given every 10 h
- a dose of 100 mg given every hour
- a dose of 1 mg given every 36s.

The effect of the choice between these three options is considerable. The first option would result in a very high plasma concentration initially (perhaps toxic), therapeutic concentrations for a certain period of time and very low concentrations (perhaps subtherapeutic) before the next dose. Such fluctuations may be suitable for certain drugs (e.g. concentration-dependent antibiotics). The third option would result in constant therapeutic plasma concentrations throughout the dosing period (as with a constant infusion), but would be impractical for long-term therapy.

So, the dosing interval and the magnitude of the dose given at each time will determine the fluctuations in plasma concentrations. Most importantly, if you suspect that the clearance of a drug may be decreased as a result of liver or renal disease, then D/T can be manipulated to compensate for the decrease in drug clearance, so that plasma drug concentrations can be kept within the therapeutic range. If you estimate that drug clearance may be decreased by 50%, then D/T will need to be decreased by 50%. Taking the above example of a D/T required of 100 mg/h (in normal animals), a D/T of 50 mg/h could be achieved by halving the dose (keeping the interval constant) or doubling the dosing interval (keeping the dose constant). Usually, since clearance is expected to be halved, the dosing interval is doubled rather than the dose halved.

Important clinical syndromes in which pharmacokinetic knowledge is critical

Liver disease/failure

Liver disease may affect the following pharmacokinetic variables.

- Bioavailability of oral drugs
- Binding of drugs to serum albumin (if hepatic albumin production decreases)
- Metabolism of prodrugs to active metabolites
- Hepatic metabolism and/or clearance of drugs.

There are no satisfactory indices of liver dysfunction in veterinary laboratory medicine that can be used to predict the magnitude of changes in hepatic clearance of drugs.

For drugs that have high plasma protein binding and are predominantly cleared by the liver, liver disease would be expected to result in an increase in the volume of distribution of the drug and decrease drug clearance. Thus, loading doses may need to be increased and dosing intervals may need to be lengthened to compensate for these changes. Close clinical monitoring will be required to aid individualization of the dose regimen and to match changes to the patient's needs.

Whether the use of certain drugs should be avoided in animals experiencing liver dysfunction is controversial. Ultimately it depends on whether that drug leads to toxicity at concentrations close to therapeutic concentrations and whether alternative drugs are available.

The effect of liver disease on drug disposition is discussed further in Chapter 3 on Adverse Drug Reactions.

Renal disease/failure

Renal disease may affect the following processes.

- Glomerular filtration of drugs
- Active tubular secretion of drugs
- Passive reabsorption of drugs
- Total body water
- Plasma albumin concentration
- Protein binding in the presence of uremia

There are few indices of renal dysfunction in veterinary laboratory medicine that can be used to predict the magnitude of changes in renal clearance of drugs. Although blood (plasma/serum) urea and creatinine are commonly used to assess renal function, they may not be appropriate indicators of renal clearance of drugs. In human medicine estimates of creatinine clearance are used to predict renal drug clearance.

For drugs that are predominantly cleared by the kidneys, renal disease would be expected to decrease drug clearance. Dosing intervals may need to be increased to compensate for these changes.

Whether the use of certain drugs should be avoided in animals experiencing renal dysfunction is also controversial. Ultimately it depends on whether that drug leads to toxicity at concentrations close to therapeutic levels and whether alternative drugs are available.

THERAPEUTIC DRUG MONITORING AS AN AID IN THERAPEUTIC MANAGEMENT OF CERTAIN DISEASES

Therapeutic drug monitoring (TDM) involves the collection of blood from an animal receiving drug treatment, analysis of drug concentrations in collected plasma and comparison of those plasma drug concentrations with a standard range. TDM gives veterinarians another tool to optimize drug therapy in an individual patient.

TDM has certain limitations for veterinarians in private practice as:

- additional expense to the client is involved
- blood samples must be taken at pharmacokinetically appropriate times after dosing
- results must be interpreted and applied to target the drug concentration appropriately. Many veterinarians find the calculations inhibiting.

TDM is also not the 'pharmacokinetic' answer to every veterinarian's question about drug therapy as:

- only certain drugs can be monitored
- the standard 'therapeutic' range for such drugs is usually extrapolated from humans and may not be an appropriate range for small animals nor for the disease being treated
- it is only a tool, the results of which must be considered in conjunction with other patient factors.

Table 2.2 Drug groups for which TDM may be considered

Drug group	Drug
Aminoglycosides	Gentamicin Amikacin
Anticonvulsants	Some benzodiazepines (including diazepam) Phenobarbital, primidone Potassium bromide
Cardiorespiratory drugs	Digoxin Lidocaine Procainamide Quinidine Theophylline
Psychotherapeutic drugs	Lithium carbonate
Thyroid hormone	

Once the drug concentration present in the sample is known, dose rates can be altered to achieve the desired plasma concentration:

$$\text{New dose} = \frac{\text{Desired concentration}}{\text{Old dose} \times \text{Measured concentration}}$$

TDM may be considered for certain drug groups, as listed in Table 2.2, with the following characteristics:

- pharmacokinetic variability
- narrow therapeutic index
- therapeutic and adverse effects related to drug concentration
- either desired therapeutic effect is difficult to monitor or drug is used to prevent an adverse event (e.g. seizures, arrhythmias).

CONCLUSION

Although veterinarians can usually do little to influence the bioavailability, volume of distribution, clearance and half-life of a drug, drug therapy can be individualized for small animal patients by adjusting dose and dosing interval. This chapter has introduced the pharmacokinetic principles involved in adjusting dose and dosing interval to individualize therapy for companion animal patients.

FURTHER READING

Adams HR (ed.) 2001 Veterinary pharmacology and therapeutics, 8th edn. Iowa State University Press, Ames, IA

Blodinger J (ed.) 1983 Formulation of veterinary dosage forms. Marcel Dekker, New York

Brunton LL, Lazo JS, Parker KL (eds) 2005 Goodman and Gilman's the pharmacological basis of therapeutics, 11th edn. McGraw-Hill, New York

Burton ME (ed.) 2006 Applied pharmacokinetics and pharmacodynamics: principles of therapeutic drug monitoring, 4th edn. Lippincott Williams and Wilkins, Baltimore, MD

Gibaldi M 1991 Biopharmaceutics and clinical pharmacokinetics, 4th edn. Lea and Febiger, Philadelphia, PA

Katzung BG (ed.) 2007 Basic and clinical pharmacology, 10th edn. Lange Medical Books/McGraw-Hill, New York

Neal MJ 2005 Medical pharmacology at a glance, 5th edn. Blackwell, Oxford

Pratt WB (ed.) 1990 Principles of drug action: the basis of pharmacology, 3rd edn. Churchill Livingstone, New York

Rowland M, Tozer TN 1995 Clinical pharmacokinetics: concepts and applications, 3rd edn. Williams and Wilkins, Baltimore, MD

Speight TM, Holford NHG (eds) 1997 Avery's drug treatment: a guide to properties, choice, therapeutic use and economic value of drugs in disease management, 4th edn. Adis International, Auckland, New Zealand

Walsh CT, Schwartz-Bloom RD 2005 Levine's pharmacology: drug actions and reactions, 7th edn. Taylor and Francis, London

APPENDIX: PHARMACOKINETIC EQUATIONS FOR CALCULATING PARAMETERS FROM DOSE ADMINISTRATION EXPERIMENTS

In order to determine the pharmacokinetic parameters of a drug, experiments are conducted whereby subjects are given a drug, and blood samples are collected at various time points after administration. The concentration of the drug in plasma is then measured. By plotting concentration versus time, several important parameters can be derived that help determine, for example, the dosing regimen for a drug. Some undergraduate veterinary courses require students to perform these types of calculations and postgraduate students may also need to be able to assess such data. Therefore basic methods for calculating various pharmacokinetic parameters are given below.

- Plot the natural logarithm of plasma concentrations against time on linear graph paper or plot plasma concentrations against time on semilog paper.
- If the plot is linear then the area under the curve (AUC) can be calculated using equation 3 below. If the plot is *not* linear, AUC can only be calculated using either differential calculus or the trapezoid method (see Fig. 2.2). An exponential decline in drug concentration is described by first-order kinetics and assumes a single compartment model (i.e. the drug appears to be in one compartment in the body or immediately distributed to all compartments).
- The rate at which the concentration declines is described by the constant λ (which is the slope at the change in concentration when concentration is plotted as natural logs).
- The concentration at any time is related to the maximum concentration by the equation:

$$C_t = C_{max} \cdot e^{-\lambda t}$$

If the plot is not linear (e.g. concave curve initially then becomes linear) this indicates that the drug has not been distributed to the tissues instantly, i.e. there are two (or more compartments), and this can be solved with a biexponential equation which is beyond the scope of this chapter. Assuming there is a linear plot from when the dose is given (time 0 for IV or complete, rapid IM injections or after rapid absorption or after infusion turned off):

1. **Elimination half-life ($t_{1/2}$)**

   Calculate $t_{1/2}$ from the graph (time it takes for a concentration anywhere along the graph to halve).

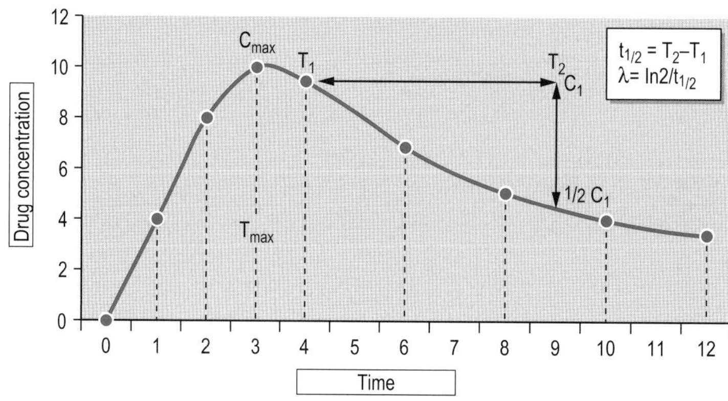

Fig. 2.2 **Estimation of area under the curve: trapezoidal rule. Observed drug concentration is plotted against time after oral administration of a drug formulation. Key features of this graph include: C_{max} (maximum concentration observed); T_{max} (time at which maximum concentration observed); elimination half-life ($t_{1/2}$) (time for concentration to halve, i.e. fall from C_1 to $1/2C_1$): elimination rate λ (rate of change of concentration).**

2. **Elimination rate constant λ**
   To calculate λ:

$$\lambda = \frac{\ln 2}{t_{1/2}} = \frac{0.69}{t_{1/2}}$$

3. **Area under the curve (AUC)**
   To calculate **AUC** (area under the curve), when the drug is given as an IV bolus and assuming the excretion is exponential use the formula:

$$AUC = \frac{C_0}{\lambda}$$

where C_o = the plasma concentration at time zero.

When the drug is given PO or by IV infusion over time calculate the AUC in the absorption/infusion phase (while the plasma concentration is increasing) by the trapezoid method (see Fig. 2.2) and ADD this to the AUC in the terminal phase as calculated by the formulae above. In this case C_o is the highest concentration reached after absorption/infusion. In Figure 2.2, the AUC from zero time to the last observed value can be estimated by adding the areas formed by the triangle between zero time and the first observation to each trapezoid under the curve formed between consecutive observations. The accuracy of the area estimate clearly improves as the number of observations increases.

$$\text{AUC(zero to last observed value)} = \tfrac{1}{2}(C_1 + C_0)(t_1 - t_0) + \tfrac{1}{2}(C_2 + C_1)(t_2 - t_1) \ldots + \tfrac{1}{2}(C_n + C_{n-1})(t_n - t_{n-1})$$

where C is concentration, t is time and the subscript refers to sequence of the observation.

To estimate the total AUC from zero time to infinity, by extrapolation, the area beyond the last observed value is estimated by dividing the value of the last observation of drug concentration C_n by the elimination rate constant (λ).

$$AUC_{(\text{zero to infinity})} = AUC_{(\text{zero to last observed value})} + C_n/\lambda$$

4. **Clearance**

$$Cl = \frac{D}{AUC}$$

where D = total dose given.

Note that if the drug is given orally or there is incomplete absorption from an intramuscular injection, D has to be adjusted to take into account the bioavailability (see point 6).

$$\text{Thus: } Cl = \frac{D.F}{AUC}$$

If the drug is given by infusion over a period of time, D = total amount given over the period of infusion.

5. **Volume of distribution**

$$V_d = \frac{D}{C_0}$$

This also needs to be adjusted for bioavailability if the drug is given orally. Thus:

$$Vd = \frac{D.F}{C_0}$$

6. **Bioavailability**

$$F = \frac{AUC_{oral}}{AUC_{IV}}$$

Note that in the latter equation you need to use trapezoids to calculate the AUC while the oral dose is being absorbed (where the plasma concentration is increasing).

If the dose given was different for the oral and IV data this needs to be corrected for.

7. **Infusion rate or dose rate**
   $R_0 = C_{ss} \times Cl$ (= Css × V × λ) where C_{ss} = plasma concentration at steady state (as the therapeutic plan should aim for the effective or therapeutic plasma concentration). If the dose is not given IV then the equation becomes:

$$R_0 = \frac{C_{ss} \times Cl}{F}$$

8. **Renal clearance**

$$Cl_{renal} = \frac{U \times C_{ur}}{C}$$

where U = urine flow rate (mL/min),
C_{ur} = concentration of drug in urine (mg/mL),
C = concentration of drug in plasma (mg/mL) (use the average of the plasma concentration at the beginning and end of the urine collection period).

9. **Calculating the plasma concentration at a particular time (t) before steady state is achieved**

$$C_t = C_{ss} \times (1 - e^{-\lambda t})$$

where Css = plasma concentration at steady state and Ct = plasma concentration at time t.

10. **Dose rate (Ro) would be required to reach a given plasma concentration (Ct) in a given time (t)**

$$R_0 = C_{ss} \times Cl \text{ (see above)}$$

Thus:

$$C_{ss} = \frac{R_0}{Cl}$$

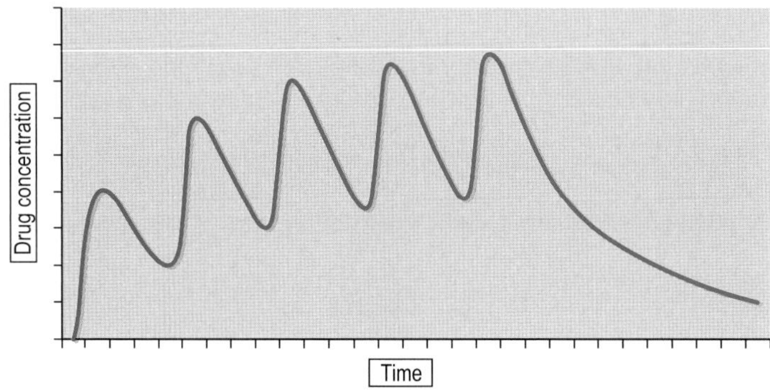

Fig. 2.3 **Multiple dose drug accumulation to steady state. Oral administration of five doses given at a dosage interval equal to the elimination half-life. After 4–5 doses, steady state is reached. Key features of the plot of drug concentration against time include: accumulation; fluctuation of drug concentration (peak and trough); dosing interval.**

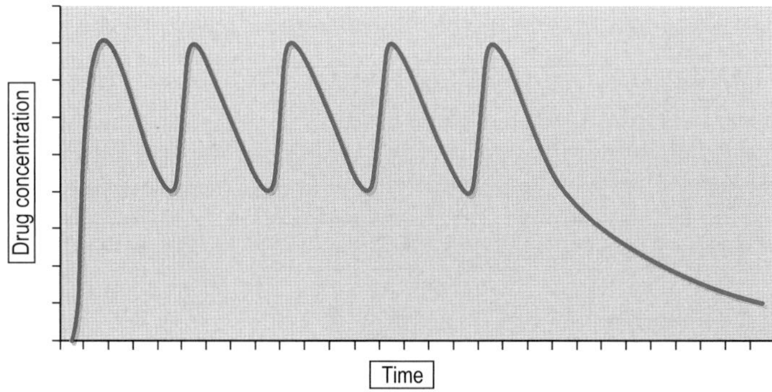

Fig. 2.4 **Loading dose (2 × maintenance dose) followed by maintenance dose every half-life. Steady state achieved after loading dose.**

Substituting Ro/Cl for Css we get:

$$C_t = \frac{R_0}{Cl} \times (1 - e^{-\lambda t})$$

Thus:

$$R_0 = \frac{C_t \times Cl}{(1 - e^{-\lambda t})}$$

11. To calculate the loading dose (LD) required to reach a desired plasma concentration

$$LD = \frac{V_{ss}}{F} \times C_{ss}$$

where V_{ss} = volume of distribution at steady state and C_{ss} = desired plasma concentration at steady state. Then the maintenance dose (MD) required:

$$MD = LD - LDe^{-\lambda t}$$

12. **Or to calculate the dosing interval required to maintain a plasma concentration at steady state** (see Figs 2.3 and 2.4)

$$C_{ss} = \frac{AUC}{\tau}$$

where τ = the dosing interval.

3

Adverse drug reactions

Jill E Maddison and Stephen W Page

An adverse drug reaction (ADR) (also called an adverse drug event (ADE) or adverse reaction) can be defined as 'an unintended or unexpected effect on animals, human beings or the environment, including injury, sensitivity reactions or lack of efficacy associated with the clinical use of a veterinary medicine (which includes pharmaceutical, biological and pesticide products)'. Generally the causality of adverse drug reactions is uncertain, making it more accurate to refer to 'suspected ADRs'. However, not all unwanted clinical phenomena encountered in practice are related to use of veterinary medicines and it is therefore important to differentiate between ADRs and adverse events (AEs) that are defined as 'untoward occurrences that may be present during treatment with a veterinary medicine but which do not necessarily have a causal relationship with this treatment' (adapted from Edwards & Aronson 2000). An algorithm describing the logical process of classification of untoward observations is presented in Figure 3.1. The study of adverse drug reactions, especially during postmarketing surveillance, is now termed pharmacovigilance – the science and activities relating to the detection, assessment, understanding and prevention of adverse drug reactions.

In veterinary medicine, ADRs in dogs and cats that are most frequently reported to spontaneous reporting schemes involve vaccines, antimicrobial drugs, nonsteroidal anti-inflammatory drugs, ectoparasiticides, anthelmintics and anesthetic agents. These are also the most common therapeutic or prophylactic agents used in these species so the higher incidence of ADRs related to these agents will reflect usage patterns, with the role of increased ADR potential more difficult to separate.

CLASSIFICATION OF ADVERSE DRUG REACTIONS

The A–F mnemonic classification of suspected ADRs described by Edwards & Aronson (2000) is also relevant to veterinary practice and usefully highlights that ADRs may not only be related to or independent of dose but may also occur over an extended (even intergenerational) time period. The greater the period between exposure and the adverse outcome, the more important is vigilance and a prepared mind.

Type A (augmented) ADRs are expected but exaggerated pharmacological or toxic responses to a drug. This may be an exaggeration of the intended response to the drug, a secondary response affecting an organ other than the target organ but predictable based on the pharmacology of the drug, or a toxic response.

Most ADRs of this type are attributable to differences in drug disposition that lead to higher plasma free drug concentrations as a result, for example, of increased drug absorption, organ failure, reduced protein binding (more likely due to decreased plasma protein than to displacement by another drug), hepatic enzyme induction or inhibition, or inappropriate dosage of a nonlipid-soluble drug in an obese dog. They are usually dose dependent and avoidable if sufficient drug and patient information is available.

A second class of ADRs is described as Type B (bizarre) reactions. These are unexpected or aberrant responses that are unrelated to the drug's pharmacological effect. They are not dose dependent and are unpredictable and idiosyncratic. Type B ADRs include allergic reactions, direct toxic effects on organs that are associated with actions unrelated to any desired therapeutic effect (the mechanisms for which may be complex and obscure) and aberrant responses in different species.

There are four further categories of ADR that are less commonly encountered in veterinary practice but which nevertheless do occur and should be recognized so that minimization or preventive strategies can be employed.

Type C (chronic) ADRs occur only during prolonged treatment programs, as for example the induction of iatrogenic hyperadrenocorticism with chronic use of prednisolone or other corticosteroid.

Type D (delayed) ADRs may be manifested some time after treatment. Second cancers developing in patients treated with alkylating agents such as cyclophosphamide would be included here as would the human ADR of clear cell adenocarcinoma of the vagina in the daughters of women (wrongfully) administered diethylstilbestrol for maintenance of pregnancy in the 1950s and 1960s.

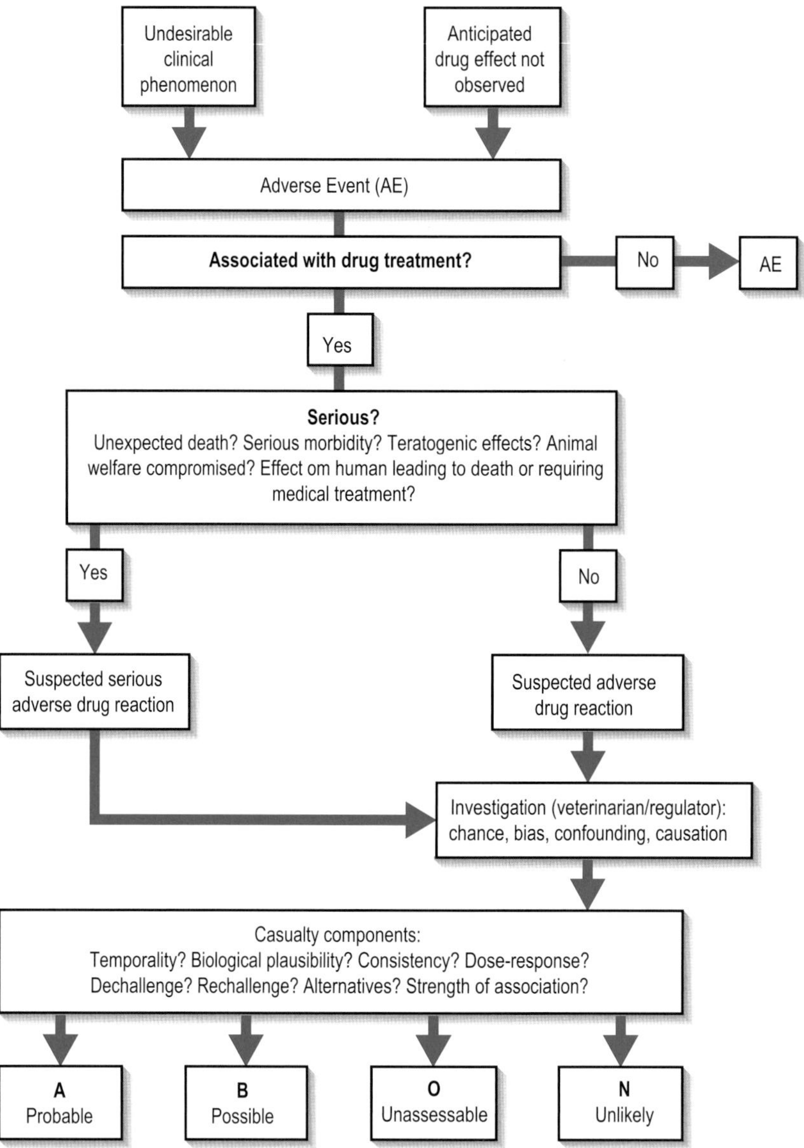

Fig. 3.1 Adverse event classification.

Type E (end of treatment) ADRs occur when drug treatment is terminated suddenly. Examples include withdrawal seizures on terminating anticonvulsant therapy and adrenocortical insufficiency subsequent to cessation of chronic administration of glucocorticoids.

Type F (failure of treatment) ADRs can be particularly informative if thoroughly investigated. There can be a multitude of reasons for treatment failure and a direct drug-related cause is unusual.

Table 3.1 provides a summary of many factors to be considered when faced with antibacterial drug failure. A similar list can readily be prepared for other drug categories.

INCIDENCE OF ADVERSE DRUG REACTIONS

The incidence of ADRs in veterinary medicine is difficult to evaluate. In human medicine it has been estimated that 3–5% of all hospitalized patients are admitted because of an ADR. Some studies give a wide variety of

Table 3.1 Apparent treatment failure: antibacterial example

Diagnosis Condition not of bacterial origin (noninfectious, other infectious – viral, protozoal, etc.)
Therapeutic goals Unrealistic objective (bacterial eradication vs disease control)
Pathophysiology Progression of underlying disease Poor management of mixed infection (e.g. mixed aerobic and anaerobic infection)
Host factors Predisposing factors uncorrected Impaired immune function (e.g. failure of passive transfer of colostral immunoglobulins) Nutritional deficits
Pharmaceutical factors Substandard product (expired, inappropriate storage)
Treatment Compliance Misadministration (e.g. animal avoided treatment, oral dosage regurgitated, injection misdirected)
Pharmacology Inappropriate drug selection Poor correlation of in vitro susceptibility and clinical outcome (e.g. in vitro rapid growth vs slower growth in vivo) Inappropriate dosage regimen (inadequate dose rate, route, frequency, duration, PK-PD mismatch) Pharmacokinetic issues (esp. changes in absorption, distribution and clearance) Impaired perfusion and penetration (BBB, abscess, edema, swollen milk ducts, etc.) Interaction with concurrent medication
Supportive therapy Omission of concurrent supportive measures (nutrition, hydration, nursing, abscess drainage, sequestrum removal)
Microbial factors Toxin elaboration Drug resistance Reinfection Bacterial dormancy (e.g. nongrowth phase) Bacterial L-forms Phenotypic tolerance (e.g. small colony variants) Dense bacterial loads in infected tissue Biofilm formation Superinfection (bacteria or fungal)
Epidemiology External bacterial challenge unabated
Toxicology Adverse drug reaction or interaction
Failure of investigation Incomplete history and physical examination (e.g. confounding factors not elucidated) Inappropriate samples collected

estimates from 1.5% to 35% of patients developing an ADR while hospitalized. On the basis of the number of reported ADRs and the number of prescriptions, it has been calculated that the average medical practitioner in the USA reports one ADR every 336 years (Etmina et al 2004). There are few studies in the veterinary literature that estimate incidence of ADRs or reporting rates but the situation is unlikely to be significantly better.

One author has concluded that the answer to the question 'How often do ADRs occur?' is 'It depends – on how intensively one searches, on what one means by an ADR and on the group of patients in whom one looks' (Kramer 1981).

Difficulties in diagnosing adverse drug reactions

One of the great challenges in determining the incidence of ADRs is the difficulty in accurate identification of ADRs. Appropriate diagnosis of an ADR is heavily dependent on the expertise of the attending clinician and the quality of the information available. Even experienced clinicians have difficulty in determining causality and experts have been shown to agree less than 50% of the time when assigning causality to an ADR.

The clinical signs of an ADR are almost always nonspecific and rarely if ever pathognomonic for an ADR. In human medicine the most common symptoms of ADRs (e.g. nausea/vomiting, diarrhea, abdominal pain, rash, pruritus, drowsiness, headache) are also reported in 80% of healthy patients on no medication. A similar situation may also exist in veterinary medicine. An examination of the US Center for Veterinary Medicine Freedom of Information summaries for seven NSAIDs reveals that concurrent placebo-treated dogs display similar incidences of the most commonly encountered adverse signs: vomiting, diarrhea/soft stool and inappetence. In addition, lethargy, dermatitis, pyrexia, abdominal pain and even death were reported in the placebo group. A recent UK study of ill health following vaccination of dogs (Edwards et al 2004) revealed a similar incidence of reported signs of ill health in recently vaccinated and unvaccinated dogs. Surprisingly, the reported incidence of signs of ill health was 19% and 25% in the 2-week period prior to questionnaire completion for recently vaccinated and unvaccinated dogs respectively. Placebo administration in humans causes an increase in the percentage of patients with symptoms and the number of symptoms per patient. Although a true placebo effect presumably does not exist in animals, veterinarians are reliant on the observations of owners who may be subject to various conscious or subconscious factors that may influence their interpretation of their pet's behavior.

Other factors that contribute to difficulties in determining whether a true ADR has occurred include multiple medications, underlying pathology and the assumption that it is the active principle of a medication that is responsible for the ADR. Many reactions are due to excipients (for example, the change in excipient in phenytoin tablets from calcium sulfate to lactose led to an epidemic of toxicity in humans due to increased bioavailability of the active substance; the use of ethylene glycol as a solvent infamously led to the Elixir Sulphanilamide tragedy) and some may be due to degradation products formed during storage (for example, tetra-ethyl pyrophosphates in some organophosphate preparations).

Even though all new drugs are intensively evaluated before release onto the market, evaluation before registration cannot assure the safety of a drug. Premarketing clinical trials, although examining up to several thousand animals, are usually too small, conducted for too short a period of time and conducted in a select and nonrepresentative population to detect rare or delayed ADRs. It is sobering to realize that the upper boundary of the 95% confidence interval in a study in which no adverse drug reactions are observed in 10,000 treated patients is 3/10,000. Clearly, the absence of detectable ADRs does not mean that no ADRs can be expected. If the clinical signs caused by the drug reaction also occur spontaneously in the untreated population, then a larger number of patients must be observed in order to attribute the reaction to the drug. In addition, it is difficult to include in trials all groups of animals including different breeds, the aged, the young, diseased animals and others that may have a high risk of developing an ADR. Hence, postmarketing surveillance or pharmacovigilance of drug ADRs is very important in assuring drug safety, detecting unusual and uncommon ADRs and identifying individuals or populations at higher risk.

Postmarketing drug surveillance (pharmacovigilance)

Postmarketing surveillance of adverse drug reactions occurs in various forms: phase IV clinical trials, spontaneous reporting schemes, intensive monitoring within hospitals (uncommon in veterinary medicine), analysis of health registers (more relevant to human medicine) and prospective studies. ADR reports rarely indicate the need to remove the drug from the market but such reports may lead to changes in dose rate, additional labelling or further clarification of labelling, additional warnings, precautions and contraindications and formulation changes.

Phase IV clinical trials may be conducted by the manufacturer after marketing approval, take place under usual clinical use of the drug and usually do not include a control group. However, it has been demonstrated in human medicine that despite the relatively large size of the cohorts monitored in phase IV studies, spontaneous reporting methods were more likely to detect previously unsuspected ADRs.

Spontaneous ADR reporting schemes can involve reporting of suspected ADRs by practitioners and animal owners through a variety of mechanisms: case reports in the literature, submissions to ADR reporting centers (which may or may not involve regulatory authorities, depending on the country) and reporting directly to the manufacturer. In many countries, manufacturers are now required to report ADRs to appropriate regulatory authorities. Spontaneous reporting schemes are relatively inexpensive and potentially draw data from all patients taking the drug. However, underreporting is a serious disadvantage – it is estimated that more than 95% of ADRs go unreported.

The ADR reporting rate is low within the medical profession and almost certainly even lower within the veterinary profession. Even in countries where ADR reporting is mandatory, the reporting rate by medical practitioners remains low. An analysis of the attitudes of medical practitioners in South Africa to ADR reporting revealed that there were differences in reporting rates between groups within the profession (a larger number of medical specialists reported ADRs compared with general practitioners). Surgical specialists did not report any ADRs during the study (Robins et al 1987). The major reasons identified for failure to report ADRs were: the belief of the medical practitioners that unusual or serious reactions were infrequent; common or trivial ADRs did not warrant reporting; apathy; being too busy to fill in the paperwork. Fear of personal consequences (criticism and medicolegal action) was not deemed to be an important impediment to reporting. The authors concluded somewhat pessimistically that 'the prognosis is poor (for improved ADR reporting) and it appears that, like all else which passes between doctors and their patients, ADRs will continue to remain largely outside the reach of an external agency'.

Similar studies have not been undertaken within the veterinary profession but there is no reason to assume that the attitudes of veterinarians to ADR reporting are radically better than those of their medical colleagues.

While complacency in reporting is widespread, an examination of those factors associated with an increased rate of reporting reveals that the likelihood of reporting is related to:

- novelty of the reaction
- severity of the reaction
- limited time of the drug on the market, often called the Weber effect (Weber 1984) after a study of NSAID ADRs in the UK which revealed that ADR reports peaked within 2 years and thereafter declined
- media coverage, also known as the Panorama effect from the effect of coverage by the BBC Panorama program on increases in ADR reports (Martin et al 2005). Certainly media attention to reported carpro-

fen ADRs in the US led to inundation of the FDA with ADR reports
- litiginousness of owner.

It is clear that the numbers of reports of suspected ADRs are incomplete and highly variable. Furthermore, there is both overascertainment (attribution of an adverse reaction to a drug when in truth it is not related) and underascertainment (failure to recognize that an adverse outcome is in truth an adverse drug reaction). Because of these important factors which influence the numerator and because the total number of times the drug is administered (the denominator) is unknown, it is not possible to calculate accurate rates of adverse reactions and there is no way to determine whether a given number of reports is smaller or larger than would be expected by chance. However, the value of spontaneous reporting programs is in **signal detection,** permitting hypotheses to be raised that can then be tested: some hypotheses will prove valid and others will not be confirmed. Pharmaco-epidemiology is the new discipline that has arisen to specialize in raising and testing such hypotheses.

Despite the variable frequency of reporting of suspected ADRs by veterinarians, spontaneous reporting programs have been successful in identifying a number of potentially serious ADRs that have led to publication of precautions, label changes and drug withdrawals, all allowing improved veterinary therapeutics. Examples include:

- anaphylactoid shock in cats following use of an ophthalmic combination antibiotic preparation containing bacitracin. Recommended to either avoid use or be prepared to manage the rare occurrences of this potentially lethal ADR (USA)
- carbon monoxide poisoning in dogs and cats undergoing anesthesia. Investigations revealed that CO can be produced when anesthetic gases interact with desiccated CO_2 absorbents. Use of low gas flow rates, avoidance of desiccation or regular change of soda lime seems to prevent this serious ADR (USA)
- soon after commercialization, ivermectin use in dogs of the collie and related breeds was associated with adverse neurological signs and led to label warnings (USA)
- extra-label repeated oral use of carprofen in the cat (according to dosage regimens recommended for the dog) has been associated with a number of deaths. Reminiscent of past experiences with aspirin, which has a much longer elimination half-life in cats than dogs, it is clear that the dog is not always a good surrogate for the cat. Since these experiences were reported, label changes have appeared warning against repeated dosing of cats. Single-dose parenteral use remains a safe and effective practice (UK)
- labeled use of NSAIDs (including carprofen, etodolac, deracoxib and meloxicam) in dogs was associated with a variety of adverse systemic signs and led to label warnings and Client Information Sheets (USA)
- the introduction of a palatable dosage form of carprofen was associated with reports of accidental ingestion by dogs (UK)
- reports of toxicity in dogs receiving the antibabesial drug diminazene highlighted the need for veterinary supervision (South Africa)
- permethrin intoxication has been reported in cats following ingestion of concentrated topical 'spot on' formulations intended for use in dogs. Label changes have since been made more strenuously warning against extra-label use in cats (USA, UK, Australia, Sweden)
- deaths in dogs following bathing in diazinon was reported. Investigation revealed that the diazinon dip concentrate contained inadequate stabilizer, allowing the formation of toxic byproducts. The product was subsequently withdrawn (Australia)
- extra-label use of fipronil in rabbits for control of mite infestations has been associated with deaths and led to a warning to the profession to avoid this use pattern (Australia)
- accidental ingestion by dogs of horse anthelmintic pastes containing trichlorfon or moxidectin has led to a number of deaths. While arguably a case of misuse, labels have been amended to warn against allowing dogs access to this horse product (Australia, UK)
- adverse gastrointestinal and neurological reactions by cats to an anthelmintic preparation containing praziquantel, pyrantel and febantel led to a change of formulation (removal of febantel) and a reduction in the frequency of ADR reports (Australia)
- severe hepatobiliary disease and death were reported in a number of dogs administered a combination of diethylcarbamazine and cyromazine per os, leading to product recall by the manufacturer (Australia)
- use of a combination drug product for canine otitis externa containing gentamicin, betamethasone and clotrimazole was associated with deafness, which was reversible if the product was flushed from the ear when deafness was first noted. A prominent warning was added to the label (USA)
- occasional reports of unexpected aggressive behavior by dogs treated with acepromazine led to label warnings (USA)
- serious adverse reactions by dogs to anthelmintic preparations containing dichlorophen and toluene led to label warnings (USA)
- keratoconjunctivitis sicca (KCS) was reported in dogs following use of the NSAID etodalac (USA)

- blindness due to retinal degeneration was associated with the use of enrofloxacin in cats. Risk factors included high doses or plasma concentrations, rapid IV infusion, prolonged course of treatment and age. An incidence of 1/122,414 cats treated has been calculated (Wiebe & Hamilton 2002) (USA)
- injection site sarcomas were identified in cats following administration of a variety of products, predominantly inactivated adjuvanted vaccines (USA, UK).

Spontaneous reports are also constant reminders of the low frequency but expected adverse drug reactions that may be rarely encountered by individual practitioners – for example, anaphylactic reactions to routine vaccination, vomiting and diarrhea associated with almost any orally administered preparation.

IDENTIFICATION OF ADVERSE DRUG REACTIONS

Any drug has the potential to affect an individual patient adversely. The justification for using a drug is the favorable ratio of anticipated benefits to potential risks. In life-threatening situations, use of a drug with a narrow therapeutic ratio may be warranted whereas the use of such a drug to treat trivial problems is more difficult to justify.

Accurate identification of an ADR is often difficult and it may go undetected if the clinical signs induced are indistinguishable from those of common disease syndromes. A clinician should always be alert to the possibility that the clinical abnormalities that an animal has presented with or has developed during the course of an illness are due to the treatment rather than the disease process itself.

When an association is observed between the administration of a drug and an adverse reaction, the following considerations can assist the decision on likely causality.

1. The **strength** of the association. To illustrate with an historic example, John Snow (the father of epidemiology) observed in 1854 that the death rate from cholera was 14 times higher in those who obtained their drinking water from the grossly polluted Southwark and Vauxhall Company compared with those supplied with sewage-free water by the Lambeth Company.
2. The **consistency** of the association. Has the same adverse event been repeatedly observed by different clinicians at different times?
3. The **specificity** of the association. Is the observed adverse event peculiar to situations where the drug is used or can the same syndrome have multiple causes?
4. The **temporality** of the association. Did drug treatment precede the event and has sufficient time elapsed to account for the particular phenomenon? It is particularly important to avoid the error of logic that would have one hastily conclude *post hoc ergo propter hoc* – after this, therefore because of this.
5. The **biological gradient** of the association. Is there evidence of a dose–response effect? In general, causality is strengthened by evidence that the likelihood of occurrence of an event increases with higher dose rates. This of course is more pertinent to Type A than Type B ADRs.
6. The **plausibility** of the association. Is there a biologically plausible mechanism of action for the adverse event that requires the presence of the drug?
7. The **coherence** of the association. Do the details of the event fit the pathophysiological state observed?
8. **Experimental evidence** (rechallenge and dechallenge). Does the event recur when the patient is rechallenged with the drug? Does discontinuation of the drug lead to abatement of the adverse effects?
9. **Analogy.** Is the observed event similar to well-described effects associated with the class of drugs to which the suspected drug belongs?
10. **Alternative hypothesis.** Is there a more valid alternative explanation?
11. **Quality.** How complete, reliable and rigorous is the evidence of the suspected adverse event?

It is important to remain critical and objective when determining likelihood of drug causality and to include, amongst the considerations outlined above, those sources of variability in clinical response to treatment presented in Chapter 1 and summarized below, including compliance, medication errors and possible confounding by comorbidities or concurrent medications (including prescription and over-the-counter medications, conventional and complementary and alternative medicines).

Having thoroughly evaluated the adverse experience, a preliminary assessment of causality can be made according to the classification recommended by the European Agency for the Evaluation of Medicinal Products (EMEA) and being adopted worldwide. There are four categories of causality in this system.

A: Probable. At a minimum, strength, plausibility, coherence, temporality, quality and absence of an alternative hypothesis should support the association of drug and event.

B: Possible. The above criteria do not all support causality, but one plausible hypothesis associates drug exposure with the observed events.

O: **Unclassified.** There is insufficient information available on which to reasonably draw any conclusion.

N: **Unlikely to be drug related.** Sufficient information is available and investigation has established beyond reasonable doubt that the suspected drug is not causally related to the observed events.

Causality categorization is generally open to change as further relevant information becomes available, including the benefits derived from additional reports and further pathophysiological or pharmacoepidemiological studies.

FACTORS THAT INFLUENCE TYPE A ADVERSE DRUG REACTIONS

It is important to understand the factors that modify the effects of drugs and their dosage in order to anticipate when a patient may be at increased risk of a Type A ADR. Many factors modify the effects of drugs in the individual patient. Some factors result in qualitative differences in the effects of the drug and may preclude its safe use in that patient. Other factors may produce a quantitative change in the usual effects of the drug that can be offset by appropriate adjustment in dose. Factors that may be important in modifying the effects of a drug in an individual include the following.

Species

In veterinary medicine we have to deal with animals of different species, different ages and, within one species, animals that may vary enormously in weight, e.g. a 2 kg chihuahua versus a 80 kg rottweiler. Therefore in order to individualize dosing regimens it is particularly important that we are aware of particular species peculiarities in drug metabolism, the effect of body size on dosing recommendations and, most importantly, that we understand that drug doses cannot necessarily be extrapolated between cats and dogs even if they are of similar weights.

Species differences in drug disposition may occur due to differences in absorption (due to differences in the anatomy of the gastrointestinal tract), differences in metabolism, distribution and excretion as well as many other factors.

Dogs versus cats

Of particular relevance to small animal clinical pharmacology are the potential differences between cats and dogs in how they handle drugs.

Although cats and dogs are physiologically similar in many respects and dosing regimens recommended for dogs can frequently be extrapolated to cats, there are some important differences in drug disposition between the two species that can have a profound influence on dosing recommendations. The majority of differences relate to pharmacokinetic differences in drug metabolism. However, differences in hemoglobin structure, receptors and behavioral differences may also account for differences in drug disposition between the two species.

Absorption and distribution

The kinetics of drug absorption appear to be similar in dogs and cats regardless of the route of administration. There are minor differences in factors that influence drug distribution between dogs and cats. For example, cats have a smaller blood volume per kg (66–70 mL/kg bodyweight) than dogs (90 mL/kg) and therefore plasma drug concentrations may differ between the two species for drugs which are confined to the plasma compartment. As understanding of drug transport proteins increases, further species differences may become evident.

Metabolism

Cats tend to be deficient in some glucuronyl transferases which are important for glucuronidation. They have substantially reduced ability to conjugate drugs such as acetominophen and aspirin with glucuronic acid. As a result hepatic clearance of aspirin in the cat is very prolonged, leading to a half-life of 37.5 hours compared with 8.5 hours in dogs. However, the drug can be used safely provided the dosage interval is appropriately extended. In contrast, acetaminophen is extremely toxic to cats and cannot be used under any circumstances because alternative metabolic pathways to glucuronidation produce toxic metabolites. Other drugs which are metabolized more slowly in cats include dipyrone, chloramphenicol, morphine and hexachlorophene.

This is not a problem for all drugs that are glucuronidated as cats are only deficient in certain families of glucuronyl transferases. A drug normally metabolized by glucuronidation may have a wide safety margin or the drug may be metabolized by a different route in cats (although this can result in toxicity for some drugs such as acetaminophen). For example, sulfation is well developed in cats compared to dogs and acetylation, which is deficient in dogs, appears to be well developed in cats.

Other drugs displaying pharmacokinetic differences include succinylcholine, which is metabolized more slowly in the cat than in the dog, presumably because of reduced blood pseudocholinesterase activity.

Dogs have a significantly reduced ability to acetylate drugs. Where this pathway is responsible for drug inactivation, e.g. sulfonamides, the drug will have a longer duration of action than in other species.

Hemoglobin

Another species difference which may raise the risk of adverse reactions in cats compared to dogs is the increased susceptibility of feline hemoglobin to oxidation and therefore methemoglobinemia. There are a number of proposed mechanisms postulated to explain this, including the different structure of feline hemoglobin, lower concentrations or activities of intracellular repair enzyme and differences in intracellular concentrations of glutathione-conjugating enzymes. Drugs affecting oxidative processes include the sulfonamides, nitrofurans and sulfones.

Receptors

Differences between dogs and cats with respect to drug receptor distribution and affinity have been described, with morphine representing the archetypal example. In addition to a slower rate of biotransformation due to the deficiency of glucuronidation in the cat, differences observed in the pharmacodynamic effects of morphine in the cat compared to the dog include CNS stimulation (CNS depression in the dog), centrally mediated emesis at much reduced sensitivity of the cat compared to the dog (dog requires dose 1/740 that of cat) and pupillary dilation (miosis in the dog). However, at a dose rate of 0.1 mg/kg subcutaneously (compared with 0.1–2 mg/kg in the dog), morphine provides effective analgesia in the cat.

Various receptors in the vomiting center, the chemoreceptor trigger zone (CRTZ), the vestibular pathways and the periphery (e.g. gut) are involved in the vomiting reflex. Species differ in the relative importance of some neurotransmitter–receptor systems related to vomiting and this has an impact on the efficacy of antiemetics. For example, apomorphine, a D_2-dopamine receptor agonist, is a potent emetic agent in dog and man but not in cat, monkey, pig, horse or domestic fowl. This suggests that D_2-dopamine receptor antagonists such as metoclopramide might not be very useful as antiemetic agents in the cat.

In contrast, xylazine, an α_2-adrenergic agonist, is a more potent emetic agent in the cat than the dog, suggesting that α_2-adrenergic antagonists, e.g. prochlorperazine (Stemetil), might be more useful antiemetic agents than D_2-dopamine receptor antagonists. Cytotoxic drug-induced emesis has been shown to be mediated by 5-HT_3 receptors in the CRTZ of the cat in contrast to the dog where visceral and vagal afferent 5-HT_3 receptors are activated.

Histamine receptors have not been demonstrated in the CRTZ of the cat. Studies based on eliminating the emetic response to parenterally administered compounds by lesioning the CRTZ suggest that the CRTZ may be less sensitive to emetic compounds in the cat than in the dog. Alternatively, other sites for the origin of emesis may be more sensitive in the cat than the dog.

Other drug effects

Other examples of drugs which have different effects in cats compared to dogs include febantel (which induces emesis much more readily in cats than dogs) and digitalis glycosides (the cat is less tolerant than the dog, presumably because of increased sensitivity of feline cardiac Na^+,K^+-ATPase to inhibition). Cats are more susceptible to aminoglycoside neurotoxicity than other species.

Behavioral differences

The grooming behavior of cats increases the likelihood that topically applied medications will be ingested. Advantage can be taken of this behavior by applying medications intended for ingestion to accessible parts of the cat's body (for example, anthelmintic or antibiotic paste preparations). However, cats are at greater risk of exposure to purposefully or adventitiously applied topical toxicants such as disinfectants (particularly phenolics that are principally candidates for glucuronidation) or pesticides. Indeed, concentrated preparations of permethrin applied topically to cats can be lethal when ingested.

Drugs which should not be used or used cautiously in cats and those which have a different toxicity profile to dogs are listed in Tables 3.2 and 3.3.

Table 3.2 Drugs not recommended for use in cats

Acetominophen (paracetamol)	Methemoglobinemia and Heinz body anemia
Apomorphine	Significant CNS depression
Azathioprine	Bone marrow suppression
Benzocaine	Methemoglobinemia Laryngeal edema
Cisplatin	Fatal, acute pulmonary edema
Propylthiouracil	Lethargy Weakness Anorexia Bleeding diathesis
Phenytoin	Sedation Ataxia Anorexia Dermal atrophy
Scopolamine	Tendency to cause behavioral changes
Sodium phosphate enemas	Depression Ataxia Vomiting Bloody diarrhea
Permethrin (high concentration products)	Hyperesthesia, generalized tremors, muscle fasciculations, hyperthermia, seizures, death

Table 3.3 Drugs which are therapeutically useful in cats but which may have different toxicity/activity profiles than in dogs	
Aspirin	Hyperpnea Hypersensitivity Hyperthermia
Chloramphenicol	Anemia
Digoxin	Vomiting Anorexia Bradycardia Arrhythmias
Doxorubicin	Renal failure
Enrofloxacin	Blindness
Furosemide	Dehydration Hypokalemia
Griseofulvin	Leukopenia and thrombocytopenia Nonreversible ataxia
Ketoconazole	Dry hair coat Weight loss
Lidocaine	Myocardial and CNS depression
Megestrol acetate	Mammary hypertrophy and neoplasia Cystic endometritis Diabetes mellitus
Methimazole	Anorexia Vomiting Self-induced facial excoriation Bleeding diathesis Hepatopathy Serious hematological side effects
Metronidazole	Disorientation Ataxia Seizures Blindness
Opioids Morphine derivatives (excluding meperidine [pethidine], butorphanol and buprenorphine)	Inconsistent sedation Increased risk of excitation
Organophosphates	Acute toxicity – hypersalivation, vomiting, diarrhea, muscle tremors Chronic or delayed toxicity – paresis or paralysis which may or may not be reversible
Tetracyclines	Hepatic lipidosis Increased ALT activity Ptyalism Anorexia
Thiacetarsamide	Drug fever Respiratory distress Fulminant pulmonary edema

Body size and percentage fat

Metabolic rate (estimated by O_2 consumption) is more closely related to body surface area than bodyweight so it has been suggested that small animals within a species may require a higher dose per kg than larger animals, when scaling is more closely linked to metabolic rate. This is particularly relevant to dogs where the body size within the species covers such a large range. Where there is a narrow therapeutic range for the drug, this factor can become very important. The dose of a drug with a narrow therapeutic ratio (e.g. digoxin, cytotoxic drugs) is usually calculated on body surface area rather than bodyweight. There can be a large difference in the calculated dose for dogs of extreme size (small or large) when weight or body surface areas are used. For drugs with a wide margin of safety such accurate dosing may not be clinically important. However, for drugs with a narrow margin of safety, failure to calculate the dose appropriately can result in toxicity or reduced therapeutic efficacy.

Another consideration when adjusting dosages for body size is the fat component of the bodyweight. Drug dosages are usually expressed per unit weight within a particular species. One should attempt to estimate the appropriate lean bodyweight and use this to calculate an appropriate dosage for nonlipid-soluble drugs even if using body surface area. Drugs which have a narrow margin of safety and are not lipid soluble include digoxin and the aminoglycoside antibiotics. For lipid-soluble drugs, increased body fat can act as a sink and reservoir, leading to protracted drug elimination if metabolism to a more water-soluble form is not involved.

Age

Neonates have a reduced capability for drug biotransformation and have underdeveloped hepatic and renal excretory mechanisms. Hence the increased sensitivity to, and prolonged recovery from, barbiturate anesthetics that may be observed in dogs and cats younger than 4 months. Other factors that influence drug disposition in the pediatric patient include increased gastrointestinal permeability, differences in body water and protein binding (greater percentage of body water, less extensive protein binding) and increased blood–brain barrier permeability.

Older animals may have reduced hepatic or renal function, less body water and reduced lean body mass and therefore often require lower doses of drugs compared to younger animals. However, it is important to be aware that the aging process varies greatly between individuals. Patient-specific physiological and functional characteristics are probably more important than age per se in predicting the predisposition to ADRs in patients.

Sex

During pregnancy or lactation, caution should be observed in administration of drugs that might affect the fetus or neonate. Drugs that should be avoided or used with caution in pregnant animals include corticosteroids, cytotoxic drugs, griseofulvin, ketoconazole, prostaglandins, salicylates, sex hormones, tetracyclines and live vaccines. Drugs which may adversely affect lactation, causing agalactia, include atropine, bromocriptine and furosemide. Adverse drug reactions occur more commonly in female humans but it is not known if this phenomenon occurs in domestic animals.

Pathology

Dosage recommendations are usually based on pharmacokinetic data obtained from healthy animals under controlled conditions even though many drugs will be given to diseased animals. Drug absorption, distribution, metabolism and excretion may be adversely affected by pathology of various organs, in particular the gastrointestinal tract, liver and kidney. Adjustment in dosage may be required, depending on changes in volume of distribution and clearance as influenced by the site of metabolism and route of elimination of the particular drug.

Drugs and the liver

The liver is the major site of metabolism of many drugs and thus the clinician is rightly concerned about the safety of administering drugs to patients with hepatic disease. Hepatocellular dysfunction can alter the bioavailability and disposition of a drug as well as influencing its pharmacological effects. In addition, the impact of hepatic pathology on drug disposition can relate to the effect of the clinical consequences of liver disease such as anorexia, pyrexia, hypoproteinemia and jaundice.

Hepatic extraction and the first-pass effect

When a drug is absorbed across the gut wall, it is delivered via portal blood to the liver prior to entry into the systemic circulation. Drug metabolism most commonly occurs in the liver prior to the drug reaching the systemic circulation although it can also occur in gut wall and portal blood. The liver may also excrete the drug into bile, allowing enterohepatic recycling.

The effect of first-pass elimination on bioavailability (the proportion of administered dose that reaches the systemic circulation unchanged) is expressed as the extraction ratio $ER = \frac{CL_{liver}}{Q}$ where CL_{liver} is clearance by the liver and Q is hepatic blood flow. This equation would predict that if clearance of a drug by the liver is reduced because of hepatocellular dysfunction causing reduced drug metabolism or decreased biliary excretion, then the ER will be reduced and systemic availability of the drug will rise when the drug is given orally. The equation also predicts that if hepatic blood flow is reduced then ER will also increase.

Studies in horses have demonstrated that acute submaximal exercise increases the elimination half-life of bromosulfan, possibly due to decreased splanchnic and hepatic blood flow. Whether this has clinical relevance for animals that are exercised to a far greater degree than the 'normal' pet is unknown.

Hepatic diseases that are accompanied by substantial intrahepatic or extrahepatic shunting (such as cirrhosis, congenital portacaval shunts) will result in *increased* bioavailability of drugs with high extraction ratios such as verapamil, pethidine, propranolol and several tricyclic antidepressants. Clearance of drugs which have intermediate extraction ratios such as aspirin, codeine and morphine may also be affected. Clearance of these drugs will also be prolonged by poor hepatic perfusion (e.g. in heart failure, in shock and with propranolol administration). Liver blood flow also tends to be reduced in older patients. In contrast, there will be little change in bioavailability of drugs that are poorly extracted by the liver (such as diazepam, theophylline, tolbutamide and warfarin) in patients with intra- or extrahepatic shunting. For these drugs altered hepatic metabolism is a more important factor in altering the pharmacokinetics of the drug.

Metabolism

The enhanced effects of drugs in patients with liver disease is primarily due to decreased drug metabolism. Fortunately, glucuronidation, a common method by which lipid-soluble drugs are metabolized in dogs, appears to be relatively unaffected by hepatic disease.

If a drug undergoes significant first-pass metabolism, a much larger dose of the drug is needed when it is given orally than when it is given by other routes. In addition, marked individual variations may occur in the extent of first-pass metabolism that can result in variable systemic availability and unpredictable effects when the drug is given orally. Serious hepatic dysfunction can reduce the first-pass effect of drugs that undergo substantial first-pass metabolism resulting in increased systemic availability. Examples of drugs that undergo substantial first-pass metabolism include aspirin, lidocaine (never given orally as its metabolites are believed to contribute to central nervous systemic toxicity), morphine, omeprazole, propranolol, salbutamol and verapamil. The increase in systemic availability increases the risk of toxic effects if the drug has a narrow therapeutic index and prolongs the duration of action of the drug.

Hepatic metabolism can produce toxic metabolites that lead to ADRs, for example halothane (trifluoroacetic acid), methoxyflurane (fluoride), cyclophosphamide (acrolein) and acetaminophen (*N*-acetyl-*p*-benzoquinone imine).

Drug effects on hepatic enzymes

Several drugs can influence the activity of the cytochrome P450 (or CYP) enzymes that constitute the major group of hepatic metabolizing enzymes. Four of the CYP isoenzymes are known to have a role in the metabolism of 95% of all drugs in man and 50–70% of drugs may be substrates for just one isoenzyme, CYP3A4 (the canine ortholog of which is CYP3A12). Several drugs can induce hepatic enzyme activity, increasing the metabolism of concurrently administered drugs and thereby influencing their activity. The best known of these drugs is phenobarbital but other drugs or substances with this capability include carbamazepine, polycyclic aromatic hydrocarbons in charcoal grilled meat and cigarette smoke, dexamethasone, phenytoin, primidone and rifampin. Although enzyme induction usually decreases the plasma concentration of drugs, if the affected drug has an active metabolite, enzyme induction can result in increased metabolite concentration and possibly an increase in drug toxicity.

Cimetidine and ethanol inhibit P450 isoenzymes and can therefore reduce the metabolism of drugs given concurrently that undergo hepatic metabolism. Other drugs that can inhibit one or several CYP isoenzymes include ciprofloxacin, clarithromycin, valproic acid, amiodarone, chloramphenicol, fluconazole, fluoxetine, miconazole, omeprazole, quinidine, cyclopsorin A and diltiazem. Imidazoles (e.g. ketoconazole, miconazole, clotrimazole) are potent inhibitors of fungal and mammalian cytochrome CYP enzymes. Ketoconazole alters the disposition and extends the duration of activity of methylprednisolone and may increase the plasma concentrations of cisapride and cyclosporin. Erythromycin can also inhibit CYP3A4 and can cause a clinically significant increase in plasma carbamazepine concentration. Marbofloxacin has been demonstrated to alter theophylline metabolism in dogs; the authors speculated that this could be clinically significant in dogs with renal impairment.

Natural remedies

An area of potential drug interaction which has yet to be fully explored involves interactions between dietary supplements, natural or herbal remedies and conventional western drugs. For example, diltiazem bioavailability was significantly increased due to inhibition of both intestinal and hepatic metabolism in rats fed *Ginko biloba* leaf extract, one of the herbal dietary supplements most widely used in Japan. Other natural products that have been reported to interact with drugs include ginseng, glucosamine, melatonin and St John's wort.

Although competitive inhibition between many hepatic metabolizing enzymes can be demonstrated in vitro, such interactions are usually not of practical significance in vivo. The inactivation of most drugs in vivo exhibits first-order kinetics (the rate of elimination is directly proportional to drug concentration – see Chapter 2) rather than zero-order or saturation kinetics (the rate of elimination is constant independent of plasma concentration due to saturation of the metabolizing enzyme at relatively low concentrations of drug). Thus the activity of enzymes is usually not rate limiting. In addition, drug concentrations are usually well below those required to saturate drug-metabolizing enzymes, which minimizes competition between substrates. However, significant mutual inhibitions of drug metabolism can be expected for drugs that usually exhibit saturation kinetics such as ethanol, phenytoin and salicylate.

Hepatotoxicity

Drugs that have been reported to directly cause hepatic toxicity in dogs include primidone, phenobarbital (rarely), rifampin, triazole antifungals such as ketoconazole, carprofen and mebendazole. Antimicrobial drugs which are believed to potentially accumulate in hepatic disease and may cause toxicity include chloramphenicol, lincosamides, macrolides, metronidazole, sulfonamides and tetracyclines.

Clinical effects of hepatic disease and their effect on drug pharmacokinetics

The clinical signs and pathological changes that occur as a result of hepatic disease can include anorexia, fever, jaundice and hypoproteinemia. These pathophysiological changes can alter drug disposition in the patient and should be kept in mind when medicating patients. The important isoenzyme CYP3A4 is reported to be decreased to 40–50% of control levels in rats with protein malnutrition and reduced metabolism of drugs that are a substrate for this isoenzyme, such as clarithromycin, has been demonstrated. Protein malnutrition in rats has also been shown to reduce metabolism of doxorubicin. Malnourishment in humans can cause altered hepatic oxidative drug biotransformations and conjugates as well as other changes that affect drug pharmacokinetics such as delayed or reduced absorption, reduced protein binding, fluctuations in volume of distribution and reduced elimination of renally excreted drugs. Short-term starvation has been shown to significantly prolong half-life and reduce hepatic clearance of phenazone in neonatal calves and similar effects may be possible in dogs and cats.

Fever may reduce metabolism of some drugs. Significant decreases in several hepatic enzymes have been demonstrated in febrile greyhounds although the clinical relevance of these findings is not known.

Patients with biliary tract obstruction appear to have an increased susceptibility to septic complications which could manifest as antimicrobial drug inefficacy. One possible explanation is the finding that biliary obstruction has been shown to reduce hepatic killing and phagocytic clearance of bacteria in rats. A logical clinical consequence of this could be that the clinician should only choose bactericidal antimicrobial drugs when treating patients with cholestatic disease.

The effects of altered plasma protein concentrations in patients with hepatic disease are complex. For drugs that have high plasma protein binding and are predominantly cleared by the liver, liver disease would be expected to increase the volume of distribution of the drug and decrease drug clearance. However, reduced protein binding due to lowered albumin levels associated with advanced hepatic disease may actually increase hepatic clearance and therefore compensate for reduced hepatic metabolism (if this is occurring). Increased serum globulin levels may occur in inflammatory hepatic disease or when the hepatic reticuloendothelial system is compromised. In these circumstances, increased protein binding (and therefore decreased systemic availability) can occur for some basic drugs such as lidocaine due to increased production of acute-phase proteins.

Conclusion

Unfortunately there are no satisfactory valid indices of liver dysfunction in veterinary or human clinical laboratory medicine that can be used to predict the magnitude of changes in hepatic clearance of drugs. In general, when administering drugs that are extensively metabolized by the liver, such as benzodiazepines, NSAIDS and opioids, to patients with liver disease, careful clinical observations are needed, with consideration of dosage interval prolongation. Use of barbiturates and several cytotoxic drugs (which have a narrow therapeutic index) such as cyclophosphamide, dacarbazine, thiotepa and asparaginase should be avoided in patients with liver disease.

Whether the use of certain drugs should be avoided in animals experiencing liver dysfunction is controversial. Ultimately it depends on whether that drug leads to toxicity at concentrations close to therapeutic concentrations (i.e. those drugs with a low therapeutic index) and whether other available drugs are suitable alternatives.

Table 3.4 gives examples of drugs that should be avoided or used with caution in patients with hepatic disease.

Renal dysfunction

The degree to which impaired renal function affects drug elimination is determined by the fraction of the dose that is excreted by the kidneys. Some drugs are nephrotoxic (e.g. aminoglycosides, amphotericin). The potential for nephrotoxicity is increased in patients with pre-existing renal disease and patients that are dehydrated due to water/sodium loss or diuretic (especially furosemide) usage. For example, the propensity for NSAID toxicity is increased when renal blood flow is reduced. Restoration of renal function is recommended prior to use of NSAIDs.

Table 3.4 gives examples of drugs that should be avoided or used with caution in patients with renal disease.

Altered cardiovascular function

Drug absorption and distribution may also be adversely affected by cardiac insufficiency. Regional blood flow will be altered in cardiovascular disease, resulting in the brain and heart receiving more blood and the kidney, skeletal muscle and splanchnic organs receiving less. Infiltrative gut disease will alter the absorption of orally administered drugs. Dehydration or acidosis may alter the absorption and distribution of drugs. For example, a dehydrated animal is unlikely to absorb drugs or fluids

Table 3.4 Examples of drugs that should be avoided or used with caution in patients with hepatic or renal disease

Drug class	Avoid*/hepatotoxic† or use with caution in liver disease	Avoid*/nephrotoxic† or use with caution in renal disease
Antimicrobial drugs	Chloramphenicol Chlortetracyclines* Erythromycin estolate* Flucytosine Griseofulvin Ketoconazole Lincosamides Macrolides Metronidazole Sulfonamide-trimethoprim*† Sulfonamides Tetracyclines	Aminoglycosides*† Amphotericin*† Fluoroquinolones Lincomycin Naficillin Nalidixic acid Nitrofurantoin Polymyxins† Sulfonamide-trimethoprim Sulfonamides Tetracyclines (except doxycycline)
Anesthetics (general/local)/ sedatives/anticonvulsants	Anticonvulsants Barbiturates*† Chlorpromazine Diazepam† Halogenated anesthetics Ketamine Lidocaine Propofol	Acepromazine Chlorpromazine Ketamine Methoxyflurane*† Procainamide
Cardiac drugs	β-blockers Lidocaine Quinidine	Angiotensin-converting enzyme inhibitors*† Cardiac glycosides Procainamide
Diuretics		Spironolactone Thiazides
Anti-inflammatories/ analgesics	Butorphanol Corticosteroids Meclofenamic acid Phenylbutazone Polysulfated glycosaminoglycan	Nonsteroidal anti-inflammatories*† Pethidine Polysulfated glycosaminoglycan
Cytotoxic drugs	Doxorubicin	Cisplatin*† Doxorubicin*† Fluorouracil Methotrexate*†
Miscellaneous	Doxapram Heparin Suxamethonium	Allopurinol Doxapram Gallamine Piperazine

from subcutaneous sites at the same rate as a well-hydrated animal.

Pharmacogenomic differences

Pharmacogenomics is the study of the effect of genetic and genomic differences between individuals on the pharmacological behavior of drugs. Genetic variability in the proteins responsible for drug transport, biotransformation (the enzymes of phase I and II processes) and receptors can be heritable and is determined by specific changes in the nucleotide sequences of specific genes. Genes in which particular nucleotide differences are present in at least 1% of the population are termed polymorphic. While heritable differences in a number of important hepatic enzymes have been well known in humans for decades, the application of pharmacogenomics to the dog is very recent, with even fewer studies in cats. In dogs CYP2B11 and CYP2D15 appear to be polymorphic, with the former enzyme, which metabolizes propofol, showing a 14-fold difference in activity amongst mixed breed dogs and the latter enzyme, that metabolizes celecoxib, being present in extensive and poor beagle phenotypes. Other important pharmacogenomic differences are summarized below.

N-acetyltransferase

A comprehensive study of the canine genome found that dogs and other canids do not possess the genes that code for cytosolic arylamine N-acetyltransferase (NAT). The absence of this gene and gene product renders the dog at increased risk of sulfonamide toxicity as NAT is a key enzyme in sulfonamide detoxification. By contrast with dogs, a study in cats has shown that while most species have at least two genes that code for NAT (NAT1 and NAT2), the cat has only one gene that codes for a NAT1-like enzyme.

Thiopurine S-methyltransferase

Thiopurine S-methyltransferase (TPMT) activity has been shown to be polymorphic in both cats and dogs. The clinical significance of this variability in enzyme activity is that TPMT is a key enzyme in the metabolism and inactivation of thiopurine analogs such as azathioprine and 6-mercaptopurine. Low TPMT activity increases the risk of myelosuppression in treated animals while high TPMT activity can be associated with poor antineoplastic efficacy.

Immune response genes

It has been hypothesized that variation in response to vaccines (for example, rabies and parvovirus vaccines) may be related to genomic differences in immune response genes of the major histocompatibility complex, consistent with the observation of unique breed-related haplotypes (Day 2006).

P-glycoprotein

P-glycoprotein (P-gp) or multidrug resistance protein 1 (Mdr1) is a member of the ATP binding cassette (ABC) superfamily of transmembrane transport proteins and in the dog is encoded by the gene *Mdr1*. P-gp is an important drug efflux transporter that has a significant impact on the gastrointestinal absorption, distribution, metabolism, excretion and toxicity of its substrates. Mutations of *Mdr1* have been observed in 10 dog breeds (see Table 3.5), with dogs that are homozygous for the *mdr1-1*Δ allele displaying nonfunctional P-gp. The pharmacological impact of homozygous mutants is the ability of ivermectin to pass the blood–brain barrier and achieve toxic concentrations within the brain two orders of magnitude higher than in dogs with functional P-gp. The identification of this mutation in collies and related breeds finally explains the well-known sensitivity of these breeds to the macrocyclic lactone class of parasiticides.

Table 3.5 P-glycoprotein polymorphism in dogs

Dog breed distribution of *mdr1-1*Δ	P-gp substrates
Collie	Acepromazine[a]
Australian shepherd	Butorphanol[a]
Border collie	Dexamethasone[a]
English shepherd	Digoxin[a]
German shepherd	Doramectin[a]
Long-haired whippet	Doxorubicin[a]
McNab	Doxorubicin[a]
Old English sheepdog	Ivermectin[a]
Shetland sheepdog (shelty)	Ketoconazole[c] (inhibitor)
Silken windhound	Loperamide[a]
	Mexiletine[a]
	Moxidectin[a]
	Ondansetron[c]
	Progesterone[c]
	Quinidine[b] (inhibitor)
	Selamectin[a]
	Vinblastine[b]
	Vincristine[a]

a Clinical evidence or **b** nonclinical evidence in dogs that these drugs can cause adverse effects if recipient is homozygous for *mdr1-1*Δ. **c** Possible substrate for canine P-gp.
Neff et al 2004; Schwab et al 2003; Mealey 2006.

Drug interactions

A drug interaction can occur if one member of a class of drugs alters the intensity of the pharmacological effects of another drug given concurrently. The net result of a drug interaction may be: enhancement of effects of one or other drug (hence increasing the risk of an ADR occurring); development of totally new effects not seen when either drug is used alone; inhibition of effect of one drug by another; no change in the net result despite the kinetics or metabolism of one or both drugs being substantially altered.

Drug interactions may be classified as:

- **pharmaceutical** – interactions that occur prior to administration (for example, mixing of a base and an acid for systemic or enteral use, such as a penicillin and an aminoglycoside). Most pharmaceutical interactions result in inactivation of one or both drugs. Rarely, a toxic interaction can arise
- **pharmacokinetic** – defined as an alteration in the absorption, distribution, metabolism or excretion of one drug by another. This is the most common type of drug interaction
- **pharmacodynamic** – where the drug affects the action or effect of the other drug.

Drug interactions can involve: direct chemical or physical interaction; interactions in gastrointestinal absorption; competition between drugs for protein-binding sites; interactions at receptor sites; interaction due to accelerated metabolism; inhibition of metabolism; alteration of renal excretion; and alteration of pH or electrolyte concentrations. While many drug interactions lead to increased risk of ADRs, other interactions may be beneficial, as for example when probenecid is combined with penicillin or clavulanic acid with amoxicillin.

Summary

From the above discussion it is apparent that the potential for the occurrence of a Type A ADR is higher in animals with organ dysfunction, particularly renal, hepatic or cardiac; in very young or very old animals; in animals to whom a number of drugs and other substances are administered concurrently; in species for which safe use of the drug or class of drugs has not been established; and in obese or cachectic patients. In general, type A ADRs should be avoidable if the above factors are considered and dosage regimens are altered appropriately.

TYPE B ADVERSE DRUG REACTIONS (HYPERSENSITIVITY)

Type B ADRs are unrelated to dose, are hard to predict and therefore difficult to avoid. The major example of idiosyncratic ADRs or Type B ADRs is allergic or hypersensitivity reactions. Drug hypersensitivity reactions are more common in patients with a prior history of allergic reactions to the drug or atopic patients but they can occur in any individual.

Penicillin-induced hypersensitivity is the best characterized drug-induced hypersensitivity in small animals. Other drugs that have been reported to cause allergic reactions include sulfonamides, doxorubicin, penicillamine, dipyrone and quinidine. In human medicine, allergic drug reactions account for approximately 5–10% of ADRs.

Any component of a drug preparation may induce a hypersensitivity reaction and microbiological contamination may also stimulate one. Drug hypersensitivity should be considered in the differential diagnosis of any apparently immune-mediated disease, e.g. polyarthropathy, hemolytic anemia and vesicular/ulcerative dermatitis.

Allergic drug reactions may occur as a result of a number of different immunological mechanisms including immediate hypersensitivity (Type I), cytotoxic hypersensitivity (Type II), immune complex formation (Type III) and delayed hypersensitivity (Type IV). However, the pathophysiology of many drug reactions eludes precise characterization and some immune reactions are a result of a combination of mechanisms.

Relatively few drugs are responsible for inducing allergic drug reactions as most drugs are not capable of forming covalent bonds with proteins, a requisite step to render a molecule immunogenic. The drug/drug metabolite–protein complex must have multiple antigenic combining sites to stimulate a drug-specific immune response and to elicit an allergic reaction. For those drugs that are capable of inducing an immunological response, it is generally the metabolites of the drug that are chemically reactive and easily form covalent bonds with macromolecules.

For example, the principal reactive product of penicillin appears to be the penicilloyl moiety resulting from the cleavage of the lactam ring. Hydroxylamine metabolites, formed from oxidation of the para-amino group of sulfonamide drugs, are capable of covalently binding to protein and are believed to be involved in allergic reactions to this class of drug. Doberman pinschers appear to be at increased risk of sulfonamide hypersensitivity. This has been postulated to be at least partially related to a decreased ability to detoxify hydroxylamine metabolites.

Cross-reactivity to other apparently unrelated drugs can occur if the particular portion of the drug molecule which is acting as the hapten also occurs in pharmacologically disparate groups of drugs. For example, the sulfamyl group is present in sulfonamide antimicrobial drugs as well as in furosemide, thiazide diuretics, the sulfonyl-urea group of oral hypoglycemic agents, e.g. glipizide, and some coxibs. Thus an animal that has a reaction to a sulfonamide may also react to these seemingly unrelated drugs.

Drug hypersensitivity may manifest in different ways. Acute anaphylaxis is associated with IgE and mast cell degranulation. It is characterized by one or all of the following clinical signs: hypotension, bronchospasm, angioedema, urticaria, erythema, pruritus, pharyngeal and/or laryngeal edema, vomiting and colic. The main shock or target organ for anaphylactic reactions varies between species, e.g. hepatic veins are the main target in dogs and the bronchi, bronchioles and pulmonary vein in cats. Drug-induced anaphylaxis will generally be apparent within minutes to hours of drug administration.

A systemic allergic reaction may also occur with drug use related to deposition of immune complexes in tissues and activation of complement. Clinical signs include lymphadenopathy, neuropathy, vasculitis, nephritis, arthritis, urticaria and fever. Various hematological perturbations may occur related to drug-induced antibody production resulting in hemolytic anemia, thrombocytopenia and rarely agranulocytosis. Cutaneous reactions may also occur related to development of immune complex deposition or delayed hypersensitivity.

Prior exposure to the drug is not essential as hypersensitivity may develop over the course of repeated drug administration. In humans, 5–7 days is required for drug–drug hypersensitivity to develop in a patient previously unexposed to the drug.

Allergic drug reactions should be managed by withdrawing the drug and treating with corticosteroids if needed. Adrenaline and fluid therapy may be needed for acute anaphylactic reactions.

Pseudoallergic drug reactions

Drug reactions may occur that resemble drug allergies but do not have an immunological basis. These reactions are often termed anaphylactoid reactions and do not require prior exposure to the drug. They occur most frequently when a drug is given rapidly intravenously. Anaphylactoid reactions may be due to nonspecific release of mediators of hypersensitivity or can be due to the direct effects of the drug on tissues.

Acute cardiovascular collapse can be induced by intravenous administration of chloramphenicol, aminoglycosides, tetracyclines and propylene glycol. Intravenous precipitation of water-insoluble drugs can also cause acute collapse. Direct release of hypersensitivity mediators can occur particularly with administration of iodinated contrast media, some intravenous anesthetics and opiates (e.g. morphine), polymyxin and thiamine. Administration of drugs in hypotonic solutions or some organic vehicles can cause erythrocyte lysis leading to acute hemolytic reactions which are not immunologically mediated. Nonimmunologically mediated drug fevers have also been reported, most frequently with penicillins and cephalosporins in dogs and tetracyclines in cats. In humans, aspirin and other nonsteroidal anti-inflammatory drugs can induce anaphylactoid reactions through interference with arachidonic acid metabolism.

REPORTING SUSPECTED ADVERSE DRUG REACTIONS

When faced with a suspected adverse drug reaction, the primary responsibility of the clinician is management of the patient's clinical situation. However, another important responsibility is to allow the collective experience with the implicated veterinary medicine to be evaluated. Veterinary clinicians should ensure that all suspected adverse drug reactions are reported to both the manufacturer of the suspected product and the local regulatory agency. It is only when reporting frequencies are high that valid assessments of the roles of suspected drugs in adverse events can be determined, risk factors identified, the veterinary profession alerted and appropriate remedial actions implemented.

Information required

While each country and regulatory agency may have a unique reporting form (which should be obtained, completed and returned to both the manufacturer and the responsible agency if possible) the following details are commonly requested.

1. Reporting veterinarian's name, address and telephone number
2. Owner's name or case identity
3. Suspected product details
   - Full name of product
   - Batch number
   - Expiry date
   - Manufacturer
4. Animal details
   - Species
   - Breed
   - Age
   - Sex
   - Weight
   - Concurrent clinical problems
5. Treatment details
   - Reason for treatment/diagnosis
   - Administered by whom
   - Dose regimen (route, dose rate, frequency and duration)
   - Date(s) and time(s) of treatment
   - Number treated
6. Reaction details
   - Time between treatment and onset of reaction
   - Description of the reaction, management and any specific or supportive treatment
   - Concurrent treatments
   - Possible contributing factors
   - Outcome of suspected adverse reaction (number affected, number dead, etc.)

All countries

Although not always mandatory, it is recommended that all suspected adverse drug reactions should be reported to the manufacturer(s) of the suspected product(s) and the local regulatory authority. Contact details of the manufacturer should be present on the product label. Details of a number of regulatory authorities and other groups interested in receipt of spontaneous reports are set out below.

Australia

For veterinary pharmaceutical, biological and pesticide products:
APVMA (Australian Pesticides and Veterinary Medicines Authority), Adverse Experience Reporting Program, Co-ordinating Veterinarian, PO Box E240, Kingston ACT 2604, Australia
Tel: 61-2-6210-4806
Fax: 61-2-6210-4813
Website: www.apvma.gov.au; http://www.apvma.gov.au/qa/aerp.shtml

Canada

For veterinary pharmaceutical products:
Veterinary Drugs Directorate, Health Products and Food Branch, Health Canada Holland Cross Complex, Ground Floor, 14–11 Holland Avenue, Ottawa, Ontario K1A 0K9, Canada, Address Locator – 3000A
Tel: 1-877-VET-REAC (1-877-838-7322)
Fax: 1-613-946-1125
Email: pharmacovigilance-vet@hc-sc.gc.ca
Website: www.hc-sc.gc.ca/dhp-mps/vet/advers-react-neg/index_e.html

For veterinary biological products:
Canadian Food Inspection Agency, Veterinary Biologics Section, 2 Constellation Crescent (Floor 8), Ottawa, Ontario K1A 0Y9, Canada
Tel: 1-613-221-7566
Fax: 1-613-228-6612
Website: www.inspection.gc.ca/english/anima/vetbio/info/vb315e.shtml

For veterinary topical pesticide products:
Director, Pest Management Regulatory Agency, 2250 Riverside Drive, Ottawa, Ontario K1A 0K9, Canada
Tel: 1-800-267-6315; 1-613-736-3799
Website: www.pmra-arla.gc.ca/english/legis/aer-e.html

New Zealand

For veterinary pharmaceutical, biological and pesticide products:
Agricultural Compounds and Veterinary Medicines (ACVM) Group, New Zealand Food Safety Authority, PO Box 2835, Wellington, New Zealand
Tel: 04-463-2550
Fax: 04-463-2566
Website: www.nzfsa.govt.nz/acvm/publications/forms/adrform.htm

South Africa

For suspected adverse reactions observed during use of a veterinary medicinal product:
Department of Pharmacology and Toxicology, Faculty of Veterinary Science, University of Pretoria, Private Bag X04, Onderstepoort, South Africa
Tel: 27-012-529-8239
Fax: 27-012-529-8304
Email: rgehring@op.up.ac.za
Report form: www.nda.agric.za/act36/Stock Remedies.htm

United Kingdom

For veterinary pharmaceutical, biological and pesticide products:
Department for Environment, Food and Rural Affairs (DEFRA), Veterinary Medicines Directorate, Suspected Adverse Reaction Surveillance Scheme, FREEPOST KT4503, Woodham Lane, New Haw, Addlestone, Surrey KT15 3BR, UK
Tel: 44-01932-338427
Fax: 44-01932-336618
Website: www.vmd.gov.uk/General/Adverse/adverse.htm

United States of America

For veterinary pharmaceutical products:
Center for Veterinary Medicine, ADE Reporting System, US Food and Drug Administration, 7500 Standish Place, Rockville, MD 20855-2773, USA
Tel: 1-888-FDA-VETS
Website: www.fda.gov/cvm/adetoc.htm

For topically applied external pesticide products:
Document Processing Desk-6(a)(2), Office of Pesticide Programs-7504P, US Environmental Protection Agency, Ariel Rios Building, 1200 Pennsylvania Avenue NW, Washington, DC 20460-0001, USA
Tel: 1-800-858-PEST (1-800-858-7378)
Website: www.epa.gov/pesticides/fifra6a2/

For veterinary biological products:
Center for Veterinary Biologics, 510 South 17th Street, Suite 104, Ames, IA 50010, USA
Tel: 515-232-5785; 1-800-752-6255
Fax: 515-232-7120
Email: cvb@aphis.usda.gov
Website: www.aphis.usda.gov/vs/cvb/html/adverseeventreport.html

REFERENCES

Day MJ 2006 Vaccine side effects: fact or fiction. Vet Microbiol 117: 51-58

Edwards DS, Henley WE, Ely ER, Wood JLN 2004 Vaccination and ill-health: a lack of temporal association and evidence of equivalence. Vaccine 22: 3270-3273

Edwards IR, Aronson JK 2000 Adverse drug reactions: definitions, diagnosis and management. Lancet 356: 1255-1259

Etmina M, Carleton B, Rochaon PA 2004 Quantifying adverse drug events. Are systematic reviews the answer? Drug Safety 27: 757-761

Kramer MS 1981 Difficulties in assessing the adverse effects of drugs. Br J Clin Pharmacol 11: 105S

Martin RM, May M, Gunnell D 2005 Did intense adverse media publicity impact on prescribing of paroxetine and the notification of

suspected adverse drug reactions? Analysis of routine databases, 2001–2004. Br J Clin Pharmacol 61: 224-228
Mealey KL 2006 Adverse drug reactions in herding-breed dogs: the role of p-glycoprotein. Comp Cont Ed 28: 23-33
Neff MW, Robertson KR, Wong AK et al 2004 Breed distribution and history of canine mdr1-1Δ, a pharmacogenetic mutation that marks the emergence of breeds from the collie lineage. Proc Nat Acad Sci USA 101: 11725-11730
Robins AH, Weir M, Biersteker EM 1987 Attitudes to adverse drug reactions and their reporting among medical practitioners. S Afr Med J 72: 131
Schwab M, Eichelbaum M, Fromm MF 2003 Genetic polymorphisms of the human MDR1 drug transporter. Annu Rev Pharmacol Toxicol 43: 285-307
Weber JCP 1984 Epidemiology of adverse reactions to nonsteroidal antiinflammatory drugs. Adv Inflamm Res 6: 1-7
Wiebe V, Hamiltion P 2002 Fluoroquinolone-induced retinal degeneration in cats. JAVMA 221: 1568-1571

FURTHER READING

Anderson JA, Adkinson F 1987 Allergic reactions to drugs and biological agents. JAMA 258: 2891
Boothe DM 1990 Drug therapy in cats: mechanisms and avoidance of adverse drug reactions. JAVMA 196: 1297
Bukowski JA, Wartenberg D 1996 Comparison of adverse drug reaction reporting in veterinary and human medicine. JAVMA 209: 40
Cribb AE 1989 Idiosyncratic reactions to sulfonamides in dogs. JAVMA 195: 1612
Davis LE 1984 Hypersensitivity reactions induced by antimicrobial drugs. JAVMA 185: 1131
Edwards IR 1987 Adverse drug reaction monitoring: the practicalities. Med Tox 2: 405
Hanley JA, Lippman-Hand A 1983 If nothing goes wrong, is everything all right? Interpreting zero numerators. JAMA 259: 1743-1745
Hill AB 1965 The environment and disease: association or causation? Proc Roy Soc Med 58: 295-300
Hoskins JD, Hubbert WT, Selig JO et al 1982 A questionnaire for the clinical assessment of veterinary adverse drug reactions. Cornell Vet 72: 3
Johnson JM 1992 Reasonable possibility: causality and postmarketing surveillance. Drug Inf J 26: 553
Ndiritu CG, Enos LR 1977 Adverse reactions to drugs in a veterinary hospital. JAVMA 171: 335
World Health Organization 2002 The importance of pharmacovigilance. Safety monitoring of medicinal products. World Health Organization, Geneva

4

The pharmacology of the autonomic nervous system

Matthias J Kleinz and Ian Spence

The investigation of the autonomic nervous system has played a central role in the development of modern pharmacology and formed the basis for establishing fundamental pharmacodynamic principles that govern drug actions. At the same time, the identification and characterization of the major transmitter pathways in the autonomic nervous system, using classic isolated organ preparations (e.g. guinea pig ileum), was the initial step towards the development of a plethora of drugs that modify autonomically controlled body functions such as the regulation of the cardiovascular system, respiratory system and gastrointestinal tract. It therefore comes as no surprise that drugs modulating autonomic function in humans, e.g. antihypertensives and antiasthmatics, have some of the largest markets for therapeutic agents worldwide. For these obvious reasons autonomic pharmacology occupies a large section in most general pharmacology texts and the increasingly widespread use of such classes of drugs in veterinary practice requires adequate presentation of autonomic nervous system pharmacology in textbooks written for veterinarians.

As a result, this chapter aims to outline the important basic features of the autonomic nervous system and its pharmacology and proceeds to discuss in detail those topics directly relevant to small animal therapeutics. A reference guide to the clinical use of drugs acting on the autonomic nervous system forms the end of the chapter.

Due to the widespread impact of autonomic regulator pathways on a multitude of organ systems, many drugs that interact with the autonomic nervous system are also described in more detail in other chapters.

ANATOMICAL ORGANIZATION OF THE AUTONOMIC NERVOUS SYSTEM

The autonomic nervous system (ANS) comprises one of two efferent components of the peripheral nervous system (PNS). As a part of the PNS, the ANS is responsible for the efferent innervation of all tissues apart from skeletal muscle, which itself is innervated by the somatic nervous system. The predominantly involuntary control of organ function by the autonomic nervous system is modulated by neuronal networks which are located mainly in the brainstem and spinal cord.

The organization of the efferent arm of the somatic nervous system is essentially uniform. The ANS, on the other hand, is divided into the sympathetic and parasympathetic nervous systems. This division is also reflected in the anatomical origin of sympathetic and parasympathetic outflow from either thoracolumbar or craniosacral segments of the central nervous system (CNS) respectively. The parasympathetic outflow to all autonomically regulated organs except the bladder, rectum and genitals (supplied by the pelvic ganglia) originates from the nuclei of four cranial nerves. These are the occulomotor nerve (III, structures of the eye), facial and glossopharyngeal nerves (VII, IX, salivary glands and nasopharynx) and the vagus nerve (X, thoracic and abdominal viscera). Figure 4.1 schematically illustrates the basic anatomical organization of the ANS.

Another important organizational characteristic that distinguishes the ANS from the somatic nervous system is the presence of a neuronal chain of one preganglionic and one postganglionic neurone in the ANS supplying the target organs, compared to a single somatic motor neurone innervating skeletal muscle fibers. This has some pharmacological importance, as certain drugs act on postganglionic neurones located in autonomic ganglia to modulate postganglionic ANS neurotransmission. The only exception to this 'two-neurone' rule of ANS organization is the sympathetic innervation of the adrenal medulla. The catecholamine-secreting chromaffin cells of the adrenal medulla are modified sympathetic postganglionic neurones, which therefore receive sympathetic input only from preganglionic sympathetic axons.

The cell bodies of preganglionic neurones are located in the sympathetic and parasympathetic nuclei of the brain and spinal cord. Postganglionic neurone cell bodies are located mainly in the paravertebral or prevertebral ganglia (sympathetic outflow) and in cranial, cervical and pelvic ganglia or in small ganglia

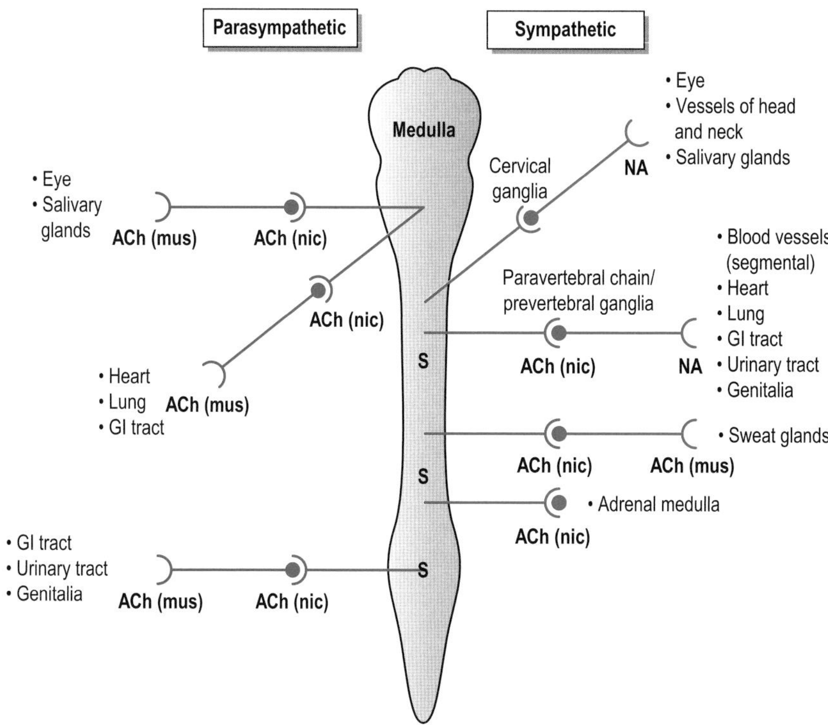

Fig. 4.1 The basic anatomical organization of the ANS.

closely associated to the target organs (parasympathetic outflow).

There is considerable species variation in the detailed anatomy of the ANS. For example, the way in which sympathetic postganglionic neurones are aggregated into the prevertebral ganglia – the celiac, superior mesenteric and inferior mesenteric – varies considerably between species. Similarly, the exact level of the spinal cord at which different sacral parasympathetic nerves exit to supply fibers to the pelvic ganglia also shows considerable variation. These differences have obvious implications in surgical situations but there is no established evidence that they alter responses to pharmacological agents. Having said this, it is perhaps worth pointing out that there has never, to the authors' knowledge, been a systematic examination of this question.

A third part of the ANS is the enteric nervous system (ENS), which does not simply fit into the general division of the ANS in sympathetic versus parasympathetic nervous system terms. The ENS is a network of interconnected neurones and ganglia localized in the wall of the gastrointestinal tract, which has considerable integrative potential and regulates gastrointestinal function via local reflex pathways. Nevertheless, neurones in both Auerbach's (myenteric) and Meissner's (submucosal) plexus receive modulatory input from the sympathetic and parasympathetic systems. It is in the ENS that a large number of novel, nonclassical ANS neurotransmitters (e.g. 5-HT, NO, ATP, VIP) have been discovered over the last 40 years and, together with classical sympathetic and parasympathetic afferents and efferents, they make up what is emerging as the gut–brain axis.

PHYSIOLOGICAL AND PHARMACOLOGICAL ORGANIZATION OF THE AUTONOMIC NERVOUS SYSTEM

The ANS carries all the neuronal output from the CNS apart from the motor innervation of skeletal muscle. The ANS controls essential physiological processes such as smooth muscle tone, exocrine and to some extent endocrine secretion, cardiac performance and energy metabolism.

Despite opposing effects of the sympathetic and parasympathetic nervous system on the smooth muscle tone of gut and bladder and on the heart's force of contraction, it is an inappropriate oversimplification to assume that the sympathetic and parasympathetic systems are strict physiological opponents. This is illustrated by the fact that a number of important organs are the target for either sympathetic or parasympathetic afferents. Sweat glands and blood vessels receive sympathetic innervation alone. The muscarinic acetylcholine (ACh) receptors on the vascular endothelium, which can cause vasodilation by inducing production of the endothelium-dependent relaxing factor nitric oxide (NO), have no parasympathetic neuronal input. The ciliary muscle of the eye and the smooth muscle of the bronchi receive only parasympathetic innervation. Salivary glands are innervated by sympathetic and parasympathetic fibers but both deliver prosecretory stimuli.

The sympathetic nervous system has an important role in tuning autonomic processes for the 'fight-and-flight' state and the parasympathetic nervous system contributes to the 'rest-and-digest' state. Under less extreme physiological everyday conditions, however, both systems jointly contribute to the maintenance of homeostasis. This fact has been highlighted by the discovery of a multitude of mechanisms that mediate presynaptic and postsynaptic modulation of one system by the other.

The most important biochemical distinction between the two major parts of the autonomic nervous system relates to the distribution of different neurotransmitters. Generally, transmission from preganglionic to postganglionic neurones is mediated by ACh acting on nicotinic ACh receptors present in both sympathetic and parasympathetic autonomic ganglia. Postganglionic transmission at sympathetic target organ synapses is mediated by noradrenaline (norepinephrine) acting on either α- or β-adrenoceptors. In the parasympathetic nervous system, on the other hand, postganglionic transmission occurs via release of ACh which activates muscarinic ACh receptors present on the postsynaptic membrane.

In addition to these two principal transmitters, a variety of other substances are synthesized, stored and may be released from autonomic nerve endings. These so-called nonadrenergic and noncholinergic (NANC) transmitters are summarized in Table 4.1. From a pharmacological perspective this knowledge of other mediators is only just starting to have an impact on clinical applications (e.g. potential use of 5-HT, substance P and VIP antagonists as antidiarrhea agents).

NEUROTRANSMISSION IN THE AUTONOMIC NERVOUS SYSTEM

Table 4.1 illustrates the increasing number of putative transmitters in the ANS besides the classic neurotransmitters acetylcholine, noradrenaline (norepinephrine) and adrenaline (epinephrine). These new transmitter systems may in future lead to new therapeutic approaches in ANS pharmacology, which is particularly interesting, as some novel transmitter systems have a more discrete distribution within the ANS, with the potential to present very selective pharmacological targets with a reduced risk of unwanted adverse effects. However, the most detailed knowledge of the process involved in ANS neurotransmission is available for the cholinergic (acetylcholine) and the catecholaminergic (noradrenaline/norepinephrine, adrenaline/epinephrine) transmitter pathways, which will therefore be discussed in more detail.

Neurotransmission at both cholinergic and catecholaminergic synapses is initiated by depolarization of the presynaptic axon terminal upon the arrival of an action potential. This results in an influx of Ca^{2+} ions, which in turn initiates a series of protein–protein interactions leading to the fusion of synaptic vesicles with the cell membrane of the presynaptic axon terminal and the release of their neurotransmitter contents into the synaptic cleft. The transmitter then diffuses through the synaptic space and binds to specific receptors on the postsynaptic membrane, initiating a response in the postsynaptic neurone. This general concept of neurotransmission at chemical synapses, where presynaptic neurotransmitter release causes the activation of specific postsynaptic receptors, applies to both cholinergic and catecholaminergic synapses. Pharmacologically important differences do, however, exist between the mechanisms by which the neurotransmitter is removed from the synaptic cleft and recycled in the presynaptic terminal in cholinergic and catecholaminergic synapses.

THE PARASYMPATHETIC NERVOUS SYSTEM – CHOLINERGIC SYNAPSES

The general process of cholinergic neurotransmission is the same at nicotinic and muscarinic synapses. The activation of distinct subtypes of postsynaptic acetylcholine receptors by the neurotransmitter acetylcholine is responsible for the different effects on target organs. In cholinergic nerve terminals, acetylcholine is synthesized from choline, which is taken up into the nerve terminal via a specific transporter, and acetyl-coenzyme-A, a product of carbohydrate intermediate metabolism. Transporter-mediated uptake of choline into the nerve terminal presents the rate-limiting step of this synthetic pathway which is catalyzed by the enzyme choline-acetyltransferase. ACh is then pumped into secretory vesicles via a transporter and stored until action potentials arriving at the nerve terminal induce Ca^{2+}-mediated fusion of secretory vesicles with the presynaptic membrane and neurotransmitter release, a process which underlies presynaptic regulation by M_2 ACh receptors and α_2-adrenoceptors. ACh then diffuses across the synaptic cleft to bind postsynaptic receptors. Ultimately, acetylcholinesterase, a specific hydrolytic enzyme, is responsible for the degradation of ACh in the synaptic cleft. After ACh hydrolysis, choline is taken up into the nerve terminal again where it is recycled.

Table 4.1 Neurotransmitters in the mammalian ANS

Substance	Location	Receptors	Cellular response	Pharmacological effects
Established neurotransmitters				
Acetylcholine	Sympathetic and parasympathetic ganglia	nAChR	Increased cation conductance (mainly Na^{2+} and K^+)	Stimulation of sympathetic and parasympathetic ganglia
	Parasympathetic postganglionic synapses (gastric and salivary glands)	M_1	$G_{q/11}$, PLCβ activation, Ca^{2+}↑	CNS excitation, gastric and salivary gland secretion
	Parasympathetic postganglionic synapses (heart, smooth muscle)	M_2	Activation of inhibitory G-protein (G_i), cAMP↓	Cardiac inhibition, presynaptic inhibition of adrenergic synapses
	Parasympathetic postganglionic synapses (gastric and salivary glands, gastrointestinal (GI) and ocular smooth muscle, vascular endothelial cells)	M_3	$G_{q/11}$, PLCβ activation, Ca^{2+}↑	Gastric and salivary gland secretion, GI smooth muscle constriction, ocular accommodation, indirect vasodilation (NO release)
	ENS	nAChR, M_1	Increased cation conductance (mainly Na^+ and K^+, fast postsynaptic excitatory potentials), $G_{q/11}$, PLCβ activation, Ca^{2+}↑ (slow postsynaptic excitatory potentials)	Increased glandular secretion and motility
	Skeletal neuromuscular junction	nAChR	Increased cation conductance (mainly Na^+ and K^+)	Muscle contraction
Noradrenaline (norepinephrine)	Sympathetic postganglionic synapses (vascular, bronchial, GI, GI sphincter, uterus, bladder sphincter, seminal tract and iris (radial) smooth muscle, liver)	α_1	$G_{q/11}$, PLCβ activation, Ca^{2+}↑	Smooth muscle constriction, relaxation of GI smooth muscle, constriction of GI sphincters, increased glycogenolysis
	Sympathetic postganglionic neurone endings, neurones of brainstem nuclei	α_2	G_i, cAMP↓	Presynaptic inhibition of noradrenaline release, blood vessel dilation and GI smooth muscle relaxation (indirect), inhibition of sympathetic outflow in CNS
	Sympathetic postganglionic synapses in the heart	β_1	Activation of stimulatory G-protein (G_s), cAMP↑	Positive inotropic and chronotropic actions
	Sympathetic postganglionic synapses (vascular, bronchial, GI, uterus, bladder and ciliary and seminal tract smooth muscle), skeletal muscle, liver	β_2	G_s, cAMP↑	Smooth muscle relaxation, increased muscle mass, speed of contraction and glycogenolysis
	Sympathetic postganglionic synapses in adipocytes and skeletal muscle	β_3	G_s, cAMP↑	Induces lipolysis and thermogenesis
Dopamine	Sympathetic postganglionic synapses in blood vessels and renal tubular epithelial cells	D_1-like ($D_{1,5}$)	G_s, cAMP↑, PLCβ/PKC activation	Vasodilation, induces renal Na^+ excretion
	Sympathetic postganglionic neurone endings	D_2-like ($D_{2,3,4}$)	G_i, cAMP↓	Presynaptic inhibition of noradrenaline release, vasodilation

Table 4.1 Neurotransmitters in the mammalian ANS (*continued*)

Substance	Location	Receptors	Cellular response	Pharmacological effects
Putative transmitters				
Adenosine triphosphate	Sympathetic ganglia	P2X	Increased cation conductance	Ganglionic stimulation
	Sympathetic postganglionic neurone endings	P2X	Increased cation conductance	Presynaptic stimulation of NA release
	Sympathetic postganglionic neurone endings	P2Y	$G_{q/11}$, PLCβ activation, $Ca^{2+}\uparrow$	Presynaptic stimulation of NA release
	Sympathetic and parasympathetic postganlionic synapses	P2Y	$G_{q/11}$, PLCβ activation, $Ca^{2+}\uparrow$	Smooth muscle contraction
	ENS, inhibitory motorneurones	P2Y	$G_{q/11}$, PLCβ activation, $Ca^{2+}\uparrow$	Circular smooth muscle relaxation
	ENS, inhibitory motorneurones	P2X	Increased cation conductance	Stimulation of inhibitory motorneurones
	ENS, intrinsic sensory neurones	P2X	Increased cation conductance	Depolarization
	ENS, intrinsic sensory neurones	P2Y	Ca^{2+}-dependent potassium conductance	Hyperpolarization
Calcitonin gene-related peptide	Peripheral unmyelinated afferent sensory neurones in heart, lung, GI tract, bladder	CGRP	NANC neurotransmission in the efferent direction	Smooth muscle relaxation, increased glandular secretion, positive chronotropic and inotropic action, neurogenic inflammation
	Sympathetic and parasympathetic ganglia	CGRP	G_i, cAMP↓	Inhibition of nAChR signaling
Carbon monoxide (CO)	Parasympathetic postganglionic synapses, ENS, autonomic ganglia	Soluble guanylate cyclase	cGMP↑	Smooth muscle relaxation
Endocannabinoids (anandamide, 2-arachidonylglycerol)	Parasympathetic preganglionic synapses, ENS	CB_1,CB_2	G_i, cAMP↓, increased K^+ conductance	Presynaptic inhibition of neurotransmitter release (predominantly ACh), reduced GI motility and secretion
Endogenous opioids (enkephalins, endorphins, dynorphins)	ENS secretomotor neurones	μ (MOP), κ (KOP), δ (DOP)	G_i, cAMP↓, increased K^+ conductance	Reduced GI motility
	Autonomic effector synapses in the heart	μ (MOP), κ (KOP), δ (DOP)	G_i, cAMP↓, increased K^+ conductance, inhibition of L-type Ca^{2+} channels	Negative chronotropic and inotropic actions
5-HT (serotonin)	Parasympathetic preganglionic synapses, ENS	5-HT_3	Increased cation conductance	Depolarization of postganglionic neurones, promotes GI motility and secretion
	Parasympathetic preganglionic synapses, ENS	5-HT_4	G_s, cAMP↑	Smooth muscle contraction, promotes GI and secretion
Gamma-amino butyric acid	ENS inhibitory neuromuscular synapses	$GABA_A$, $GABA_B$	Increased anion conductance (A), G_i, cAMP↓, activation of inwardly rectifying K^+ channels (B)	Hyperpolarization
Galanin	ENS secretomotor neurones and intrinsic sensory neurones	GAL_1, GAL_2, GAL_3	G_i, cAMP↓	Modulates gastrointestinal motility and secretion
	Parasympathetic postganglionic neurone endings in the heart	GAL_1, GAL_2, GAL_3	G_i, cAMP↓	Presynaptic inhibition of neurotransmitter release (predominantly ACh), indirect positive inotropic and chronotropic actions
Gastrin-releasing peptide (GRP)	Parasympathetic postganglionic synapses	BB_2	$G_{q/11}$, PLCβ activation, $Ca^{2+}\uparrow$	Increased GI motility and pancreatic insulin secretion, modulates gastric acid secretion

Table 4.1 Neurotransmitters in the mammalian ANS (*continued*)

Substance	Location	Receptors	Cellular response	Pharmacological effects
Neuropeptide Y (NPY), peptide YY (PYY), pancreatic polypeptide (PP)	Sympathetic postganglionic synapses	Y_1	G_i,cAMP↓	Vasoconstriction
	Parasympathetic postganglionic neurone endings	Y_2	G_i,cAMP↓	Reduced parasympathetic neurotransmitter release, negative inotropic actions
	Sympathetic postganglionic neurone endings	Y_2	G_i,cAMP↓	Modulation of sympathetic neurotransmitter release, reduction of gastric acid secretion, reduction in vasoconstriction
Nitric oxide (NO)	Endocrine cells (adrenal gland), autonomic nervous system synapses	Synaptobrevin, synaptotagmin	Formation of synaptobrevin-synaptotagmin complex	Promotes exocytosis of neurotransmitter vesicles
	Autonomic effector synapses in heart, lung, intestine and blood vessels	Soluble guanylate cyclase, nitrosylated cytoplasmatic proteins and transcription factors	cGMP↑	Smooth muscle relaxation
Nociceptin	Sympathetic and parasympathetic postganglionic neurone endings	NOP	G_i, cAMP↓, increased K^+ conductance	Presynaptic inhibition of neurotransmitter release, effects on multiple organ systems
Pituitary adenylate-cyclase activating peptide (PACAP)	ENS secretomotor neurones	PAC_1	G_s, cAMP↑	Reduced GI motility
Substance P and related tachykinins	Parasympathetic baroreceptor afferents	NK_1	$G_{q/11}$, inhibition of sympathetic and activation of parasympathetic preganglionic neurones	Vasodilation
	Autonomic afferent neurones in the respiratory system and GI tract	NK_1, NK_2	$G_{q/11}$, PLCβ activation, Ca^{2+}↑, activation of parasympathetic preganglionic neurones	Smooth muscle contraction, increased glandular secretion
	ENS intrinsic neurones and interneurones	NK_1, NK_2, NK_3	$G_{q/11}$, PLCβ activation, Ca^{2+}↑	Cotransmission in ENS secretomotor neurones, increased GI motility
	Sympathetic and parasympathetic ganglia	NK_1	Allosteric modification of nAChR	Inhibition of nAChR signaling
Vasoactive intestinal peptide (VIP)	ENS secretomotor neurones	$VPAC_1$, $VPAC_2$	G_s, cAMP↑	Reduced GI motility
	Parasympathetic postganglionic synapses (heart, vasculature, lung)	$VPAC_1$, $VPAC_2$	G_s, cAMP↑	Positive inotropic and chronotropic actions, coronary vasodilation, bronchodilation

PLCβ, phospholipase Cβ; IP3, inositol triphosphate; DAG, diacylglycerol; PKC, protein kinase C; cAMP, cyclic adenosine monophosphate; cGMP, cyclic guanosine monophosphate; GI, gastrointestinal; SM, smooth muscle; NANC, non-adrenergic non cholinergic.

Figure 4.2 shows the general process of neurotransmission at a cholinergic nerve terminal.

Table 4.2 summarizes clinically important pharmacological agents that can interfere with the various stages of the cholinergic transmission process (only one example is given in each case and further examples are discussed below).

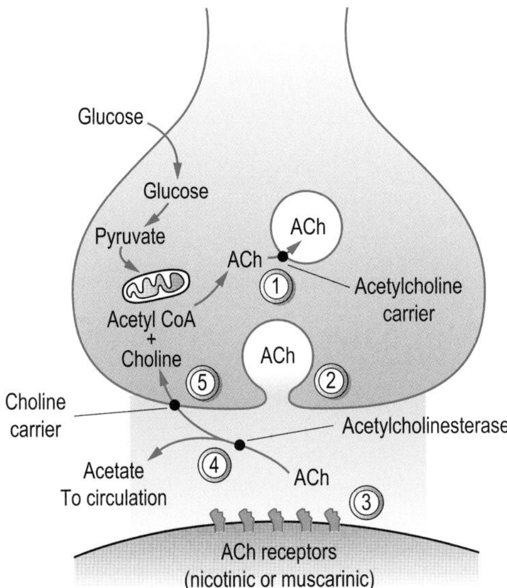

Fig. 4.2 **Schematic diagram of a generalized cholinergic synapse (not to scale). The transport of precursors and the metabolism of acteylcholine (ACh) are essentially the same at nicotinic and muscarinic junctions. The circled numbers refer to Table 4.2.**

Cholinergic neurotransmission

Cholinergic neurotransmission is the result of binding of ACh, released from presynaptic nerve terminals, to acetylcholine receptors. Acetylcholine receptors can be divided into two fundamentally different classes with further subtypes: nicotinic (a1–a10) and muscarinic (M_1–M_5) acetylcholine receptors. These two subclasses were originally defined based on their responses to the alkaloids nicotine (from *Nicotiana tabacum*, a South American flowering plant) and muscarine (from *Amanita muscaria*, a poisonous mushroom). Subsequently it has become clear that nicotinic and muscarinic receptors have very distinct pharmacological properties and physiological roles. These major differences are summarized in Table 4.3.

Vascular actions of acetylcholine

Many, perhaps all, blood vessels possess receptors for ACh. This is curious as few, if any, vessels receive cholinergic innervation and physiologically, ACh is not circulating in the bloodstream. Thus the presence of muscarinic ACh receptors and their effect on vascular tone are of pharmacological rather than physiological interest. Acting on muscarinic receptors present on vascular endothelial cells rather than vascular smooth muscle, ACh and other muscarinic agonists cause the release of endothelium-derived relaxing factors (predominantly nitric oxide, NO). The gaseous transmitter NO diffuses into the vascular smooth muscle layer where it leads to the activation of soluble guanylate cyclase, the formation of cyclic guanosine monophosphate (cGMP) and thus induces smooth muscle relaxation.

Table 4.2 Cholinergic transmission

Transmission step	Agent	Effect	Affected transmission step in Fig. 4.2
Vesicle loading	Vesamicol	Block of ACh uptake into secretory vesicles, neurotransmitter depletion	1
Vesicle fusion	Botulinum toxin	Irreversible block of ACh release	2
	Tick toxin (*Ixodes holocyclus*)	Reversible block of ACh release	2
Postsynaptic binding	Tubocurarine	Nondepolarizing block of neurotransmission at the neuromuscular junction (nicotinic)	3
	Suxamethonium	Depolarizing block of neurotransmission at the neuromuscular junction (nicotinic)	3
	Hexamethonium	Block of neurotransmission at autonomic ganglia (nicotinic)	3
	Atropine	Block of neurotransmission at target organs (glands, cardiac muscle, smooth muscle) (muscarinic)	3
Breakdown of transmitter	Neostigmine	Block of neurotransmitter breakdown by acetylcholinesterase resulting in amplification/ prolongation of postsynaptic response	4
Uptake of choline	Hemicholinium	Blocks reuptake of choline into the presynaptic nerve ending	5

ACh, acetylcholine.

Table 4.3 Basic properties of cholinergic receptors

	Nicotinic	**Muscarinic**
Receptor type	Ligand-gated ion channel	G protein-coupled receptor
Ligand receptor interaction	Binding of two ACh molecules required to cause receptor activation	Receptor activated by a single ACh molecule
Receptor response to ligand binding	Channel opening, increased cation conductance (mainly Na^+, K^+)	Receptor associates with heterotrimeric G proteins
Cellular response	Depolarization	Activation of second messenger pathways (cAMP, IP_3/DAG, Ca^{2+}, depending on receptor subtype)
Time from ligand binding to response	<1 ms	~400 ms
Localization	Neuromuscular junction, autonomic ganglia, secretory cells of adrenal medulla	Parasympathetic postganglionic synapses, sympathetic postganglionic synapses (sweat glands)

IP_3, inositol triphosphate; DAG, diacylglycerol; cAMP, cyclic adenosine monophosphate; GI, gastrointestinal; SM, smooth muscle; ACh,acetylcholine.

Table 4.4 Nicotinic receptors

Receptor	**Location**	**Membrane response**	**Functional response**	**Agonists**	**Antagonists**
α1 (muscle type)	Neuromuscular junction	Increased cation conductance (mainly Na^+, K^+)	Excitatory postsynaptic potential, skeletal muscle constriction	ACh, CCh, suxamethonium	Tubocurarine, conotoxin, α bungarotoxion
α3 (ganglion type)	Autonomic ganglia, secretory cells of the adrenal medulla	Increased cation conductance (mainly Na^+, K^+)	Stimulation of postganglionic autonomic neurones (sympathetic and parasympathetic)	ACh, CCh, nicotine	Trimetaphan, mecamylamine hexamethonium

ACh, acetylcholine; CCh, carbamylcholine (carbachol).

Drugs affecting nicotinic receptors

Nicotinic ACh receptors are pentameric proteins, which function as cation-selective ligand-gated ion channels at postsynaptic membranes of autonomic ganglia (sympathetic and parasympathetic), at the neuromuscular junction and in CNS synapses.

Based on molecular studies, 10 nicotinic receptor subtypes have been identified (a1–a10), two of which have an important established role in mediating cholinergic neurotransmission in the peripheral nervous system. a1 (the muscle type nicotinic receptor) mediates cholinergic neurotransmission at the neuromuscular junction and a3 (the ganglion type nicotinic receptor) mediates cholinergic transmission in autonomic ganglia and at sympathetic synapses that innervate secretory cells of the adrenal medulla. Pharmacologically, the two major classes of nicotinic receptors can be distinguished using selective agonists and antagonists, which are presented in Table 4.4.

Nicotinic agonists

Nicotinic agonists have no important role in veterinary therapeutics. The stereotypical nicotinic agonist – nicotine itself – is used as a recreational stimulant by many people via various routes of administration. After administration of doses commonly used for this purpose there is little or no effect on peripheral nicotinic synapses. The general stimulatory effect of small doses of nicotine is the result of nicotine promoting the release of a large number of CNS neurotransmitters. This stimulating effect of low-dose nicotine is reversed when nicotine is administered at higher doses. Peripheral effects include tachycardia, increased arterial pressure and reduction of gastrointestinal motility. The light-headed feeling experienced by naive smokers is due to stimulation of nicotinic receptors located on sensory nerve fibers, principally chemoreceptors in the carotid body. Nicotine is quite toxic (0.5–1.0 mg/kg in mammals) and higher doses can cause serious adverse reactions and even death.

Suxamethonium (succinylcholine), is a selective agonist of the nicotinic muscle type receptor. It dissociates readily from the nicotinic receptor but is not metabolized by acetylcholinesterase. It can be used as a short-acting neuromuscular blocking agent as continuous activation of the ACh receptors results in functional antagonism. It is sporadically used in dogs and cats during anesthesia and for the diagnosis of malignant hyperthermia.

Nicotinic antagonists

Nicotinic antagonists fall into two distinct groups: ganglion blockers and peripheral muscle relaxants. The differences between the nicotinic receptors at autonomic ganglia and those at the neuromuscular junction mentioned above form the basis of the distinct pharmacodynamic actions of these two classes of drugs. Generally, ganglion blockers have little or no effect on transmission at the neuromuscular junction.

The prototypic ganglion blocker is hexamethonium, which causes a fall in blood pressure as the result of blockade of sympathetic ganglia that mediate some control on arterial and venous blood pressure. Hexamethonium in the past was used as an antihypertensive agent but has been superseded by β-blockers and other antihypertensive treatments. Trimetaphan, another ganglion blocker, is now only occasionally used in human medicine for controlled hypotension during surgery.

The prototypic peripheral muscle relaxant is curare. This is not a pure substance but a mixture of alkaloids from the South American vine *Chondodendron tomentosum*. The main active constituent, *d*-tubocurarine, was isolated at the beginning of the last century and many synthetic agents are now available. Some of the older peripheral muscle relaxants, including tubocurarine and gallamine, have mild ganglion-blocking activity.

The group of antinicotinic peripheral muscle relaxants used in veterinary medicine can be further subdivided into nondepolarizing (pancuronium, atracurium besylate, vecuronium) or depolarizing (suxamethonium/succinylcholine, see above) agents. Nondepolarizing peripheral muscle relaxants bind to nicotinic receptors at the motor endplates, acting as classic competitive antagonists with no intrinsic activity, thereby inhibiting neuromuscular transmission. Depolarizing peripheral muscle relaxants act as agonists at the nicotinic receptors of the neuromuscular junction that cause muscle paralysis by inducing sustained depolarization as a result of extremely slow dissociation of the receptor–ligand complex.

The neuromuscular blockade produced by nondepolarizing blockers can be reversed with anticholinesterases. The neuromuscular blockade produced by depolarizing blockers cannot be reversed by this method. This latter point is rarely a problem as depolarizing blockade is very short-lived as suxamethonium is a substrate for circulating pseudocholinesterases.

Drugs affecting muscarinic receptors

Muscarinic receptors generally mediate the effects of acetylcholine release at postsynaptic parasympathetic synapses, causing predominantly smooth muscle constriction and glandular secretion. The only sympathetic effect mediated by muscarinic receptors is the stimulation of sweat glands by atypical cholinergic postganglionic sympathetic nerves. As opposed to nicotinic receptors, which are ligand-gated ion channels, muscarinic receptors belong to the class of seven transmembrane-spanning G protein-coupled receptors (7TMs) which, depending on the subtype, can affect a plethora of intracellular target molecules including ion channels, protein kinases and transcription factors. Based on their genetic sequence, five subtypes of muscarinic receptors (M_1–M_5) can be distinguished and the functional role of the three most important ones (M_1–M_3) has been well characterized. The major characteristics of these receptor subtypes are presented in Table 4.5.

Muscarinic agonists

Muscarinic agonists are often referred to as parasympathomimetics as their action resembles generalized stimulation of the parasympathetic system. Examples of such agents include, of course, muscarine but also other choline esters related to acetylcholine, such as bethanechol and pilocarpine. These compounds are agonists at both muscarinic and nicotinic receptors that do, however, display higher potency at muscarinic receptors.

Depending on their potency and selectivity for muscarinic receptors, parasympathomimetics induce cardiac slowing and reduce cardiac output and their action on endothelial M_3 receptors contributes to a pronounced reduction in arterial blood pressure. They increase the tone of all smooth muscle apart from vascular smooth muscle and smooth muscle forming the urinary bladder sphincter, resulting in increased gastrointestinal motility, bronchoconstriction, miosis and support of bladder emptying. In combination with their prosecretory effects on exocrine glands (bronchial, salivary, lacrimal, sweat), the bronchoconstriction induced by muscarinic agonists can severely impair respiratory function.

Generally parasympathomimetics are polar quarternary ammonium compounds with a linked ester group. These chemical properties limit their bioavailability and prevent them from crossing the blood–brain barrier. Less polar compounds which cross the blood–brain barrier more easily, such as pilocarpine, display central

Table 4.5 Muscarinic receptors

Receptor	Location	Cellular response	Functional response	Agonists	Antagonists
M_1	Gastric and salivary glands, CNS	Activation of $G_{q/11}$/PLCβ/IP_3/DAG, Ca^{2+}↑, K^+conductance↓	Glandular secretion↑, CNS excitation	ACh, CCh	Atropine, pirenzepin
M_2	Heart, GI, smooth muscle	Activation of G_i, cAMP↓, K^+conductance↑	Cardiac inhibition, neural inhibition, central muscarinic effects	ACh, CCh	Atropine, gallamin
M_3	Exocrine glands, SM of the eye and GI tract, vascular endothelium	Activation of $G_{q/11}$/PLCβ/IP_3/DAG, Ca^{2+}↑	Glandular secretion↑, GI SM constriction, ocular accommodation, vasodilation	ACh, CCh	Atropine

PLCβ, phospholipase Cβ; IP_3, inositol triphosphate; DAG, diacylglycerol; cAMP, cyclic adenosine monophosphate; GI, gastrointestinal; SM, smooth muscle; ACh,acetylcholine; CCh, carbamylcholine (carbachol).

effects causing tremor and hypothermia via activation of M_1 receptors in the brain. The procognitive effects of central M_1 receptor activation by selective M_1 agonists have led to the investigation of such compounds as antidementia drugs in humans. Modifications of the basic chemical structure of muscarinic agonists as outlined above have yielded drugs with increased cholinesterase resistance and higher selectivity for muscarinic receptors (acetylcholine versus bethanechol).

Whilst muscarine has no clinical applications, other M-selective parasympathomimetic drugs (e.g. bethanechol) have limited clinical use in situations of reduced smooth muscle tone such as hypomotility disorders of the gut and reduced bladder tone.

Pilocarpine, a nonpolar tertiary ammonium compound, which is readily absorbed via mucous membranes, can be used for the treatment of increased intraocular pressure (glaucoma) (see Chapter 25). Pilocarpine is not approved for veterinary use in the US or UK but can be applied topically to the eye in companion animals as extra-label use or under the requirements of the UK/European prescribing cascade. It predominantly constricts the smooth muscle of iris and ciliary body, leading to improved drainage of aqueous humor via the drainage angle. In the past another parasympathomimetic, arecoline, was used to aid removal of intestinal parasites in dogs. However, the clinical use of arecoline has been superseded by newer, safer and more efficacious anthelmintics (see Chapter 10).

Muscarinic antagonists

Antimuscarinic agents are competitive antagonists at muscarinic acetylcholine receptors. The general lack of M-receptor subtype selectivity of these parasympatholytic drugs helps to explain the similar responses seen after administration of muscarinic antagonists, which include the reversal of parasympathetic cardiac inhibition, mydriasis, bronchial, biliary and urinary tract smooth muscle relaxation, inhibition of exocrine glandular secretions and, at higher doses, reduction in GI motility.

Antagonists of M acetylcholine receptors such as the plant alkaloids atropine (*Atropa belladonna*, deadly nightshade) and hyoscine (*Hyoscyamus niger*, thorn apple) share a similar basic chemical structure with acetylcholine, but the replacement of the acetyl side chain by a bulky aromatic group results in high affinity but abolished intrinsic activity at M-receptors. Compared to parasympathomimetics, muscarinic antagonists are nonpolar tertiary amines which are readily absorbed and cross the blood–brain barrier. Atropine, for example, the archetypal muscarinic antagonist, is widely distributed but not readily metabolized in most species (the exception is rabbits which, as a consequence, can safely eat deadly nightshade) and therefore has a long duration of action.

Atropine is clinically used as an anesthetic premedication to manage bradycardia and excessive bronchial secretion associated with the use of anesthetics and opioids. Atropine and other muscarinic antagonists are also used for the treatment of organophosphate and carbamate toxicity. Organophosphate and carbamate pesticides inhibit cholinesterase, causing excessive generalized parasympathetic neurotransmission. Atropine plays an important role in the symptomatic relief of these intoxication states, the lack of M subtype selectivity being advantageous as it causes antagonism of anticholinergic effects in all parts of the parasympathetic system.

Other muscarinic antagonists occasionally used in veterinary medicine include propantheline bromide, hyoscine and isopropamide in antiemetic and antidiarrheal preparations (see Chapter 19) or for management of bradyarrhythmias (see Chapter 17).

Ipratropium, a quaternary ammonium compound, is under scrutiny as an inhalant for cats with asthma.

Limited systemic uptake makes it a safe candidate to induce bronchial smooth muscle relaxation without the risk of generalized parasympathetic actions. The drug is, however, not approved for the use in small animals in the US and UK. Short-acting muscarinic antagonists such as tropicamide are occasionally used as topical applications in the eye (see Chapter 25).

Cholinesterase inhibitors

As indicated above, the inactivation of ACh at cholinergic synapses following release of this neurotransmitter involves the breakdown of ACh by synaptic acetylcholinesterase. Together with butyrylcholinesterase, another closely related serine hydrolase with ubiquitous tissue and plasma distribution, acetylcholinesterase not only terminates synaptic transmission but also reduces the circulating levels of acetylcholine to virtually zero, making acetylcholine a pure neurotransmitter. Both cholinesterases are equally inhibited by a number of naturally occurring and synthetic substances with similar chemical structure to acetylcholine, which as a common mode of action transfer an acetyl (short-acting anticholinesterases, i.e. edrophonium), carbamyl (medium-duration anticholinesterases, i.e. neostigmine) or phosphate (irreversible anticholinesterases, i.e. parathion) onto the catalytic site of the enzyme to block hydrolytic activity. The difference in affinity of acetyl, phosphate and carbamyl groups to this site determines the duration of action of various anticholinesterases.

The clinical uses of these cholinesterase inhibitors are very limited as the consequences of inhibiting these enzymes are widespread central and peripheral parasympathomimetic effects that are difficult to control. These effects include enhanced transmitter activity at postganglionic parasympathetic synapses (bradycardia, bronchoconstriction, glandular secretion, gastrointestinal hypermotility), depolarization block of the neuromuscular junction, neurotoxicity and, if compounds can cross the blood–brain barrier, initial excitation and convulsions followed by depression.

There is, however, one important clinical use in veterinary medicine. The short-acting drug edrophonium is used to aid the diagnosis of myasthenia gravis, an autoimmune disease in which antibodies directed against muscle-type nicotinic receptors cause impaired cholinergic transmission at the neuromuscular junction, resulting in muscle weakness. Medium-duration anticholinesterases such as neostigmine and pyridostigmine are used in the clinical management of the disease in combination with immunosuppressants.

Irreversible anticholinesterases such as parathion and dichlorvos, which in some parts of the world are still used as insecticides, can be the source of intoxication in domestic animals.

THE SYMPATHETIC NERVOUS SYSTEM – CATECHOLAMINERGIC SYNAPSES

Catecholaminergic neurotransmission mediates the various actions of sympathetic nervous system activation at postganglionic nerve terminals, which predominantly regulate smooth muscle tone in a number of organs and control cardiac function. Neurotransmitters synthesized in catecholaminergic nerve terminals are generally the catecholamines noradrenaline (norepinephrine), dopamine and adrenaline (epinephrine), which are synthesized from the amino acid precursor L-tyrosine via a single enzymatic cascade. Out of these three, noradrenaline (norepinephrine) is by far the most important neurotransmitter in the autonomic nervous system. As a result, postganglionic sympathetic synapses are usually classified as noradrenergic synapses, despite the presence of small amounts of dopamine and adrenaline (epinephrine) in sympathetic nerve endings. Dopamine, on the other hand, plays a more important role as a modulatory neurotransmitter in the CNS, while adrenaline (epinephrine), produced and secreted from chromaffin cells of the adrenal medulla, acts predominantly as a circulating hormone.

The basic synaptic processes of noradrenergic neurotransmission are similar to those in cholinergic synapses, the principal differences lying in the neurotransmitter synthesis pathways, postrelease metabolism and recycling (for details see below).

Figure 4.3 outlines the essential steps in the transmission process at a noradrenergic synapse in the PNS. Table 4.6 summarizes the drugs that can interfere with the various stages of this process.

Apart from adrenoceptor antagonists and agonists and to some extent monoamine oxidase (MAO) blockers, these drugs have little or no clinical application in veterinary medicine.

Adrenoceptors

The complex effects that sympathetic activation induces in mammalian organisms via the release of mainly a single neurotransmitter, especially the opposing effects on smooth muscle tone in different organs, can only be explained by the existence of distinct adrenoceptor subtypes. However, a detailed understanding of the nature and distribution of these catecholamine receptors lagged a long way behind the systematic classification of nicotinic and muscarinic acetylcholine receptors. Despite the fact that Sir Henry Dale had made observations suggesting the existence of such receptor subtypes (he realized that in animals pretreated with certain ergot alkaloids, adrenaline produced a paradoxical reduction in blood pressure compared to the expected increase) as far back as 1913, scientists were struggling to draw the right

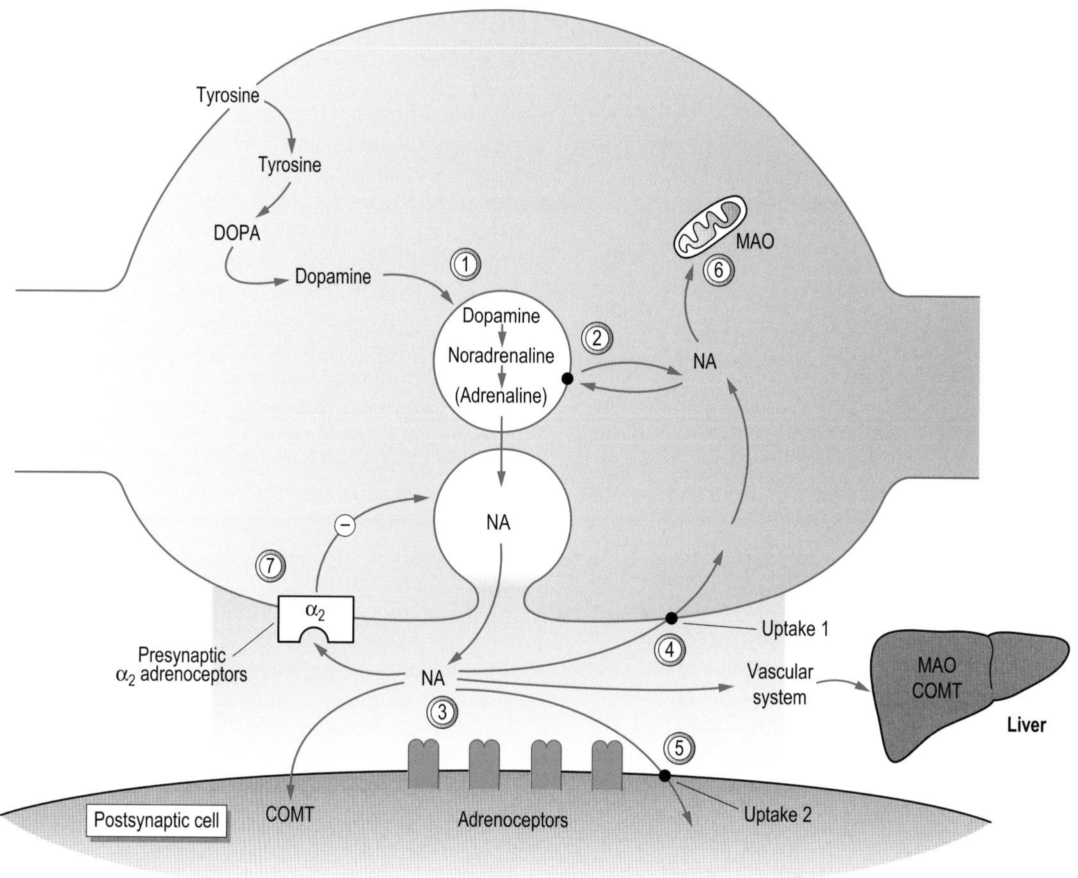

Fig 4.3 Schematic diagram of a noradrenergic varicosity (a release site of a sympathetic postganglionic nerve fiber). The circled numbers refer to Table 4.6. COMT, catechol-*O*-methyl transferase; MAO, monoamine oxidase; NA, noradrenaline (norepinephrine).

conclusions. The main reason for this was the fact that Dale studiously ignored the logical explanation for his observations as a result of his dislike for John N Langley, who had first introduced the pharmacological concept of receptor subtypes when he classified acetylcholine receptors as nicotinic and muscarinic receptors. The solution to the problem, the existence of adrenoceptor subtypes, was therefore not proposed until much later, when Raymond Ahlquist studied the effects of three different catecholamines in different tissues, observing different orders of potency for noradrenaline (norepinephrine), adrenaline (epinephrine) and the synthetic catecholamine isoprenaline.

In 1948, based on his observations, Ahlquist suggested the following classification:

- α-adrenoceptors, where noradrenaline (norepinephrine) and adrenaline (epinephrine) are much more potent than isoprenaline
- β-adrenoceptors, where isoprenaline is much more potent than noradrenaline (norepinephrine) and adrenaline (epinephrine).

In due course, the discovery of selective adrenoceptor antagonists resulted in the further subclassification of adrenoceptors into α_1 and α_2 as well as β_1, β_2 and β_3 with additional subtypes that can be identified based on molecular differences.

All adrenergic receptors are typical 7TM G protein-coupled receptors which can induce a wide range of effects by coupling to specific second messenger systems.

Table 4.7 summarizes the main characteristics of the different adrenoceptor subtypes, their tissue distribution and functional role.

Table 4.6 Noradrenergic transmission

Transmission step	Drug	Effect	Affected transmission step in Fig. 4.3
Synthesis	α-methyltyrosine/carbidopa	Block of NA synthesis via tyrosine hydroxylase/ dopa-decarboxylase	1
Synthesis	Methyldopa	Synthesis of a false transmitter (methylnorepinephrine/noradrenaline) that causes potent presynaptic inhibition via α_2-receptors	1
Neurotransmitter storage	Reserpine	Blocks uptake of NA into synaptic vesicles via VMAT. NA depletion of the presynaptic nerve terminal and transmission block	2
Postsynaptic binding (α-adrenoceptors)	Phentolamine	Specific receptor block, effect depends on site of action: prevent vasoconstriction	3
Postsynaptic binding (β-receptors)	Propranolol	Specific receptor block, effect depends on site of action: bradycardia, bronchoconstriction	3
Uptake 1	Cocaine; tricyclic antidepressants	Block of reuptake of NA via uptake 1 and lead to increased synaptic NA levels	4
Uptake 1	Indirectly acting sympathomimetics (amfetamine, ephedrine)	Compounds enter the nerve terminal via uptake 1, accumulate in synaptic vesicles (VMAT) and displace NA leading to increased NA release at sympathetic synapses	4
Uptake 2	Phenoxybenzamine	Block of NA uptake into nonneuronal cells, increased synaptic NA levels	5
MAO/COMT	MAO/COMT-blockers	Block of neurotransmitter breakdown	6
Presynaptic modulation (presynaptic α_2-adrenoceptors)	Clonidine, xylazine, medetomidine	Presynaptic inhibition of NA release	7

NA, noradrenaline (norepinephrine); MAO, monoamine oxidase; COMT, catecholamine-*O*-methyl transferase; VMAT, vesicular monoamine transporter.

Table 4.7 Adrenoceptors

Receptor	Location	Cellular response	Functional response	Agonists	Antagonists
α_1	Smooth muscle, hepatocytes	Activation of $G_{q/11}$/PLCβ/ IP_3/DAG, Ca^{2+}↑	Constriction of vascular, bronchial, uterine, vas deferens and sphincter SM, dilation of GI SM	NA > Adr > ISO, phenylephrine, metoxamine	Prazosin
α_2	Smooth muscle (vascular, GI), pancreatic islets adrenergic & cholinergic nerve terminals, brainstem	Activation of G_i, cAMP↓, K^+conductance↑	Reduced pancreatic insulin secretion, presynaptic inhibition of neurotransmitter release, reduced sympathetic CNS outflow	Adr > NA > ISO, clonidine, medetomidine, xylazine	Yohimbine, Atipamezole
β_1	Heart	Activation of G_s, cAMP↑	Increased heart rate and cardiac output	ISO > NA > Adr, dobutamine	Propranolol, atenolol
β_2	Smooth muscle, skeletal muscle, hepatocytes	Activation of G_s, cAMP↑	Dilates vascular, GI, bronchial, uterine, vas deferens, GI and urinary sphincter SM, induces skeletal muscle tremor and hypertrophy, glycogenolysis	Salbutamol, clenbuterol	Butoxamine
β_3	Skeletal muscle, adipocytes	Activation of G_s, cAMP↑	Thermogenesis, lipolysis	BRL37344	

NA, noradrenaline (norepinephrine); Adr, adrenaline (epinephrine); ISO, isoprenaline; PLCβ, phospholipase Cβ; IP_3, inositol triphosphate; DAG, diacylglycerol; cAMP, cyclic adenosine monophosphate; GI, gastrointestinal; SM, smooth muscle.

Catecholamine transmitters

All the major catecholamine transmitters – dopamine, noradrenaline (norepinephrine) and adrenaline (epinephrine) – are products/precursors of a single synthetic pathway, starting with the tyrosine hydroxylase-catalyzed conversion of tyrosine to dihydroxyphenylalanine (DOPA) as the rate-limiting step. In three further steps, the enzymes DOPA decarboxylase, dopamine β-hydroxylase and phenyethanolamine N-methyl transferase synthesize dopamine from DOPA, noradrenaline (norepinephrine) from dopamine and adrenaline (epinephrine) from noradrenaline (norepinephrine) respectively.

In mammalian tissues the predominant product of this pathway is noradrenaline (norepinephrine) and only noradrenaline (norepinephrine) (PNS) and dopamine (mainly CNS) can be regarded as true neurotransmitters whilst adrenaline (epinephrine) plays a role in sympathetic activation as a hormone released from the adrenal gland. In some organ systems of nonmammalian species (e.g. the frog heart), adrenaline (epinephrine) is a neurotransmitter.

Comparable to transmission at other chemically transmitting synapses, presynaptic catecholamine release from secretory vesicles is mediated via Ca^{2+}-dependent mechanisms. This transmitter release can be regulated by presynaptic autoinhibition via adrenoceptors (especially α_2) present on the presynaptic nerve terminal or via heterologous inhibition via acetylcholine, ATP, angiotensin II and a number of neuropeptides. Termination of transmitter action after dissociation of the neurotransmitter–receptor complex, however, is achieved by quite different mechanisms in catecholaminergic synapses.

Termination of noradrenergic neurotransmission–noradrenaline metabolism

Compared to the enzymatic processes at cholinergic synapses, the termination of noradrenergic neurotransmission is not predominantly the result of cleavage and inactivation of the neurotransmitter. Following diffusion away from receptors, noradrenaline (norepinephrine) is removed from the synaptic cleft by transporters located in both the nerve terminals and postsynaptic cells. The predominantly neuronal catecholamine transporter constitutes uptake 1, a highly specific noradrenaline reuptake mechanism with high affinity but relatively low transport rate. The ubiquitous catecholamine transporters in nonneuronal postsynaptic cells constitute uptake 2, a transporter with lower affinity yet higher transport rate for noradrenaline (norepinephrine) that also effectively carries adrenaline (epinephrine).

After reuptake into the presynaptic nerve terminal via uptake 1, noradrenaline (norepinephrine) enters the cytoplasmic neurotransmitter pool to be recycled to a large extent into synaptic vesicles. Noradrenaline (norepinephrine and other catecholamines) which are taken up into nonneuronal cells undergo enzymatic degradation by two important intracellular pathways: monoamine oxidase (MAO) and catechol-O-methyl transferase (COMT).

Monoamine oxidase is an enzyme that is abundantly expressed in neuronal cells where it attaches to the outer mitochondrial membrane, but lower levels of MAO are present in all cells. Noradrenaline (norepinephrine), adrenaline (epinephrine) and dopamine, as well as several of their metabolites and other biogenic amines such as histamine and serotonin, are all substrates for these enzymes which do, however, play a very limited role in the termination of catecholaminergic transmission in the PNS. After being taken back up into nerve terminals, only very small amounts of noradrenaline (norepinephrine) are broken down by MAO (in the periphery predominantly MAO_A). MAO does however play a more important role in terminating noradrenergic transmission in the brain, where two different forms of MAO, MAO_A and MAO_B, with different substrate preferences are expressed. MAO_A metabolizes noradrenaline (norepinephrine) and serotonin whilst MAO_B breaks down dopamine. Selegiline, a specific inhibitor of MAO_B, can be used for the treatment of behavioral disorders (see Chapter 23) and has been proposed as adjuvant treatment in pituitary-dependent hyperadrenocorticism. COMT is a more specific enzyme than MAO, accepting only catechols as substrates. It is widely expressed in neuronal and nonneuronal tissues and plays a certain role in the inactivation of circulating catecholamines.

Sympathomimetic drugs

A number of drugs mimic the actions of endogenous catecholamines. These include adrenoceptor agonists and drugs that interfere with uptake and metabolism of endogenous catecholamines and therefore are called indirect sympathomimetics (see also Fig. 4.3 and Table 4.7). In veterinary medicine, the catecholamines themselves and selective adrenoceptor agonists have some clinical importance and will be discussed in more detail below. Indirect sympathomimetics such as reserpine, amphetamines and cocaine play only minor roles as veterinary therapeutics.

Adrenoceptor agonists

Adrenoceptor agonists are synthetic compounds which have been designed by modifying the chemical structures of the endogenous catecholamines noradrenaline (norepinephrine) and adrenaline (epinephrine) and the classic synthetic adrenoceptor agonist isoprenaline, which per se show higher potencies and affinities for certain adrenoceptor subtypes (see above). These chemical modifications have yielded a number of compounds with high selectivity for adrenoceptor subtypes which can therefore selectively mimic specific physiological effects of sympathetic nervous system activation.

The predominant pharmacological effects of selective agonists at adrenoceptor subtypes can be deduced from the physiological role of these receptors in mediating sympathetic target organ control summarized in Table 4.7.

Selective α_1-adrenoceptor agonists such as phenylephrine, oxymetazoline and phenylpropanolamine mainly induce constriction of vascular smooth muscle, resulting in an increase in arterial blood pressure and reflex bradycardia, constriction of the radial muscle of the iris and closure of the sphincter of the urinary bladder and their main clinical use is accordingly. Phenylephrine is used to induce mydriasis for ophthalmological examination and surgery and phenylpropanolamine is the standard treatment for urinary incontinence. The α_1 effects of adrenaline (epinephrine) on vascular smooth muscle justify its use as a blocking agent that increases the tissue half life of local anesthetics and it can be used in emergency situations for the treatment of anaphylactic shock.

The selective α_2-adrenoceptor agonists clonidine, xylazine and medetomidine have strong central and peripheral inhibitory effects on the presynaptic release of noradrenaline (norepinephrine) and as a result xylazine and medetomidine are widely used as sedative analgesics in veterinary medicine. This sedation can be antagonized by selective α_2-adrenoceptor antagonists such as atipamezole. Initially these compounds can induce peripheral vasoconstriction which is eventually overcome by the central and peripheral presynaptic effects on noradrenaline (norepinephrine) release.

Selective β-adrenoceptor agonists are mainly used clinically for their selective effects on cardiac β_1-adrenoceptors. The selective compound dobutamine is used as a diagnostic tool because of its positive inotropic effects in the dobutamine stress test for the diagnosis of systolic myocardial dysfunction in dogs with heart failure. It is also used to support cardiac function in states of shock. The nonselective β-adrenoceptor agonist isoprenaline has a clinical role in the emergency treatment of atrioventricular block.

Compounds such as clenbuterol, salbutamol and terbutaline, which dilate smooth muscle by selectively activating β_2-adrenoceptors are used as bronchodilators for the treatment of allergic asthma and as tocolytic agents (agents that reduce contractility of uterine smooth muscle) in veterinary obstetrics. β_2-adrenoceptor agonists lead to skeletal muscle hypertrophy and increased speed of contraction which has resulted in the use of such compounds as doping agents in humans and animals and as growth promoters in meat production.

The mixed α- and β-adrenoceptor effects (overall increase in peripheral vascular resistance and positive inotropic actions) of the endogenous catecholamine adrenaline (epinephrine) make it one of the most important drugs in emergency treatment of cardiogenic and anaphylactic shock and cardiac arrest.

Indirect sympathomimetics

Indirectly acting sympathomimetics such as reserpine, amphetamines and cocaine play a very limited clinical role. Amphetamines are powerful, orally active CNS stimulants that also cause release of catecholamines from peripheral sites – nerves and the adrenal medulla. They have been used clinically in humans as appetite suppressants in the past. The only recognized indication in humans now is the management of attention deficit hyperactivity disorder (ADHD), although considerable controversy surrounds this use. Amphetamines and cocaine are mainly used as recreational drugs. Methylphenidate and dexamphetamine are sometimes used for behavioral modification in animals (see Chapter 7).

Adrenoceptor antagonists

α-Adrenoceptor antagonists

Drugs that block α-adrenoceptors clinically are mainly used for their relaxing effects on vascular smooth muscle which results in a reduction in peripheral resistance and a fall in blood pressure.

Nonselective α-adrenoceptor antagonists such as phenoxybenzamine (binds covalently to the receptor leading to long-lasting receptor blockade, also blocks ACh and 5-HT receptors) and phentolamine (competitive antagonist at all α-adrenoceptors) have strong hypotensive effects and cause reflex tachycardia. This tachycardia is augmented by the stimulatory effects of α_2-adrenoceptor blockade on noradrenaline (norepinephrine) release from cardiac sympathetic nerve terminals. Selective α_1-antagonists such as prazosin and doxazosin reduce blood pressure with a less pronounced sympathetic reflex to the heart.

Clinical uses of phenoxybenzamine and phentolamine in veterinary medicine include the management of hypertension associated with pheochromocytoma, relaxation of the internal bladder sphincter in cases of reflex dyssynergia/functional urethral obstruction (phenoxybenzamine) and the management of hypertension associated with *Ixodes holocylus* toxicity (phenoxybenzamine).

Prazosin has clinical applications in the management of heart failure in dogs as it results in a significant reduction of cardiac afterload. This is discussed in more detail in Chapter 17.

The selective α_2-receptor antagonist atipamezole is commonly used as an antidote for the central sedative and analgesic effects of medetomidine and xylazine.

Ergot alkaloids such as ergotamine, bromocriptine and cabergoline, which are partial agonists at α-adrenoceptors, can have effects on vascular tone depending on the level of basal sympathetic stimulation. In veterinary medicine they are mainly used for their effects in the reproductive tract which are mediated via the activation of α-adrenoceptors and dopamine receptors.

β-Adrenoceptor antagonists

β-Adrenoceptor blockers are used extensively in human therapeutics in the management of hypertension due to their potential to induce slow-onset reduction of blood pressure by reducing cardiac output, reducing the release of renin from the juxtaglomerular cells of the kidney and inhibiting central sympathetic activity. The main veterinary application of β-blockers is their use as antidysrhythmic drugs for the treatment of supraventricular tachyarrhythmia in cats and dogs. Furthermore, the use of β-blockers can be indicated in treating hypertension associated with renal failure and hyperthyroidism. Despite their negative inotropic effects, β-blockers have been shown to improve survival in human patients with heart failure and recently have been suggested as treatment for heart failure in cats and dogs. More detail on the use of β-blockers in the treatment of cardiovascular disease can be found in Chapter 17.

The prototype of these agents is propranolol, a nonspecific β-blocker affecting both β_1 and β_2 receptors which, alongside the desired effects on heart and vasculature, can therefore induce bronchoconstriction. This is a potential problem in patients with asthma. Alternatively, the use of selective β_1-adrenoceptor antagonists such as atenolol can prevent these unwanted side effects. Nonselective blockers of β_1 or β_2 receptors with partial agonist properties (oxprenolol, alprenolol) in future may provide the clinical advantage that they support cardiac function at rest but block the detrimental effects of excessive sympathetic activation in heart failure.

The topical administration of β-blockers to the eye is commonly used to treat glaucoma. Their application results in the inhibition of β_2-mediated relaxation of the ciliary muscle, thus facilitating drainage of aqueous humor via the canal of Schlemm and reducing intraocular pressure (see Chapter 25).

DRUGS ACTING ON THE AUTONOMIC NERVOUS SYSTEM AND THEIR CLINICAL APPLICATION

Cholinergic agonists (parasympathomimetics)

Bethanechol

Clinical applications

Bethanechol can be used in cases of paralytic ileus following surgery and for the treatment of nonobstructive urinary retention. Approved veterinary drugs are not available in the USA and UK, but approved human preparations can be used for extra-label use and under the requirements of the UK/European prescription cascade.

Mechanism of action

Bethanechol directly stimulates muscarinic acetylcholine receptors. It has negligible nicotinic activity when used at therapeutic doses. It has a longer duration of activity than ACh as it is more resistant to cholinesterase-mediated hydrolysis.

Formulations and dose rates

Bethanechol chloride is supplied as tablets for oral use and in solution for parenteral use.

DOGS
- 5–25 mg PO q.8 h

CATS
- 2.5–7.5 mg q.8 h

Pharmacokinetics

There is no information on the pharmacokinetics of bethanechol in dogs and cats. In humans it is poorly absorbed from the gastrointestinal tract. After oral dosing, onset of action is 30–90 min; after subcutaneous dosing onset of action is 5–15 min. The duration of action can persist for up to 6 hours after oral dosing and 2 hours after subcutaneous dosing. Subcutaneous administration results in a greater stimulatory effect on the urinary tract than oral dosing. Bethanechol does not cross the blood–brain barrier. The metabolic and elimination fate of bethanechol is unknown.

Adverse effects

- Adverse effects are usually mild and may include vomiting, diarrhea, salivation and anorexia.
- Overdosage may result in cardiovascular signs (bradycardia, arrhythmia, hypotension) and bronchoconstriction.

Known drug interactions

- Bethanechol should not be used concurrently with other cholinergic drugs or anticholinesterase agents.
- Quinidine, procainamide, adrenaline (epinephrine) and other sympathomimetic amines and atropine can antagonize the effects of bethanechol.

Cholinergic antagonists (parasympatholytics)

Pilocarpine

See Chapter 25.

Atropine

Clinical applications

Atropine can be used as an anesthetic premedication to reduce salivation and respiratory tract secretions. It may also be used to treat bradyarrhythmia (see Chapter 17). It is used as an antidote to organophosphate and carbamate toxicity, to treat overdoses of cholinergic agents (see also Chapter 10) and muscarinic mushroom intoxication (fly agaric and other mushrooms belonging to the Amanita, Omphaletus, Belotus and Clitocybe genera). No approved veterinary formulations are available in the USA and UK.

Mechanism of action

Atropine is a competitive antagonist at postganglionic muscarinic acetylcholine receptors. Low doses result in inhibition of salivation, bronchial secretion and sweating. Moderate doses cause pupillary dilation and tachycardia, and inhibit pupil accommodation. High doses decrease gastrointestinal and urinary tract motility. Very high doses will inhibit gastric acid secretion.

Formulations and dose rates

DOGS AND CATS

Preanesthetic and treatment of bradycardia

- 0.022–0.044 mg/kg

Treatment of cholinergic toxicity

- 0.2–2.0 mg/kg: give one-quarter dose IV and remainder SC or IM

Pharmacokinetics

Atropine sulfate is well absorbed after oral, IM and endotracheal administration as well as inhalation. Peak effect occurs 3–4 min after IV administration. It is well distributed throughout the body and crosses into CNS, across the placenta and into milk (in small quantities). Atropine undergoes hepatic metabolism and is eliminated via the kidney. Approximately 30–50% of the dose is excreted unchanged into urine. The plasma half-life in humans is reported to be 2–4 hours.

Adverse effects

Atropine is contraindicated in patients with:

- narrow angle glaucoma
- thyrotoxicosis-induced tachycardia
- cardiac insufficiency-associated tachycardia
- gastrointestinal obstruction
- paralytic ileus
- myasthenia gravis (unless used to reverse adverse muscarinic effects).

It should be used with extreme caution in patients with known or suspected gastrointestinal infections (see Chapter 19) and autonomic neuropathy.

Adverse effects that may occur with high or toxic doses include:

- alimentary – dry mouth, dysphagia, constipation, vomiting
- genitourinary – urinary retention
- CNS – ataxia, seizures, stimulation or drowsiness
- ophthalmic – blurred vision, photophobia, cycloplegia, pupillary dilation
- cardiac – sinus tachycardia (high doses), bradycardia (initially and at very low doses), hypertension, hypotension, arrhythmias.

Known drug interactions

Atropine sulfate is physically incompatible with noradrenaline (norepinephrine) bitartrate, methohexitone and sodium bicarbonate.

Tropicamide

See Chapter 25.

Propantheline bromide

See Chapter 19.

Isopropamide

See Chapter 19.

Nicotinic antagonists

Nondepolarizing muscle relaxants

EXAMPLES

Atracurium besylate (Tracrium®), pancuronium bromide (Pavulon®), vecuronium bromide (Norcuron®).

Clinical applications

Nondepolarizing muscle relaxants are used to enhance muscle relaxation during surgery and to facilitate mechanical ventilation. They should not be used on conscious animals. Appropriate equipment for endotracheal intubation and to provide controlled mechanical ventilation must be available when they are used. No approved veterinary formulations are available in the USA and UK.

Mechanism of action

Nondepolarizing muscle relaxants bind competitively to cholinergic receptors at the neuromuscular junction, resulting in muscle paralysis. Since antagonism is competitive, nondepolarizing neuromuscular blockade can be reversed using cholinesterase inhibitors, which act to increase the local concentration of acetylcholine. Atracurium has one-quarter to one-third the potency of pancuronium, which is variably reported to be one-third as potent or as potent as vecuronium.

Formulations and dose rates

Nondepolarizing muscle relaxants should only be used by veterinarians familiar with their use and the reader should consult textbooks of anesthesiology for further information. Since the use of nondepolarizing muscle relaxants results in the paralysis of respiratory muscles, endotracheal intubation and intermittent positive pressure ventilation are mandatory. As a note of caution, it should be considered that neuromuscular blocking drugs alter many of the parameters that are used to assess anesthetic depth; for example, the eye assumes a central position, jaw tone is absent and palpebral and pedal reflexes are lost. Careful monitoring of anesthetic depth is essential to ensure that the patient is not conscious while paralyzed.

DOGS AND CATS

Atracurium
- 0.2–0.5 mg/kg IV initial dose, increments of 0.1–0.2 mg/kg if required

Pancuronium
- 0.05–0.1 mg/kg IV initial dose, increments of 0.01 mg/kg if required

Vecuronium
- 0.05–0.1 mg/kg IV initial dose, increments of 0.04 mg/kg if required or 0.06 mg/kg/h as an infusion

Pharmacokinetics

The onset of muscle relaxation after IV administration occurs within 3–5 min for atracurium, 2–3 min for pancuronium and within 2 min for vecuronium. The duration of action is quite variable but as a general guide atracurium lasts for 20–35 min, pancuronium for 30–45 min and vecuronium for approximately 25 min.

A variety of factors can influence the intensity and duration of neuromuscular blockade. Hypokalemia, hypocalcemia and hypermagnesemia tend to potentiate the blockade, as does respiratory acidosis. Body temperature also may influence blockade. However, the effect of temperature on the actions of these drugs (and on neuromuscular function itself) is complex. There are a number of reports of hypothermia causing reduced blockade but other reports of enhancement. In an intact system the degree of block seems to be reduced with hypothermia but the duration is prolonged.

The response to nondepolarizing drugs is also altered in a number of neurological disorders. Patients with myasthenia gravis have fewer acetylcholine receptors and are consequently more sensitive to nondepolarizing muscle relaxants. Conversely, patients with denervating injuries or conditions may be resistant to nondepolarizing drugs since the number of acetylcholine receptors is increased. However, ACh receptors which appear with denervation are not necessarily located to respond to ACh released from nerve terminals.

For atracurium, recovery times do not change after maintenance doses are given so predictable blocking effects can be achieved if the drug is given at regular intervals. Unlike for other nondepolarizing muscle relaxants, rate of onset and duration of drug action for atracurium are not impaired in patients with hepatic and renal failure and hepatic shunts. In contrast, additional doses of pancuronium may slightly increase the magnitude of neuromuscular blockade and significantly increase the duration of action.

Pancuronium and vecuronium are partially metabolized by the liver followed by renal and biliary excretion. Prolonged recovery times may occur in patients with renal or hepatic disease. Atracurium may be a better choice in such patients since its elimination does not depend on renal or hepatic function. Atracurium undergoes spontaneous degradation at physiological pH and temperature, a process known as Hofmann elimination. In addition, the drug is hydrolyzed by nonspecific esterases.

Adverse effects

- Pancuronium has mild vagal blocking activity and may also stimulate the release of catecholamines from adrenergic nerve endings. Thus heart rate and blood pressure tend to rise.
- Atracurium may cause adverse effects related to histamine release, i.e. hypotension, tachycardia and bronchoconstriction. However, such adverse effects are unlikely if the drug is administered slowly intravenously and a dose of 0.5 mg/kg is not exceeded.
- Histamine release is not a problem with the isomer of atracurium, cisatracurium.
- Laudanosine, a breakdown product of Hofmann elimination of atracurium, is a theoretical concern. High concentrations have been associated with CNS excitation and seizures; however, such concentrations are unlikely to develop following administration of clinical doses of atracurium.
- Vecuronium does not cause histamine release and is free from ganglion-blocking or vagolytic activity. It

is therefore the most cardiostable of the nondepolarizing neuromuscular blockers commonly used in veterinary anesthesia.

Known drug interactions

- Nondepolarizing neuromuscular blockade can be reversed by administration of cholinesterase inhibitors such as edrophonium and neostigmine. Anticholinesterase treatment causes ACh to accumulate not only at the neuromuscular junction but also at muscarinic sites, resulting in bradycardia and increased bronchial and salivary secretions. For this reason a parasympatholytic such as atropine is administered in conjunction with neostigmine.
- The neuromuscular blocking action of these drugs can be enhanced by procainamide, quinidine, verapamil, aminoglycosides, lincosamides, thiazide diuretics, isoflurane and halothane.
- Few studies have reported positive and negative interactions between the administration of loop diuretics, e.g. furosemide (frusemide) and nondepolarizing neuromuscular blockers.
- Succinylcholine may enhance the onset of action and neuromuscular effects.

Depolarizing muscle relaxants

EXAMPLES

Succinylcholine chloride (Scoline®).

Clinical applications

Succinylcholine is used primarily to facilitate endotracheal intubation in cats, in which it has a rapid onset and short duration of action. No approved veterinary formulations are available in the USA and UK.

Mechanism of action

Succinylcholine is an ultra-short-acting depolarizing muscle relaxant, which binds to motor endplate cholinergic receptors to produce depolarization. Since the depolarization is sustained, the electrical activity of the motor endplate is lost, leading to paralysis. Transient muscle fasciculations may be seen to precede neuromuscular blockade, which persist as long as sufficient amounts of drug remain at the endplate.

Formulations and dose rates

Succinylcholine should only be used by veterinarians familiar with its use and the reader should consult textbooks of anesthesiology for further information. As for the nondepolarizing muscle relaxants, intermittent positive pressure ventilation is essential.

Dogs: 0.3 mg/kg IV

Cats: 1 mg/kg IV

Pharmacokinetics

After IV administration, muscle relaxation occurs rapidly, within 30–60 seconds. The duration of action varies in different species. In cats muscle relaxation lasts for approximately 5 min while in dogs it lasts for 20–30 min as dogs are relatively deficient in pseudocholinesterase.

Succinylcholine is extensively metabolized by the enzyme pseudocholinesterase and only a fraction of the administered dose reaches the neuromuscular junction. Levels of pseudocholinesterase may be reduced in liver disease, malnutrition and renal failure, leading to a more prolonged duration of effect. Diffusion of drug away from the active site as the serum concentration declines also contributes to the short duration of action. Succinylmonocholine, the main metabolite, has weak neuromuscular blocking activity (one-twentieth of the activity of succinylcholine). A proportion of the drug, approximately 10%, is excreted unchanged in urine.

Adverse effects

- Succinylcholine is structurally similar to acetylcholine and is capable of stimulating nicotinic receptors in parasympathetic and sympathetic ganglia, as well as muscarinic receptors in the sinoatrial node of the heart. Consequently, various cardiovascular effects are possible, including bradycardia, tachycardia, hypotension and hypertension. Arrhythmias have also been reported.
- During succinylcholine-induced depolarization there is an efflux of potassium ions into the extracellular compartment. The resulting increase in serum potassium concentration is not normally significant. However, in patients with burn injuries, major trauma and neurological conditions in which denervation occurs, the elevation in potassium may be sufficient to cause life-threatening cardiac arrhythmias. This is largely a consequence of an increase in the number of acetylcholine receptors. Muscle contracture may also develop if succinylcholine is used under these circumstances.
- Unlike other skeletal muscles, the extraocular muscles have more than one motor endplate on each cell. As a result, depolarization by succinylcholine produces a state of contracture that raises intraocular pressure. This agent is therefore contraindicated in patients with penetrating eye injuries. Intracranial and intragastric pressures may also rise as a consequence of muscle fasciculations.
- Succinylcholine will trigger malignant hyperthermia in susceptible animals.
- Additional adverse effects include muscle soreness and myoglobinuria.

Known drug interactions

- Drugs that inhibit cholinesterase enzymes, including edrophonium, neostigmine and organophosphate pesticides, will prolong the duration of depolarizing neuromuscular blockade (whilst they reduce the duration of action of nondepolarizing muscle relaxants).
- The neuromuscular blocking action of succinylcholine can be enhanced by furosemide (frusemide), oxytocin, β-blockers, quinidine, lidocaine (lignocaine) and isoflurane.
- Intravenous procaine competes for the pseudocholinesterase enzyme and therefore may prolong succinylcholine's effects.
- Intravenous cyclophosphamide decreases plasma pseudocholinesterase levels and may also prolong succinylcholine's effects.
- Thiazide diuretics and amphotericin B may cause electrolyte imbalances and may increase the effect of succinylcholine.
- Diazepam may reduce the duration of action.

Cholinesterase inhibitors

EXAMPLES

Neostigmine, edrophonium chloride.

Clinical applications

Neostigmine is approved for the treatment of myasthenia gravis and reversal of nondepolarizing muscle relaxants. Edrophonium chloride is approved for reversal of nondepolarizing muscle relaxants and as a diagnostic medication for the diagnosis of myasthenia gravis. The pharmacodynamic profile of cholinesterase inhibitors also allows their use in the treatment of bladder and gut hypomotility. An approved veterinary formulation of neostigmine for this indication is only available for large animals in the US.

Mechanism of action

Cholinesterase inhibitors are competitive reversible antagonists of the enzyme cholinesterase which is responsible for the breakdown of acetylcholine at cholinergic synapses (ganglionic, postganglionic and neuromuscular) and the termination of cholinergic neurotransmission. Cholinesterase inhibitors therefore lead to increased levels of acetylcholine and prolonged transmission in cholinergic synapses, an action which is mainly used in the treatment of disorders of neuromuscular transmission (myasthenia gravis) and the antagonism of nondepolarizing neuromuscular blockade. Because the actions of cholinesterase inhibitors also affect ANS synapses, causing strong parasympathomimetic actions, coadministration with parasympatholytics such as atropine is recommended.

Formulations and dose rates

DOGS AND CATS

Neostigmine

- 0.1 mg/kg IV initial dose, repeated after 5 min if required for the reversal of muscle relaxation
- 0.5 mg/kg oral q.8 h to treat myasthenia gravis

Edrophonium

- 0.5–1 mg/kg IV initial dose for the reversal of muscle relaxation
- 0.1–0.5 mg/kg IV for myasthenia gravis diagnosis

Pharmacokinetics

The polar quaternary ammonium structure of these drugs reduces their oral bioavailability and their ability to penetrate the blood–brain barrier, making intravenous administration the route of choice. After intravenous administration neostigmine actions can be observed as soon as 2 min after infusion and, with a bolus dose, last for ~30 min.

Adverse effects

The major unwanted side effect of cholinesterase inhibitors is the unwanted augmentation of cholinergic neurotransmission at postganglionic autonomic synapses via activation of muscarinic acteylcholine receptors, resulting in hypersalivation, increased bronchial secretions, bronchoconstriction, gut hypermotility, bradycardia, hypotension and excessive sweating.

Known drug interactions

Administration of cholinesterase inhibitors with the antiparasitic drug levamisole can result in strong symptoms of parasympathetic activation.

Adrenergic agonists

Adrenaline (epinephrine)

Clinical applications

Adrenaline (epinephrine) has several uses. Topically applied adrenaline (epinephrine) can be used to control hemorrhage from skin and mucous membranes. The effects of injected adrenaline (epinephrine) on vascular tone are, however, complex. It causes both constriction (of skin vessels) and dilation (of skeletal muscle vessels). Cerebral vessels that have no sympathetic innervation are not directly affected by adrenaline (epinephrine).

The vasoconstrictor actions of adrenaline (epinephrine) are useful in several situations apart from emergency hemostasis. They also help to relieve acute allergic reactions (anaphylactic shock). Adrenaline (epinephrine) reduces blood flow and thus alleviates edema of the glottis, which is often the cause of death in allergic reactions to bites and stings. It also relaxes bronchial smooth muscle, as well as reducing blood flow and hence congestion in the lungs.

The reduced blood flow to mucous membranes is also exploited to relieve the symptoms of allergic rhinitis. Ephedrine and pseudoephedrine have similar but weaker vasoconstrictive actions and are often used for this purpose.

Vasoconstrictor actions are also the reason why adrenaline (epinephrine) is often coadministered with local anesthetics when these are given by injection. Here adrenaline (epinephrine) functions both to prolong the action of the local anesthetic and to prevent the escape of high concentrations into the systemic circulation with the attendant risk of causing cardiac arrhythmia.

Very occasionally adrenaline (epinephrine) is used in cardiovascular emergencies – acute severe hypotension and cardiac arrest. It may be useful in the short term but it often masks the progress of the underlying problem and should be used cautiously. It is also proarrhythmogenic and increases the workload of the heart so other catecholamines such as dopamine and dobutamine are usually preferred (see Chapter 17).

No approved veterinary formulations are available in the USA or UK.

Formulations and dose rates

Adrenaline (epinephrine) is available in an injectable formulation as 0.1 mg/mL (1:10000) and 1 mg/mL (1:1000) solutions.

DOGS AND CATS

- *Cardiac resuscitation*: 0.05–0.5 mg (0.5–5 mL) of 1:10000 solution intratracheally, IV or intracardially
- *Anaphylaxis:* 0.02 mg/kg IV. Dose may be doubled and given intratracheally
  - Dilute 1 mL of 1:1000 solution in 10 mL saline and give 1 mL/5 kg IV or IM. May repeat q.5–15 min
- *Feline asthma:* 0.1 mL of 1:1000 solution SC or IV
  - Dilute 1 mL of 1:1000 solution in 10 mL saline and give 1 mL/10 kg IV or IM. May repeat q.5–15 min

Pharmacokinetics

Adrenaline (epinephrine) is well absorbed from IM and SC sites; absorption can be enhanced by massaging the injection site and absorption is slightly faster from IM sites compared to SC. Onset of action after IV administration is immediate and after SC administration within 5–10 min. Oral administration is not effective as it is rapidly metabolized in the gut. Adrenaline (epinephrine) crosses the placenta and enters milk but does not cross the blood–brain barrier.

Action is terminated by uptake and metabolism in sympathetic nerve endings. It is also metabolized in liver and other tissues by MAO and catechol-O-methyltransferase (COMT) to yield inactive metabolites.

Adverse effects

Adverse effects associated with adrenaline (epinephrine) administration include:

- anxiety
- tremor
- excitability
- vomiting
- hypertension
- arrhythmias.

Repeated injections can cause necrosis at the injection site.

Contraindications and precautions

- Contraindicated in narrow angle glaucoma, during halothane anesthesia, during labor and in patients with heart disease and heart failure.
- When combined with local anesthetics, it should not be administered to small body appendages as the ensuing vasoconstriction can cause tissue hypoxia, necrosis and slough.
- Use with caution in patients with:
  - hyperthyroidism
  - diabetes mellitus
  - hypertension.

Known drug interactions

- In solution, adrenaline (epinephrine) hydrochloride is incompatible with aminophylline, hyaluronidase, sodium bicarbonate and warfarin sodium.
- Adrenaline (epinephrine) should not be used concurrently with other sympathomimetic drugs.
- Some antihistamines (e.g. diphenhydramine, chlorphenamine (chlorpheniramine)) and levothyroxine may potentiate the effects of adrenaline (epinephrine).
- The concomitant use of β-blockers may potentiate hypertension and antagonize the bronchodilatory and cardiostimulatory effects of adrenaline (epinephrine).
- Nitrates, α-blocking agents and diuretics may abolish or reduce the pressor effects of adrenaline (epinephrine).
- Use of adrenaline (epinephrine) concurrently with drugs that sensitize the myocardium to arrhythmias (e.g. halothane, digoxin) may increase the risk of arrhythmias.
- Use of oxytocin concurrently with adrenaline (epinephrine) or other sympathomimetic drugs can cause postpartum hypertension.

Phenylpropanolamine

Clinical applications

Phenylpropanolamine is one of the mainstays of treatment of urinary incontinence in the bitch. Stimulation of α-adrenoceptors on the smooth muscle of the bladder sphincter and pelvic urethra results in increased tone of smooth muscle cells and improvement of the sphincter function.

Formulations and dose rates

Oral formulations of phenylpropanolamine for veterinary use are available as capsules or as syrup.

DOGS
- 1 mg/kg q.8 h

CATS
- 1–1.5 mg/kg q.12 h

Adverse effects
A number of studies have reported aggression, anorexia, cardiac arrhythmia, hypertension and diarrhea as a result of using phenylpropanolamine in animals.

Contraindications and precautions
Because phenylpropanolamine is not a selective α-adrenoceptor agonist but shows some residual potency at β-adrenoceptors, its use is contraindicated in pregnant and lactating animals.

Known drug interactions
When used in combination with β-adrenoceptor blockers, especially nonselective β-adrenoceptor blockers, phenylpropanolamine can cause a strong increase in peripheral vascular resistance.

During anesthesia with inhalation narcotics such as halothane and isoflurane, phenylpropanolamine can induce cardiac arrhythmia.

Dobutamine
Clinical applications
Dobutamine is an apparently β_1-selective adrenoceptor agonist which clinically is used as a positive inotrope in the treatment of heart failure and as an emergency treatment for cardiogenic shock. It is also used as a diagnostic treatment for the early detection of myocardial systolic dysfunction.

Mechanism of action
The apparent β_1-selective effects of dobutamine, showing mainly positive inotropic actions in the heart, are based on partly opposing actions of the constituents of naturally occurring racemic dobutamine. (+)Dobutamine is a nonselective β-adrenoceptor agonist and also a potent antagonist at α_1-adrenoceptors, whilst (–)dobutamine shows very low potency at β-adrenoceptors but has strong α_1 mimetic effects. This results in balancing out of the α_1-adrenoceptor actions of the isomers whilst some local vascular α_1 effects result in physiological antagonism of β_2 actions, leading to an apparently β_1-selective pharmacodynamic profile of dobutamine.

As a result, the predominant effect of dobutamine treatment is a strong increase in cardiac contraction force which, compared to the effects of adrenaline and isoprenaline, is accompanied by only very sparse positive chronotropic actions.

Pharmacokinetics
The plasma half-life of dobutamine is extremely low in dogs (~2min) and the drug therefore needs to be infused intravenously at a rate of 2–20 μg/kg/min. The plasma half-life in cats is higher and the recommended infusion rate is <10 μg/kg/min.

Adverse effects
Dobutamine, especially when administered in high doses, can result in a sharp blood pressure increase and cardiac arrhythmia.

Known drug interactions
Dobutamine can induce vasoconstriction and a sharp increase in blood pressure when used in combination with β-adrenoceptor blockers.

Clenbuterol, salbutamol, terbutaline
See Chapter 17.

Dopamine
See Chapter 17.

Ephedrine
Ephedrine is a natural product that has been used in Chinese traditional medicine for more than 2000 years. It has essentially the same actions as adrenaline (epinephrine) but with the following differences: lower potency, oral efficacy, longer duration of action, more pronounced CNS effects. In human medicine it is used principally for the relief of the symptoms of allergic reactions (especially as a nasal decongestant for the treatment of allergic rhinitis). In veterinary medicine it is used to increase the tone of the internal bladder sphincter in cases of urinary incontinence. It has also been occasionally used for bronchoconstriction and could theoretically be used parenterally as a pressor agent in shock.

Mechanism of action
The mechanism of action of ephedrine is thought to be similar to that of the amphetamines, i.e. it causes release of noradrenaline (norepinephrine) thus stimulating catecholaminergic receptors. Ephedrine has a more potent

CNS effect than adrenaline (epinephrine). Prolonged or excessive use can result in a reduced response (tachyphylaxis) as a result of depletion of noradrenaline (norepinephrine) from storage sites.

Formulations and dose rates

Ephedrine is available in tablets or capsules in some countries and in formulations appropriate for parenteral use.

DOGS
- *Urinary incontinence:* 4 mg/kg PO q.8–12 h or 12.5–50 mg/dog
- *Bronchoconstriction:* 1–2 mg/kg q.8–12 h
- *Vasopressor:* 0.75 mg/kg IM, SC. Repeat as needed

CATS
- *Urinary incontinence:* 2–4 mg/kg PO q.8–12 h
- *Bronchoconstriction:* 2–5 mg/cat
- *Vasopressor:* 0.75 mg/kg IM, SC. Repeat as needed

Pharmacokinetics
Ephedrine is rapidly absorbed after oral, IM or SC administration. It is thought to cross the blood–brain barrier and the placenta. It is metabolized in the liver as well as being excreted unchanged in the urine. Urine pH can alter excretion characteristics, with the half-life increasing with increased pH.

Adverse effects
- Restlessness and irritability
- Tachycardia
- Hypertension
- Anorexia

Contraindications and precautions
- Contraindicated in severe cardiovascular disease, particularly if associated with arrhythmias.
- Use with caution in patients with:
  - glaucoma
  - prostatic hypertrophy
  - hyperthyroidism
  - diabetes mellitus
  - cardiac disease
  - hypertension.
- Effect on fertility, pregnant animals or fetuses is not known.

Known drug interactions
- Ephedrine should be administered cautiously with other sympathomimetic agents.
- Concurrent treatment with NSAIDs, tricyclic antidepressants and ganglionic blocking agents can increase risk of hypertension.
- Ephedrine should not be administered within 2 weeks of a patient receiving a monoamine oxidase inhibitor, e.g. selegiline.
- Halothane increases the risk of ephedrine-induced arrhythmias.
- Urinary alkalinizers such as sodium bicarbonate and acetazolamide may reduce urinary excretion and therefore prolong ephedrine's action.
- Concurrent use of ephedrine and β-blockers may decrease the action of both drugs.
- Concurrent use of digoxin increases the risk of arrhythmias.

Isoprenaline (isoproterenol)
See Chapter 17.

Xylazine, medetomidine
See Chapter 6.

Adrenergic antagonists

Phenoxybenzamine/phentolamine
Clinical applications
Phenoxybenzamine and phentolamine are used in human and veterinary medicine to treat pheochromocytoma, a tumor of the adrenal medulla that results in a massive increase in the levels of circulating catecholamines. Phenoxybenzamine is also used to relax the internal bladder sphincter in cases of reflex dyssynergia and to reduce blood pressure in patients affected by the paralysis tick, *Ixodes holocyclus*.

Mechanism of action
Phenoxybenzamine (a haloalkylamine derivative) noncompetitively blocks α-adrenoceptors as a result of stable binding to the receptor or nearby structures. It has no effect on β-adrenoceptors.

Phentolamine is a competitive α-adrenoceptor blocker. As a result of α-adrenoceptor blockade, phenoxybenzamine and phentolamine can cause hypotension, particularly if administered rapidly IV or administered to a patient whose cardiovascular system is under pronounced sympathetic tone, e.g. during hypovolemia. They will decrease hypertension in patients with pheochromocytoma. They cause relaxation of the nictitating membrane and increased cutaneous blood flow, and block pupillary dilation. They reduce internal urethral sphincter tone in dogs and cats.

Both drugs also block α_2-adrenoceptors, which can ultimately result in increased availability of catecholamines, leading to β_1-adrenoceptor stimulation and therefore paradoxical sympathomimetic effects on the heart.

Formulations and dose rates

Phenoxybenzamine is available as capsules (10 mg) and as a parenteral formulation in some countries.

DOGS
- *Detrusor areflexia:* 0.25 mg/kg PO q.8–12 h or 0.5 mg/kg q.24 h
- *Hypertension associated with pheochromocytoma:* 0.2–1.5 mg/kg PO q.12 h for 10–14 days prior to surgery; start at low end of dosage range and increase until desired blood pressure is reached
- *Management of hypertension associated with* Ixodes holocyclus *toxicity:* 1.0 mg/kg IV as 0.1% solution over 10–15 min

CATS
- *Detrusor areflexia:* 0.5 mg/kg PO initially, increasing to a maximum of 10 mg/cat

Pharmacokinetics

Little is known about the pharmacokinetics of these drugs in dogs and cats. In humans phenoxybenzamine is variably absorbed after oral administration with a relatively low bioavailability of 20–30%. The activity of orally administered phentolamine is less than 30% of an intravenously administered dose. There is a slow onset of drug action (several hours), which increases over several days after regular dosing. The serum half-life in humans is approximately 24 hours. Effects persist for 3–4 days after discontinuation of the drug.

Phenoxybenzamine is very lipid soluble. It is metabolized (dealkylated) in the liver and excreted in bile and urine. It causes local irritation and therefore can only be administered intravenously or orally.

Adverse effects

- Hypotension
- Tachycardia
- Miosis
- Increased intraocular pressure
- Nausea and vomiting
- Nasal congestion
- Inhibition of ejaculation

Known drug interactions

- α-Adrenoceptor blockers will prevent the sympathomimetic effects of α-adrenergic agonists.
- If administered concurrently with a drug that has α- and β-adrenergic effects, e.g. adrenaline (epinephrine), hypotension and tachycardia will be exacerbated.

Atipamezole, yohimbine

See Chapter 6.

Prazosin

See Chapter 17.

Propranolol, atenolol

See Chapter 16.

FURTHER READING

Bishop Y 2004 The veterinary formulary, 6th edn. Pharmaceutical Press, London

Katzung BG 2006 Basic and clinical pharmacology, 10th edn. Appleton and Lange, Stanford, CT

Rang HP, Dale MM, Ritter JM, Flower R 2007 Rang and Dale's pharmacology, 6th edn. Churchill Livingstone, Edinburgh

The green book: database of approved animal drug products in the USA. Available online at: http://dil.vetmed.vt.edu/GreenBook/

Anesthetic agents

Patricia Pawson and Sandra Forsyth

INHALATIONAL ANESTHETICS

INTRODUCTION

Anesthesia can be defined as a state of unconsciousness in which there is a reduced sensitivity and response to noxious stimuli. Anesthetic agents, such as the inhalation anesthetics, are able to induce this state through reversible and controlled depression of CNS function. General anesthesia is made up of three components:

- unconsciousness
- analgesia
- muscle relaxation.

Inhalation anesthetics are not particularly effective analgesics and vary in their ability to produce muscle relaxation; hence if they are used alone to produce general anesthesia, high concentrations are necessary. If inhalation anesthetics are used in combination with specific analgesic or muscle-relaxant drugs the inspired concentration of inhalation agent can be reduced, with an associated decrease in adverse effects. The use of such drug combinations has been termed balanced anesthesia.

GENERAL CLINICAL APPLICATIONS

Anesthesia is indicated when painful surgical or diagnostic procedures are to be performed, to minimize patient suffering and operator risk and to facilitate the procedure through immobilization of the patient. Inhalation anesthetics are unusual drugs in that they are administered and subsequently removed from the body as the patient breathes. The concentration of agent inspired can be adjusted from one minute to the next and, for the most part, this translates into rapid and predictable changes in anesthetic depth. Thus inhalation anesthetics are well suited to the maintenance phase of anesthesia.

The administration of these agents requires special apparatus that incorporates a source of carrier gas, usually oxygen, a source of anesthetic and a breathing system to convey the gases to the patient. This method of administration, in particular the provision of supplemental oxygen, allows optimum oxygenation of the patient. Furthermore, if the trachea is intubated, ventilation can be assisted or controlled should the need arise. The main disadvantage of inhalation anesthetics is the potential for environmental pollution. Chronic low-level exposure to waste anesthetic gases has been linked to a number of health problems.

PHYSIOLOGICAL PRINCIPLES

Anesthetics are a diverse group of drugs with markedly different chemical structures, ranging from simple inorganic molecules such as nitrous oxide to more complex organic agents like the barbiturates. This led early investigators to conclude that the mode of action is nonspecific, dependent on physicochemical properties.

Anesthetic potency is closely correlated to lipid solubility and it has been suggested, therefore, that anesthetics interact with a hydrophobic site on the cell membrane, either the lipid bilayer itself or the hydrophobic domain of a membrane protein. These two possible sites of action have given rise to two main theories of anesthesia: the lipid theory and the protein theory.

According to the earlier **lipid theory**, anesthetic agents dissolve in the lipid bilayer, thereby altering the physical properties of the cell membrane. Volume expansion and increased fluidity of the membrane have been proposed as possible mechanisms of altered function. It has been hypothesized that these alterations in the membrane interfere with the activity of ion channels or receptor proteins. Anesthesia can be reversed by increasing hydrostatic pressure, a process known as 'pressure reversal'. This phenomenon is consistent with the volume expansion theory, since hydrostatic compression of membrane lipids will oppose volume expansion.

However, there are problems with the lipid theory. Relatively mild elevations in temperature (≈1°C) produce increases in the volume and fluidity of the cell membrane comparable to those induced by clinical concentrations of anesthetics. Furthermore, some anesthetic agents display stereo-selectivity, implying that an interaction between drug and receptor occurs. The 'cut-off' phenomenon further supports the idea that anesthetics interact with a discrete receptor site. Increasing the chain length of a hydrocarbon-based anesthetic increases its lipid solubility and therefore its anesthetic potency.

However, beyond a certain size, additional increases in chain length decrease potency despite further increases in lipid solubility.

These problems with the volume expansion hypothesis lend support to the **protein theory** of anesthesia, which has gained widespread acceptance in recent years. According to this theory, anesthetic agents interact with protein targets to modify central synaptic transmission. Clinically relevant concentrations of many anesthetics have been shown to modify the activity of ion channels and receptor proteins. Both pre- and postsynaptic effects have been identified.

Many anesthetics have been shown to reduce presynaptic neurotransmitter release, largely through inhibition of voltage-gated calcium channels, while postsynaptic effects include depression of excitatory neurotransmission or potentiation of inhibitory neurotransmission. The main inhibitory neurotransmitter in the brain is γ-aminobutyric acid, or GABA. Two types of GABA receptor have been identified: $GABA_A$ receptors, which open chloride channels, and $GABA_B$ receptors, which are linked to potassium channels. $GABA_B$ receptors are largely unaffected by general anesthetic agents. However, enhanced activation of $GABA_A$ receptors appears to be a mechanism common to many anesthetics, including both injectable and volatile agents.

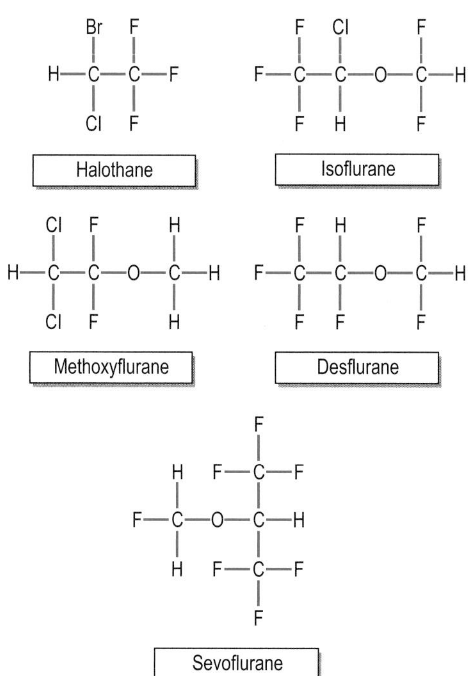

Fig. 5.1 Chemical structure of the volatile anesthetics.

INHALATION ANESTHETIC AGENTS

EXAMPLES

Halothane, isoflurane, desflurane, sevoflurane, methoxyflurane, nitrous oxide

General chemical structure

The majority of inhalation anesthetics in common use are halogenated organic substances, either hydrocarbons or ethers (Fig. 5.1). In general terms, halogenation has been shown to increase anesthetic potency while improving stability. Nitrous oxide is an example of an inorganic inhalation anesthetic.

General physical properties

Inhalation anesthetics can be classed as either vapors or gases. According to this classification a gas exists in the gaseous state at room temperature and sea-level pressure, while a vapor exists as a liquid under similar standard conditions. The most commonly used inhalation agents are vapors which must therefore be converted to the gaseous phase before addition to the carrier gas. These agents are frequently described as the volatile anesthetics. Nitrous oxide is one of the few anesthetic gases in clinical use.

There are several different ways of quantifying the amount of anesthetic vapor or gas in a mixture:

- concentration (volume %)
- partial pressure (mmHg)
- mass (mg or g).

In clinical practice concentrations of inhalation agents are frequently quoted since vaporizers are calibrated to deliver anesthetic as a percentage of total gas flow. Anesthetic agent analyzers used in monitoring tend also to use concentrations.

A vapor or gas can also be described in terms of the partial pressure it exerts. Pressure originates when randomly moving molecules of gas or vapor collide with other molecules or with the walls of the container. In a mixture of gases, the pressure exerted by an individual vapor or gas is termed its partial pressure. A difference in partial pressure is required if molecules of gas or vapor are to diffuse between compartments or phases, e.g. from alveolar air to blood. Less commonly, anesthetic gases or vapors are quantified as mass. It is possible to convert from mass to volume since a mole of any gas (i.e. a gram molecular weight) will occupy a volume of 22.4 L under standard conditions.

Vapor pressure

Molecules of liquid and gas are in constant random motion. At a liquid–gas interface some molecules will pass from the liquid into the gaseous state, while others return to the liquid. The former transition is known as vaporization. In a closed container and at a constant temperature, vaporization of liquid will proceed until an equilibrium is reached at which there is no further net movement of molecules between phases. At equilibrium, the gaseous phase is said to be saturated and the pressure exerted by the molecules of vapor is termed the saturated vapor pressure. Thus, vapor pressure gives an indication of the ease with which a volatile anesthetic evaporates. The higher the vapor pressure, the more volatile the anesthetic.

The saturated vapor pressure also dictates the maximum concentration of vapor that can exist at a given temperature. The higher the saturated vapor pressure, the greater the concentration of volatile agent that can be delivered to the patient. To determine the maximum concentration, vapor pressure is expressed as a percentage of barometric pressure at sea level, i.e. 760 mmHg. For example, halothane has a saturated vapor pressure of 244 mmHg at 20°C; therefore the maximum concentration of halothane that can be delivered at this temperature is 32% ($244/760 \times 100 = 32\%$). Desflurane has the highest vapor pressure (664 mmHg at 20°C) of the agents currently used and the maximum achievable concentration of this agent approaches 90%. Anesthetic gases such as nitrous oxide do not need to undergo vaporization and can therefore exist over the full range of concentrations, i.e. 0–100%.

In theory, a low saturated vapor pressure might restrict the usefulness of a volatile anesthetic, if therapeutic concentrations cannot be achieved. However, this is not a limitation for the volatile agents in current use.

Solubility

Molecules of anesthetic gas and vapor are able to dissolve in liquids and solids. Thus, if molecules of anesthetic are present in a mixture of gases overlying a liquid they will diffuse into the liquid, i.e. they will dissolve. This process will continue until an equilibrium is reached at which there is no net movement of anesthetic molecules between the two phases. At equilibrium, the partial pressure exerted by the anesthetic in the gas phase will equal the partial pressure of anesthetic in the liquid phase. However, the total number of anesthetic molecules in each compartment will not be equal.

The number of particles or volume of an individual gas in a mixture of gases is simply proportional to its partial pressure. However, the number of particles or volume of gas that dissolves in a solvent at a given temperature is dependent also on solubility.

According to Henry's law:

$$V = S \times P$$

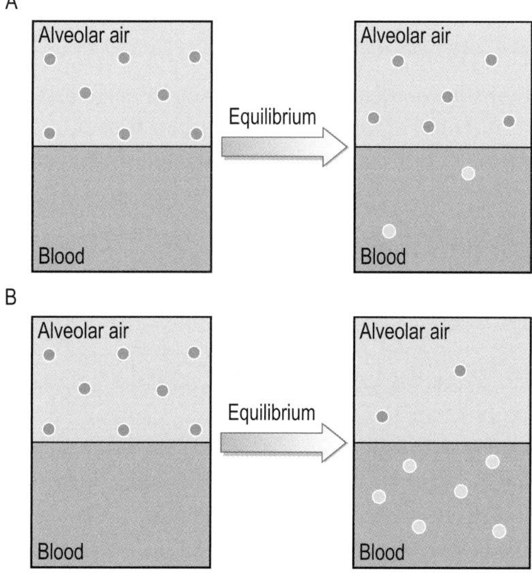

Fig. 5.2 Partition of anesthetic molecules between alveolar air and blood. (A) For an anesthetic agent that is poorly soluble in blood, equilibrium is reached when relatively few molecules have dissolved. The partial pressure of anesthetic at equilibrium will be relatively high. (B) For an anesthetic agent that is highly soluble in blood, equilibrium is not reached until a large number of molecules have dissolved. In this case the partial pressure of anesthetic at equilibrium will be relatively low.

where:

V = volume of gas
P = partial pressure of gas
S = solubility coefficient of gas in solvent.

For an anesthetic gas or vapor that is poorly soluble in a solvent such as blood, equilibrium will be reached when relatively few molecules have dissolved. The partial pressure at which equilibrium occurs will be relatively high. Conversely, for an agent that is highly soluble in blood there will be a large number of molecules in the liquid phase at equilibrium and partial pressure will be relatively low (Fig. 5.2).

Partition coefficients

Partition coefficients are used to describe the solubility of inhalation anesthetics in a variety of different solvents. A partition coefficient is simply the ratio of the concentration of anesthetic in one phase or solvent compared to another. The coefficients of most clinical relevance are the blood:gas and oil:gas partition coefficients. The blood:gas partition coefficient is an important determinant of the speed of anesthetic induction and recovery. It describes the partition of an agent between a gaseous phase, such as alveolar air, and the blood.

The greater the blood:gas partition coefficient, the greater the solubility in blood. The oil:gas partition coefficient has been correlated to anesthetic potency – the higher the coefficient, the more potent the agent.

The solubility of anesthetics in other tissues or in components of a breathing system, such as rubber, may also be relevant.

General pharmacokinetics

The aim in using inhalation anesthetics is to achieve a partial pressure of anesthetic in the brain sufficient to depress central nervous system (CNS) function and induce general anesthesia. Thus, anesthetic depth is determined by the partial pressure of anesthetic in the brain. To reach the brain, molecules of anesthetic gas or vapor must diffuse down a series of partial pressure gradients, from inspired air to alveolar air, from alveolar air to blood and from blood to brain.

Inspired air → Alveolar air → Blood → Brain

At each interface, diffusion proceeds until equilibrium is reached and the partial pressures equalize. Gas exchange at the level of the alveoli is an efficient process and molecules of anesthetic rapidly equilibrate between alveolar air and blood. Equilibration between the blood and the brain is equally rapid. Thus, the partial pressure of anesthetic in the brain closely follows the partial pressure of anesthetic in arterial blood, which in turn closely follows the partial pressure of anesthetic in the alveoli. Expressed in a different way, this means that anesthetic depth is largely determined by the partial pressure of anesthetic in the alveoli.

The rate of change of anesthetic depth

Factors that produce a rapid change in alveolar partial pressure of anesthetic will produce a rapid change in anesthetic depth, appreciated clinically as a rapid induction and recovery. The most important factors are listed below and can be broadly divided into those that affect delivery of anesthetic to the alveoli and those that affect removal of anesthetic from the alveoli:

- inspired concentration
- alveolar ventilation
- solubility of anesthetic in blood
- solubility of anesthetic in tissues
- cardiac output.

Certain pathophysiological factors such as mismatching of ventilation and perfusion may also influence the uptake of anesthetic by altering the alveolar-to-arterial partial pressure gradient.

Inspired concentration of anesthetic

A high inspired concentration of anesthetic is associated with rapid induction of anesthesia, since increased delivery of anesthetic to the alveoli induces a rapid rise in alveolar partial pressure of anesthetic. Conversely, the lower the inspired concentration, the more rapid the recovery.

A number of factors may influence the inspired concentration. The saturated vapor pressure of an agent imposes a limit on the maximum concentration that can be delivered at a given temperature. However, for most inhalation agents, this limit far exceeds the concentrations required for clinical use. Some inhalation anesthetics are soluble in rubber or plastic and may therefore be absorbed by components of the breathing system, effectively reducing the inspired concentration.

For the volatile agents, the setting on the vaporizer is an important determinant of inspired concentration, although other factors such as the fresh gas flow and the nature and volume of the anesthetic breathing system will also exert an influence. For rebreathing anesthetic systems such as the circle, fresh gas flow is low relative to system volume. In addition, expired gases contain variable amounts of anesthetic. These factors serve to delay changes in inspired concentration instigated by altering the vaporizer setting.

Alveolar ventilation

An increase in alveolar ventilation is associated with a more rapid induction of anesthesia. As for a high inspired concentration, delivery of anesthetic to the alveoli is increased and the rise in alveolar partial pressure is rapid. Conversely, hypoventilation will slow both induction and recovery.

Many analgesic and anesthetic drugs, including the inhalation agents, will depress ventilation and thereby influence subsequent anesthetic uptake. Similarly, increases in physiological dead space associated with rapid shallow breathing serve to reduce alveolar ventilation. On the other hand, intermittent positive pressure ventilation tends to increase alveolar ventilation, allowing for more rapid changes in alveolar partial pressure of anesthetic.

Solubility in blood

Inhalation agents that are poorly soluble in blood, i.e. have low blood:gas partition coefficients, produce more rapid induction of anesthesia. More rapid recovery and more rapid rate of change of anesthetic depth are also features of such agents.

The rise in alveolar partial pressure of anesthetic at induction can be described by plotting a graph of alveolar partial pressure, expressed as a percentage of inspired partial pressure, against time (Fig. 5.3). For an agent of low blood solubility (Fig. 5.3A), equilibration between alveolar air and blood occurs rapidly when relatively few molecules of anesthetic have diffused into the blood. Furthermore, since the majority of anesthetic molecules

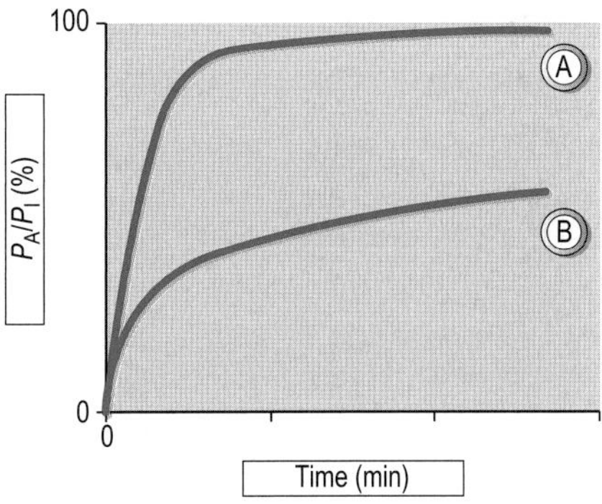

Fig. 5.3 **The rise in alveolar partial pressure of anesthetic (P_A) towards the inspired partial pressure (P_I) for an agent of (A) low and (B) high solubility in blood.**

remain within the alveoli, the alveolar partial pressure at equilibration approaches the partial pressure of anesthetic in the inspired gas. The result is a rapid rise in alveolar partial pressure and therefore rapid induction of anesthesia. In contrast, for an agent that is highly soluble in blood (Fig. 5.3B) more anesthetic molecules must diffuse from the alveoli into the blood before equilibration is reached. As a result, the partial pressure of anesthetic in the alveoli at equilibrium is very much less than that in the inspired gas. Consequently, the rise in alveolar partial pressure is slowed and induction delayed.

Cardiac output

A high cardiac output tends to slow anesthetic induction. An increase in blood flow through the lungs serves to maintain the diffusion gradient between the alveoli and blood. Therefore, more molecules of anesthetic diffuse out of the alveoli, slowing the rise in alveolar partial pressure of anesthetic. The influence of cardiac output is evident in clinical cases. Induction is frequently slowed in excited patients but occurs more rapidly in animals with reduced cardiac output, e.g. in hypovolemia or shock.

Solubility in tissues

A faster induction and recovery are associated with anesthetic gases and vapors that are poorly soluble in the tissues. At induction, tissue uptake lowers the venous partial pressure of anesthetic, thereby restoring the diffusion gradient between alveolar air and blood. In turn, this maintains the movement of anesthetic molecules out of the alveoli, slowing the rise in alveolar partial pressure. For inhalation anesthetics that are relatively insoluble in the tissues, these effects are minimal. However, for more soluble agents, tissue uptake may considerably reduce venous and thus alveolar partial pressures.

A rapid fall in alveolar partial pressure is required for a swift recovery. If significant quantities of inhalation agent reside in the tissues at the end of anesthesia, transport of this agent back to the alveoli will serve to slow the fall in alveolar partial pressure and recovery will be delayed.

Metabolism and elimination

Inhalation anesthetics are eliminated primarily through the lungs, i.e. they are exhaled. Nonetheless, these agents are not totally inert and undergo biotransformation, primarily in the liver, to a variable degree. Metabolism might be expected to promote recovery from anesthesia. However, for the newer inhalation agents any contribution to recovery is slight. Of more direct importance is the potential production of toxic metabolites. The generation of such intermediates does not require exposure to high concentrations of inhalation agent and so this form of toxicity is a hazard to the anesthetist (or indeed anyone working in a contaminated environment) as well as the patient.

Anesthetic potency: minimum alveolar concentration

The potency of a drug is a measure of the quantity of that drug that must be administered to achieve a given effect; the more potent the drug, the less is required. In the case of inhalation anesthetics potency is described by the minimum alveolar concentration (MAC). The MAC value is the minimum alveolar concentration of anesthetic that produces immobility in 50% of patients exposed to a standard noxious stimulus. The lower the MAC, the more potent the anesthetic. The MAC is inversely correlated to the oil:gas partition coefficient. Thus a very potent inhalation anesthetic will have a low MAC and a high oil:gas partition coefficient.

MAC values vary slightly between species and may also be modified by other factors such as body temperature and age (Table 5.1). Many of the drugs included in anesthetic protocols, including sedatives, analgesics and injectable anesthetics, reduce the MAC of inhalation anesthetics.

General side effects

Central nervous system effects

All inhalation anesthetics induce reversible dose-dependent depression of the CNS. However, the volatile agents do not possess specific analgesic activity.

Most inhalation agents vasodilate the cerebral vasculature, thereby increasing cerebral blood flow and raising intracranial pressure. Such changes are unlikely to be significant in normal patients. However, if

Table 5.1 Sources of variation in minimum alveolar concentration (MAC) that occur within a species

Factors that decrease MAC	Factors that increase MAC
Hypothermia	Hyperthermia
Hyponatremia	Hypernatremia
Pregnancy	CNS stimulants, e.g. amfetamine
Old age	
CNS depressants, e.g. sedatives, analgesics, injectable anesthetics	
Severe anemia	
Severe hypotension	
Severe hypoxia	
Extreme respiratory acidosis (P_aCO_2 > 95 mmHg)	

intracranial pressure is already raised, e.g. by an intracranial mass, further increases in pressure may severely compromise cerebral perfusion and thus oxygen delivery. Most inhalation anesthetics will also reduce the metabolic rate and oxygen requirement of the brain and it is the balance between supply and demand that governs overall safety.

Cardiovascular effects

All inhalation anesthetics cause dose-dependent depression of the cardiovascular system. At clinical concentrations some agents tend to affect the heart more than the vessels, while for others depression of vascular tone is the predominant effect. Inhalation agents may also sensitize the myocardium to catecholamine-induced arrhythmias. This detrimental effect is influenced by the chemical structure of the agent, hydrocarbons being more arrhythmogenic than ethers.

Respiratory effects

All volatile anesthetics depress ventilation in a dose-dependent fashion. As the inspired concentration of agent is increased, tidal volume falls, followed by reductions in respiratory rate. These changes lead to retention of carbon dioxide and the arterial partial pressure of carbon dioxide (P_aCO_2) rises accordingly. In the conscious patient such a change would stimulate increased ventilation but this reflex is depressed by inhalation anesthetics. For most agents, respiratory arrest is likely at alveolar concentrations of between two and three times MAC. Variations in the degree of respiratory depression induced by different volatile anesthetics are relatively small.

Hepatic effects

Mild and transient hepatic dysfunction may be associated with all the volatile anesthetics, probably as a result of reduced blood flow and oxygen delivery. More severe hepatocellular damage occurs rarely and is usually associated with the use of halothane.

Renal effects

All inhalation anesthetics will reduce renal blood flow and thus glomerular filtration rate. Direct nephrotoxicity is a potential adverse effect of those agents that undergo extensive metabolism to free fluoride ions, e.g. methoxyflurane.

Skeletal muscle effects

All halogenated volatile anesthetics can trigger malignant hyperthermia, a potentially life-threatening myopathy that occurs in susceptible individuals. Susceptibility is conferred genetically and is most common in rapidly growing breeds of pig, such as the landrace, large white and pietrain. However, the syndrome has been reported in other species, including the dog and cat. It may also be triggered by stress, and in wild species the term 'capture myopathy' has been used.

The mechanism of malignant hyperthermia is not fully understood but involves a marked elevation in the concentration of intracellular calcium. This causes widespread muscle contracture. Lactic acidosis rapidly ensues as oxygen supply fails to meet demand. The resultant cell membrane damage leads to electrolyte disturbances, particularly hyperkalemia, that serve to compound the problem. Clinical signs include muscle rigidity, hyperthermia, tachycardia and tachypnea progressing to dyspnea. The condition is rapidly fatal and treatment must be instituted at an early stage if it is to be successful. Inhalation anesthesia should be terminated immediately and, if available, dantrolene should be given (2–5 mg/kg IV). This muscle relaxant, which inhibits the release of calcium from the sarcoplasmic reticulum, has been used to prevent as well as treat malignant hyperthermia. Symptomatic treatments should also be instituted, including aggressive body cooling, intravenous fluids, ventilation with 100% oxygen and administration of bicarbonate to correct the acidosis and hyperkalemia.

Special considerations

Hazards to people

Many adverse health effects, ranging from dizziness and headaches to spontaneous abortion and congenital abnormalities, have been attributed to chronic exposure to waste anesthetic gases, particularly halothane and nitrous oxide. While experimental studies have largely failed to confirm this association, measures to minimize the exposure of operating room personnel to waste anesthetic gases would seem sensible.

Environmental concerns

Halogenated anesthetics are closely related to the chlorofluorocarbons (CFCs). CFCs release free chlorine, which destabilizes and destroys ozone. The volatile anesthetics are also capable of releasing free chlorine but, unlike the CFCs, they are extremely unstable and the vast majority of anesthetic molecules will be destroyed before reaching the ozone layer.

Nitrous oxide is classed as a 'greenhouse gas'. While it does not directly affect the ozone layer, reaction with oxygen yields nitric oxide and this agent does contribute to ozone destruction. Furthermore, nitrous oxide is quite stable, persisting in the atmosphere for many years.

Halothane

Clinical applications

Halothane was first introduced into anesthetic practice in the 1950s. At that time it was much safer than the existing inhalation anesthetics and rapidly gained popularity. In human anesthesia it has since been superseded by even safer agents, although its use in veterinary practice is still widespread.

Halothane is used primarily to maintain anesthesia following induction with an injectable agent. It may also be used to induce anesthesia if injectable drugs are considered inappropriate, e.g. where intravenous access is difficult or there are contraindications to the use of specific injectable induction agents. It is licensed for use in most companion animal species.

Pharmacokinetics

Chemical and physical properties

Halothane is a halogenated hydrocarbon (see Fig. 5.1). It is a liquid at room temperature and sea-level pressure and therefore is classed as an anesthetic vapor. It is nonflammable but is degraded by ultraviolet light and is therefore supplied in dark bottles. Addition of a preservative, thymol, further slows decomposition. Unfortunately thymol, which is less volatile than halothane, tends to accumulate within vaporizers and can potentially cause malfunction.

Solubility

Halothane has a moderately low blood:gas partition coefficient, although not as low as many of the newer agents (Table 5.2). The low solubility in blood results in a moderately rapid induction, recovery and rate of change of anesthetic depth. Solubility in tissues such as muscle and fat is quite high (fat:gas partition coefficient = 51), but not markedly greater than for other agents. High tissue solubility tends to slow induction and recovery.

The oil:gas partition coefficient for halothane is high, implying high potency, and this is confirmed by a low MAC value of approximately 0.9% in the dog.

Metabolism and elimination

In people, the rate of metabolism of halothane is 20–25%. In other words, 75–80% of the inspired halothane is exhaled unchanged. Halothane is metabolized by the cytochrome P450 system in hepatocytes. The major products of oxidative metabolism are trifluoroacetic acid and inorganic chloride and bromide. Under anaerobic conditions, reductive metabolism may occur, bromide and fluoride ions being among the products.

Increases in the rate of metabolism have been observed following prolonged exposure to halothane, even at low

Table 5.2 Some physical and pharmacokinetic properties of the inhalation anesthetics

Inhalation agent	Vapor pressure at 20°C (mmHg)	Volume of vapor per volume of liquid (mL)	Blood:gas partition coefficient	Oil:gas partition coefficient	Fat:gas partition coefficient	Approximate MAC values (%/vol)	Approximate rate of metabolism (%)
Halothane	244	227	2.5	224	51	0.87 dog 1.14 cat	20–25
Isoflurane	240	195	1.5	91	45	1.3 dog 1.6 cat	0.17
Desflurane	681	210	0.42	19	27	7.2 dog 9.79 cat	0.02
Sevoflurane	170	183	0.68	47	48	2.36 dog 2.58 cat	3.0
Methoxyflurane	23	207	15	970	902	0.29 dog 0.23 cat	50
Nitrous oxide	–	–	0.47	1.4	1.08	222 dog 255 cat	0.004

doses. This is clearly a concern for operating theater staff.

Adverse effects

Central nervous system effects

Halothane induces dose-dependent depression of the CNS without significant analgesia.

It is a particularly potent cerebral vasodilator while reducing metabolic oxygen consumption to a lesser degree. The tendency to raise intracranial pressure and potentially impair perfusion exceeds the ability to reduce cerebral oxygen requirement. Thus halothane should be avoided in patients with elevated intracranial pressure.

Cardiovascular effects

Halothane reduces cardiac output at clinically useful concentrations, primarily through direct depression of myocardial contractility. Changes in heart rate, if they occur, are slight. Arterial blood pressure falls, primarily as a consequence of decreased cardiac output. In addition, halothane sensitizes the myocardium to the arrhythmogenic effects of catecholamines and is the most potent of the inhalation anesthetics in this regard.

Respiratory effects

Halothane is possibly less depressant than some of the other agents available. It also produces bronchodilation and has been considered the agent of choice in patients with increased airway resistance, although some of the newer agents may be equally effective.

Hepatic effects

Halothane reduces blood flow in both the hepatic artery and the hepatic portal vein. Mild hepatic damage can arise as a result of the reduced blood flow and consequent hepatocyte hypoxia. Such changes are unlikely to result in clinical signs, although increases in liver enzymes have been observed. A rare and potentially fatal syndrome of fulminant hepatic failure has been described in people (termed 'halothane hepatitis'). The mechanism of hepatic injury is incompletely understood. Metabolites of halothane are believed to form conjugates with hepatic proteins, initiating an immune-mediated hepatic necrosis. According to an experimental model developed in rats, a metabolite generated under hypoxic conditions may be responsible. However, more recent work conducted in humans has implicated the oxidative metabolite trifluoroacetic acid. All volatile anesthetics possessing a $-CF_3$ group are capable of metabolism to trifluoroacetic acid. However, halothane undergoes more extensive metabolism than the newer volatile agents and so the potential for toxicity is greater.

Renal effects

Halothane, like all agents, will reduce renal blood flow and glomerular filtration rate. Direct nephrotoxicity has not been recorded since fluoride is not an important metabolite.

Skeletal muscle effects

Of the volatile anesthetics, halothane is the most potent trigger for malignant hyperthermia and should never be used in susceptible individuals. It produces moderate muscle relaxation as a result of CNS depression. Shivering, not necessarily related to body or environmental temperature, is occasionally seen during recovery.

Contraindications and precautions

Halothane should be avoided in patients:

- with a space-occupying intracranial lesion or raised cerebrospinal fluid pressure
- with cardiac dysfunction, especially cardiomyopathy or dysrhythmias
- with hepatic disease
- susceptible to malignant hyperthermia.

Known drug interactions

- It has been suggested that halothane may reduce the ability of the liver to metabolize concurrently administered drugs. This is not simply an effect on metabolism, and other factors such as reduced liver blood flow may contribute.
- Metabolism of halothane may be enhanced by microsomal enzyme inducers, such as phenobarbital.
- Calcium channel and β-adrenergic blocking agents will augment the negative inotropic effect of halothane.
- All inhalation anesthetics, including halothane, potentiate the action of nondepolarizing neuromuscular blocking drugs.

Isoflurane

Clinical applications

Isoflurane is used increasingly in veterinary practice and offers a number of advantages over halothane. As for halothane, it is used primarily for maintenance of anesthesia but can also be used for induction. However, it is not well suited to mask induction and its rather unpleasant odor frequently causes breath holding.

Isoflurane is licensed for use in most companion animals, including dogs, cats and horses. It has also proved to be a popular anesthetic in more unusual pets, including small mammals, reptiles and birds, and is also licensed in these species.

Pharmacokinetics

Chemical and physical properties

Isoflurane is a halogenated ether (see Fig. 5.1). It is a nonflammable and stable anesthetic vapor. It is not degraded by ultraviolet light and the inclusion of preservatives is unnecessary.

Solubility

Isoflurane has a lower blood:gas partition coefficient than halothane (see Table 5.2) and is therefore associated with a more rapid induction, recovery and rate of change of anesthetic depth. The oil:gas partition coefficient is also lower and this reflects the lower potency and higher MAC of isoflurane (≈1.3% in the dog). Solubility in tissues such as fat is slightly less than for halothane.

Metabolism and elimination

In people, the rate of metabolism of isoflurane is extremely low, less than 0.2%, and virtually all the isoflurane inhaled is exhaled unchanged. What metabolism there is occurs in the liver and the main products are trifluoroacetic acid and inorganic fluoride ions.

Adverse effects

Central nervous system effects

Isoflurane produces less cerebral vasodilation than halothane, while still reducing metabolic oxygen consumption. The reduced oxygen requirement is usually sufficient to compensate for any tendency towards impaired oxygen delivery. Thus, isoflurane is preferred over halothane when anesthetizing patients with elevated intracranial pressure. Furthermore, isoflurane, unlike halothane, does not impair the responsiveness of the cerebral circulation to carbon dioxide and hyperventilation can be used to lower intracranial pressure in isoflurane-anesthetized patients.

Cardiovascular effects

Isoflurane does depress myocardial contractility, but to a lesser degree than halothane. Heart rate tends to increase slightly so that at light-to-moderate levels of anesthesia, cardiac output is often maintained. Isoflurane, like halothane, frequently causes arterial blood pressure to fall. However, decreased vascular resistance, rather than reduced cardiac output, is the main mechanism involved.

As a halogenated ether, isoflurane is associated with a much lower incidence of arrhythmias than halothane.

Respiratory effects

Isoflurane depresses ventilation to a greater extent than halothane; therefore arterial partial pressure of carbon dioxide is likely to rise. Bronchodilation is a potentially beneficial side effect.

Hepatic effects

Although isoflurane decreases hepatic portal vein blood flow, hepatic arterial blood flow is increased. The overall effect is a reduction in hepatic blood flow of lesser magnitude than that seen with halothane. Consequently hepatic injury related to hepatocyte hypoxia is less likely to occur. Trifluoroacetic acid is a potential metabolite of isoflurane and a condition similar to halothane hepatitis has been reported in humans, although the incidence is extremely low.

Renal effects

Metabolism of isoflurane is minimal; therefore very little fluoride is generated and renal toxicity is unlikely. As for halothane, renal blood flow and glomerular filtration rate may be reduced.

Skeletal muscle effects

Isoflurane can trigger malignant hyperthermia in susceptible individuals. It produces good muscle relaxation and may maintain better muscle blood flow than halothane.

Contraindications and precautions

Absolute contraindications are few:

- patients susceptible to malignant hyperthermia.

Known drug interactions

Isoflurane potentiates nondepolarizing neuromuscular blocking drugs to a greater extent than halothane.

Sevoflurane

Clinical applications

Sevoflurane is a recently introduced agent that is gaining popularity in veterinary anesthesia. It has many features in common with isoflurane but is less potent. Unlike isoflurane, it lacks a pungent odor and is said to be pleasant to inhale, rendering it suitable for mask induction.

Pharmacokinetics

Chemical and physical properties

Sevoflurane is a halogenated ether (see Fig. 5.1). It is stable and nonflammable.

Sevoflurane reacts with the alkaline carbon dioxide absorbents commonly used in rebreathing anesthetic systems to yield a potentially toxic product, compound A ($CF_2{=}C[CF_3]{-}O{-}CH_2F$). A variety of factors can influence the generation of compound A and production appears to be increased by:

- high environmental temperatures
- high concentrations of sevoflurane
- the use of baralyme rather than soda lime
- low fresh gas flows
- the use of absorbent that has been previously exposed to sevoflurane.

While compound A causes renal failure in rats at relatively low concentrations, its toxicity in humans and other species, including dogs, has not been established. Despite the lack of evidence most authors recommend that a minimum fresh gas flow of 2 L/min be used when sevoflurane is delivered via a rebreathing system.

Solubility

Sevoflurane has a very low blood:gas partition coefficient associated with a rapid onset of action. This is an added advantage if sevoflurane is to be used for mask induction. Recovery is also rapid but may be slowed slightly by a relatively high solubility in tissues, particularly fat.

Sevoflurane has a lower oil:gas partition coefficient than isoflurane and is therefore less potent, having a MAC value of approximately 2.3% in the dog.

Metabolism and elimination

Approximately 3% of sevoflurane is metabolized in the liver, inorganic fluoride being the main product. Intrarenal metabolism to fluoride is minimal (compare methoxyflurane).

Adverse effects

Many of the pharmacological effects of sevoflurane are qualitatively and quantitatively similar to those of isoflurane.

Central nervous system effects

Sevoflurane reduces cerebral metabolic rate but also causes cerebral vasodilation, thereby increasing intracranial pressure. The responsiveness of the cerebral vasculature to carbon dioxide is maintained.

Cardiovascular effects

Sevoflurane, like isoflurane, produces mild depression of myocardial contractility, systemic vascular resistance and arterial blood pressure. It may be less likely to increase heart rate than isoflurane and vasodilation may not be so prominent. However, these differences are not marked. Sevoflurane has low arrhythmogenicity.

Hepatic effects

As for isoflurane, sevoflurane decreases hepatic portal vein blood flow but increases hepatic arterial flow. Although sevoflurane has two $-CF_3$ groups, trifluoroacetic acid is not an important metabolite (free fluoride is generated instead) and sevoflurane-induced hepatitis has not been reported.

Renal effects

Increased serum concentrations of fluoride, approaching nephrotoxic levels, have been documented in people anesthetized with this agent. However, renal damage has not been reported despite the now widespread use of sevoflurane in human anesthesia. Intrarenal production of fluoride may be a more significant cause of nephrotoxicity than fluoride generated by hepatic metabolism (compare methoxyflurane).

Generation of potentially nephrotoxic compound A is an additional concern when rebreathing anesthetic systems are used.

Although sevoflurane-induced renal damage has not been documented it would seem sensible to avoid this agent in patients with pre-existing renal impairment.

Desflurane

Clinical applications

Desflurane was first synthesized in the 1960s, along with enflurane and isoflurane. It was not pursued further at that time, since its low potency was considered a disadvantage. Its properties have since been re-examined and desflurane is a relatively recent introduction to the field of human anesthesia, where it has gained favor as an anesthetic for day-case surgery. As yet it is not widely used in veterinary anesthesia.

Pharmacokinetics

Chemical and physical properties

Desflurane is a fluorinated ether (see Fig. 5.1). Its structure is similar to that of isoflurane, differing only in the substitution of a fluorine atom for chlorine. It is non-flammable and stable.

The vapor pressure of desflurane is exceptionally high; in fact, its boiling point (22.8°C) is close to room temperature. Standard vaporizers are unable to deliver a predictable concentration of desflurane and an electronic, temperature-controlled, pressurized vaporizer must be used to ensure a reliable output.

Volatile anesthetics that possess an $-O-CHF_2$ group, i.e. desflurane and isoflurane, can react with the carbon dioxide absorbent soda lime to generate carbon monoxide. This reaction is most likely with desflurane. Recommendations to limit carbon monoxide production include regular replacement of used soda lime and flushing of rebreathing circuits with oxygen for a couple of minutes prior to use, especially if the circuit has not been used for a couple of days.

Solubility

Desflurane has the lowest blood:gas partition coefficient of the volatile anesthetics currently available, i.e. it is relatively insoluble in blood. This factor, coupled with a low solubility in tissues, accounts for the more rapid rate of onset, recovery and change of anesthetic depth associated with this agent.

However, the oil:gas partition coefficient is low, hence the low potency and high MAC of desflurane (7.2% in the dog).

Metabolism and elimination

A further desirable feature of desflurane is its low rate of biotransformation. In people, as little as 0.02% of the inhaled dose of desflurane undergoes metabolism.

Adverse effects

Central nervous system effects

Desflurane is typical of the inhalation anesthetics, reducing cerebral metabolic rate while increasing cerebral blood flow and thereby intracranial pressure. As for isoflurane and sevoflurane, the responsiveness of the cerebral vasculature to carbon dioxide is maintained. In addition, desflurane may have an unfavorable effect on CSF pressure, which tends to increase.

Cardiovascular effects

Cardiac output is frequently maintained at clinically useful concentrations, as it is for isoflurane and sevoflurane. Rapid increases in the inspired concentration of desflurane may elevate plasma levels of catecholamines leading to increases in heart rate and arterial blood pressure. Despite this, desflurane does not appear to sensitize the myocardium to adrenaline (epinephrine)-induced arrhythmias.

Respiratory effects

Desflurane produces dose-dependent depression of respiratory function. High inspired concentrations cause airway irritation, coughing, breath holding and laryngospasm in people and so this agent is not suitable for mask induction.

Hepatic and renal effects

Although desflurane undergoes limited biotransformation, trifluoroacetic acid is a potential metabolite. Cases of desflurane-induced hepatitis have been reported although the incidence is extremely low. Desflurane causes minimal depression of renal blood flow and there is no evidence of nephrotoxicity.

Methoxyflurane

Methoxyflurane was once a popular inhalation agent, used primarily in small animal anesthesia. However, it has been largely superseded by newer, safer agents. Today it is mainly of interest as an example of a less than ideal volatile anesthetic.

Pharmacokinetics

Chemical and physical properties

Methoxyflurane is a halogenated ether (see Fig. 5.1). It is nonflammable but unstable and so an antioxidant preservative must be included. It has an unusually low vapor pressure (see Table 5.2) so does not readily evaporate. This feature may limit the usefulness of an inhalation anesthetic, i.e. if a therapeutic vapor concentration cannot be achieved. In this case the impact of low vapor pressure is largely offset by the high potency of methoxyflurane.

Solubility

The blood:gas partition coefficient for methoxyflurane is high, so induction, recovery and rate of change of anesthetic depth are slowed. This is compounded by a high solubility in the tissues, particularly fat.

Furthermore, methoxyflurane has a high solubility in rubber and will dissolve in components of the breathing system.

Methoxyflurane is an extremely potent inhalation anesthetic as indicated by its very high oil:gas partition coefficient and extremely low MAC value – 0.29% in the dog.

Metabolism and elimination

Methoxyflurane undergoes extensive hepatic biotransformation and as much as 50% of the inhaled agent is metabolized in people. The main metabolites are fluoride, dichloroacetic acid and oxalic acid. Recent studies have shown that methoxyflurane also undergoes significant metabolism to fluoride within the kidney itself.

Adverse effects

The side effects of methoxyflurane are typical of the older inhalation agents such as halothane.

Central nervous system effects

Methoxyflurane is an extremely potent anesthetic. Some authors suggest that it also possesses analgesic properties that extend into the recovery period, but it is unclear if this simply reflects the delayed recovery from this agent.

Cardiovascular effects

Like halothane, methoxyflurane depresses myocardial contractility, reducing cardiac output and arterial blood pressure. It is also capable of sensitizing the heart to adrenaline (epinephrine)-induced arrhythmias, but this effect is much less common than with halothane.

Renal effects

Free fluoride, the main metabolite of methoxyflurane, is potentially nephrotoxic. Traditionally the risk of nephrotoxicity has been correlated to plasma fluoride concentrations, which reflect hepatic metabolism. However, methoxyflurane also undergoes metabolism to fluoride within the kidney and this intrarenal production of fluoride appears to be a key factor in the development of nephrotoxicity (compare sevoflurane).

High-output renal failure has been recorded in people anesthetized with methoxyflurane. In dogs anesthetized with this agent increased serum concentrations of fluoride have been documented; however, reports of renal damage are limited to dogs given additional nephrotoxic drugs, such as nonsteroidal anti-inflammatories.

Known drug interactions

As for halothane, metabolism of methoxyflurane may be enhanced by microsomal enzyme inducers such as phenobarbital.

Nitrous oxide

Clinical applications

Nitrous oxide is used primarily as an adjunct to anesthesia induced and maintained by other agents. It is not sufficiently potent to be used alone; however, its use at relatively high inspired concentrations may be advantageous in selected patients. Nitrous oxide is unusual in having analgesic properties, but inspired concentrations of 50% and greater are needed if it is to contribute significantly to analgesia and anesthesia. This inevitably reduces the inspired concentration of oxygen and an upper limit of 66% inspired nitrous oxide (or minimum 33% inspired oxygen) should be observed to avoid hypoxemia.

The main indication for using nitrous oxide is as part of a balanced anesthetic technique, i.e. its use allows a reduction in the inspired concentration of the more potent volatile agent with an associated decrease in adverse effects. Nitrous oxide may also be useful at induction: its addition to the inspired gases speeds the onset of anesthesia.

Pharmacokinetics

Chemical and physical properties

Nitrous oxide (N_2O) is an example of an anesthetic gas. It is nonirritant and nonflammable, although it can support combustion. It is supplied in cylinders as a liquid under increased pressure (approximately 50 atmospheres – 5000 kPa). Cylinders must be weighed to determine the quantity of nitrous oxide remaining, since a pressure gauge will not accurately reflect the contents of the cylinder. Pressure gauges measure the pressure of the gas overlying the liquid phase and this will not change until all the liquid has evaporated, i.e. the pressure gauge will indicate that the cylinder is full until it is almost empty.

Solubility

If nitrous oxide is used in combination with a second agent, such as halothane, the speed of anesthetic induction is increased. Two factors contribute to this. Nitrous oxide has a very low blood:gas partition coefficient (see Table 5.2); therefore any contribution to anesthesia by nitrous oxide is extremely rapid in onset. More importantly, since nitrous oxide is used in high concentrations, uptake from the alveoli of a relatively large volume of nitrous oxide has a concentrating effect on the second agent and the alveolar partial pressure of that agent rises more rapidly as a result. This has been termed the second gas effect.

The inclusion of nitrous oxide in the inspired gas mixture may cause expansion of gas-filled spaces within the body. This effect is rarely important in normal animals, with the possible exception of adult ruminants. However, it may be significant in situations where a closed gas space contributes to cardiovascular or respiratory compromise, e.g. pneumothorax or gastric dilation and volvulus. The use of nitrous oxide in such patients is contraindicated. Expansion of such air-filled spaces arises because nitrous oxide diffuses in more rapidly than nitrogen can diffuse out and this is primarily a consequence of nitrogen's extremely low solubility in blood (blood:gas partition coefficient for nitrogen = 0.015).

This unequal exchange of nitrous oxide and nitrogen may also lead to complications at the end of anesthesia when the nitrous oxide is turned off and the patient is breathing room air. Nitrous oxide diffuses out of the blood and back into the alveoli more rapidly than nitrogen can diffuse from the alveoli into the blood. This tends to reduce the alveolar oxygen concentration, leading to diffusion or dilutional hypoxia. To avoid this complication patients should be maintained on oxygen for approximately 10 min after the nitrous oxide has been turned off.

The oil:gas partition coefficient of nitrous oxide is very low and this is associated with its low potency and high MAC value. In fact, the MAC is so high (>200%) that it cannot be achieved, hence nitrous oxide is used as an adjunct to anesthesia, not as the sole agent.

Metabolism and elimination

Nitrous oxide is extremely stable and undergoes virtually no metabolism. Reduction to nitrogen, mediated by anaerobic intestinal bacteria, occurs to a limited extent.

Adverse effects

Central nervous system effects

Nitrous oxide has analgesic properties and has recently been shown to be an *N*-methyl-D-aspartate (NMDA) receptor antagonist. This receptor is crucial in the development of central sensitization, whereby pain sensitivity is enhanced following tissue injury or inflammation. As an NMDA receptor antagonist nitrous oxide may limit the development of enhanced pain sensitivity following surgery.

Nitrous oxide increases cerebral blood flow and thereby intracranial pressure, although this effect appears to be more prominent when nitrous oxide is used alone than when it is used in combination with other agents.

Cardiovascular effects

Nitrous oxide is capable of producing direct myocardial depression. However, this action is balanced by indirect stimulation, mediated via activation of the sympathetic nervous system. As a result any impact on cardiovascular function is slight. Unfortunately, enhanced sympathetic activity may be associated with a greater incidence of adrenaline (epinephrine)-induced arrhythmias.

Respiratory effects

Direct respiratory depression is mild. Indeed, some authors suggest that nitrous oxide may actually increase pulmonary ventilation when it is combined with a volatile agent such as halothane or isoflurane. Expansion of gas-filled spaces is an additional factor that may contribute to ventilatory depression in some patients.

Inclusion of nitrous oxide in the inspired gas mixture will inevitably lower the arterial partial pressure of oxygen, primarily as a result of the reduced inspired oxygen concentration. This may be significant in animals with impaired alveolar gas exchange due, for example, to pulmonary disease or ventilation/perfusion mismatching. Reduced arterial oxygenation may also be relevant where oxygen delivery is compromised, e.g. in anemic patients. Development of diffusion hypoxia may be an additional concern.

Bone marrow suppression

Prolonged exposure to nitrous oxide leads to inactivation of a number of vitamin B_{12}-dependent enzymes that are required for DNA synthesis. Folate deficiency develops secondary to this. Bone marrow suppression results, with reduced production of both red and white blood cells. A polyneuropathy may also occur as a consequence of impaired myelin formation. These effects are unlikely to develop in patients anesthetized for less than 10 hours. However, they may be a concern for people working in a contaminated environment such as a polluted operating theater.

Other effects

- Nitrous oxide has little or no effect on renal or hepatic function and is a relatively mild trigger for malignant hyperthermia.
- Nitrous oxide may be teratogenic and should be avoided in pregnant patients.

Contraindications and precautions

The use of nitrous oxide is contraindicated in patients with the following conditions.

- Raised intracranial pressure
- Pneumothorax
- Gastric dilation and volvulus
- Intestinal obstruction
- Lung pathology
- Anemia

INJECTABLE ANESTHETICS

Injectable agents are used to provide anesthesia for a range of diagnostic and therapeutic procedures in small animals. Typically, injectable anesthetics are used to induce anesthesia before maintenance with an inhalational agent. In general the injectable anesthetics provide a rapid and calm induction with a smooth transition to inhalational anesthesia.

Injectable anesthetics, administered by intramuscular injection or intermittent intravenous bolus, have also been used to maintain anesthesia for procedures of short duration. These methods of administration have a number of drawbacks. Intubation and provision of oxygen are not routine and this may result in hypoventilation, airway obstruction and hypoxia. Depth of anesthesia is not easily controlled and once the agent is administered, the patient must redistribute or metabolize the drug to recover.

More recently there has been increased interest in the intravenous infusion of injectable anesthetics, either alone or in combination with analgesic drugs. This has been termed total intravenous anesthesia (TIVA). During TIVA the patient is typically intubated and breathes oxygen-enriched gas, as during inhalational anesthesia. However, the lack of environmental pollution is a major advantage. Furthermore, if drugs with a suitable pharmacokinetic profile are selected (i.e. rapid metabolism and elimination), anesthetic depth can be adjusted by altering the rate of infusion.

INJECTABLE ANESTHETIC AGENTS

EXAMPLES

Thiopental, alphaxalone, propofol, etomidate, ketamine, tiletamine/zolazepam, pentobarbital

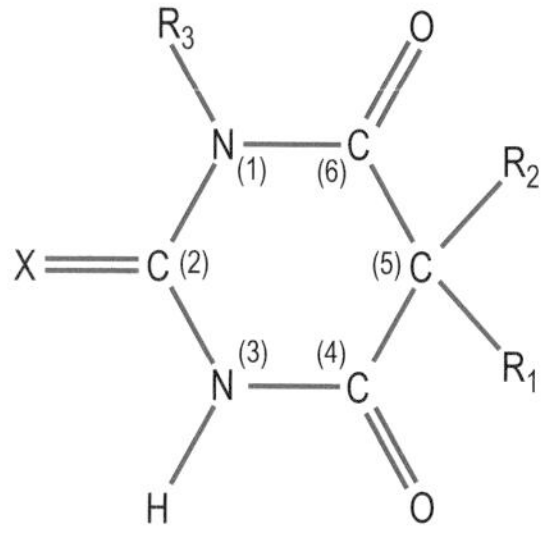

Fig. 5.4 **Basic structure of the barbiturates.**

Chemical structure

The injectable anesthetic agents are a diverse group of unrelated chemicals. Thiopental and pentobarbital belong to the barbituric acid group, which are classified according to either duration of action or chemical substitutions on the parent molecule. Thiopental is an ultra-short-acting agent providing less than 15–20 min of anesthesia after a single dose. Pentobarbital is classified as a short-acting barbiturate, although it provides anesthesia for 30–90 min after a single dose.

The barbiturates are derived from barbituric acid and share a common basic structure (Fig. 5.4). Pentobarbital is an oxybarbiturate having an oxygen atom at the carbon 2 position (i.e. X=O). If this oxygen atom is replaced by sulfur (X=S), a thiobarbiturate such as thiopental is produced. This modification reduces the time to onset and duration of action of the drug. Methohexital is a third barbiturate anesthetic that is no longer widely used. It is an oxybarbiturate with a methylated nitrogen in position 1 (i.e. X=O, R_3=CH_3). This methylation also produces a drug with a more rapid onset and shorter duration but unfortunately also confers unwanted excitatory side effects.

Ketamine and tiletamine are dissociative anesthetic agents, so-called because in humans they produce a sense of dissociation from the body and the environment. The remaining injectable anesthetics are an unrelated group. Alphaxalone is a steroidal anesthetic, propofol an alkylphenol and etomidate an imidazole anesthetic agent.

General physical properties

The barbiturates, ketamine, tiletamine and etomidate have asymmetrical carbon atoms resulting in isomers with varying potency. Other than etomidate, which is available as a single active dextrorotatory isomer, all other isomeric anesthetic agents are manufactured as racemic mixtures. Potency is dependent upon the concentration of active isomer, whereas side effects may be produced by either form of the molecule.

General pharmacokinetics

Intravenously administered injectable anesthetics produce a rapid smooth transition to unconsciousness because, provided an adequate dose is given, the animal passes through the first excitatory phases of anesthesia within a matter of seconds. There are several factors that determine the plasma (brain) concentration required to produce anesthesia, the speed of onset and the duration of anesthetic effect. The dose of drug administered has an effect, as does the route of administration and, for some intravenously administered drugs, the speed of injection. After intravenous administration the injectable agents are rapidly delivered to the brain and other organs with high perfusion. There is simultaneous uptake by other tissues, which is slower and of longer duration.

For agents that rely on redistribution for recovery (thiopental), peak muscle uptake corresponds to a lightening of anesthesia that occurs about 10–15 min after administration. Recovery from agents with a shorter duration of action (alphaxalone, propofol, etomidate) is due to a combination of redistribution and rapid metabolism. The injectable anesthetics are ultimately biotransformed in the liver and other tissues and eliminated in the urine and/or bile. The rate of transformation varies with species, age, the physical condition of the animal and the presence or absence of concurrently administered drugs.

Mechanism of action

Studies have demonstrated that most injectable anesthetic agents produce anesthesia by enhancing γ-aminobutyric acid (GABA)-mediated neuronal transmission, primarily at $GABA_A$ receptors. GABA is an inhibitory neurotransmitter found throughout the CNS. On binding to postsynaptic $GABA_A$ receptors, it causes an increase in chloride conductance that results in cellular hyperpolarization. Hyperpolarization inhibits or depresses neuronal function. These receptors, in addition to binding GABA, also bind benzodiazepines (diazepam, midazolam), barbiturates, etomidate, propofol and probably alphaxalone.

The dissociative anesthetic agents (ketamine and tiletamine) do not produce a 'true' anesthetic state and they do not appear to have an affect at the GABA receptor. They induce a dissociative state and analgesia by acting as antagonists of the excitatory amino acid glutamate at NMDA receptors. The NMDA receptor is linked to a calcium ion channel and by regulating calcium entry is able to amplify excitatory signals. Ketamine (and probably tiletamine) can block the channel, thus preventing ion movement. Ketamine and tiletamine are not generally administered as sole agents but are combined with CNS depressants such as α_2-agonists (xylazine, medetomidine) or benzodiazepines (diazepam, zolazepam, midazolam) to produce an anesthetic state.

General side effects

Central nervous system effects

Injectable anesthetics induce reversible dose-dependent depression of the CNS. Most injectable agents decrease cerebral blood flow, cerebral metabolic oxygen requirements and intracranial pressure in the presence of both normal and raised intracranial pressure. The dissociative agents are the exception to this, having the opposite effect.

Of the injectable agents, only the dissociative anesthetics provide significant analgesia. If agents with minimal analgesic activity are used surgery cannot be undertaken without excessive CNS depression. Ideally these agents should be combined with specific analgesic drugs (e.g. opioids), thereby allowing surgery to be performed at lighter planes of anesthesia.

Cardiovascular effects

The injectable agents have a variable effect on the cardiovascular system. In general, these agents cause dose-dependent cardiovascular depression with a decrease in blood pressure, myocardial contractility and/or peripheral vascular resistance. At low doses the injectable agents have only a small effect on cardiovascular parameters but as the dose is increased depression of myocardial function and vascular tone may be severe. Etomidate is much less depressant than the other agents, having a negligible effect on cardiovascular parameters.

Respiratory effects

All injectable agents can cause respiratory depression of variable severity. At low doses this depression may be mild to moderate, depending upon the agent administered, with hypoventilation increasing as the dosage of drug increases. Apnea may occur at surgical planes of anesthesia with some agents. Apnea at induction of anesthesia is also commonly encountered with the injectable agents. The duration of apnea depends upon the agent administered, the rate of drug administration when given intravenously, the physical condition of the animal and whether other respiratory depressant drugs (e.g. opioids) have been given concurrently. In the animal breathing room air, hypoxia can be a consequence of hypoventilation, recumbency and vascular changes induced by the injectable agents.

Hepatic and renal effects

Large doses of some agents have been implicated in the development of hepatic damage but in general at clinical doses the injectable agents do not have a direct effect on hepatic and renal function. However, hepatic and renal function may be compromised when reduced blood flow occurs secondary to anesthetic-induced hypotension. The injectable agents are metabolized in the liver, with the metabolites excreted in urine or bile, and a decrease in hepatic or renal function may prolong the action of these agents.

Skeletal muscle effects

The injectable agents, other than the dissociative anesthetics, provide some degree of muscle relaxation. Muscle rigidity can be profound with the dissociative agents when they are used as the sole agent. Relaxation is markedly improved with the addition of an α_2-agonist or benzodiazepine. The injectable agents, with the exception of ketamine and tiletamine, have been safely administered to patients susceptible to malignant hyperthermia.

Other effects

The injectable agents cross the placenta and depress the fetus. Generally the agents that are rapidly metabolized by the dam are also rapidly removed by the neonate although the duration of effect in the young can be longer because of immature hepatic and renal function. Maintenance of anesthesia with injectable agents for a cesarean section is not recommended.

General guidelines for administration of injectable anesthetic agents

In general the dose of injectable agent required to produce anesthesia is reduced in sedated, compromised, old and pediatric patients. In healthy animals individual variation in dose requirements also exists. For this reason the calculated dose of intravenous agent is not given as a single bolus but is administered to effect. Typically the calculated dose is drawn up, one-quarter to half of the dose is given as a bolus and the depth of anesthesia is assessed after 20–30 seconds. Further increments, of a quarter-dose or less, can be given as required until the desired level of anesthesia is achieved. Administration of the entire calculated dose may not be necessary.

Thiopental

Clinical applications

Thiopental is an ultra-short-acting thiobarbiturate that is usually given for induction before gaseous anesthesia but may be administered as the sole agent for short procedures that are minimally painful.

Following thiopental administration, induction and transition to inhalational anesthesia are smooth and rapid in the premedicated animal. However, if an inadequate dose is given to an unsedated or poorly sedated animal, excitement and hypertonus may be seen.

Emergence from anesthesia is rapid after a single dose but can be prolonged in the animal that has received multiple doses. Recovery may also be prolonged by hypothermia, compromised organ function and concurrently administered sedative, analgesic and inhalational anesthetic agents. Emergence may also be delayed in emaciated patients. Recovery is generally smooth in the sedated animal but excitement may be seen in the absence of sedation.

Mechanism of action

Thiopental enhances GABA-mediated inhibition of synaptic transmission by opening membrane chloride channels, causing cellular hyperpolarization. Thiopental does not act directly on the $GABA_A$ receptor or the chloride channel but binds to an allosteric site that increases GABA action and prolongs the duration of chloride-channel opening.

Formulations and dose rates

Thiopental is manufactured as a sodium salt that is soluble in water and 0.9% saline. For use in small animals, sufficient water or saline is added to make a solution of 1.25–5% (2.5% is most commonly used). The whitish-yellow crystalline powder is stable with a long shelf-life but once in solution, it is stable for only about 2 weeks at room temperature. The aqueous solution is strongly alkaline and is incompatible with acidic drugs and oxidizing substances such as analgesics, phenothiazines (e.g. acepromazine), adrenaline (epinephrine) and some antibiotics and muscle relaxants.

- The dosage of thiopental required for induction of anesthesia in the unpremedicated animal is approximately 20–25 mg/kg IV. To avoid excitement during induction, one-half of this calculated dose must be given as a bolus. Additional quarter-doses may be required to obtain the necessary depth of anesthesia.
- Premedication is preferred and reduces the induction requirement by 50–75%, i.e. to a dose of 10–12.5 mg/kg. An initial bolus dose of one-quarter to one-half of the calculated dose should be given, depending upon the depth of sedation.
- A single dose of thiopental provides anesthesia for about 10–15 min.
- Intravenous diazepam (0.25–0.5 mg/kg) given just before thiopental administration reduces the barbiturate requirements to 5–10 mg/kg and reduces the duration of effect to about 5–10 min.
- An unusual aspect of thiopental use is that the administration of a 2.5% rather than a 5% solution markedly reduces the total dose of drug needed to induce anesthesia.
- Because of its strong alkalinity, thiopental can cause severe tissue reactions and must only be given by the intravenous route.

Pharmacokinetics

Thiopental is highly lipid soluble and after intravenous administration, concentrations sufficient to induce unconsciousness occur in less than 30 seconds. The thiopental concentration in all highly perfused organs (brain, heart, liver, kidneys) is initially high but rapidly falls. Muscle concentration of thiopental rises for about 20 min then begins to fall but fat continues to accumulate thiopental for a further 3–6 hours. Uptake by muscle is the dominant cause for the rapid fall in plasma thiopental and peak muscle uptake corresponds to a lightening of anesthesia that occurs about 10–15 min after administration. Uptake by fat and hepatic metabolism also account for some of the initial fall in plasma concentration.

Once the brain concentration falls below the effective threshold, consciousness returns. Because redistribution is the major factor causing recovery, prolonged anesthesia can be seen with repeated doses as uptake sites become saturated with drug. Drug that has been redistributed to the tissues subsequently returns to the plasma and is gradually metabolized by the liver into inactive compounds that are excreted by the kidneys. The patient may appear groggy during this 'hangover' period as significant quantities of drug remain. Sighthounds (greyhound, Afghan, saluki, whippet, borzoi) may sleep 2–4 times longer than other breeds of dog because of a deficiency in the hepatic enzyme required to cleave the sulfur molecule from the thiopental, the first step in metabolism.

Thiopental is a weak acid. The ratio of ionized to unionized drug will be influenced by plasma pH. Low plasma pH, i.e. acidemia, will increase the concentration of unionized drug. Since it is the unionized drug that is active, this may enhance the anesthetic effect.

Thiopentone is highly protein bound (80–85%) and an enhanced anesthetic effect is also possible in severely hypoproteinemic patients or when other highly protein-bound drugs (e.g. NSAIDs) are given concurrently. Uremia may also augment the anesthetic effect by displacing protein-bound drug.

Adverse effects

Central nervous system effects

- Thiopental produces a dose-dependent decrease in cerebral oxygen requirements, cerebral blood flow and intracranial pressure (ICP). The decrease in cerebral oxygen requirements follows the neuronal depression produced by thiopental and the fall in blood flow occurs as a result of the decrease in demand for oxygen. The effect of thiopental on ICP makes this agent useful in patients with raised ICP (head trauma, brain tumor, hydrocephalus).
- Thiopental is also an anticonvulsant, making it safe in patients with epilepsy and those undergoing myelography.

Cardiovascular effects

- Thiopental reduces blood pressure in a dose-dependent manner. Peripheral vasodilation is the main mechanism involved and a compensatory rise

in heart rate frequently occurs. In healthy animals the resulting hypotension is not severe but in patients with congestive heart failure or hypovolemia, hypotension can be profound.
- Administration of thiopental can be associated with ventricular dysrhythmias and bigeminy is occasionally seen. These arrhythmias do not appear to progress to anything more serious and cease shortly after the induction dose is given. During halothane anesthesia thiopental reduces the threshold for adrenaline (epinephrine)-induced cardiac arrhythmias. However, thiopental does not increase sympathetic tone and is suitable for induction of hyperthyroid cats provided that heart failure is not present.
- The intravenous injection of greater than 2.5% thiopental in small animals may result in thrombophlebitis and intra-arterial administration will cause arteriospasm and ischemic tissue necrosis. Perivascular injection can cause tissue necrosis and sloughing. When extravasation is suspected 0.5–2 mL of lidocaine (lignocaine) without adrenaline (epinephrine) should be infused around the area. Lidocaine (lignocaine) is an acidic solution and this helps neutralize the alkalinity of the barbiturate. More importantly, it induces a localized vasodilation that promotes uptake of the drug. Infiltration of the area with saline to further dilute the barbiturate will also help.

Respiratory effects
- Thiopental produces dose-dependent respiratory depression with a reduction in both rate and tidal volume. Transient postinduction apnea is frequently seen. Thiopental depresses sensitivity of the respiratory center to carbon dioxide and the apnea is probably due to high plasma concentrations that are present after a bolus administration. Ventilation should be assisted until spontaneous breathing resumes.
- During light thiopental anesthesia the laryngeal reflexes remain strong and laryngospasm at intubation may be seen in cats. Arytenoid function is minimally depressed during light thiopental anesthesia, making this agent useful for assessment of laryngeal paralysis.

Hepatic effects
- High doses of thiopental can induce hepatic dysfunction, but low doses appear to be safe even in patients with liver damage.
- Thiopental is metabolized in the liver and a prolonged recovery can be anticipated in the patient with liver disease.

Renal effects
- When hypotension develops secondary to deep or prolonged thiopental anesthesia a reduction in renal blood flow occurs that can impair renal function.
- Uremia may enhance the effect of thiopental and the drug should be avoided or used with care in patients with raised blood urea concentrations.

Other effects
- Thiopental easily diffuses across the placenta and depresses the neonate during cesarean section. Alternative induction agents with a shorter duration of action should be considered for this surgery.
- Thiopental decreases intraocular pressure and can be administered to patients with glaucoma, penetrating eye injury, deep corneal ulcer or descemetocele.
- Engorgement of the reticuloendothelial system with blood after thiopental administration makes it unsuitable for splenectomy, liver biopsy and tonsillectomy.
- Thiopental appears to reduce packed cell volume (PCV) to a greater extent than other injectable agents.
- Anaphylactic reactions to thiopental have been reported, although such reactions appear to be rare.

Contraindications and precautions
Thiopental should be avoided or used with caution in the following patients.
- Hypovolemic and septic patients
- Patients with cardiac disease, especially dysrhythmias
- Uremic patients
- Patients with liver disease
- Patients undergoing splenectomy and liver biopsy
- Sighthounds
- Emaciated patients

Known drug interactions
- The dosage of thiopental required to induce anesthesia is variably reduced by the prior or concurrent administration of sedatives and opioids. If α_2-agonists are used for premedication the induction dose may be reduced by 50% or more.
- Phenobarbital treatment stimulates hepatic microsomal enzyme activity and hastens the metabolism of thiopental in greyhounds; this effect may occur in other breeds also.

Propofol

Clinical applications
Propofol is a very short-acting alkylphenol that is typically used to induce anesthesia prior to maintenance with an inhalational agent. Induction of anesthesia is rapid and generally smooth. The transition to

inhalational anesthesia must be prompt to ensure that the animal does not recover from propofol before an adequate quantity of inhalant is absorbed. Propofol, administered intravenously by intermittent bolus or variable rate infusion, can also be used to maintain anesthesia. For painful procedures specific analgesic drugs such as opioids should be incorporated into the protocol. Recovery from propofol anesthesia is generally rapid with minimal postoperative confusion or excitement. Recovery time is slightly longer in the cat and may be significantly delayed in this species if propofol is given by infusion.

Propofol is useful in the patient undergoing cesarean section because fetal depression is minimal if more than 18–20 min elapse between administration and delivery of the neonate. Induction of anesthesia followed by preparation of the surgical site usually ensures that sufficient time has elapsed at delivery for the neonate to be minimally depressed by propofol. As in adults, kittens take longer to recover than puppies after delivery.

Propofol has an anticonvulsant action and has been used to control status epilepticus in patients resistant to first-line therapies. Low infusion rates have also been used to provide sedation of dogs in an intensive care setting. In people antiemetic and antipruritic properties are also recognized and propofol has been shown to relieve the pruritus associated with epidural or spinal administration of opioids.

Mechanism of action

Propofol appears to activate the $GABA_A$ receptor by binding to a different site from thiopental but resulting in the same opening of chloride channels, causing cellular hyperpolarization.

Formulations and dose rates

Propofol is a substituted isopropylphenol that is insoluble in water but forms a 1% aqueous emulsion with 10% soyabean oil, 2.25% glycerol and 1.25% egg phosphatide. It is a slightly viscous, milky-white isotonic solution with a pH of 7–8.5. The emulsion can support bacterial growth, so asepsis during administration and storage is necessary. It is recommended that the contents of a vial should be discarded after 6 hours. If storage of propofol is necessary then the vial contents should be aspirated into a sterile syringe and capped with a needle or collected into a plain sterile vacutainer and used as soon as possible. There are reports of sepsis developing in patients that have been exposed to contaminated propofol. Propofol is compatible with lactated Ringer's solution and 5% dextrose but should not be mixed with blood or plasma.

- The dosage of propofol recommended to induce anesthesia in unpremedicated animals is 6.5 mg/kg in dogs and 8 mg/kg in cats. Following premedication the recommended doses are 4 and 6 mg/kg respectively in dogs and cats. However, the drug should be administered 'to effect' and smaller doses may be adequate, especially in compromised patients and those that have been premedicated with α_2-agonists.
- The period of anesthesia is short and a single dose will provide 2–10 min of unconsciousness.
- Complete recovery after a single dose occurs within 15–20 min in the dog and 30 min in the cat.
- To prolong anesthesia, small boluses of 0.5–2 mg/kg can be given as required or alternatively an infusion of 0.2–0.5 mg/kg/min can be administered. Stepwise reduction in the infusion rate is recommended for anesthetics of long duration. The use of propofol for maintenance of anesthesia is not recommended in cats as recovery may be prolonged. Delayed recovery following infusion has also been reported in greyhounds.
- An infusion rate of 0.1 mg/kg/min can be used to provide sedation in the dog.
- Propofol is ineffective given by either the intramuscular or subcutaneous route.

Pharmacokinetics

Propofol is extremely lipid soluble and so has a rapid onset, with unconsciousness occurring in less than 30 seconds. The drug is also highly protein bound; therefore patients with hypoproteinemia may require a lower dose for induction of anesthesia.

Recovery is rapid and is due to a combination of redistribution and metabolism. The latter involves hydroxylation followed by glucuronidation and sulfation. The resulting conjugates are excreted in urine. Cats have reduced glucuronidase activity, which might explain the longer duration of action in this species. The clearance of propofol is high; in fact, it exceeds hepatic blood flow, which would indicate that other tissues take part in its biotransformation. The kidney may be important and there is evidence of uptake by the lungs in cats. In people there is little evidence of altered pharmacokinetics in the presence of severe hepatic or renal impairment. Clinical experience suggests that this is also the case in dogs, although prolonged recoveries are likely in cats with hepatic lipidosis and other liver diseases. Clearance may also be influenced by the concurrent administration of sedatives, opioid analgesics (e.g. fentanyl) and other anesthetics.

Adverse effects

Central nervous system effects

- Propofol causes a decrease in cerebral blood flow, cerebral metabolic oxygen requirement and intracranial pressure. These effects should make it a useful agent in the patient with raised ICP (head trauma, cerebral neoplasia) but it may also reduce cerebral perfusion secondary to a fall in systemic blood pressure.
- Propofol is equal to or more potent than thiopental as an anticonvulsant, making it suitable for the patient with epilepsy or the animal undergoing myelography.

- Excitatory phenomena, including muscle twitching and rigidity, paddling and opisthotonus, are occasionally seen at induction. These reactions are believed to be subcortical in origin and are usually transient. Treatment is rarely required. Diazepam (0.2–0.5 mg/kg IV) would seem to be a logical treatment but is not always effective. Some authors recommend low doses of ketamine (0.25 mg/kg IV).

Cardiovascular effects

- Propofol causes a greater depression of blood pressure than other injectable anesthetics but these effects are of short duration. In people, systolic and diastolic pressures fall within 2 min of injection but return almost to normal values by 5 min. The fall in blood pressure is due to decreases in myocardial contractility and systemic vascular resistance without a compensatory rise in heart rate. It is thought that propofol impairs the baroreceptor response to low blood pressure. Hypotension can be minimized by using low doses of propofol and administering slowly to effect. However, this agent should still be used cautiously in patients with hypovolemia or impaired cardiac function.
- Although generally propofol is considered to have minimal effects on heart rate, profound bradycardia is occasionally seen.
- Despite some evidence that propofol decreases the cardiac threshold for adrenaline (epinephrine)-induced dysrhythmias most authors do not consider it to be inherently arrhythmogenic.

Respiratory effects

- The most frequent side effect associated with propofol administration is apnea at induction. This side effect appears to be most common and severe when the drug is given rapidly and in some patients may last for several minutes. Decreases in both respiratory rate and tidal volume commonly occur, resulting in a rise in arterial partial pressure of carbon dioxide. Hypoxia is also possible in the patient breathing room air.
- Recovery after propofol anesthesia is rapid and this allows early restoration of airway reflexes, which is beneficial in patients at risk of upper airway obstruction.

Skeletal muscle effects

- Myoclonus is occasionally seen (see CNS effects) but propofol does not trigger malignant hyperthermia.

Other effects

- Propofol decreases intraocular pressure and may be given to the patient with glaucoma, penetrating eye injury, deep corneal ulcer or descemetocele.
- Allergic reactions have not been reported despite the fact that propofol is a potentially allergenic molecule.
- If given repeatedly, i.e. on several consecutive days, propofol can induce oxidative injury in feline red blood cells causing Heinz body formation, diarrhea, anorexia and malaise. In addition, recovery times may be prolonged.
- Accidental perivascular injection of propofol does not result in irritation or tissue reaction.
- Pain on intravenous injection is common in people but is rarely recognized in animals. It may be more likely when propofol is injected into smaller veins.
- Propofol causes no significant endocrine effect, no change in the coagulation profile or platelet count and no significant effect on gastrointestinal motility.
- Propofol may have antioxidant effects similar to vitamin E.

Contraindications and precautions

Propofol should be avoided or used with caution in the following patients.

- Hypovolemic or hypotensive patients
- Cats that require multiple anesthetics

Alphaxalone (± alphadolone)

Alphaxalone ± alphadolone (Saffan®), alphaxalone (Alfaxan®-CD).

Clinical applications

Alphaxalone (± alphadolone) may be administered as the sole agent for short-term anesthesia or for induction before gaseous anesthesia in cats. Saffan® should not be administered to dogs because severe histamine release may result. Alfaxan®-CD does not induce histamine release and has recently been licensed for use in dogs.

Induction of anesthesia with alphaxalone (± alphadolone) is rapid and usually smooth. Facial and peripheral muscular twitching may be seen initially but good muscle relaxation follows. There is a rapid return to consciousness after a single or multiple doses; however, muscle tremors, paddling and opisthotonus may occur during recovery. If a cat is stimulated during recovery more vigorous movement and excitement may be seen. This generally ceases when the stimulation stops. These side effects can be minimized if the cat is sedated before induction and is recovered in a quiet area. Excitement during recovery is less frequently seen after Alfaxan®-CD anesthesia.

Mechanism of action

The mechanism of action of alphaxalone ± alphadolone is believed to be via binding to or near the $GABA_A$ receptor and enhancing chloride conductance causing cellular hyperpolarization. Alphaxalone ± alphadolone may also activate chloride channels independently of GABA.

Formulations and dose rates

There are currently two different formulations of alphaxalone. A combination of alphaxalone and alphadolone is manufactured as a clear solution containing 9 mg/mL alphaxalone and 3 mg/mL alphadolone (Saffan®). Cremophor EL (polyoxyethylated castor oil) is used as a solvent. The solubility of alphaxalone in Cremophor EL is enhanced by the addition of alphadolone, which has only weak hypnotic properties. The Cremophor EL-based drug forms a viscid solution with a pH of about 7. It is isotonic with blood and miscible with water. Cremophor EL causes mild-to-moderate histamine release in the cat and marked histamine release in the dog.

Alphaxalone is also marketed as a 'ready-to-use' 10 mg/mL solution in hydroxylpropyl-β cyclodextrin, buffered to pH 7 by sodium phosphate (Alfaxan®-CD). This solution contains no preservatives. The recommended shelf-life after opening varies in different countries (up to 7 days) but generally the solution should be used as quickly as possible.

- The alphaxalone/alphadolone combination should only be used in cats. The dosage is expressed as milligrams of total steroid per kilogram. A dosage of 9 mg/kg IV provides 10–15 min of anesthesia.
- Anesthesia can be prolonged by administering small boluses of 2–3 mg/kg as needed or by providing an infusion of 0.2–0.25 mg/kg/min.
- It can also be given by the intramuscular route. An IM dose of 9 mg/kg produces light sedation and 12–18 mg/kg produces light-to-moderate anesthesia.
- The response following intramuscular administration can be variable unless the injection is given deep into the muscle. Because of the large volumes required with intramuscular administration, several sites may be necessary.
- Alphaxalone ± alphadolone is ineffective when given by the subcutaneous route because of rapid metabolism.
- The alphaxalone solution that lacks Cremophor EL, i.e. Alfaxan®-CD, can be used in cats and dogs. The dosage of alphaxalone required for endotracheal intubation is 1–3 mg/kg IV in dogs and 5 mg/kg in cats. Anesthesia can be prolonged by administering small boluses of approximately 1 mg/kg as needed (approximately every 10 minutes) or by providing an infusion of 0.10–0.18 mg/kg/min. Doses at the higher end of the range are required in cats and unpremedicated patients.

Pharmacokinetics

After intravenous administration, alphaxalone ± alphadolone produces muscle relaxation within 9 seconds and unconsciousness within 30 seconds. Intramuscular injection takes about 6–12 min to have an effect and lasts about 15 min. Alphaxalone is not highly protein bound (30–50%) and hypoproteinemia has only a small effect on the dosage required to induce anesthesia. After IV administration a rapid fall in plasma drug concentration occurs as a result of hepatic metabolism and redistribution. Once plasma and brain concentrations fall below the effective threshold, recovery from anesthesia occurs. Because degradation is the major factor causing termination of anesthesia, accumulation is minimal and multiple doses can be given without prolonging the duration of recovery. Metabolites are excreted in urine.

Adverse effects

Central nervous system effects

- The cerebral depression produced by alphaxalone ± alphadolone is similar to that of thiopental. Cerebral metabolic oxygen requirement, cerebral blood flow and intracranial pressure are all decreased, making this agent useful in the patient with cerebral disease.
- Disturbing a cat during recovery can result in paddling and twitching, and violent convulsant-like activity may occur with rough handling.

Cardiovascular effects

- Alphaxalone ± alphadolone decreases arterial blood pressure in a dose-dependent manner. The fall in blood pressure appears to be due to a decrease in myocardial contractility and stroke volume. Heart rate usually increases and central venous pressure falls. Low doses (≤5 mg/kg) of alphaxalone have a mild transient effect on blood pressure, whereas larger doses (10 mg/kg) cause a moderate hypotension that persists for up to 40 min after a single dose. Clinical doses (8–9 mg/kg) of the alphaxalone/alphadolone combination cause the greatest decrease in blood pressure and the decrease may last for over 60 min. Much of the cardiovascular depression associated with alphaxalone ± alphadolone may be due to the Cremophor EL base rather than the active ingredients, as alphaxalone in cyclodextrin appears to produce less cardiovascular depression. In the cat alphaxalone ± alphadolone provides some protection against adrenaline (epinephrine)-induced cardiac arrhythmias.
- Perivascular administration of alphaxalone ± alphadolone does not cause any irritation or pain.

Respiratory effects

- Respiratory depression is minimal after alphaxalone ± alphadolone administration. Transient postinduction apnea can occur but is considered rare.

Other effects

- Cremophor EL causes marked histamine release and hypotension in dogs, making alphaxalone ± alphadolone unsuitable for anesthesia in this species.
  - In cats Cremophor EL also appears to cause histamine release, although it is less severe than that seen in dogs.

  - Edema or hyperemia of ears and paws are commonly encountered but these are of little clinical significance. There are rare reports of necrosis of the appendages.
  - Of more concern are the reports of pulmonary and laryngeal edema. These adverse events are potentially fatal but the incidence is low. Prompt treatment with corticosteroids and antihistamines may be required and in the case of laryngeal edema, a patent airway should be established and maintained.
  - Alphaxalone in cyclodextrin is not associated with histamine release.
- Despite being steroidal anesthetics, alphaxalone and alphadolone have no significant endocrine effect.
- Alphaxalone ± alphadolone crosses the placenta but depression of kittens appears to be minimal if the total dose is kept below 6 mg/kg.

Contraindications and precautions

Alphaxalone ± alphadolone should be avoided or used cautiously in the following patients.

- Cremophor EL-based drug should not be administered to dogs
- Cremophor EL-based drug should not be administered to cats with asthma or mast cell tumors
- Hypovolemic and hypotensive patients
- Patients with heart disease

Known drug interactions

- Premedication may prolong and smooth the recovery period. It also variably reduces the dose required for induction of anesthesia.
- Antihistamines will reduce the side effects associated with Cremophor EL administration.

Etomidate

Clinical applications

Etomidate can be used to induce anesthesia prior to maintenance with an inhalant. Alternatively it can be used as a maintenance agent for nonpainful procedures of short duration. It has fewer adverse cardiovascular effects than other injectable anesthetics and is frequently recommended in patients that are hemodynamically unstable. Fetal transfer is poor and there is less depression of the neonate than with other agents, making this agent useful in the patient requiring cesarean section. It has a wide safety margin, with a therapeutic index of 16 in dogs.

Mechanism of action

Etomidate produces dose-dependent cortical depression. It activates the $GABA_A$ receptor, which opens chloride channels, resulting in cellular hyperpolarization.

Formulations and dose rates

Etomidate is a carboxylated imidazole. Commercial preparations contain only the active dextrorotatory isomer. It has a pH-dependent ring structure that is water soluble at low pH but becomes lipid soluble at physiological pH. There are two formulations available. One preparation contains etomidate dissolved in 35% propylene glycol (Hypnomidate®). It forms a clear hypertonic solution that does not support bacterial growth. The other preparation contains etomidate in an aqueous emulsion of 10% soyabean oil, 2.25% glycerol and 1.25% egg phosphatide (Etomidate-Lipuro®). It is milky white, slightly viscous and does support bacterial growth. There is no bacteriostatic agent in either preparation and any unused drug should be discarded. Etomidate is currently unlicensed for use in animals.

- The recommended induction dose for etomidate is 0.5–2 mg/kg IV in the premedicated animal. As with other induction agents, the drug should be given to effect rather than as a single bolus.
- Etomidate should not be administered in the absence of sedation because excitatory side effects are commonly seen.
- Anesthesia can be maintained for short periods with etomidate given at a rate of 0.05–0.15 mg/kg/min in premedicated animals. Prolonged infusion is not recommended. It may be associated with adverse effects including adrenocortical suppression and hemolysis.

Pharmacokinetics

Etomidate is moderately lipid soluble and in the dog approximately 76% protein bound. After IV administration it induces unconsciousness in less than 30 seconds. Anesthesia lasts for 5–10 min and recovery is rapid. Termination of anesthesia is due to redistribution and rapid hydrolysis by hepatic microsomal enzymes and plasma esterases. The hepatic extraction ratio for etomidate is about 0.5 and a decrease in hepatic blood flow has a moderate effect on metabolism; however, clearance in patients with intrinsic liver disease is unchanged. The inactive metabolites are excreted mainly in the urine.

Adverse effects

Central nervous system effects

- Etomidate decreases cerebral metabolic oxygen requirement, cerebral blood flow and intracranial pressure. Cerebral metabolic oxygen requirements ($CMRO_2$) are decreased because neuronal function is depressed by etomidate. The decrease in cerebral blood flow is due to direct cerebral vasoconstriction and is independent of the fall in $CMRO_2$. Because etomidate has a minimal effect on arterial blood pressure, cerebral perfusion pressure is better maintained than with thiopental and propofol.
- Etomidate has anticonvulsant properties and is capable of controlling status epilepticus.
- Etomidate is tolerated well by the patient with cerebral disease or epilepsy and those undergoing myelography.

- Excitatory effects such as muscle twitching and paddling are not uncommon following administration of an induction dose of etomidate. Similar reactions are occasionally reported during recovery. These effects have been attributed to disinhibition of subcortical areas. Premedication appears to reduce the incidence of such phenomena.

Cardiovascular effects

- Etomidate produces minimal cardiovascular changes. After an induction dose of etomidate systemic vascular resistance and arterial blood pressure may decline slightly. Heart rate, myocardial contractility and cardiac output are generally well maintained. At higher doses (about 4 mg/kg IV), heart rate may also decrease. Cardiovascular parameters are also maintained at preanesthetic values during an etomidate infusion.
- Etomidate is not arrhythmogenic and is well tolerated in animals with rhythm disturbances.
- Because it produces minimal cardiovascular depression, etomidate may be the preferred induction agent in hemodynamically unstable patients. It has been recommended in cases that are hypovolemic (e.g. following trauma or gastric dilation and volvulus) or that have low cardiac output due to impaired myocardial contractility or dysrhythmia. However, when choosing to use etomidate in such patients its effects on adrenal steroidogenesis should not be overlooked (see endocrine effects below).

Respiratory effects

- Etomidate produces minimal respiratory depression. Tidal volume may fall transiently but minute volume tends to be maintained by an increase in respiratory rate. In a study conducted in dogs breathing room air a dose of 1.5 mg/kg IV caused minimal alteration in arterial blood gases. A higher dose of 3.0 mg/kg increased P_aCO_2 slightly and produced transient hypoxemia. The respiratory depression seen with etomidate appears to be dependent on dose and rate of injection, with slower rates causing less respiratory depression.

Hepatic effects

- In people, cirrhosis does not appear to delay clearance of etomidate, which is rapidly hydrolyzed by a combination of hepatic microsomal enzymes and plasma esterases. It has therefore been recommended as an induction agent in small animal patients with hepatic disease. However, etomidate infusions have been shown to decrease hepatic blood flow in the dog by inducing hepatic arterial vasoconstriction.

Renal effects

- In the small number of studies carried out, etomidate appeared to have no effect on renal function. However, etomidate formulated in propylene glycol can induce intravascular hemolysis and hemoglobinuria, especially when given as an infusion. The hemoglobin load compromises renal filtering ability, and fluid administration should be instituted to maintain renal perfusion.

Endocrine effects

- Etomidate can inhibit adrenal steroid synthesis. Following administration of a single induction dose, adrenocortical function may be suppressed for up to 6 hours in the dog. The significance of this effect in healthy patients is unclear but it is likely to be detrimental in patients with pre-existing impaired adrenocortical function, i.e. those on long-term steroid therapy or with hypoadrenocorticism. Adequate adrenocortical function is also crucial in the response to severe trauma and sepsis and the use of etomidate in such patients has been questioned. Where adrenal insufficiency is a concern, supplemental steroids should be administered.
- Infusion of etomidate is likely to result in more prolonged adrenocortical suppression and in people has been linked to increased mortality. Prolonged infusion of etomidate, for sedation or anesthesia, is no longer recommended.

Other effects

- Intravascular hemolysis has been reported after single doses and infusions of etomidate formulated in propylene glycol.
- Accidental perivascular injection of etomidate is not irritating and tissue reactions do not result.
- Pain on injection is reported in people, especially when small veins are used.

Contraindications and precautions

Etomidate should be avoided or used with caution in the following patients.

- Unpremedicated patients
- Animals with hypoadrenocorticism
- Animals on long-term steroid therapy
- Patients with sepsis, septic shock or severe trauma
- Critical patients requiring long-term sedation

Ketamine

Clinical applications

Ketamine can be used to induce anesthesia prior to maintenance with a gaseous agent. Alternatively, it can be used to induce and maintain anesthesia for procedures of short-to-moderate duration. Ketamine causes marked muscle rigidity and is rarely administered as the sole agent. It is usually combined with an α_2-agonist such as medetomidine or a benzodiazepine such as diazepam.

Ketamine does not produce a true anesthetic state but induces dissociation from the environment with analgesia and sensory loss. It does not suppress laryngeal and pharyngeal reflexes and swallowing persists to a variable degree, even when ketamine is combined with other drugs. An active swallow reflex should not be equated with an ability to protect the airway and the trachea should be intubated as with other anesthetic agents. Increased muscle tone and open eyes are additional features of the dissociative state.

More recently there has been an increased interest in the use of ketamine as an analgesic. As an NMDA receptor antagonist it is able to reverse the enhanced pain sensitivity that frequently accompanies major trauma or surgical injury. Subanesthetic doses, usually administered by infusion, may be beneficial in sensitized individuals especially when combined with more conventional analgesics such as opioids and NSAIDs.

Mechanism of action

Unlike other injectable anesthetics, ketamine has no effect at the $GABA_A$ receptor. Its main effects, i.e. dissociative anesthesia and analgesia, result from an antagonistic action at the NMDA receptor.

Formulations and dose rates

Ketamine belongs to the cyclohexamine group of dissociative injectable agents. It is a water-soluble acidic drug (pH of solution is 3.5–4.1) that should not be mixed with alkaline solutions. It exists as two optical isomers and is manufactured as the racemic mixture. The S(+) isomer produces greater CNS depression and analgesia but less muscular activity compared to the R(–) isomer.

- Ketamine should not be used alone to produce anesthesia in mammalian species, especially dogs. It should be combined with other sedative-type drugs to reduce the incidence of muscle rigidity and seizures.
- Assessment of anesthetic depth is more difficult when ketamine is used. Typical dissociative effects, such as increased muscle tone, an open eye and active reflexes, would indicate inadequate depth of anesthesia if a conventional anesthetic agent were administered. Therefore care is needed in deciding when additional drugs are required.

INTRAVENOUS KETAMINE AND BENZODIAZEPINE COMBINATIONS

- Ketamine 5–10 mg/kg + diazepam/midazolam 0.25–0.5 mg/kg in dogs and cats.
- Equal volumes of ketamine (100 mg/mL) and diazepam/ midazolam (5 mg/mL) can be mixed and administered slowly to effect. Approximately 1 mL/10 kg of the mixture (0.25 mg/kg diazepam/midazolam + 5 mg/kg ketamine) will produce anesthesia of short duration sufficient to allow endotracheal intubation. Administration of twice this dose produces 15–20 min of anesthesia.

INTRAMUSCULAR KETAMINE AND BENZODIAZEPINE COMBINATIONS

- Midazolam 0.2 mg/kg + ketamine 5–10 mg/kg.
- This combination can be used to produce 20–30 min of heavy sedation to light anesthesia in cats.

INTRAVENOUS KETAMINE AND α_2-AGONIST COMBINATIONS IN CATS

- Medetomidine 40 μg/kg + ketamine 1.25–2.5 mg/kg ± butorphanol 0.1 mg/kg.
- α_2-agonist and ketamine combinations are licensed for intravenous use in cats and produce 20–30 min of anesthesia.

INTRAMUSCULAR KETAMINE AND α_2-AGONIST COMBINATIONS

Dogs

- Medetomidine 40 μg/kg + ketamine 5–7.5 mg/kg.
- Medetomidine 25 μg/kg + butorphanol 0.1 mg/kg + ketamine 5 mg/kg.
- Xylazine 1 mg/kg + ketamine 10–20 mg/kg.

Cats

- Medetomidine 80 μg/kg + ketamine 2.5–7.5 mg/kg.
- Medetomidine 80 μg/kg + butorphanol 0.4 mg/kg + ketamine 5 mg/kg.
- Xylazine 1 mg/kg + ketamine 10–20 mg/kg.
- Combinations with an α_2-agonist (± butorphanol) provide 30–50 min of anesthesia when administered IM. Use of xylazine may be associated with a slightly shorter duration whereas higher doses of ketamine may extend the effect. The α_2-agonist (± butorphanol) can be given first, followed 10–20 min later by the ketamine. This practice allows time for the patient to vomit before anesthesia is induced and is recommended when xylazine is used in cats. Alternatively drugs can be combined in the same syringe and administered concurrently. Use of atipamezole to reverse the α_2-agonist is not recommended following ketamine use in the dog.

INTRAMUSCULAR KETAMINE AND PHENOTHIAZINE COMBINATIONS

- Low doses of ketamine (2–3 mg/kg) may be combined with acepromazine and opioid and administered IM (or SC) to premedicate or sedate painful or fractious cats.

USE OF KETAMINE AS AN ANALGESIC

- Ketamine 0.1–1 mg/kg IV or 1–2.5 mg/kg IM in dogs and cats.
- Ketamine 2–10 μg/kg/min as an IV infusion ± 0.5 mg/kg as a loading dose in dogs.
- Supplemental analgesia of short duration, e.g. sufficient for a dressing change, can be produced by administration of an IV bolus or IM dose of ketamine. To achieve a more prolonged effect in sensitized canine patients an IV infusion can be given, usually in combination with opioid analgesics. The use of analgesic ketamine infusions has not been reported in the cat. Administration of analgesic doses of ketamine to anaesthetized patients may be associated with respiratory depression and respiratory parameters should be monitored carefully.

Pharmacokinetics

Ketamine rapidly crosses the blood–brain barrier to induce anesthesia; however, the onset time is slower than with thiopental. After intramuscular or subcutaneous injection, 10–15 min elapse before sedation or anesthesia develops. The duration of anesthesia is dose dependent and lasts for 5–15 min after a single intravenous dose. Termination of anesthesia is due to redistribution from the brain and plasma to other tissue.

Ketamine is metabolized in the liver, producing a number of metabolites. Some, e.g. norketamine, have anesthetic activity. Induction of hepatic enzymes occurs with chronic administration of ketamine and higher doses may be required when it is given repeatedly. Hepatic dysfunction can prolong the action of ketamine and the drug should be used with caution in patients with a hepatopathy.

Ketamine and its metabolites, including norketamine, are excreted in urine. Despite this, diuresis does not enhance elimination although a prolonged effect may be seen in animals with renal insufficiency. Prolonged recoveries may also occur after multiple doses, intramuscular or subcutaneous administration and following the concurrent use of other sedative and anesthetic agents.

Adverse effects

Central nervous system effects

- Ketamine increases cerebral blood flow and thereby raises intracranial pressure. Combination with a benzodiazepine lessens the rise in ICP. The provision of intermittent positive pressure ventilation (IPPV) to prevent hypercapnia may also attenuate this response.
- Ketamine can induce seizures, especially if used alone in dogs. Seizures have also been reported following the administration of atipamezole to dogs anesthetized with a combination of an α_2-agonist and ketamine. It is possible that early reversal of the α_2-agonist leaves the ketamine action unopposed by a suitable sedative. Although anticonvulsant effects have also been documented it would seem sensible to avoid ketamine in patients with epilepsy and those undergoing myelography.
- Adverse emergence reactions with excitement, hallucinatory behavior, ataxia and increased muscle activity are occasionally seen during recovery from ketamine, used alone or in combination with a benzodiazepine. Sedative premedication reduces the incidence and severity of such side effects.

Cardiovascular effects

Ketamine has a two-fold effect on the cardiovascular system.

- It has a direct depressant effect on myocardial function and an indirect stimulatory effect mediated by increased sympathetic nervous system activity. Normally the latter action dominates and heart rate, cardiac output and arterial blood pressure all increase slightly after ketamine administration. Peripheral vascular resistance is usually unchanged. These stimulating effects may be diminished or prevented by the concurrent administration of other drugs. Of these, the benzodiazepines have the least effect and α_2-agonists and halothane the greatest effect.
- Ketamine alone appears to have an antiarrhythmic effect but concurrent administration of halothane reduces the cardiac threshold for adrenaline (epinephrine)-induced arrhythmias.
- Overall, ketamine appears to produce minimal cardiovascular depression and can be administered to many patients with cardiovascular disease. Occasionally critically ill patients appear to decompensate when ketamine is given. If catecholamine stores have been depleted, e.g. patients in end-stage shock, further increases in sympathetic activity are not possible and the direct depressant effects of ketamine may be unmasked. A similar phenomenon may occur if sympathetic antagonists such as propranolol are given concurrently.

Respiratory effects

- Transient respiratory depression occurs and hypoxia is possible in the animal breathing room air. The severity of the respiratory depression is dependent on the dose administered and the concurrent administration of other sedative and anesthetic agents. The benzodiazepines cause little additional respiratory depression whereas the α_2-agonists, opioids and inhalational agents can cause greater depression.
- An apneustic respiratory pattern, whereby the patient breath-holds on inspiration, has been described but is not frequently seen in small animals.

Hepatic effects

- Ketamine appears to have no effect on hepatic function.
- Ketamine is metabolized in the liver and hepatic dysfunction can result in a prolonged action.

Renal effects

- Ketamine appears to have no direct effect on the kidney but anesthetic-induced hypotension can result in compromised renal function.
- Animals with renal or postrenal disease can have a prolonged recovery time.

Skeletal muscle effects

- Ketamine alone can induce extreme muscle tone and spontaneous movement that is reduced by the concurrent use of a sedative.

- Increased motor activity, hyperreflexia and secondary hyperthermia may be seen during recovery following use of ketamine alone and sometimes following use of ketamine/benzodiazepine combinations. Because of the effect on muscle tone, ketamine has the potential to induce malignant hyperthermia.

Other effects

- Ketamine causes hypersalivation and increased bronchial secretions. In the past, concurrent administration of atropine has been advocated but this is no longer routinely recommended as tachycardia and an increase in myocardial oxygen requirement may result.
- Intraocular pressure rises after ketamine administration and the drug should be avoided in animals with glaucoma, penetrating eye injury, deep corneal ulcer or descemetocele.
- Because the eye remains open corneal drying may occur and application of an ocular lubricant is recommended.
- Accidental perivascular injection does not result in tissue necrosis but does cause a painful reaction. Pain may also be evident on intramuscular injection.

Contraindications and precautions

Ketamine should be avoided in the following patients.

- Patients that have a pre-existing tachycardia and those in which tachycardia would be detrimental
- Patients with elevated sympathetic tone, e.g. hyperthyroidism and pheochromocytoma
- Patients with hypertrophic cardiomyopathy
- Patients with raised ICP (e.g. due to an intracranial mass or head trauma)
- Epileptic patients or those undergoing myelography
- Patients with glaucoma, deep corneal ulcer or descemetocele
- Patients susceptible to malignant hyperthermia

Tiletamine-zolazepam

Clinical applications

Tiletamine-zolazepam can be administered for sedation or anesthesia of short-to-moderate duration or for induction before gaseous anesthesia. Separately tiletamine and zolazepam do not have ideal sedative or anesthetic properties but together they produce dissociative anesthesia, muscle relaxation and some analgesia.

Induction is smooth when given by any route provided that an adequate dose is administered. Analgesia is adequate for minor procedures such as wound sutures and cat castrations but not for major surgery such as ovariohysterectomy or castration in dogs. About 40% of animals retain some muscular tone.

Mechanism of action

Tiletamine probably has the same action as ketamine at the NMDA receptor and zolazepam enhances the action of GABA.

Formulations and dose rates

Tiletamine HCl belongs to the cyclohexamine group of dissociative agents and zolazepam is a benzodiazepine related to diazepam and midazolam. The combination is manufactured as a lyophilized powder that can be added to water, saline or 5% dextrose for reconstitution. The resulting solution is clear with a pH of 2.0–3.5.

The powder has a long shelf-life but the solution should be discarded after 4 days if stored at room temperature or 14 days if stored in a refrigerator.

- A 100 mg/mL solution contains 50 mg tiletamine and 50 mg zolazepam. The dosage and route recommended by the manufacturer for the cat are 9.7–15.8 mg/kg IM and for the dog 6.6–13.2 mg/kg IM. The recommended dose is high, producing a prolonged recovery, and the drug can be given by the intravenous and subcutaneous routes also.
- Smaller doses than recommended are effective but the actual dose appears to vary.
- In the USA, Telazol® administered at 2.5 mg/kg IM produces heavy sedation to light anesthesia in cats and excitement is not seen at lower doses. However, Zoletil® administered at 2.5 mg/kg IM produces excitement in young, healthy cats and a dose of 5 mg/kg IM is required to produce sedation or anesthesia.
- In geriatric or compromised animals a lower dose can be given for sedation.

Pharmacokinetics

After intravenous administration the onset of unconsciousness is less than 30–60 seconds. After IM administration, an effect can be seen in less than 2–5 min and a peak effect is seen in about 10 min. The duration of anesthesia after IM or SC administration is dose dependent, with low doses (2–5 mg/kg) providing sedation-anesthesia for approximately 15–20 min. A single IV dose lasts 10–20 min and full recovery takes 3–5 hours.

Recovery is initially due to redistribution and an infusion or several boluses prolong the duration of recovery. The drug is ultimately eliminated after hepatic metabolism and metabolites of both tiletamine and zolazepam are reported to be excreted by the kidneys.

Adverse effects

Very little work has been carried out to investigate the effects of tiletamine-zolazepam in small animals. It can probably be assumed that many of the effects of this drug will be similar to those of a ketamine and diazepam combination.

Central nervous system effects

- Tiletamine-zolazepam should be avoided in patients with raised ICP and cerebral disease because tiletamine can increase ICP, cerebral blood flow and metabolic oxygen requirements of the brain.
- Tiletamine as a sole agent can cause seizures and it would be wise to avoid this agent in patients with epilepsy or those undergoing myelography.
- Excitement, purposeless muscle activity and hyperthermia are common on recovery unless a sedative is given. These side effects are more commonly seen in dogs than cats; however, cats generally resent handling during recovery.
- Large or repeated doses prolong recovery and also decrease the quality of recovery.

Cardiovascular effects

- Tiletamine increases sympathetic tone, which causes a stimulatory effect on the heart, with increased contractility, tachycardia and increased potential for cardiac arrhythmias.
- Premature ventricular contractions may be seen after tiletamine-zolazepam administration; however, the arrhythmogenic dose of adrenaline (epinephrine) is not reduced in patients that receive both halothane and tiletamine-zolazepam.

Respiratory effects

- Tiletamine-zolazepam causes dose-dependent respiratory depression with a minimal effect seen at low doses.
- Other respiratory effects that have been reported include apnea, dyspnea and pulmonary edema.

Other effects

- Prolonged recovery, ataxia and sudden death have been seen in cats.
- Hyperthermia, prolonged and turbulent recovery, convulsions and death have been reported in dogs.
- Tiletamine-zolazepam crosses the placenta and depresses the fetus and because of its long duration of action is not recommended for cesarean section.
- Some animals show a pain response when the drug is given by the IM or SC route.

Contraindications and precautions

Tiletamine-zolazepam should be avoided or used with care in patients with the following conditions.

- Patients that have a pre-existing tachycardia and those in which tachycardia would be detrimental
- Patients with elevated sympathetic tone, e.g. hyperthyroidism and pheochromocytoma
- Patients with hypertrophic cardiomyopathy
- Patients with raised ICP (e.g. due to an intracranial mass or head trauma)
- Epileptic patients or those undergoing myelography
- Patients with glaucoma, deep corneal ulcer, penetrating eye injury or descemetocele
- Patients susceptible to malignant hyperthermia
- Patients requiring cesarean section

Further contraindications listed by the manufacturers include:

- pancreatitis
- renal insufficiency or failure
- pregnancy.

LOCAL ANESTHETICS

The first local anesthetic to be used was cocaine, which was introduced into human clinical practice in the 1880s as an ophthalmic anesthetic. Cocaine's addictive nervous system actions were soon discovered but it was still used until procaine was synthesized in the early 1900s. Lidocaine (lignocaine) is probably the agent most commonly used today. Other agents used in veterinary practice include mepivacaine, bupivacaine, proxymetacaine and prilocaine. Procaine is still used occasionally.

Clinical applications

Local anesthetics are used (as implied by their name) to desensitize a localized or regional area. They may be administered topically (spray, ointment) or infiltrated subcutaneously, around nerves, into joints or into the epidural space. In veterinary medicine they are often used in association with chemical restraint for relatively short, minor procedures or to provide additional analgesia in anesthetized patients undergoing major surgery.

Examples of local anesthetic use include:

- topical anesthesia of the larynx to assist endotracheal intubation, particularly in cats
- topical anesthesia of the eye to assist in removal of foreign bodies
- inclusion in 'shotgun' ear preparations to reduce pain and swelling associated with the inflammatory process
- subcutaneous infiltration to provide analgesia for minor procedures such as suturing, removal of small skin tumors and skin biopsies
- peripheral nerve blocks to provide regional analgesia of the head or limbs (e.g. for dental work or surgery of the forelimb)
- interpleural administration via a chest drain to provide analgesia after thoracic trauma or surgery
- intra-articular administration to provide analgesia prior to or following surgical exploration of joints
- epidural administration to provide regional analgesia of the caudal abdomen, hindlimb and perineum

(e.g. for cesarean section or hindlimb orthopedic procedures)
- intravenous regional administration to provide analgesia for surgery of the distal limbs.

In addition, infusions of the local anesthetic lidocaine have a sparing effect on the MAC of volatile anesthetics and have been used as an adjunct to general anesthesia. Infusions are also occasionally used to treat pain that is resistant to conventional analgesic therapies. Furthermore, lidocaine is an important antiarrhythmic and is a drug of choice in the treatment of malignant ventricular arrhythmias (see Chapter 17).

Mechanism of action

An electrically excitable cell, such as a nerve fiber, is able to generate an action potential in response to membrane depolarization. This activity is dependent on the function of voltage-gated ion channels in the cell membrane. At rest there is a potential difference across the cell membrane of approximately 60–90 mV, the intracellular environment being negative relative to the extracellular environment. During excitation, membrane depolarization opens voltage-activated sodium channels allowing sodium ions to flow into the cell, down a concentration gradient. This influx of positive charge produces further depolarization (i.e. the interior becomes less negative) and an action potential is generated. Two events serve to restore the resting membrane potential. Delayed opening of voltage-activated potassium channels produces an outward current of positive ions. In addition, the sodium channels are inactivated. These ion currents also require concentration gradients, which are restored by the sodium–potassium pump.

Local anesthetics inhibit both the initiation and conduction of action potentials by preventing the inward sodium current. They bind to receptors within the sodium channel to block the flow of ions. Access to the binding site cannot be gained through the external opening of the ion channel. The local anesthetic must first diffuse through the axon membrane and then enter the ion channel via the opening on the internal surface of the membrane. Alternatively the drug can reach the ion channel by diffusing directly through the membrane.

Local anesthetics can potentially block impulse conduction in all types of nerve fiber but differences in sensitivity exist. Small-diameter fibers are more sensitive than large-diameter fibers and a myelinated neurone will block more readily than an unmyelinated neurone of similar size. Thus nociceptive afferents (Aδ and C fibers) are more susceptible than motor neurones and in theory it is possible to achieve analgesia without loss of motor function. Autonomic nerve fibers are also very sensitive to the effects of local anesthetic. Another factor that influences susceptibility is the discharge rate of an axon and rapidly firing axons are blocked most readily. This form of use-dependence can be related to the functional state of the ion channel. The channel is more susceptible when in the open state since this improves access to the binding site. Sensory fibers, including nociceptive afferents, have a high firing rate and this serves to enhance their susceptibility to local anesthetics.

Formulations and dose rates

A large number of different local anesthetic preparations are available for topical anesthesia.

- EMLA cream (eutectic mixture of local anesthetic) contains a mixture of lidocaine (2.5%) and prilocaine (2.5%). It can be used to provide topical anesthesia of the skin prior to venepuncture. After application the skin should be covered with an occlusive dressing. Sixty min may be required for the maximum effect to develop.
- A clear solution of 2% lidocaine administered by a metered dose spray is available for topical anesthesia of the larynx. Each spray contains 2–4 mg of lidocaine. Lidocaine is also available as a 1% gel to facilitate procedures such as urethral catheterization.
- A 0.5% solution of proxymetacaine is commonly used to desensitize the cornea.

Local anesthetics are also available as aqueous solutions for injection (e.g. 5% procaine, 2% lidocaine, 2% mepivacaine, 0.5% bupivacaine, 0.2% ropivacaine).

- Bupivacaine, mepivacaine and ropivacaine have an asymmetrical carbon and exist as optical isomers. Racemic mixtures of bupivacaine and mepivacaine are used most frequently in veterinary medicine; however, the S isomer of bupivacaine is available separately and is less toxic. Ropivacaine is only available as the S enantiomer.
- Some formulations of lidocaine contain low concentrations of adrenaline (epinephrine) and therefore produce a localized vasoconstriction. This serves to reduce systemic absorption of the local anesthetic, thereby prolonging its duration of effect and reducing the risk of systemic toxicity. Such preparations should not be used for intravenous regional analgesia. Neither are they recommended for desensitization of an extremity such as a digit.

Local anesthetic techniques

In small animal patients lidocaine and bupivacaine are the most popular agents for local anesthetic techniques (see Table 5.3). Mepivacaine is occasionally used. Ropivacaine is a newer agent that is gaining popularity in human anesthesia and reportedly causes less motor blockade. Other texts should be consulted for a description of the techniques themselves (see Further reading).

To reduce the risk of systemic toxicity, total doses of 6 mg/kg lidocaine, 5 mg/kg mepivacaine or 2 mg/kg bupivacaine should not be exceeded in dogs. Toxic

Table 5.3 Uses of local anesthetics

Drug	Topical	Infiltration	Peripheral nerve block	Intravenous regional analgesia	Epidural
Procaine		+	+		
Proxymetacaine	+				
Lidocaine	+	+	+	+	+
Prilocaine	+				
Mepivacaine		+	+		+
Bupivacaine		+	+		+
Ropivacaine		+	+		+

doses may be lower in cats and doses should not exceed 4 mg/kg lidocaine, 2.5 mg/kg mepivacaine or 1.5 mg/kg bupivacaine. Toxicity is additive and if combinations of local anesthetics are used the dose of individual drugs should be reduced accordingly.

Infiltrative block

- 0.5–2% lidocaine or 0.125–0.5% bupivacaine or 1.0–2.0% mepivacaine
- Solutions containing adrenaline (epinephrine) should not be used to desensitize extremities
- Dilution with 0.9% sodium chloride is recommended to minimize the overall dose

Peripheral nerve blocks

- 0.5–2.0% lidocaine or 0.125–0.5% bupivacaine or 1.0–2.0% mepivacaine
- 0.25–2.0 mL per site

Intra-articular analgesia

- Up to 1 mL/4.5 kg of 2% lidocaine or 0.5% bupivacaine
- Mepivacaine may cause less tissue irritation and has also been recommended for intra-articular use

Interpleural blockade

- 1–2 mg/kg 0.25% bupivacaine in dogs (0.5 mg/kg in cats)

Intravenous regional analgesia in dogs (Bier block)

- 2.5–5 mg/kg lidocaine without adrenaline (epinephrine) is injected into a superficial vein distal to a tourniquet
- The tourniquet must be removed within 60–90 min
- Bupivacaine is more cardiotoxic than lidocaine and should not be used

Lumbosacral epidural

- In dogs 1 mL/4.5 kg of 2% lidocaine or 0.5% bupivacaine
- In cats 1 mL/4.5 kg of 2% lidocaine or 1 mL/7 kg of 0.5% bupivacaine

A

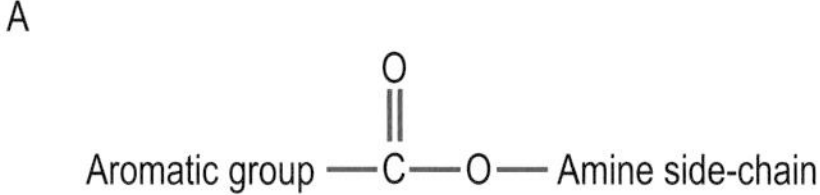

B

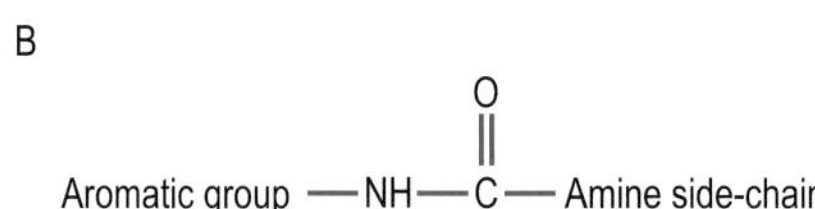

Fig. 5.5 Basic chemical structure of (A) an ester-linked and (B) an amide-linked local anesthetic.

- The total volume of drug injected epidurally should not exceed 6 mL in dogs or 1.5 mL in cats

Pharmacokinetics

Most local anesthetics share a common chemical structure comprising a lipophilic aromatic ring linked to a hydrophilic amine side chain by an ester or amide bond (see Fig. 5.5). The amphiphilic nature of the molecule is important in conferring both lipid- and water-soluble characteristics. The linkage also has an impact on the biotransformation of the drug and local anesthetics can be classified as being ester or amide linked.

Most local anesthetics are weak bases and are largely ionized at physiological pH. Only unionized drug is sufficiently lipid soluble to diffuse through the axon membrane to reach the binding site within the ion channel. Therefore a drug that is less ionized at physiological pH will have a faster onset than a highly ionized drug (see Table 5.4). This explains the slow onset time of bupivacaine (20–30 min) compared to lidocaine (10–15 min). Once the drug gains access to the channel it is the ionized form that binds most avidly to the receptor. The degree of ionization can be influenced by the pH of the tissues. Inflammation tends to lower pH and this can increase ionization sufficiently to interfere with drug activity.

The lipid solubility of a local anesthetic is correlated to potency: the more lipid soluble the agent, the greater the potency. Protein binding is variable (see Table 5.4).

Table 5.4 A comparison of the pharmacology of commonly used local anesthetics

Drug	Onset	Duration (min)	pK_a	Unionized fraction (%) at pH 7.4	Protein binding (%)
Ester linked					
Procaine	Intermediate	45–60	8.9	3	6
Amide linked					
Lidocaine	Rapid	60–120	7.9	25	70
Mepivacaine	Rapid	90–180	7.6	39	77
Bupivacaine	Slow	240–480	8.1	15	95
Ropivacaine	Slow	240–480	8.1	15	94

Local anesthetics that are highly protein bound, e.g. bupivacaine, tend to have a longer duration of action. It is presumed that an agent that binds readily to plasma proteins will likewise have a high affinity for the receptor protein within the ion channel.

Ester-linked local anesthetics, e.g. procaine and proxymetacaine, undergo rapid hydrolysis by plasma cholinesterase enzymes and typically have a short duration. Most of the commonly used agents, including lidocaine, bupivacaine, mepivacaine and ropivacaine, are amide linked and are metabolized by hepatic microsomal enzymes. The precise metabolic pathway varies but frequently involves dealkylation followed by hydrolysis. Impaired hepatic function is likely to extend the duration of amide-linked drugs and increase the risk of toxicity.

Adverse effects

Systemic toxicity is associated with high plasma concentrations of local anesthetic and typically follows administration of an excessive dose or inadvertent intravascular injection.

Central nervous system effects

- The CNS is particularly sensitive to the toxic effects of local anesthetics. Excessive plasma concentrations initially produce excitatory signs such as restlessness, agitation and muscle twitching. With increasing concentrations, seizures develop. These excitatory signs are believed to result from the selective depression of cortical inhibitory pathways.
- If plasma concentrations rise further, generalized CNS depression, with unconsciousness and respiratory arrest, ensues. Local anesthetic-induced seizures should be treated with intravenous diazepam. Measures to protect the airway and support ventilation may also be required.

Cardiovascular effects

- The cardiovascular system is generally more resistant to signs of toxicity than the CNS. Local anesthetics act directly on the heart to depress automaticity, conduction velocity and myocardial contractility. At low plasma concentrations the resultant antiarrhythmic effect may be beneficial but as the concentration rises cardiac output is reduced. In addition, some local anesthetics, particularly lidocaine, cause vasodilation and profound hypotension can develop. These effects may be compounded by autonomic nervous system blockade.
- Bupivacaine is more cardiotoxic than either lidocaine or ropivacaine. Its optical isomers also differ in terms of cardiotoxicity. The S isomer has fewer adverse effects and is available separately for use in people.
- Caution must be exercised with local anesthetic–adrenaline (epinephrine) combinations, as prolonged vasoconstriction of an extremity can result in ischemic necrosis. These combinations should therefore never be used in the penis or near vessels supplying the digits or tail.

Other effects

- Some adverse effects can be related to the technique used. For example, epidural administration of local anesthetic can produce a range of complications depending on the nature of the nerves affected. Blockade of the sacral parasympathetic nerves can cause urinary retention. Sympathetic blockade is associated with peripheral vasodilation and if widespread, this will depress blood pressure. Interference with conduction in motor nerves can cause hindlimb weakness or paralysis and if the local anesthetic migrates as far cranially as the cervical spinal segments, hypoventilation is possible.
- Allergic reactions have been reported but are considered rare. The ester-linked local anesthetics are considered more allergenic than the amide-linked drugs. Methylparaben, a preservative included in some local anesthetic preparations, is also allergenic.
- High doses of prilocaine have been linked to methemoglobinemia. A metabolite, *o*-toluidine, is believed to be responsible.

FURTHER READING

American College of Veterinary Anesthesiologists 1996 Commentary and recommendations on control of waste anesthetic gases in the workplace. JAVMA 209: 75-77

Clarke KW 1999 Desflurane and sevoflurane: new volatile anesthetics. Vet Clin North Am Small Animal Pract 29: 793-810

Dobromylskij P, Flecknell PA, Lascelles BD, Pascoe PJ, Taylor P, Waterman-Pearson A 2000 Management of postoperative and other acute pain. In: Flecknell P, Waterman-Pearson A (eds) Pain management in animals. WB Saunders, London: 81-145

Franks NP, Lieb WR 1994 Molecular and cellular mechanisms of general anesthesia. Nature 367: 607-614

Hall LW, Taylor PM 1994 Anaesthesia of the cat. Baillière Tindall, London

Hird JFR, O'Sullivan J 1994 Anesthetic pollution and the COSHH regulations. J Small Animal Pract 35: 57-59

Kästner SBR 2007 Intravenous anaesthetics. In: Seymour C, Duke-Novakovski T (eds) BSAVA Manual of canine and feline anaesthesia and analgesia. British Small Animal Veterinary Association, Gloucester: 133–149

Martin JL 2005 Volatile anesthetics and liver injury: a clinical update of what every anesthesiologist should know. Can J Anesthesia 52: 125-129

Mathews NS 2007 Inhalant anaesthetics. In: Seymour C, Duke-Novakovski T (eds) BSAVA Manual of canine and feline anaesthesia and analgesia. British Small Animal Veterinary Association, Gloucester: 150–155

McKelvey D, Hollingshead KW 2000 Anesthetic agents and techniques. In: Small animal anesthesia and analgesia, 2nd edn. Mosby, St Louis, MO: 109-142

Morgan GE, Mikhail MS, Murray MJ 2002 Inhalational anesthetics. In: Clinical anesthesiology, 3rd edn. Lange Medical Books, New York: 127-150

Short CE, Bufalari A 1999 Propofol anesthesia. Vet Clin North Am Small Animal Pract 29: 747-778

Skarda RT 1996 Local and regional anesthetic and analgesic techniques: dogs. In: Thurmon JC, Tranquilli WJ, Benson GJ (eds) Lumb and Jones' veterinary anesthesia, 3rd edn. Williams and Wilkins, Baltimore, MD: 426-447

Steffey EP 2001 Inhalation anesthetics. In: Adams HR (ed.) Veterinary pharmacology and therapeutics, 8th edn. Iowa State University Press, Ames, IA: 185-212

Stoelting RK 1999 Nonbarbiturate induction drugs. In: Pharmacology and physiology in anesthetic practice, 3rd edn. Lippincott Williams and Wilkins, Philadelphia, PA

Stoelting RK 1999 Local anesthetics. In: Pharmacology and physiology in anesthetic practice, 3rd edn. Lippincott Williams and Wilkins, Philadelphia, PA

Weir CJ 2006 The molecular mechanisms of general anaesthesia: dissecting the $GABA_A$ receptor. Cont Educ Anaesthesia Crit Care Pain 6: 49-53

Wingfield WE, Ruby DL, Buchan RM, Gunther BJ 1981 Waste anesthetic gas exposures to veterinarians and animal technicians. JAVMA 178: 399-402

6

Sedatives

Patricia Pawson

INTRODUCTION

A confusing array of terms has been used to describe sedative-type drugs. According to one system of classification, drugs may be divided into tranquilizers, sedatives and hypnotics. Tranquilizers relieve anxiety without causing undue drowsiness, while sedatives make the patient drowsy. Hypnotic agents induce or facilitate sleep. Some authors have condensed this system into two groups: the tranquilizers and the sedative-hypnotics.

In human medicine, the nomenclature has focused on the clinical application of drugs. Thus, anxiolytics are drugs used primarily to relieve anxiety. The terms neuroleptic and more recently antipsychotic have been adopted to describe tranquilizers used in the treatment of psychoses. However, in veterinary medicine the word neuroleptic is frequently applied to any sedative or tranquilizer.

Such classifications are not always useful and some drugs will fall into more than one category depending on the dose used. One distinction worth making is that between the tranquilizers and the sedative-hypnotics. Increasing the dose of a tranquilizer, such as a phenothiazine, will not cause a loss of consciousness. However, if the dose of a sedative-hypnotic, such as an α_2-agonist, is increased, a state of profound central nervous system (CNS) depression resembling anesthesia may be induced. For simplicity the term sedative has been used throughout this chapter to describe all tranquilizer, sedative or hypnotic drugs.

GENERAL CLINICAL APPLICATIONS

Sedatives may be used to relieve anxiety or to provide chemical restraint. They facilitate the handling of patients, allowing thorough examination, positioning for radiography, etc. Sedatives are also used for preanesthetic medication. Their use renders the patient more tractable, thereby improving staff safety and assisting the placement of intravenous catheters.

There are benefits for the patient too! By reducing fear and anxiety prior to induction of anesthesia, the potential for catecholamine-induced dysrhythmias is reduced. Generally, the quality of anesthetic induction and recovery is improved by sedatives, there being less risk of excitement. In addition, the dose of induction agent required is reduced.

Many sedative drugs do not possess analgesic activity and will therefore not have an effect in animals that are in pain or are subject to painful procedures. In these cases the sedative should be combined with an opioid analgesic, a practice termed neuroleptanalgesia. Such combinations have a number of advantages and their use is to be recommended even in the nonpainful patient. The sedative and opioid act synergistically to enhance sedation; thus lower doses are required and the risk of adverse effects is reduced. In addition, the sedative may counteract some of the undesirable effects of the opioid, such as vomiting or excitement.

Where high doses of a very potent opioid are combined with a sedative the degree of CNS depression may be sufficient to permit minimally invasive surgery. Such combinations have been termed 'neuroleptanesthetics'. They are generally associated with a greater incidence of adverse effects and should be distinguished from neuroleptanalgesic combinations. There is further discussion of the use of opioids to induce anesthesia in Chapter 5.

The sedatives used in veterinary medicine fall into four main categories.

- Phenothiazines
- Butyrophenones
- Benzodiazepines
- α_2-adrenergic agonists

RELEVANT PHYSIOLOGY

Many of the drugs used in the practice of anesthesia, including sedatives, exert their effects through the modification of chemical transmission in the CNS. Central synaptic mechanisms are basically similar to those occurring in the periphery; however, the complexity of interneuronal connections in the brain makes the prediction of drug effects far more difficult. A large number of neurotransmitters have been identified in the CNS, including:

- glutamate
- γ-aminobutyric acid (GABA)
- glycine

- noradrenaline (norepinephrine)
- dopamine
- 5-hydroxytryptamine
- acetylcholine
- histamine.

Glutamate, GABA and glycine

Glutamate, GABA and glycine are amino acid transmitters. Glutamate is the principal excitatory amino acid transmitter in the CNS. It acts at four main types of receptor: NMDA, AMPA, kainate and metabotropic receptors. NMDA and metabotropic receptors are involved in the development of adaptive responses that modulate synaptic transmission, known collectively as synaptic plasticity. These responses have a role in both physiological (e.g. learning) and pathological processes (e.g. facilitation of central nociceptive transmission in chronic pain states). The dissociative anesthetic ketamine blocks the channel associated with the NMDA receptor (see p. 104).

The principal inhibitory neurotransmitter in the CNS is GABA. There are two types of GABA receptor: $GABA_A$ and $GABA_B$. The benzodiazepines owe their sedative action to facilitation of this inhibitory neurotransmitter, binding to a discrete site on the $GABA_A$ receptor.

Glycine is primarily an inhibitory transmitter found in the gray matter of the spinal cord. However, it is also a coagonist for NMDA receptors and in this context may be considered excitatory.

Noradrenaline (norepinephrine)

Noradrenergic transmission in the CNS appears to be important in control of alertness and mood and in the regulation of blood pressure. As in the periphery, adrenoceptors are recognized and further divided into subtypes, i.e. α_1, α_2, β_1, β_2 and β_3. While noradrenaline (norepinephrine) appears to have an inhibitory effect on individual brain cells, mediated primarily via β-receptors, excitatory effects may also be observed at both α- and β-receptors. The α_2-adrenoceptor agonists owe their sedative action to effects on central noradrenergic transmission.

Dopamine

Dopamine, a precursor of noradrenaline (norepinephrine), has a role in the control of movement and in aspects of behavior. There are two families of dopamine receptor: D_1 and D_2. The D_2 group appears more important in the CNS and comprises D_2, D_3 and D_4 receptors. The D_1 group is subdivided into D_1 and D_5 receptors. The sedative action of the phenothiazines and the butyrophenones has been ascribed to dopamine antagonism, primarily at the D_2 family of receptors. Since dopaminergic neurones are also involved in the production of nausea and vomiting, these drugs have additional antiemetic activity.

5-Hydroxytryptamine

Various functions have been attributed to 5-hydroxytryptamine (5-HT). These include the regulation of sensory pathways and the control of mood, wakefulness, feeding behavior and vomiting. An equally large number of receptor types and subtypes have been identified, although receptors belonging to the $5\text{-}HT_1$, $5\text{-}HT_2$ and $5\text{-}HT_3$ groups are probably the most important in the CNS. While none of the veterinary sedatives act principally on 5-HT pathways, the phenothiazines and butyrophenones have mild $5\text{-}HT_2$ blocking effects.

Acetylcholine

Functions associated with acetylcholine in the CNS include arousal, learning, memory and motor control. Muscarinic receptors appear to be more important, although nicotinic receptors are also present. The effects of acetylcholine are mostly excitatory, although inhibition may be seen at some central muscarinic receptors.

Histamine

Histaminergic pathways have been described in the brain, and H_1, H_2 and H_3 receptors have been identified. The central functions of histamine are poorly understood, although involvement in the control of wakefulness seems likely, since H_1-receptor antagonists induce sedation as a side effect. The phenothiazines have variable H_1-receptor blocking activity.

CLASSES OF SEDATIVE/TRANQUILIZER

Phenothiazines

EXAMPLES

Acepromazine, chlorpromazine, promethazine, promazine, prochlorperazine.

Clinical applications

Phenothiazines may be classed as tranquilizers, neuroleptics or antipsychotics. Acepromazine is the drug most commonly used and is licensed for use in the dog and cat in most countries. It is used to facilitate the handling or restraint of patients and is often employed as a premedicant prior to general anesthesia.

Low doses of acepromazine have a general calming effect. Increasing the dose will induce a degree of sedation, which is more apparent in dogs than cats. However, the dose–response curve reaches a plateau, after which further increases in dose simply prolong the duration of action and increase the incidence of adverse effects.

Phenothiazines do not possess analgesic activity and must be combined with an analgesic, usually an opioid, if sedation is to be achieved in painful patients. The antiemetic effects of phenothiazines are of benefit in such combinations.

Phenothiazines are also considered to be antiarrhythmic and will protect the myocardium against adrenaline (epinephrine)-induced fibrillation.

Some phenothiazines, such as prochlorperazine, are used principally for their antiemetic properties. Others, for example promethazine, are used primarily for their potent antihistamine activity.

Mechanism of action

The sedative and antiemetic actions of phenothiazines are due to antagonism of dopamine, primarily at D_2 receptors. Additional side effects of the phenothiazines can be attributed to their antagonistic activity at other receptors, including α_1-adrenergic receptors, H_1-histaminergic receptors and muscarinic cholinergic receptors.

Formulations and dose rates

DOGS AND CATS

Acepromazine

- 0.01–0.1 mg/kg IV, IM or SC in dogs and cats
- 1–3 mg/kg PO

The total dose of acepromazine administered parenterally should not exceed 3 mg. This maximum dose should be reduced to 2 mg in giant breeds, which appear to be particularly sensitive to the effects of acepromazine. Doses at the lower end of the range should also be used in brachycephalic breeds and when the drug is used for preanesthetic medication or is administered IV.

Chlorpromazine

- 0.05–1.1 mg/kg IM
- 3 mg/kg PO

Promazine

- 2.2–4.4 mg/kg IM

Pharmacokinetics

Phenothiazine is the parent compound of all drugs in this group. The chemical structure of acepromazine is 2-acetyl-10-(3-dimethylaminopropyl) phenothiazine.

Acepromazine is well absorbed following intramuscular injection, but less so from subcutaneous sites. Time to full effect is approximately 30 min following IM injection but is less if the intravenous route is used. Duration of action is dose dependent and doses at the higher end of the clinical range will produce 4–6 h of sedation.

An oral preparation is available (10 mg and 25 mg tablets); however, oral bioavailability is low and somewhat variable (20–55%). Higher doses are necessary if this route is used and the effect is difficult to predict. A dose that is ineffective in one patient may cause profound and prolonged sedation in another.

Acepromazine is very lipophilic and is widely distributed throughout the body. The degree of protein binding is high.

Phenothiazines, including acepromazine, are metabolized by hepatic microsomal enzymes. Oxidation to sulfoxides and glucuronide conjugation are the most important metabolic pathways. Prolonged duration of action may be observed in patients with impaired liver function. Metabolites, which are inactive, are excreted primarily in urine.

Adverse effects

Central nervous system effects

- Since dopamine is also important in motor control, high doses of phenothiazines may cause extrapyramidal signs such as restlessness, rigidity, tremor and even catalepsy.
- Acepromazine is widely believed to lower the seizure threshold, and is frequently avoided in patients that are likely to convulse for any reason. However, clinical studies have failed to demonstrate a significant proconvulsant effect.
- An additional central effect is the modification of thermoregulatory mechanisms at the level of the hypothalamus, which may lead to hypothermia. This effect is compounded by peripheral vasodilation and is particularly significant in small patients with large surface area-to-volume ratios.

Cardiovascular effects

- The main cardiovascular effect of phenothiazines, such as acepromazine, is peripheral vasodilation and a consequent fall in blood pressure. This effect is mediated predominantly through α_1-adrenergic blockade; however, depression of central vasomotor centers and a direct action on vascular smooth muscle may also contribute. The hypotension is generally well tolerated in healthy animals but may be precipitous in hypovolemic or shocked patients.
- Marked hypotension has also been described in excessively fearful dogs given acepromazine. In such cases it is hypothesized that α_1-adrenergic blockade prevents the usual vasopressor action of circulating adrenaline (epinephrine), thereby unmasking β_2-mediated vasodilation in skeletal muscle and leading to so-called 'orthostatic' hypotension.
- Severely hypotensive patients will appear collapsed and tachycardic with weak, thready pulses. Aggressive intravenous fluid therapy forms the mainstay of

treatment, with severely affected cases requiring sympathomimetic drugs in addition. Sympathomimetics that act primarily at α_1-receptors, such as phenylephrine, are preferred. Clearly adrenaline (epinephrine), with its β_2-receptor activity, is contraindicated.
- There have been reports of bradycardia and even sinoatrial arrest in dogs following administration of very high doses of acepromazine. However, clinically relevant doses have little effect on heart rate in the majority of patients. Fainting associated with high levels of vagal tone (sometimes termed vasovagal syncope) has been described in brachycephalic breeds, particularly boxers, given acepromazine. In these cases collapse is attributed to the combined effects of peripheral vasodilation and bradycardia. Treatment involves the administration of an anticholinergic drug such as atropine and supportive fluid therapy. To prevent vasovagal syncope in susceptible breeds, lower doses of acepromazine are recommended and many sources suggest concomitant administration of an anticholinergic drug.

Respiratory effects
- Acepromazine causes minimal changes in respiration. While slight reductions in respiratory rate may occur, minute respiratory volume is generally unchanged.
- Acepromazine has been recommended to calm patients with mild-to-moderate airway obstruction related to tracheal collapse or laryngeal paralysis. However, a recent study has demonstrated that it may impair arytenoid motion and this may be relevant in patients anesthetized to facilitate assessment of laryngeal function.

Gastrointestinal effects
- Phenothiazines have a spasmolytic action on the gut and will reduce gastrointestinal motility in the dog. This effect is believed to result from anticholinergic activity and other anticholinergic effects such as a decrease in salivation have been reported.

Other effects
- As a group the phenothiazines exhibit variable antihistamine activity. This property is most prominent in promethazine, a potent H_1-receptor antagonist.
- Acepromazine is much less active in this respect; nevertheless, it may still interfere with the results of intradermal allergy testing and should be avoided in such cases.
- Acepromazine causes a fall in hematocrit that is most likely due to sequestration of red blood cells in sites such as the liver and spleen.
- Acepromazine may also transiently reduce platelet numbers and aggregatory function.

Contraindications and precautions
Contraindications to the use of acepromazine include the following.
- Hypovolemia and shock
- Patients with a history of seizures

In addition, phenothiazines should be used with caution, i.e. reduced doses, in the following cases.
- Patients with cardiac dysfunction
- Patients with hepatic dysfunction
- Young, old or debilitated patients
- Brachycephalic breeds, especially boxers
- Giant breeds

Known drug interactions
- The CNS-depressant effects of phenothiazines will potentiate the CNS-depressant effects of concomitantly administered drugs. Thus a greater degree of sedation is achieved when acepromazine is combined with an opioid analgesic, even in nonpainful patients. Likewise, the induction and maintenance doses of a variety of general anesthetic agents are reduced when acepromazine is used as a premedicant. This sparing effect is in the order of 30% if typical clinical doses are used.
- The use of adrenaline (epinephrine) is contraindicated in patients treated with phenothiazines, for the reasons discussed above.
- Phenothiazines are mild cholinesterase inhibitors and may therefore enhance the action of depolarizing neuromuscular blocking drugs and ester-linked local anesthetics, such as procaine.
- In addition, they may potentiate the toxicity of organophosphates.

Butyrophenones

EXAMPLES

Fluanisone (with fentanyl, Hypnorm®), droperidol (Droleptan®, with fentanyl Leptan®, Innovar-Vet®), azaperone.

Clinical applications
Butyrophenones may be classed as tranquilizers, neuroleptics or antipsychotics. They are similar to the phenothiazines in many respects.

Azaperone is employed almost exclusively in pigs, as a sedative/premedicant or to reduce fear and aggression in recently mixed groups of pigs. It is not recommended for use in small animals.

Fluanisone and droperidol are both marketed in combination with fentanyl, although availability and licensing of these combinations are not universal. They induce a state of neuroleptanalgesia, i.e. sedation with profound analgesia. The fluanisone–fentanyl combination can be used as a sedative or premedicant in rabbits and rodents. Following its use, anesthesia is generally induced with a benzodiazepine, such as diazepam or midazolam. The droperidol–fentanyl combination is a similar product used primarily in dogs. Neither combination can be recommended for use in the cat since unwanted CNS stimulation may occur. The use of fluanisone and droperidol as sole agents is also not advised.

The butyrophenones are potent antiemetic agents and are particularly effective in inhibiting opioid-induced vomiting.

Similarly to phenothiazines, butyrophenones provide protection against adrenaline (epinephrine)-induced arrhythmias.

Mechanism of action

As for the phenothiazines, the sedative and antiemetic effects of the butyrophenones are primarily mediated by antagonism of dopamine. α-Adrenergic antagonism accounts for the cardiovascular effects of these agents.

Formulations and dose rates

Dogs

Innovar-Vet®

Innovar-Vet® contains 0.4 mg/mL fentanyl and 20 mg/mL droperidol.

- 0.05–0.1 mL/kg IM

Hypnorm®

Hypnorm® contains 0.315 mg/mL fentanyl citrate (equivalent to 0.2mg fentanyl base) and 10 mg/mL fluanisone.

- 0.5 mL/kg IM

Rabbits, rats and mice

- 0.2–0.5 mL/kg IM or IP for sedation or premedication

Guinea pigs

- 1 ml/kg IM or IP for sedation or premedication

Intravenous administration of butyrophenones is not recommended.

Adverse effects

Central nervous system effects

- Extrapyramidal signs such as muscle tremors and rigidity may be observed if high doses are used.
- Excitement reactions have also been seen, especially after intravenous administration. To avoid such effects the intravenous route should not be used and patients should be left undisturbed until sedation has developed.
- Hallucinations and dysphoria have been reported in people treated with butyrophenones but it is not clear if animals experience such unpleasant sensations.
- Occasionally, animal patients exhibit unexpected aggression or excitement following the use of these agents but it is difficult, if not impossible, to establish if this is a consequence of dysphoria. For this reason most authors suggest that butyrophenones should only be used in combination with other drugs.

Cardiovascular effects

Cardiovascular effects are similar to those induced by the phenothiazines.

- Peripheral vasodilation occurs as a result of α_1-adrenergic blockade and possibly a degree of central vasomotor depression.
- Hypotension may result, but is generally less marked than that seen with an equipotent dose of a phenothiazine. Nonetheless, butyrophenones should be avoided in hypovolemic patients.
- Combinations with fentanyl induce bradycardia but this is primarily an opioid effect. It can be minimized by premedication with an anticholinergic, such as atropine or glycopyrrolate.
- Butyrophenones are generally considered to be antiarrhythmic. However, droperidol has been shown to exert a proarrhythmic effect in people through prolongation of the QT interval.

Respiratory effects

- While high doses of butyrophenones will slow respiratory rate, low-to-moderate doses tend to increase it, causing a fall in P_aCO_2.
- This finding prompted the suggestion that butyrophenones might antagonize the respiratory-depressant effects of opioids. If this effect does occur its significance is questionable, since the overall action of the droperidol–fentanyl combination is respiratory depression and raised P_aCO_2.

Gastrointestinal effects

- Butyrophenone and fentanyl combinations may cause salivation and defecation. These effects are likely to be mediated by the opioid fentanyl and can be reduced by anticholinergic premedication.

Contraindications and precautions

- Shock and hypovolemia
- Patients with a history of seizures
- Butyrophenone–fentanyl combinations should also be avoided in patients with significant respiratory disease and renal or hepatic dysfunction.

Known drug interactions

- Butyrophenones potentiate the action of other CNS-depressant drugs such as general anesthetics and analgesics.
- Concomitant use of adrenaline (epinephrine) is contraindicated.

Benzodiazepines

EXAMPLES

Diazepam, midazolam, zolazepam (combined with tiletamine in Telazol®, Zoletil®).

Clinical applications

Benzodiazepines are classed primarily as anxiolytic drugs although high doses may cause sedation and hypnosis. A wide range of benzodiazepines are available for use in people. However, they are not used as frequently for chemical restraint and premedication in veterinary patients and are not specifically licensed for use in animals.

Benzodiazepines do not induce reliable sedation in normal healthy animals and, indeed, their anxiolytic action may increase excitement and render patients more difficult to handle. However, in very young, very old and critically ill patients benzodiazepines may produce effective sedation and their relative lack of adverse effects is an advantage in such 'high-risk' groups. They have also been used to calm distressed or restless patients in the postoperative period. It should be emphasized, however, that benzodiazepines lack analgesic activity and should not be used to compensate for inadequate pain control.

Benzodiazepines may be used to induce general anesthesia in combination with other agents, typically the dissociative anesthetics. The anticonvulsant and muscle-relaxant properties of the benzodiazepines counteract some of the less desirable effects of the dissociative drugs, reducing muscle tone and decreasing the incidence of seizures. A preparation that combines the dissociative anesthetic tiletamine with zolazepam is available in some countries (see Chapter 5).

Benzodiazepines may be used specifically for their anticonvulsant action and diazepam is a drug of choice in the treatment of status epilepticus (see Chapter 16). The ability to relax skeletal muscles may also have specific indications such as the treatment of tetanus and relief of urethral spasm. Benzodiazepines will stimulate appetite in a number of species and this property has proved clinically useful in anorexic cats (see Chapter 19).

All actions of the benzodiazepines can be reversed by the specific benzodiazepine antagonist flumazenil.

Mechanism of action

The sedative and anticonvulsant properties of the benzodiazepines have been attributed to the potentiation of the inhibitory neurotransmitter GABA at $GABA_A$ receptors. These receptors are linked to chloride channels, opening of which causes hyperpolarization and a reduction in membrane excitability. Benzodiazepines combine with a regulatory site on the $GABA_A$ receptor, thereby facilitating the binding of GABA and enhancing its effect. Endogenous ligands for the benzodiazepine receptor are believed to occur but the identity or function of such agents has not been clearly established.

Endogenous benzodiazepines may have a role in the pathophysiology of hepatic encephalopathy and the benzodiazepine antagonist flumazenil has been shown to reverse the signs of this condition in a proportion of cases.

Formulations and dose rates

Diazepam

Dogs

- 0.1–0.5 mg/kg IV
- 2–10 mg/dog PO q.8 h for muscle relaxation

Cats

- 0.05–0.4 mg/kg IV
- 1.25–5 mg/cat PO q.8 h for muscle relaxation

Doses at the lower end of the range are used for sedation/premedication (0.1–0.25 mg/kg) and appetite stimulation, while higher doses may be required to control seizures (0.5 mg/kg).

Midazolam

Dogs

- 0.05–0.2 mg/kg IV or IM
- 0.2 mg/kg/h IV continuous infusion

Cats

- 0.05–0.2 mg/kg IV or IM

Zolazepam

Doses of Telazol® or Zoletil® are quoted in milligrams per kilogram of combined product.

Dogs and cats

- 2–4 mg/kg IV for induction of anesthesia
- 2.5–5 mg/kg IM for sedation

The manufacturers recommend higher intramuscular doses of up to 15 mg/kg to produce heavy sedation or anesthesia in dogs and cats.

Pharmacokinetics

The chemical structures of the benzodiazepines are as follows.

- Diazepam: 7-chloro-1-methyl-5-phenyl-2,3-dihydro-1 *H*-1,4-benzodiazepin-2-one
- Midazolam: 8-chloro-6-(2-fluorophenyl)-1-methyl-4 *H*-imidazo (1,5-α)(1,4)benzodiazepine

Most of the benzodiazepines have a high oral bioavailability and oral administration may be preferred for long-term therapy. In dogs, reported values for the oral bioavailability of diazepam range from 74% to 100%, while a figure of 89% has been quoted for midazolam.

Diazepam is insoluble in water; therefore, solutions for injection are prepared using propylene glycol, sodium benzoate in benzoic acid and ethanol. These solvents are irritant and may cause pain and thrombophlebitis following intravenous injection. The intramuscular and subcutaneous routes are not recommended, since absorption is erratic and injection causes considerable pain. A less irritant emulsion preparation of diazepam (Diazemul®) is available in some countries but may have slightly reduced bioavailability.

Midazolam is water soluble by virtue of its pH-dependent ring structure. At a pH of less than 4 the midazolam ring is open and the drug is water soluble. However, at higher pH values, including physiological pH, the ring closes, conferring a high degree of lipid solubility. To ensure water solubility, commercial preparations are buffered to an acid pH (3.5). Therefore, irritant solvents are not required and the drug can be administered by intramuscular as well as intravenous injection. Bioavailability following intramuscular injection is of the order of 90%.

Benzodiazepines are lipophilic drugs and this is reflected in their high volumes of distribution, e.g. 3.0 L/kg for midazolam in the dog. They readily cross blood–brain and placental barriers.

Benzodiazepines are highly bound to plasma proteins: over 90% binding has been reported for diazepam in a range of species.

Benzodiazepines are metabolized in the liver by a number of pathways, including demethylation, hydroxylation and glucuronide conjugation. Some metabolites of diazepam in the dog, such as *N*-desmethyldiazepam (or nordiazepam) and oxazepam, are pharmacologically active, accounting for the more prolonged effect of this benzodiazepine. Resedation 6–8 h after the initial dose of diazepam has been reported and has been attributed to enterohepatic recycling of these metabolites. Midazolam is metabolized to hydroxymidazolams, which are relatively inactive.

Elimination half-lives for diazepam and midazolam in the dog have been estimated as 3.2 h and 77 min respectively. Excretion of conjugated metabolites occurs primarily via the urine, with a small proportion (≈10%) excreted in bile.

Adverse effects

- Generally, clinical doses of benzodiazepines have a minimal effect on respiratory and cardiovascular systems. However, high doses will cause slight reductions in blood pressure and cardiac output.
- In addition, benzodiazepines may enhance the depressant effects of other concomitantly administered drugs, such as the respiratory depressant effects of the opioid analgesics.
- Acute nephrotoxic effects have not been reported.
- Fulminant hepatic failure has been reported in cats treated with repeated oral doses of diazepam; consistent risk factors could not be identified.
- Flumazenil, a benzodiazepine antagonist, is the treatment of choice should overdose occur. Other supportive measures may be indicated, i.e. support the circulation with intravenous fluids, maintain the airway, provide supplemental oxygen and ventilate if required.
- Adverse cardiovascular effects, such as dysrhythmias, have been reported following the rapid intravenous injection of diazepam and have been attributed to the propylene glycol base. Slow intravenous injection is recommended to minimize such effects and also to limit the development of thrombophlebitis.

Teratogenic effects

- Congenital abnormalities have been reported in babies born to women given diazepam during the first trimester of pregnancy. While a direct causal relationship has not been established, these agents are best avoided in early pregnancy.

Dependence and tolerance

- Dependence and tolerance are features of long-term benzodiazepine use in people. Physical signs of withdrawal, such as nervousness, loss of appetite and tremor, have also been documented in animals. Tolerance, whereby an increasing dose of benzodiazepine is required to produce the desired effect, is not as marked as with drugs like the barbiturates. The mechanism by which it occurs is poorly understood.

Contraindications and precautions

Absolute contraindications are few, but benzodiazepines should be used with caution in the following cases.

- Patients with hepatic encephalopathy, especially those with portosystemic shunts
- Patients during early pregnancy

Known drug interactions

- Benzodiazepines will potentiate the CNS-depressant effects of barbiturates and propofol, allowing a reduction in the dose of these agents required to induce anesthesia.
- The CNS effects of opioid analgesics, including respiratory depression, are also enhanced.
- Concurrent therapy with drugs that inhibit microsomal enzymes may impair elimination of benzodiazepines, thereby extending the duration of action. For example, erythromycin is reported to prolong midazolam-induced sedation while cimetidine may impede the elimination of diazepam.

Special considerations

Diazepam will adsorb on to plastic surfaces, so should not be stored in plastic syringes, giving sets or fluid bags.

It is not miscible with other drugs or solutions, although in practice it is frequently mixed in the same syringe with ketamine prior to administration.

Benzodiazepine antagonists

EXAMPLE

Flumazenil

Clinical applications

Flumazenil has been used in people to reverse benzodiazepine-induced sedation and to treat overdose. It is effective in dogs and cats but as yet is not widely used.

Formulations and dose rates

Dogs and cats

- *Flumazenil:* up to 0.1 mg/kg IV

In one study, doses of 0.075–0.1 mg/kg effectively reversed the signs of diazepam (2 mg/kg) and midazolam (1 mg/kg) overdose in dogs. From this, the authors suggested that 1 part flumazenil is required to reverse the effects of 26 parts diazepam or 13 parts midazolam.

Pharmacokinetics

Flumazenil has a relatively short duration of action (approximately 60 min), so repeated administration may be required.

Adverse effects

Flumazenil is a specific antagonist and is capable of reversing benzodiazepine effects without causing additional complications.

α2-Adrenoceptor agonists

EXAMPLES

Xylazine, detomidine, romifidine, medetomidine.

Clinical applications

α_2-Adrenoceptor agonists may be classed as sedative-hypnotics and have additional muscle-relaxant and analgesic properties. They are widely used for chemical restraint and premedication in small and large animals. The level of sedation induced by α_2-agonists is generally more predictable than that achieved with agents such as the phenothiazines or benzodiazepines. Nonetheless, failures do occur, especially in frightened, painful or excited patients in noisy surroundings.

While α_2-agonists are considered more reliable sedatives, they also exert quite profound effects on other body systems and their use should generally be limited to the young, healthy patient.

Sedation is to some extent dose dependent, increasing doses producing a state of deep sleep or hypnosis. However, the dose–response relationship does reach a plateau, beyond which further increases in dose simply serve to enhance side effects and prolong the duration of action.

Analgesia induced by α_2-agonists is most evident when doses at the higher end of the range are used. Good sedation can be achieved at relatively low doses if the α_2-agonist is combined with an opioid such as pethidine (meperidine) or butorphanol, since sedative and analgesic effects are synergistic.

α_2-Agonists have also been used as premedicants in a variety of anesthetic protocols. They produce a marked reduction in the requirement for both injectable and inhalation anesthetics and care is needed to ensure that overdose does not occur. They have proved popular in combination with the dissociative anesthetic ketamine and there is a rationale for such combinations. The muscle-relaxant properties of the α_2-agonist counteract the rigidity that is a feature of ketamine anesthesia and also promote a smooth recovery, while the sympathomimetic action of ketamine may moderate some of the unwanted cardiovascular effects of the α_2-agonist.

Another factor contributing to the popularity of α_2-agonists is the availability of specific α_2-receptor antagonists. These agents can be used to reverse α_2-induced sedation, allowing a more rapid recovery. This feature has proved particularly useful in the sedation of wildlife. However, there is some evidence that not all α_2-agonist effects are antagonized to the same degree, reversal of cardiopulmonary effects requiring higher doses than reversal of sedation.

Currently there are four α_2-agonists approved for use in veterinary medicine. In most countries detomidine is only licensed for use in the horse. Xylazine, medetomidine and romifidine are generally licensed for use in cats and dogs but are used in a much wider range of species, including small mammals.

Mechanism of action

α_2-Adrenoceptors are found both centrally and peripherally in pre- and postsynaptic locations. Presynaptic α_2-receptors serve as prejunctional inhibitory receptors, i.e. they reduce release of the neurotransmitter noradrenaline (norepinephrine), thereby exerting a sympatholytic effect (Fig. 6.1). Conversely, activation of postsynaptic α_2 receptors triggers a sympathomimetic response more typical of α_1-adrenoceptor activation.

The sedative, analgesic and muscle-relaxant properties of the α_2-agonists are mediated at central α_2-receptors. The primary mechanism involves a decrease in noradrenaline (norepinephrine) release and thereby

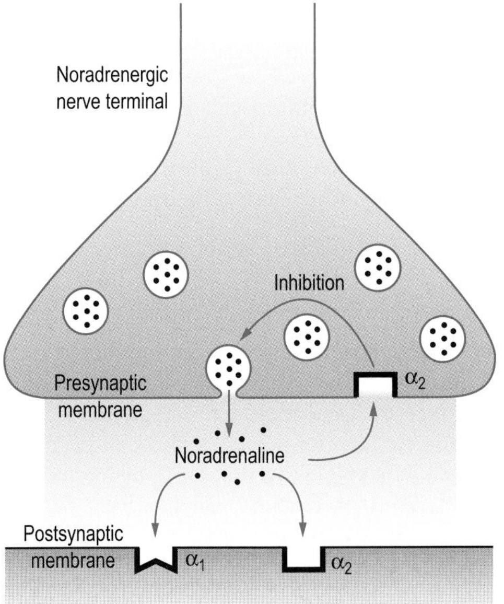

Fig. 6.1 α_2-Receptors are located on both the pre- and postsynaptic membranes. Activation of postsynaptic α_2-receptor initiates a response similar to that following α_1-receptor stimulation, while activation of presynaptic α_2-receptors serves to reduce further noradrenaline (norepinephrine) release.

inhibition of impulse transmission. Sedation has been attributed to depression of neurones in the locus ceruleus, a region of the lower brainstem through which impulses are transmitted to the forebrain and limbic system.

α_2-Adrenoceptors are G protein-coupled receptors linked to the cAMP second messenger system. Activation of the α_2-receptor inhibits adenylate cyclase and thereby reduces cAMP. Other effector mechanisms include opening of potassium channels and reduced calcium entry. Three different α_2-adrenoceptor subtypes have been identified: α_{2a}, α_{2b} and α_{2c}. Recent studies have clarified the role of individual subtypes; for example, α_{2a}-adrenoceptors appear to mediate sedation, analgesia and hypotension while the α_{2b}-adrenoceptor mediates vasoconstriction and hypertension (i.e. postsynaptic α_2-adrenoceptors are probably of the α_{2b} subtype).

The α_2-agonists in veterinary use are not truly specific to α_2-receptors and most exert some α_1 effects in addition. Medetomidine is the most selective, having an α_2:α_1 selectivity ratio of 1620:1. Romifidine, detomidine and xylazine are much less selective, having α_2:α_1 ratios of 340:1, 260:1 and 160:1 respectively. In addition, some α_2-agonists (detomidine and the dextrorotatory isomer of medetomidine) also activate imidazoline receptors.

Formulations and dose rates

Xylazine

Dogs
- 1–3 mg/kg IV, IM (preferred) or SC

Cats
- 3 mg/kg IM

Medetomidine

Dogs
- 10–40 μg/kg in dogs IV, IM or SC

Cats
- 40–80 μg/kg in cats IM or SC

Lower doses, 2–10 μg/kg IM, will produce sufficient sedation for premedication when combined with an opioid. Lower doses should also be used if the drug is to be administered intravenously.

Romifidine

Dogs
- 40–120 μg/kg IM, IV or SC

Cats
- 200–400 μg/kg IM or IV

As for medetomidine, lower doses may be effective if combined with an opioid.

Pharmacokinetics

The chemical structures of the α_2-agonists are as follows.

- Xylazine: 2-(2,6-dimethyl phenylamino)-4*H*-5,6-dihydro-1,3-thiazine
- Medetomidine: 4-(2,3-dimethylphenyl)ethyl-1 *H*-imidazole

Medetomidine is a racemic mixture of two optical isomers: dexmedetomidine and levomedetomidine. Dexmedetomidine is the active enantiomer and has a potency approximately twice that of the racemic mixture (i.e. approximately half the dose is required). Dexmedetomidine is likely to be available separately in the near future.

For optimum activity, α_2-agonists should be administered by intravenous or intramuscular injection. They are generally active within 3–5 min following intravenous administration but may take 10–20 min to reach full effect if the intramuscular route is used. Bioavailability of xylazine following intramuscular injection ranges from 52% to 90% in the dog. Absorption from subcutaneous sites is very variable and this route is not recommended. The duration of effect varies according to the drug used and also the dose. A single standard dose of xylazine will produce sedation of 30–40 min duration, while medetomidine and romifidine have a longer action, lasting for 60–90 or 60–120 min respectively. Higher doses have more prolonged effects and for all α_2-agonists, complete recovery may take several hours.

α_2-Agonists undergo extensive first-pass metabolism and so activity is poor following oral administration. These drugs may, however, be absorbed through the oral and pharyngeal mucosa and sedation has been reported after squirting α_2-agonists into the mouths of fractious patients.

These agents have also been administered into the epidural space to achieve analgesia. This results primarily from inhibition of nociceptive transmission at the level of the dorsal horn cells in the spinal cord, although local anesthetic-like effects have also been described following epidural administration of xylazine. Systemic side effects are generally less evident if this route is used but they do still occur. Duration of action is extended. In a study conducted in dogs, epidural administration of 15 μg/kg medetomidine produced analgesia for 4–8 h.

α_2-Agonists are lipid-soluble drugs that are therefore widely distributed. Medetomidine is very lipophilic and has a high volume of distribution, 2.8 L/kg in the dog and 3.5 L/kg in the cat. The volume of distribution of xylazine is slightly less, ranging from 1.9 to 2.7 L/kg. α_2-Agonists are not extensively bound to plasma proteins.

Xylazine is metabolized by hepatic mono-oxygenases. Hydroxylated metabolites undergo glucuronide conjugation (except in cats), prior to excretion in the urine. The elimination half-lives for xylazine and medetomidine in the dog are respectively 30 min and 1–1.6 h.

Adverse effects

Central nervous system effects

- α_2-Agonists appear to have both anti- and proconvulsant effects. This may be related, at least in part, to dose. Low doses of dexmedetomidine have been shown to raise the seizure threshold, whereas high doses tend to lower it. In addition, low doses may have neuroprotective properties. Convulsions have been reported following inadvertent intracarotid injection of xylazine and this may reflect high plasma concentrations in blood reaching the brain.
- Alterations in body temperature, both increased and decreased, have been reported in animals sedated with α_2-agonists. In small animal patients, centrally mediated hypothermia appears to be the predominant finding.
- There are anecdotal reports of dogs responding unexpectedly, and in some cases aggressively, to touch, despite appearing heavily sedated. A similar phenomenon is recognized in the horse and studies in this species indicate that α_2-agonists may induce a degree of cutaneous hypersensitivity.

Cardiovascular effects

- The α_2-agonists exert profound effects on the cardiovascular system, even when low doses are used. Indeed, the hemodynamic effects of IV medetomidine have been shown to be almost maximal at doses of 5 μg/kg in the dog. Similarly for romifidine, increasing the dose beyond 25 μg/kg IV appears to produce little additional alteration in cardiovascular function.
- Bradycardia is common and heart rates frequently fall by 50% or more following administration of sedative doses. This effect has been attributed to a central decrease in sympathetic drive and thereby a predominance of vagal tone, although a baroreceptor response to hypertension may also contribute.
- Bradycardia may also be accompanied by alterations in rhythm. Sinus arrhythmia, sinoatrial block and first-, second- and third-degree atrioventricular blocks occur not infrequently.
- Effects on vascular tone and thereby arterial blood pressure are complex. Activation of peripheral postsynaptic α_2- and α_1-receptors (NB: α_2-agonists are not specific) leads to vasoconstriction. In contrast, activation of central and peripheral presynaptic α_2-receptors tends to cause vasodilation through reductions in noradrenaline (norepinephrine) release and sympathetic outflow.
- The balance of these effects influences blood pressure. Theoretically, the vasoconstrictive effects predominate initially, resulting in a period of hypertension. This is followed by a more sustained fall in arterial blood pressure as the central effects become more important. Studies conducted in experimental dogs have confirmed the biphasic nature of the blood pressure response to intravenous medetomidine or romifidine. The extent of the hypertensive phase is variable, being influenced by the dose and the route of administration. It is more evident if the α_2-agonist is administered intravenously and if high doses are used. These studies have also confirmed that arterial blood pressure subsequently falls below baseline values, although hypotension (i.e. mean arterial blood pressure less than 80 mmHg) was not seen at the doses used.
- Despite causing relatively little direct myocardial depression, α_2-agonists cause a marked reduction in cardiac output, primarily as a consequence of bradycardia, although increased afterload may contribute. Central venous pressure tends to increase as a result. Anticholinergics, such as atropine and glycopyrrolate, have been recommended to both prevent and treat α_2-agonist induced bradycardias. However, their use is questionable since they tend to cause tachycardia and extend the hypertensive phase, thereby producing further reductions in cardiac

output. Reversal with a specific α_2-receptor antagonist is a more appropriate treatment for severe α_2-agonist-induced bradycardia.

- The influence of α_2-agonists on catecholamine-induced arrhythmias is controversial. Early studies showed that xylazine reduced the threshold for adrenaline (epinephrine)-induced arrhythmias in anesthetized dogs. However, a later study, investigating the effects of xylazine and medetomidine, failed to demonstrate a proarrhythmic effect with either agent. The effect of dexmedetomidine on cardiac rhythm is less contentious. Studies have demonstrated an antiarrhythmic effect, possibly mediated through interaction with imidazoline receptors.

Respiratory effects

The respiratory effects of α_2-agonists vary in severity between species.

- In dogs and cats, minute ventilation tends to fall, primarily as a consequence of reduced respiratory rate, but changes in arterial blood gases are usually slight. A proportion of patients appear cyanotic and this has been observed in the absence of major reductions in the arterial partial pressure of oxygen. It has been suggested that the cyanosis reflects venous desaturation as a consequence of increased oxygen extraction by the tissues. Whatever the cause, such patients should receive supplemental oxygen.
- More severe alterations in arterial blood gases, including overt hypoxemia, have been documented in ruminants, particularly sheep, sedated with α_2-agonists. Mismatching of pulmonary ventilation and perfusion is the most likely cause. Acute pulmonary edema has also been reported following xylazine use in small ruminants. Although the mechanism is unknown, factors such as pre-existing pathology, pulmonary hypertension, altered capillary permeability and free radical generation may contribute.
- Anecdotal reports suggest that acute pulmonary edema may occur, albeit infrequently, in small animal patients as well.

Gastrointestinal effects

- Vomiting is a frequent occurrence following intramuscular administration of α_2-agonists. It is most common with xylazine, especially in cats, in which the incidence may approach 50%. It is mediated centrally through direct activation of receptors in the chemoreceptor trigger zone.
- Overall, α_2-agonists depress gastrointestinal motility and prolong gut transit times. This parasympatholytic effect has been attributed to reduced release of acetylcholine from cholinergic nerve terminals innervating the gastrointestinal tract. Reductions in salivary and gastric secretions may also occur.
- In dogs, xylazine has been shown to reduce gastroesophageal sphincter tone, which may increase the risk of gastric reflux.
- Gastric distension is an additional adverse effect that has been recorded in large breed dogs. It is not clear how it arises. It may simply be a consequence of gastrointestinal atony leading to accumulation of gas or alternatively aerophagia may be involved.

Endocrine effects

- α_2-Agonists exert a variety of effects on endocrine function. Of most significance are reductions in the release of insulin and antidiuretic hormone. Inhibition of insulin release is mediated via α_2-receptors on the β-cells of the pancreas and the result is hyperglycemia and glycosuria. Pancreatitis has been observed in experimental cats following repeated IM administration of high doses of romifidine. The mechanism involved is not clear.
- Diuresis also occurs, primarily as a consequence of reduced ADH release, although glycosuria may contribute.
- Transient alterations in growth hormone, testosterone, prolactin and FSH have also been reported.

Effects in pregnancy

- Uterine contractility may be modified by α_2-agonists. The effects of medetomidine in the pregnant bitch appear to be dose dependent. While low doses decrease uterine electrical activity, higher doses ($\geq$40 μg/kg) have a transient stimulatory effect.
- Definitive evidence that α_2-agonists increase the incidence of abortion or obstetrical complications is lacking. Nonetheless, their use in pregnant patients cannot be recommended.

Contraindications and precautions

α_2-Adrenoceptor agonists can only be recommended for use in young healthy patients. Contraindications include the following.

- Patients with myocardial disease or reduced cardiac reserve
- Hypotension and shock
- Respiratory disease
- Hepatic insufficiency
- Renal dysfunction
- Diabetes mellitus
- Any sick/debilitated patient
- Pregnancy.

Romifidine may increase blood urea concentrations in cats and attention to fluid balance is recommended.

Known drug interactions

- α_2-Agonists act synergistically with opioid analgesics. The use of such combinations allows the dose

Table 6.1 Suggested doses of specific antagonists for reversal of selected α2-agonists in the dog and cat

	Dog (mg/kg)			Cat (mg/kg)		
	To reverse xylazine	To reverse medetomidine	To reverse romifidine	To reverse xylazine	To reverse medetomidine	To reverse romifidine
Atipamezole	0.2	0.05–0.2 (5 × medetomidine dose)	0.2 (approx. 1.7 × romifidine dose)	0.2	0.1–0.2 (2.5 × medetomidine dose)	0.4 (equal to romifidine dose)
Yohimbine	0.10–0.15	–	–	0.1–0.2	0.5	–
Tolazoline	0.5–1	–	–	2	–	–

of α_2-agonist to be reduced without compromising the quality of the sedation.

- In addition, α_2-agonists greatly reduce the required dose of intravenous and inhalation anesthetics, by 50% or more in some cases. Since they also tend to slow the circulation it is relatively easy to overdose a patient with the induction agent. Thus if α_2-agonists are used for premedication, the induction drug should be given slowly and at a much reduced dose.
- Fatalities have been documented in horses sedated with detomidine that concurrently received intravenous potentiated sulfonamides. This interaction has not been reported following the use of other α_2-agonists.

Special considerations

- α_2-Agonists can be absorbed through mucous membranes or broken skin and so should be handled with care. Should inadvertent self-administration occur, medical attention should be sought immediately, since serious CNS disturbance can result.

α2-Adrenoceptor antagonists

EXAMPLES

Yohimbine (Antagonil®, Yobine®), atipamezole (Antisedan®), tolazoline (Tolazine®).

Clinical applications

α_2-Adrenoceptor antagonists are used to reverse the sedation induced by α_2-agonists, allowing a more rapid recovery. Unfortunately, not all properties of the α_2-agonists are reversed equally and higher doses may be required to fully antagonize the adverse cardiopulmonary effects of these drugs.

Atipamezole is the most specific of the α_2-antagonists available. It is generally licensed to reverse medetomidine in dogs and cats but has been used to antagonize other α_2-agonists. Yohimbine and tolazoline have been used primarily to reverse xylazine-induced sedation.

Formulations and dose rates

Atipamezole

Dogs and cats: 0.05–0.4 mg/kg IM

Yohimbine

Dogs and cats: 0.1–0.11 mg/kg IV to reverse xylazine

The actual dose required depends on the species and also which α_2-agonist is being reversed (Table 6.1).

Adverse effects

- A number of adverse effects have been documented following administration of α_2-antagonists to dogs and cats. These are generally transient and include apprehension or excitement, muscle tremors and in some cases hypersalivation and vomiting.
- Convulsions have also been recorded but primarily in patients that have been treated with ketamine. This dissociative anesthetic, if unopposed by a suitable sedative, is capable of inducing seizures, especially in dogs.
- Hypotension and tachycardia may occur if atipamezole is injected rapidly intravenously; the intramuscular route is therefore preferred for this antagonist.
- Tolazoline is the least specific of the antagonists. In particular, it behaves as an agonist at H_2-histamine receptors and signs including nausea, abdominal pain, diarrhea and gastrointestinal bleeding have been recorded in humans.

Contraindications and precautions

- Patients with renal dysfunction
- Patients with a history of seizures
- Dogs that have also received ketamine

FURTHER READING

Cullen LK 1996 Medetomidine sedation in dogs and cats: a review of its pharmacology, antagonism and dose. Br Vet J 152: 519-535

England GCW, Flack TE, Hollingworth E, Hammond R 1996 Sedative effects of romifidine in the dog. J Small Animal Pract 37: 19-25

Greene SA, Thurmon JC 1988 Xylazine – a review of its pharmacology and use in veterinary medicine. J Vet Pharmacol Ther 11: 295-313

Gross ME, Booth NH 2001 Tranquilizers, α_2-adrenergic agonists and related agents. In: Adams HR (ed.) Veterinary pharmacology and therapeutics, 8th edn. Iowa State University Press, Ames, IA: 299-342

Hall LW, Clarke KW, Trim CM 2001 Principles of sedation, analgesia and premedication. In: Veterinary anaesthesia, 10th edn. Baillière Tindall, London: 75-112

Jackson AM, Tobias K, Long C, Bartges J, Harvey R 2004 Effects of various anesthetic agents on laryngeal motion during laryngoscopy in normal dogs. Vet Surg 33: 102-106

Johnson C 1999 Chemical restraint in the dog and cat. In Practice 21: 111-118

Murrell JC 2007 Premedication and sedation. In: Seymour C, Duke-Novakovski T (eds) BSAVA Manual of canine and feline anaesthesia and analgesia. British Small Animal Veterinary Association, Gloucester: 120-132

Murrell JC, Hellebrekers LJ 2005 Medetomidine and dexmedetomidine: a review of cardiovascular effects and antinociceptive properties in the dog. Vet Anaesth Analg 32: 117-127

Pypendop BH, Verstegen JP 1998 Hemodynamic effects of medetomidine in the dog: a dose titration study. Vet Surg 27: 612-622

Pypendop BH, Verstegen JP 2001 Cardiovascular effects of romifidine in dogs. Am J Vet Res 62: 490-495

Rang HP, Dale MM, Ritter JM, Moore PK 2003 Amino acid transmitters. In: Rang HP, Dale MM, Ritter JM, Moore PK (eds) Pharmacology, 5th edn. Churchill Livingstone, Edinburgh: 462-473

Rang HP, Dale MM, Ritter JM, Moore PK 2003 Other transmitters and modulators. In: Rang HP, Dale MM, Ritter JM, Moore PK (eds) Pharmacology, 5th edn. Churchill Livingstone, Edinburgh: 474-489

Thurmon JC, Tranquilli WJ, Benson GJ 1996 Preanesthetics and anesthetic adjuncts. In: Thurmon JC, Tranquilli WJ, Benson GJ (eds) Lumb and Jones' veterinary anesthesia, 3rd edn. Williams and Wilkins, Baltimore, MD: 183-209

7

Behavior-modifying drugs

Kersti Seksel

CLINICAL AND DIAGNOSTIC CONSIDERATIONS

Behavior-modifying drugs are increasingly forming an important part of the management of companion animal behavior problems. However, although the initial trials of psychotropic medications were conducted on animals (as early as the 1950s), most drugs in common use are not registered for this purpose in animals. Most information on behavior-modifying drugs is derived from human literature and thus cannot necessarily be extrapolated directly to other animal species.

Establishing a diagnosis

The use of drugs to treat behavior problems without a concurrent behavior modification program is unlikely to be of benefit. Some behavior problems can be managed by behavior modification alone. Drugs should always be an adjunct to behavior modification therapy, not a replacement.

Before prescribing any drug to modify an animal's behavior, it is vitally important that the veterinarian has made a diagnosis based on a thorough physical examination and behavioral history. Additionally, the symptomatic treatment of nonspecific signs such as excessive vocalization, aggression or inappropriate elimination is not acceptable and will ultimately lead to treatment failures.

Owners and veterinarians should be aware that there are no quick solutions and no magic overnight cures for behavioral disorders. In most cases, behavior problems take time to develop and will therefore take time to modify. Once behavioral modification is achieved it needs to be maintained by lifelong commitment from the owner and continued support from the veterinarian. Most behavior problems are not 'cured' but can be managed or controlled. An appropriate medical analogy is diabetes mellitus, which is not considered to be cured but can be controlled by appropriate medication combined with diet and lifestyle modification.

Assuming the diagnosis is correct, the most common reasons for apparent treatment failures when behavior-modifying medications are prescribed include:

- selection of an inappropriate medication for the behavior problem
- an inadequate length of time allowed for the treatment program to take effect
- use of medications as 'stand-alone' therapy when they should have been combined with a behavior modification program.

Client consent and compliance

Before prescribing any medication, basic pharmacodynamic and pharmacokinetic knowledge of the drug is needed. As most medications used in veterinary behavioral therapy are not registered for use in animals, it is even more important that the rationale for drug use and potential side effects should be clearly explained and the owner should give informed consent to the use of the drug on their pet. A signed consent form is recommended to ensure that a client has understood the implications of the treatment program, possible side effects and likely length of treatment required.

Client compliance is important, as many behavior-modifying drugs may take up to 6–8 weeks to reach therapeutic blood concentrations or for a clinical response to be evident. Owners should be aware that it will take time to see the desired behavioral changes. The choice of medication may be affected by the personal experience of the veterinarian, reported efficacy of case studies or trials, extrapolation from human literature, ease of medicating the animal, health status of the animal, and cost. Owners should be aware that, although one medication was not successful, either because of lack of discernible positive effects or because of unwanted side effects, an alternative medication may still prove useful.

An attempt should be made to gradually wean off medication once the desired result is achieved and maintained for a period of 2–3 months. However, there are some patients that will require lifelong medication and this should be made clear to the owner at the outset of therapy.

Clinical applications and drug classes

Behavior problems where medication has proved useful include anxiety-related problems (including fears and phobias), obsessive-compulsive behaviors, some types of aggression, abnormal sexual behavior and geriatric behavior problems.

Many classes of medication have been used in the treatment of behavior problems. These include antihistamines, antipsychotics, anxiolytics, antidepressants, anticonvulsants, mood stabilizers, β-blockers, central nervous system (CNS) stimulants, hormones, opiate antagonists, monoamine oxidase inhibitors, neuroleptics, ergot alkaloids and phenothiazines. Medications that may have anxiolytic actions include the benzodiazepines, tricyclic antidepressants (TCAs), antihistamines, azaperones, barbiturates, selective serotonin reuptake inhibitors (SSRIs) and β-blockers. Only drugs in common use will be discussed in this chapter.

Pretreatment screening

Blood tests prior to prescribing medication are strongly recommended, especially in very old or young animals or those with a previous history of medical problems. A minimum database should include a complete blood count, biochemistry panel and urinalysis. As most behavior-modifying drugs are metabolized by the liver and renally excreted, it is important to assess liver enzymes and renal function prior to starting drug treatment. It may be prudent in some cases to reassess liver and renal function approximately 4–6 weeks after starting treatment, depending on the animal, the drug and the effects observed. All animals on long-term behavior-modifying medication should be retested at least every 6–12 months.

NEUROPHYSIOLOGY AND NEUROCHEMISTRY OF BEHAVIOR

The rationale for using behavior-modifying drugs is based on their purported neurochemical actions in the brain. The drugs may act presynaptically, affecting the presynaptic action potential, synthesis, storage, metabolism, release, reuptake or degradation of the neurotransmitter. Alternatively, they may act postsynaptically, binding to or modifying receptors.

Neurotransmitters can be classed into three groups:

- amino acids, e.g. γ-aminobutyric acid (GABA), glutamate and glycine
- amines, e.g. acetylcholine (ACh) and monoamines (dopamine, serotonin and noradrenaline (norepinephrine))
- peptides, e.g. cholecystokinin (CCK), substance P and neuropeptide Y.

ACh, dopamine, serotonin, noradrenaline (norepinephrine) and GABA are particularly important in the actions and side effects of behavior-modifying drugs.

Acetylcholine

Acetylcholine is derived from choline (important in fat metabolism) and acetyl CoA (product of cellular respiration in mitochondria) by the action of choline acetyltransferase. It acts as a neurotransmitter in both the peripheral and central nervous systems. It is widely distributed in the body. ACh is present at the neuromuscular junction and is synthesized by all motor neurones in the spinal cord. It is metabolized by acetylcholinesterase to choline and acetic acid.

Cholinergic receptors (nicotinic and muscarinic) have numerous physiological (see Chapter 4) and behavioral effects. Muscarinic receptors appear to mediate the behavioral effects of arousal, learning and short-term memory. Muscarinic agonists (arecoline) and anticholinesterase drugs (physostigmine) are reported to improve performance in short-term memory while muscarinic antagonists (scopolamine) cause amnesia. Certain neurodegenerative diseases, especially dementia and parkinsonism, are thought to be associated with abnormalities in cholinergic pathways.

Many behavior-modifying drugs have anticholinergic effects. Adverse anticholinergic effects that may occur include dry mouth, dry eyes, urinary and fecal retention and pupillary dilation.

Catecholamines

Tyrosine is the precursor for the catecholamines (dopamine, noradrenaline (norepinephrine) and adrenaline (epinephrine)). Catecholaminergic neurones are found in the midbrain, hypothalamus and limbic system. They are involved in regulation of movement, mood and attention as well as visceral function (see Chapter 4). They are associated with the arousal of the autonomic nervous system. Their release during stressful or fearful episodes results in stimulation of the CNS and anxiety.

The actions of catecholamines are terminated in the synaptic cleft by selective reuptake into the axon terminal. Within the terminal they can be reused or destroyed by monoamine oxidase (MAO) and by catechol-O-methyltransferase (COMT).

Dopamine

Tyrosine hydroxylase converts tyrosine to L-dopa. Dopamine is produced from L-dopa by dopa decarboxylase in dopaminergic neurones. Dopamine is a neurotransmitter as well as precursor for noradrenaline (norepinephrine). It is degraded to 3,4-dihydroxyphenylacetic acid (DOPAC) and homovanillic acid (HVA), which are excreted in urine.

There are at least five dopaminergic pathways in the brain, with the mesolimbic-mesocortical cells in the nucleus accumbens most closely related to behavior. The nigrostriatal pathway is involved in the co-ordination of voluntary movement. Dopaminergic receptors are divided into two families (D_1 and D_2), with most known functions being mediated by the D_2 family.

Deterioration of dopaminergic neurones in the brain is responsible for diseases such as Parkinson's disease in humans. Behavioral effects of excessive dopamine activity include stereotypies observed with increased dopamine release (e.g. amfetamine) and dopamine agonists (e.g. apomorphine). In humans, abnormalities of dopaminergic neurones have also been implicated in schizophrenia – the side effects of antischizophrenic drugs include a variety of Parkinson-like movement disorders (dyskinesia).

Noradrenaline (norepinephrine)

Noradrenaline (norepinephrine) is produced by hydroxylation of dopamine by dopamine β-hydroxylase in synaptic vesicles of noradrenergic neurones. Noradrenergic cell bodies within the CNS occur in discrete clusters, mainly in the pons and medulla. The locus ceruleus is one of the most important noradrenergic clusters related to behavior. Stimulation of locus ceruleus neurones leads to an increased fear response (in monkeys).

The actions of noradrenaline are mainly inhibitory in the CNS (β-receptors) but some are excitatory (α- or β-receptors). Excitatory actions occur by direct (blockade of potassium conductances that slow neuronal discharge) and indirect methods (disinhibition, whereby inhibitory neurones are inhibited). This facilitation of excitatory transmission is thought to be responsible for the behavioral effects of arousal, attention, etc. and has been characterized most in the α_2-receptors in the locus ceruleus.

Noradrenergic transmission is thought to be important in control of mood, function of the 'reward' system, arousal, control of wakefulness and alertness and blood pressure regulation. Medications that are noradrenaline agonists cause increased arousal through activation of the reticular activating system.

Noradrenaline is converted to adrenaline (epinephrine) by phenylethanolamine *N*-methyltransferase. Adrenaline (epinephrine) acts as a neurotransmitter in the brain and is also released by the adrenal gland.

Indoleamines

The indolamines, serotonin (5-hydroxytryptamine) and melatonin (*N*-acetyl-5-methoxytryptamine), are synthesized from tryptophan. In the pineal gland, serotonin acts as the precursor for melatonin. Over 90% of serotonin in the mammalian body is found in the enterochromaffin cells in the gastrointestinal tract.

Serotonin

Serotonin is derived from tryptophan in a two-step process and its availability is the rate-limiting step in synthesis. 5-Hydroxytryptamine (5-HT) neurones are concentrated in the midline raphe nuclei in the pons and medulla, projecting diffusely to the cortex, limbic system, hypothalamus and spinal cord. Serotonin can exert inhibitory or excitatory effects and can act presynaptically or postsynaptically. Many serotonin-receptor subtypes have been identified (5-HT_{1a}, 5-HT_{1b}, 5-HT_{1d}, 5-HT_2, 5-HT_3). The exact functions of each subtype have not yet been clearly identified.

Serotonin is also thought to act as an anxiogenic neurotransmitter in the limbic system. Serotonin pathways are thought to be involved in regulation of mood, feeding behavior, sleep/wakefulness, control of sensory pathways including nociception, control of body temperature, vomiting and emotional behaviors such as aggression.

After release into the synaptic cleft the action of serotonin is terminated by reuptake into the axon terminal by a specific transporter, where it is reused or degraded by MAO, forming 5-hydroxyindolacetic acid (5-HIAA). 5-HIAA is excreted in urine and provides a measure of 5-HT turnover.

Melatonin

Melatonin is thought to play a role in diurnal cycles and sleep/wake patterns in humans. It is released mainly at night. Three MEL_1-receptor variants have been identified to date in the suprachiasmic nucleus of the hypothalamus. Melatonin is a potent inhibitor of dopamine release and its release appears to be linked with endogenous opioids. Very little is known about this neurohormone and its physiological effects. It has been shown to regulate sleep patterns in some studies in humans. Melatonin has been used to treat jet lag as well as seasonal affective disorder, self-injurious behavior and childhood depression in humans. It is freely available in the USA and some other countries, as it has been labelled a food, not a drug. However, it is not available worldwide. In a number of countries, melatonin implants have been used in the reproductive management of ruminants.

Melatonin's efficacy in companion animal medicine is unknown, although its use has been reported in the treatment of thunderstorm phobias, recurrent flank alopecia in dogs, to decrease isolation distress in chickens and in the treatment of separation anxiety in a black bear that would not hibernate. Additionally, it has been used concurrently with amitriptyline to successfully treat one case of noise phobia (especially to birdsong) in a dog. The suggested dose rate in dogs is 0.1 mg/kg PO q.24 h or as needed. Side effects in humans include sleepiness, headaches and hangover-type malaise. Melatonin should not be given concurrently with MAO inhibitors or corticosteroids in humans.

γ-Aminobutyric acid (GABA)

Glutamate is converted to GABA by glutamic acid decarboxylase. GABA is only synthesized by those neurones that use it as a neurotransmitter. It is widely distributed throughout the brain but very little is found in peripheral tissues. GABA-ergic neurones are the major inhibitory neurones in the mammalian nervous system.

GABA is the main inhibitory neurotransmitter in the cerebral cortex and limbic system. There are three types of GABA receptor. $GABA_A$ receptors occur mainly postsynaptically and are directly coupled with chloride channels, which, when opened, reduce membrane excitability. Activation of $GABA_B$ receptors alters Ca^{2+} (presynaptic) and K^+ (postsynaptic) conductance via second messengers, resulting in hyperpolarization and reduced outflow of other neurotransmitters. $GABA_C$ receptors have recently been described and are predominantly located in the retina.

Drugs that interact with $GABA_A$ receptors and channels include the benzodiazepines and barbiturates (see Chapters 7 and 16).

GABA is removed from the synaptic cleft mainly by reuptake but some is also deaminated by GABA-transaminase.

CLASSES OF BEHAVIOR-MODIFYING DRUGS

ANTIHISTAMINES

EXAMPLES

Cyproheptadine, diphenhydramine, hydroxyzine.

Clinical applications

Antihistamines are not considered first-choice options in the treatment of anxiety disorders nor for long-term treatment of anxiety. However, they have proved useful for treating inappropriate urination associated with anxiety, to reduce anxiety and motion sickness associated with car travel and to reduce excessive unexplained nocturnal activity of cats such as pacing and vocalization while the owners are at home. A short-term positive therapeutic response has sometimes been helpful in obtaining client compliance in carrying out the environmental changes needed to modify abnormal behavior, as well as improving neighborly relations.

Antihistamines may also be effective in the management of pruritus associated with anxiety. However, relatively high doses are necessary and the positive effect observed may be due to sedation. Doxepin, a tricyclic antidepressant (TCA), has proved more useful than antihistamines for the treatment of anxiety-related pruritus and self-mutilation.

There is a single case report of the successful use of cyproheptadine to treat urine spraying and masturbation in a neutered male cat. Its efficacy in the treatment of urine spraying is currently being studied. The use of cyproheptadine as an appetite stimulant in dogs and cats has also been mooted (see Chapter 19) and may result from 5-HT antagonism.

Mechanism of action

Antihistamines act by competitive inhibition of H_1 receptors. They have mild hypnotic and sedative effects. Cyproheptadine also acts as a serotonin antagonist, is an appetite stimulant and may have a calcium channel-blocking action.

Formulations and dose rates

DOGS

Cyproheptadine
- 0.3–2 mg/kg PO q.12 h (antihistamine dose)

Diphenhydramine
- 2–4 mg/kg PO q.8–12 h

Hydroxyzine
- 0.5–2.2 mg/kg PO q.8–12 h

CATS

Cyproheptadine
- 0.4–0.5 mg/kg PO q.12 h (2–4 mg/cat q.8–12 h)

Diphenhydramine
- 2–4 mg/kg PO q.8–12 h

Hydroxyzine
- 2.2 mg/kg PO q.8–12 h

Pharmacokinetics

Antihistamines are well absorbed from the gastrointestinal tract and are widely distributed throughout the body. Many antihistamines are extensively and quickly metabolized, resulting in low bioavailability after oral administration. They are excreted in urine and feces. The sedative effects are usually seen within 30–60 min and may last 4–6 h.

Adverse effects

- Mild CNS depression or sleepiness
- Anticholinergic effects
- Excitation, agitation and convulsions have been reported at therapeutic doses in humans, especially children

Contraindications and precautions

Antihistamines should be used with care or alternatives considered if the following conditions are present.
- Urinary retention
- Glaucoma
- Hyperthyroidism

Antihistamines should not be used within 2 weeks of administration of monoamine oxidase inhibitors (MAOIs).

Known drug interactions

- Concurrent use of other drugs that cause CNS depression can produce additive effects.
- MAOIs may intensify the anticholinergic effects of antihistamines.

ANTIPSYCHOTICS (NEUROLEPTICS)

Also known as major tranquilizers, antipsychotics can be divided in several groups, including phenothiazines, thioxanthenes and butyrophenones. There are also a number of miscellaneous compounds. The mechanisms of action and pharmacokinetics of these drugs are described in more detail in Chapters 5 and 6. All are dopamine antagonists.

Pharmacokinetics (general)

Most antipsychotics are readily but incompletely absorbed from the gastrointestinal tract and undergo significant first-pass metabolism. Most are highly lipid-soluble with a large volume of distribution. This may account for longer than expected duration of action. Metabolites of chlorpromazine can be excreted for weeks after discontinuation of action after long-term use in humans. Most are almost completely metabolized and very little drug is excreted unchanged.

Phenothiazines

EXAMPLES

Acetylpromazine, chlorpromazine, thioridazine.

Clinical applications

Phenothiazines have a variety of effects on the central nervous system (CNS) and the autonomic and endocrine systems because of their ability to block dopamine, α-adrenergic, muscarinic, H_1-histaminic and serotonin (5-HT_2) receptors. They are commonly used in veterinary medicine as tranquilizers for restraint and sedation (see Chapter 6) or for brief treatment of arousal (which can be agitation, alertness to excitement or hypervigilance, often associated with fear- or anxiety-provoking circumstances or excitement from anticipation). However, they are seldom used in long-term behavioral therapy because of potential extrapyramidal effects. In addition, other, more appropriate medications are available.

Acetylpromazine maleate is nonspecific in its effects. Because it decreases motor function and produces ataraxia (decreased emotional reactivity or awareness of external stimuli and indifference to stress), as well as being an antiemetic, it has been used for motion sickness and anxiety associated with car travel. The length and depth of effect are variable, depending on the animal and the environmental stimuli. This makes accurate dosing difficult. However, recent research demonstrated that acepromazine is not as effective as other medications in decreasing perioperative concentrations of stress-related hormones. Acetylpromazine and chlorpromazine have also been used in the treatment of aggression, to reduce excitement and in the treatment of anxiety-related conditions. Thioridazine was used in one case to control aberrant motor activity in a dog. The aberrant behavior observed included running around barking frantically, erratic episodes of tail and carpus chewing and apparent unprovoked aggression. However, other medications, such as TCAs and benzodiazepines, are preferred in the treatment of aggression, aberrant behavior and anxiety, as their mechanism of action is directed at the underlying neurochemical cause of the behavior rather than at blunting the behavioral response.

Formulations and dose rates

DOGS

Acetylpromazine

- 0.1–2.2 mg/kg PO q.6–24 h

Chlorpromazine

- 0.5–3.3 mg/kg PO q.6–24 h

Thioridazine

- 1.1–2.2 mg/kg PO q.12–24 h

CATS

Acetylpromazine

- 0.5–2.2 mg/kg PO as needed

Chlorpromazine

- 0.5–3.3 mg/kg PO q.6–24 h

Adverse effects

- Sedation
- Anticholinergic effects
- Hypersensitivity to noise
- Sudden aggression and excitement have been reported in dogs (acetylpromazine)
- Hypotension
- Bradycardia
- Paradoxical excitability
- Akathesia (motor restlessness, pacing, agitation reported in some animals)
- Extrapyramidal signs (ataxia, muscle tremors, inco-ordination)

Contraindications and precautions

Traditionally, phenothiazines have been contraindicated in epileptic patients because they are believed to lower the threshold to seizures. Although the evidence for this is anecdotal and far from convincing, some authors suggest that prolonged use of neuroleptics may cause seizures by stimulation of the extrapyramidal motor pathways.

Extreme caution should be exercised when approaching animals that have been given acetylpromazine as they may become more reactive to noise and startle easily. The effect of acetylpromazine on aggressive behavior is unpredictable and may depend on the level of arousal prior to medication as well as individual variation in effect. There is a large, unpredictable variation in drug effect and duration between individuals.

Fainting associated with high levels of vagal tone (sometimes termed vasovagal syncope) can occur in brachycephalic breeds, particularly boxers, given acetylpromazine. In these cases, collapse is associated with bradycardia and treatment involves the administration of an anticholinergic drug such as atropine.

Butyrophenones

EXAMPLE

Haloperidol.

Clinical applications

Haloperidol has been used in the acute treatment of aggressive and psychotic states, Huntington's chorea and Tourette's syndrome in humans, as well as in the management of nausea and vomiting associated with chemotherapy.

Haloperidol has been used experimentally in dogs, rats and monkeys. It has been reported to assist in the control of stress and therefore to prevent injuries when several species of wild African herbivore are handled at game parks. Haloperidol has been reported to have a slight effect in dogs with obsessive-compulsive disorders and certain types of aggression but dose rates have not been established. It has been used long term (up to 9 years) in the management of self-mutilation and feather-plucking in birds, with some success. It is reported to have greater efficacy in birds that mutilate soft tissue rather than just traumatize feathers.

Mechanism of action

Haloperidol is a butyrophenone-derivative antipsychotic with actions similar to the piperazine-derivative phenothiazines. Haloperidol decanoate is a long-acting form of haloperidol. The precise mechanism of action is unclear but it appears to inhibit the ascending reticular system, possibly through the caudate nucleus. It competitively blocks postsynaptic dopamine receptors in the mesolimbic dopaminergic system and increases turnover of brain dopamine. It acts mainly on D_2-receptors and has some effect on 5-HT_2 and α_1-receptors but negligible effects on D_1-receptors. There is also some blockade of α-adrenergic receptors of the autonomic system.

Formulations and dose rates

PARROTS
- 0.2–04 mg/kg PO q.12 h; start at lowest dose and increase 0.02 q2d to effect
- 1–2 mg/kg haloperidol decanoate IM q.3 weeks, lower dose for cockatoos, African greys and Quaker parrots

DOGS
- 0.05–4 mg PO q.12 h

CATS
- 0.1–1.0 mg/kg PO

Adverse effects

Decreased activity and inappetence have been reported in birds.

Contraindications and precautions

Caution should be exercised when administering haloperidol to macaws as death has been reported with its use in this species. There has also been a report of recurrent bilateral hock dislocation associated with its administration in one Quaker parakeet.

Miscellaneous antipsychotics – clozapine

Clozapine is an atypical antipsychotic and has markedly different clinical effects in humans, i.e. different humans react or respond in different or various ways to the drug.

Clinical applications

Experimentally clozapine has shown to be effective in treating aggression in animal models of self-abuse. However, its use in treating aggressive dogs has been disappointing.

Mechanism of action

Clozapine is classed as a dibenzodiazepine and seems to have minimal central antidopaminergic activity, in contrast to many antipsychotic drugs. This may account for the different clinical effects observed in humans compared with other neuroleptics used to treat schizophrenia.

Formulations and dose rates

A suggested dose in dogs is 1.0–7.0 mg/kg PO. However, reliable dose–response data have not been established in animals.

Pharmacokinetics

The pharmacokinetics of clozapine have not been determined in animals. However, in humans it is well absorbed orally and is subject to moderate first-pass metabolism. Peak blood levels occur in 2.1 h, with mean half-life of 12 h; 95% is bound to plasma proteins and it is almost completely metabolized prior to excretion.

Adverse effects

- Significant risk of agranulocytosis in humans.
- Clozapine should be used with care in patients with concurrent cardiovascular disease.
- In dogs clozapine caused excessive salivation and ataxia, and blocked avoidance behaviors.

ANTICONVULSANTS

Anticonvulsants currently have a minor role in veterinary behavioral medicine, unless a neurological problem such as epilepsy is suspected to be involved in the behavioral problem being managed. The mechanism of action and pharmacokinetics of anticonvulsants are described in Chapter 16.

EXAMPLES

Phenobarbital (phenobarbitone), carbamazepine.

Clinical applications

Phenobarbital has been used with some success to manage mild overactivity and excessive vocalization in cats. It is generally used for short-term management while environmental changes are being instituted and when other therapeutic options have been explored and proved unsuccessful.

Anticonvulsants such as phenobarbital have been used in the past to treat behavioral problems such as tail chasing or spinning in bull terriers, hyperesthesia syndrome in cats and 'rage syndrome'. However, they are generally not recommended or used for these problems now unless there is clear evidence of a neurological cause for the behavior.

Carbamazepine, an iminodiabenzyl derivative of imipramine, has been used in humans to control explosive aggressive events (episodic dyscontrol) and depression, in addition to its use in seizure control. It was reported to control some forms of fear aggression in two cats and has been used to control motor activity in dogs that may have been associated with seizures.

Formulations and dose rates

DOGS

Phenobarbital

- 1–4 mg/kg PO q.12 h or as needed up to 16 mg/kg/day

Carbamazepine

- 4–10 mg/kg/day divided q.8 h or 5–10 mg/kg q.12 h

CATS

Phenobarbital

- 1–4 mg/kg PO q. 12–24 h or as needed

Carbamazepine

- 25 mg PO q. 12–24 h or 4–8 mg/kg q. 12 h

Adverse effects

Phenobarbital

- Long-term use of phenobarbital may cause hepatotoxicity.

Carbamazepine

- Carbamazepine is mildly sedating, mildly anticholinergic and does not cause muscle relaxation in animals.
- Side effects reported in humans include ataxia, clonic-tonic convulsions and gastrointestinal upsets.
- It has been reported to cause idiosyncratic blood dyscrasias. Deaths have been reported due to aplastic anemia and agranulocytosis so careful monitoring is essential.
- Carbamazepine must be used with particular care in patients with renal, hepatic, cardiovascular or hematological disorders.

β-BLOCKERS

The mechanism of action, pharmacokinetics and side effects of β-blockers are described in detail in Chapter 17.

EXAMPLES

Propranolol, pindolol.

Clinical applications

Noradrenaline (norepinephrine) is released in fear- or anxiety-provoking situations. Blocking some of the effects of noradrenaline reduces the physical manifestations of fear and anxiety such as muscle tremors, trembling, tachycardia and altered gastrointestinal motility. As a result, β-blockers can have a calming effect on anxious animals. β-Blockers such as propranolol have been used to treat some forms of anxiety such as noise phobias in animals and stage fright in humans. However, these drugs appear to be more efficacious in humans.

Propranolol may also block brain serotonin receptors and therefore may be useful in inhibiting aggression. It has been used for this purpose in humans (e.g. treatment of violent outbursts associated with organic brain syndromes) but has not proved as successful for this purpose in companion animals. Pindolol, a partial β-agonist, reportedly has a greater serotonergic effect, so may be more effective in the treatment of aggression.

Formulations and dose rates

DOGS

Propranolol
- Small: 5 mg/dog PO q.8 h
- Large 10–20 mg/dog PO q.8 h
- 0.5–3.0 mg/kg PO q.12 h or as needed

Pindolol
- 0.125–0.25 mg/kg PO q.12 h

CATS

Propranolol
- 0.2–1.0 mg/kg PO q.8 h

Adverse effects
- Sedation and sleep disturbance have been reported in humans.
- β-Blockers should be gradually withdrawn after chronic use because of potential problems with β-receptor blockade, as this can depress myocardial contractility and excitability and cardiac decompensation may ensue.

Contraindications and precautions
- Use with care in diabetics as β-blockers may increase the likelihood of exercise-induced hypoglycemia.
- Bradycardia
- Hypotension
- Bronchospasm

OPIOID AGONISTS/ANTAGONISTS

Opioid alkaloids produce analgesia via endogenous opioid peptide receptors. The pure opioid antagonists are morphine derivatives with substitutions at the N_{17} position and have a high affinity for μ opioid receptor-binding sites.

EXAMPLES

Naloxone (antagonist), naltrexone (antagonist), hydrocodone (agonist).

Clinical applications
The opioid antagonists have been used to treat a number of stereotypies and obsessive-compulsive disorders in humans. In companion animals problems such as self-mutilation, acral lick dermatitis and tail chasing have been treated, with variable results. The rationale for treatment is the premise that opioid peptides are released during stress and activate the dopamine system, which may be responsible for compulsive behaviors. Additionally, as endogenous opioid peptides induce analgesia, it is possible that they reduce the pain that might normally inhibit self-mutilation.

Naloxone has been used as a diagnostic aid for compulsive disorders. However, its short duration of action and parenteral formulation does not make it useful in a chronic treatment program. Naltrexone is longer acting and has been used therapeutically. However, its expense usually makes long-term treatment impractical.

The opioid agonist hydrocodone has also been used successfully in some cases of self-mutilation in cats and chronic management of canine acral lick dermatitis.

Mechanism of action
See Chapter 14.

Pharmacokinetics
See Chapter 14.

Formulations and dose rates

DOGS

Naloxone
- 11–22 μg/kg SC, IM, IV or 0.5 mg q.12 h

Naltrexone
- 2.2 mg/kg PO q.12–24 h

Hydrocodone
- 0.25 mg/kg PO q.8–12 h

CATS

Naltrexone
- 2–4 mg/kg PO q.24 h (up to 25–50 mg/cat)

Hydrocodone
- 0.25–1.0 mg/kg PO q.12–24 h

Adverse effects
- Constipation is reported to be a problem in humans.
- In cats a decrease in activity has been reported.

CNS STIMULANTS - AMFETAMINES

Amfetamines appear to act centrally by promoting release of catecholaminergic neurotransmitters such as dopamine, weakly inhibit MAO and possibly act as catecholaminergic agonists.

EXAMPLES

Methylphenidate (Ritalin®), dexamfetamine.

Clinical applications

Amfetamines are used to treat attention-deficit hyperactivity disorders and narcolepsy in humans. True hyperactivity (versus overactivity) is rare in dogs. CNS stimulants have a paradoxical calming effect on truly hyperactive dogs while in normal dogs they increase excitement and activity. Lifelong medication may be needed in some cases. Amfetamines have also been used in the treatment of narcolepsy in dogs.

Mechanism of action

Amfetamines cause release of noradrenaline (norepinephrine), dopamine and serotonin from presynaptic terminals, as opposed to having direct agonist effects on postsynaptic receptors.

Pharmacokinetics

Amfetamines have a very short biological life in humans and reach higher concentrations in the brain than in blood. They are metabolized by hepatic enzymes.

Formulations and dose rates

DOGS

Methylphenidate (Ritalin®)

- Hyperkinesis: 0.2–1 mg/kg PO should lead to 15% decrease in heart rate and respiration rate in 75–90 min (for diagnosis)
- 2–4 mg/kg q.8–12 h or 5 mg PO q.12 h in small dogs to 20–40 mg PO q.12 h in large dogs
- Narcolepsy: 0.05–0.25 mg/kg PO q.12–24 h

Dexamfetamine

- Hyperkinesis: 0.2–1.3 mg/kg PO as needed
- Narcolepsy: 5–10 mg q.24 h
- 1.25 mg/dog PO as needed

CATS

Dexamfetamine

- Narcolepsy: 1.25 mg as needed

Adverse effects

- Increased heart rate
- Increased respiratory rate
- Tremors with possible hyperthermia
- Decreased appetite
- Insomnia

Contraindications and precautions

- Cardiovascular disease
- Concurrent use of MAOIs
- Hyperthyroidism
- Glaucoma
- Methylphenidate may lower the seizure threshold

Known drug interactions

Amfetamines can potentiate narcotic analgesics.

BENZODIAZEPINES

See Chapters 5 and 6 for further information.

EXAMPLES

Diazepam (Valium®), clorazepate dipotassium (Tranxene®), alprazolam (Xanax®), clonazepam (Rivitrol®), oxazepam (Serepax®), lorazepam, flurazepam.

Mechanism of action

The benzodiazepines are classified as sedative hypnotics. All benzodiazepines have structural similarity and appear to work through the same mechanisms. They potentiate the inhibitory effects of GABA by interacting allosterically with GABA-binding sites and chloride channels. However, they differ pharmacokinetically and pharmacodynamically.

Most benzodiazepines are 1,4-benzodiazepines and most contain a carboxamide group in the 7-membered heterocyclic ring structure. A substituent such as a halogen or nitro group in the 7 position is required for sedative-hypnotic activity. The structure of alprazolam includes the addition of a triazole ring at the 1,2 position. Benzodiazepines are metabolized at varying rates and some have active metabolites that are more potent than the parent compound. The long half-life of intermediate metabolites such as *N*-desmethyldiazepam (60 h in humans) accounts for the cumulative effects of many of the benzodiazepines.

The anxiolytic effects are believed to be due to the inhibitory action of benzodiazepines on neurones in the limbic system, including the amygdala, and on serotonergic and noradrenergic neurones in the brainstem.

Clinical applications

Although benzodiazepines have been used in the treatment of fear- and anxiety-related disorders in humans and companion animals, they lack behavioral specificity. The effect of benzodiazepines is dose dependent. Low doses have a sedative effect, moderate doses have an anxiolytic effect and may help with social interactions, while high doses facilitate sleep.

Tolerance to the sedative effects may develop but not usually to the anxiolytic effects. Cats appear to be particularly sensitive to the muscle-relaxant effects of benzodiazepines. This effect is independent of sedation.

Anxiety has been shown to decrease locomotion and ingestion and increase muscle tone. Therefore, treatment with benzodiazepines would be expected to counter these effects of anxiety and make animals more active.

In cats benzodiazepines have been used to treat problems such as inappropriate elimination associated with anxiety, urine marking or spraying, fear aggression and overgrooming, as well as to stimulate appetite. They have been used in dogs in the treatment of noise phobias, panic attacks and sleep disorders such as night-time waking.

Because of its short half-life in dogs, the clinical use of diazepam is limited in this species. However, it has proved useful as an adjunct in treating anxiety of short duration, for example noise phobia. Clorazepate, because of its longer half-life, may be more suitable for dogs.

In one study diazepam was reported to be effective in reducing urine spraying in 75% of cats and eliminating the problem in 43% of treated cats. It was reported to be more efficacious in males and in cats living in multicat households. However, in another study a recidivism rate of 91% was reported when medication was withdrawn.

As benzodiazepines have a disinhibiting effect, they have also been used in cases of intercat aggression to decrease the fear or anxiety of the victim. Alprazolam has been used successfully for panic attacks in humans and also in dogs in the anticipatory phase of thunderstorm phobias and separation anxiety.

Flurazepam is used to treat insomnia in humans and has been used, as has alprazolam and triazolam, to treat night-time waking or changed sleep patterns that may be associated with anxiety in companion animals. Triazolam has also been used to treat some cases of aggression in cats.

When drug therapy is no longer required gradual withdrawal from therapy is recommended by reducing the daily dose by 10–25% per week.

Formulations and dose rate

DOGS

Alprazolam

- 0.25–2.0 mg/dog q.8–12 h, or 0.02–0.1 mg/kg q.4h, or 0.125–1.0 mg/kg PO q.12 h. No more than 4 mg/day. For example, 0.5 mg to small dogs, 1.0 mg to medium dogs and 2.0 mg to large dogs q.12 h

Diazepam

- 0.5–2.0 mg/kg PO q.4–12 h or as needed

Clorazepate dipotassium

- 0.50–2.0 mg/kg q.8–24 h or 11.25–22.5 mg/dog PO q.12–24 h

There is a sustained-release formulation of clorazepate.

Clonazepam

- 0.1–0.5 mg/kg PO q.8–12 h

Oxazepam

- 0.2–0.5 mg/kg PO q.8–24 h

Lorazepam

- 0.02–0.5 mg/kg PO q.12–24 h. For example, 1 mg for small dogs, 2.0 mg for medium dogs and 4.0 mg for large dogs to start

Flurazepam

- 0.2–0.4 mg/kg PO for 4–7 days (sleep/wake cycles) or 0.1–0.5 mg/kg PO q.12–24 h (appetite stimulant)

CATS

Alprazolam

- 0.0125–0.25 mg/cat PO q.12 h or as needed, or 0.1 mg/kg q.8 h or as needed

Diazepam

- 0.2–0.5 mg/kg PO q.12–24 h

Clorazepate dipotassium

- 0.5–2.0 mg/kg PO q.12–24 h or as needed.

There is a sustained-release formulation of clorazepate.

Clonazepam

- 0.016 mg/kg PO q.6–24 h

Oxazepam

- 0.2–1.0 mg/kg PO q.12–24 h

Flurazepam

- 0.2–0.4 mg/kg PO for 4–7 days (sleep/wake cycles) or 0.1–0.2 mg/kg PO q.12–24 h (appetite stimulant)

Triazolam

- 0.03 mg/kg q.12 h or 2.5–5 mg/cat PO q.8 h

Pharmacokinetics

Diazepam is rapidly absorbed following oral administration. It is slowly and incompletely absorbed after intramuscular administration. It is highly lipid soluble and widely distributed throughout the body. Diazepam readily crosses the blood–brain barrier and is highly protein bound.

Diazepam is metabolized in the liver. The common intermediate metabolite of diazepam and clorazepate, *N*-desmethyldiazepam (nordiazepam), is in turn biotransformed to the active compound, oxazepam. Diazepam has a short half-life in dogs (2.5 h) compared with cats (5.5–20 h). Additionally, its active metabolite nordiazepam also has a short half-life in dogs (3 h versus 21 h in cats).

Adverse effects

- Diazepam affects depth perception, so cats may fall off objects or miss objects when they jump until they learn to compensate.
- Increased appetite.
- Transient ataxia. This should resolve within 3–4 days of continued use; if it doesn't the dose should be decreased or the drug withdrawn as the potential for cumulative effects and toxicity due to accumulation of the intermediate metabolite exists.
- Paradoxical hyperactivity in some cats.
- Increased affection/friendliness (can become overwhelming for the owner, especially in Oriental breeds).
- Increased vocalization in cats.

- Drug tolerance.
- Interference with memory (amnesia with intravenous dosing in humans).
- Disinhibition of suppressed behavior, e.g. aggression.
- Interference with learning conditioned responses.
- Anxiety.
- Insomnia.
- Diazepam may increase predation in cats (possibly through its effects on the lateral hypothalamus and its inhibitory effect on ACh).
- Fatal idiopathic hepatic necrosis has been reported rarely in cats.

Contraindications and precautions

- Hepatic or renal failure.
- Use with caution in aggressive animals.
- The patient must be weaned off treatment gradually if they have been dosed daily.

ANTIDEPRESSANTS

Antidepressants have been used extensively in human psychiatry and are increasingly used in the treatment of companion animal behavior problems. Although the name implies that their main clinical indication is for alleviating depression, they are also used in humans to treat problems such as agoraphobia, enuresis, narcolepsy, recurrent fears and anxieties and to decrease some types of volatile or explosive aggression. In companion animal medicine they have proved useful as part of behavior modification treatment programs.

A number of different chemical structures have been found to have antidepressant activity. The three most common types are the tricyclic antidepressants (TCAs), the selective serotonin reuptake inhibitors (SSRIs) and the monoamine oxidase inhibitors (MAOIs).

All antidepressants take about 2 weeks to produce any beneficial effects (in humans), even though their pharmacological effects are produced immediately. This suggests that secondary adaptive changes are important, such as drug modification of receptor sites.

Tricyclic antidepressants

Tricyclic antidepressants (TCAs) are closely related to phenothiazines in chemical structure, both having three linked rings. The TCAs, however, lack a sulfur constituent in the middle ring. They are less related pharmacologically. They differ principally by the incorporation of an extra atom in the central ring; thus the molecule is no longer planar.

EXAMPLES

Tertiary amines: Amitriptyline, clomipramine, doxepin, imipramine.
Secondary amines: Desipramine, nortriptyline.

Clinical applications

Medication with TCAs has proved helpful and is in fact often necessary as an adjunct to a behavior modification program in cases, especially in anxiety, that are long-standing or particularly severe.

In cats, TCAs have been recommended as part of the treatment protocol for anxiety-related disorders such as spraying/marking behavior, intercat aggression, fear aggression, overgrooming and excessive licking in obsessive-compulsive disorder. They have also proved useful in the treatment of excessive vocalization due to anxiety. Success rates of up to 80% have been reported for the treatment of urine spraying with amitriptyline. Up to a 90% success rate has been reported with clomipramine treatment for urine spraying. Additionally, clomipramine has been effective in controlling over 90% of cases of obsessive-compulsive disorder when used in combination with a behavior modification program. TCAs with strong anticholinergic activity have also been used to reduce predation in cats, as ACh is the principal neurotransmitter involved in predatory aggression.

In dogs, TCAs have been used as part of the treatment protocol in cases of dominance aggression, fear aggression, separation anxiety, obsessive-compulsive disorders, including acral lick granulomas, fears and phobias such as thunderstorm phobia, enuresis and narcolepsy.

In a double-blind placebo-controlled study, clomipramine was shown to be effective in contributing to the resolution of separation anxiety in dogs after 2 months of treatment in 70% of cases compared with less than 20% of cases where behavior modification alone was used. Other trials have reported a 50–70% improvement in licking behavior in lick granulomas and 65–100% response in the treatment of stereotypic and obsessive-compulsive disorders in dogs. TCAs are more successful when the animal presents with only one problem, as opposed to multiple behavior problems.

Amitriptyline has been used in the management of cats with lower urinary tract disease. Imipramine has been used successfully in the treatment of urethral incompetence because of its anticholinergic and α-adrenergic effects.

Doxepin and amitriptyline have considerable antihistaminergic effects so they are useful in cases where antipruritic or sedating effects are also needed.

Mechanism of action

The TCAs have five principal modes of action.

- They block reuptake of serotonin.
- They block reuptake of noradrenaline (norepinephrine).
- They have anticholinergic, antimuscarinic effects.
- They have α_1-adrenergic antagonist effects.
- They have antihistaminic effects to varying degrees.

Thus TCAs produce three major effects.

- Blocking reuptake of brain amines (antidepressant effect in humans).
- Anticholinergic (atropine-like) effects.
- Sedation.

TCAs act by inhibiting the amine (noradrenaline (norepinephrine) or serotonin) reuptake pumps, which presumably permits longer duration of action of the neurotransmitter at the receptor site. In chronic use they may cause a decrease in the number of β-adrenergic and 5-HT_2 receptors.

Prototypic drugs, imipramine and amitriptyline, are mixed noradrenaline (norepinephrine) and serotonin uptake inhibitors and have antimuscarinic, antihistaminic and α-adrenoreceptor blocking actions. Clomipramine hydrochloride is the 3-chloro analog of imipramine. It preferentially inhibits the neuronal reuptake of serotonin and noradrenaline (norepinephrine).

The precise mechanism of action of the antipruritic effects of doxepin is unknown but is thought to relate to its potent H_1 antagonist properties.

Formulations and dose rates

DOGS

Amitriptyline

- 1–4 mg/kg PO q.12–24 h

Amitriptyline is extremely bitter, so it can be difficult to administer if the tablet is broken.

Clomipramine

- 1–2 mg/kg PO q.12 h 2 weeks, then 3 mg/kg PO q.24 h; may need up to 4 mg/kg to manage some disorders

Clomipramine is approved for veterinary use in many countries. One formulation of clomipramine available, Clomicalm®, is meat flavored and generally well accepted by cats and dogs. Higher doses appear to be necessary to control obsessive-compulsive disorders than anxiety disorders.

Doxepin

- 3–5 mg/kg PO q.8–12 h (for acral lick dermatitis)
- 0.5–1 mg/kg PO q.12 h (for obsessive-compulsive disorder)

Imipramine

- 2.0–4.0 mg/kg PO q.12–24 h

Nortriptyline

- 1–2 mg/kg PO q.12–24 h

CATS

Amitriptyline

- 0.5–1.0 mg/kg PO q.24 h

Clomipramine

- 0.25–0.5 mg/kg PO q.24 h; may need up to 1 mg/kg to manage some disorders

Doxepin

- 0.5–1.0 mg/kg PO q.12–24 h

Imipramine

- 0.5–1 mg/kg PO q.12–24 h

Nortriptyline

- 0.5–2.0 mg/kg PO q.12–24 h

Generic forms of most TCAs are inexpensive and generally make a good choice (where a veterinary product is not indicated) for treatment programs that are expected to be long-standing or lifelong.

Pharmacokinetics

Tricyclic antidepressants are rapidly absorbed from the gastrointestinal tract and bind strongly to plasma albumin (90–95%). Clomipramine undergoes substantial first-pass metabolism that reduces its bioavailability to 50%. They preferentially bind hepatocytes, myocardial cells, pulmonary and brain tissue. High protein binding and relatively high lipid solubility lead to large volumes of distribution and slow elimination rates.

Most TCAs undergo significant metabolism. They are metabolized by the liver by two main routes: demethylation, followed by glucuronide conjugation. Thus, alteration of the aliphatic side chain, *N*-demethylation (tertiary amines converted to secondary amines, e.g. amitriptyline to nortriptyline), occurs first. This is followed by transformation of the tricyclic nucleus by ring hydroxylation and conjugation to form glucuronides. Monodemethylation produces active metabolites, e.g. desipramine and nortriptyline. In humans, the relative proportion of each metabolite varies between individuals. During prolonged treatment the plasma concentration of active metabolites is likely to be comparable to the parent compound, although individual variation occurs. It appears that the metabolites are more potent noradrenaline (norepinephrine) inhibitors, while the parent compound is generally more potent in inhibiting serotonin uptake.

Renal filtration is generally ineffective in eliminating the parent compounds because they are highly protein bound, very lipophilic and widely dispersed in tissues. Metabolism and inactivation by glucuronide conjugation of the hydroxylated metabolites are required for significant excretion of glucuronides in urine.

Up to 2–3 weeks or even longer is required to reach therapeutic blood levels. However, clinical effects are seen soon after administration.

Adverse effects

It should be noted that, because clomipramine is registered for use in animals, more is known about its specific effects in companion animals than those of other TCAs. However, the pharmacology of other TCAs in companion animals is expected to be similar to clomipramine.

- The most predictable side effects are short-term lethargy or sedation, mild and intermittent vomiting which is usually transient and increases or decreases in appetite.
- Anticholinergic side effects may be encountered, often, but not always, at high dose rates.
- Other side effects, which usually disappear if the dose is decreased or the medication is withdrawn, include:
  - Sedation (antihistamine effect)
  - Dry mouth (antimuscarinic effect)
  - Constipation (antimuscarinic effect)
  - Tachycardia
  - Cardiac arrhythmias
  - Ataxia
  - Decreased tear production
  - Mydriasis
  - Disturbances of accommodation.
- High doses have been associated with increased liver enzymes, hepatotoxicity and convulsions.
- A few cases of urine retention have been reported in cats after treatment with clomipramine. This effect is likely to be the result of decreased bladder muscle tone, which decreases intraluminal pressure and allows collapse of the trigone area, obstructing urinary outflow. Hence animals treated with clomipramine should be monitored daily for signs of urine retention or constipation. If urine retention or constipation occurs, drug administration should be stopped until normal urination or defecation is observed, then reinstated at a lower dose.
- Cats are more sensitive to the cardiac effects of TCAs than dogs and should be monitored closely.
- In humans, TCAs may lower the seizure threshold.
- TCAs should be used with caution in patients with hyperthyroidism or receiving thyroid supplementation as there may be an increased risk of cardiac arrhythmias.

Contraindications and precautions

- Cardiac dysrhythmias
- Urinary retention
- Concurrent use of hypertensive drugs
- Narrow angle glaucoma
- Seizures

Known drug interactions

- Concurrent MAOI administration should be avoided as it may lead to a serotonin syndrome.
- TCAs used with antithyroid medications may increase the potential risk of agranulocytosis.
- As TCAs are strongly bound to plasma protein, their effects may be temporarily enhanced by drugs that compete for protein-binding sites (e.g. aspirin, phenylbutazone).
- As hepatic metabolism is necessary for elimination, drugs such as neuroleptics and some steroids may inhibit metabolism.
- Simultaneous administration of clomipramine and cimetidine (an enzyme inhibitor) may lead to increased plasma levels of clomipramine.
- Plasma levels of certain antiepileptic drugs such as phenytoin and carbamazepine may be increased by coadministration with clomipramine.
- Clomipramine may potentiate the effects of antiarrhythmic drugs, anticholinergic agents and other CNS-acting drugs (e.g. barbiturates, benzodiazepines, neuroleptics).
- Concurrent use with sympathomimetic drugs may increase the risk of cardiac effects (arrhythmias, hypertension).

Selective serotonin reuptake inhibitors

Currently, there are at least five selective serotonin reuptake inhibitors (SSRIs) on the market worldwide for human use. As their collective name implies, they are selective for serotonin, lacking the anticholinergic and cardiovascular side effects of TCAs. They do not resemble TCAs structurally and have minimal autonomic activity. They have much improved safety and tolerability over the TCAs and MAOIs and wider therapeutic indications than depression.

EXAMPLES

Fluoxetine (Prozac®), paroxetine, sertraline, fluvoxamine, citalopram.

Clinical applications

Apart from the treatment of depression, SSRIs have been used successfully in cases of panic disorder, obsessive-compulsive disorder, posttraumatic stress disorder, chronic pain, social phobias, enuresis and eating disorders in humans.

In cats, fluoxetine and paroxetine have been used to treat urine spraying, with the reported success rate of fluoxetine being around 80% for urine spraying and anxiety-related disorders. Both have also been used to treat some types of aggression and obsessive-compulsive disorders.

In dogs, fluoxetine and sertraline have been used in the treatment of acral lick granulomas. Fluoxetine has also been used to treat obsessive-compulsive disorders, separation anxiety, generalized anxiety or global fear and dominance aggression. Paroxetine has also been used to treat generalized anxiety disorder with 50% of patients showing clinical improvement. Citalopram has been used to treat acral lick dermatitis with a satisfactory result being seen in about 2 weeks. Until recently, their high cost generally prevented SSRIs from being the drug of first choice in companion animal therapy. However, fluoxetine is now off patent and the generic forms are more affordable. They and other SSRIs are a valuable therapeutic option if the owner's financial constraints do not preclude their use. However, the mint-flavored liquid formulation is not readily accepted by some cats.

Mechanism of action

Selective serotonin reuptake inhibitors selectively inhibit serotonin reuptake in presynaptic neurones in the CNS. The therapeutic effect of SSRIs in obsessive-compulsive disorders is thought to be mediated by disinhibition of serotonin neurones in the pathway from the midbrain raphe to the basal ganglia. Similarly, the amelioration of panic disorders is thought to occur when disinhibition of the pathway to the limbic cortex and hippocampus occurs. However, activation of serotonin receptors can worsen panic or anxiety initially. This has been observed in both humans and companion animals.

Formulations and dose rates

DOGS

Fluoxetine
- 1–2 mg/kg PO q.24 h

Fluvoxamine
- 0.5–2 mg/kg PO q.24 h (up to 4 mg/kg q.12 h if necessary, increased incrementally)

Paroxetine
- 1 mg/kg q.24 h

Sertraline
- 1–3 mg/kg PO q.24 h

Citalopram
- 0.5–1 mg/kg q.24 h

CATS

Fluoxetine
- 0.5–1 mg/kg PO q. 24 h

Fluvoxamine
- 0.25–0.5 mg/kg PO q.24 h (up to 1–2 mg/kg q.12 h; increase incrementally)

Paroxetine
- 0.5–1 mg/kg PO q.24 h

Sertraline
- 0.5–1 mg/kg PO q.24 h

BIRDS

Fluoxetine
- 2.0–5.0 mg/day

Pharmacokinetics

Fluoxetine is well absorbed after oral administration, with peak plasma concentrations in humans achieved in 4–8 h. In a study in beagles, bioavailability was 70%. The presence of food alters the rate but not extent of absorption. Fluoxetine is highly protein bound (95%) in humans. It has been administered transdermally to cats. However, the relative bioavailability by this route was only 10% of that achieved after oral administration; the study did not determine the actual oral bioavailability in cats.

Fluoxetine and its major metabolite are distributed throughout the body, with highest levels found in lung and liver. CNS concentrations are detected 1 h after dosing. Fluoxetine is metabolized in the liver to a variety of metabolites. The demethylated active metabolite, norfluoxetine, has a half-life of 7–9 d at steady state, while the parent drug has a shorter half-life of 2–3 d. In humans, there is wide interpatient variation in duration of action. Liver, but not renal, impairment will increase clearance times.

Sertraline and paroxetine have similar pharmacokinetic parameters to the TCAs.

Adverse effects

- Mild sedation.
- Transient decreased appetite.
- Increased anxiety.
- Decreased sexual motivation in animals and humans.
- Nausea, lethargy, weight loss, tremors and agitation have been reported in humans.
- In humans increased liver enzymes may occur, although there are no reports of liver pathology unless the patient had prior liver disease.
- Gastrointestinal disturbances such as vomiting or diarrhea have been reported in humans.
- Drug-induced rashes have been reported in humans.

Known drug interactions

- Fluoxetine can increase the half-life of concurrently administered diazepam, although in the short term the drug combination is recommended for humans by some psychiatrists.
- Concomitant MAOI therapy can cause a serotonin syndrome. This is a very serious condition characterized by changes in mental status, hyperthermia,

agitation, myoclonus and autonomic instability, which may lead to death. At least 2 weeks should be allowed as a wash-out period between SSRI and MAOI therapy, 5 weeks for fluoxetine.
- Coadministration of TCAs can increase plasma levels of the TCA.
- Fluoxetine can enhance the effects of haloperidol (increased extrapyramidal effects), lithium (increased lithium levels), L-tryptophan (CNS stimulation, GI disturbances), TCAs (increased TCA side effects) and buspirone (increased anxiety).

Monoamine oxidase inhibitors

Monoamine oxidase inhibitors were among the first drugs to be used as antidepressants. However, they have been superseded by TCAs, which have fewer side effects. The MAOIs are classified as hydrazides or nonhydrazides depending on whether or not they have the C-N-N structure. The hydrazides appear to combine irreversibly with monoamine oxidase. Older MAOIs are nonselective inhibitors of both MAO-A and MAO-B (e.g. phenelzine), while newer types are selective for either MAO-A and reversible (e.g. moclobemide) or MAO-B (e.g. selegiline). Only selegiline has been used in veterinary medicine.

EXAMPLE

Selegiline (L-deprenyl).

Clinical applications

In humans, selegiline has been used in the treatment of Parkinson's disease. It has been used in older cats presenting with anxiety, disturbed sleep/wake cycles and excessive vocalization associated with aging. It has also been used to treat generalized anxiety, compulsive licking and several types of aggression, but higher doses seem to be required for cats than dogs.

In the USA and Australia the main behavioral use of selegiline is for canine cognitive dysfunction syndrome in old dogs. It is also useful in some anxiety problems. In Europe, the drug is used for a wider range of behavioral problems. It has been advocated in young dogs, even as young as 8 weeks, that have been diagnosed with overactivity/hyperactivity, anxiety problems, phobias, sleep disorders and stereotypies such as tail chasing. It has also been used in adult dogs with anxiety disorders that present with signs such as vomiting, diarrhea, salivation, phobias and acral lick dermatitis, as well as depressive disorders. It has been reported to be effective in reducing fear aggression but not territorial aggression. For older dogs (over 7 years of age) it has been successfully used to treat anxiety and sleep disorders, as well as cognitive dysfunction.

It may take up to 3 months to see the full behavioral benefits of selegiline, although owners have often reported improvement in their dogs within 7–10 days.

Mechanism of action

As the name implies, the MAOIs inhibit the enzyme monoamine oxidase (MAO). MAO is an intracellular enzyme, subclassified into two types, A and B, which differ in their substrate specificity and tissue distribution. MAO is widely distributed throughout the body and found in nearly all tissues. MAO-A has a substrate preference for 5-HT while MAO-B has a substrate preference for phenylethylamine. Both enzymes act on noradrenaline (norepinephrine) and dopamine. In CNS neurones, MAO plays an important role in the catabolism and inactivation of catecholamines, mainly dopamine, and to a lesser extent noradrenaline and adrenaline (epinephrine).

Monoamine oxidase inhibitors inhibit one or both forms of brain MAO, thus increasing cytosolic stores of noradrenaline, dopamine and 5-HT in nerve terminals. MAO-A is primarily responsible for noradrenaline, serotonin and tyramine metabolism, while MAO-B is more selective for dopamine metabolism.

Selegiline hydrochloride N-[(2R)-1-cyclohexylpropan-2-yl]-N-methylprop-2-yn-1-amine is a β-phenylethylamine (PEA) analog that acts as an irreversible inhibitor of MAO-B. This is thought to lead to increased synaptic occupancy of PEA and reduced catabolism of other monoamines, like dopamine, noradrenaline and tyramine. PEA seems to play a neuromodulation role for dopamine and noradrenaline.

Selegiline is thought to be a selective inhibitor of MAO-B in the dog. It is believed to also increase synthesis and release of dopamine into the synapse as well as interfering with dopamine reuptake. The secondary metabolites, including L-amfetamine and L-methamfetamine, both of which have pharmacological actions of their own, may also contribute to the behavioral effects seen; however, the extent of this is not known. Selegiline or its metabolites may also enhance the release of other neurotransmitters such as noradrenaline. Selegiline also increases the action of superoxide dismutase (SOD) and of catalase enzymes, which are both responsible for the detoxification of free radicals, particularly dopamine metabolites.

Formulations and dose rates

Selegiline

DOGS

- 0.5 mg/kg PO q.24 h; if no response after 4 weeks, 1.0 mg/kg PO q.24 h. It is generally recommended that the drug be administered in the morning

CATS

- 0.5–1.0 mg/kg PO q.24 h

Pharmacokinetics

Monoamine oxidase inhibitors are absorbed from the gastrointestinal tract. The plasma elimination half-life of selegiline is thought to be 60 min, based on intravenous administration to four dogs. Its volume of distribution is estimated to be 9.4 L/kg, suggesting that selegiline is extensively distributed to body tissues. The absolute bioavailability of an oral solution is less than 10%, suggesting poor absorption or considerable prehepatic metabolism.

Inhibition of MAO persists even after the drug is no longer detectable in plasma.

Adverse effects

- Stereotypic behaviors with overdosage.
- Gastrointestinal effects – vomiting and/or diarrhea.
- Hyperactivity or restlessness.
- Pruritus, hypersalivation, anorexia, diminished hearing and listlessness have also been reported in dogs.

Known drug interactions

Concomitant use of phenylpropanolamine, amitraz (an MAOI), ephedrine or pethidine (meperidine) or other opioids is not recommended. The mechanism of action of this drug interaction is not fully understood. However, it can be fatal.

In humans, severe CNS toxicity, including death, has been reported with the combination of TCAs or SSRIs and selegiline, although no adverse effects have been reported in field trials with dogs. It is recommended that there be a 2-week wash-out before administration of selegiline after TCA therapy. A 5-week wash-out is recommended before administration of selegiline after fluoxetine, because of the long half-life of fluoxetine and its metabolites.

AZASPIRODECANEDIONES – AZASPIRONES

EXAMPLE

Buspirone (Buspar®).

Clinical applications

Buspirone has been used to treat anxiety disorders in humans. Its anxiolytic efficacy is believed to be equivalent to the benzodiazepines. However, it has not proved effective as the sole treatment of panic disorders in humans. Interestingly, buspirone appears to be least effective in patients who have taken benzodiazepines within the 4 weeks prior to commencing buspirone treatment. Whether this is also the case in animals is unknown but should be considered when devising a treatment protocol. Buspirone is ineffective when taken irregularly. It may take 1–2 weeks for any beneficial effects to occur. Maximal effectiveness is achieved after 4–6 weeks in humans and this time frame appears to be similar in companion animals. Consequently, the use of buspirone in acute anxiety conditions is limited. Buspirone does not produce dependence.

Buspirone treatment has been advocated for anxiety-related problems of long standing in cats, including urine marking/spraying and overgrooming. Its success rate in reducing urine spraying has been reported to be about 55%, with a recidivism rate of about 50% after withdrawal of medication. It has also been used successfully for travel sickness in cats.

Advantages of buspirone in comparison to benzodiazepines include lack of sedation and a high safety margin. However, the frequency of dosing and cost can be problematic.

Because of its expense, buspirone has not been commonly used for canine behavior problems. However, it has been used in the treatment of dominance aggression and some stereotypic disorders, with limited success.

Mechanism of action

Buspirone is a potent anxiolytic with a high affinity for 5-HT_{1A} receptors. These receptors are abundant in the parts of the brain that receive projections from the 5-HT neurones of the midbrain raphe. It also binds to dopamine receptors, acting as both an agonist and an antagonist, but this is not thought to contribute to its anxiolytic effect. It has no direct effects on $GABA_A$ receptors and does not produce sedation; however, it does enhance benzodiazepine binding. It does not have anticonvulsant or muscle-relaxant activity and does not impair motor task performance.

The exact mode of action of buspirone is unclear but it is thought to produce its anxiolytic effect by acting as a partial agonist at 5-HT_{1A} receptors pre- and postsynaptically. Buspirone may act presynaptically and inhibit 5-HT release.

Formulations and dose rates

DOGS
- 1.0–2.0 mg/kg PO q.8–24 h

CATS
- 0.5–1 mg/kg PO q.8–24 h

Pharmacokinetics

Buspirone is rapidly absorbed orally but undergoes extensive first-pass metabolism via hydroxylation and dealkylation to form several active metabolites, so that bioavailability is only 4% in humans. One of its active metabolites, 1-(2-pyrimidyl)-piperazine, acts via α_2-

adrenergic receptors to increase the rate of firing of the locus ceruleus, an undesirable effect in anxiety. However, it is not known whether this limits buspirone's efficacy. In humans the half-life of buspirone is 2–4 h. Liver dysfunction decreases its clearance.

Adverse effects

- Bradycardia/tachycardia.
- Nervousness.
- Gastrointestinal disturbances.
- Stereotypic behaviors.
- Restlessness has been reported in humans.
- Caution is needed as treatment can lead to increased aggression as buspirone may decrease the inhibitory effects of fear.

HORMONES

Hormones are chemical messengers produced by endocrine glands and secreted into the bloodstream, where they act on target cells to exert specific effects. Hormonal therapy has been used in the treatment of many behavioral problems but their use is now outdated in most circumstances. The most common hormones used are the progestins and estrogens.

Progestins

EXAMPLES

Medroxyprogesterone acetate (MPA®, Depo-Provera®), megestrol acetate (Ovarid®, Suppress®).

Clinical applications

Synthetic progestins have been used traditionally in veterinary behavioral medicine to treat a variety of problems. It has been claimed that they are effective in the treatment of problems ranging from roaming, sexual perversion, raucous behavior, obsessive barking, destructiveness, hole digging, car chasing, excessive timidity and poultry killing to urine spraying and aggression.

The rationale for treatment was based on the fact that some behaviors are directly affected by male hormones and hence treatment with synthetic progestins may counteract these effects. Additionally, the sedating effects of the progestins may also have been considered useful. However, this treatment approach does not take into account the underlying cause of many of the behaviors treated. It should also be noted that the addition of female hormone may not necessarily mimic the removal of male hormone, so the effect of progestins is not necessarily due to suppression or counteraction of male hormone. Treatment failure is common and the adverse effects of progestins unacceptable. Currently, synthetic progestins should be considered as drugs of last resort, not only because of their many side effects but also because many other medications are available that directly affect the cause of the behavior problem and are therefore more effective clinically.

Progestins may be the drug of choice for some sexually dimorphic behaviors that do not respond to castration. In cats, progestins have been used to successfully treat urine marking, with 42% of cats showing decreased or cessation of spraying. Males respond significantly better than females. The success rate, therefore, is much poorer for females treated with progestins compared to treatment with anxiolytics such as fluoxetine, diazepam or buspirone. However, a similar success rate for progestin versus anxiolytic therapy is reported for males. There have been reports of successful use of progestins in the treatment of intermale aggression.

In dogs, progestins have been used to treat 'dominance' aggression, urine marking, mounting, intermale aggression (6/8 dogs responded) and pseudopregnancy.

Mechanism of action

The 21-carbon synthetic progestins medroxyprogesterone and megestrol are the most closely related pharmacologically and chemically to the natural progestin, progesterone, the precursor of estrogens, androgens and adrenocortical steroids. The physiological effects of the synthetic progestins are similar to those of the other steroid hormones (see Chapter 23).

Progesterone and its metabolites cause nonspecific depression of the CNS, act as nonspecific sedatives and have barbiturate-like activity. They are antiandrogenic and act mainly in the medial preoptic area and the anterior hypothalamus, the areas that control male sexual behavior and urine marking. Progesterone also interferes with synthesis of estrogen receptors and suppresses the production of testosterone in the reproductive tract of intact animals. However, progestins also suppress male-like behavior in castrated cats.

The behavioral and physiological effects of progestins were initially thought to be due to inhibition of 5α-steroid reductase. However, their effects are now thought to be mediated in a number of other ways, including actions on $GABA_A$ receptors to produce effects similar to those of the benzodiazepines.

Formulations and dose rates

DOGS

Megestrol acetate

- 1.1–2.2 mg/kg PO q.24 h for 2 weeks, then one-half dose for next 2 weeks then one-quarter dose for last 3 weeks

Medroxyprogesterone acetate (MPA-50)
- 5–11 mg/kg SC or IM, maximum 3 times per year

CATS

Megestrol acetate
- 2.5–10 mg PO q.24 h for 1 week, then reduce dose to minimum effective dose

Medroxyprogesterone acetate (MPA-50)
- 50 mg (females) 100 mg (males) SC or IM, maximum 3 times per year

Pharmacokinetics
Medroxyprogesterone acetate has a duration of activity of at least 30 days in cats. Megestrol is well absorbed from the gastrointestinal tract, is metabolized in the liver and has a half-life of 8 days in the dog. It is excreted mainly in urine.

Adverse effects
Multiple side effects have been reported and include the following.
- Increased appetite
- Weight gain
- Depression/lethargy
- Mammary gland hyperplasia and carcinoma
- Diabetes mellitus
- Bone marrow suppression
- Endometrial hyperplasia
- Pyometria
- Adrenocortical suppression
- Thinning and increased fragility of the skin

Contraindications and precautions
- Progestins should not be used in intact females, breeding animals and in animals with diabetes mellitus (increases insulin resistance).
- Concurrent corticosteroid use is contraindicated.

α-ADRENERGIC AGONISTS

Sympathomimetic amines produce vasoconstriction by activation of α_1-adrenoreceptors, exerting a powerful effect on skin, mucous membranes, splanchnic, hepatic and renal circulation, with little effect on cerebral and coronary blood flow.

EXAMPLES

Phenylpropanolamine, ephedrine.

Clinical applications
Adrenergic drugs are primarily used in the treatment of urinary incontinence (see Chapter 4). They have also been used as an adjunct in the treatment of urination associated with excitement, submissive urination and nocturnal urination in combination with behavior modification.

In humans, ephedrine is used as a nasal decongestant and in the management of stress incontinence in women.

Mechanism of action
Ephedrine is structurally related to noradrenaline (norepinephrine) and acts primarily through the release of catecholamines. It also has direct effects on α- and β-adrenoreceptors and inhibits MAO. It is a mild CNS stimulant. Ephedrine is nonselective and mimics the affects of adrenaline (epinephrine).

Ephedrine and phenylpropanolamine decrease urinary incontinence by increasing urethral sphincter tone in cases of urethral incompetence.

Formulations and dose rates

Ephedrine

Ephedrine is available in over-the-counter nasal decongestant preparations.

DOGS: 15–50 mg PO q.12 h or 5–15 mg q.8 h

CATS: 2–4 mg/cat PO q.8–12 h

Phenylpropanolamine

Phenylpropanolamine is available in over-the-counter weight reduction preparations.

DOGS: 1.1–4.4 mg/kg PO q.8–12 h

CATS: 12.5 mg PO q.8 h

Pharmacokinetics
In humans a substantial amount of ephedrine is excreted unchanged in urine.

Adverse effects
- Bronchodilation
- Restlessness, excitability, irritability and anxiety
- Hypertension
- Panting
- Anorexia
- Tremors
- Cardiac arrhythmias

Contraindications and precautions
- Concurrent MAOI therapy
- Glaucoma
- Prostatic hypertrophy
- Hyperthyroidism
- Diabetes mellitus
- Cardiovascular disease
- Hypertension

α-ADRENERGIC ANTAGONISTS

> **EXAMPLE**
>
> Nicergoline (Fitergol®).

Clinical applications

Currently one α-adrenergic antagonist, nicergoline, is marketed for use in companion animals. At present it is only registered for use in dogs. It is used in humans for the prevention and treatment of cerebrovascular disorders and arteriosclerotic diseases.

Although not registered for use in cats, nicergoline has been reported to be beneficial for cats that present with behavioral problems associated with aging, such as excessive vocalization and restlessness, especially at night.

Nicergoline has been recommended for dogs showing signs consistent with aging-related behavioral disorders (canine cognitive dysfunction syndrome – CCDS) and cerebral insufficiency of vascular origin. These include alteration in sleep/wake cycles and loss of learned behaviors such as housetraining. It has also been advocated in the treatment of aggression associated with aging. In the author's experience, nicergoline has alleviated these clinical signs in 70% of cases. In addition, the author has successfully used nicergoline in one 12-year-old dog that exhibited behavioral changes, possibly analogous to depression in humans, after the death of its companion dog.

Mechanism of action

Nicergoline belongs to the ergoline group of compounds and has a core structure analogous to that of natural ergot alkaloids. It is an α_1-adrenergic antagonist. In vitro studies demonstrate that it has high affinity for α_1-adrenergic receptors and only minimal affinity for α_2-adrenergic or β-adrenergic receptors.

Nicergoline has a neuroprotective effect (in rat fetuses) by blocking the toxic effects and neuronal damage induced by the vasoconstrictive effects of catecholamines during ischemic episodes. It increases the oxygen supply to the brain by causing vasodilation. Nicergoline also increases oxygen and glucose uptake of brain cells, increases cerebral blood flow, especially in ischemic episodes, stimulates memory and learning and has antithrombotic effects (inhibits platelet aggregation and platelet adhesion to endothelium). Restoration of learned conditioned responses after an hypoxic episode has been demonstrated.

Other reported effects include increased dopamine turnover. Studies have also indicated that nicergoline stimulates the turnover of secondary messengers such as inositol triphosphate, which is purported to be important in learning. This effect is more consistent with long-term use.

> **Formulations and dose rates**
>
> **DOGS**
> - 0.25–0.5 mg/kg PO q.24 h to be given in the morning for at least 30 days. Repeat monthly or as needed
>
> **CATS**
> - 0.25–0.5 mg/kg PO q.24 h in the morning. Repeat monthly or as needed

Pharmacokinetics

Nicergoline is rapidly absorbed after oral administration, with peak plasma levels in dogs attained in 1 h. It is partially metabolized on first pass through the liver and plasma levels appear to stabilize 12–15 d after commencement of treatment in rats.

Adverse effects

No definite adverse effects have been reported in any clinical trials to date. However, there is a single case report of diarrhea, vomiting and tremors in one dog. However, it was not known if this was due to the drug or coincidental.

Known drug interactions

- Nicergoline can be expected to have an additive effect if used concurrently with other vasodilators.
- Treatment should be stopped 24 h before induction of anesthesia with xylazine. Because it is an α-antagonist, nicergoline may interfere with the activity of xylazine, reducing or negating its sedative effects. Alternatively, xylazine may reduce the effectiveness of nicergoline.

PHEROMONES

Pheromones are volatile chemical messengers that are produced in exocrine glands. They are released into the environment by animals to communicate with and alter the behavior of other members of (usually) the same species. Recently, synthetic analogs of pheromones have been used in the treatment of behavior problems in cats and dogs. Pheromones for other species are in development. Cats are believed to use facial pheromones to familiarize themselves with their environment.

> **EXAMPLES**
>
> Feliway®, Dog Appeasement Pheromone® (DAP).

Clinical applications

Feliway® has been advocated for use in cases of urine spraying or anxiety in domestic cats and cheetahs. It has been reported to be help decrease intercat aggression in multicat households (one of the major causes of urine spraying). It can be used alone or concurrently with anxiolytic medication. It has been reported to successfully reduce urine spraying in over 90% of cases. As it does not involve actually medicating the cat (rather, it is applied to the environment), it has proved to be a useful and convenient tool for behavioral modification. The author recommends its use in most cases of anxiety-related problems in cats and where owners are unable to medicate their pet.

Feliway is also recommended to help cats tolerate clinical examinations during a veterinary consultation. Over 70% of veterinarians surveyed in France reported that it was helpful in these circumstances. The author has had considerable success using Feliway in the consultation room, on the examination table and on personnel involved in handling cats, to calm fractious cats.

Other uses include calming cats prior to travel by spraying the cat-carrier prior to placing the cat inside, helping cats to become familiar with a new house and in the introduction of a new cat to the household. Additionally, it appears to be useful in stimulating appetite in hospitalized cats. It has also been reported to help to control undesirable scratching behavior.

It has also been used successfully in catteries, boarding establishments and veterinary hospitals to decrease anxiety and assist cats to familiarize themselves with the novel environment.

Dog Appeasement Pheromone® has been used in dogs in the treatment of noise phobias (fireworks and thunderstorms), separation anxiety, motion sickness and helping puppies settle in to their new home. It has also been used as an adjunct to treatment with other anxiety disorders.

It has also been used successfully in boarding establishments and veterinary hospitals to help decrease anxiety, facilitate handling of dogs and assist dogs to familiarize themselves with the novel environment.

Mechanism of action

To date, five functional fractions of facial secretions of cats have been identified. The F_3 fraction of facial pheromone is thought to inhibit urine marking, enhance feeding in an unknown situation and enhance exploratory behavior in unfamiliar surroundings. The F_4 fraction is said to be an allomarking pheromone, hence familiarizing and calming the cat.

Feliway® contains a synthetic analog of the F_3 fraction of feline facial pheromone, along with a cat attractant (the alcoholic extract of the plant *Valeriana officinalis*).

Dog Appeasement Pheromone® is believed to be the synthetic analog of the appeasing pheromone that the bitch secretes in the first few days after birth which helps the attachment process of mother to pups.

Formulations and dose rates

Feliway®

Spray and diffuser are now available.

Spray: for scratching/urine marking, spray daily at a height of 20 cm (cat nose level) in 6–8 prominent locations per room, including areas that have been marked with urine. Needs to be used continuously for 21 d for scratching, 30 d for urine marking, 45 d for older cats; **for travel**: spray cat carrier 15 min prior to introducing the cat.

Diffuser: needs to be plugged in the room where the cat spends most of its time. One diffuser covers around 50 sq m and lasts approximately 1 month. In multistory houses diffusers need to be placed on each level. The product should be used continuously for 1–3 months initially depending on the problem.

DAP®

Spray, diffuser and collar are now available.

Spray (e.g. for for car travel): spray 8–10 pumps of DAP 15 min before effect is required and before introducing the dog into the car or crate. It can also be sprayed onto a bandana and tied around the dog's neck if the DAP collar is not available.

Diffuser: should be placed in the room where the dog spends most of its time. It should not be placed behind furniture or areas that the dog cannot access as many dogs prefer to lie close to the diffuser. It should not be placed under tables as this will prevent circulation through the room. One diffuser covers approximately 50–70 sq m and lasts around 30 days. In multistory houses a diffuser should be placed on each level. The diffuser should be plugged in continuously for at least 30 days..

Collar: the collar should be fitted firmly on the dog's neck (one finger between collar and neck). Each collars lasts about 1 month.

Adverse effects

- None have been reported, although some clients claim that the alcohol vehicle is irritating.
- Caution should be exercised if there are birds in the environment as they are likely to investigate anything new in the environment by sniffing.

ERGOT ALKALOIDS

EXAMPLE

Bromocriptine.

Clinical applications

Bromocriptine has been used for urine spraying in cats, with a success rate of 85% in treated males and 40% in females. It has also been used for the treatment of pseudocyesis in dogs.

Mechanism of action

Ergot alkaloids are dopamine agonists and inhibit prolactin release from the anterior pituitary gland. However, the mechanism by which bromocriptine reduces urine spraying in some cats is unknown.

Formulations and dose rates

DOGS
- 0.01–0.10 mg/kg once PO or divided twice per 24 h

CATS
- 2–4 mg/cat SC; repeat after 2–4 weeks

However, the injectable formulation is no longer available. Oral dose rates have not been determined.

Pharmacokinetics

Bromocriptine is a dopamine agonist that acts at D_1-receptor sites, particularly in the CNS. It is absorbed from the gastrointestinal tract, reaching a peak plasma level 1–2 h after dosing in humans. It is metabolized in the liver into two main metabolites and excreted in bile and feces. After a single oral dose in humans, mean elimination half-life varied from 2 to 8 h for the parent compound and from 50 to 73 h for the metabolites.

In dogs peak plasma levels are reached 3–5 h after subcutaneous injection and after 10–21 days similar levels are still seen, with total clearance after 60 days post injection. Phenothiazines can counteract the effect of bromocriptine.

Adverse effects

- Bromocriptine can cause vomiting and diarrhea, hypotension, sedation and fatigue in dogs.
- In cats bromocriptine can cause prolapse of the third eyelid and inappetence for the first 2 days of treatment.

LITHIUM

Clinical applications

Lithium is a monovalent cation that is used, particularly for acute mania in humans, as an antidepressant and an antipsychotic. It is used to control the mood swings of bipolar manic depression in humans. Lithium has been used to treat some cases of unpredictable, severe aggression in dogs. However, it has a narrow therapeutic window, so a complete blood count and biochemistry panel, electrocardiogram and thyroid function test should be run prior to commencing treatment. Additionally, regular monitoring of its plasma concentration is required. Lithium is not considered a drug of first choice for these reasons.

Mechanism of action

Lithium's mechanism of action is not understood. However, it is thought that it may act on the second messenger systems, by interfering with either cAMP formation or inisitol triphosphate formation. Its effects on neurotransmitters are complex but it is thought to enhance serotonin transmission and may also affect dopamine, noradrenaline (norepinephrine) and acetylcholine.

Formulations and dose rates

Lithium carbonate

DOGS
- 3–12 mg/kg q.12–24 h

Titrate dose by measuring plasma concentration (range 0.8–1.2 mEq/L).

Pharmacokinetics

Lithium is excreted via the kidneys in two phases, with about half excreted within 12 h and the rest over the next 1–2 weeks in humans. It therefore has a long plasma half-life and narrow therapeutic window. Plasma concentration monitoring is essential.

Adverse effects

- Adverse effects are common and include nausea, vomiting and diarrhea, tremor, polyuria leading to polydipsia, thyroid enlargement and weight gain in humans.
- Acute overdose causes confusion, convulsions, cardiac arrhythmias and death.
- Renal disease and sodium depletion increase the likelihood of lithium toxicity.

Known drug interactions

Diuretics enhance lithium's action and increase the likelihood of toxicity.

XANTHINE DERIVATIVE GLIAL CELL MODULATORS

EXAMPLE

Propentofylline (Vivitonin®, Karsivan®).

Clinical applications

Propentofylline is a neuroprotective glial cell modulator that has proved effective in clinical trials in patients with vascular dementia and those with dementia of the Alzheimer type. Some of the pathological process of Alzheimer's disease, including glial cell activation and increased production of cytokines, free radicals and glutamate, have been shown to be modulated by propentofylline.

Propentofylline has been demonstrated to improve learning and memory deficits induced by β-amyloid protein deposition. In clinical studies in humans it improved cognitive functions as well as global functions. It improves the ability of patients suffering from Alzheimer's disease and vascular dementia to cope with the routine tasks of daily life.

Similar neuropathological changes are found in the brains of senile dogs and in human patients suffering from Alzheimer's disease. In senile dogs a distinctive correlation exists between the quantity of β-amyloid accumulation and the degree of dementia. Propentofylline is recommended to improve dullness, lethargy and overall demeanor in old dogs. It is claimed to increase exercise and activity and decrease sleeplessness in dogs.

Mechanism of action

Propentofylline is a xanthine derivative. It is a selective inhibitor of adenosine uptake and phosphodiesterase that has been shown to be neuroprotective in focal ischemia. It is thought to directly interfere with the neurodegenerative process and reduce the extent of damage to brain structures. In experimental models of vascular dementia and/or Alzheimer's disease it improved cognitive functions, inhibited inflammatory processes and inhibited excessive activation of microglia, formation of free radicals, cytokines and abnormal amyloid precursor proteins (APP). Its effects are thought to be exerted via stimulation of nerve growth factor, increased cerebral blood flow and inhibition of adenosine uptake. It is thought to increase oxygen supply to the brain, inhibit platelet aggregation and make red blood cells more pliable. It also acts as an antiarrhythmic, peripheral vasodilator and diuretic.

Formulations and dose rates

DOGS

- 6–11 mg/kg divided and administered in two equal doses PO

Administer 1 h before feeding for at least 30 days, then continue indefinitely.

Pharmacokinetics

The mean half-life of propentofylline in humans is 0.74 h, with peak concentration after oral administration at about 2.2 h, and it is rapidly metabolized. Although the drug is registered for animal use in some countries, the author was unable to obtain pharmacokinetic information about propentofylline in companion animals.

Adverse effects

In humans adverse effects are mostly minor and transient and affect the digestive and nervous systems. No significant effects were seen on laboratory findings.

FURTHER READING

Crowell-Davis S L, Murray T 2006 Veterinary psychopharmacology. Blackwell, Ames, IA

Katzung BG 1998 Basic and clinical pharmacology. Appleton and Lange, Stanford, CT

Landsberg G, Hunthausen W, Ackerman L 2003 Handbook of behaviour problems of the dog and cat. Butterworth-Heinemann, Oxford

Overall KL 1997 Clinical behavioral medicine for small animals. Mosby, St Louis, MO

Rang HP, Dale MM, Ritter JM, Gardner P 1995 Pharmacology. Churchill Livingstone, New York

8

Antibacterial drugs

Jill E Maddison, A David J Watson and Jonathan Elliott

PRINCIPLES OF ANTIBACTERIAL THERAPY

History

Antibacterial drugs are chemical substances that suppress the growth of microbes and may eventually destroy them. They are produced by either natural fermentation or chemical synthesis. Those derived from substances produced by various microbial species (bacteria, fungi, actinomycetes) are known as 'antibiotics' but not all antibacterial agents are antibiotics: some are produced solely by chemical synthesis, e.g. sulfonamides and fluoroquinolones.

It had long been known that the application of various moldy materials to wounds and infections assisted healing but the possibility that this effect was due to microbes was not recognized until the late 19th century. The observations, developmental work and clinical endeavors of Fleming, Chain and Florey heralded the start of the revolution in antibiosis in the 20th century. But the clinical use of antibiotic agents in effect represents the practical, controlled and directed application of phenomena that occur naturally and continuously in soil, sewage, water and other natural habitats of microbes.

Although Erhlich described the concept of 'magic bullets' for treatment of syphilis in 1909, the modern era of chemotherapy began in 1935 with the clinical use of Prontosil (sulfonamide-chrysoidin). The 'golden age' arrived in 1941 with commercial production and clinical use of penicillin. As a result of subsequent developments, many previously fatal bacterial infections can now be treated successfully but the widespread use of antibacterial agents has resulted in substantial problems, including the emergence and dissemination of drug-resistant pathogens and increasing health-care costs as new drugs are developed to counteract bacterial resistance.

Aims of therapy

The goal of antibacterial therapy is to help the body eliminate infectious organisms without toxicity to the host. It is important to recognize that the natural defense mechanisms of a patient are of primary importance in preventing and controlling infection. Examples of natural defenses against bacterial invasion are:

- the mucociliary escalator in the respiratory tract
- the flushing effect of urination
- the normal flora in the gastrointestinal tract.

All such mechanisms can be affected by disease or therapeutic interventions.

Once microbial invasion occurs, various host responses serve to combat the invading organisms, including:

- the inflammatory response
- cellular migration and phagocytosis
- the complement system
- antibody production.

The difficulty of controlling infections in immunocompromised patients emphasizes that antibacterial therapy is most effective when it supplements endogenous defense mechanisms rather than when acting as the sole means of control.

Adverse effects

Antibacterial agents are not without the potential for toxicity to the host and may cause:

- direct host toxicity (aminoglycosides, peptides)
- toxic interactions with other drugs
- interference with protective effects of normal host microflora (by suppressing obligate anaerobes, for example)
- selection or promotion of drug resistance (see below)
- tissue necrosis at injection sites (tetracyclines)
- impairment of host immune or defense mechanisms (chloramphenicol)
- reduced phagocytosis, chemiluminescence and chemotactic activity of neutrophils (tetracyclines)
- inhibition of phagocytosis (aminoglycosides)
- hypersensitivity reactions (penicillins, sulfonamides)
- hepatic microsomal enzyme induction or inhibition that interferes with their own metabolism as well as that of concurrent medications (chloramphenicol)
- residues in animal products for human consumption (all antibacterials).

Therefore it is imperative that antibacterial agents be used prudently; that is, only when an infectious process is either identified definitively or considered most probably present and the infection is believed likely to progress without medical therapy.

Because of the theoretical and possibly practical potential for some antibacterials to reduce protein production (e.g. aminoglycosides, chloramphenicol, lincosamides, macrolides, tetracyclines), concurrent antibacterial medications need to be selected carefully when immunizing animals, especially with nonadjuvant killed vaccines (which generally induce a lesser immune response than adjuvant killed or attenuated live vaccines).

Selection or promotion of resistance

Although many previously fatal bacterial infections can now be treated successfully with antibacterial drugs, the widespread use of these agents has resulted in other problems, such as emergence of antibacterial-resistant pathogens and the resultant rising health-care costs as new drugs are developed to counteract drug resistance.

Antibacterial agents do not cause bacteria to become resistant but their use preferentially selects resistant populations of bacteria. Some genes that code for resistance have been identified in bacterial cultures established before antibacterial agents were used. Indeed, the ability of micro-organisms to produce antibiotics depends on the presence of mechanisms to overcome their effects. These mechanisms are not infrequently transferable to other organisms.

Antibacterial drug resistance can emerge in various ways, the most clinically important being R (resistance) plasmids. R plasmids are cytoplasmic genetic elements that can transfer drug resistance to previously susceptible bacteria. This can occur between species and genera and may involve genes that impart resistance to various unrelated antibacterial agents.

Acquired resistance is not a problem in all bacterial species. For example, Gram-positive bacteria (with some exceptions, including *Staphylococcus* spp) are often unable to acquire R plasmids (and thus acquire resistance through mutation, a slower process), whereas resistance is an increasing problem in many Gram-negative pathogens such as the Enterobacteriaceae.

The intestine is a major site of transfer of antibacterial resistance. This is particularly important when antibacterial agents are used in animals managed intensively and in contact with fecal material, an enormous reservoir of intestinal bacteria.

Nosocomial infections

In veterinary hospitals, nosocomial infection (infection acquired during hospitalization) by resistant bacteria is an emerging problem, though apparently neither as prevalent nor as serious as that currently experienced in human hospitals. Bacteria most frequently implicated in veterinary hospitals have been *Klebsiella, Escherichia, Proteus* and *Pseudomonas* spp.

Factors predisposing to nosocomial infections include age extremes (young or old), severity of disease, duration of hospitalization, use of invasive support systems, surgical implants, defective immune responses and prior antibacterial drug use.

The drugs with greatest potential to suppress components of the endogenous flora that normally prevents colonization by pathogenic enteric bacteria are those most active against obligate anaerobic bacteria (chloramphenicol, lincosamides, penicillins) and those undergoing extensive enterohepatic recycling (chloramphenicol, lincosamides, tetracyclines). Agents generally lacking this effect include aminoglycosides, fluoroquinolones and sulfonamides with and without trimethoprim. Cephalosporins are a major risk factor for nosocomial enterococcal infection in humans.

Hypersensitivity

Hypersensitivity reactions to antibacterial agents are reported less frequently in veterinary medicine than in human patients, where they constitute 6–10% of all drug reactions. To induce an allergic response, drug molecules must be able to form covalent bonds with macromolecules such as proteins. Bonding with the protein carrier enables reaction with T lymphocytes and macrophages. The reactive moiety is usually a drug metabolite, e.g. the penicilloyl moiety of penicillins and the sulfonamide metabolite hydroxylamine.

- Hypersensitivity reactions depend on the combination of antigen and antibody and are usually not dose related. The first episode cannot be anticipated, although atopic individuals reportedly have a greater tendency to develop drug allergies.
- Hypersensitivity reactions have been reported most frequently in veterinary patients with cephalosporins, penicillins and sulfonamides.
- Doberman pinschers appear to have an increased risk of sulfonamide hypersensitivity, possibly due to delayed sulfonamide metabolism. Other breed predispositions have not been reported.
- The probability of an anaphylactoid reaction (i.e. direct histamine release that is not immunologically mediated) is increased with penicillin preparations containing methylcellulose as a stabilizer.

Drug hypersensitivity may manifest in different ways.

- **Acute anaphylaxis** is associated with IgE-triggered mast cell degranulation and characterized by one or more of the following signs: hypotension, bronchospasm, angioedema, urticaria, erythema, pruritus,

pharyngeal and/or laryngeal edema, vomiting and colic.
- A drug-related systemic allergic reaction may also occur with **deposition of immune complexes** in tissues and activation of complement. Clinical consequences include lymphadenopathy, neuropathy, vasculitis, nephritis, arthritis, urticaria and fever.
- Various hematological perturbations may follow **drug-induced antibody production**, namely hemolytic anemia, thrombocytopenia or rarely neutropenia.
- **Cutaneous reactions** may be caused by immune complex deposition or delayed hypersensitivity.

Allergy to antibacterial agents will only occur if there has been previous exposure to that drug or a related substance (including earlier doses in the current regimen). However, certain anaphylactoid substances in formulations may not require previous exposure to elicit hypersensitivity reactions and these reactions will probably recur every time the drug or related substance is administered. It might not be feasible to confirm this clinically, though, because of concerns of discomfort or danger to the patient.

Treatment of drug hypersensitivity involves discontinuation of the drug and, if anaphylaxis is present, treatment with adrenaline (epinephrine), corticosteroid, antihistamine and intravenous fluids as warranted.

Factors affecting the success of antibacterial therapy

Bacterial susceptibility

Various factors need to be considered in susceptibility testing. The minimum inhibitory concentration (MIC) is the concentration of drug that must be attained at the infection site to achieve inhibition of bacterial replication.

In general, if bacteria are not susceptible to a drug in vitro they will be resistant in vivo. (Exceptions exist: resistance may be overcome by high concentrations achieved in urine or with topical application of some agents.) If a pathogen is sensitive to a drug in vitro the drug *may* be effective in vivo, depending on a variety of pharmacological, host and bacterial factors.

Distribution to the site of infection (pharmacokinetic phase)

To be effective, an antibacterial agent must be distributed to the site of infection and come into contact with the infecting organism in adequate concentrations of the active drug form.

For most, but not all, tissues antibacterial drug distribution is *perfusion limited*.This means that, in tissues with adequate blood supply, free (unbound) drug concentrations achieved in plasma are directly related to or equal to the concentration in the extracellular (interstitial) space. However, drug distribution to the CNS, eye, epithelial lining of the lung (bronchial secretions), prostate and mammary gland is *permeability limited*, as the lipid membrane forms a barrier to drug diffusion (Table 8.1). Contrary to popular belief, most antibacterial drugs reach therapeutically adequate concentrations in bone and synovial fluid, although some drugs achieve higher concentrations in bone than do others.

Bacteria that locate intracellularly (*Bartonella, Brucella, Chlamydophila, Mycobacterium, Rickettsia*) will not be affected by antibacterial agents that remain in the extracellular space. *Staphylococcus* is facultatively intracellular and may sometimes resist treatment because of intracellular survival. Drugs that accumulate in leukocytes and other cells include fluoroquinolones, lincosamides and macrolides but aminoglycosides and β-lactams do not achieve effective intracellular concentrations.

An infectious/inflammatory process often adversely affects the distribution of a drug in vivo. An exception is inflammation of the meninges (meningitis), which reduces the normal barrier between blood and cerebrospinal fluid (CSF), so that antibacterial agents that normally cannot cross this barrier reach the CSF. This breakdown of barriers by inflammation does not occur to an appreciable extent with the blood–prostate barrier and blood–bronchus barrier.

Effective antibacterial concentrations may not be achieved in poorly vascularized tissues, e.g. the extremities during shock, sequestered bone fragments or heart valves.

Favorable environmental conditions

Local factors that restrict access of antibacterial agents to the site of infection include abscess formation, pus and necrotic debris (inactivates aminoglycosides and sulfonamides) and edema fluid. The presence of foreign material in an infected site markedly reduces the likelihood of effective antibacterial therapy; in an attempt to phagocytose and destroy the foreign body, phagocytes degranulate, depleting intracellular bactericidal substances. These phagocytes are then relatively inefficient in killing bacterial pathogens. In addition, foreign material in a wound can protect bacteria from antibacterial drugs and phagocytosis as the bacteria can form a biofilm (glycocalyx) at the site of infection.

Unfavorable environmental conditions may slow bacterial growth, thus rendering them less susceptible to antibacterials like the penicillins and cephalosporins that act by inhibiting cell wall synthesis and require actively dividing cells to exert their bactericidal effects.

These factors highlight the importance of creating an environment conducive to wound healing and anti-

Table 8.1 Physicochemical properties of antibacterial drugs and effects on tissue distribution

Polar (hydrophilic) drugs of low lipophilicity		Drugs of moderate to high lipophilicity			Highly lipophilic molecules with low ionization
Acids	*Bases*	*Weak acids*	*Weak bases*	*Amphoteric*	
β-Lactamase inhibitors Cephalosporins Penicillins	Aminoglycosides – amikacin – gentamicin – neomycin – streptomycin – tobramycin Polymyxins Spectinomycin	Sulfonamides	Lincosamides – clindamycin – lincomycin Macrolides – azithromycin – clarithromycin – erythromycin – spiramycin – tilmicosin – tylosin Trimethoprim	Tetracyclines (except doxycycline, minocycline)	Chloramphenicol Fluoroquinolones – ciprofloxacin – enrofloxacin – marbofloxacin – norfloxacin – orfloxacin Lipophilic tetracyclines (doxycycline, minocycline) Metronidazole Rifampicin
These drugs: • Do not readily penetrate 'natural body barriers' so that effective concentrations are not always achieved in CSF, milk and other transcellular fluids • Adequate concentrations may be achieved in joints, pleural and peritoneal fluids • Penetration may be assisted by acute inflammation • Weak acids (cephalosporins, penicillins) may diffuse into prostate in small concentrations but easily diffuse back to plasma		**These drugs:** • Cross cellular membranes more readily than polar molecules so enter transcellular fluids to a greater extent • Weak bases will be ion-trapped (concentrated) in fluids that are more acidic than plasma, e.g. prostatic fluid, milk, intracellular fluid if lipophilic enough to penetrate (e.g. erythromycin) • Penetration into CSF and ocular fluids is affected by plasma protein binding as well as lipophilicity – sulfonamides and trimethoprim penetrate effectively whereas lincosamides, macrolides and tetracyclines do not, probably due to efflux pumps • Azalides (azithromycin, clarithromycin) have prolonged half-life due to extensive uptake to, and slow release from, tissues. They penetrate phagosomes and phagolysomes well and have extensive tissue distribution as a result of their concentration in macrophages and neutrophils • Tetracyclines do not achieve high concentrations in prostate			**These drugs:** • Cross cellular barriers very readily • Penetrate into difficult transcellular fluids such as prostatic fluid and bronchial secretions • However, chloramphenicol and tetracyclines don't reach high concentrations in prostate • All penetrate CSF except tetracyclines and rifampicin which do not, probably due to efflux pumps • All penetrate into intracellular fluids

Modified from Watson ADJ, Maddison JE, Elliott J 1998 Antibacterial drugs. In: Gorman NT (ed.) Canine medicine and therapeutics, 3rd edn. Blackwell, Oxford: 53–72.

bacterial action, including appropriate surgical drainage and wound cleansing.

Lowered pH and oxygen tension can also adversely affect activity of various antibacterial agents. For example, the lethal action of penicillins depends on autolytic enzyme activity in bacteria that is impaired by low pH. Penicillins in general are not much affected by an acidic environment but activity is diminished in the presence of hemoglobin. Low pH also results in marked loss of activity of erythromycin, clindamycin and fluoroquinolones. An anaerobic environment decreases the effectiveness of aminoglycosides, whereas metronidazole has no activity against aerobic bacteria.

Environmental conditions can be manipulated to enhance antibacterial activity. For example, in lower urinary tract infections it is desirable for urine to be acidic when using tetracyclines and alkaline when using aminoglycosides.

The ability of a molecule to penetrate membranes increases with decreasing electrostatic charge; thus antibacterial drugs that are weak acids work best in an acidic environment and those that are weak bases work best in an alkaline environment.

High lipid solubility (see Table 8.1) will facilitate penetration of antibacterial drugs generally, including into devitalized tissue and phagocytic cells.

Client compliance

As with all drug therapy, antibacterials will not be effective unless administered correctly to the patient. As discussed in Chapter 1, it is important to maximize the likelihood that a client will administer drugs at the right dose and dosing interval. Undesirable consequences of poor compliance include inadequate response to treatment, increased costs and creation of doubt in the client's mind about the effectiveness of the drug and the clinician. Strategies to enhance client compliance are discussed in Chapter 1.

Factors influencing the clinician's choice of antibacterial drug

Antibacterial agents should only be used if a bacterial infection has been diagnosed definitively or is strongly suspected and the natural course is considered likely to be progressive without medical therapy. It is irrational to prescribe antibacterials for every clinical problem and in lieu of a diagnosis. Although ideally culture and susceptibility testing should be performed before initiating antibacterial therapy, this is often not practical for economic reasons. If possible, the clinician should perform a Gram stain on exudate, urine or an aspirate from the infected site to determine if Gram-positive or Gram-negative bacteria are present. But financial and time constraints in practice may even preclude this. The clinician should then choose a drug based on the organisms most likely to be pathogens at that site (see Table 8.2). If therapy fails or the infection immediately recurs once therapy has ceased, culture and susceptibility testing are strongly recommended.

The clinician should also consider possible involvement of other factors that can impair therapy, such as the presence of urinary calculi or a foreign body, lack of appropriate surgical drainage, impairment of body defense mechanisms or an underlying nonbacterial etiology. In these circumstances, even a well-chosen antibacterial drug may be ineffective unless additional measures are taken.

Regardless of whether drugs are selected on the basis of susceptibility testing, smear examination or deduction, it is often apparent that a number of drugs are potentially effective against the pathogen. Several factors should be considered in choosing from these alternatives.

- **The width of antibacterial spectrum.** Drugs that are more selective are generally to be preferred as they are less likely to disrupt the normal microflora. Furthermore, habitual reliance on broad-spectrum antibacterial agents indicates a low standard of diagnosis on the part of the clinician.
- **Bactericidal versus bacteriostatic activity.** Bactericidal drugs are often favored because they may be more effective when host defenses are impaired but there is probably little difference in efficacy between bactericidal and bacteriostatic drugs for treating noncritical infections in otherwise healthy patients.
- **Cost.** The cost of some drugs may preclude their use, especially in large dogs. It may then be necessary to choose a cheaper alternative despite possibly lower efficacy. This decision should be made in consultation with the client.
- **Toxicity.** Most of the antibacterial drugs in common use are relatively safe when correct dosages are employed. However, one should be aware of the potential for adverse effects of any drug used, e.g. sulfonamide hypersensitivity in dobermans, gentamicin nephrotoxicity, the gastrointestinal effects of erythromycin. Also, be aware of measures that may ameliorate adverse reactions, such as giving doxycycline orally with food.
- **Intercurrent disease.** The presence of kidney or liver disease may increase toxic risks with some drugs, either because they further damage these organs or because impaired excretion or metabolism allows the drug or its metabolites to accumulate to toxic levels.
- **Pregnant or neonatal patients.** Particular care may be necessary in these patients because of known or suspected adverse effects and the necessity to individualize dose regimens accordingly.

Route of administration of antibacterial agent

Often there is a choice of routes of administration, although some drugs (such as aminoglycosides) must be given parenterally if systemic activity is desired. Other factors influencing route selection include the characteristics of the disease being treated, likely treatment duration, the patient's temperament and owner's capability.

- **Topical administration** is valuable for disorders of eye and ear and some skin or gut infections. High drug concentration may be achieved locally in this way and some drugs too toxic for routine systemic administration (bacitracin, neomycin, polymyxins) can be useful topically.
- **Oral administration** is adequate in most infections and is usually preferable for home treatment. Some owners find it easier to administer drugs orally with food but the potential adverse effects of ingesta on systemic drug availability should be considered (Table 8.3). If in doubt, administration on an empty stomach (no food for 1–2 h before and after dosing) is recommended, as the most common outcome of drug–ingesta interactions is impaired systemic drug availability.
- **Parenteral administration** is not routinely advantageous but can be useful for fractious, unconscious or vomiting patients, or those with oral/pharyngeal/esophageal pain or dysfunction. Intramuscular (IM)

Table 8.2 Suggested antibacterial drug selection for canine and feline infections

Diagnosis	Common organisms (less common)	Suggested drugs
Pyoderma, pustular dermatitis		
Dogs	*Staphylococcus* (secondary *Escherichia, Proteus, Pseudomonas*)	Amoxicillin-clavulanate, cephalosporin, cloxacillin/flucloxacillin
Cats	*Streptococcus, Pasteurella, Staphylococcus*	Amoxicillin-clavulanate, lincosamide, doxycycline, cephalosporin
Bite wounds, traumatic and contaminated wounds		
Dogs	*Staphylococcus, Streptococcus, Pasteurella*, anaerobes	Amoxicillin-clavulanate, cephalosporin
Cats	Anaerobes, *Pasteurella, Actinomyces*	Penicillin G, clindamycin, doxycycline, amoxicillin, cephalosporin
Anal sac inflammation, abscessation		
	Escherichia, Enterococcus, (*Clostridium, Proteus*)	Amoxicillin-clavulanate, chloramphenicol, sulfonamide-trimethoprim
Otitis externa		
	Staphylococcus, Malasezzia, Pseudomonas, Proteus	Topical: aminoglycoside, polymyxin, fluoroquinolone, chloramphenicol, ticarcillin
Otitis media, otitis interna		
	Staphylococcus, Pseudomonas, Proteus	Amoxicillin-clavulanate, fluoroquinolone, chloramphenicol, ticarcillin
Conjunctivitis		
Dog	*Staphylococcus, Streptococcus, Escherichia, Proteus*	Topical: neomycin-polymyxin-bacitracin, chloramphenicol, gentamicin
Cats	Viruses, *Chlamydophila, Mycoplasma*, 2° bacteria	Tetracycline, chloramphenicol
Infectious tracheobronchitis		
Dogs	*Bordetella*, viruses, secondary bacteria (*Mycoplasma?*)	Sulfonamide-trimethoprim, doxycycline, chloramphenicol
Bacterial pneumonia*, pyothorax*		
Dogs	Single or mixed Gram-negative aerobes and/or anaerobes	Amoxicillin-clavulanate, fluoroquinolone + metronidazole
Cats	Various anaerobes, *Pasteurella*, other Gram-negative aerobes, *Actinomyces*	Amoxicillin-clavulanate, fluoroquinolone + metronidazole
Periodontitis, gingivitis, ulcerative stomatitis		
	Anaerobes and mixed aerobes	Penicillin G, amoxicillin, metronidazole ± spiramycin, doxycycline, clindamycin
Small intestine bacterial overgrowth/antibiotic-responsive diarrhea		
	Escherichia, Enterococcus, Staphylococcus, Clostridium	Tetracycline, tylosin, metronidazole
Cholecystitis, cholangitis		
Dogs	*Escherichia, Salmonella*, anaerobes	Amoxicillin-clavulanate, chloramphenicol, fluoroquinolone + metronidazole
Cats	Coliforms	Amoxicillin-clavulanate, chloramphenicol, fluoroquinolone
Lower urinary tract infection, pyelonephritis*		
Dogs	*Escherichia, Proteus, Staphylococcus, Streptococcus, Klebsiella, Pseudomonas, Enterobacter*	Amoxicillin-clavulanate, sulfonamide-trimethoprim, cephalosporin, fluoroquinolone
Prostatitis		
Dogs	*Escherichia, Proteus, Staphylococcus, Streptococcus, Klebsiella, Pseudomonas, Enterobacter*	Sulfonamide-trimethoprim, fluoroquinolone
Mastitis*		
	Escherichia, Staphylococcus, Streptococcus	Chloramphenicol, amoxicillin-clavulanate, fluoroquinolone
Osteomyelitis*		
	Staphylococcus (possibly with *Streptococcus, Escherichia, Proteus, Pseudomonas*, anaerobes)	Amoxicillin-clavulanate, lincosamide, cloxacillin/ flucloxacillin, fluoroquinolone, cephalosporin
Discospondylitis		
	Staphylococcus (*Streptococcus, Aspergillus*)	Cloxacillin/flucloxacillin, lincosamide, cephalosporin, amoxicillin-clavulanate
Septic arthritis*		
	Staphylococcus, Streptococcus (anaerobes, coliforms)	Cloxacillin/flucloxacillin, amoxicillin-clavulanate
Septicemia*, bacterial endocarditis*		
	Various aerobes or anaerobes	Fluoroquinolone + penicillin G or metronidazole, gentamicin + cephalosporin or cloxacillin/flucloxacillin
Toxoplasmosis		
	Toxoplasma gondii	Clindamycin, sulfonamide + pyrimethamine
Feline infectious anemia		
	Mycoplasma haemofelis (formerly *Haemobartonella felis*)	Doxycycline, enrofloxacin

'Anaerobes' here signifies bacterial species that are obligate anaerobes, while 'aerobes' denotes aerobic and facultatively anaerobic bacteria. Culture and susceptibility testing should be performed, if possible, prior to initiating therapy for those conditions marked by * and in all other conditions if initial empirical antimicrobial therapy is unsuccessful.

Table 8.3 Suggested administration of oral antibacterial drugs in dogs in relation to feeding[a]

Category	Drugs or drug groups
Better when fasting Drug absorption may be impaired by ingesta. Fasting means no food for at least 1–2 h before and 1–2 h after dosing	Azithromycin Cefradine Most erythromycin preparations Most fluoroquinolones[b] Lincomycin Most penicillins# Rifampicin Most sulfonamides Most tetracyclines
Better with food Drug availability is improved, or gastrointestinal upsets are reduced by ingesta	Cefadroxil Chloramphenicol palmitate (in cats) Doxycycline* Ibafloxacin Metronidazole* Nitrofurantoin*
No restriction needed	Cefalexin Chloramphenicol capsules and tablets Chloramphenicol palmitate (in dogs) Clarithromycin Clindamycin Hetacillin Spiramycin

[a] Data from human studies except: cefadroxil, cefalexin, chloramphenicol, clarithromycin, enrofloxacin, ibafloxacin, penicillins.
[b] Enrofloxacin availability is reduced by ingesta in dogs. Effects of ingesta on fluoroquinolones are generally mild but absorption may be delayed slightly; avoid dairy foods.
Effect on amoxicillin is mild.
* Food may reduce gut irritation without hindering absorption importantly.

or subcutaneous (SC) administration may be equally satisfactory in these instances. The intravenous (IV) route should be considered if maximum plasma drug concentrations are desired immediately after dosing, as with life-threatening infections, or in shocked or hypotensive patients where poor tissue perfusion may impede drug absorption after administration by other routes.

Dosage and frequency of administration

Dosing regimens for commonly used antibacterial drugs are suggested in Table 8.4 and are based on the mode of action of each drug (concentration or time dependent), the susceptibility of the target pathogen and the pharmacokinetics of the drug. The ideal regime may vary with the case, depending on the susceptibility of the pathogen, tissue penetration of the drug and degree of immunocompetence of the patient. Smaller doses may suffice in lower urinary tract infections using drugs excreted in high concentration in urine but larger or more frequent doses may be required for relatively resistant pathogens or infections in areas where drug penetration is poor.

Assessment and duration of therapy

In acute infections, it is usually evident within 2–3 days whether treatment is having the desired effect. An inadequate response should prompt re-evaluation of the diagnosis and treatment. If underdosing or poor tissue penetration is suspected, an increased dose rate and/or frequency of administration of the same drug might be appropriate. Otherwise, selection of a different drug is warranted. For the majority of uncomplicated and acute infections in dogs and cats, treatment for 4–5 days up to a week seems adequate.

With chronic infections, it may take longer to determine whether treatment is being effective and prolonged administration is usually required. This can be explained by existing tissue damage, impaired blood supply and compromised local immunity. Treatment for 4–6 weeks or more is generally required when bacterial infections are chronic. Similarly prolonged treatment is also advised for pyoderma, prostatitis, pyelonephritis, recurrent lower urinary tract infections, septic arthritis, osteomyelitis, septicemia, pneumonia, bacterial endocarditis and antibiotic-responsive diarrhea.

Combination antibacterial therapy

Combination antibacterial therapy is only indicated in certain specific circumstances (except sulfonamide-trimethoprim and β-lactam plus β-lactamase inhibitor). Bacteriostatic and bactericidal drugs should not generally be used in combination. The disadvantages of combination chemotherapy include increased cost and increased risk of toxicity.

The primary indications for using combinations include:

- mixed bacterial infections
- to delay emergence of resistance in certain specific circumstances
- severe infections where the etiology is unknown (ensure selected drugs are compatible)
- life-threatening infections prior to availability of susceptibility data
- unusual pathogens, including *Mycobacterium*, *Rhodococcus* and fungi.

Examples of antibacterial combinations sometimes used in small animal practice include: a fluoroquinolone with metronidazole (capable of penetrating difficult body barriers and efficacy against Gram-negative aerobes, obligate anaerobes, penicillinase-producing *Staphylococcus*, most Gram-positive aerobes except *Streptococ-*

Table 8.4 Dosage regimens for antibacterial drugs in dogs and cats

Drug	Route	Dose
Penicillins		
Narrow spectrum		
Penicillin G, Na, K	IV, IM, SC	20,000–40,000 U/kg q.6–8 h
Penicillin G, procaine	IM, SC	20,000 U/kg q.12–24 h
Penicillin G, benzathine	IM	40,000 U/kg every 3–5 days
Penicillin V	PO	10 mg/kg q.8 h
Antistaphylococcal		
Cloxacillin, flucloxacillin	PO	10–40 mg/kg q.6–8 h
Dicloxacillin	PO	10–40 mg/kg q.8 h
Aminopenicillins		
Amoxicillin	PO, IV, IM, SC	10–20 mg/kg q.8–12 h
Ampicillin	IV, IM, SC, PO	10–20 mg/kg q.6–12 h
Amoxicillin-clavulanate (e.g. *Synulox®*, *Clavulox®*)	PO, IM, SC	12.5–25 mg/kg q.8–12 h
Antipseudomonal		
Carbenicillin	IV, IM, SC	50 mg/kg q.6–8 h
Ticarcillin	IV, IM, SC	50–75 mg/kg q.6–8 h Infusion: 15–25 mg/kg given over 15 min, then at constant rate of 7.5–15 mg/kg/h
Ticarcillin-clavulanate (*Timentin®*)	IV	Dogs: 40–110 mg/kg IV q.6–8 h Cats: 40–75 mg/kg IV q.6–8 h
Cephalosporins and cephamycins		
First generation		
Cefachlor	PO	10–25 mg/kg q.8–12 h
Cefadroxil (e.g. *Cefa-Tabs®*)	PO	10–30 mg/kg q.8–12 h
Cefalexin (e.g. *Keflex®*, *Ceporex®*)	PO	Dogs: 20–40 mg/kg q.8–12 h Cats: 22–50 mg/kg q.8–12 h
Cefazolin	IV, IM	10–30 mg/kg q.4–8 h
Cefapirin	IV, IM, SC	10–30 mg/kg q.6–8 h
Second generation		
Cefotetan	IV	30 mg/kg q.6–8 h
Cefoxitin	IV, IM, SC	10–30 mg/kg q.6–8 h
Cefuroxime (*Zinacef®*)	IV, IM, SC	20–50 mg/kg q.8–12 h
Third generation		
Cefixime	PO	5–12.5 mg/kg q.12 h
Cefotaxime	IV, IM, SC	20–80 mg/kg q.6–8 h
Cefovecin (*Convenia®*)	SC	8 mg/kg (repeated every 14 days depending on indication)
Cefpodoxime proxetil (*Simplicef®*)	PO	5–10 mg/kg q.12–24 h
Ceftazidime	IV, IM	20–50 mg/kg q.8–12 h
Ceftiofur (*Naxcel®*)	SC	2.2–4.4 mg/kg q.12–24 h
Ceftriaxone	IV, IM	15–50 mg/kg q.12–24 h
Third generation antipseudomonal		
Cefoperazone	IV, IM	22 mg/kg q.6–12 h
Aminoglycosides		
Amikacin	IV, IM, SC	10 mg/kg q.8 h
Gentamicin	IV, IM, SC	6 mg/kg q.24 h
Neomycin	PO	10 mg/kg q.6 h
Streptomycin	PO IM, SC	20 mg/kg q.6 h 10 mg/kg q.12 h
Tobramycin	IV, IM, SC	1–2 mg/kg q.8 h
Fluoroquinolones		
Ciprofloxacin	PO	5–15 mg/kg q.12 h
Difloxacin	PO	5–10 mg/kg q.24 h
Enrofloxacin	PO, IM, SC	Dogs: 2.5–10 mg/kg q.12 h Cats: 2.5–5.0 mg/kg q.12 h
Ibafloxacin	PO	2–5 mg/kg q.24 h
Norfloxacin	PO	5–20 mg/kg q.12 h
Marbofloxacin	PO	2.75–5.5 mg/kg q.24 h
Orbifloxacin	PO	2.5–7.5 mg/kg q.24 h

Table 8.4 Dosage regimens for antibacterial drugs in dogs and cats (*continued*)

Drug	Route	Dose
Tetracyclines		
Chlortetracycline	PO	20 mg/kg q.8 h
Doxycycline	PO, IV	5–10 mg/kg q.12 h
Minocycline	PO	5–15 mg/kg q.12 h
Oxytetracycline	PO	20 mg/kg q.8 h
	IV, IM	10 mg/kg q.12 h
Tetracycline	PO	20 mg/kg q.8 h
	IV, IM	10 mg/kg q.12 h
Azalides, lincosamides and macrolides		
Clindamycin (e.g. *Antirobe*®)	PO, IV, IM, SC	Dogs: 10–20 mg/kg q.12 h
		Cats: 12.5–25 mg/kg q.12 h (the higher dose is needed for toxoplasmosis, in most other infections 50 mg/cat is adequate)
Lincomycin	PO	10–20 mg/kg q.8–12 h
	IV, IM	10 mg/kg q.12 h
Erythromycin	PO	10–20 mg/kg q.8–12 h
Tylosin (e.g. *Tylan*®)	PO	10 mg/kg q.8 h
	IV, IM	5–10 mg/kg q.12 h
Azithromycin	PO	Dogs: 10 mg/kg q.24 h
		Cats: 5 mg/kg q.24–48 h
Clarithromycin		2.5–10 mg/kg q.12 h
Sulfonamides		
Sulfadiazine-trimethoprim	PO, IV, IM, SC	30 mg/kg q.12–24 h
Sulfadimethoxine-ormetoprim	PO	50 mg/kg loading, 25 mg/kg q.24 h
Miscellaneous		
Chloramphenicol	PO, IV, IM, SC	Dogs: 50 mg/kg q.8 h
		Cats: 50 mg/cat q.12 h
Clofazimine	PO	Dogs: 4–8 mg/kg q.24 h
		Cats: 4–8 mg/kg q.24 h or 25–50 mg/cat q.24 h
Florfenicol	IM, SC (not IV)	25–50 mg/kg q.8 h
Furazolidone	PO	2.2–20 mg/kg q.8–24 h
Metronidazole	PO	10–20 mg/kg q.12–24 h
Nitrofurantoin	PO	4 mg/kg q.6–8 h
Rifampicin (Rifampin)	PO	10–20 mg/kg q.12 h (max. 600 mg daily)

cus and several atypical bacteria); an aminoglycoside plus amoxicillin-clavulanate (efficacy against Gram-negative aerobes, obligate anaerobes, penicillinase-producing *Staphylococcus* and Gram-positive aerobes but with some limitations in penetrating difficult body barriers); an antipseudomonal penicillin such as ticarcillin or piperacillin, plus an aminoglycoside such as gentamicin, to delay the emergence of resistance when treating pseudomonal infections.

Adjunctive treatments

Many bacterial infections are not cured by systemic antibacterial drug therapy alone and require additional specific or supportive measures.

- Fluid therapy may be crucial to correct acid–base imbalances, tissue perfusion deficits and dehydration and to maintain the patient while antibacterial therapy is undertaken.
- Surgery may be needed to remove infected implants, sequestra, necrotic tissue, calculi or foreign material or to establish drainage from the site.
- In lower urinary tract infections the antibacterial activity of the selected drug may be improved by modifying the urine pH, using sodium bicarbonate orally for alkalinization or ammonium chloride orally for acidification.
- Fever is common in more severe infections and may benefit the patient by inhibiting proliferation of pathogens. Antipyretic treatment is usually not warranted and may obscure the natural course of the disease or the response to antibacterial treatment. On the other hand, sustained hyperthermia exceeding 41°C can be detrimental and warrants intervention (cool baths, cool water enemas) to quickly reduce body temperature to safe levels.
- Glucocorticoid administration is potentially deleterious in animals with sepsis because it may suppress the host's defenses and mask signs of infection.

Nonetheless, in some circumstances administering a shorter-acting glucocorticoid (such as hydrocortisone) topically or prednisolone systemically for a few days can help by suppressing an acute inflammatory response that may be causing pain or discomfort and provoking self trauma, as with skin or ear infections.

Prophylactic antibacterial treatment

Prophylactic antibacterials in surgery

Perioperative prophylactic use of antibacterial drugs in surgery is not indicated for routine, clean surgery where no inflammation is present, the gastrointestinal, reproductive or respiratory systems have not been invaded and aseptic technique has not been broken.

Perioperative antibacterial prophylaxis is indicated after dental procedures in which there has been bleeding (almost all), patients with leukopenia (viral, drug-induced), contaminated surgery and surgery where the consequences of infection would be disastrous (e.g. orthopedic), there is major tissue trauma (e.g. major thoracic and abdominal surgery) or the surgical time exceeds 90 min.

If antibacterial agents are used prophylactically, they should be administered before the procedure so that adequate concentrations are present in blood and tissue at the time of surgery; for maximum effect the drug must be present in the wound when bacterial contamination occurs. IV administration 20–30 min prior to surgery is currently recommended as this gives the highest tissue concentrations at the time of surgery. Timings of initial and subsequent doses of perioperative antibiotics depend on the pharmacokinetics of the selected drug in the patient undergoing anesthesia and concomitant fluid therapy. The advantages of perioperative antibacterial prophylaxis are minimal if the drug is first administered any later than 3–5 h after contamination.

Note that acute toxicity on cardiovascular or neuromuscular function is most likely after IV administration and drugs should be injected slowly. Anesthetic and sedatives agents may interact to increase the likelihood of adverse reactions; β-lactams are the safest drugs in this respect.

The drug chosen should be appropriate in relation to the likely contaminating pathogen. In small animal practice this may include penicillinase-producing *Staphylococcus* (from the patient or the surgeon), so that nonpotentiated penicillins such as amoxicillin are not suitable. If contamination by intestinal bacteria is suspected or confirmed, drugs that are effective against obligate anaerobes and Gram-negative aerobes should be chosen (see Fig. 8.25).

Chemoprophylaxis is not usually continued for longer than 24 h post surgery and in some institutions a postoperative dose of antibacterial is only administered if surgery time exceeds 90 min.

Other prophylactic uses of antibacterial agents

Prophylactic use of antibacterial agents has been important in controlling certain infectious diseases, primarily in intensively managed production animals. Metaphylaxis refers to treating the whole group when only a proportion shows clinical signs.

Potential disadvantages include:

- toxicity
- encouragement of selection of drug resistance
- residues in edible animal products
- cost.

Principles of successful prophylaxis include the following.

- Medication should be directed against a specific pathogen or disease condition.
- Target organism should be one that does not readily develop drug resistance.
- Duration should be as short as possible consistent with efficacy.
- Should only be used where efficacy is clearly established.
- Dosage should be the same as used therapeutically.

CLASSIFICATION OF ANTIBACTERIAL DRUGS

Bactericidal versus bacteriostatic

Antibacterial agents are often described as bacteriostatic or bactericidal. However, this classification only really applies under strict laboratory conditions, is inconsistent against all bacteria and becomes more arbitrary in clinical cases.

Bacteriostatic drugs

Bacteriostatic drugs (chloramphenicol, lincosamides, macrolides, sulfonamides, tetracyclines, trimethoprim) temporarily inhibit the growth of organisms but the effect is reversible once the drug is removed. For these drugs to be clinically effective, the drug concentration at the site of the infection should be maintained above the MIC throughout the dosing interval. Many bacteriostatic drugs can be bactericidal if drug exposure is sufficiently high or prolonged. Although traditionally bacteriostatic drugs have been avoided in serious infections, evidence from human studies suggests that clindamycin, a bacteriostatic drug, might be preferred for the treatment of staphylococcal and streptococcal infections as it inhibits the toxic shock syndrome that can occur when bactericidal drugs are used.

Bactericidal drugs

Under ideal laboratory conditions, bactericidal drugs (aminoglycosides, cephalosporins, fluoroquinolones, metronidazole, penicillins, potentiated sulfonamides) cause the death of the microbe. These are preferred in infections that cannot be controlled or eradicated by host mechanisms, because of the nature or site of the infection (e.g. bacterial endocarditis) or because of reduced immunocompetence of the host (e.g. patient with immunosuppressive illness or receiving immunosuppressive therapy). However, successful clinical outcomes are reported in humans with Gram-positive meningitis, endocarditis and osteomyelitis treated with bacteriostatic drugs such as clindamycin. For Gram-positive infections, the susceptibility of the organism and the ability of the drug to penetrate and concentrate in infected tissue are often more important predictors of a successful clinical outcome than whether the drug is bactericidal or bacteriostatic.

Bactericidal drugs are further classified as time-dependent or concentration-dependent drugs. **Time-dependent drugs** (penicillins and cephalosporins) are slowly bactericidal. Plasma levels should be above MIC for as long as possible during each 24-hour period although no strict guidelines on the exact percentage of time required have been established. For these drugs there is little or no advantage (regarding proportion of pathogens killed or duration of postantibiotic effect) in achieving a peak plasma concentration (C_{max}) greater than 2–4 times MIC.

For **concentration-dependent drugs** (aminoglycosides and fluoroquinolones) the peak concentration achieved (aminoglycosides, fluoroquinolones) and/or the area under the plasma concentration versus time curve (fluoroquinolones) predicts antibacterial success. For these drugs the higher the peak plasma concentration:

- the greater the proportion of target bacteria killed
- the longer the postantibiotic effect.

For this second group the C_{max}/MIC ratio is predictive of treatment success; optimal regimens achieve a ratio greater than 8 : 1.

Classification based on mechanism of action

Major categories of antibacterial agents exert their antibacterial action through one of four mechanisms.

- Inhibition of cell wall synthesis – bacitracin, cephalosporins, penicillins, vancomycin
- Inhibition of cell membrane function – polymyxins
- Inhibition of protein synthesis – aminoglycosides, chloramphenicol, lincosamides, macrolides, tetracyclines
- Inhibition of nucleic acid synthesis or prevention of repair – fluoroquinolones, metronidazole, rifampicin, sulfonamides, trimethoprim

Classification based on antibacterial spectrum

The veterinary student and clinician cannot hope to remember all details of antibacterial activity for each antibacterial drug. However, it is useful to have a reasonable understanding of the broad patterns for each drug class, particularly where drug classes are invariably inactive against particular groups of bacteria. For example, aminoglycosides and those fluoroquinolones currently available are inactive against obligate anaerobes while some narrow-spectrum penicillins (e.g. penicillin G, aminopenicillins) are inactive against penicillinase-producing *Staphylococcus* spp.

The term broad spectrum has traditionally ignored obligate anaerobes, resulting in confusion in the minds of practitioners about the spectrum of various drugs relevant to clinical infections. An alternative approach is to consider the activity of antibacterial drugs on the basis of their activity against four groups of bacterial pathogens: Gram-positive aerobes, Gram-negative aerobes, Gram-positive anaerobes and Gram-negative anaerobes. However, this is not particularly helpful in small animal practice as (a) Gram-negative and Gram-positive anaerobes do not differ greatly in their antibacterial susceptibility and any differences are difficult to predict, and (b) this classification ignores the differences in susceptibility pattern between penicillinase-producing *Staphylococcus* spp and other Gram-positive aerobes. Therefore antibacterial drugs are discussed here in relation to activity against the following four quadrants:

- Gram-positive aerobes
- *Staphylococcus* spp (in small animal medicine most clinically relevant infections are penicillinase producing)
- Gram-negative aerobes
- obligate anaerobes.

Note that in this context, the term aerobe includes the many bacteria that are facultative anaerobes such as the Enterobacteriaceae family (*E. coli* et al), *Pasteurella* and Vibrioaceae family.

The general spectrum of activity of each drug class is depicted in the text in the section entitled 'Antibacterial spectrum' as illustrated in Figure 8.1. The patterns shown here reflect the susceptibility of broad bacterial groups to the drugs as they are used clinically, i.e. they reflect acquired resistance patterns in addition to the intrinsic susceptibility of the organisms.

In addition, there are the atypical bacterial species which do not Gram stain and fall outside the above classification. These include *Bartonella, Chlamydophila, Mycobacterium, Mycoplasma* and *Rickettsia*.

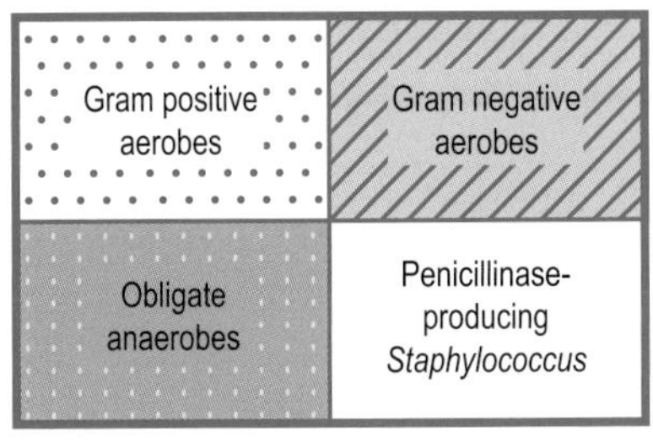

Excellent activity against most, although not necessarily all, pathogens in this quadrant

Good activity against many pathogens in this quadrant but some important pathogens may be resistant

Moderate activity against pathogens in this quadrant–unpredictable resistance patterns

No useful activity against most pathogens in this quadrant, although there may be some individual exceptions–refer to individual drug information

Fig. 8.1 **Antimicrobial spectrum chart and key.**

β-LACTAM ANTIBIOTICS

PENICILLINS

Mechanism of action

Penicillin G is derived from various *Penicillium* molds. Discovery of the penicillin nucleus, 6-aminopenicillanic acid, led to production of various semisynthetic penicillins. Those penicillins have been synthesized in an attempt to improve the spectrum, activity and stability of the parent compound. Many of the newer penicillins are modifications of ampicillin. For example, substitution of a carboxy group for the amino group of ampicillin on the acyl side chain produced carbenicillin and ticarcillin.

Bacteria differ from animal cells by possessing a rigid outer layer, the cell wall. The bacterial cell possesses an unusually high internal osmotic pressure. Injury to the cell wall or inhibition of its synthesis may result in cell lysis. The peptidoglycan component of the cell wall is essential to the integrity of the bacterial envelope. It consists of alternating units of *N*-acetylglucosamine and *N*-acetylmuramic acid, crosslinked by short strands of peptides. Almost all bacteria have cell membrane-binding proteins called penicillin-binding proteins (PBP). The PBPs are enzymes (transpeptidases, carboxypeptidases, endopeptidases) involved in the terminal stages of assembling the cell wall by crosslinking the peptidoglycan layer and reshaping the cell wall during growth and division. Binding of transpeptidase PBPs causes inhibition of peptidoglycan synthesis. The final step in the action of β-lactams probably involves inactivation of an inhibitor of autolytic enzymes in the cell wall.

Penicillins are structural analogs of D-alanyl-D-alanine and bind with high affinity to those PBPs involved in cell wall synthesis. However, other PBPs act as β-lactamases and thus inactivate penicillins and cephalosporins. Bacteria have 3–6 PBPs and different PBPs possess different affinities for different drugs. The antibacterial activity of each β-lactam is dependent on its ability to bind one of the PBPs that form or maintain cell wall structure while avoiding destructive PBPs. PBPs are under chromosomal control and mutations can alter their number and affinity for different β-lactam drugs. The antibacterial spectrum of any penicillin depends primarily on its stability against bacterial β-lactamases but also its ability to reach the PBP on the cell membrane and its binding affinity for the target PBP.

Differences in susceptibility of Gram-positive and Gram-negative bacteria to penicillins result from structural differences in cell walls, differences in receptor sites (PBPs) and binding affinity for the target PBP, the relative amount of peptidoglycan present (Gram-positive bacteria possess far more) and to the different types of β-lactamase produced by bacteria. In Gram-negative bacteria the outer portion of the cell wall is a lipopolysaccharide and lipoprotein bilayer membrane, which may hinder the passage of drugs through the cell wall. All penicillins tend to be ionized at physiological pH so will not diffuse through the lipid bilayer of the Gram-negative outer membrane. The large hydrophobic groups on the narrow-spectrum penicillins (e.g. penicillin G) hinder their passage through the porins in most Gram-negative outer membranes. Substitution with more hydrophilic amino groups (e.g. ampicillin, amoxicillin) in place of the benzyl group allows the molecule to penetrate this barrier and so broadens the spectrum of activity. In contrast, Gram-positive organisms have a thin outer layer exterior to the peptidoglycan layer, which β-lactams can rapidly penetrate.

Penicillins affect growing cells and have little influence on those that are dormant, so they should not be administered with bacteriostatic agents. The antibacterial action of penicillin is greatest during the periods of rapid bacterial multiplication. Penicillins (and cephalosporins) are time-dependent killers; thus the time for which plasma concentrations remain above MIC is the best predictor of treatment success and frequent dosing or depot formulations are therefore required.

Mechanisms of resistance

Resistance to β-lactams is mediated by induced β-lactamase production or by intrinsic means. β-lactamases are a diverse group of enzymes that hydrolyze the cyclic amide bond of the β-lactam ring and render it inactive. They were isolated from bacteria before β-lactam antibiotics were developed commercially and therefore have intrinsic activity in the bacteria.

The β-lactamases are generally secreted extracellularly in large amounts by Gram-positive bacteria; relatively small quantities are strategically produced in the periplasmic space in Gram-negative bacteria. Bacteria that produce β-lactamases include *Enterobacter*, *Escherichia, Klebsiella, Proteus, Pseudomonas* and *Staphylococcus*,

Different bacteria produce different types of β-lactamase. Staphylococcal β-lactamase is called penicillinase. Production of β-lactamases is widespread among common Gram-negative primary and opportunistic pathogens.

In Gram-positive bacteria, especially *Staphylococcus*, resistance to penicillin G is mediated mainly by production of penicillinases that are plasmid mediated and excreted extracellularly as inducible exoenzymes. Penicillinase is induced during treatment, which may explain treatment failure in a patient with a strain of *Staphylococcus intermedius* that is sensitive to penicillin in vitro.

The inherent resistance to penicillin G of many Gram-negative bacteria results from low bacterial permeability, lack of PBPs and various β-lactamase enzymes. In Gram-negative bacteria, β-lactamase may be chromosomally mediated or plasmid-mediated and may be inducible or constitutive (i.e. part of the normal make-up of the organism). Plasmid-mediated β-lactamase causes high-level resistance whereas those that are chromosomally mediated are present at low levels and only sometimes contribute to resistance. Resistance may also occur by production of an impermeable outer membrane through mutations in the porin structure. *Pseudomonas,* for example, is innately resistant to most penicillins because the porins in its outer membrane are small and very difficult for many drugs to pass through.

Efforts to overcome bacterial resistance caused by β-lactamase production proceed along two lines. One seeks to modify the β-lactam nucleus so that the antibiotic is stable in the presence of penicillinase; cloxacillin is an example of this. The other searches for substances that inhibit β-lactamase and can be coupled with the penicillin (or cephalosporin) to protect the drug from destruction by β-lactamases; clavulanic acid and sulbactam, two products of this approach, are discussed later in this chapter.

Pharmacokinetics

Penicillins in general:

- are able to achieve concentrations adequate to kill or inhibit susceptible bacteria in most tissue fluids, though high doses may be required to obtain adequate concentrations in joint, pleural and peritoneal cavities
- are generally excluded from CNS, prostate and eye
- are charged at physiological pH and lipid insoluble, so do not readily enter living cells
- show enhanced entry across biological membranes and through blood–brain and blood–CSF barriers in the presence of inflammation (this does not apply to the prostate or blood–bronchus barrier)
- may reach concentrations in inflamed tissues that exceed plasma concentrations
- undergo minimal hepatic metabolism, except for ampicillin
- are eliminated by glomerular filtration and renal tubular secretion: 60–100% of drug is excreted in urine unchanged, resulting in very high concentrations in urine. Urine:plasma ratios are of the order of 200–300:1
- cross the placenta slowly
- are not all stable in gastric acid; some have to be given parenterally
- may have their systemic availability after oral administration delayed and/or reduced by ingesta (e.g. with cloxacillin and ampicillin but less so with amoxicillin)
- have a time-dependent mode of bacterial killing, so that plasma concentrations should be maintained above the MIC of the pathogen for as long as possible throughout the dosing interval.

Adverse effects

- Penicillins in general have a very wide therapeutic ratio as mammalian cells do not possess a cell wall. Most toxic effects are related to hypersensitivity, usually immediate in onset. This may manifest as local reactions at the site of injection (swelling, edema, pain) or systemic reactions such as urticaria and skin rashes or anaphylaxis and collapse. Hypersensitivity reactions have been recorded in most domestic species and can be fatal. They are much less common after oral administration. If an animal is allergic to one form of penicillin it will react to other forms.
- Penicillins can induce gastrointestinal superinfection in many species in which fermentation in the cecum is an important part of the digestive process. Thus penicillins should never be given to guinea-pigs, ferrets, rabbits and hamsters by any route.
- Many of the acute reactions to penicillins reported in animals are in fact due to the toxic effects of the potassium or procaine with which the penicillin has been combined. Potassium penicillin G should be injected slowly. At high doses, procaine injected IM can cause nervous excitement (ataxia, excitability,

seizures), particularly in horses. The risk is greater if there has been some dissociation of procaine from penicillin. Procaine benzylpenicillin (procaine penicillin) should be stored in the refrigerator (high temperatures increase dissociation), should not be used past the expiry date and repeated use of the same injection site should be avoided.

Known drug interactions

- Penicillins are often said to be synergistic with aminoglycosides against many Gram-positive bacteria except those showing high-level aminoglycoside resistance. Such synergism may even be seen with penicillinase-producing *Staphylococcus aureus*.
- Narrow-spectrum penicillins such as penicillin G are synergistic with drugs that bind β-lactamase enzymes, including cloxacillin, clavulanate and some cephalosporins.

CLASSES OF PENICILLINS

Narrow-spectrum penicillins

EXAMPLES

Benzylpenicillin (penicillin G), phenoxymethyl-penicillin (penicillin V), phenethicillin (semisynthetic).

Antibacterial spectrum (Fig. 8.2)

- Narrow-spectrum penicillins are active specifically against Gram-positive aerobes, facultative aerobes and obligate anaerobes.
- They are ineffective against most Gram-negative aerobes and facultative anaerobes, except possibly *Escherichia* and *Klebsiella* at the high concentrations achieved in urine.
- They are active against several fastidious Gram-negative bacteria (which grow on blood agar or enriched medium but not on McConkey agar), including *Pasteurella* (isolates from small animals but not from farm animals) and *Haemophilus*.

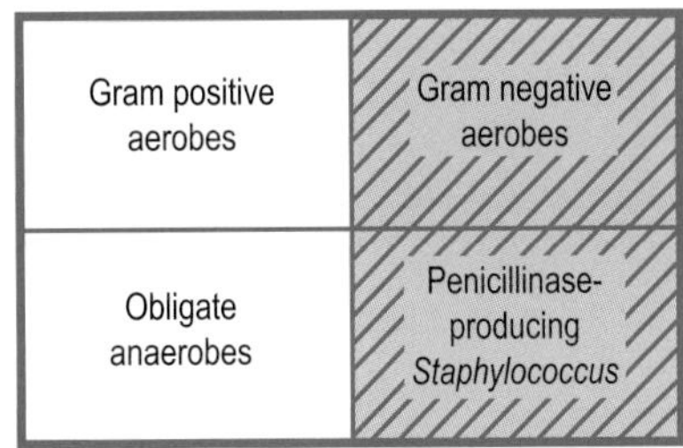

Fig. 8.2 **Antibacterial spectrum for narrow-spectrum penicillins.**

- They have good activity against all obligate anaerobes except β-lactamase producing strains of *Bacteroides*.
- Most *Staphylococcus intermedius* isolates (the common 'staph' in dogs and cats) are now resistant.
- *Actinobacillus*, *Borrelia*, *Brucella*, *Haemophilus* and *Leptospira* are moderately susceptible although this may vary due to acquired resistance.
- Enterobacteriaceae (including *Proteus*), *Bacteroides fragilis*, *Bordetella*, most *Campylobacter* and *Nocardia* are resistant.

Clinical applications

Conditions for which a narrow-spectrum penicillin is still the drug of choice in small animals include clostridial diseases, listeriosis, actinomycosis, anaerobic infections (abscess, fight wound, pyothorax) and β-hemolytic streptococcal infections.

Route of administration

Oral

- Penicillin G is rapidly hydrolyzed by gastric acid, resulting in only 20–30% absorption (though may still give therapeutic urinary concentrations against susceptible organisms if adequate doses are given).
- Penicillin V is more acid stable, resulting in 40–50% absorption.
- Phenethicillin is resistant to gastric acid hydrolysis.

Parenteral

- Penicillin G is complexed with sodium or potassium salts for parenteral administration. This gives high concentrations of short duration with IV administration and lower concentrations of longer duration after IM administration.
- Penicillin G is complexed with procaine or benzathine for IM administration. Both formulations result in incomplete and delayed absorption of the penicillin component. The availability of penicillin from procaine formulations is greater than from benzathine formulations.
- Plasma and tissue concentrations with procaine penicillin G are satisfactory for 12–24 h for most penicillin-sensitive organisms.
- Benzathine penicillin persists for up to 7 days but only organisms that are very sensitive to penicillin will be inhibited by the low tissue concentrations achieved. The persistence of drug residues at the injection site has led to problems in setting safe withdrawal periods for this formulation for food-producing animals and it has disappeared from many European markets.
- The international standard unit used in some forms of penicillin is 1 mg penicillin G = 1667 IU.

Antistaphylococcal penicillins

EXAMPLES

Cloxacillin, dicloxacillin, flucloxacillin, methicillin, oxacillin.

Antibacterial spectrum (Fig. 8.3)

- The spectrum of the antistaphylococcal penicillins is similar to the natural narrow-spectrum penicillins (although potency is less than that of penicillin G) except that they are resistant to staphylococcal β-lactamase.
- They have no activity against Gram-negative bacteria.
- Unlike natural penicillins, they have little activity against enterococci (*Enterococcus faecalis* and *E. faecium*).
- Activity against anaerobes is variable; for example, *Clostridium* are susceptible to cloxacillin but *Bacteroides* are not.

Clinical applications

- Staphylococcal skin infections in dogs
- Surgical prophylaxis, especially for orthopedic procedures
- Treatment of osteomyelitis, discospondylitis

Route of administration

Antistaphylococcal penicillins other than methicillin can be given orally, although some inactivation by gastric acid does occur. They are best given on an empty stomach. Methicillin is rarely used in domestic animals.

Aminopenicillins

EXAMPLES

Amoxicillin, ampicillin, hetacillin.

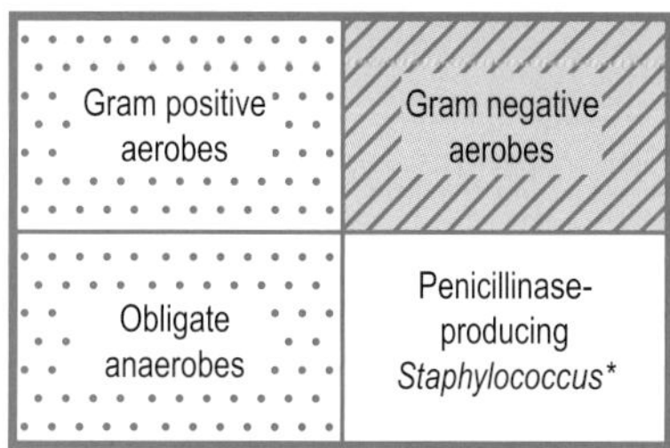

Fig. 8.3 **Antibacterial spectrum for antistaphylococcal pencillins.**

Antibacterial spectrum (Fig. 8.4)

- The aminopenicillins were developed in the 1960s as broad-spectrum penicillins. They are slightly less active against Gram-positive and anaerobic bacteria than penicillin G but have greater activity against Gram-negative bacteria. Enhanced Gram-negative activity is due to increased binding affinity to PBP1b and PBP3 and enhanced ability to penetrate the outer cell membrane of many Gram-negative species.
- Emergence of many resistant strains of Gram-negative bacteria and increasing prevalence of *Klebsiella pneumoniae, Pseudomonas aeruginosa* and *Enterobacter* spp as pathogens (which are intrinsically nonsusceptible to aminopenicillins) mean that their classification as broad-spectrum antibacterial drugs is now misleading.
- Aminopenicillins are as sensitive to hydrolysis by Gram-positive or Gram-negative β-lactamases as penicillin G and therefore are not active against penicillinase-producing *Staphylococcus* or Gram-negative bacteria that produce β-lactamases.

Clinical applications

- The relatively high prevalence of acquired resistance has limited the role of nonpotentiated aminopenicillins in small animal practice.
- They are used for soft tissue infections in dogs and cats provided *Staphylococcus* is not suspected to be involved.
- They are useful for treating cat abscesses.
- Treatment of uncomplicated urinary tract infections can be successful as such high concentrations of drug are achieved in urine but amoxicillin-clavulanate might be a better choice.
- Aminopenicillins may also be useful in some enteric infections.
- Amoxicillin in combination with metronidazole and omeprazole has been used for treatment of *Helicobacter* gastritis.
- Aminopenicillins should not be used for surgical prophylaxis as *Staphylococcus* are common pathogens.

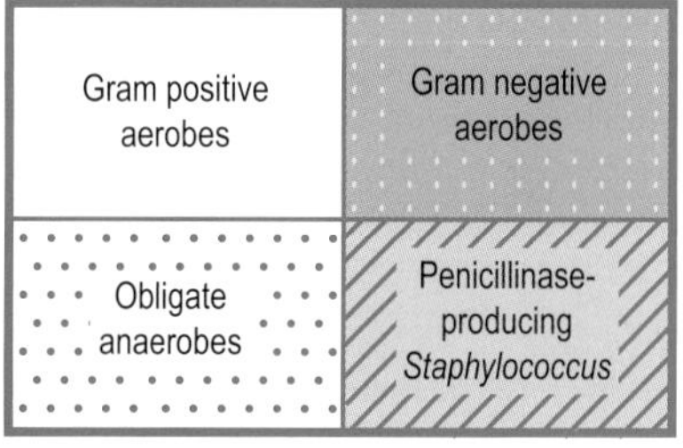

Fig. 8.4 **Antibacterial spectrum for aminopenicillins (nonpotentiated).**

Route of administration

Aminopenicillins are acid stable and may be given orally. However, ampicillin absorption is affected by food (30–50% decrease in bioavailability). Amoxicillin is less affected (20% decrease) but some studies suggest that food delays absorption, so it is probably best given on an empty stomach.

Adverse effects

Broad-spectrum penicillins have greater potential to disturb normal flora than the narrow-spectrum penicillins because they undergo biliary excretion and have activity against obligate anaerobes. However, despite widespread use of these drugs, there is little evidence of adverse effects in dogs and cats.

Antipseudomonal penicillins

EXAMPLES

Carboxypenicillins (carbenicillin, ticarcillin), ureidopenicillins (azlocillin, mezlocillin, piperacillin).

Antibacterial spectrum (Figs 8.5, 8.6)

- The antipseudomonal penicillins were developed to improve the Gram-negative spectrum of penicillin, particularly against *Pseudomonas aeruginosa*. Increased activity against these organisms is achieved through increased binding affinity for PBP3 and improved penetration through the bacterial cell wall.
- Most *Klebsiella, Citrobacter* and *Serratia* and all *Enterobacter* enterococci are resistant.

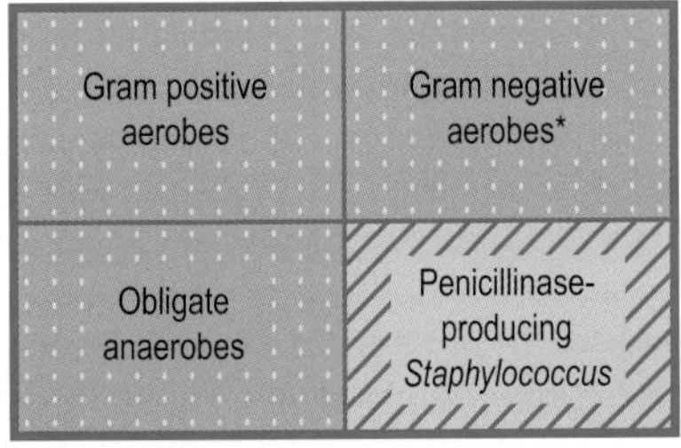

*excellent activity against P. aeruginosa

Fig. 8.5 Antibacterial spectrum for carbencillin and ticarcillin.

Gram positive aerobes	Gram negative aerobes*
Obligate anaerobes	Penicillinase-producing *Staphylococcus*

*excellent activity against Pseudomonas

Fig. 8.6 Antibacterial spectrum for piperacillin.

- Ticarcillin is less active than azlocillin and piperacillin. It has a similar spectrum to carbenicillin but is 2–4 times more active against *P. aeruginosa.*
- Azocillin, mezlocillin and piperacillin are described as extended-spectrum antipseudomonal penicillins. This results from their interaction with PBPs other than those that bind aminopenicillins as well as their resistance to some species-specific chromosomal β-lactamases and increased penetration of Gram-negative bacteria. They have greater activity against Gram-negative bacteria, particularly *Klebsiella* and *P. aeruginosa,* than carbenicillin as well as increased activity against *Bacteroides fragilis.*
- Piperacillin is more active than azocillin and mezocillin. It inhibits over 95% of *P. aeruginosa* isolates and many Enterobacteriaceae and is active against many anaerobes.
- Antipseudomonal penicillins are susceptible to staphylococcal β-lactamase and to some common Gram-negative β-lactamases. Ticarcillin is available in various markets in combination with a clavulanate salt which extends its activity against β-lactamase producing *Staphylococcus* and Gram-negative bacteria.
- Combined use with an aminoglycoside is recommended in any serious pseudomonal infection to delay emergence of resistance and increase bacterial kill, as a degree of immunosuppression is often present in these patients.

Clinical applications

- The most common veterinary application for these drugs is topical treatment of otitis externa due to *P. aeruginosa* resistant to other drugs.
- They may also be used for systemic treatment infections by *Pseudomonas* spp, usually in combination with an aminoglycoside to delay the emergence of resistance.
- When combined with clavulanate (see below), ticarcillin is effective against many β-lactamase producing strains of otherwise resistant Gram-negative bacteria and *Staphylococcus.*

Route of administration

Carbenicillin, ticarcillin and piperacillin must be given parenterally and high doses are required. Ticarcillin and piperacillin can also be dissolved and used aurally to treat otitis externa caused by *Pseudomonas.*

β-LACTAMASE INHIBITORS

Clavulanic acid

Mechanism of action

Clavulanic acid is a β-lactam drug (the first natural β-lactam containing oxygen ever identified) that has little intrinsic antibacterial activity but irreversibly binds and inactivates many different β-lactamases. It is a natural product of *Streptomyces clavuligerus*. It readily penetrates Gram-positive and Gram-negative bacteria. The potassium salt is used in drug formulations.

Mechanisms of resistance

Emergence of resistance to clavulanic acid has not been reported as a clinical problem in bacteria isolated from animals. However, a variety of resistance mechanisms have emerged in human bacterial isolates.

Antibacterial spectrum (Figs 8.7, 8.8)

- Addition of clavulanate to amoxicillin and, more recently ticarcillin (a human-approved formulation only), enhances the in vitro spectrum of activity of these drugs considerably.
- Amoxicillin-clavulanate, in contrast to amoxicillin alone, has activity against penicillinase-producing *Staphylococcus* and has enhanced activity against Gram-negative pathogens.
- Most anaerobes, including *Bacteroides fragilis*, are susceptible.
- Susceptibility of some *Escherichia* and *Klebsiella* can be variable because of poor penetration.
- *Enterobacter*, *Citrobacter*, *Pseudomonas aeruginosa*, *Serratia* and methicillin-resistant *Staphylococcus* are resistant.

Gram positive aerobes	Gram negative aerobes
Obligate anaerobes	Penicillinase-producing *Staphylococcus**

* MRSA are resistant

Fig. 8.7 Antibacterial spectrum for amoxicillin-clavulanate.

Gram positive aerobes	Gram negative aerobes
Obligate anaerobes	Penicillinase-producing *Staphylococcus**

* MRSA are resistant

Fig. 8.8 Antibacterial spectrum for ticarcillin-clavulanate.

Clinical applications

- Amoxicillin-clavulanate has many applications in small animal practice because of its broad spectrum and excellent activity against *Staphylococcus*. It is often the drug of first choice for infections in skin, soft tissue and urinary tract and for surgical prophylaxis.
- A combination of ampicillin and sulbactam (another β-lactamase inhibitor) is available in some countries and has similar uses.
- Ticarcillin-clavulanate is effective against many β-lactamase producing strains of otherwise resistant Gram-negative bacteria and also *Staphylococcus*. However, treatment outcomes in human infections have been disappointing, possibly because of induction of β-lactamases by the clavulanate component.
- The indication for ticarcillin-clavulanate is usually for systemic treatment of susceptible *Pseudomonas aeruginosa* infections resistant to other less expensive and more convenient antibacterials.

Route of administration

- Amoxicillin-clavulanate can be given PO (tablets or drops), IM or SC. Some SC injections have been associated with tissue reactions such as sterile abscess formation.
- Ampicillin-sulbactam is given IM or SC.
- Ticarcillin-clavulanate is administered IV.

Pharmacokinetics

Clavulanate is well absorbed orally and absorption is unaffected by ingesta. It penetrates poorly into milk and CSF (in the absence of significant inflammation) and poorly across the blood–prostate and blood–bronchus barriers (regardless of the degree of inflammation). Excretion is primarily by glomerular filtration, producing high clavulanate concentrations in urine. Formulations for use in dogs and cats provide 1.25 mg potassium clavulanate for every 5 mg of amoxicillin. The half-life of clavulanate is shorter than amoxicillin because of extensive metabolism.

Special considerations

Clavulanate is highly moisture sensitive, so precautions must be taken to ensure dryness, including the use of dry syringes for injection.

CEPHALOSPORINS AND CEPHAMYCINS

Mechanism of action

Cephalosporins were developed from cephalosporin C, a natural product of *Cephalosporium acreminium*. Cephamycins are related drugs derived from *Streptomyces* spp or are synthetic derivatives. These antibacterials are related structurally to benzylpenicillin and have a β-lactam ring. Like penicillins, they inhibit cell wall synthesis by preventing cross-linking of peptidoglycan. However, unlike many penicillins, cephalosporins are resistant to β-lactamase produced by *Staphylococcus* spp. By convention, cephalosporins discovered before 1975 were spelled with a 'ph' and those discovered after 1975 with an 'f' but the recommended international nonproprietary names have been changed now so that they are all spelled with an 'f'.

Mechanisms of resistance

Resistance to cephalosporins can occur due to reduced permeability, enzymatic inactivation or absence of specific PBPs. Constitutive and acquired resistance caused by periplasmic β-lactamases against the different cephalosporins defines the different cephalosporin classes.

Extracellular expression of β-lactamases and efflux pumps has to some extent limited the use of the newer cephalosporins in human medicine. Outbreaks of resistant nosocomial infections have occurred in hospitals. Some mutants have altered outer membrane permeability as well as drug pump efflux activity and may show cross-resistance to aminoglycosides, chloramphenicol, fluoroquinolones, tetracyclines and trimethoprim. Plasmid-mediated acquired resistance has also been described.

Classification of cephalosporins

Cephalosporins are divided into first-, second-, third- and fourth-generation groups plus antipseudomonal cephalosporins (Table 8.5). Some of the drugs listed in Table 8.5 are actually cephamycins (e.g. cefoxitin, cefotetan, latamoxef) but they are included there as cephalosporins because they have very similar properties.

All groups include drugs that can be given parenterally and oral preparations are also available for most first-generation and a few third-generation drugs.

Spectrum of activity (Figs 8.9–8.11)

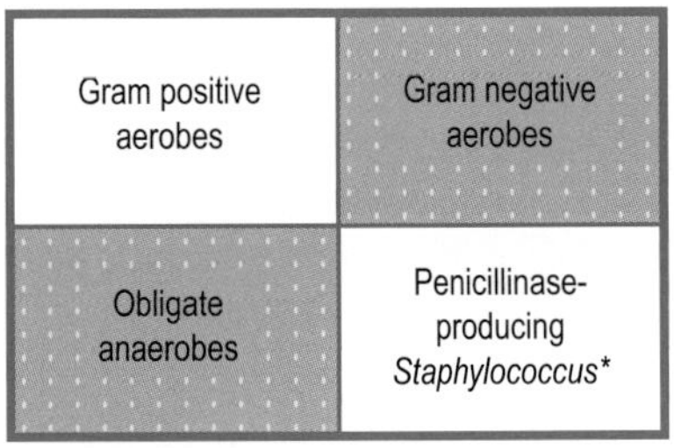

Gram positive aerobes	Gram negative aerobes
Obligate anaerobes	Penicillinase-producing *Staphylococcus**

* MRSA are resistant

Fig. 8.9 Antibacterial spectrum for first-generation cephalosporins.

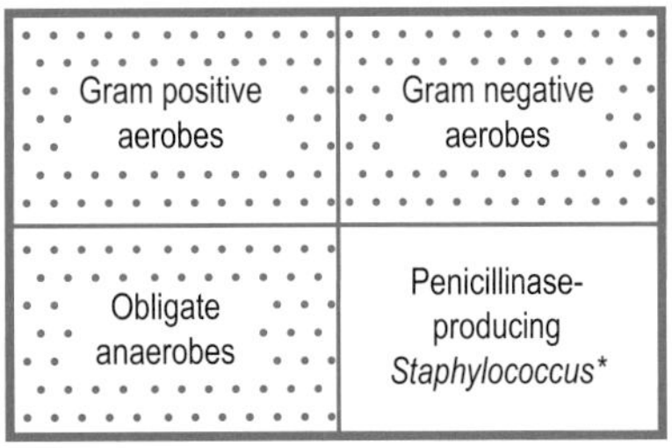

Gram positive aerobes	Gram negative aerobes
Obligate anaerobes	Penicillinase-producing *Staphylococcus**

* MRSA are resistant

Fig. 8.10 Antibacterial spectrum for second-generation cephalosporins.

Gram positive aerobes	Gram negative aerobes
Obligate anaerobes	Penicillinase-producing *Staphylococcus**

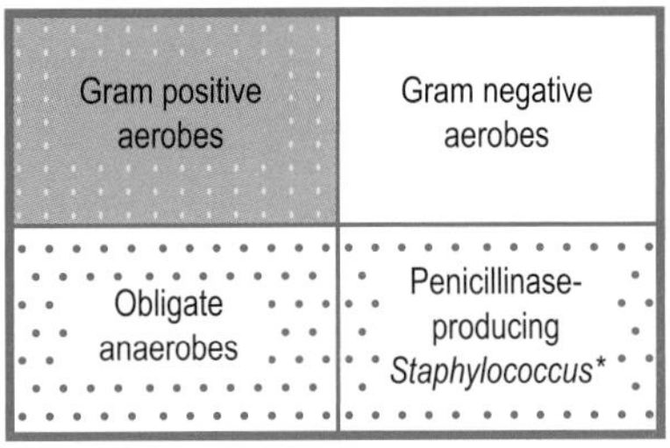

* Varies from moderate to good depending on individual drug
MRSA are resistant

Fig. 8.11 Antibacterial spectrum for third-generation cephalosporins.

Clinical applications

First-generation

- Skin infections caused by *Staphylococcus*
- Soft tissue infections due to susceptible organisms
- Urinary tract infections (but not prostate)
- Osteomyelitis
- Discospondylitis
- Bacterial conjunctivitis (cefalonium)

Second-generation

- Similar to orally active cephalosporins in dogs and cats.
- In human medicine and some veterinary institutions, the human-approved formulation cefuroxime is used for surgical prophylaxis, particularly for orthopedic surgery because of good activity against appropriate opportunistic pathogens.

Third-generation

- Because of cost, availability of cheaper alternatives and the potential to select for resistant bacteria, third-generation cephalosporins should be reserved in small animal practice for serious infections caused by Gram-negative aerobic and facultatively anaerobic bacteria, especially Enterobactericaceae.
- They may also be indicated for the treatment of urinary tract infections caused by otherwise resistant bacteria.

Table 8.5 Classification and spectrum of activity of cephalosporins

Generation	Drugs	Spectrum
First-generation	*Parenteral* Cefacetrile Cephalothin Cefapirin Cefazolin Cefradine *Oral* Cefadroxil Cefalexin Cefaloglycin Cefradine *Ophthalmic* Cefalonium	The antibacterial spectrum of the first-generation cephalosporins is similar for all drugs within this group. Their only major advantages over aminopenicillins are their excellent activity against penicillinase-producing *Staphylococcus* and generally greater activity against *Pasteurella* • Good activity against Gram-positive bacteria including β-lactamase producing *Staphylococcus* • Methicillin-resistant *Staphylococcus* are resistant • Moderate activity against Gram-negative aerobes • Resistant bacteria of clinical importance include *Bordetella, Campylobacter, Pseudomonas aeruginosa* and *Rhodococcus equi* • Acquired resistance common among Gram-negative bacteria, particularly Enterobacteriaceae, but rare in Gram-positive bacteria • Activity against obligate anaerobes unpredictable and less than for most penicillins
Second-generation (all parenteral)	Cefaclor Cefamandole Cefotetan Cefoxitin Cefuroxime	*Moderate Gram-positive and Gram-negative activity* • Moderately active against Gram-positive bacteria • Broader activity against Gram-negative bacteria than first-generation cephalosporins but not *Pseudomonas aeruginosa* • Most of the group have only moderate activity against obligate anaerobes except cefoxitin which has excellent activity
Third-generation	*Parenteral* Cefmenoxime Cefotaxime cefquinome Ceftiofur Ceftizoxime Ceftazidime Ceftriaxone Cefovecin Latamoxef *Oral* Cefetamet Cefixime Cefpodoxime proxetil	*Decreased Gram-positive but increased Gram-negative activity* • Good activity against many Gram-positive bacteria including *Streptococcus* but not *Enterobacter* • The parenteral drugs have moderate–good activity against *Staphylococcus* but oral agents are largely inactive • Susceptible Gram-negative bacteria include *Escherichia, Klebsiella, Proteus, Pasteurella, Haemophilus, Actinobacillus, Salmonella* • Activity against *Proteus* and *Pseudomonas* varies between drugs • Variable activity against obligate anaerobes – *Clostridium* and *Fusobacterium* are susceptible but *Bacteroides* are often resistant to some but not all drugs (e.g. cefovecin has good activity)
Third-generation antipseudomonal (all parenteral)	Cefoperazone Cefsulodin Ceftazidime	• High activity against *Pseudomonas aeruginosa* • Otherwise generally less active than other third-generation drugs
Fourth-generation (all parenteral)	Cefepime Cefpirome	*Increased Gram-positive and Gram-negative activity* • High activity against Enterobacteriaceae • Moderate activity against *Pseudomonas aeruginosa* • Enhanced activity against *Staphylococcus* • *Enterococcus* resistant • Variable resistance amongst obligate anaerobes – *Clostridium perfringens* susceptible, *Bacteroides* and *Clostridium difficile* resistant

- Ceftriaxone's long half-life, good CNS penetration and activity against *Borrelia burgdorferei* have made it a potential choice for treating Lyme disease.
- There are currently no indications for the use of ceftiofur in small animals, although it is used increasingly in large animal practice because of its zero drug withdrawal time. It is used extensively to treat acute undifferentiated bovine pneumonia, neonatal septicemia in foals, respiratory and systemic infections in swine and to control *Escherichia* infections in poultry.

There are no approved human formulations of ceftiofur but the impact on bacterial resistance of widespread use of a third-generation cephalosporin in food-producing animals may be of concern.

- Cefovecin (*Convenia*®) is registered in some markets for use in canine skin and soft tissue infections associated with *Staphylococcus intermedius*, β-hemolytic streptococci, *Escherichia* and *Pasteurella multocida*; canine urinary tract infections associated with *Escherichia* and Proteus spp; feline skin and soft tissue infections associated with *Pasteurella multocida*, *Fusobacterium* spp, *Bacteroides* spp, *Prevotella oralis*, β-hemolytic streptococci and *Staphylococcus intermedius*; and feline urinary tract infections associated with *Escherichia.*

Antipseudomonal parenteral cephalosporins

- These drugs are used in human medicine to treat septicemias caused by *Pseudomonas* and other Gram-negative pathogens in neutropenic patients.
- They have had limited use to date in veterinary medicine but cefoperazone could be useful in small animal practice to treat serious infections, especially against Enterobacteriaceae such as *Pseudomonas aeruginosa,* not susceptible to less expensive agents or if aminoglycosides are excluded due to potential toxicity.

Fourth generation

- Uses in human medicine include treatment of nosocomial or community-acquired lower respiratory tract infections, bacterial meningitis and urinary tract infections.
- As they have particular value in human therapeutics, they are unlikely to be used much in domestic animals in the near future.

Pharmacokinetics

The pharmacokinetic features and toxicity of the cephalosporins and cephamycins are similar to those of penicillins except that they cross the placenta well. In addition, they can be used in patients that are hypersensitive to penicillins although about 5% of human patients show cross-reactivity between cephalosporins and penicillins.

They are primarily excreted by the kidney (with a few exceptions). Some penetrate the CSF well but not the orally active drugs. Elimination is relatively rapid for most except cefovecin.

Oral cephalosporins

The pharmacokinetic features of the oral cephalosporins are similar to those of aminopenicillins. They are rapidly and largely absorbed after oral administration in dogs and cats, though poorly and erratically absorbed in horses and ruminants. Effects of ingesta on systemic availability vary (see Table 8.2).

Cephalosporins are largely confined to extracellular fluids and pass poorly across biological membranes, although inflammation enhances passage across some membrane barriers.

Most orally active cephalosporins have short half-lives (usually less than 1 h) and are excreted largely unchanged in urine.

Parenteral cephalosporins

Most parenteral cephalosporins are rapidly and well absorbed after IM or SC injection. IV formulations are licensed for human but not veterinary use.

Most half-lives are short (usually less than 1 h) and excretion is largely renal, although some hepatic metabolism occurs for some of these drugs. The exception is cefovecin which has a very long elimination half-life following subcutaneous administration. Half-life at the registered dose is 5.5 days in dogs and 6.9 days in cats. The antimicrobial activity of cefovecin following a single injection lasts up to 14 days.

Other routes

Cefalonium (Cepravin®) is available in some markets as an ophthalmic ointment for treatment of bacterial conjunctivitis in dogs and cats. It is available as an intramammary in the treatment of mastitis in cattle.

Adverse effects

- Adverse reactions to cephalosporins are uncommon. Allergic reactions are rare and in humans 95% of allergic reactions are not cross-reactive with penicillin.
- Vomiting and diarrhea may occur in monogastric animals; administering the drug with a meal may alleviate this.
- While it has been demonstrated that cephalosporins, particularly cefalothin, have the potential to cause nephrotoxicity, the risk of this adverse effect appears minimal when conventional dosages are given to patients with normal renal function.
- Some of these drugs (cefamandole, cefoperazone, latamoxef) have been implicated in causing bleeding problems in humans. The significance of this for animal patients is unclear as veterinary use of these drugs is limited but caution would seem advisable in patients receiving anticoagulant therapy or those with warfarin-type rodenticide toxicity.
- In vitro, cephalosporins have synergistic or additive activity with aminoglycosides against some bacteria including Enterobacteriaceae such as *Pseudomona aeruginosa*. However, concurrent use of cephalosporins with other potentially nephrotoxic drugs (e.g. aminoglycosides or amphotericin B) is controversial; they could cause additive nephrotoxicity, though this

interaction has only been well documented with cefaloridine (no longer marketed).

- Furosemide could theoretically increase the nephrotoxic potential of cephalosporins but this has not been reported clinically.
- Some parenteral cephalosporins such as ceftazidime may cause pain when administered IM or SC. Sterile abscesses or other local tissue reactions may occur but are uncommon. Thrombophlebitis may occur after IV administration.
- Except for cefotaxime, cephalosporins may cause false-positive urine glucose determinations when using cupric sulfate solution (Benedict's solution, Clinitest®). Tests using glucose oxidase (Tes-Tape®, Clinistix®) are not affected.
- When using Jaffe's reaction to measure blood or urine creatinine, cephalosporins other than cefotaxime and ceftazidime in high doses may cause falsely increased values.
- On rare occasions, ceftazidime causes false-positive Coombs' tests and increases prothrombin times.

CARBAPENEMS

Imipenem

Antibacterial spectrum (Fig. 8.12)

Imipenem is a β-lactam antibacterial classified as a carbapenem that has the widest activity of all individual antibacterial drugs. It is active against almost all clinically important aerobic and anaerobic Gram-positive or Gram-negative cocci and rods. *Nocardia* and *Brucella* are susceptible. MRSA is resistant.

Resistance

Resistance during therapy has been commonly reported in *Pseudomonas aeruginosa* and attributed to reduced membrane permeability due to alterations in outer membrane proteins.

Gram positive aerobes	Gram negative aerobes
Obligate anaerobes	Penicillinase-producing *Staphylococcus**

* MRSA are resistant

Fig. 8.12 **Antibacterial spectrum for imipenem.**

Clinical applications

Imipenem is used in human medicine to treat hospital-acquired infections caused by multiple-resistant Gram-negative bacteria, or mixed aerobic and anaerobic infections, including those in immunocompromised hosts. Veterinary use is rarely warranted but could be considered for serious and multiresistant bacterial infections when single-agent treatment is sought or when less expensive antibiotics are ineffective or pose unacceptable risks.

Pharmacokinetics

Imipenem is available as a fixed-dose combination with cilastatin. Imipenem is not absorbed after administration PO. Following IV administration it is widely distributed to extracellular fluid and reaches therapeutic concentrations in most sites in humans, including the CSF in meningitis. Bioavailability after IM administration in humans is about 95% for imipenem and 75% for cilastatin. In dogs bioavailability of imipenem after SC administration is complete. Imipenem crosses the placenta and passes into milk.

Imipenem is almost exclusively eliminated renally, after being metabolized in renal tubules by a dipeptidase. Cilastatin prevents this process so that active drug is excreted into the urine in large amounts. Cilastatin does not affect systemic pharmacokinetic behavior but may protect against proximal tubular necrosis, which can occur when imipenem is used alone. Half-life in patients with normal renal function is 1–3 h on average.

Adverse effects

- The most common adverse effects in humans are gastrointestinal disturbances and cutaneous hypersensitivity reactions.
- Seizures and tremors have occurred in a small percentage of patients, associated with high doses, renal failure or underlying neurological abnormality.
- Infusion reactions such as thrombophlebitis or gastrointestinal toxicity after rapid infusion have been reported.

Known drug interactions

- Additive or synergistic antibacterial effects may occur against some bacteria when imipenem is used with an aminoglycoside.
- Antagonism of antibacterial effects may occur if used with other β-lactam antibacterials.
- Synergy may occur against *Nocardia asteroides* when used in combination with trimethoprim-sulfonamide.
- Chloramphenicol may antagonize the antibacterial efficacy of imipenem.

PEPTIDE ANTIBIOTICS

Glycopeptides

EXAMPLES

Avoparcin, teicoplanin, vancomycin.

Mechanism of action

Glycopeptides inhibit synthesis of cell well peptidoglycan and inhibit bacterial cell membrane permeability. They also affect bacterial RNA synthesis. Vancomycin has had limited use in veterinary medicine because of high cost and the need for continuous IV infusion. However, the emergence of MRSA infections in animals has resulted in its greater use in veterinary practice. Teicoplanin may be more useful as it has slightly better activity, can be administered IM and has a long half-life. Avoparcin was used extensively as a growth promoter in poultry but has been withdrawn from most markets because it may select for vancomycin-resistant enterococci which may be a source of infection for immunocompromised patients.

Antibacterial spectrum (Fig. 8.13)

Teicoplanin and vancomycin are bactericidal to most Gram-positive aerobes and anaerobes as well as penicillinase-producing *Staphylococcus*. Most Gram-negative bacteria are resistant.

Clinical applications

Vancomycin

- Vancomycin is important in human medicine for treating multidrug-resistant infections. It should not be used in veterinary patients unless it is the only alternative, when serious infections are resistant to other antibiotics.
- The most common indication would be MRSA infections or multidrug-resistant *Enterococcus*.

Gram positive aerobes	Gram negative aerobes
Obligate anaerobes	Penicillinase-producing *Staphylococcus**

* Including MRSA

Fig. 8.13 Antibacterial spectrum for vancomycin and teicoplanin.

- It is used to treat pseudomembranous colitis due to *Clostridium difficile* in humans and may have a similar application in animals, including rabbits and hamsters.

Teicoplanin

- Teicoplanin has advantages over vancomycin as it requires less frequent dosing, can be given IM and has reduced potential for ototoxicity or nephrotoxicity.
- Teicoplanin is used in human medicine to treat serious infections, such as septicemia, endocarditis, bone and joint infections caused by Gram-positive bacteria resistant to other drugs, cystitis due to multidrug-resistant enterococci and catheter-associated staphylococcal infections in neutropenic patients.
- Selection for resistant bacteria is a problem and there is evidence that teicoplanin may be less active in vivo than predicted in vitro.

Pharmacokinetics

Vancomycin

- Vancomycin is poorly absorbed after PO administration. After IV administration penetration into tissues is adequate but relatively poor. It distributes into CSF if the meninges are inflamed.
- Half-life in dogs is shorter than in humans: 2 h vs 6 h.
- Most vancomycin is excreted by glomerular filtration with a small amount in bile.
- Dosage alteration (based on monitoring plasma drug concentrations) is required in patients with renal failure.

Teicoplanin

- No pharmacokinetic studies have been reported in small animals.
- It is not absorbed after PO administration in humans but absorption after IM injection is excellent.
- Half-life in humans is 45–70 h after IV administration.
- Penetration is poor across difficult body barriers.
- Elimination is almost entirely renal.

Route of administration

Vancomycin

- Vancomycin should not be administered IV rapidly or as a bolus as thrombophlebitis, severe hypotension and cardiac arrest (rare) have been reported. Administer it over at least 30 min in a dilute solution.
- IM, SC or IP routes should not be used.
- PO administration can be used to treat enteric infections (*C. difficile* colitis).

Teicoplanin

- Teicoplanin is administered IM but can also be given by rapid IV injection.

Adverse effects

- Toxicity information is only available for humans.
- Nephrotoxicity and otoxicity are potential but uncommon with vancomycin. They are rare with teicoplanin and usually only occur in patients also receiving an aminoglycoside.
- Skin rashes and hypersensitivity reactions have been reported with both drugs in humans.
- Reversible neutropenia has been reported in humans treated with vancomycin especially if given at high doses for prolonged periods.
- PO administration of vancomycin may cause nausea and inappetence.

Bacitracin

Bacitracin inhibits the formation of bacterial cell wall peptidoglycan by complexing directly with the pyrophosphate carrier and inhibiting the dephosphorylation required for its regeneration. Bacitracin has activity against Gram-positive organisms but causes nephrotoxicity if given systemically and so is restricted to topical and ophthalmic use in combination with polymyxin and/or neomycin.

ANTIBACTERIALS ACTING BY INHIBITING CELL MEMBRANE FUNCTION

The cytoplasmic membrane of certain bacteria (and fungi) can be more readily disrupted by certain agents than the cell membranes in animals. Therefore selective chemotherapeutic activity is possible, even though the drugs involved have a narrow therapeutic index. These antibacterials induce chemical instability in cell membranes, altering their permeability and causing cells to lose their osmotic integrity. This is similar to a detergent action.

Examples of agents acting in this manner are polymyxins and certain antifungal agents (amphotericin B, imidazoles, triazoles). The latter are discussed in Chapter 9.

Polymyxins

Mechanism of action and resistance

Polymyxins (including colistin, or polymyxin E) are cationic, surface-active agents that disrupt the structure of cell membrane phospholipids and increase cell permeability by a detergent-like action. Gram-negative bacteria are much more sensitive than Gram-positive bacteria because they contain more phospholipid in their cytoplasm and outer membranes. Acquired resistance is rare but can occur with *Pseudomonas aeruginosa* as a result of decreased bacterial permeability.

Antibacterial spectrum

Polymyxins are highly active against many Gram-negative bacteria, including *Pseudomonas aeruginosa* but not *Proteus*. Activity against *P. aeruginosa* is reduced in vivo by calcium at physiological concentrations.

Clinical applications

Although polymyxins can be given parenterally, the incidence of serious nephro- and neurotoxicity is such that they are only indicated in small animal medicine when other effective, nontoxic drugs are not available. Therefore they are generally only used in topical or ophthalmic medications, often in combination with bacitracin and neomycin or tetracycline.

ANTIMICROBIALS AFFECTING BACTERIAL PROTEIN SYNTHESIS

AMINOGLYCOSIDES AND AMINOCYCLITOLS

EXAMPLES

Aminoglycosides: amikacin, framycetin (in ocular and aural preparations only), gentamicin, kanamycin, neomycin, streptomycin, tobramycin
Aminocyclitols: spectinomycin

Members of this group continue to be important for treating serious Gram-negative infections. All inhibit bacterial protein synthesis and suffer the disadvantage of multiple types of resistance and several potential side effects.

Mechanism of action

Aminoglycosides cause irreversible inhibition of bacterial protein synthesis, although the exact mechanism for this is unknown. The agent must penetrate the cell envelope to exert its effect; this happens partly as an active process and partly by passive diffusion. Penetration of the cell envelope can be enhanced by drugs that interfere with cell wall synthesis, such as penicillins. Because active transport is an oxygen-dependent process, aminoglycosides are inactive against anaerobes and against facultative anaerobes growing under anaerobic conditions, as in abscesses.

Aminoglycosides bind to receptors on the 30S subunit of bacterial ribosomes and induce misreading of the genetic code on the messenger RNA template. This results in incorporation of incorrect amino acids into the peptide and thus inhibition of ribosomal protein synthesis. The extent and type of misreading vary because different aminoglycosides interact with different proteins. Streptomycin acts at a single site but other aminoglycosides act at several.

Other actions of aminoglycosides include interference with the cellular electron transport system, induction of RNA breakdown, inhibition of translation, effects on DNA metabolism and damage to cell membranes.

Mechanisms of resistance

Resistance to aminoglycosides, often plasmid-mediated, can develop rapidly. The mechanisms involved include:

- mutation of the organisms, resulting in altered ribosomes that no longer bind the drug
- reduced permeability of the bacteria to the drug
- inactivation of the drug by bacterial enzymes.

Bacteria may acquire the ability to produce enzymes (phosphotransferases, acetyltransferases, adenyltransferases) that modify aminoglycosides at exposed hydroxyl or amino groups to prevent ribosomal binding. This is the principal type of resistance among Gram-negative enteric bacteria, is usually plasmid-controlled and is very important clinically and epidemiologically.

Bacterial strains with reduced permeability, and consequently two- to fourfold increases in MIC, may be selected during treatment with an aminoglycoside and show cross-resistance to all other drugs within the group. This may only be important in neutropenic patients.

Deletion or alteration of receptor protein on 30S subunits because of chromosomal mutation is less important than plasmid-mediated resistance, except for streptomycin, where a single-step mutation imparting high-level resistance can occur readily even during treatment.

Antibacterial spectrum (Fig. 8.14)

- Predominantly active against Gram-negative aerobic bacteria.
- *Staphylococcus* are usually susceptible to aminoglycosides but most other Gram-positive aerobes are not; β-hemolytic *Streptococcus* are reasonably susceptible to gentamicin but not to neomycin, streptomycin or kanamycin. Resistance may emerge during treatment.
- Some *Mycobacterium* and *Mycoplasma* are susceptible.
- In potency, the spectrum of activity and stability to enzymes of plasmid-mediated resistance is: amikacin > tobramycin ≥ gentamicin > neomycin = kanamycin > streptomycin.
- Streptomycin is the most active against *Mycobacterium* and the least active against other microbes.

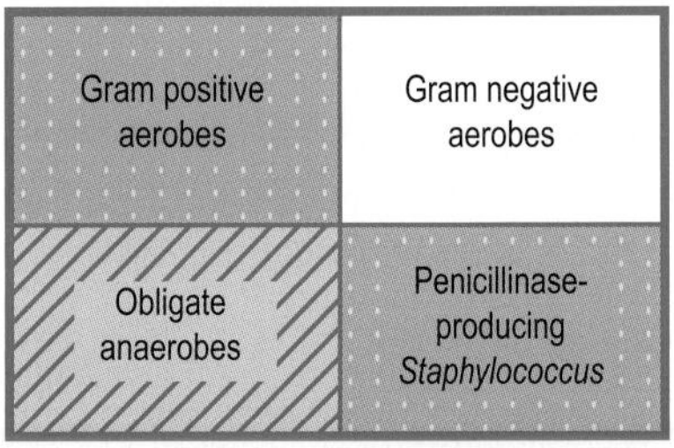

Gram positive aerobes	Gram negative aerobes
Obligate anaerobes	Penicillinase-producing *Staphylococcus*

Fig. 8.14 Antibacterial spectrum for aminoglycosides.

Pharmacokinetics

- Aminoglycosides are not significantly absorbed from the gut, so must be given parenterally to treat systemic infections.
- All have poor tissue penetration (including CNS and eye) as they are highly hydrophilic.
- They are eliminated almost exclusively by glomerular filtration.
- Half-lives are short in plasma (40–60 min) but much longer (>30 h) for tissue-bound drug.
- Aminoglycosides have a prolonged postantibiotic effect; so plasma concentrations do not need to continuously exceed the MIC of the target organism. Once-daily dosing is now recommended to reduce toxicity.
- The bactericidal action of aminoglycosides is enhanced in an alkaline medium and may be reduced by acidity secondary to tissue damage.
- All aminoglycosides bind to and are inactivated by pus.

Adverse effects

Adverse effects of the aminoglycosides may be enhanced by concurrent administration of diuretics, which may deplete extracellular fluid and increase circulating aminoglycoside concentrations.

Nephrotoxicity

All aminoglycosides can cause renal toxicity to some degree. They bind to the brush border of proximal renal tubular cells, accumulate in lysosomes and inhibit lysosomal phospholipase. Toxicity correlates with the degree of tubular reabsorption of the drug and the degree to which phospholipid metabolism in proximal tubular cells is inhibited. Therefore gentamicin, which undergoes the greatest reabsorption and interferes most potently with phospholipid metabolism, has the greatest nephrotoxic potential. Amikacin is the least nephrotoxic. Toxicity is cumulative and transport of the drug into proximal tubular cells is a saturable process. Hence giving the total daily dose in a single injection is less toxic than dividing the dose. Aminoglycosides also compete with calcium in mitochondria and decrease glomerular permeability and the diameter of endothelial fenestrae.

Nephrotoxicity is reversible if recognized early. Factors that increase the risk of nephrotoxicity include:

- renal dysfunction (more common in older patients)
- age (young animals are at greater risk)
- dehydration
- fever and sepsis
- concurrent treatment with other potentially nephrotoxic drugs (especially nonsteroidal anti-inflammatory drugs in dehydrated patients; see Chapter 13)
- concurrent treatment with a diuretic
- hypokalemia
- frequent low-dose administration (i.e. SID dosing is less toxic than dosing many times a day).

Feeding prior to administration of the drug may reduce nephrotoxicity by saturating drug receptor sites with protein. The dose or treatment interval should be altered if significant risk factors exist; regimens with increased time interval and fixed dose cause less toxicity than those having reduced dose and fixed interval. Renal function should be monitored during treatment in 'at-risk' patients (check urine specific gravity, protein and glucose). Therapeutic drug monitoring is recommended in these patients; plasma trough drug concentrations should be 0.5–2 μg/mL before the next dose for gentamicin and tobramycin and <6 μg/mL for amikacin.

Ototoxicity

Vestibular and/or auditory dysfunction can occur with any aminoglycoside. Streptomycin and gentamicin predominantly produce vestibular effects (although deafness due to gentamicin has been known to occur); amikacin, neomycin and kanamycin have auditory effects; tobramycin affects both equally. Topical application to ruptured tympanic membrane may result in ototoxicity. Cats appear more susceptible than dogs to aminoglycoside ototoxicity.

Neuromuscular blockade

This is uncommon but may occur at high doses. It mostly occurs in association with anesthesia or administration of other neuromuscular blocking agents. Patients with myasthenia gravis are particularly susceptible. Aminoglycosides inhibit prejunctional release of acetylcholine by blocking nerve terminal calcium entry through N-type calcium channels.

Cardiac effects

All aminoglycosides, if given by rapid IV injection, slow the heart, reduce cardiac output and lower blood pressure through an effect on calcium channels. These changes are of minor significance but should be kept in mind, particularly if administering aminoglycosides IV in an anesthetized patient.

Neomycin

- Nephrotoxicity prevents systemic use but can be administered PO to suppress gastrointestinal bacteria and ammonia production in small animals with hepatic encephalopathy.
- Also used topically in ophthalmic, aural and skin preparations, usually in combination with other antibacterials.
- Activity against *Staphylococcus* is good (hence its use topically).

Streptomycin

- First aminoglycoside developed; use restricted now due to the degree of resistance that has developed and ototoxicity.
- Plasmid-mediated streptomycin resistance is commonly linked with sulfonamide, ampicillin and tetracycline resistance genes.
- Chromosomal mutations arise commonly; it is therefore usually combined with other drugs to delay emergence of resistance.
- Streptomycin is the least active aminoglycoside, except against *Mycobacterium.*
- Used in treatment of leptospirosis to eliminate the renal carrier state.
- There is no evidence in companion animal species that streptomycin-penicillin combinations are synergistic or more efficacious than either drug used alone.
- Cats are particularly sensitive to the ototoxic effects of streptomycin.

Kanamycin

Kanamycin is inferior in activity to other more recent aminoglycosides and is therefore not much used clinically.

Framycetin

Framycetin is used in some ophthalmic and aural preparations (e.g. Canaural®).

Gentamicin

- Spelt with an 'i' not a 'y', unlike others in the group, as it is a product of *Micromonospora purpurea* not a *Streptomyces* sp.
- Probably now the most commonly used aminoglycoside for severe infections caused by Gram-negative aerobic bacteria.

- Little resistance 10 years ago but resistant strains are emerging, particularly in some referral centers. These are mainly detected in dogs with oft-treated ear infections.
- Gentamicin has little activity against *Mycobacterium*.

Tobramycin

- Very similar antibacterial spectrum to gentamicin; some cross-resistance occurs but is unpredictable.
- More active against *Pseudomonas*.

Amikacin

- Amikacin is resistant to most enzymes that inactivate other aminoglycosides, particularly important in treating serious *Pseudomonas* and other Gram-negative infections in immunosuppressed patients.
- Can be administered for 2–3 weeks at recommended doses with less risk of nephrotoxicity than with gentamicin.

Spectinomycin

Is an aminocyclitol rather than an aminoglycoside but has many similar properties.

- Lacks most of the toxic effects of the aminoglycosides.
- Is usually bacteriostatic but may be bactericidal at higher concentrations (e.g. 4 × MIC).
- Has limited clinical application because resistance develops readily.
- Is marketed in combination with lincomycin, which marginally enhances activity against *Mycoplasma*.

TETRACYCLINES

The tetracycline group of drugs were first developed in the late 1940s.

EXAMPLES

Chlortetracycline, doxycycline, minocycline, oxytetracycline, tetracycline.

Mechanism of action

Like the aminoglycosides, tetracyclines inhibit protein synthesis by binding to the 30S subunit of bacterial ribosome and interfering with RNA-protein translation. Access to ribosomes is by:

- passive diffusion through hydrophilic pores in the outer cell membrane
- energy-dependent active transport through the inner cytoplasmic membrane. This involves a periplasmic protein carrier. Unlike aminoglycosides, this step does not depend on membrane potential; therefore tetracyclines can work in anaerobic and hyperosmolar environments.

Tetracyclines also bind to mammalian 80S ribosomal subunits and inhibit protein synthesis in the host but with much less affinity. However, host protein synthesis in rapidly dividing cells may be impaired at high doses, resulting in an antianabolic effect. Selective toxicity is dependent on mammalian cells lacking the transporter molecule so they do not accumulate the drug in the same way that bacterial cells do.

Mechanism of resistance

Acquired resistance to tetracyclines is widespread, usually plasmid-mediated, and often involves interference with both active transport of tetracyclines into, and increased efflux out of, bacterial cells. Another major mechanism is ribosomal protection where a cytoplasmic protein protects against inhibition of protein synthesis. At least 12 different genetic determinants for tetracycline resistance have been described, coding for several mechanisms of drug resistance such as efflux, ribosomal protection or chemical modification.

Antibacterial spectrum (Fig. 8.15)

- Tetracyclines have activity against many Gram-positive and Gram-negative aerobic bacteria but acquired resistance limits their activity against many species, such as *Staphylococcus*, *Enterococcus*, Enterobacteriaceae including *Enterobacter*, *Escherichia*, *Klebsiella*, *Proteus* and *Salmonella*.
- *Mycobacterium*, *Proteus vulgaris*, *Pseudomonas aeruginosa* and *Serratia* are resistant.
- Anaerobes show variable susceptibility.
- Atypical bacterial species (*Rickettsia*, *Borrelia*, *Chlamydophila* and *Mycoplasma*) are generally susceptible, though some *Mycoplasma* (*M. bovis*, *M. hyopneumoniae*) are resistant.

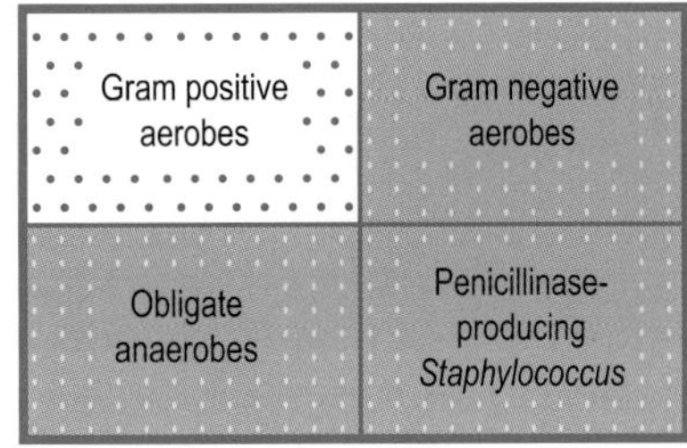

Fig. 8.15 Antibacterial spectrum for tetracyclines.

Differences in activity between different members of the group are generally minor and are primarily due to pharmacokinetic factors rather than differences in susceptibility.

Clinical applications

- In veterinary medicine tetracyclines are used most frequently for atypical bacterial diseases due to *Chlamydophila* (particularly in cats), *Borrelia, Rickettsia* and *Mycoplasma.*
- Tetracyclines are the drugs of choice for *Ehrlichia canis* and *Rickettsia rickettsii* infections.
- Brucellosis is commonly treated with tetracyclines in combination with rifampicin or streptomycin.
- Tetracyclines are used to treat bacterial overgrowth of the small intestine and antibiotic-responsive diarrhea (other common drug choices are tylosin and metronidazole; this appears to be based on the clinician's preference rather than empirical data).
- Tetracyclines have anti-inflammatory properties that are independent of their antibacterial action, particularly in the case of doxycycline and minocycline.

Pharmacokinetics

All tetracyclines are absorbed following oral dosing, although absorption may be erratic – oxytetracycline has the worst absorption, doxycycline and minocycline the best. The drug's ability to chelate calcium and other divalent cations correlates with bioavailability. Systemic availability after oral administration is impaired by food, dairy products and antacids containing aluminum, magnesium and calcium.

Tetracyclines vary in lipid solubility and this largely determines their distribution and rate of excretion (see Table 8.1). They enter most tissues and body fluids with the exception of CSF; the degree to which they enter the CNS and CSF is related to their lipid solubility and presence of efflux pumps. Minocycline and doxycycline are more lipid soluble than other tetracyclines but are also more highly protein bound.

Tetracylines, except minocycline and doxycycline, are excreted unchanged in urine. All are concentrated in the liver and undergo biliary excretion and enterohepatic recycling (which prolongs half-lives to 6–10 h and provides some rationale for using them in bacterial cholangitis), although the major route of elimination, except for minocycline and doxycycline, is renal. Doxycycline elimination in humans involves both renal and biliary mechanisms but in dogs bile may be the predominant route.

Preparations used in small animals include oral preparations (capsules, syrup, paste), injectable preparations and ophthalmic ointment.

Adverse effects

- Gastrointestinal disturbances are not uncommon, especially in cats. Other adverse effects in cats can include anorexia, fever and depression.
- Esophageal strictures resulting from incomplete swallowing of oral doxycycline tablets have been reported. As a precaution it is recommended that animals be given a small amount of water by syringe or a small amount of food following administration, or butter be placed on the nose to encourage swallowing.
- Tetracyclines are irritant and may cause vomiting after oral administration and tissue damage at injection sites. This is particularly true for oxytetracycline, especially long-acting preparations.
- Fatal anaphylaxis has occasionally been recorded.
- Rapid IV injection is likely to cause the patient to collapse (probably related to the vehicle).
- Tetracyclines have been reported to induce dose-related functional changes in renal tubules in several species. This may be exacerbated by dehydration, hemoglobinuria, myoglobinuria, toxemia or another nephrotoxic drug.
- Severe renal tubular damage has been attributed to the administration of outdated or incorrectly stored preparations.
- Severe liver damage has been reported following overdosage of tetracyclines in animals with pre-existing renal failure.
- Fatal nephrotoxicosis has been reported after accidental administration of two doses of 130 mg/kg.
- Superinfection is a risk with most tetracyclines because appreciable amounts remain unabsorbed in the bowel and they are actively excreted into bile. This is especially true in the horse where the lipophilic tetracyclines minocycline and doxycycline have such a high potential for causing digestive disturbances that they should be avoided.
- Serious adverse effects have been reported in hamsters and guinea-pigs but tetracyclines appear to be safe for rabbits.
- Tetracyclines may accumulate in renal failure and their antianabolic effect could exacerbate azotemia in renal failure, so dosage should be modified in patients with renal failure. The exception is doxycycline, the elimination of which is not affected. Doxycycline is therefore the tetracycline of choice for patients with renal disease.
- The antianabolic effects of tetracyclines may cause azotemia, potentially exacerbated by corticosteroids.
- Tetracyclines chelate with calcium pyrophosphate in teeth and bone. This causes hypoplasia of dental enamel, discoloration of developing teeth and slower bone development. This may not occur with doxycycline.

- Tetracyclines should not be used in pregnant animals because of their antianabolic effects.

CHLORAMPHENICOL

Originally isolated from *Streptomyces venezuelae*, chloramphenicol was the first broad-spectrum antibacterial developed (1947). It is now produced synthetically.

Mechanism of action

Chloramphenicol is a nonionized, highly lipophilic compound. It enters bacterial cells by passive or facilitated diffusion and binds primarily to the 50S ribosomal subunit but may also bind to the 30S subunit. As a result bacterial protein synthesis is inhibited.

Chloramphenicol can also bind to the mammalian ribosome (70S) that resembles bacterial ribosomes and interfere with mitochondrial protein synthesis. This is particularly relevant in erythropoietic cells.

Resistance

Resistance is commonly plasmid-mediated and occurs as a result of enzymatic inactivation by several types of chloramphenicol transacetylase.

Antibacterial spectrum (Fig. 8.16)

- Chloramphenicol is bacteriostatic for most Gram-positive and many Gram-negative aerobic bacteria but can be bactericidal against some very sensitive bacteria.
- Acquired resistance occurs in many species, especially where chloramphenicol is in common use. *Pseudomonas aeruginosa, Escherichia, Klebsiella, Enterobacter, Salmonella* and *Proteus* now show patterns of plasmid-mediated resistance. However, the current level of acquired resistance is difficult to predict, as chloramphenicol is not used in food animals in many countries and is now used much less frequently than previously in small animals.

Gram positive aerobes	Gram negative aerobes
Obligate anaerobes	Penicillinase-producing *Staphylococcus*

+ *Chlamydophila, Rickettsia are susceptible*

Fig. 8.16 Antibacterial spectrum for chloramphenicol.

- All anaerobic bacteria are inhibited by chloramphenicol at usual therapeutic concentrations.
- Chloramphenicol suppresses growth of *Rickettsia* and *Chlamyophila* but clinical efficacy against *Mycoplasma* infections is often disappointing, even though *Mycoplasma* often seem susceptible in vitro.
- *Mycobacterium* and *Nocardia* are resistant.

Clinical applications

- In many countries, use of chloramphenicol in any form, including topical and ophthalmic preparations, is prohibited in food-producing animals. This is because chloramphenicol, even in minute doses, is associated with an idiosyncratic fatal aplastic anemia in some humans.
- In small animals, chloramphenicol is often regarded now as the drug of first choice only for bacterial infection of the chambers of the eye.
- There is mixed opinion as to whether chloramphenicol is a drug of choice for bacterial CNS infections but it does achieve high levels in the CNS and has a very broad spectrum. However, many other drugs also effectively cross the blood–brain barrier in the presence of meningitis and may be more effective and, perhaps most importantly, are bactericidal.
- Chloramphenicol may be indicated for anaerobic infections, prostatitis and salmonellosis.
- As chloramphenicol is usually bacteriostatic, it should not be used in immunocompromised patients or where bactericidal treatment is preferable.
- Chloramphenicol is best avoided in anemic animals.
- Avoid using chloramphenicol in cats with renal failure.

Pharmacokinetics

- Well distributed throughout the body, including CNS and eye.
- Attains higher concentrations in CSF than other antibacterials (30–50% of plasma concentrations in the absence of meningitis) and concentrations in CNS are maintained longer than in plasma.
- Eliminated primarily by hepatic glucuronide conjugation in the dog: only 5–10% is excreted unchanged in the urine.
- In the cat, more than 25% is excreted in the urine because of reduced ability to glucuronidate drugs.
- Elimination half-life is similar in both species: 4 h following IV administration, 7–8 h following PO administration.
- Drug from tablets and capsules is readily absorbed orally.
- In fasted cats chloramphenicol suspensions (palmitate ester) administered PO produce lower blood drug concentrations than provided by solid dosage

forms (this difference is not observable in dogs). Since many sick cats given chloramphenicol are inappetent, tablets rather than suspension should be given.
- Parenteral formulations are sodium succinate solution (which has an excellent bioavailability regardless of route) and aqueous suspension (gives lower plasma concentrations, maximum concentration 6 h after injection). Parenteral routes are only used in patients for whom oral dosing is impossible.
- Chloramphenicol should not be given to young animals (ill-equipped with metabolizing enzymes) and avoided in adults with liver disease.

Adverse effects
- Reversible, dose-related nonregenerative anemia can occur in dogs and cats. Cats may be more susceptible but the increased prevalence is probably related to overdosing of cats if using the dog dosing schedule, which is approximately five times higher per kilogram (see Table 8.4).
- Idiosyncratic fatal aplastic anemia has not been reported in small animals.
- Chloramphenicol inhibits hepatic microsomal enzymes, thus prolonging effects of drugs such as barbiturates and phenytoin. The inhibition is irreversible and therefore long lasting.
- Chloramphenicol may also theoretically interfere with antibody production in active immunization procedures.

Related drugs
Thiamphenicol is a chloramphenicol analog with a range of activity similar to chloramphenicol, although it is generally 1–2 times less active. It has equal activity against *Haemophilus, Bacteroides fragilis* and *Streptococcus*. It differs pharmacokinetically in that it is not eliminated by hepatic glucuronidation and is excreted unchanged in urine, so elimination is unaffected by liver disease. Unlike chloramphenicol, thiamphenicol does not cause aplastic anemia in humans.

Florfenicol is a structural analog of thiamphenicol which has greater in vitro activity against pathogenic bacteria than chloramphenicol and thiamphenicol. It is also active against some bacteria that are resistant to chloramphenicol, especially enteric bacteria. Florfenicol is not susceptible to inactivation by chloramphenicol transacetylases; thus some organisms that are resistant to chloramphenicol through this mechanism are susceptible to florfenicol.

In dogs florfenicol is poorly absorbed after SC administration. It has a half-life of less than 5 h. The drug is well absorbed in cats after PO and IM administrations with a similar elimination half-life. It should not be given IV. Florfenicol can cause dose-related bone marrow suppression but has not been reported to cause fatal aplastic anemia in humans.

Florfenicol shows promise as a replacement for other broad-spectrum antibacterials such as sulfonamides and tetracyclines that have been associated with toxicity and residue concerns in food animals. Currently it is approved for use only in cattle, aquaculture and pigs. In cattle it is used to treat infectious conjunctivitis and respiratory disease caused by bacteria like *Pasteurella* and *Haemophilus*.

MACROLIDES AND LINCOSAMIDES

These groups of antibacterials are structurally distinct but considered together because they have many common properties.

EXAMPLES

Macrolides: azithromycin, clarithromycin, erythromycin, spiramycin, tilmicosin, tulathromycin, tylosin.
Lincosamides: clindamycin, lincomycin.

Mechanism of action and resistance
The mechanism of action of the macrolides and lincosamides is similar to that of chloramphenicol, acting on the 50S ribosomal subunit. Chromosomal resistance develops fairly readily to both these drug groups and plasmid-mediated resistance is common.

Resistance is the result of methylation of adenine residues in the 23S ribosomal RNA of the 50S ribosomal subunit, which prevents drug binding to the target. There is usually complete cross-resistance between lincomycin and clindamycin and cross-resistance between lincosamides and macrolides is common.

Antibacterial spectrum (Figs 8.17–8.20)
- Active against Gram-positive aerobic bacteria, *Mycoplasma* and *Bartonella henselae* (cat scratch disease).

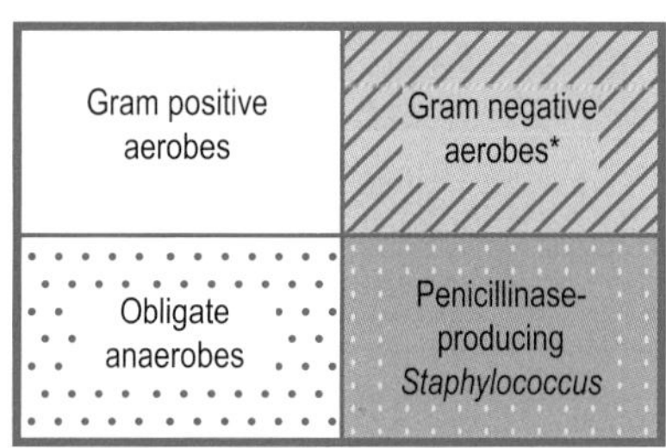

Fig. 8.17 Antibacterial spectrum for lincomycin, *Campylobacter spp. are susceptible.

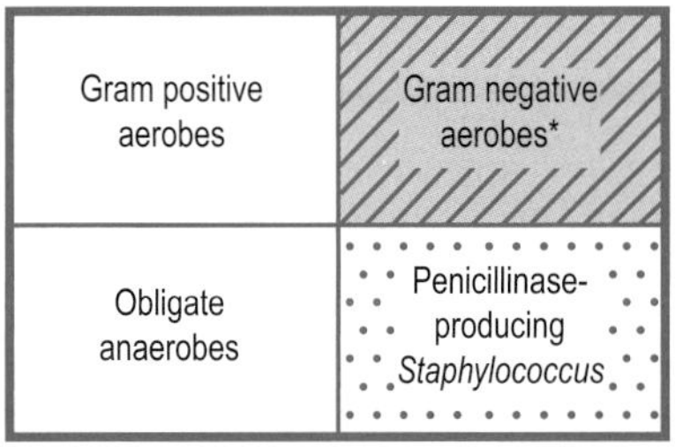

Gram positive aerobes	Gram negative aerobes*
Obligate anaerobes	Penicillinase-producing *Staphylococcus*

+ *Toxoplasma* and *Neospora*

* Campylobacter are susceptible

Fig. 8.18 Antibacterial spectrum for clindamycin.

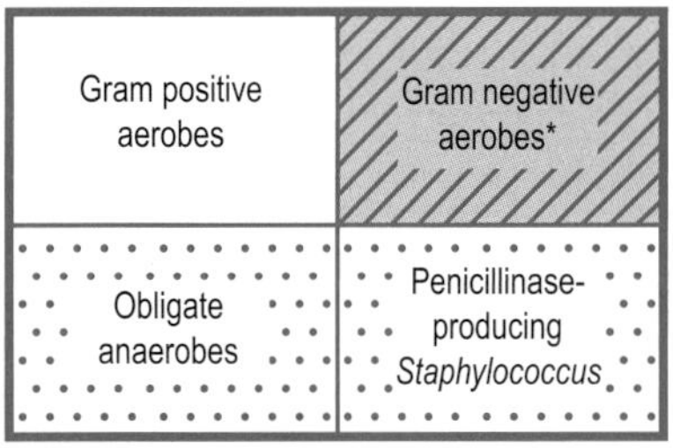

Gram positive aerobes	Gram negative aerobes*
Obligate anaerobes	Penicillinase-producing *Staphylococcus*

* Campylobacter are susceptible

Fig. 8.19 Antibacterial spectrum for erythromycin.

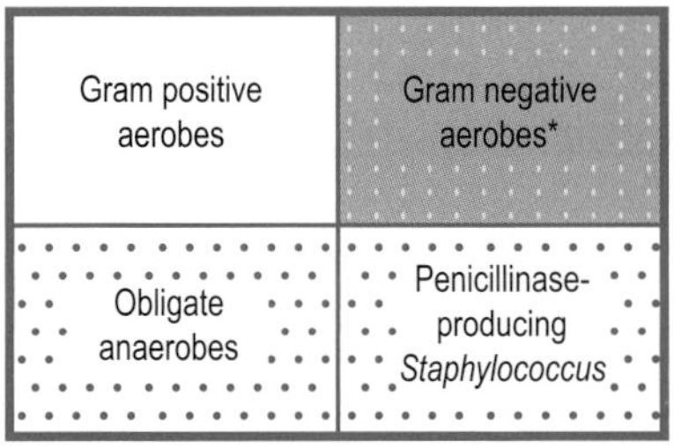

Gram positive aerobes	Gram negative aerobes*
Obligate anaerobes	Penicillinase-producing *Staphylococcus*

+ atypical *Mycobacteria* spp.

* Campylobacter are susceptible

Fig. 8.20 Antibacterial spectrum for azithromycin.

- Good activity against anaerobic bacteria.
- Virtually all aerobic Gram-negative bacteria are resistant because of drug impermeability and methylation of the ribosomal binding site but *Campylobacter jejuni* is an exception.
- Erythromycin and lincomycin are more effective against *Staphylococcus* than aminopenicillins but not as effective as antistaphylococcal penicillins, cephalosporins and amoxicillin-clavulanate.

Pharmacokinetics

Macrolides and lincosamides have high lipid solubility and wide distribution in the body and across cellular barriers. They are usually bacteriostatic but erythromycin can be bactericidal at high concentrations. Because of their basic nature, ion-trapping occurs in milk and prostatic fluid where the transcellular pH is lower than the blood. Ion-trapping also occurs inside cells since intracellular pH is lower than extracellular fluid pH. Concentrations in CSF are relatively low (20% of plasma concentrations) due to extensive plasma protein binding and relatively rapid elimination. Concentrations achieved in bone are also relatively low (10–20% of plasma concentrations) although this can still be clinically effective.

Lincosamides are well absorbed from the intestine of nonherbivores. They are eliminated mainly by hepatic metabolism, although about 20% is eliminated in active form in the urine.

Adverse effects

The major toxic effect of lincosamides is their ability to cause serious and fatal diarrhea in humans, horses, rabbits and other herbivores. The diarrhea is due to overgrowth of *Clostridium difficile* because of destruction of competing anaerobic flora in the colon. However, lincosamides are relatively nontoxic to dogs and cats.

Erythromycin frequently causes gastrointestinal upsets in dogs, mainly vomiting. It appears to mimic the effects of the hormone motilin as well as acting on presynaptic cholinergic neurones to stimulate gastric, pyloric and duodenal contractions. Low doses are prokinetic but higher doses used in antibacterial therapy stimulate vomiting.

Lincomycin

The combination of lincomycin with spectinomycin appears to give marginally enhanced activity against *Mycoplasma* in vitro and is convenient for treating *Mycoplasma* and *Chlamydophila* infections in catteries.

Lincomycin and clindamycin penetrate well into all tissues, including bone, and have therefore been popular for treating osteomyelitis. Concentrations in the extracellular fluid of bone depend on blood supply. However, at adequate dose rates most antibacterial drugs attain therapeutically acceptable concentrations in bone and synovial fluid, although some achieve higher concentrations in bone than others. The important features of treatment of osteomyelitis include the need for high local concentrations of bactericidal drugs, prolonged treatment, especially in chronic infections and surgical removal of necrotic bone. Bacteriostatic agents like lincosamides are thus not a particularly good choice.

Clindamycin

- Clindamycin is more potent than lincomycin against all pathogens.

- It is especially active against obligate anaerobes.
- Clindamycin is indicated for *Toxoplasma* and *Neospora* infections although in human medicine sulfadiazine and pyrimethamine remain the drugs of choice for toxoplasmosis.
- Clindamycin is one of several suitable drugs for treating chronic rhinosinusitis in cats.
- Clindamycin is commonly combined with an aminoglycoside in human medicine to treat or prevent mixed aerobic-anaerobic bacterial infections such as those associated with intestinal perforation. The combination has additive effects against a wide range of bacteria.
- Clindamycin reportedly has synergistic effects with metronidazole against *Bacteroides fragilis.*
- Combinations of clindamycin with macrolides or chloramphenicol are antagonistic in vitro.

Erythromycin

- Erythromycin is the drug of choice for treatment of *Campylobacter jejuni* infections.
- It is one of the drugs of choice for treatment of *Mycoplasma* infections.
- Erythromycin has greater activity against *Staphylococcus* than lincomycin but not clindamycin.

Tylosin

- Tylosin has a similar spectrum of activity to erythromycin. It is less active against bacteria but more active against many *Mycoplasma.*
- Tylosin is often prescribed for feline respiratory tract infections and may be effective because of activity against *Mycoplasma*, *Chlamydophila* and Gram-positive bacteria.
- Tylosin is used to treat bacterial overgrowth of the small intestine and antibiotic-responsive diarrhea (other common choices are tetracyclines and metronidazole; selection seems to be based on clinician's preference rather than empirical data).
- Tylosin should not be used in horses.

Spiramycin

- Spiramycin is less active against bacteria than erythromycin in vitro but more active in vivo because of exceptional ability to concentrate in tissues.
- It is marketed in some countries in combination with metronidazole, mainly for treatment of oral infections in dogs and cats.

Azithromycin and clarithromycin

- These azalides, derivatives of erythromycin, have greater potency and a wider spectrum of activity, particularly against Gram-negative aerobes.
- Both have very useful activity against many *Mycobacteria, Bartonella, Borrelia, Brucella, Leptospira, Campylobacter* and *Helicobacter* and have very good activity against *Chlamydophila* and *Toxoplasma.*
- They may be suitable for PO administration once daily.
- Both drugs are concentrated in phagocytes and phagolysosomes.
- Both are expensive but may be affordable for small individuals such as cats.

ANTIMICROBIALS AFFECTING NUCLEIC ACID SYNTHESIS

SULFONAMIDES AND POTENTIATORS

The sulfonamides are one of the oldest recognized group of antibacterial agents – they preceded penicillin by 3 years. Since then, emergence of resistance has decreased the usefulness of sulfonamides alone but in the 1970s potentiation of sulfonamides by the addition of trimethoprim or other potentiators (baquiloprim, ormetoprim, pyrimethamine) resulted in a resurgence in their use.

The major advantage of the sulfonamides is their low cost compared to other antibacterial drugs (provided they are clinically effective).

EXAMPLES

Systemically acting sulfonamides: sulfadiazine, sulfadimidine, sulfadoxine, sulfatroxazole
Sulfonamides poorly absorbed from the gut: phthalysulfathiazole, sulfasalazine
Topical: sulfacetamide

Mechanism of action

Sulfonamides are structural analogs of *para*-aminobenzoic acid (PABA) and thus act as competitive antagonists in microbial cells. Microbes need PABA to form dihydrofolic acid, a precursor of folic acid. Folic acid is required for purine and pyrimidine synthesis and hence nucleic acid synthesis. Sulfonamides not only block formation of folic acid – they are incorporated into the precursors, forming a pseudometabolite that is reactive and antibacterial. Mammalian cells are not susceptible to sulfonamides as they absorb and use preformed folic acid, resulting in a wide therapeutic index. The combination of sulfonamides with trimethoprim or other diaminopyrimidines potentiates their activity.

Trimethoprim enters bacteria and inhibits bacterial dihydrofolic acid reductase, thus acting on the same metabolic pathway as sulfonamides. Therefore the combination has synergistic activity. The binding affinity of trimethoprim is very much greater for the bacterial enzyme than for mammalian enzyme; therefore selective bacterial toxicity occurs.

Sulfonamides do not appear to antagonize the bactericidal effects of penicillins but should not be used with procaine benzylpenicillin (procaine penicillin), as procaine is an analog of PABA and will antagonize sulfonamide's antibacterial action.

Mechanisms of resistance

Chromosomally mediated resistance develops slowly and gradually and results from impairment of drug penetration, production of an insensitive dihydropteroate synthase or hyperproduction of PABA. Plasmid-mediated resistance is far more common and can involve impairment of drug penetration or production of additional, sulfonamide-resistant, dihydropteroate synthetase enzymes. The R-factor genes that control sulfonamide resistance are commonly linked with those that control streptomycin resistance.

Extensive use of sulfonamides has resulted in widespread resistance in bacteria isolated from animals and cross-resistance within the group is complete.

Antibacterial spectrum (Fig. 8.21)

Sulfonamides on their own are bacteriostatic. When combined with trimethoprim, they may be bactericidal. Potentiated sulfonamides are now generally used more commonly than sulfonamides alone, especially in small animal medicine, and the following discussion relates especially to sulfonamide-trimethoprim.

- Sulfonamide-trimethoprim inhibits:
  - Gram-negative and Gram-positive aerobic bacteria, especially *Nocardia*, for which they are the preferred choice
  - anaerobes? Opinions vary. If necrotic tissue is present, thymidine and PABA antagonize their antibacterial effect
  - some protozoa.
- Synergism between trimethoprim and the sulfonamide results in up to 40% of bacteria that are resistant to one component being susceptible to the combination.
- When sulfonamides are combined with pyrimethamine they have greater antiprotozoal activity against *Toxoplasma* and *Neospora,* for example.
- Sulfonamide-trimethoprim is not effective against *Pseudomonas aeruginosa* or *Proteus.*
- Different sulfonamides may show quantitative but not necessarily qualitative differences in activity.
- Trimethoprim-sulfonamide may be the treatment of choice for *Pneumocystis* pneumonia.
- *Mycobacterium, Mycoplasma, Rickettsia* and spirochetes are resistant.

Gram positive aerobes	Gram negative aerobes
Obligate anaerobes	Penicillinase-producing *Staphylococcus*

+ *Toxoplasma, Neospora, Coccidia, Isospora, Chlamydophila, Nocardia, Cryptosporidium* spp.

Fig. 8.21 Antibacterial spectrum for trimethoprim-sulfonamides.

Clinical applications

- *Toxoplasma* infection (combined with pyrimethamine).
- *Chlamydophila* infection.
- *Nocardia* infection (with or without trimethoprim).
- *Bordetella bronchiseptica* infection (kennel cough).
- Prostatic infections (concentrations in prostatic tissue are 10× greater than in plasma).
- Poorly absorbed sulfonamides can be used to treat gastrointestinal infections, including coccidiosis (phthalysulfathiazole), or idiopathic ulcerative colitis (sulfasalazine).
- Topical sulfonamides are used in ophthalmic and skin preparations.

Pharmacokinetics

Most sulfonamides are rapidly absorbed orally. They distribute widely to all body tissues and body fluids, including synovial fluid and CSF. They exist predominantly in the nonionized form in biological fluids and diffuse well through cell membranes and barriers. Freely diffusible sulfonamides (e.g. sulfadiazine) cross the blood–brain barrier and have excellent penetration into prostate and eye (see Table 8.1). Sulfonamides are weak acids, trimethoprim is a weak base.

In animals, the half-lives of sulfonamides and trimethoprim differ (in contrast to humans) but the combination is clinically effective as there is a relatively broad range of drug ratio over which synergism occurs.

Sulfonamides are extensively metabolized and excreted primarily by renal excretion; therefore large amounts of drug are present in urine. Trimethoprim is more lipid soluble than sulfonamides and reaches higher concentrations in lungs and prostate.

Sulfonamides are bound to plasma proteins to an extent varying from 15% to 90%. There are differences between species in binding of individual sulfonamides. Extensive protein binding (>80%) increases half-life. In any one species the extent of protein binding, apparent volume of distribution and half-life vary widely between sulfonamides.

In most species, sulfonamides undergo acetylation prior to renal elimination but in the dog they are eliminated by glucuronidation and renal filtration. They are also excreted in milk, feces, bile, sweat and tears. The acetyl derivative of most sulfonamides (except sulfapyrimidines) is less soluble in water than the parent compound and may increase the risk of damage to renal tubules due to precipitation.

Renal elimination involves glomerular filtration of free drug, active carrier-mediated proximal tubular excretion of nonionized unchanged drug and metabolites and passive reabsorption of nonionized drug from distal tubular fluid. The extent of reabsorption is determined by the pKa of the sulfonamide and the pH of the distal tubular fluid. Urinary alkalinization increases both the fraction of the dose eliminated unchanged in urine and the solubility of sulfonamides in urine.

Topical wound powders containing sulfonamides are not useful because blood, pus and tissue breakdown products impede antibacterial effectiveness and wound healing can be delayed.

Adverse effects

Hypersensitivity reactions (dogs)

Abnormalities that may occur with hypersensitivity reactions to sulfonamides include polyarthritis and fever, cutaneous eruptions, thrombocytopenia, leukopenia and hepatitis.

The sulfonamide molecule is too small to be immunogenic. It is thought that hypersensitivity reactions occur because of hydroxylamine metabolites that are formed from oxidation of the *para*-amino group. These are cytotoxic and capable of binding covalently to protein.

Doberman pinschers are predisposed to sulfonamide hypersensitivity. This may be because of a reduced ability to detoxify hydroxylamine groups compared with mixed-breed dogs. Also, dobermans and other breeds of dogs commonly affected with von Willebrand's disease (Scottish terriers, German shepherds) may not tolerate sulfonamides well. These drugs probably should be avoided in dobermans.

Keratoconjunctivitis sicca (KCS)

This may occur with prolonged use of some sulfonamides. It is probably most often associated with sulfasalazine, as this drug is used for long-term treatment of ulcerative colitis. However, KCS has also been reported within the first week of treatment in a small proportion of dogs treated with trimethoprim-sulfadiazine. The dogs all weighed less than 12 kg, suggesting that care should be taken with dose calculations for smaller dogs.

Renal effects

Crystalluria, hematuria and urinary tract obstruction can occur as a result of concentration of sulfonamides in renal tubules and acid pH. Ensure that animals receiving sulfonamides are well hydrated.

Excessive salivation

Cats often foam at the mouth if given oral sulfonamide drugs, particularly if enteric-coated tablets are broken.

Other effects

- Trimethoprim-sulfonamides have been reported to cause idiosyncratic severe hepatic necrosis on rare occasions.
- Aplastic anemia and thrombocytopenia may occur but are rare.
- It has been postulated but not proven that trimethoprim-sulfonamides are a risk factor for acute pancreatitis.
- Sulfonamides at high doses (30 mg/kg twice daily) can profoundly alter thyroid physiology. They cause decreased iodinization of colloid and decreased concentrations of thyroxine and thyronine. Clinically relevant decreased thyroid function is apparent by 3 weeks of therapy and will return to normal within 3 weeks of therapy being discontinued.

FLUOROQUINOLONES

The fluoroquinolones are synthetic antibacterial agents derived from the 4-quinolone molecule, which was first synthesized in the early 1960s. Nalidixic acid, the first quinolone marketed for clinical use, had limited effectiveness because of poor absorption, narrow spectrum of activity and toxicity. The first fluoroquinolone, norfloxacin, developed in the early 1980s, had greater absorption, better antibacterial activity and reduced toxicity.

EXAMPLES

Ciprofloxacin, danofloxacin, difloxacin, enrofloxacin, marbofloxacin, norfloxacin, orbifloxacin, sarafloxacin.

Mechanism of action

Fluoroquinolones specifically inhibit topoisomerase II (also referred to as DNA gyrase), an enzyme that controls the supercoiling of bacterial DNA by catalyzing the cleavage/reunion of the two strands in the DNA molecule. This is the major target of fluoroquinolones in Gram-negative bacteria. Binding of fluoroquinolones to DNA gyrase disrupts enzyme activity, resulting in rapid cell death. The mechanism of action against Gram-positive bacteria is not well understood but the primary target may be topoisomerase IV, which also catalyzes changes in coiling.

The bactericidal action of fluoroquinolones is rapid and concentration-dependent. The more the concentration exceeds the MIC, the greater the bactericidal effect and the less the likelihood of selecting resistant pathogens. However, activity is inhibited at very high concentrations through direct inhibition of RNA synthesis and can be antagonized by protein synthesis inhibitors (chloramphenicol) and RNA synthesis inhibitors (rifampicin).

Mechanisms of resistance

Clinically important fluoroquinolone resistance is chromosomally mediated. There are three mechanisms by which it can occur: decreased permeability of the bacterial cell wall, activation of an efflux pump which actively transports the drug out of the cell and mutation of DNA topoisomerase II or IV that alters drug-binding sites. This latter mechanism is the most important. Cross-resistance between the fluoroquinolones frequently occurs. In addition, some mutations that alter permeability or activate the efflux pump also confer resistance to other antimicrobials such as cephalosporins and tetracyclines.

Selection of resistant organisms is related to the concentration of drug at the site of infection; the higher the concentration, the fewer resistant bacteria. The high concentrations of fluoroquinolones achieved in urine and gut following oral dosage tend to prevent the emergence of low-level resistant mutants but treatment of infections in other sites may be associated with development of resistance. Because resistance is chromasomally mediated, it is stable and not energy dependent. Resistant bacteria have the potential to persist even after removal of drug from their environment. Therefore repeated exposure to sublethal concentrations of drug can select for high-level, stable resistance. There have been reports of increasing patterns of resistance to ciprofloxacin and enrofloxacin amongst several bacteria, including *Staphylococcus aureus, Pseudomonas aeruginosa, Escherichia* and other Gram negatives.

Plasmid-mediated resistance that targets DNA gyrase has not been clinically demonstrated and may only become apparent after several decades of intense drug use. Because fluoroquinolones are important for treating certain serious Gram-negative infections, it is prudent to suggest that use of these drugs should ideally be supported by culture and susceptibility test data whenever possible.

Antibacterial spectrum (*Fig. 8.22*)

- Highly active against Gram-negative aerobes.
- Lower, but often useful, activity against Gram-positive aerobes, though the 'prudent use' principle would argue for choice of a narrower spectrum agent instead.
- Active against all aerobic enteric Gram-negative bacilli and all aerobic bacterial gut pathogens.
- Better activity against *Pseudomonas* than with antipseudomonal penicillins, cephalosporins or gentamicin; activity is similar to that of tobramycin.
- Active against 90–100% of bacterial isolates from urine (where concentrations are 10–20-fold higher than in plasma) including methicillin-resistant *Staphylococcus.*
- Active against *Brucella, Chlamydophila, Mycobacterium* and *Mycoplasma.*
- Penetrate intracellularly, thus potentially effective against intracellular bacteria. Concentrate in phagolysosomes, enhancing intracellular killing.
- Variable activity against *Streptococcus.*

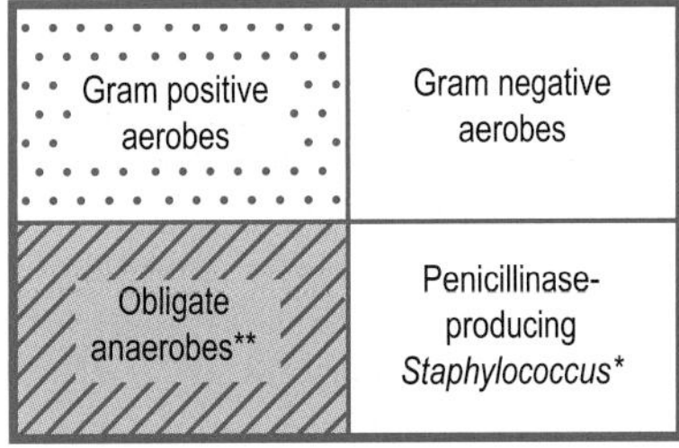

+ *Brucella, Mycoplasma, Chlamydophila, Rickettsia, Mycobacterium* spp.

* MRSA may be susceptible

Fig. 8.22 **Antibacterial spectrum for fluoroquinolones. **New fluoroquinolones that have anti-anaerobic activity may reach the veterinary market in the future.**

- Rarely synergistic or antagonistic in combination with other antibacterial drugs.
- Fluoroquinolones currently in the veterinary market are relatively inactive against obligate anaerobic bacteria. However, newer fluoroquinolones with anti-anaerobic activity (such as trovafloxacin) have been developed and used in human medicine. Similar drugs may reach the veterinary market in the future.

There are some differences in antibacterial spectrum between individual fluoroquinolones. Norfloxacin is less active than newer fluoroquinolones against *Pseudomonas*. Ciprofloxacin has greater activity against multidrug-resistant Gram-negative bacteria such as *Pseudomonas*, various *Mycoplasma* and intracellular pathogens such as *Brucella* and *Mycobacterium*. Enrofloxacin, the first 'veterinary' fluoroquinolone, has greater absorption after oral administration than ciprofloxacin but less antipseudomonal activity.

Clinical applications

Fluoroquinolones are important drugs for treating serious Gram-negative infections and should not be used routinely and nonselectively for small animal infections. Possible indications for use as drug of first choice include the following.

- Urinary tract infections caused by *Pseudomonas*
- Bacterial prostatitis in dogs
- Serious Gram-negative systemic infections
- Osteomyelitis caused by Gram-negative aerobes
- Saprophytic *Mycobacterium* infection in cats
- Deep granulomatous pyoderma
- Serious bacterial respiratory tract infections
- Management of neutropenic, febrile patients on cancer chemotherapy
- Otitis externa due to Gram-negative infections (following culture and susceptibility testing).

Pharmacokinetics

Fluoroquinolones are rapidly absorbed after oral administration in monogastric animals; absorption is complete (80–100%) for enrofloxacin, less so for ciprofloxacin (50–70%) and norfloxacin (40%). Administration with food may delay the time to peak plasma concentration but does not alter the concentration achieved. Administration with compounds that contain metal ions will adversely affect plasma fluoroquinolone concentrations.

Low protein binding, low ionization and high lipid solubility result in large volumes of distribution and good penetration into CSF, bronchial secretions, bone, cartilage and prostate. Concentrations achieved in respiratory and genitourinary tract secretions are higher than plasma concentrations and prostatic concentrations may be 2–3 times higher than in plasma.

The major metabolite of enrofloxacin is ciprofloxacin but the amount of ciprofloxacin produced varies between and within species. Elimination may be renal, hepatic or both, depending on the drug. Enrofloxacin undergoes predominantly renal elimination, for difloxacin it is fecal and marbofloxacin is excreted in both urine and feces.

The elimination half-life varies with the drug but is usually sufficiently long (8–12 h) to permit once-daily dosing. A postantibiotic effect (continued suppression of bacterial growth following removal of the drug) of a few minutes to several hours occurs with fluoroquinolones against most Gram-negative and some Gram-positive bacteria. The duration of the postantibiotic effect depends on the pathogen, the concentration of the drug above MIC and the duration of exposure.

Urinary drug concentrations are substantially in excess of MIC values for virtually all susceptible pathogens, exceeding plasma concentrations by several hundred times and remaining high for 24 h after administration.

Adverse effects

- Adverse effects with fluoroquinolones are uncommon. Vomiting, inappetence or diarrhea may occur occasionally. Facial erythema and edema have been reported rarely, as have tremors and ataxia.
- Seizures have been reported rarely in animals with CNS disorders, with high doses and with concurrent use of nonsteroidal anti-inflammatory drugs.
- An apparent species-specific toxicity is acute retinal degeneration in cats treated with enrofloxacin. Blindness often results but some cats may regain vision. The daily and total doses of enrofloxacin administered and duration of treatment in affected cats seem highly variable. However, the blindness does appear to be dose related and doses in cats should not exceed 5 mg/kg/day. It has been postulated that the relatively open blood–brain barrier of cats combined with the lipophilic properties of enrofloxacin predispose cats to accumulating high concentrations of the drug in the CNS. The risk may be higher in cats with urinary tract infections and concomitant renal failure and care should be taken with dosage in geriatric cats or those with liver or renal impairment. It is not clear whether other fluoroquinolones can also cause blindness.
- Fluoroquinolones should not be used in young animals as they cause erosion of articular cartilage (in dogs more than cats and large dogs especially). The mechanism of cartilage damage may be related to chelation of magnesium in joints. Lesions have been documented in dogs given five times the recom-

mended dose and occur within 1–2 days of beginning administration. It is recommended that fluoroquinolones be avoided in large breed dogs up to 18 months of age (12 months for medium breeds, 9 months for small breeds). If a fluoroquinolone must be used because there is no suitable alternative, strict exercise restriction (especially for large breed dogs) and use of chondroprotectives (see Chapter 13) are advised.

METRONIDAZOLE

Mechanism of action and resistance

Metronidazole is bactericidal to anaerobic bacteria, probably in a concentration-dependent manner. After entry into the cell it undergoes reduction to produce unstable intermediates, some of which have antibacterial activity. These cause extensive breakage of DNA strands and inhibit the DNA repair enzyme, DNAase-1. This reduction reaction occurs under anaerobic conditions and is insufficient to produce active metabolites in aerobic bacteria. Hence metronidazole is only active against those bacteria that are anaerobic. It is also active against many protozoa but the mechanisms involved are incompletely understood. Resistance is rare among susceptible bacteria and involves reduced intracellular drug activation.

Antibacterial spectrum (Fig. 8.23)

Metronidazole is bactericidal for many Gram-positive and most Gram-negative obligate anaerobes; its activity is equal to that of benzylpenicillin and of clindamycin. It has no effect on aerobic bacteria. It is active against *Balantidium coli, Entamoeba histolytica, Giardia* and *Trichomonas. Campylobacter* are moderately susceptible. *Helicobacter pylori* are commonly susceptible but the susceptibility of animal-derived *Helicobacter* spp has not been established. Resistance is rare amongst susceptible species.

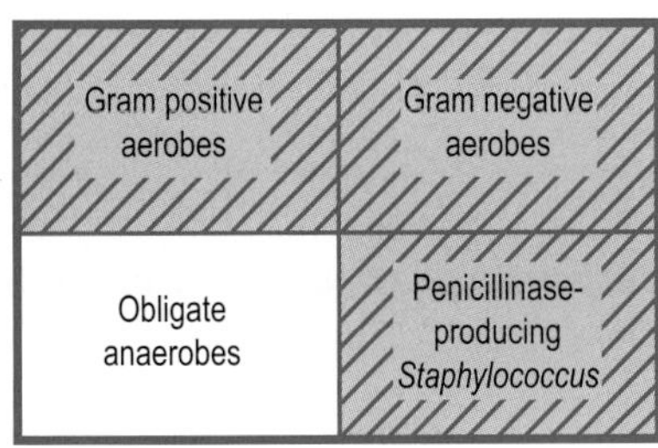

+ *Giardia, Entomoeba histolytica, Trichomonas* and *Balantidium coli.*

Fig. 8.23 Antibacterial spectrum for metronidazole.

Clinical applications

- Gastrointestinal infections with *Balantidium coli, Entamoeba histolytica, Giardia, Trichomonas* or anaerobic bacteria.
- Mouth infections, periodontal disease, ulcerative gingivitis – sometimes used in combination with spiramycin for these.
- Bacterial overgrowth of the small intestine and antibiotic-responsive diarrhea (other common drug choices are tylosin and tetracyclines; choice appears to reflect the clinician's preference rather than empirical data).
- Anaerobic soft tissue infections, especially where good tissue penetration is important.
- In combination with a fluoroquinolone for serious sepsis of unknown etiology or spillage of intestinal contents.
- Metronidazole has some inhibitory action on cell-mediated immunity which may partly account for its beneficial effects in some cases of diarrhea.

Pharmacokinetics

Metronidazole is relatively well absorbed after oral administration PO and absorption is enhanced in dogs by administration with food (in contrast to humans, in whom absorption is delayed). Bioavailability is high but varies individually from 50% to 100%. Metronidazole HCl powder is available for injection IV.

Metronidazole is highly lipophilic and achieves excellent penetration of tissues, including bone, CNS and abscesses. It is extensively oxidized and conjugated in the liver to less active metabolites but about two-thirds of the dose is excreted in the urine, mostly in an active form. Elimination half-life is reported to be 4–5 h in dogs compared with 6–8 h in humans.

Adverse effects

- Adverse effects are uncommon but vomiting, nausea or inappetence may occur.
- Dose-related neurotoxicity has been reported in dogs given 67–129 mg/kg/day for 6–12 days. Signs included severe ataxia, positional nystagmus, seizures and head tilt.
- Cats often salivate profusely after administration of metronidazole.
- Inappetence has been noted in horses.
- A marginal and contentious carcinogenic effect has been observed in some laboratory studies. As a result metronidazole and other nitroimidazoles are no longer used in food-producing animals in some countries.
- Metronidazole may be teratogenic and therefore should not be used during pregnancy, especially in the first 3 weeks, unless the benefits to the mother outweigh potential risks to the fetus.

RIFAMPICIN (RIFAMPIN)

This synthetically modified antibiotic product of *Streptomyces mediterranei* has been an important component of the treatment of tuberculosis in humans.

Mechanism of action and resistance

Rifampicin acts by inhibiting RNA polymerase, which catalyzes the transcription of DNA to RNA. Gram-negative bacteria are relatively impermeable to the drug.

Chromosomal mutation leading to high-level resistance develops readily in most bacteria. The mechanism involves development of stable changes in RNA polymerase that prevent binding. Because the mutation rate is high, rifampicin should always be used in combination with another antibacterial drug. Resistance to rifampicin is not transferable and there is no cross-resistance with other antibacterials.

Antibacterial spectrum (Fig. 8.24)

Rifampicin is bactericidal and has a wide spectrum of activity, including the following.

- Gram-positive aerobic bacteria, particularly *Staphylococcus spp* and *Rhodococcus equi.*
- *Brucella* and some other fastidious organisms are susceptible but Gram-negative bacteria more generally are resistant.
- Gram-positive and Gram-negative anaerobic bacteria are inhibited at low concentrations, including *Bacteroides fragilis.*
- *Chlamydophila* and *Rickettsia* are susceptible.
- *Mycobacterium tuberculosis*: activity is high against this organism but most other mycobacteria are resistant.
- Some protozoa.
- Some fungi and poxviruses (although this activity is thought to be of no clinical value).

Gram positive aerobes	Gram negative aerobes**
Obligate anaerobes	Penicillinase-producing *Staphylococcus**

* MRSA may be susceptible

** Brucella and other fastidious organisms may be susceptible

Fig. 8.24 **Antibacterial spectrum for rifampicin. *MRSA may be susceptible.**

Clinical applications

- Rifampicin is primarily used in small animal practice to treat chronic granulomatous skin infections in dogs.
- It is used in combination with erythromycin to treat *Rhodococcus equi* infections in foals.

Pharmacokinetics

Absorption after oral administration is good and peak blood concentration occurs within 2–4 h. Rifampicin has excellent tissue penetration and is effective against intracellular bacteria. Penetration into CSF is poor but enhanced by inflammation. Penetration into phagocytic cells is excellent. Half-life is about 8 h in dogs.

Rifampicin is acetylated in the liver to a bioactive metabolite. The metabolite and unchanged drug are excreted primarily in bile but a proportion may be excreted in urine. Rifampicin can induce hepatic microsomal enzymes, which may result in increased elimination rate with time. The metabolism of other drugs, such as barbiturates, ketoconazole, theophylline and corticosteroids, may be increased. Urine, feces, sweat and tears may be colored red-orange.

Adverse effects

There is a greater prevalence of toxicity to rifampicin in dogs than in humans. Approximately 20% of dogs develop increases in hepatic enzyme concentrations in blood and may progress to clinical hepatitis. This may be fatal in dogs with a history of liver disease.

NITROFURANS

EXAMPLES

Nitrofurantoin, furazolidone.

Mechanism of action

The antibacterial effect of nitrofurans results from poorly characterized reduction products that derived from degradation of the drug by bacterial nitroreductase enzymes. One mechanism by which these reduction products kill bacteria is by disrupting codon–anticodon interactions, which prevents mRNA translation. The mechanism of action against susceptible protozoa has not been determined.

Antimicrobial spectrum, clinical applications and clinical pharmacology

Nitrofurantoin

Nitrofurantoin has broad antibacterial activity but its use in small animals is limited to treatment of lower urinary tract infections.

- Nitrofurantoin has activity against several Gram-negative and some Gram-positive aerobic bacteria

including many isolates of *Escherichia, Klebsiella, Enterobacter, Enterococcus, Staphylococcus* and *Salmonella.*
- It has little or no activity against most strains of *Proteus* and no activity against *Pseuodmonas.*
- Nitrofurans have moderate activity against anaerobic bacteria and are most active in anaerobic conditions. Some aerobic bacteria that are resistant under aerobic conditions are susceptible when tested under anaerobic conditions.
- Nitrofurantoin is rapidly absorbed from the gut. It is rapidly eliminated (drug appears in the urine within 30 min of administration) and therapeutic blood concentrations cannot be maintained. Half-life in humans with normal renal function averages 20 min. Approximately 40–50% of the drug is eliminated unchanged in the urine.
- Adverse effects reported in small animals include gastrointestinal disturbances and hepatopathy.

Furazolidone

- Furazolidone has antiprotozoal and antibacterial activity. It is active against *Giardia, Trichomonas* and many coccidia as well as several Gram-negative aerobic bacteria.
- It is used clinically in small animals to treat enteric infections caused by these organisms.
- The degree to which furazolidone is absorbed has not been definitely established.
- Adverse effects are uncommon but may include anorexia, vomiting, abdominal cramps and diarrhea.

CLOFAZIMINE

Clofazimine is a phazine dye that binds to DNA and may inhibit its function as a template. It is used in humans as part of multidrug protocols to treat leprosy. Clofazimine is used in cats to treat *Mycobacterium lepraemurium* and other nontuberculous mycobacterial infections. The clinical pharmacology of the drug and its adverse effect profile have not been well documented in small animals. In humans the adverse effect of most concern is dose-related skin, eye and body fluid discoloration (pink to brownish black) that occurs in most patients and can persist for months to years after the drug is discontinued. This effect has been reported to occur in animals. Hepatoxicity has been reported in a dog.

SUMMARY OF ACTIVITY/INACTIVITY OF ANTIBACTERIAL DRUGS

Drugs	Quadrant	Quadrant	Drugs
Aminopenicillins Cephalosporins Lincosamides/macrolides Penicillin G	Gram positive aerobes	Gram negative aerobes	Cephalosporins (2nd and 3rd generation) Aminoglycosides Fluoroquinolones Ticarcillin-clavulanate
Aminopenicillins Chloramphenicol Clindamycin Metronidazole Penicillin G	Obligate anaerobes	Penicillinase-producing *Staphylococcus*	Amoxicillin-clavulanate Antistaphylococcal penicillins Cephalosporins (1st and 2nd generation) Fluoroquinolones Rifampicin Vancomycin

Fig. 8.25 Summary of drugs with excellent activity against most, although not necessarily all, pathogens in each quadrant.

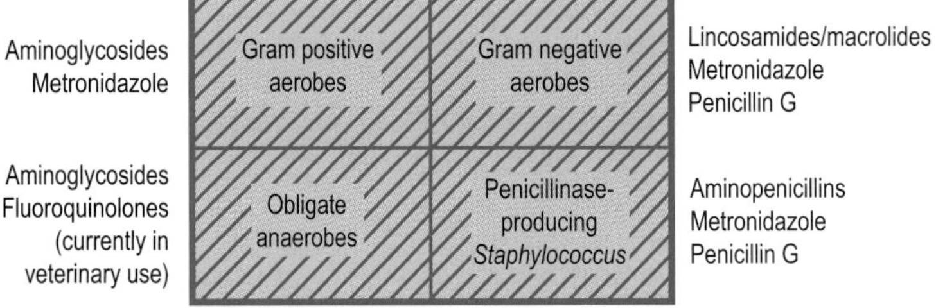

Fig. 8.26 Summary of drugs with no useful activity against most pathogens in each quadrant, although there may be some individual exceptions.

9

Systemic antifungal therapy

Joseph Taboada and Amy M Grooters

INTRODUCTION

Fungal pathogens have assumed an increasingly important role in human disease in the past three decades as immunocompromise associated with bone marrow transplantation, organ transplantation and human immunodeficiency virus infection has become more prevalent. The need for more effective and less toxic options for the treatment of systemic mycoses in human patients has prompted a search for new agents that selectively target the fungal cell wall and for new ways to increase the efficacy and safety of traditional antifungal agents, such as amphotericin B and the azoles. As a result, veterinarians now have access to a rapidly expanding armamentarium of compounds with high efficacy and low toxicity for the treatment of mycotic infections in small animal patients.

Targets for antifungal drug therapy

Historically, progress in the development of antifungal drugs has been slow in comparison to antibacterial agents. One important reason for this delay is that, as eukaryotic organisms, fungi contain few drug targets that are not also present in mammalian cells, making the search for agents with selective fungal toxicity difficult. The vast majority of traditional antifungal drugs target ergosterol, an essential component of the fungal cell membrane. The selectivity of these drugs is based on their greater affinity for ergosterol in the fungal cell membrane than for cholesterol in the mammalian cell membrane and limits, but does not eliminate, their potential for toxicity to mammalian cells. The ideal antifungal agent would be one that targets structures present in fungal pathogens that are absent in other eukaryotic cells. The fungal cell wall, a structure that is both unique and essential to fungi, would seem to be such a target. For this reason, compounds that interfere with the synthesis of important fungal cell wall components such as glucan, chitin and mannoproteins have become a focus in the development of new antifungal agents.

AMPHOTERICIN B

Amphotericin B, a polyene antibiotic, acts by binding to ergosterol in the fungal cell membrane, disrupting membrane stability and quickly causing cell death. Because of its efficacy against a broad spectrum of yeast and filamentous fungal pathogens, amphotericin B has traditionally been the treatment of choice for invasive fungal infections in human and small animal patients. However, its application has been hindered by nephrotoxicity, which limits the total dose that can be administered and prevents its use in patients with underlying renal dysfunction. However, the use of novel delivery systems has been effective in reducing nephrotoxicity and improving organ-specific delivery of amphotericin B.

Clinical applications

- Initial treatment of choice for rapidly progressive systemic mycoses in which oral triazoles are unlikely to act quickly enough.
- Initial therapy for dogs with cryptococcal meningitis in which case it may be combined with flucytosine as well as fluconazole.
- Treatment of systemic mycoses that fail to respond to azole therapy.
- Treatment of animals with mycotic gastrointestinal disease such as pythiosis or zygomycosis in which persistent vomiting precludes the administration of oral medications.
- Treatment of blastomycosis, histoplasmosis, cryptococcosis, coccidioidomycosis, candidiasis, sporotrichosis and pythiosis.

Mechanism of action

Amphotericin B binds to ergosterol in the fungal cell membrane, causing depolarization and increased membrane permeability, leakage of cell contents and cell death. The clinical usefulness of this drug is based on its greater affinity for ergosterol in the fungal cell membrane than for cholesterol in the mammalian cell membrane. In addition to its fungicidal action, there is convincing evidence that amphotericin B has significant immunomodulatory effects, which may play an important role in its antifungal activity. The results of both in vitro and in vivo studies suggest that amphotericin B is a powerful macrophage activator, potentiating their phagocytic, tumoricidal and microbicidal actions. One important mechanism for this potentiation appears to be enhancement of macrophage-killing activity via nitric oxide-dependent pathways mediated by amphotericin-induced production of tumor necrosis factor (TNF)-α and interleukin (IL)-1. In addition, amphotericin B has been shown to augment the macrophage oxidative burst induced by TNF-α.

Formulations and dose rates

Amphotericin B deoxycholate (Fungizone®)

Amphotericin B deoxycholate, a lyophilized preparation of amphotericin B combined with deoxycholate and sodium phosphate buffer to form a micellar suspension for injection, is the traditional formulation of amphotericin B. It is relatively inexpensive but its usefulness in small animal patients has been limited by cumulative dose-dependent nephrotoxicity.

Amphotericin B deoxycholate is most often administered intravenously. An appropriate dose should be diluted in 5% dextrose and administered over a period of time ranging from 10 min to 4–5 h. However, longer infusion times should be used in debilitated animals and those that demonstrate infusion-related side effects. Cats are more susceptible than dogs to the nephrotoxic effects of amphotericin B and a lower dose must therefore be administered. Care should be exercised if amphotericin B is to be used in a patient with pre-existing renal disease. Although the amount of drug administered per dose is usually not altered, the total cumulative dose that can be tolerated by these patients may be lower.

DOGS

- 0.25–0.75 mg/kg, IV, three times weekly to a cumulative dose of 4–8 mg/kg, or until azotemia develops. In particularly severe mycoses some dogs may require and tolerate IV doses of 1 mg/kg, with cumulative doses up to 12 mg/kg. The lower cumulative doses are generally recommended when amphotericin B is used concurrently with an azole antifungal

CATS

- 0.1–0.25 mg/kg, IV, three times weekly to a cumulative dose of 4–6 mg/kg

Subcutaneous administration

Subcutaneous administration of amphotericin B has been described as a means to decrease nephrotoxicity while increasing the cumulative dose that can be administered. The following protocol has been used successfully to treat cryptococcosis in dogs and cats: 0.5–0.8 mg/kg of amphotericin B diluted in 400 mL (cats) or 500–1000 mL (dogs) of 0.45% NaCl/2.5% dextrose and administered subcutaneously 2–3 times per week to a cumulative dose of 8–26 mg/kg. Sterile abscesses may occur following subcutaneous administration of amphotericin B at concentrations greater than 20 mg/L. Such concentrations are at times unavoidable when treating large dogs.

Pharmacokinetics

Amphotericin B is poorly absorbed from the gastrointestinal tract and must therefore be administered parenterally. Following intravenous administration, amphotericin B is highly bound (>90%) to plasma proteins (primarily lipoproteins). The drug is rapidly cleared from the plasma and binds to cholesterol-containing membranes in local tissues, where it is metabolized. Highest concentrations are found in the kidney, liver, spleen and lung, with low concentrations in cerebrospinal fluid (CSF), eye, bone and urine. Amphotericin B will cross inflamed pleura and synovium; however, drug levels achieved in these spaces are approximately half those found in plasma. The metabolic fate of amphotericin B is unknown. It exhibits a biphasic elimination in humans, with an initial plasma half-life of 24–48 h, followed by a longer terminal half-life of more than 15 days, probably related to its very slow release from tissues. Little unmetabolized (parent) amphotericin B is excreted in urine or bile.

Adverse effects

- The therapeutic usefulness of amphotericin B in small animal patients is significantly limited by cumulative dose-related nephrotoxicity, which is attributable to both vasoconstrictive and tubulotoxic effects.
- Vascular side effects are manifested as decreased glomerular filtration rate (GFR) and renal blood flow (which may eventually lead to azotemia).
- Tubular effects are directed primarily at the distal tubule, resulting in impaired urinary acidification, decreased urinary concentrating ability and potassium wasting. Tubular and vascular side effects are thought to be related. Disruption of tubular cell integrity results in increased delivery of chloride ions to the distal tubule with subsequent decreased GFR and renal blood flow resulting from tubuloglomerular feedback. This feedback is amplified by sodium depletion and suppressed by sodium loading.
- Saline diuresis or furosemide administration prior to amphotericin B infusion have been shown to blunt its effect on renal blood flow and their use should be considered in patients at high risk for nephrotoxicity.
- Because the development of nephrotoxicity is common, serum blood urea nitrogen (BUN), creatinine and potassium should be evaluated prior to each treatment in animals receiving amphotericin B. If azotemia develops, treatment should be discontinued until values have normalized.
- To avoid exacerbation of nephrotoxicity, animals should be well hydrated prior to administration of amphotericin B.

- Infusion-related side effects such as pyrexia, tremors, nausea and vomiting may occur in some animals during intravenous administration of amphotericin B. These effects can be diminished by pretreating patients with an antihistamine (e.g. diphenhydramine, 2 mg/kg IV or PO), aspirin (10 mg/kg PO), or a physiological dose of a glucocorticoid prior to subsequent infusions.
- Other potential side effects include thrombophlebitis, hypomagnesemia, cardiac arrhythmias and non-regenerative anemia.

Contraindications and precautions

Amphotericin B should be used with caution in animals that have pre-existing renal disease. In azotemic animals with systemic mycoses that are not immediately life-threatening, the use of triazole antifungal agents should be considered instead of amphotericin B for initial treatment.

Known drug interactions

- Because amphotericin B deoxycholate is solubilized in a phosphate-containing buffer, it should not be diluted in calcium-containing fluids.
- The use of amphotericin B with other nephrotoxic drugs (such as aminoglycosides) should be avoided.

Amphotericin b lipid complex (ABLC; Abelcet®)

The use of novel delivery systems has been effective in reducing toxicity and improving organ-specific delivery of many drugs, including amphotericin B. The development of liposomal-encapsulated and lipid-complexed preparations of amphotericin B has reduced its nephrotoxicity and increased its uptake by specific tissue sites. There are currently three novel formulations of amphotericin B marketed for clinical use in human patients: amphotericin B lipid complex (Abelcet®), amphotericin B colloidal dispersion (Amphotec®) and liposome-encapsulated amphotericin B (AmBisome®). These formulations offer an improved therapeutic index, in part because they increase the drug's uptake by tissues such as the liver and lungs, preventing its accumulation in the kidneys. Of the three formulations, amphotericin B lipid complex (Abelcet®) has been the most extensively evaluated in small animals.

Clinical applications

Clinical trials in human patients have documented the efficacy and improved therapeutic index of lipid-complexed amphotericin B for the treatment of many common fungal pathogens, including *Candida, Aspergillus, Cryptococcus, Histoplasma, Blastomyces* and *Coccidioides immitis*. In small animal patients, ABLC has been used successfully for the treatment of blastomycosis, coccidioidomycosis, histoplasmosis, cryptococcal meningitis, protothecosis and pythiosis.

Mechanism of action

The improved therapeutic index of ABLC has been demonstrated in numerous animal studies. In dogs receiving multiple doses, ABLC was determined to be 8–10 times less nephrotoxic than conventional amphotericin B. This decreased nephrotoxicity can be attributed to several factors.

- Lipid binding results in reduction of amphotericin-induced direct tubular toxicity.
- Lipid binding reduces the amount of free amphotericin in solution.
- Lipid complexes provide the opportunity for selective transfer of amphotericin from its lipid carrier to ergosterol in the fungal cell membrane.
- Binding of lipid-complexed amphotericin to high-density lipoproteins results in decreased uptake by renal cells.

In human studies, lipid-based products significantly reduced the risk of all-cause mortality by an estimated 28% compared with conventional amphotericin B. The primary reduction in toxicity was related to reduced nephrotoxicity. Infusion-related toxicities were not significantly different from conventional amphotericin B.

In animal studies the primary reason for increased efficacy is reduced toxicity, allowing higher cumulative doses to be obtained. The increased efficacy of ABLC may also be due to the rapid uptake of lipid complexes by the reticuloendothelial (RE) system. As a result, the drug is able to target sites of inflammation and organs of the RE system, such as the liver, spleen and lungs. Once at the target site, lipases from either fungal or inflammatory cells may release the amphotericin B from its lipid complex, allowing it to bind to and disrupt the fungal cell membrane.

Formulations and dose rates

ABLC is diluted in 5% dextrose to a concentration of 1 mg/mL and infused intravenously over 1–2 h. As with traditional amphotericin, serum creatinine, BUN and potassium should be checked prior to each administration. Preloading with saline fluids to protect from nephrotoxicity does not appear to be necessary when administering ABLC.

DOGS

- 2–3 mg/kg of ABLC IV 3 days per week for a total of 9–12 treatments, to a cumulative dose of 24–27 mg/kg

CATS

- 1 mg/kg 3 days per week for a total of 12 treatments to a cumulative dose of 12 mg/kg

FLUCYTOSINE

Flucytosine is a synthetic fluorinated pyrimidine antifungal drug that was first synthesized as a cytosine analog for use as an antineoplastic compound. It is classed as a nucleoside analog.

Clinical applications

- When used alone, flucytosine has weak therapeutic activity and limited clinical application.
- The drug is synergistic with amphotericin B and is used almost exclusively as an adjunct to amphotericin B in the treatment of cryptococcosis.
- It is effective against *Candida* spp but resistance develops rapidly, making it less than ideal.

Mechanism of action

The activity of flucytosine is attributed to disruption of protein synthesis by inhibition of RNA synthesis in the fungal cell. Flucytosine enters fungal cells via cytosine permease, an enzyme that is lacking in mammalian cells. Once inside the fungal cell, flucytosine is converted to 5-fluorouracil.

Formulations and dose rates

Flucytosine is administered orally. It is generally administered concurrently with amphotericin B.

DOGS

- 25–50 mg/kg PO q.6–8 h

CATS

- 25–50 mg/kg PO q.6–8 h

Pharmacokinetics

Flucytosine has high oral bioavailability. It is widely distributed and crosses the blood–brain barrier. Only about 2–4% of the drug is bound to plasma proteins. Absorbed drug is freely filtered via glomerular filtration and excreted unchanged in the urine. Significant prolongation of the half-life can be expected in animals with renal impairment.

Adverse effects

- The most common adverse effects include diarrhea, anorexia and vomiting.
- Dose-dependent bone marrow suppression manifesting as neutropenia, thrombocytopenia or pancytopenia is a less common but more significant toxicity.
- Hypersensitivity resulting in cutaneous eruption and rash has been reported.
- In cats, seizures and aberrant behavior have been noted.

Contraindications and precautions

- Flucytosine is contraindicated in patients with a known hypersensitivity.
- Extreme care should be used in patients with renal dysfunction or in patients with pre-existing disease affecting the bone marrow.
- Flucytosine should not be used in pregnant animals.

Known drug interactions

Flucytosine has been shown to be synergistic with amphotericin B, but amphotericin B-associated decreases in GFR may result in increased toxicity.

AZOLE ANTIFUNGALS

EXAMPLES

The azoles are classified as imidazoles (miconazole, econazole, clotrimazole and ketoconazole) or triazoles (fluconazole, itraconazole and voriconazole) according to whether they contain, respectively, two or three nitrogen atoms in the five-member azole ring. Ketoconazole and itraconazole have similar pharmacological profiles but fluconazole is unique because of its comparatively small molecular size and low lipophilicity. Voriconazole has a pharmacological profile that is similar to itraconazole in some respects but to fluconazole in others.

Clinical applications

The azole class has become the initial treatment of choice for all but the most rapidly progressing and most severe systemic fungal infections. A major advantage of azole therapy has been the ability to treat endemic mycoses such as histoplasmosis and blastomycosis on an outpatient basis with oral medication. The azoles act much more slowly than the polyenes, making them less useful for severely affected patients or patients with rapidly progressive systemic mycoses.

Ketoconazole has a more significant effect on host cholesterol metabolism than the other azole antifungal agents and has been used (with limited success) as an inhibitor of corticosteroid biosynthesis in the treatment of canine hyperadrenocorticism.

Mechanism of action

The azoles are a rapidly expanding class of antifungal agents that act by inhibiting ergosterol biosynthesis, thus interfering with fungal cell membrane function by causing depletion of ergosterol and accumulation of lanosterol and other 14-methylated sterols (Fig. 9.1). The azole antifungal agents inhibit cytochrome P450-dependent 14-sterol demethylase, a cytochrome P450

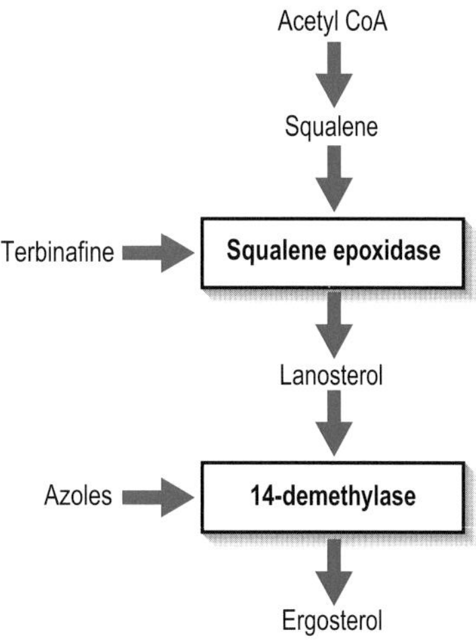

Fig. 9.1 **Sites of enzyme inhibition by antifungal drugs in the ergosterol biosynthesis pathway.**

enzyme that is necessary for the conversion of lanosterol to ergosterol. Similar interaction in mammalian cells with enzymes dependent on cytochrome P450 mediates some of the major toxic effects.

The imidazoles are much more potent inhibitors of mammalian cell cytochrome P450 than the triazoles. The triazoles also owe their antifungal activity at least in part to inhibition of cytochrome P450-dependent 14-methyl sterol demethylase. Other antifungal effects of less clear significance include inhibition of endogenous respiration, toxic interaction with membrane phospholipids and inhibition of morphogenetic transformation of yeasts to the mycelial forms. Some of the azole antifungal drugs, especially itraconazole and ketoconazole, are potent immunosuppressive agents, suppressing T-lymphocyte proliferation in vitro. In addition, ketoconazole has anti-inflammatory properties that are probably mediated through inhibition of 5-lipoxygenase activity.

Pharmacokinetics

Ketoconazole and itraconazole are weak bases that require an acid environment for maximum oral absorption. The oral bioavailability of itraconazole in the capsule form is 2–3 times higher when taken with food. However, the solution formulation of itraconazole is not significantly affected by the degree of gastric acidity and is best administered to a fasted animal.

Fluconazole is not affected by gastric pH and food does not affect oral bioavailability. After treatment is begun, steady state is not achieved for itraconazole and fluconazole for 6–21 days. This may account for the clinical lag time that is often noted when animals with systemic fungal infections are treated with these drugs. A loading dose of double the standard dose can be given for the first 3 days of treatment to reduce the time until steady-state concentrations are attained.

Ketoconazole and itraconazole are extensively bound to plasma proteins (>99%), but because of their lipophilicity, both drugs distribute well throughout most tissues while concentrations in urine and CSF are typically very low. Neither drug crosses the blood–brain or blood–ocular barriers well. Despite this, CNS, prostatic and ocular fungal infections respond well to treatment with itraconazole.

Itraconazole is concentrated in the skin with delivery via sebum. Sebum concentrations are 5–10 times higher than plasma concentrations and detectable amounts persist for up to 14 days after the drug is discontinued. Detectable concentrations can be found in the hair and stratum corneum for up to 4 weeks. This property makes itraconazole ideal for treating dermatophytes and other fungal infections with significant cutaneous manifestations.

Fluconazole is minimally protein bound, highly water soluble and distributes similarly to free water. High concentrations can be found in urine, CSF and ocular fluids and the drug crosses the blood–brain, blood–prostate and blood–ocular barriers well.

Ketoconazole and itraconazole are extensively metabolized in the liver and excreted in bile and, to a lesser extent, in urine. By contrast, fluconazole is minimally metabolized and approximately 80% is excreted unchanged in urine; consequently, the dose of fluconazole should be reduced in patients with decreased GFR.

Voriconazole has excellent oral bioavailability and can be administered either orally or intravenously. It has also been shown to penetrate the anterior and posterior segments of the eye following topical or oral administration in humans, rabbits and horses. Voriconazole is eliminated by hepatic metabolism, with less than 2% excreted unchanged in the urine. Because consumption of a high-fat meal decreases its oral bioavailability, voriconazole should not be given with food.

Adverse effects

- Most adverse effects of the azole antifungal agents are dose related and are similar across the class. Ketoconazole is the least well tolerated and fluconazole appears to be the best.
- Dose-related gastrointestinal side effects such as anorexia and vomiting are most common, especially in cats. When seen, splitting or reducing the dose may be of benefit.
- Azole-induced anorexia in cats is also often ameliorated by the use of appetite stimulants such as oxazepam or cyproheptadine.

- Hepatotoxicity is a potentially severe side effect that is seen most often with ketoconazole and less often with the triazoles.
- Patients being treated with azole antifungals should periodically have liver enzymes monitored.
- Hepatotoxicity is rare after the first 2–3 months of therapy.
- Asymptomatic increases in transaminase activities are common. They are seen in about half of animals treated with itraconazole and a smaller number of animals treated with fluconazole. Increases appear to correlate well with serum concentrations of the drug. Asymptomatic increases in transaminase activities are not usually indicative of clinically significant hepatotoxicity and thus do not necessitate changes in therapy unless the animal is also anorectic, vomiting, depressed, has abdominal pain or other evidence of hepatic dysfunction. Enzyme concentrations will often return to normal without dose adjustment or other intervention.
- Cutaneous reactions are occasionally seen, especially with itraconazole use. More severe reactions such as erythema multiforme or toxic epidermal necrolysis are rare.
- Thrombocytopenia has been associated with ketoconazole and fluconazole use.
- A unique toxicity to ketoconazole is suppression of adrenal and testicular steroid production.
- Adrenal insufficiency is possible with ketoconazole use.
- Voriconazole is well tolerated by most human patients, but adverse effects that have occasionally been reported include reversible visual disturbances, dermatopathies, elevations in liver enzymes and, rarely, hepatic failure.

Contraindications and precautions

- The azoles (especially ketoconazole) are potentially teratogenic and should not be used in pregnant animals without weighing the risk to the fetus against the severity of the fungal infection.
- Ketoconazole should not be used in thrombocytopenic patients or in patients with hepatic disease, whereas the triazoles are not absolutely contraindicated but should be used with great caution in such circumstances.
- Midazolam and cisapride should not be used concurrently with azole antifungals as fatal drug reactions have been noted in humans.
- Metabolism of a number of drugs may be altered by azole antifungal therapy (see below).

Known drug interactions

- Azole inhibition of hepatic microsomal enzymes can lead to increased concentrations of drugs such as ciclosporin, digoxin, phenytoin, quinidine, sulfonylureas, midazolam, cisapride and warfarin when these drugs are coadministered.
- Antacids, H_2-receptor antagonists and proton-pump inhibitors may reduce gastric acidity and result in decreased oral bioavailability of ketoconazole and itraconazole.

Ketoconazole

Clinical applications

Ketoconazole was the first orally active azole available commercially and became one of the most frequently used antifungal agents in veterinary medicine. The poor selective toxicity of ketoconazole, however, does not allow high enough doses to be used to adequately treat many systemic fungal infections. Efficacy is generally less than that seen with the polyene antifungals or the triazoles. Ketoconazole is generally less expensive than the triazole antifungal agents. However, this can be misleading when treating systemic fungal infections because longer treatment courses, lower efficacy and increased likelihood of relapse often result in substantially higher total costs for therapy over time compared to itraconazole or fluconazole. Ketoconazole has been effective as a sole therapeutic agent in the management of blastomycosis, histoplasmosis, cryptococcosis and coccidioidomycosis. However, with the possible exception of coccidioidomycosis, ketoconazole is probably not as effective for these infections as amphotericin B. Ketoconazole can be used in conjunction with amphotericin B when managing systemic infections, allowing lower doses of amphotericin B to be used and thus limiting nephrotoxicity.

Formulations and dose rates

DOGS

- 5–20 mg/kg PO q.12 h
- The higher doses are often needed to treat systemic fungal infections, especially if CNS involvement is suspected. The lower doses are often adequate for treating coccidioidomycosis

CATS

- 5–10 mg/kg PO q.12 h
- Higher doses are often needed but are rarely tolerated.

Itraconazole

Clinical applications

Itraconazole is more effective than ketoconazole and can be used as a sole agent in the management of most systemic mycoses. Itraconazole appears to be more effective than fluconazole in most situations and is the treatment of choice for blastomycosis and most other systemic mycoses in dogs. Itraconazole has proved very effective as a sole treatment agent for histoplasmosis in cats. It has historically been an important treatment for systemic aspergillosis in humans, but has not proved to be very effective in dogs and cats for this purpose. We have found high-dose itraconazole combined with terbinafine to be variably effective in treating dogs with pythiosis, despite the fact that *Pythium insidiosum* does not contain significant concentrations of membrane ergosterol.

When treating most systemic fungal infections, there is a lag between the initiation of treatment and clinical improvement. In severely affected animals consideration should be given to the concurrent administration of amphotericin B and itraconazole, especially during this lag period. Itraconazole is a less toxic, more efficacious alternative to griseofulvin for treating dermatophytes and to potassium iodide for treating sporotrichosis.

Formulations and dose rates

DOGS
- 5–10 mg/kg PO or IV q.24 h
- Dogs with blastomycosis should be treated with 5 mg/kg as there is no added benefit to increasing the dose and side effects are dose dependent. Dogs with other systemic fungal infections may require 10 mg/kg

CATS
- 10 mg/kg PO or IV q.24 h
- Anorexia and gastrointestinal side effects are less apparent when the dose is divided into two daily doses

Pharmacokinetics
Pharmacokinetic studies in healthy humans and cats have demonstrated increased absorption of itraconazole after administration of the oral solution in comparison to capsules. Concentrations of itraconazole are typically low in urine and CSF and it does not cross the blood–brain, blood–prostate or blood–ocular barrier well. However, despite this fact, fungal infections involving the CNS, prostate or eye often respond well to itraconazole therapy, perhaps because its liphophilicity allows even small amounts of the drug that move across inflamed barriers to accumulate in these lipid-laden tissues.

Adverse effects
Dose-related local ulcerative dermatitis, caused by a cutaneous vasculitis, is seen in approximately 5–10% of dogs given high (10 mg/kg) oral doses of itraconazole. When recognized early, the vasculitis usually resolves shortly after the drug is discontinued and rarely recurs if lower doses are reinstituted. If not recognized early, however, the vasculitis can result in catastrophic cutaneous and subcutaneous necrosis and sloughing.

Fluconazole

Clinical applications
Fluconazole can be used similarly to itraconazole although it appears to be slightly less efficacious for many systemic fungal infections. The drug's metabolism and its low lipophilicity and small molecular size may allow increased drug concentrations and efficacy in the management of central nervous system, prostatic and urinary tract infections. However, controlled studies in humans do not indicate a major advantage. Fluconazole appears to be the treatment of choice for cryptococcosis. The marketing of a generic formulation of fluconazole in the USA has substantially reduced the cost of treatment, making fluconazole the most cost-effective antifungal agent in many circumstances.

Formulations and dose rates

DOGS
- 2.5–10 mg/kg PO or IV q.24 h

CATS
- 10 mg/kg PO or IV q.24 h
- 50 mg/cat < 3.2 kg, 100 mg/cat > 3.2 kg for cryptococcosis

Clotrimazole

Clotrimazole is one of the oldest imidazole antifungal drugs.

Clinical application
Clotrimazole has proved to be very effective as an intranasal infusion in the treatment of nasal aspergillosis.

Formulations and dose rates

Clotrimazole has very poor oral bioavailability and is thus used as a topical preparation. A 1% solution of clotrimazole in polyethylene glycol is infused through the nares into the nasal cavity and nasal sinuses. A large Foley catheter is used to occlude the internal nasal choanae by placing the balloon of the catheter into the nasopharynx in a retrograde manner via the oral cavity. Two smaller Foley catheters can be used to occlude the external nares. The drug is infused into the nasal cavity (60 mL per side in medium to large-breed dogs) of the anesthetized patient and allowed to sit for 1 h. Rotating the head after each 15 min has been recommended to enhance drug distribution.

A 1% solution in propylene glycol is available commercially. Although used safely in many cases, this preparation has been implicated in the induction of pharyngeal inflammation and edema in one dog that developed upper airway obstruction. However, other factors associated with case management probably contributed.

Pharmacokinetics

As previously mentioned, clotrimazole has very poor oral bioavailability. Less than 3% is absorbed from mucosal surfaces and less than 0.5% is absorbed through the skin. Most of the absorbed drug is metabolized on first pass through the liver.

Adverse effects

- Pharyngeal and upper airway irritation is a potential complication. Care should be taken to allow all of the solution to drain from the nasal cavity by keeping the head tilted ventrally over the edge of the table for a short period of time after the procedure. In addition, gauze sponges should be packed into the pharynx during the procedure to catch any of the solution that may leak from the nasopharynx.
- In dogs with cribriform invasion, clotrimazole may cause CNS irritation, which may result in seizures.

NEW TRIAZOLES

The emergence in human patients of azole-resistant fungal pathogens (zygomycetes, dematiaceous fungi, *Candida krusei, C. glabrata*, some strains of *C. albicans, Trichosporon* spp, *Fusarium* spp, *Scedosporium* spp and some *Aspergillus* spp) has prompted a search for new triazoles with greater potency and a wider spectrum of activity. The first of these new-generation triazoles to undergo clinical evaluation are voriconazole, posaconazole, ravuconazole and albaconazole. Of these, only voriconazole has achieved FDA approval and is currently available for clinical use in humans in the USA. Both voriconazole and posaconazole are approved for medical clinical use by the European Union.

Voriconazole

Voriconazole (Vfend®, Pfizer) is a fluconazole derivative that has demonstrated potent activity against many common opportunistic and endemic fungal pathogens in both laboratory animals and humans, with the notable exception of zygomycosis caused by pathogens in the order Mucorales. In human patients, voriconazole is indicated for the treatment of invasive aspergillosis, esophageal candidiasis and infections caused by *Scedosporium apiospermum* and *Fusarium* spp. Although there are no reports to date of the clinical use of voriconazole in veterinary patients, its pharmacokinetic behaviour in the dog has been described. Its expected clinical applications include the treatment of localized fungal infections that are often poorly responsive to itraconazole (such as pheohyphomycosis and mycetoma) and the topical treatment of fungal keratitis in horses. It may also be considered an alternative to amphotericin B for the treatment of systemic aspergillosis, disseminated hyalohyphomycosis and endemic mycoses. Unfortunately, its high expense significantly limits its use in veterinary patients.

The recommended dose of voriconazole in human patients is 6 mg/kg q.12 h for 24 h, followed by 4 mg/kg q.12 h thereafter. Voriconazole has excellent oral bioavailability and can be administered either orally or intravenously. It has also been shown to penetrate the anterior and posterior segments of the eye following topical or oral administration in people and horses. A recent study in healthy horses showed that a 1% voriconazole solution applied topically to the eye was well tolerated and is a reasonable choice for future clinical studies of equine fungal keratitis.

Posaconazole

Posaconazole (Noxafil®, Schering-Plough), a highly potent itraconazole analog, is arguably the most broad-spectrum azole to be approved by the FDA. Data from in vitro studies, animal studies and clinical trials support its activity against a wide variety of fungal pathogens, including *Candida* spp (including azole-resistant species), *Aspergillus* spp, *Fusarium* spp, *Scedosporium* spp, dematiaceous fungi and the causative agents of the endemic mycoses.

In addition, posaconazole is the first azole to show significant efficacy for the treatment of zygomycosis caused by molds in the order Mucorales. In clinical trials, posaconazole has been shown to be as effective as liposomal amphotericin B and voriconazole for the treatment of refractory aspergillosis. The anticipated clinical applications of posaconazole in human patients include the treatment of invasive fungal infections that are resistant to itraconazole (e.g. aspergillosis, zygomycosis, pheohyphomycosis, fusariosis and scedosporiosis), refractory endemic mycoses (e.g. coccidioidomcyosis, histoplasmosis and cryptococcosis) and azole-resistant candidiasis. Posaconazole was approved in the European Union in October 2005 for the treatment of certain serious invasive fungal infections and it was released in Germany in November 2005. It was approved by the FDA in September 2006 for treatment of aspergillosis and candidiasis.

Albaconazole

Albaconazole (Uriach & Co, Barcelona, Spain) is a new broad-spectrum triazole that has good in vitro activity against azole-resistant yeasts, as well as *Aspergillus* spp and *Scedosporium* spp. Interestingly, albaconazole has been reported to induce parasitic cure in a dog model of Chagas disease (caused by the protozoan *Trypano-*

soma (Schizotrypanum) cruzi). It is currently in phase II clinical trials for the treatment of vulvovaginal candidiasis and phase I trials for the treatment of systemic mycoses.

GRISEOFULVIN

Griseofulvin, produced by *Penicillium griseofulvum*, is a fungistatic drug used to treat dermatophytosis caused by species of *Microsporum* and *Trichophyton*. Although griseofulvin has traditionally been considered the drug of choice for systemic therapy of dermatophytosis in dogs and cats, it has been replaced to some degree by itraconazole, which is often better tolerated (especially in cats) and may be more efficacious for the treatment of *M. canis*.

Clinical applications

Griseofulvin is indicated and approved in many countries for systemic treatment of dermatophytic infections of the skin, hair and claws in dogs and cats.

Mechanism of action

Griseofulvin acts by disrupting mitosis, nucleic acid synthesis and cell wall synthesis.

Formulations and dose rates

Close monitoring of the complete blood count is important during griseofulvin administration, especially when using the higher end of the dose range.

DOGS

Microsize preparation*
- 20–50 mg/kg/day PO divided q.12 h

Ultramicrosize preparation
- 5–20 mg/kg/day PO divided q.12 h

CATS

Microsize preparation*
- 20–50 mg/kg/day PO divided q.12 h

Ultramicrosize preparation
- 5–20 mg/kg/day PO divided q.12 h

* Should be administered with a fatty meal to maximize absorption

Pharmacokinetics

Following absorption from the gastrointestinal tract, griseofulvin is deposited in the stratum corneum, with highest concentrations in the outermost layers. Because it is also deposited in keratin precursor cells, new hair or nail growth is resistant to infection.

Oral absorption of griseofulvin is limited by its poor water solubility. However, absorption from the gastrointestinal tract can be enhanced by administration of griseofulvin with a fatty meal or as a polyethylene glycol (PEG) formulation. The particle size of the drug also affects absorption, with the ultramicrosize formulation absorbed about 1.5 times as well as the microsized formulation.

Metabolism of griseofulvin occurs in the liver by oxidative demethylation and glucuronidation to 6-desmethylgriseofulvin (an inactive metabolite). Less than 1% of the drug is excreted unchanged in the urine.

Adverse effects

- The most common side effects associated with griseofulvin therapy are vomiting, diarrhea and anorexia. These can be minimized by decreasing the daily dose and/or dividing it into two or three administrations.
- In general, toxicities associated with griseofulvin administration occur more often in cats than in dogs.
- Bone marrow suppression (usually manifested as neutropenia) may occur as an idiosyncratic reaction, especially in kittens. For this reason, griseofulvin should not be used in kittens under 8 weeks of age, with many authors recommending a minimum age of 12 weeks. In addition, neutropenic reactions are more common in cats infected with feline immunodeficiency virus (FIV). Consequently, FIV testing should be performed prior to initiation of griseofulvin therapy and cats that are FIV positive should receive an alternative therapy (such as itraconazole or terbinafine).
- Other reported side effects of griseofulvin administration include hepatotoxicity and neurological signs.
- In general, adverse reactions to griseofulvin therapy occur more often in Himalayan, Abyssinian, Persian and Siamese cats than in other breeds.
- Griseofulvin is also a potent teratogen and its use is contraindicated in pregnant animals or those that may be bred within a month of therapy. It may also inhibit spermatogenesis.

Contraindications and precautions

Griseofulvin should not be administered to pregnant animals, kittens less than 12 weeks of age or cats that are FIV positive.

Known drug interactions

Phenobarbital may decrease blood concentrations of griseofulvin by inducing hepatic microsomal enzymes.

Therefore, dosage adjustments may be necessary when griseofulvin is administered concurrently with phenobarbital.

ALLYLAMINES

Terbinafine

Terbinafine (Lamisil®) is a synthetic antifungal agent of the allylamine class that inhibits squalene epoxidase, a complex membrane-bound enzyme system that is not part of the cytochrome P450 superfamily. The allylamines were discovered by chance during research into novel central nervous system drugs. Naftifine, a topical allylamine, was the first drug discovered in the class. Terbinafine is an analog that was developed in an attempt to optimize the antifungal properties of naftifine.

Clinical applications

Terbinafine has been most extensively studied for the treatment of dermatophytes. There are few clinical studies of terbinafine use in veterinary patients with other fungal infections. In the cat the drug shows great promise in the treatment of dermatophytes. In humans the drug is most extensively used in the treatment of onychomycosis, dermatophytosis and tinea infections. Pharmacoeconomically, it is considered the drug of choice for treating dermatophyte infections in humans. It also has shown good efficacy when used to treat sporotrichosis. Systemic mycoses are typically less responsive than the superficial mycoses.

Terbinafine is sometimes combined with itraconazole for the treatment of mycotic infections that are traditionally difficult to treat medically, such as pheohyphomycosis, hyalohyphomycosis, systemic aspergillosis, pythiosis and lagenidiosis.

Mechanism of action

Terbinafine is a potent inhibitor of squalene epoxidase, an enzyme important in the synthesis of ergosterol at a site much earlier in the pathway than the 14-demethylation of lanosterol inhibited by the azole antifungal drugs (see Fig. 9.1). The end result of the inhibition of squalene epoxidase in fungi is ergosterol deficiency in the cell membrane and intracellular squalene accumulation. In some species of fungi there is only modest reduction in the ergosterol content so the significant inhibition of fungal cell growth associated with the drug's use is primarily thought to be associated with the accumulation of squalene. In others, ergosterol inhibition appears to be more important. The accumulation of squalene appears to be an important factor that imparts a fungicidal activity to terbinafine.

Formulations and dose rates

DOGS
- 5–10 mg/kg q.24 h when combined with itraconazole for treatment of deep fungal infections
- 30–40 mg/kg q.24 h for treatment of dermatophytosis

CATS
- 5–10 mg/kg q.24 h when combined with itraconazole for treatment of deep fungal infections
- 30–40 mg/kg q.24 h for treatment of dermatophytosis

Pharmacokinetics

Orally administered terbinafine is well absorbed (>70%). The absorption does not appear to be significantly affected by food. The drug is highly lipophilic, metabolized extensively in the liver and widely distributed to the tissues, especially to adipose tissue, the dermis, epidermis and nails. Terbinafine is delivered to the skin primarily through sebum and, like itraconazole, remains in the skin in high concentrations for weeks after the drug has been discontinued. Doses necessary to maintain fungicidal concentrations of terbinafine in the hair of cats are twofold to sixfold higher than doses necessary in humans. The higher end of the dose range (30–40 mg/kg) is necessary to treat cutaneous fungal infections in cats effectively.

Elimination is primarily via hepatic metabolism but, unlike the azole antifungal drugs, the cytochrome P450 system is largely unused in the process so the disposition of drugs whose metabolism involves these enzyme systems is not altered in the same manner as is seen with the azoles. Hepatic metabolism results in a large number of inactive metabolites, many of which are then excreted by the kidney. There does not appear to be renal excretion of active terbinafine.

Adverse effects

Adverse effects are relatively rare but have not been well studied in veterinary patients. They include the following.
- Mild-to-moderate gastrointestinal signs
- Hepatotoxicity (rare)
- Neutropenia or pancytopenia (rare)

Contraindications and precautions

None known but it has been suggested that the dosage should be reduced in humans with hepatic or renal dysfunction.

Known drug interactions

- Cimetidine decreases terbinafine clearance.
- Rifampicin (rifampin) increases its clearance.

ANTIFUNGAL AGENTS THAT TARGET THE FUNGAL CELL WALL

Because of their potential for greater selective toxicity, compounds that interfere with the synthesis of important fungal cell wall components (glucan, chitin and mannoproteins) have recently become a focus in the development of new antifungal agents.

β-glucan synthase inhibitors

Echinocandins and pneumocandins represent a class of antifungal agents (the lipopeptides) that hold perhaps the greatest promise for changing the way in which systemic mycoses are treated in the next decade. These fungicidal compounds act by inhibiting β-glucan synthase, blocking the synthesis of 1,3-β-D-glucan, a structural fungal cell wall component that is not present in mammalian cells. Recently, a new generation of echinocandins with improved water solubility, enhanced potency and an expanded spectrum of antifungal activity has been developed. Because of their poor oral bioavailability, these drugs can only be administered intravenously. The primary limitation of this class of antifungals is their ineffectiveness against *Cryptococcus neoformans*, which contains very little glucan synthase. In general, the echinocandins are well tolerated and are associated with relatively few adverse effects in humans.

Caspofungin (Cancidas®, Merck), the first of the β-glucan synthase inhibitors to gain FDA approval, is a broad-spectrum parenteral formulation that has potent activity against *Aspergillus* and *Candida* species. In addition, it is highly effective for the treatment of *Pneumocystis carinii* (*jiroveci*) pneumonia because of its ability to prevent development of the cyst form, in which glucans are a major structural wall component. In human patients, caspofungin is indicated for the treatment of invasive aspergillosis and candidiasis. Its clinical niche is similar to that of the newer formulations of amphotericin B, but with fewer side effects, and with fewer drug interactions than the azoles. In veterinary patients, caspofungin is indicated for the treatment of systemic aspergillosis, pythiosis, lagenidiosis and refractory endemic mycoses other than crytococcosis. Unfortunately, its expense renders it unavailable to the vast majority of small animal patients.

Micafungin (Mycamine®, Astellas Pharma) is a similar echinocandin that has been approved by the FDA for the treatment of oroesophageal candidiasis and the prevention of candidal infections in neutropenic patients.

Anidulafungin (Pfizer) is an echinocandin with a spectrum of activity similar to that of caspofungin. It has been evaluated in clinical trials for the treatment of oroesophageal candidiasis, candidemia and invasive candidiasis and is currently under FDA review.

Chitin synthase inhibitors

Nikkomycins are competitive inhibitors of chitin synthase that have been most extensively evaluated for their activity against *Coccidioides immitis*, a fungal pathogen with high chitin content. One member of this group, **Nikkomycin Z**, was found to be highly effective for the treatment of coccidioidomycosis in animal models. Unfortunately, the spectrum of activity of nikkomycins for other systemic mycoses is limited and as a result, this class of antifungals is no longer being developed.

Lufenuron (Program®) is a chitin synthase inhibitor of the benzoylphenyl urea class. It has been evaluated for the treatment of pulmonary coccidioidomycosis in 17 dogs treated with 5–10 mg/kg once daily for 16 weeks. Clinical and radiographic improvement was noted in most of these dogs. However, because spontaneous remission may occur in infected dogs without treatment, it is unclear whether or not the clinical improvement was attributable to lufenuron administration. Dogs with disseminated coccidioidomycosis have not responded well to lufenuron therapy. A recent in vitro study showed that lufenuron had no antifungal activity against isolates of *Coccidioides immitis* and *Aspergillus fumigatus*. Lufenuron is not recommended for the treatment of systemic mycoses in veterinary patients.

FURTHER READING

Barrett JP, Vardulaki KA, Conlon C et al 2003 A systematic review of the antifungal effectiveness and tolerability of amphotericin B formulations. Clin Ther 25: 1295-1320

Boothe DM, Herring I, Calvin J et al 1997 Itraconazole disposition after single oral and intravenous and multiple oral dosing in healthy cats. Am J Vet Res 58: 872-877

Chen A, Sobel JD 2005 Emerging azole antifungals. Expert Opin Emerg Drugs 10: 21-33

Clode AB, Davis JL, Salmon J et al 2006 Evaluation of concentration of voriconazole in aqueous humor after topical and oral administration in horses. Am J Vet Res 67: 296-301

Davidson AP 2005 Coccidioidomycosis and aspergillus. In: Ettinger SJ, Feldman EC (eds) Textbook of veterinary internal medicine, 6th edn. Elsevier, Philadelphia, PA: 690-699

De Marie S 1996 Liposomal and lipid-based formulations of amphotericin B. Leukemia 10(suppl 2): S93-S96

Greene CE, Watson ADJ 1998 Antifungal chemotherapy. In: Greene CE (ed.) Infectious diseases of the dog and cat, 2nd edn. WB Saunders, Philadelphia, PA: 357-361

Groll AH, De Lucca AJ, Walsh TJ 1998 Emerging targets for the development of novel antifungal therapeutics. Trends Microbiol 6: 117-124

Gupta AK, Katz HI, Shear NH 1999 Drug interactions with itraconazole, fluconazole and terbinafine and their management. J Am Acad Dermatol 41: 237-249

Hay RJ 1999 Therapeutic potential of terbinafine in subcutaneous and systemic mycoses. Br J Dermatol 141(suppl 56): 36-40

Herbrecht R, Nivoix Y, Fohrer C et al 2005 Management of systemic fungal infections: alternatives to itraconazole. J Antimicrob Chemother 56(suppl 1): i39-i48

Hiemenz JW, Walsh TJ 1996 Lipid formulations of amphotericin B: recent progress and future directions. Clin Infect Dis 22(suppl 2): S133-S144

Hodges RD, Legendre AM, Adams LG et al 1994 Itraconazole for the treatment of histoplasmosis in cats. J Vet Intern Med 8(6): 409-413

Jacobs GJ, Medleau L, Calvert C, Brown J 1997 Cryptococcal infection in cats: factors influencing treatment outcome and results of sequential serum antigen titers in 35 cats. J Vet Intern Med 11: 1-4

Johnson LB, Kauffman CA 2003 Voriconazole: a new triazole antifungal agent. Clin Infect Dis 36: 630-637

Keating GM 2005 Posaconazole. Drugs 65: 1553-1567; discussion 1568-1559

Krawiec DR, McKiernan BC, Twardock AR et al 1996 Use of amphotericin B lipid complex for treatment of blastomycosis in dogs. JAVMA 209: 2073-2075

Legendre AM, Rohrbach BW, Toal RL et al 1996 Treatment of blastomycosis with itraconazole in 112 dogs. J Vet Intern Med 10: 365-371

Malik R, Craig AJ, Wigney DI et al 1996 Combination chemotherapy of canine and feline cryptococcosis using subcutaneously administered amphotericin B. Aust Vet J 73: 124-128

Medleau L, Jacobs GJ, Marks MA 1995 Itraconazole for the treatment of cryptococcosis in cats. J Vet Intern Med 9: 39-42

Moriello KA 2004 Treatment of dermatophytosis in dogs and cats: review of published studies. Vet Dermatol 15: 99-107

Morrison VA 2005 Caspofungin: an overview. Expert Rev Anti Infect Ther 3: 697-705

Olsen JW 1992 The use of liposomal amphotericin B in mycotic and algal diseases in the dog (abstract). 10th ACVIM Forum, p. 808

Perfect JR, Marr KA, Walsh TJ et al 2003 Voriconazole treatment for less-common, emerging, or refractory fungal infections. Clin Infect Dis 36: 1122-1131

Taboada J, Grooters AM 2005 Systemic mycoses. In: Ettinger SJ, Feldman EC (eds) Textbook of veterinary internal medicine, 6th edn. Elsevier, Philadelphia, PA: 671-690

Torres HA, Hachem RY, Chemaly RF et al 2005 Posaconazole: a broad-spectrum triazole antifungal. Lancet Infect Dis 5: 775-785

Wiederhold NP, Lewis RE 2003 The echinocandin antifungals: an overview of the pharmacology, spectrum and clinical efficacy. Expert Opin Investig Drugs 12: 1313-1333

10

Antiparasitic drugs

Stephen W Page

INTRODUCTION

Helminth, arthropod and protozoal infections of companion animals continue to cause significant morbidity and mortality in dogs and cats and frequently present a zoonotic hazard with public health implications. Infection occurs frequently despite the availability and use of a number of very potent and selective antiparasitic drugs (Table 10.1). This highlights the fact that, in addition to the type of drug selected, the way in which drugs are used and integrated with other approaches to parasite control is critical to successful and sustained management of parasite infection. This chapter provides information on the clinical pharmacology of the major antiparasitic drugs together with a summary of the most important epidemiological and public health considerations associated with the parasites of dogs and cats.

PUBLIC HEALTH CONSIDERATIONS

Close contact of humans with dogs and cats as true companions in an aging and increasingly immunocompromised human population has increased the importance and likelihood of transmission of parasitic infections with zoonotic potential. As well as direct transmission of parasitic diseases from dogs and cats to humans, the diagnosis of a specific parasitosis in dogs and cats is frequently a warning or signal that humans too may be exposed to a common source of infection. The list of parasitoses is growing in size and many known associations with human disease are identified in the Appendix to this chapter (p. 245). Veterinarians should include discussion of public health implications of diagnosed parasite infections with clients wherever appropriate, providing advice concerning measures to minimize or exclude the possibility of transmission. Antiparasitic drug use in dogs and cats has the potential to select resistant parasites. If resistant parasites can be transmitted to humans then treatment of infected humans may be jeopardized. Dogs are the major reservoir of *Leishmania infantum* and the public health implications of use of pentavalent antimonial drugs and other agents that are also used in humans have been raised as an issue for consideration when selecting the most appropriate therapy of leishmaniosis in dogs.

APPARENT INEFFICACY

When interventions to treat parasite infections do not meet the therapeutic objective it is important to investigate and find the cause, rather than to simply assume drug failure and change to an alternative drug. Common causes of apparent inefficacy include:

- incorrect diagnosis
- inappropriate or unrealistic therapeutic objective (e.g. the animal may have had a lethal infection and could not have been expected to respond to treatment; control of clinical signs may be possible when eradication of infection is unlikely)
- inappropriate drug prescribed (target disease agent resistant or not inherently susceptible)
- incorrect dose regimen recommended or implemented (inadequate dose rate, frequency or duration of treatment)
- compliance failure (a large category that includes insufficient mixing of suspensions, inadequate application of externally applied products, incorrect dosing frequency and many more)
- reinfection by continuous or intermittent exposure (very common with many parasites such as fleas, *Trichuris* and *Giardia*)
- insufficient supplementary specific or supportive treatment (e.g. with *Babesia* infection, *Toxoplasma* uveitis, tick paralysis, flea allergy dermatitis, adult heartworm infection)
- multiple infection (e.g. concurrent infection with ticks, *Babesia* and *Ehrlichia* spp)
- physiological or pathological conditions (e.g. gut stasis and piperazine may allow ascarids to recover from drug exposure, increased gut motility may not allow sufficient time for drug absorption)
- underlying disease (e.g. immunodeficiency and infections with *Pneumocystis* or *Demodex* spp)
- drug interactions (e.g. corticosteroids and praziquantel, piperazine and pyrantel)
- drug resistance
- out-of-date or incorrectly stored product.

Knowledge of the actual cause of apparent inefficacy permits appropriate revisions to the therapeutic plan to be made, elevating the chances of future success.

Table 10.1 Antiparasitic drugs approved for use or reported as efficacious in dogs and cats

Species of approval	Active constituents
Endoparasiticidal drugs	
Dog and cat	Dichlorophen[1,2,4]; disophenol[1]; epsiprantel[1,4]; flubendazole[1]; ivermectin[1,2,4]; levamisole hydrochloride[1,2]; milbemycin oxime[1,2,3,4]; moxidectin[1,3]; niclosamide[1,2]; oxibendazole[1]; piperazine (adipate, citrate, dihydrochloride, phosphate)[1,2,3,4]; praziquantel[1,2,3,4]; pyrantel embonate#[1,2,3,4], selamectin[1,3,4]
Dog only	Abamectin[1]; diethylcarbamazine citrate[1]; febantel[1,2,3,4]; melarsomine dihydrochloride[1,4]; fenbendazole[1,2,3,4]; mebendazole[1,2]; nitroscanate[2,3]; oxantel embonate#[1,2]; thiacetarsamide sodium[1]
Cat only	Emodepside[1,3]
Approved only in other species	Albendazole (sheep, cattle)[1,2,3,4]; oxfendazole (sheep, cattle)[1,2,3]; triclabendazole (sheep, cattle)[1,2,3]
Ectoparasiticidal drugs	
Dog and cat	Bioallethrin (d-trans-allethrin)[2,4]; carbaryl[1,2,4]; citronella oil[1,4]; cypermethrin[1,2]; cythioate[1]; diazinon[1,2,4]; diethyltoluamide[1]; di-N-propyl isocinchomeronate[1,2,4]; eucalyptus oil[1,4]; fenthion[1,2]; fipronil[1,2,3,4]; imidacloprid[1,2,3,4]; d-limonene[4]; lufenuron[1,2,3,4]; malathion (maldison)[1]; melaleuca oil[1]; metaflumizone[3], S-methoprene[1,2,3,4]; N-octyl bicycloheptene dicarboximide[1,2,4]; nitenpyram[1,2,3,4]; permethrin* (cis : trans 25 : 75 or 40 : 60)[1,2,3,4]; phenothrin[4]; piperonyl butoxide[1,2,4]; propoxur[1,2,3]; pyrethrins[1,2,4]; pyriproxyfen[1,2,4]; rotenone[1,4]; selamectin[1,3,4], sulfur[1,4]; temephos[1]; tetramethrin[4]
Dog only	Amitraz[1,2,3,4]; bendiocarb[1]; benzyl benzoate[4]; chlorfenvinphos[1,2]; chlorpyrifos[1,2,4]; lambda cyhalothrin[4]; deltamethrin[2,3]; dichlorvos[2,4]; flumethrin[1,2]; lindane (benzene hexachloride or BHC)[2,4], pyriprole[3]
Approved for other indications or in other species	Macrocyclic lactone injections and oral solutions: doramectin (sheep, cattle, pigs)[1,2,3,4], ivermectin (sheep, cattle, pigs)[1,2,3,4], moxidectin (sheep and cattle)[1,2,3,4]
Antiprotozoal drugs	
Dog and cat	Clindamycin[1,2,3,4]; metronidazole[1,2,3] (± spiramycin); sulfonamide-trimethoprim[1,2,3,4]; doxycycline[1,2,3,4]
Dog only	Diminazene[2]; febantel[1,2,3,4]; fenbendazole[1,2,3,4]; imidocarb dipropionate[2,4]; isometamidium chloride[2]; trypan blue[2]
Approved only in other species	Diclazuril (poultry, pigs, sheep)[1,2,3,4]; ronidazole (pigeons)[1,2]; toltrazuril (poultry)[1,2,3]; ponazuril (horses)[4]; decoquinate (poultry, cattle)[2,4]; nitazoxanide (horse)[4]

1 Australia (APVMA 2006); 2 South Africa (IVS 2006); 3 UK (NOAH 2007); 4 USA (CVP 2007).
Embonate is the British Approved Name (BAN) and International Non-proprietary Name (INN) and is synonymous with pamoate, the US Approved Name (USAN).
* Concentrated permethrin products can be lethal to cats.

SELECTIVE TOXICITY

In an address to the International Congress of Medicine in 1913 [*Lancet*, August 16, pp 445–451] Nobel Laureate Paul Ehrlich described in detail for the first time the special characteristics of selective antiparasitic chemotherapy. He noted that 'if we can succeed in discovering among [the chemoreceptors of parasites] a grouping which has no analogue in the organs of the body, then we should have the possibility of constructing the ideal remedy'. Amongst the examples described by Ehrlich, trypan blue as a remedy for babesiosis and arsenic as an antiparasitic treatment remain in use today. Trypan blue exemplifies many of the characteristics of an ideal remedy but arsenic has little selectivity for parasites over hosts and the margin of safety is low.

Since Ehrlich's time there has been a continuous search for antiparasitic agents with high efficacy against parasites and high safety for the host. In many (but not all) parasitoses ideal remedies have been identified and introduced. However, the longevity of ideal remedies is eventually threatened by the emergence of resistance and the need for discovery of new antiparasitic agents with novel modes of action remains important. Use of comparative genomic, proteomic and bio-informatic tools is allowing significant progress to be made in the discovery of new targets for parasite control. There are a multitude of parasite physical and pharmacological peculiarities that have been and can be exploited in the development of selectively toxic drugs.

- The surface area-to-volume ratio of parasites is vastly higher than that of the host.
- Ion channels that are either unique to parasites (e.g. the GluCl is present in invertebrates but not vertebrates) or have distinct structural, physiological and pharmacological characteristics (e.g. nAChR, VGCC of platyhelminths, voltage-gated sodium channels of arthropods).
- Motoneurones of invertebrates are unmyelinated (unlike those of vertebrates).

- Muscle fibers in arthropods are innervated by excitatory synapses (l-glutamate) and inhibitory nerves (GABA).
- Cholinergic nerves or arthropods are concentrated in the CNS.
- Nematodes have cholinergic excitatory and GABA-inhibitory synapses at the neuromuscular junctions as well as in the central ventral cords.
- Selective uptake and concentration of arsenicals, antimonials and aromatic diamidines by trypanosomes.
- Enzymes unique to parasites
  - The aromatic amino acids phenylalanine and tryptophan are made in bacteria, plants and protozoa that contain apicoplasts or plastid remnants from shikimic acid (3,4,5-trihydroxycyclohex-1-ene-1-carboxylic acid). Mammals cannot synthesize the benzene ring and obtain these amino acids from dietary sources. Glyphosate (a herbicide with promising antiprotozoal activity) inhibits the biosynthesis of chorismic acid by inhibiting the sixth enzyme of the shikimate pathway (5-enolpyruvyl shikimate 3-phosphate synthase (EPSP synthase)), preventing aromatic amino acid, folate and ubiquinone synthesis.
  - Apicoplasts contain a Type II or dissociable fatty acid synthase (FAS) pathway, while animals use a dissimilar Type I FAS pathway.
  - Isoprenoid synthesis by the apicoplast utilizes the nonmevalonate isopentenyl diphosphate biosynthesis pathway while animals use the nonhomologous mevalonate pathway.
- Differential enzyme activity kinetics favor selectivity (e.g. ODC).
- Absence of de novo synthesis of purines in parasitic protozoa.
- Complete dependence of trypanosomes on glycolysis of host glucose for energy: trypansomes have no cytochromes, citric acid cycle or generation of ATP.
- Entamoeba use pyrophosphate in place of ATP as cofactor for phosphofructokinase.
- Insect hormones (juvenile hormone, ecdysone) necessary for development and metamorphosis.
- Kinetoplasts of trypanosomes contain DNA but lack histones, making the DNA more vulnerable to disruption than nuclear DNA of mammals.
- Organelles unique to parasites with parasite-specific functions (acidocalcisomes of trypanosomatids and apicomplexa; apicoplasts of apicomplexa; glycosomes of trypanosomes; hydrogenosomes of trichomonads; mitosomes of Entamoeba).

Key characteristics of selective toxicity are described for a number of antiparasitic agents in Table 10.2. Selective toxicity may arise from pharmaceutical, pharmacokinetic and pharmacodynamic factors alone or in combination. Parasites that are located outside the body (either on the skin or in the gastrointestinal tract) can be exposed selectively to antiparasitic agents that are not absorbed. Absorption can be controlled by intrinsic properties of the agent or its salts or by the delivery system. For agents that are absorbed, selectivity is improved if the target of antiparasitic activity has no counterpart in the host or if the host analog is unlikely to be exposed to biologically active concentrations as a result of pharmacokinetic factors, that may include barriers to distribution (such as the blood–brain barrier or protein or tissue binding) and rapid metabolic biotransformation and excretion.

INTERNAL PARASITICIDES

BENZIMIDAZOLES

The modern era of selectively toxic anthelmintics commenced in 1961 with the introduction of tiabendazole

Text continued on p. 205

Table 10.2 Selective toxicity

Mechanism	Parasite receptor	Susceptible parasite group	Antiparasitic agents	Antiparasitic action	Comments on selective toxicity*
Electron transport	NADP/ubiquinone	Arthropod	Rotenone	Antagonist Inhibits electron transport between NADH and ubiquinone	PK: low GI absorption, rapid metabolism PD: no selectivity
	Atovaquone-binding domain of cytochrome b	Protozoa (apicomplexa)	Atovaquone	Antagonist Inhibits binding of ubiquinone to cytochrome bc_1	PK: little selectivity: high protein binding PD: differences in binding sites, with mammalian site 100-fold less sensitive

Table 10.2 Selective toxicity (*continued*)

Mechanism	Parasite receptor	Susceptible parasite group	Antiparasitic agents	Antiparasitic action	Comments on selective toxicity*
	Cytochrome b	Protozoa (*Eimeria* and *Hepatozoon*)	Decoquinate	Antagonist Potent inhibitor of *Eimeria* NADH or succinate-induced mitochondrial respiration	PK: poor oral bioavailability PD: no effect on in vitro mammalian mitochondrial respiration
	Inner mitochondrial membrane (proton ionophores)	Helminth (some nematode and cestode spp)	Niclosamide, disophenol, dichlorophen	Antagonist Uncouple oxidative phosphorylation	PK: low oral bioavailability; high protein binding PD: no selectivity
Enzyme	Acetylcholinesterase	Helminth (nematodes), arthropods	Chlorpyrifos, diazinon, fenthion, malathion, carbaryl, propoxur	Antagonist Inhibition of OP and carbamate hydrolysis	PK: dermal barrier; rapid metabolic inactivation by host PD: no selectivity
	Chitin synthesis complex	Arthropods (especially insects)	Lufenuron	Antagonist Inhibition of chitin synthesis and cuticle formation (not via inhibition of chitin synthase)	PK: low selectivity PD: chitin not present in mammals
	Dihydrofolate reductase (DHFR)	Protozoa	Trimethoprim, pyrimethamine	Antagonist Inhibits conversion of dihydrofolate to tetrahydrofolate, blocking 1-carbon transfers involved in purine, pyrimidine and methionine synthesis as well as metabolism of serine, glycine, histidine and glutamate	PK: low selectivity; high bioavailability PD: increased lipid solubility of pyrimethamine associated with 2000-fold greater affinity for protozoal DHFR than mammalian DHFR. Mammalian DHFR upregulated in response to inhibition
	Dihydropteroate synthase (DHPS)	Protozoa	Sulfonamides	Antagonist Inhibits synthesis of dihydropteroate from p-amino benzoic acid (PABA) and 6-hydroxymethyl-7,8-pterin pyrophosphate	PK: low selectivity; high bioavailability PD: mammals do not synthesize folate and have no DHPS
	Hypoxanthine-guanine phosphoribosyl transferase (HGPRT)	Protozoa (especially trypanosomatids)	Allopurinol	Agonist (subversive) Allopurinol is converted to the inosine monophosphate (IMP) analog, thence via sequential reactions to the ATP derivative and finally incorporated into RNA where function is blocked	PK: rapidly metabolized by xanthine oxidase to oxypurinol which is not a substrate for HGPRT PD: mammalian HGPRT has low affinity for allopurinol

Table 10.2 Selective toxicity (*continued*)

Mechanism	Parasite receptor	Susceptible parasite group	Antiparasitic agents	Antiparasitic action	Comments on selective toxicity*
	Mixed-function oxidases	Arthropods	Piperonyl butoxide, MGK 264	Antagonist Synergize pyrethrin and SP antiparasitic agents by inhibition of metabolic inactivating enzymes	PK: dermal barrier PD: no selectivity
	Ornithine decarboxylase (ODC)	Protozoa (especially trypanosomatids)	Eflornithine (DFMO, DL-α-difluoro methyl ornithine)	Antagonist Trypanosomes are fully dependent on intrinsic polyamine biosynthesis. DFMO irreversibly inhibits ODC resulting in inhibition of biosynthesis of trypanothione and the polyamines putrescine, spermidine and spermine	PK: low oral bioavailability and rapid excretion PD: ODC turnover in mammals is 100-fold faster than in trypanosomes
	Phosphofructokinase	Protozoa (especially trypanosomatids)	Antimonials	Antagonist Inhibition of PFK prevents phosphorylation of fructose-6-phosphate, resulting in decreased fructose-1,6-diphosphate, lower aldolase activity, and energy depletion	PK: low selectivity, high bioavailability PD: differences in enzyme affinity
	Pyruvate:ferrodoxin oxidoreductase (PFOR)	Protozoa (especially anaerobic flagellates)	Metronidazole (MNZ)	Agonist (subversive) Under anaerobic conditions in trichomonads and *Giardia*, MNZ can accept electrons to form cytotoxic anions	PK: rapid and extensive metabolism PD: PFOR is not present in mammals. Cytotoxic anions produced only under anaerobic conditions
	Sterol 14α-demethylase	Protozoa (especially trypanosomatids)	Azoles (albaconazole, itraconazole)	Antagonist Inhibition of sterol 14-demethylase (that removes the 14-methyl group from lanosterol) prevents the subsequent synthesis of ergosterol	PK: low selectivity, preferred agents are well absorbed with long residence time PD: mammals do not synthesize ergosterol, and azoles have lower affinity for the mammalian enzyme

Table 10.2 Selective toxicity (*continued*)

Mechanism	Parasite receptor	Susceptible parasite group	Antiparasitic agents	Antiparasitic action	Comments on selective toxicity*
	Trypanothione reductase	Protozoa (especially trypanosomatids)	Nifurtimox, antimonials	Agonist Nifurtimox is a subversive substrate of TR, reduced in single electron steps to form radical ions that react with molecular oxygen, regenerating nifurtimox while deranging intracellular redox potential	PK: variable bioavailability PD: TR is unique to trypanosomatids and accepts only positively charged conjugates in contrast to mammalian glutathione reductase which accepts only negatively charged glutathione disulfide
Ion channel	GABA-gated Cl^- channel	Helminth (nematode)	Piperazine	Agonist Cl^- channels opened, leading to muscle cell hyperpolarization and flaccid paralysis	PK: mammalian $GABA_A$ receptors protected by blood–brain barrier PD: receptor differences
	GABA-gated Cl^- channel	Arthropod (insects, some acarines)	Fipronil, pyriprole, lindane	Antagonist Cl^- channels blocked, leading to hyperexcitation of arthropod neurotransmission	PK: mammalian $GABA_A$ receptors protected by blood–brain barrier PD: receptor differences
	Glutamate-gated Cl^- channel	Helminth (nematode), arthropod	Ivermectin, selamectin, moxidectin, milbemycin	Agonist Increased ion channel opening and Cl^- flux resulting in muscle hyperpolarization and flaccid paralysis	PK: mammalian $GABA_A$ sensitive but protected by BBB PD: GluCl channels not present in mammals
	Glutamate-gated Cl^- channel	Arthropod (insects, some acarines)	Fipronil	Antagonist Chloride channel blocked	PK: mammalian $GABA_A$ sensitive but protected by BBB PD: GluCl channels not present in mammals
	Nicotinic acetylcholine receptor (nAChR) (Na^+ K^+ channel)	Helminth (nematode)	L subtype: levamisole, pyrantel N subtype: oxantel	Agonist Depolarization of parasite neuro-muscular membrane leading to spastic paralysis	PK: dermal barrier (IMI), low GI absorption (embonate salts of pyrantel and oxantel) PD: receptor differences
	Nicotinic acetylcholine receptor (nAChR) (Na^+ K^+ channel)	Arthropod (especially insect)	Imidacloprid (IMI), nitenpyram	Agonist Hydrophobic neonicotinoids (NN) rapidly penetrate insect CNS to act at postsynaptic ACh receptor	PK: dermal barrier (IMI) PD: receptor subtype differences; lower affinity of unprotonated NN for mammalian receptor. Receptor selectivity ratio of 500–600
	Voltage-gated Ca^{2+} channel (VGCC)	Helminth (cestode, trematode)	Praziquantel, epsiprantel	Agonist Act via the platyhelminth $Ca_v\beta$var subunit of the VGCC to increase Ca^{2+} influx resulting in rapid and sustained muscular contraction	PK: little selectivity; praziquantel has high bioavailability PD: receptor unique to susceptible parasites

Table 10.2 Selective toxicity (*continued*)

Mechanism	Parasite receptor	Susceptible parasite group	Antiparasitic agents	Antiparasitic action	Comments on selective toxicity*
	Voltage-gated Na^+ channel	Arthropod	Pyrethrins, pyrethroids (permethrin, cypermethrin, deltamethrin, flumethrin), metaflumizone	Agonist Act at binding site 7 (pyrethrins) or possibly 9 (metaflumizone) to slow opening and closing of Na^+ channels, blocking fast inactivation, causing membrane depolarization and repetitive after-discharges	PK: dermal barrier; metabolic inactivation PD: (pyrethins/oids) less sensitive receptors, temperature dependence. Combined PK + PD selectivity ratio of >2000. Do block mammalian $GABA_A$ and other receptors
G protein-coupled receptor	Latrophilin receptor (GPCR)	Helminth (nematode)	Emodepside	Agonist Inhibition of pharyngeal pumping and somatic muscle cell paralysis	PK: little selectivity; high dermal bioavailability in cats PD: receptor differences assumed
	Octopamine receptor (GPCR)	Arthropod (acarine)	Amitraz	Agonist Stimulates octopaminergic neurotransmission via GPCR	PK: dermal barrier PD: absence of octopaminergic pathways in mammals. α_2-agonist and MAOI in mammals
Nuclear receptor	Juvenile hormone (JH) receptor	Arthropod (insect)	S-methoprene, pyriproxyfen	Agonist JH mimics, maintain high JH activity and inhibit metamorphosis	PK: dermal barrier, rapid metabolism PD: JH not present in mammals
Tubulin	β-tubulin	Helminth (various nematode, cestode, trematode spp), protozoa (*Giardia*)	Benzimidazoles and prodrugs: albendazole, febantel, fenbendazole	Antagonist Inhibits tubulin polymerization in susceptible helminths and protozoa	PK: low oral bioavailability PD: less avid binding to mammalian β-tubulin. Receptor selectivity ratio of 25–400
	α-tubulin	Protozoa (apicomplexa and trypanosomatid)	Trifluralin (herbicide with possible application as antiparasitic drug)	Antagonist Inhibits tubulin polymerization in plants, apicomplexa and trypanosomatids	PK: low oral bioavailability PD: less avid binding to mammalian α-tubulin
DNA	Kinetoplast DNA (kDNA)	Protozoa (trypanosomatid)	Aromatic diamidines	Antagonist Interact electrostatically with RNA and kDNA leading to structural disorganization and unwinding	PK: absorption and distribution impacted by cationic form PD: kDNA unprotected by histones and more sensitive. Off-target effects include increased cholinergic activity
	Giardia DNA	Protozoa (*Giardia*)	Quinacrine	Antagonist Intercalation of giardial DNA inhibiting nucleic acid function	PK: absorbed rapidly and widely distributed with extended elimination PD: reduced uptake by mammalian cells

* PK pharmacokinetic factors; PD pharmacodynamic factors.

by Merck & Co., the first of a large number of benzimidazoles. Use was initially for ruminants, quickly followed by applications in other species, including humans. Indeed, benzimidazoles remain widely used (especially in humans) for the control of a large number of important helminth and protozoal infections.

Mechanism of action

The benzimidazoles bind to β-tubulin, with a 25–400-fold greater inhibition constant for nematode tubulin compared with that of mammals. Tubulin is a protein subunit of the microtubules that have a fundamental and ubiquitous role in the mitotic spindle. Benzimidazole-specific binding sites on β-tubulin lead to local unfolding of the protein with the resulting abnormal conformation inhibiting further polymerization of α- and β-tubulin subunits to form microtubules and in rapidly dividing cells, this results in a lethal effect. However, in nondividing cells, a variety of effects on homeostatic mechanisms is elicited, often leading to nonlethal expulsion of nematodes from their sites of predilection. At higher concentrations, benzimidazoles have a variety of nonspecific effects on nematodes, e.g. the inhibition of fumarate reductase. Depending on specific molecular characteristics, the spectrum of antiparasitic activity of the benzimidazoles can include nematodes, cestodes, trematodes and certain protozoa.

Pharmacokinetics

All benzimidazoles have low aqueous solubility and absorption from the gastrointestinal tract is poor. Absorption can be significantly improved by coadministration with a fatty meal. Drug that is absorbed is subject to hepatic biotransformation and excretion in either feces (most benzimidazoles) or urine (albendazole). Systemic clearance of benzimidazoles in dogs and cats is rapid and enteric clearance is related to gut transit time. Because of the mode of action of the benzimidazoles, optimal efficacy is time dependent and related to duration of exposure and normally only observed after repeated doses, generally for 3–5 days, depending on the sensitivity of the target parasite and the dose rate administered. Indeed, single doses at high dose rates can be effective, as can prolonged daily low-dose administration. However, studies of the pharmacokinetics of fenbendazole in dogs have shown that systemic availability is not linearly related to dose – higher doses did not result in commensurately higher blood levels.

Adverse effects

- Although there is a great deal of selectivity in the mode of action of the benzimidazoles, particularly because of the poor systemic availability, rapidly dividing cells are at risk of toxicity if exposure is sufficient. Thus extremely elevated doses of benzimidazoles are known to variously affect hematopoietic stem cells, intestinal epithelium and hair growth.
- Some but not all benzimidazoles have the potential to be teratogenic. Teratogenic effects are dose and species dependent and are observed only if exposure takes place during critical times of embryogenesis. Of the benzimidazoles used in companion animals, fenbendazole and febantel via their sulfoxide metabolite (oxfendazole), as well as albendazole, have been shown to be teratogenic under particular circumstances.

Tiabendazole

2-(4-thiazolyl)-1 H-benzimidazole.

Clinical applications

Tiabendazole is little used but does appear useful in the treatment of *Strongyloides* infections of dogs and cats and is an active constituent in some preparations for otoacariasis.

Formulations and dose rates

For *Strongyloides felis* and *S. canis* control tiabendazole is administered at 50 mg/kg PO for 3–5 days, repeated as necessary. For *S. tumefaciens* a dose rate of 125 mg/kg q.24 h for 3 days has been reported. At these dose rates, adverse effects are likely.

Oxibendazole

[5-propoxy-1 H-benzimidazol-2-yl]carbamic acid methyl ester.

Clinical applications

Oxibendazole was described by Smith Kline & French in 1968. Its principal applications are in combination with diethylcarbamazine (DEC) for daily administration to dogs for control of *Toxocara canis, Ancylostoma caninum* and *Trichuris vulpis* and, in combination with praziquantel, as a single-dose product for control of canine ascarids, hookworm, whipworm and tapeworm.

Formulations and dose rates

See Table 10.3.

Adverse effects

Hepatotoxicity has been associated with the use of the oxibendazole-DEC combination, presumed to result from exposure to the oxibendazole component.

Table 10.3 Internal parasiticide spectrum of activity

Class	Active constituent(s) (administered orally unless otherwise stated)	Dose rate (mg/kg)	Species	Heartworm: L3/4/5	Heartworm: Adults	Heartworm: Microfilariae (L1)	Roundworms: T canis	Roundworms: TP/TM canis	Roundworms: T cati	Roundworms: T leonina	Hookworms: A caninum	Hookworms: A tubaeforme	Hookworms: A braziliense	Hookworms: U stenocephala	W: T vulpis	Tapeworm: Dipylidium	Tapeworm: Taenia spp	Tapeworm: Echinococcus	Tapeworm: Spirometra	Other
OP	Dichlorvos (resin pellet)	27–33	D				✓			✓	✓			✓	✓					
OP	Dichlorvos (tablet)	10	D,C				✓		✓	✓	✓	✓	✓	✓						
OC	Dichlorophen	220	D,C													✓	✓			
PIP	Diethylcarbamazine citrate	6-6.6	D	✓																
PIP	Diethylcarbamazine citrate	55–110	D,C				✓		✓	✓										
CES	Epsiprantel	5.5 2.75	D C													✓	✓			
BZ	Febantel	10–15	D				✓		✓	✓	✓	✓		✓	✓					
BZ	Fenbendazole	25–100	D,C				✓	✓	✓	✓	✓	✓	✓	✓	✓		✓			G, Lw
BZ	Flubendazole	22	D,C				✓		✓	✓	✓	✓	✓	✓	✓		✓			
ML	Ivermectin	0.006	D	✓	+[1]	+														
ML	Ivermectin	0.022	C	✓								✓	✓							
IT	Levamisole	7.5–10	D,C		+	+	+			+	+		+							
BZ	Mebendazole	22	D,C				✓		✓	✓	✓	✓		✓	✓		✓			
As	Melarsomine IM injection	2.5	D		✓															
ML	Milbemycin oxime	0.5/2.0	D/C	✓		+	✓		✓	✓	✓	✓			✓					
ML	Moxidectin	0.003	D	✓		+														
ML	Moxidectin SC injection[2]	0.5	D	✓							✓			✓						
MIS	Nitroscanate	50	D				✓			✓	✓		✓	✓		✓	✓			
PIP	Piperazine (various salts)	45–100	D,C				✓		✓	✓										
CES	Praziquantel IM injection Topical	5/20 5–7 8	D,C D,C C													✓	✓	✓	✓	
THP	Pyrantel (embonate)	5/20	D/C				✓		✓	✓	✓	✓	✓	✓						
ML	Selamectin topical	6	D,C	✓		+	✓	+	✓		+	✓								FSOLTN
As	Thiacetarsamide IV injection	2.2	D		✓															
Combination products																				
DEP	Emodepside	3	C						✓	✓		✓				✓	✓	✓		
CES	Praziquantel topical	12																		
IT CES	Levamisole HCl + Niclosamide	4.2–5 100	D,C				✓		✓	✓	✓	✓	✓	✓		✓	✓			
ML IGR	Milbemycin oxime + Lufenuron	0.5 10	D	✓			✓			✓	✓				✓					F
ML	Moxidectin	2.5/10	D	✓			✓			✓	✓		✓	✓	✓					FDSOL
NN	Lmidacloprid topical	1/10	C	✓					✓	✓		✓	✓	✓						OF
BZ CES	Oxibendazole + Praziquantel	22.5 5	D,C				✓		✓	✓	✓	✓		✓	✓	✓	✓	✓		

Table 10.3 Internal parasiticide spectrum of activity (*continued*)

Class	Active constituent(s) (administered orally unless otherwise stated)	Dose rate (mg/kg)	Indications																	
				Heartworm			*Roundworms*				*Hookworms*				*W*	*Tapeworm*				*Other*
			Species	*L3/4/5*	*Adults*	*Microfilariae (L1)*	*T canis*	*TP/TM canis*	*T cati*	*T leonina*	*A caninum*	*A tubaeforme*	*A braziliense*	*U stenocephala*	*T vulpis*	*Dipylidium*	*Taenia spp*	*Echinococcus*	*Spirometra*	
BZ CES ML	Oxibendazole + Praziquantel + Abamectin	22.5 5 0.01	D	✓			✓			✓	✓			✓	✓	✓	✓	✓		
THP BZ CES	Pyrantel (embonate) + Febantel + Praziquantel	5/20 25 5	D				✓			✓	✓		✓	✓	✓	✓	✓	✓		G
THP THP	Pyrantel (embonate) + Oxantel (embonate)	5 20	D				✓			✓	✓		✓	✓	✓					
THP BZ	Pyrantel (embonate) + Febantel	5 15	D				✓			✓	✓		✓	✓	✓					
THP ML	Pyrantel (embonate) + Ivermectin	5 0.006	D	✓			✓			✓	✓		✓	✓						
THP CES	Pyrantel (embonate) + Niclosamide monohydrate	20 169	C						✓	✓		✓	✓	✓		✓	✓			
THP CES	Pyrantel (embonate) + Praziquantel	20 5	C						✓	✓		✓	✓	✓		✓	✓			
THP THP CES	Pyrantel (embonate) + Oxantel (embonate) + Praziquantel	5 20 5	D				✓			✓	✓		✓	✓	✓	✓	✓	✓		

ABBREVIATIONS: ✓ approved claim, + efficacy established but claim not currently approved. TP transplacental, TM transmammary, D *Demodex*, F fleas, G *Giardia*, S *Sarcoptes*, L lice, Lw lungworm, O *Otodectes*, T ticks, N nasal mite, P prevention, W whipworm, As arsenical, CES cestocide, DEP depsipeptide, IGR insect growth regulator; IT imidazothiazole, MIS miscellaneous, ML macrocyclic lactone, NN neonicotinoid; OC organochlorine, OP organophosphate, PIP piperazine, THP tetrahydropyrimidine; 1 ivermectin control of adult heartworm in dogs associated with progressive arterial disease; 2 6–12 months protection of heartworm disease, hookworm control at time of treatment only.

Mebendazole

[5-benzoyl-1 H-benzimidazol-2-yl]carbamic ester methyl ester.

Clinical applications

Mebendazole was patented by Janssen Pharmaceutica of Belgium in 1971 and has been used widely in dogs and cats for the control of nematodes (3-day regimen) and *Taenia* spp (5-day regimen).

Formulations and dose rates

See Table 10.3.

Adverse effects

The acute oral LD_{50} of mebendazole in dogs and cats exceeds 640 mg/kg. However, idiosyncratic hepatotoxicity has been described in dogs receiving routine use rates and at 33 mg/kg for 5 days.

Flubendazole

[5-(4-fluorobenzoyl)-1 H-benzimidazol-2-yl]carbamic acid methyl ester.

Clinical applications

Flubendazole is the *para*-fluoro analog of mebendazole and was first described by Janssen Pharmaceutica in 1971. The efficacy and safety profiles are similar to those of mebendazole, although it appears more active against *Trichuris vulpis* and in some species flubendazole is better tolerated and use has not been associated with hepatotoxicity. Experimental formulations of flubendazole administered parenterally have shown a high level of efficacy against macrofilarial parasites such as *Dirofilaria immitis*.

Formulations and dose rates

See Table 10.3.

Table 10.4 Extra-label uses of fenbendazole

Parasite	*Dose of fenbendazole*
Aelurostrongylus abstrusus	25–50 mg/kg PO q.12 h 14 days 50 mg/kg PO q.24 h 3 days
Angiostrongylus vasorum	50 mg/kg PO q.24 h 3 weeks
Crenosoma vulpis	50 mg/kg PO q.24 h 3–14 days
Encephalitozoon cuniculi	(20 mg/kg PO q.24 h 4 weeks – rabbit study)
Eucoleus (Capillaria) aerophila *Pearsonema (Capillaria)/plica*	25–50 mg/kg PO q.12 h 10–14 days
Filaroides hirthi/osleri	50 mg/kg PO q.24 h 10–21 days
Giardia	50 mg/kg PO q.24 h or 25 mg/kg PO q.12 h 3–5 days
Lagochilascaris major	50 mg/kg PO q. 24 h, 3 days
Mesocestoides metacestodes	50–100 mg/kg PO q.24 h 28 days
Ollulanus tricuspis	50 mg/kg PO q.24 h 3 days
Paragonimus kellicotti	25–50 mg/kg PO q.12 h 14 days
Schistosoma/Heterobilharzia	40–50 mg/kg PO q.24 h 10 days

Fenbendazole

[5-(phenylthio)-1 H-benzimidazol-2-yl]carbamic acid methyl ester.

Clinical applications

Fenbendazole was described by Hoechst in 1973 and retains an important role in the chemotherapy of parasites of dogs. Fenbendazole has a broad spectrum of activity that includes prevention of transplacental transmission of *T. canis* if administered at 25 mg/kg PO daily from day 40 of pregnancy until 2 days post partum. Other approved clinical applications are set out in Table 10.3. However, extra-label uses that have been described are listed in Table 10.4.

Adverse effects

Rare cases of bone marrow hypoplasia and thromboischemic pinnal necrosis have been reported.

Albendazole

[5-(propylthio)-1 H-benzimidazol-2-yl]carbamic acid methyl ester.

Clinical applications

Albendazole was developed in 1973 by Smith Kline & French and has had an important and continuing role as an antiparasitic agent in ruminants and humans. Despite the fact that it has never been approved for use in dogs or cats, it has a number of applications for the control of unusual parasites. Bioavailability of albendazole is increased by concurrent fatty meals (2.6-fold), administration of praziquantel (4.5-fold) or of dexamethasone (twofold).

Albendazole has perhaps the broadest spectrum of activity of the benzimidazoles, being active against a variety of nematodes, trematodes, cestodes and protozoa of companion animals.

Formulations and dose rates

Pearsonema (Capillaria) plica	50 mg/kg PO q.12 h 10–14 days
Filaroides hirthi/osleri	25 mg/kg PO q.12 h 5 days
Trichinella spiralis	50 mg/kg PO q.12 h 7 days – tissue stages
Paragonimus kellicotti	25 mg/kg PO q.12 h 14 days
Giardia intestinalis	25 mg/kg PO q.12 h 2–3 days (dog) or 5 days (cat)

Adverse effects

Albendazole should be used cautiously as it is potentially teratogenic and its use has uncommonly been associated with bone marrow toxicosis in dogs.

Febantel

[[2-[(methoxyacetyl)amino]-4-(phenyl-thio) phenyl] carbonimidoyl]biscarbamic acid dimethyl ester).

Formulations and dose rates

Febantel is available in combination with other anthelmintics to provide a wider spectrum of activity. Dose rates and available products are presented in Table 10.3. It should be noted that a dose rate of 15 mg/kg is recommended in dogs and cats less than 6 months of age, and 10 mg/kg for those older than 6 months.

Clinical applications

Febantel is a pro-benzimidazole, developed by Bayer in 1975. It is biotransformed in the liver to the anthelmintically active metabolites fenbendazole and fenbendazole sulfoxide (oxfendazole).

Adverse effects

While usually well tolerated, cats appear more likely than dogs to manifest adverse signs after treatment, most commonly vomiting and diarrhea.

NICOTINIC ANTHELMINTICS

The nicotinic anthelmintics include the tetrahydropyrimidines (pyrantel and oxantel) and the imidazothiazole, levamisole.

Mechanism of action

Nicotinic anthelmintics act selectively on parasite nicotinic acetylcholine receptors (nAChR), producing depolarization and spastic paralysis, while leaving host receptors unaffected. A number of receptor subtypes have been identified which are differentially expressed by different parasites. Levamisole and pyrantel are most active at the L-subtype and oxantel is active at the N-subtype. Concurrent administration of pyrantel and oxantel may have therapeutic advantages, increasing spectrum of activity and reducing potential for resistance development. Interestingly, it has been observed that, when exposed to high doses, some parasites recover, apparently as a result of receptor desensitization. This observation implies that lower doses (perhaps repeated or sustained) may potentially have greater therapeutic effect.

Pyrantel

1, 4, 5, 6-tetrahydro-1-methyl-2-[2-(2-thienyl)ethenyl] pyrimidine.

Clinical applications

Pyrantel was first described in 1965 by researchers from Pfizer who had searched for cyclic amidines with suitable pharmacokinetic properties (especially duration of action) for use as an anthelmintic. Pyrantel is principally available in formulations for dogs and cats as the embonate salt, which contains 34.7% pyrantel base.

In addition to the applications set out in Table 10.3, pyrantel has been used successfully for the treatment of *Physaloptera* spp in dogs. Activity of pyrantel appears to be synergized by coadministration with febantel, when increased activity against *Ancylostoma caninum* and *Trichuris vulpis* has been observed.

Formulations and dose rates

See Table 10.3.

Pharmacokinetics

Pyrantel embonate has low aqueous solubility and low systemic availability, which increases the margin of safety and efficacy against gut parasites. The margin of safety of soluble salts (e.g. the tartrate or citrate) is much reduced and toxicity has been reported.

Adverse effects

- Pyrantel embonate is well tolerated by most dogs. Daily administration of 20 mg/kg for 3 months was not associated with any adverse effects.
- A low incidence (1.4%) of vomiting was recorded in puppies given 33 mg/kg.

Contraindications and precautions

Efficacy may be reduced if administered to dogs with diarrhea, presumably resulting from reduced gut transit time.

Known drug interactions

Based on opposing modes of action, coadministration of piperazine can be expected to antagonize the anthelmintic effects of pyrantel.

Oxantel

3-[2-(1,4,5,6-tetrahydro-1-methyl-2-pyrimidinyl)ethenyl]phenol.

Clinical applications

Oxantel is the *m*-oxyphenol analog of pyrantel with particular anthelmintic activity against *Trichuris* spp. It is most frequently encountered as the embonate salt which contains 35.8% oxantel base.

Pharmacokinetics

Oxantel embonate has low aqueous solubility and little (around 8–10%) is absorbed, permitting the drug to reach the lower gut at sufficient concentrations to be effective against whipworm.

Levamisole

(–)-(S)-2,3,5,6-tetrahydro-6-phenylimidazol[2,1-b]thiazole].

Clinical applications

Levamisole, the levorotatory and biologically active isomer of the racemic tetramisole, was discovered by Janssen Pharmaceutica in 1966 and developed as a broad-spectrum anthelmintic for use in a variety of mammalian and avian species. While widely used as an antiparasitic agent in ruminants, with a number of immunomodulatory uses still under development in humans and other species (see Chapter 12), levamisole has not found wide application as an anthelmintic in dogs and cats, principally because of the narrow therapeutic index.

Levamisole is available for both parenteral and oral administration, usually as the phosphate and hydrochloride salts respectively, although the limited use is almost exclusively per os because of concerns with toxicity when used parenterally.

Specific clinical applications and related dose rates

In both cats and dogs an oral dose rate of 5 mg/kg levamisole HCl is effective in the control of infection with roundworm (*Toxocara* spp and *Toxascaris leonina*) and hookworm (*Uncinaria stenocephala* and *Ancylostoma* spp). Levamisole is not effective against *Trichuris vulpis*. In a small number of dogs, extended use of levamisole for 2–4 weeks has shown some success in the treatment of infection with *Spirocera lupi* and *Oslerus* (*Filaroides*) *osleri*. In cats, levamisole has also been found to be effective for the treatment of *Aelurostrongylus abstrusus* infection. In dogs, levamisole HCl (2.5 mg/kg daily for 14 days, followed by 5.0 mg/kg for 14 days and then a final 14 days at 10.0 mg/kg) was widely used in the past as a microfilaricide for *Dirofilaria immitis* after adult worms (macrofilaria) had been removed. Levamisole administered at 5 mg/kg for 5–10 days to dogs with *Dipetalonema repens* microfilaremia led to sustained amicrofilaremia, first apparent at 3 days. It appeared that levamisole may not only be microfilaricidal but adulticidal as well.

Pharmacokinetics

Levamisole is rapidly absorbed from all routes of administration, with peak blood levels occurring within an hour followed by rapid metabolism and depletion principally via urinary excretion, with an elimination half-life of approximately 4 h.

Adverse effects

Adverse effects associated with the use of levamisole include:

- vomiting (sometimes in as many as 20% of dogs and prevented by pretreatment with atropine)
- nervous signs (panting, apprehensiveness and shaking)
- supraventricular premature contractions
- less frequently, hemolytic anemia (after protracted use), bleeding and thrombocytopenia.

Known drug interactions

Although levamisole is cholinomimetic and it has been suggested that concurrent use of cholinesterase inhibitors such as the organophosphates should be avoided, there is no evidence of any adverse interaction with concurrent use of these antiparasitic agents.

MACROCYCLIC LACTONE PARASITICIDES

Endectocides (avermectin-milbemycin class)

The avermectins were first isolated in 1976 from the actinomycete *Streptomyces avermitilis*, cultured from a soil sample collected near a golf course in Japan. The avermectins were quickly characterized as extremely potent anthelmintics with unexpected activity against arthropods (insects, mites and ticks). Although the milbemycins had already been described in 1973 and activity against agriculturally important mites defined, their activity against nematodes was only investigated after the anthelmintic properties of the avermectins were published. It soon became apparent that both avermectins and milbemycins were important members of a single class with a common mode of action. Structurally, they all share a 16-membered macrocyclic ring, giving rise to the class name. The avermectins are disaccharides (ivermectin, doramectin) or monosaccharides (selamectin), while the milbemycins (milbemycin oxime and moxidectin) have no sugar substituents.

The macrocyclic lactones (MLs) have become an important class of parasiticide in agriculture, animal health and human health. In the latter case, ivermectin has been used extensively and safely for the treatment of onchocerciasis, the cause of 'river blindness' in large areas of Africa.

Mechanism of action

In both arthropods and nematodes, exposure to MLs results in lethal paralysis following opening of chloride ion channels in cell membranes of peripheral nerve tissues, leading to hyperpolarization. The target site has been well characterized as a glutamate-gated Cl^- channel that is present in both neuronal and muscle membranes of many invertebrates but which is not present in mammals. Actions on nematode muscle include the paralysis of the pharyngeal pump, necessary for food intake, resulting in starvation. A combination of neural and muscular effects is probably involved in the biological activity of the MLs. An absence of binding sites in cestodes and trematodes renders these parasites insensitive to the action of the MLs. The reason why adult filarial parasites (for example, *Dirofilaria immitis*) are not susceptible to the lethal effects of the MLs is unclear but may be associated with adult-specific expression and distribution of less susceptible chloride channel subunits.

The MLs are also agonists of GABA-gated Cl^- channels of invertebrates and vertebrates where they are located in the CNS. In part, the selectivity of action of the MLs is due to the protection of the mammalian CNS from exposure by the blood–brain barrier conferred by the transmembrane transport pump, P-glycoprotein (responsible for drug efflux) expressed within brain capillary endothelial cells. Animals with increased sensitivity to ivermectin (for example, collies) have been shown to be deficient in P-glycoprotein in both the CNS and intestinal epithelium.

Adverse effects

- Generally the MLs are particularly safe even at elevated doses. However, a toxicosis syndrome has been described, especially in particularly sensitive animals, notably collies and related breeds and in kittens. Likelihood of toxicity is related to the selected drug, the dose rate and the recipient animal's predisposition.

- Administration of some MLs to microfilaria-positive dogs has also been associated with adverse effects, generally milder than those encountered with the use of DEC, although deaths have been reported.

Resistance

Resistance has not yet been reported among the parasites of dogs and cats but is widely encountered in endoparasites of ruminants, including sheep, goats and cattle.

Resistance to both avermectins (ivermectin) and milbemycins (moxidectin) is reduced by administration of the calcium channel inhibitor verapamil, indicating that at least one mechanism involves active drug efflux out of target parasites by the drug transporter P-glycoprotein.

Precautions

- Use in collies and other breeds with reduced or absent P-glycoprotein activity.
- Use in microfilaremic dogs.
- Missed doses in heartworm prevention.

AVERMECTINS

Ivermectin

22,23-dihydro-avermectin B_{1a}; 22,23-dihydroavermectin B_{1b}.

Ivermectin contains at least 80% 22,23-dihydroavermectin B_{1a} and not more than 20% 22,23-dihydroavermectin B_{1b} and was first commercialized in 1981.

Pharmacokinetics

Ivermectin is absorbed rapidly after oral administration of tablets or chewable dosage forms, with peak plasma concentrations noted at 4–10 h. Maximum concentrations increase in direct proportion to dose, indicating a linear relationship between dose and bioavailability. The drug is widely distributed, with a V_d of 2.4 L/kg, and is eliminated with a half-life of approximately 1.8 days. Similar pharmacokinetics are present in the cat, with T_{max} reported to be 5.5 h and no detectable ivermectin by day 5 after treatment.

Clinical applications and dose rates

Indication	Dose
DOGS	
D. immitis precardiac stages	0.006 mg/kg PO monthly
D. immitis adults after repeated monthly treatments[#]	
Extra-label applications (not for sensitive dogs including collies)	
D. immitis microfilaria	0.050 mg/kg
96% of 121 dogs became amicrofilaremic after a single dose (90% within 3 weeks) and the remainder after repeated doses.	
Sarcoptes scabiei	0.2–0.3 mg/kg PO, SC
Otodectes cynotis	
Demodex canis (repeated every 2–3 weeks)	
Pneumonyssoides	
Eucoleus and *Pearsonema* (*Capillaria*) spp	
T. vulpis	
T. canis (not *T. leonina*)	
A. caninum	
A. braziliense	
U. stenocephala	
Angiostrongylus vasorum	
Physaloptera rara	
D. reconditium	
T. canis prevention of transmission to puppies	0.3 mg/kg SC to pregnant bitches on gestation days 0, 30, 60 and postgestation day 10
Demodex canis	0.3–0.6 mg/kg PO daily for 2 months
Filaroides osleri (repeated every 2 weeks)	0.4 mg/kg
CATS	
D. immitis precardiac stages	0.024 mg/kg PO monthly
A. tubaeforme	
A. braziliense	
Sarcoptes	0.2–0.4 mg/kg PO, SC
Notoedres	
Otodectes	
T. cati	0.3 mg/kg SC
Cheyletiella spp	
Lynxacarus radovskyi	
Aelurostrongylus abstrusus	0.4 mg/kg SC

[#] Heartworm adulticidal activity of monthly ivermectin has been associated with deterioration of radiographic signs and should be applied carefully and with appropriate monitoring in symptomatic and asymptomatic dogs.

Adverse effects

Dogs

- The acute oral LD_{50} of ivermectin in beagles is 80 mg/kg and the highest no-effect dose is 2 mg/kg with single doses and 0.5 mg/kg for daily doses for 14 days.

- The acute toxic syndrome includes mydriasis, depression, tremors, ataxia, stupor, emesis, salivation and coma. Convulsions and seizures are not usually associated with ivermectin toxicosis.
- Some dog breeds are particularly sensitive to ivermectin, most notably certain collies, with adverse effects noted at doses as low as 0.1 mg/kg and death at 0.2 mg/kg. Pharmacogenomic testing of the presence of P-glycoprotein mutations is available in some countries.
- The characteristic toxic syndrome at dose rates that exceeded the recommended dose rate has also been observed in individual cases in an Old English sheepdog, Australian shepherds, German shepherd, West Highland white terrier, border collies, Australian blue heeler, Jack Russell terrier, labrador, pit bull terrier and samoyed. These occurrences serve to emphasize that clinical caution and vigilance are indicated whenever using products in an extra-label fashion.
- In dogs with circulating microfilariae, administration of ivermectin has been associated with vomiting, salivation, diarrhea and depression and occasionally death.
- Occasionally, apparent mild hypersensitivity reactions are seen within 24 h of treatment of *Sarcoptes scabiei* infections with ivermectin injection.

Cats

- The no-effect dose in cats is reported to be approximately 0.75 mg/kg PO. However, many cases of toxicosis have been reported at dose rates in excess of 0.5 mg/kg.
- Adverse effects have been reported in kittens receiving 0.3–0.4 mg/kg SC or PO.

Selamectin

(5Z,25S)-25-cyclohexyl-4′-O-de(2,6-dideoxy-3-O-methyl-a-L-*arabino*-hexopyranosyl)-5-demethoxy-25-de(1-methylpropyl)-22,23-dihydro-5-hydroxyimino avermectin A_{1a}.

Selamectin is the most recently discovered, developed and commercialized of the MLs and the only ML to have approved indications for both internal and external parasites of dogs and cats. It was selected for development on the basis of safety in sensitive collies and activity against *Ctenocephalides felis*, a parasite otherwise relatively resistant to the ML class.

Pharmacokinetics

After topical application the systemic bioavailability of selamectin is approximately 4% and 74% and the plasma elimination half-life 14 and 69 hours in the dog and cat respectively. The prolonged elimination appears to result from sustained release from selamectin depots in an undetermined extravascular site. The differences in bioavailability between dogs and cats are thought to result from differences in transdermal flux which is expected to be much higher in cats combined with possible oral intake following grooming behavior of cats. A study of topical administration in male and female beagles has described significantly higher AUC and lower clearance in female dogs compared with male dogs. The clinical significance of this observation is unclear as the link between plasma selamectin concentration and efficacy has not been reported and is unlikely to be a simple relationship or common to all target parasite species. The disposition of radiolabeled selamectin has been investigated in fleas fed on treated calf blood. Dose-dependent concentration of selamectin was observed in the sub- and supra-esophageal ganglia of the flea brain, regions rich in glutamate-gated chloride channels. Interestingly, ivermectin concentrations in fleas similarly treated were significantly lower, consistent with the differential toxicity of selamectin and ivermectin to fleas.

Clinical applications and dose rates

DOGS

6 mg/kg topically monthly:
- *Dirofilaria immitis*, precardiac stages
- *Ctenocephalides* spp, adulticidal, ovicidal and larvicidal
  - administered to pregnant bitches at 40 and 10 days prior to parturition and 10 and 40 days after parturition prevented infection in both puppies and dams
- *Otodectes cynotis*
- *Sarcoptes scabiei*
- *Linognathus setosus*
- *Trichodectes canis*
- *Heterodoxus spiniger*
- *Toxocara canis*, adults
  - administered to pregnant bitches at 40 and 10 days prior to parturition and 10 and 40 days after parturition reduced transplacental and lactogenic transmission to puppies
- *Dermacentor variabilis* (treatment fortnightly for first month)

CATS

6 mg/kg topically monthly:
- *D. immitis*, precardiac stages
- *Ctenocephalides* spp, adulticidal, ovicidal and larvicidal
- *Otodectes cynotis*
- *Sarcoptes scabiei*
- *Felicola subrostrata*
- *Toxocara cati*
- *Ancylostoma tubaeforme*

Contraindications and precautions

Approximately 1% of cats may experience transient localized alopecia at the site of application, with or without inflammation, following treatment.

Doramectin

25-cyclohexyl-5-O-demethyl-25-de(1-methylpropyl)-avermectin A_{1a}.

Doramectin is available for use in pigs, cattle, deer and sheep but is not approved for use in dogs and cats. The plasma disposition of doramectin following subcutaneous or oral administration is similar to that described for ivermectin. Compared with oral administration, C_{max} is lower and occurs later while AUC is higher after SC injection. In both cases the elimination half-life is approximately 3–4 days. Experimental studies have demonstrated that administration of doramectin at 1 mg/kg SC to pregnant bitches on day 55 of gestation prevented lactogenic transmission of *Ancylostoma caninum* and if given to dams on days 40 and 55 of gestation, reduced *Toxocara canis* worm burdens in their puppies by 99%. Recently, there have been a number of descriptions published of successful treatment and prevention of tick infestation in dogs, canine generalized demodicosis (0.3–0.6 mg/kg SC q.7–14 d) and notoedreic mange in cats.

MILBEMYCINS

Milbemycin oxime

Not less than 80% 5-didehydromilbemycin A_4; not more than 20% 5-didehydromilbemycin A_3.

Clinical applications and dose rates

DOGS

0.5 mg/kg PO monthly:

- *Dirofilaria immitis*, precardiac stages
- *D. immitis*, microfilariae
- Adult *Ancylostoma caninum*
- *Toxocara canis*
- *Trichuris vulpis*

0.5–1 mg/kg PO once weekly for 3 consecutive weeks:

- *Pneumonyssoides caninum*

0.5–1 mg/kg PO daily for 90+ days:

- Generalized demodicosis

2 mg/kg PO once weekly, three treatments:

- *Sarcoptes scabiei* (two studies, 71% and 100% of dogs with negative scrapings)

Single doses up to 1.2 mg/kg are ineffective against *Uncinaria stenocephala*

CATS

0.5 mg/kg PO monthly:

- *Dirofilaria immitis*, precardiac stages

Also available as an aural solution containing 0.1% milbemycin oxime for the treatment of *Otodectes cynotis* in dogs and cats.

Adverse effects

- Similar to ivermectin; the margin of safety in ML-sensitive collies is 10–20 times.
- Use in microfilaremic dogs has resulted in depression, salivation, coughing, tachypnea and emesis, with severity somewhat correlated with magnitude of microfilarial concentration.

Moxidectin

5-O-demethyl-28-deoxy-25-(1,3-dimethyl-1-butenyl)-6,28-epoxy-23-(methoxyimino)-(6R,23E,25S(E))-milbemycin B.

Moxidectin is a single compound produced by chemical modification of nemadectin, the principal component of the LL28249 antibiotic complex derived from *Streptomyces cyaneogriseus* subspecies *noncyanogenus*, first isolated from an Australian soil sample.

Pharmacokinetics

After oral administration moxidectin is absorbed rapidly with T_{max} at 2–3 h. The high lipophilicity of moxidectin facilitates its deposition in adipose tissue, which acts as a drug reservoir contributing to the long persistence of moxidectin. The volume of distribution is 12.2 L/kg and elimination half-life 19 d (by comparison, the same parameters for ivermectin are 2.4 L/kg and 1.8 d). Following topical application, moxidectin is absorbed and distributed systemically and is slowly eliminated from the plasma as manifested by detectable moxidectin concentrations in plasma throughout treatment intervals of 1 month.

Clinical applications and dose rates

DOGS

0.003 mg/kg PO monthly:

- *Dirofilaria immitis*, precardiac stages

1 mg/kg PO to pregnant bitch on day 55 of pregnancy:

- *Ancylostoma caninum*, prevention of lactogenic transmission

0.4 mg/kg PO q.24 h, 2–7 months (extra-label).

- Canine generalized demodicosis. High rates of clinical and parasitological cure reported after 2–7 months of treatment.

Sustained-release subcutaneous injection:

- Sustained protection from *Dirofilaria immitis*, precardiac stages for 6–12 months, dependent on dose rate, with a single SC dose of 0.17 mg/kg providing 180 days protection in a controlled study. Based on geometric worm count reduction compared with untreated dogs, efficacy against *A. caninum* and *U. stenocephala* was greater than 90% for 4 and 3 months respectively.

Adverse effects

- Adverse reactions occur infrequently. Doses of 1.120 mg/kg (300 times the recommended dose) have elicited no significant effects.
- Collies have received 20 times dose rate without untoward effects.
- However, respiratory failure requiring treatment with intermittent positive pressure ventilation has been reported in a young male collie, confirming that at least some collies may have an increased susceptibility to moxidectin, as this breed does to the macrocyclic lactone class as a whole.

CYCLO-OCTADEPSIPEPTIDES

The cyclo-octadepsipeptides are the most recent novel class of antiparasitic drug to become available for use in veterinary medicine.

Emodepside

The anthelmintic activity of the 24-membered cyclo-octadepsipeptides was first observed in tests of the compound PF1022A against *Ascaridia galli* in chickens. PF1022A is a natural secondary metabolite of *Mycelia sterilia*, a fungus which belongs to the microflora of the leaves of *Camellia japonica*. Emodepside, a semisynthetic derivative of PF1022A, acts on specific heptahelical transmembrane G protein-coupled receptors named depsiphilins, members of the latrophilin receptor class, where latrotoxin from the venom of the black widow spider is the defining ligand. Extracellular binding by emodepside to the N-terminus of the receptor initiates a presynaptic signal transduction cascade that involves the mobilization and activation of second messengers diacylglycerol (DAG), UNC-13 and synaptobrevin, leading in turn to the release of a final unknown transmitter (or modulator) that acts postsynaptically to induce inhibition and flaccid paralysis of the pharyngeal and somatic musculature of nematodes.

Pharmacokinetics

Following topical application of emodepside to cats, it is rapidly absorbed transdermally with detectable levels in blood within 2 h. Maximum concentration is reached at approximately 40 h. A second delayed peak is evident after about 4 d, indicating that emodepside may be released and redistributed from a tissue storage site, most likely fat. The elimination half-life has been reported as 8.3 d. Treatment every month can be expected to lead to a minor level of accumulation.

Clinical applications and dose rates

CATS

The efficacy of emodepside for treatment of feline gastrointestinal nematodes has been extensively studied. The spectrum of activity includes larval and adult stages of *Toxocara cati, Toxascaris leonina* and *Ancylostoma tubaeforme*. Emodepside is currently only available as a topically applied product in combination with praziquantel. Dose rates and spectrum of activity are presented in Table 10.3. Studies in 7-week-old kittens, 7-month-old adult cats, pregnant and lactating cats at elevated dose rates have not revealed any adverse effects. Oral administration of the formulated topical product is associated with salivation and vomiting. The oral and dermal acute LD_{50} in rats is greater than 500 and 2000 mg/kg respectively.

CESTOCIDES

Apart from the rare occurrence in dogs and cats of infection with cystic larval stages or metacestodes (especially those of *Spirometra* and *Mesocestoides*), adult intestinal cestodes seldom cause any adverse clinical signs, despite, in some species, the presence of many tens of thousands of parasites.

The decision to treat is frequently based on the following factors.

- *Public health considerations.* Humans can be directly infected by the eggs of *Echinococcus* spp, resulting in significant morbidity and not infrequently death.
- *Esthetics.* Other zoonotic infections (such as that associated with *Dipylidium caninum*) are transmitted by the intermediate host (in this case usually *Ctenocephalides felis*)while dogs and cats provide the principal reservoir of infection. Although not very pathogenic, treatment of this cestode and many others may be undertaken on esthetic grounds.
- *Transmission to food animals.* Treatment may be directed by the possible transmission from companion animals to food-producing animals, whereby metacestodes (for example, hydatid cysts of *E. granulosus*) in edible tissues may lead to carcass condemnation and substantial financial loss.
- *Pathogenicity.* While intestinal infections are usually asymptomatic, infections of other organ systems (e.g. lungs, mesenteric vasculature, peritoneal cavity) can be associated with significant morbidity.

When selecting a compound for use against intestinal cestodes, consideration should be given to the importance of activity against both scolex (the point of attachment) and proglottids (the chain of segments). If activity is confined to the latter, then there will be only a temporary interruption to the passage of eggs. Of course, drug use should be combined with measures to prevent reinfection by ensuring intermediate hosts are unavailable. Refer to the Appendix for details of sources of infection.

Bunamidine hydrochloride

N,N-dibutyl-4-(hexyloxy)-1-naphthalene-carboxyimidamide.

Clinical applications

- *Taenia* spp
- *Dipylidium caninum*
- *Spirometra erinacei*
- *Mesocestoides lineatus*

Bunamidine is not uniformly efficacious even at elevated dose rates against *Echinococcus granulosus*.

Formulations and dose rates

DOGS: 25–50 mg/kg PO
CATS: 25–50 mg/kg PO

Pharmacokinetics

Bunamidine is absorbed from the gastrointestinal tract, reaching peak concentrations in plasma in 3–8 h. It is extensively metabolized by the liver and excreted principally in the feces. Anthelmintic activity is significantly reduced in the presence of food, which should therefore be withheld for at least 3 h before treatment. Factors that elevate systemic exposure, e.g. crushing tablets to permit intraoral absorption, exercise or liver disease that may decrease first-pass biotransformation, increase the likelihood of hepatic, neuromuscular or cardiac toxicity.

Mechanism of action

Studies of *Hymenolepis* spp reveal that bunamidine may have two complementary modes of action that lead to death of sensitive tapeworms. The tapeworm tegument is disrupted, causing decreased glucose uptake and increasing glucose efflux. In addition, the fumarate reductase system is disrupted, leading to a reduction in generation of ATP. The major action is exerted on the proglottids and not uncommonly the scolex may survive exposure to restrobilate.

Adverse effects

- Bunamidine hydrochloride is irritant to the buccal mucosa and tablets, which are usually coated with lactose or other suitable substance, should therefore be given whole.
- Vomiting and diarrhea are not infrequently encountered.
- Rare idiosyncratic deaths in dogs have been associated with hepatic dysfunction.
- In both dogs and humans bunamidine can be cardiotoxic, thought to result from sensitization of the myocardium to catecholamines, resulting in ventricular fibrillation and heart failure. Adverse cardiovascular events (including death in approximately 1 in 2000 cases) are more common in working dogs than more sedate urban dogs and appear to be dose related.
- It has been recommended that excitement and exertion be avoided for up to 2 d after treatment.

Dichlorophen

2,2′-dihydroxy-5,5′dichlorodiphenylmethane.

Dichlorophen is a narrow-spectrum cestocide first described in the 1940s, still available for treatment of dogs and cats but little used. It is practically insoluble in water and little absorption is presumed to follow oral administration.

Clinical applications

Efficacy is restricted to *Taenia* spp, with poor to no activity against *Echinococcus* spp and *Dipylidium caninum*. Against these and other species, dichlorophen may act against the strobilus, leaving the scolex to generate new proglottids. The mechanism of action is thought to be similar to that of the salicylanilides, involving the uncoupling of oxidative phosphorylation. In susceptible species, death appears swiftly, with disintegrated cestodes eliminated within 8 h of dosing.

Formulations and dose rates

Recommended dose rate in both dogs and cats is 200 mg/kg PO.

Adverse effects

- In cats, hyperesthesia, ataxia, salivation and inappetence have been reported at the recommended dose.
- In dogs, vomiting and diarrhea are not infrequently described.
- The minimum lethal dose in mammals is between 2000 and 3000 mg/kg.

Niclosamide

2′,5-dichloro-4′-nitrosalicylanilide.

Niclosamide was the first commercialized salicylanilide that emerged from a search for new anthelmintics based on structural modifications of dichlorophen and has been in use since 1960. Like dichlorophen, it is practically insoluble in water. Unlike other salicylanilides, the little drug that is absorbed (around 2%) is metabolized quickly to glucuronide conjugates and excreted renally.

Mechanism of action

Niclosamide, in common with other salicylanilides, is a hydrogen ionophore that translocates protons across the inner membrane of mitochondria, resulting in the uncoupling of oxidative phosphorylation from electron transport, inhibiting the production of ATP. These effects are observed in isolated mitochondria of helminths and mammals. Selective toxicity is conveyed by the minimal systemic absorption combined with the protective influence of protein binding.

Clinical applications

- *Taenia* spp
- *Dipylidium caninum*
- *Joyeuxiella pasqualei* (at a fivefold elevation in dose)
- No reliable echinococcal activity
- Niclosamide is active as a molluscicide and is widely used for control of the freshwater snails that are intermediate hosts of *Schistosoma* spp.

Formulations and dose rates

Recommended dose rate is 100–157 mg/kg PO.

Adverse effects

Adverse reactions are usually confined to transient vomiting and diarrhea.

Praziquantel

2-(cyclohexylcarbonyl)-1,2,3,6,7,11*b*-hexahydro-4H-pyrazino[2,1*a*]isoquinolin-4-one.

The introduction of praziquantel in 1975 was a significant milestone in antiparasitic chemotherapy of cestode infections. For the first time a safe, highly effective, broad-spectrum drug was available, active in a single dose by oral or parenteral administration. Praziquantel remains a key component of programs in animals to control parasites of zoonotic importance (especially *Echinococcus* spp) and in humans for the control of schistosomiasis, limited only by the emergence of resistance.

Clinical applications and dose rates

Activity at the recommended dose rate of 5 mg/kg PO:

- *Taenia* spp
- *Dipylidium caninum*
- *Joyeuxiella pasqualei* (some reports that 25mg/kg q 6w may be necessary)
- *Echinococcus granulosus*
- *Echinococcus multilocularis*
- *Mesocestoides corti*
- *Hymenolepis diminuta*

Activity requiring elevated dose rates or repeated treatment program:

Spirometra erinacei	7.5 mg/kg q.24 h for 2 days or single dose of 20–30 mg/kg
S. erinacei sparganosis (metacestode infection)	20 mg/kg mebendazole q.24 h for 21 days followed by praziquantel 5 mg/kg q.24 h for 21 days, cycle repeated for 3 months
Nanophyetus salmincola	10 mg/kg
Platynosomum fastosum	20 mg/kg
Paragonimus kellicotti	25 mg/kg q.8 h for 2 days
Pharyngostomum cordatum	30 mg/kg
Diphyllobothrium latum	35 mg/kg
Schistosoma spp	50 mg/kg
Heterobilharzia spp	50 mg/kg

Praziquantel is also available as an injection for SC or IM administration to dogs and cats at a dose rate of 5–7 mg/kg.

A topical spot-on preparation (4% w/v praziquantel) is available for cats (with or without the anthelmintic emodepside), administered at a dose rate of 8 mg/kg.

Mechanism of action

Exposure of cestodes and susceptible trematodes to praziquantel is followed by rapid influx of Ca^{2+}, consistent with an effect of praziquantel on the β-subunit of voltage-gated calcium channels (VGCC). The presence or absence of the $Ca_v\beta$var subunit of the VGCC in a given organism is consistently correlated with the presence or absence of sensitivity to praziquantel, suggesting that this may be the site of action. Susceptible species (platyhelminths, but not *Fasciola* spp) display both spastic and tetanic muscular contractions and rapid vacuolization of the tegument. The vacuoles enlarge and coalesce, allowing leakage of glucose, lactate and amino acids. The damage to the tegument allows the exposure of previously concealed parasite antigens, leading to attack of damaged parasites by the host immune system, ultimately resulting in parasite death.

Pharmacokinetics

Praziquantel is rapidly absorbed after oral administration, with maximum concentrations in plasma of dogs observed within 1–2 h. Absorption from the gastrointestinal tract is significantly improved in humans by administration with food, more so with a high carbohydrate meal than with a high content of lipids. A similar enhancement of absorption should be anticipated in dogs and cats.

Praziquantel is widely distributed to all tissues, including the CNS, with higher concentrations in liver, bile and kidney. The drug is extensively metabolized and is rapidly excreted, principally in the urine, where almost no parent drug is detected but a variety of inactive metabolites, including glucuronides and sulfates, are present.

Efficacy may be reduced by concurrent administration of corticosteroids, phenytoin or carbamazepine which have been reported to decrease praziquantel plasma concentration. Plasma concentrations have been shown to be increased by concurrent high carbohydrate meal or by administration of cimetidine which inhibits various CYP isoforms. It has been observed that the efficacy of praziquantel against *Echinococcus* may be adversely affected by coinfection with *Spirometra erinacei*. Further investigation is necessary to confirm the nature of this apparent interaction. Praziquantel has been shown to increase the bioavailability of coadministered albendazole.

Adverse effects

- Administration of tablets to dogs and cats at dose rates up to 150 mg/kg has generally been well tolerated.
- While lethargy was occasionally observed, the principal adverse effect was vomiting, which is considered to prevent further exposure and more serious signs developing.
- The margin of safety was considered to be greater than fivefold for both oral and parenteral preparations (compared with the usual dose rate of 5 mg/kg).
- The administration of injectable praziquantel to cats at 20 times the labeled rate resulted in high mortality.
- Transient injection site pain is the most frequent adverse effect following injection.
- Ingestion of the topical product may lead to excessive salivation in cats, presumed to be due to the bitter flavor of praziquantel.
- Occasionally use of praziquantel may be associated with transient vomiting, drowsiness and staggering gait.

Epsiprantel

2-(cyclohexylcarbonyl)-4-oxo-1,2,3,4,6,7,8,12*b*-octahydropyrazino[2,1*a*]benzazepine.

Clinical applications

Epsiprantel has a high level of activity against enteric cestodes: *Taenia* spp and *Dipylidium caninum*. High levels of activity against mature infections of *Echinococcus* spp have been reported, but this use has not been approved.

Mechanism of action

The mode of action of epsiprantel is thought to be similar to that of praziquantel.

Pharmacokinetics

Epsiprantel is practically insoluble in water. Systemic availability after oral administration is negligible.

Formulations and dose rates

DOGS: 5.5 mg/kg PO
CATS: 2.75 mg/kg PO

Adverse effects

- In cats, no significant adverse effects were observed in animals given 40 times the recommended dose rate daily for 4 d.
- Similarly in dogs, no significant adverse effects were observed after daily administration of 500 mg/kg PO for 14 d.
- Use in animals less than 7 weeks of age is not recommended.

ARSENICALS

Inorganic or organic arsenical compounds have had traditional use as parasiticides for some centuries and recently arsenic trioxide has been approved for use in humans for the treatment of certain leukemias. Arsenicals are generally nonspecific in their toxicity, with only a small margin of safety. Trivalent arsenic (As^{3+}) is the principal active (toxic) form, acting on the sulfhydryl groups of proteins to change or inhibit their function. For example, a number of mitochondrial respiratory enzymes are particularly sensitive to arsenic, resulting in inhibition of energy-linked reduction of NAD.

Thiacetarsamide sodium

Disodium salt of 2,2′-[[[4-(aminocarbony) phenyl]-arsinidene]bis(thio)]bisacetic acid.

Clinical applications

Thiacetarsamide sodium, an organic trivalent arsenical containing 17.8% As^{3+}, was first described in 1930 and was, from its first clinical description in dogs in 1947 until recently, the mainstay of *Dirofilaria immitis* adulticidal treatment.

Thiacetarsamide has been used successfully in cats but cats are particularly sensitive to worm displacement and thromboembolism, and treatment protocols have not been finalized.

Formulations and dose rates

- 2.2 mg/kg by careful IV injection, q.12 h for 2 d. Efficacy is improved if four injections are administered within 36 h
- Expected efficacy is in the range of 50–100% reduction in adult heartworm
- If adverse effects prevent completion of the four-dose program, treatment should be repeated in full when the dog has recovered and at least 2 weeks later. Retreated dogs will not necessarily experience adverse effects again

Pharmacokinetics

Following IV administration of thiacetarsamide, the plasma half-life of arsenic is 177 min, with a volume of distribution of 2.2 L/kg and mean residence time of only 75 min. Some 50% and 85% of the administered dose is eliminated within 24 h and 48 h respectively, principally in the feces. Arsenic is widely distributed, with significant binding to erythrocytes, and concentrations are highest in liver and kidney, target organs of toxicity. The active form of the drug is not clear but it does not appear to be arsenic per se, as orally administered thiacetarsamide providing equivalent blood arsenic concentrations to IV drug is not effective. Efficacy against macrofilariae appears to be more related to the duration of exposure to a minimum effective drug concentration rather than to short periods of high concentrations. Efficacy is also related to the age of heartworms (infections 2 or 24 months of age are better controlled than those between these ages) and their sex (female worms are much more tolerant than males).

Adverse effects

- Around 15% of dogs can be expected to react adversely. The most serious effects include pulmonary thromboembolism, hepatotoxicity, nephrotoxicity and perivascular inflammation and necrosis. Common signs include:
  - vomiting
  - anorexia
  - icterus
  - lethargy
  - fever.
- Thiacetarsamide is irritant if injected perivascularly and will cause local tissue necrosis.

Contraindications and precautions

Thiacetarsamide should not be administered to dogs with severe heartworm disease.

Special considerations

- To minimize the impact of pulmonary thromboembolism, after treatment dogs should be rested.
- Microfilariae are not eliminated by thiacetarsamide and appropriate treatment (commonly an ML) should be instituted.

Melarsomine hydrochloride

[4-[(4,6-diamino-1,3,5-triazon-2-yl)amino] phenyldithioarsenite of di(2-aminoethyl) dihydrochloride.

Clinical applications

Melarsomine is used as a *Dirofilaria immitis* macrofilaricide in dogs. Use in cats has not been defined, although the dog dosage regimen appears inappropriate.

Melarsomine dihydrochloride contains 14.9% As^{3+} and is believed to provide a greater degree of convenience, efficacy and safety for macrofilarial control than thiacetarsamide if used strictly as directed. However, serious adverse reactions have been reported when the drug is not used according to the manufacturer's strict guidelines in relation to clinical staging of the patient. This may relate to the greater efficacy of melarsomine in killing adult heartworms in comparison with thiacetarsamide, resulting in increased risk of thromboembolism.

Formulations and dose rates

2.5 mg/kg IM (into lumbar muscles), two doses on alternate sides 24 h apart. In dogs with advanced clinical signs of dirofilariosis (class 3), an alternative regimen has been recommended, whereby a single IM dose of 2.5 mg/kg (which is expected to kill around 50% of worms) is followed, when the condition of the dog improves 1–2 months later, by the standard protocol.

Pharmacokinetics

Following melarsomine injection into the lumbar epaxial musculature of dogs, the drug is rapidly absorbed, reaching maximum blood arsenic concentrations in around 11 min. The terminal elimination half-life is approximately 3 h, with a mean residence time of 7 h. These parameters compare very favorably with those of thiacetarsamide and demonstrate that parasite exposure to arsenic will be significantly longer after treatment with melarsomine.

Macrofilarial efficacy appears to be related to sustained exposure to blood arsenic concentrations of at least 0.1 mg/L. Melarsomine dosage regimens provide such a pharmacokinetic profile, resulting in high and reproducible efficacy. Indeed, 90% of male and 10% of female worms are killed in response to a single injection.

Adverse effects

- Direct toxicity of melarsomine is unusual. However, the margin of safety is low, with deaths observed in heartworm-negative dogs given 7.5 mg/kg.
- Signs of pulmonary thromboembolism; as noted above, there may be greater risk of thromboembolism occurring compared to thioacetarsamide treatment, especially if patients are not appropriately clinically staged and the manufacturer's guidelines in relation to patient management prior to melarsomine treatment are not followed strictly.
- Pain and swelling at injection site.

Contraindications and precautions

- Because the hazards of treatment are related to the health status of the pulmonary and cardiovascular systems and their ability to cope with worm emboli, patient evaluation before treatment is vital. Patient evaluation algorithms are detailed on product leaflets and should be closely observed.
- Melarsomine should not be administered to dogs with severe heartworm disease.

Special considerations

- In cases of suspected arsenic intoxication, administration of dimercaprol (BAL, British anti-Lewisite) at 3 mg/kg IM may reverse the signs if administered early. However, it is expected that dimercaprol will reduce the efficacy of melarsomine.
- To minimize the impact of pulmonary thromboembolism, dogs should be rested after treatment.
- Microfilariae are not eliminated by melarsomine and appropriate treatment (commonly an ML) should be instituted.
- Refer to current Guidelines for the Diagnosis, Prevention and Management of Heartworm (*Dirofilaria immitis*) Infection in Dogs (www.heartwormsociety.org).

MISCELLANEOUS ANTHELMINTICS

Piperazine

Hexahydropyrazine.

Clinical applications

Piperazine has particular utility against ascarid infection.

Mechanism of action

Piperazine acts as a γ-aminobutyric acid (GABA) agonist, causing chloride channel opening, neural hyperpolarization and flaccid paralysis of susceptible parasites. Affected worms are then expelled from their predilection sites by normal enteric movements. In the absence of peristaltic waves, worms may recover from paralysis and resume their parasitic state.

Formulations and dose rates

Piperazine is available as a number of salts:

Piperazine hexahydrate	(44% piperazine base)
Piperazine adipate	(37% piperazine base)
Piperazine citrate	(35% piperazine base)
Piperazine sulfate	(46% piperazine base)
Piperazine dihydrochloride	(50% piperazine base)

Usual use rates are 45 mg piperazine base (or 100 mg piperazine hexahydrate equivalents)/kg bodyweight PO in both dogs and cats.

Pharmacokinetics

In humans piperazine is rapidly absorbed and eliminated after oral administration, being detected in urine within 30 min, reaching peak concentrations within 1–8 h and being undetectable after 24 h.

Adverse effects

At recommended use rates vomiting, diarrhea, inappetence and depression may occur.

In addition, a dose-related neurological syndrome has been described that includes ataxia, muscular weakness, intention tremor of the head and neck, head pressing, epileptiform seizures, hyperesthesia, tetanic spasms, slow pupillary light reflex and lethargy. Symptomatic and supportive treatment is usually quickly successful.

Known drug interactions

Since they have opposing modes of action, coadministration of pyrantel can be expected to antagonize the anthelmintic effects of piperazine.

Diethylcarbamazine citrate

N,*N*-diethyl-4-methyl-1-piperazinecarboxamide dihydrogen citrate.

Clinical applications and dose rates

Since the first description of oral prophylaxis against *D. immitis* infection in 1962, diethylcarbamazine (DEC) has been used for prevention of heartworm establishment. At a dose rate of 6.6 mg/kg q.24 h. PO, DEC is active against third-stage larvae and the molt from third to fourth stage. At 22 mg/kg/day (higher than usual prophylactic dose rates) there is useful activity against fourth-stage larvae and possibly young adults.

DEC is also used for treatment of ascarids in dogs and cats at a dose of 50–100 mg/kg PO and has been reported at 100 mg/kg as suitable for control of fourth-stage and adult *B. malayi* in cats.

Mechanism of action

Diethylcarbamazine (DEC) is a piperazine derivative but with a mode of action distinct from that of piperazine, at least for the first larval stage (microfilaria) of filarial parasites. In contrast to its activity in vivo against microfilaria, DEC has no activity in vitro. It appears to activate an innate immune response, after having inhibited production of PGI_2 and PGE_2 by host endothelial cells, with consequent vasoconstriction and aggregation of host granulocytes and platelets about the microfilariae.

Pharmacokinetics

DEC is rapidly absorbed after oral administration with C_{max} at 3 h, widely distributed, extensively metabolized in the liver by N-dealkylation and N-oxidation and eliminated in urine.

Adverse effects

An acute anaphylaxis-like syndrome involving hepatic vein constriction and hypovolemic shock can result from administration of DEC to dogs with *Dirofilaria immitis* microfilaremia. Toxicity is normally noted from 30 min to 3 h after treatment. While many dogs will recover spontaneously, seriously affected cases can die without intervention

Toluene

Methylbenzene.

Toluene is a flammable hydrocarbon distillation product of petroleum with uses as both a fuel additive in motor vehicles and an anthelmintic in dogs and cats.

Clinical applications

Dogs: *Toxocara canis*, *Toxascaris leonina*, *Ancylostoma caninum*, *Uncinaria stenocephala*
Cats: *Toxocara cati*, *Toxascaris leonina*, *Ancylostoma tubaeforme*, *Uncinaria stenocephala*

Formulations and dose rates

0.22 mL/kg PO

Adverse effects

- Possibly because of its solvent effect, toluene is irritant to mucous membranes and skin. It is available in capsules that, if bitten, can cause oral mucosal irritation, leading to copious salivation.
- Margin of safety is narrow with little selective toxicity.
- The oral LD_{50} in the rat is 7.5 g/kg.

N-butyl chloride

1-chlorobutane.

A highly flammable organochlorine used as both a butylating agent in organic syntheses and an anthelmintic in dogs and cats.

Clinical applications

Dogs: *Toxocara canis*, *Toxascaris leonina*, *Ancylostoma caninum*, *Ancylostoma braziliense*, *Uncinaria stenocephala*
Cats: *Toxocara cati*, *Ancylostoma tubaeforme*

Formulations and dose rates

Animals should not be fed for 18–24 h prior to treatment and treatment should be followed in 30–60 min by administration of a cathartic such as magnesium oxide (milk of magnesia) to aid worm expulsion.
Dogs and cats: 300–1200 mg/kg PO

Adverse effects

The oral LD_{50} in the rat is 2.7 g/kg. Adverse reactions other than vomiting are rarely encountered.

Dichlorvos

O,O-dimethyl-O-2,2-dichlorovinyl phosphate.

An anticholinesterase compound.

Clinical applications

Dogs: *Toxocara canis*, *Toxascaris leonina*, *Ancylostoma caninum*, *Uncinaria stenocephala*, *Trichuris vulpis*
Cats: *Toxocara cati*, *Toxascaris leonina*, *Ancylostoma tubaeforme*, *Uncinaria stenocephala*

Formulations and dose rates

Tablets: 11 mg/kg PO
Resin pellets: 27–33 mg/kg administered, of which 10–12 mg/kg is released and available

Nitroscanate

4-(4-nitrophenoxy)phenyl isothiocyanate.

Clinical applications

Nitroscanate is active against ascarids, hookworms, *Taenia* spp and *Dipylidium caninum*, although the mechanism of action is not known.

Adverse effects

Approximately 10% of dogs vomit after administration. However, the margin of safety is otherwise high with an acute oral LD_{50} in the dog of more than 10,000 mg/kg. Efficacy and safety are improved if coadministered with food and efficacy is further enhanced if the drug is micronized.

Use in cats is not advised, with vomiting, inappetence and posterior paresis being reported.

EXTERNAL PARASITICIDES

Perhaps because of the visibility of external parasites and their effects (both psychological and physical) on humans in close contact, external parasiticides are among the most widely used and misused drugs in dogs and cats. Without professional advice from veterinarians concerning the most appropriate treatment and control programs, continued failures of long-term management can be expected. External parasiticides alone can never be expected to completely control infection as they must be combined with measures to ensure that sources of reinfection are eliminated.

Typical claims are summarized in Table 10.5. It should be emphasized that label directions take priority and must be followed. In many countries (e.g. Australia and the USA) most external parasiticides must be used only as labeled; even veterinarians are not permitted by law to deviate from labeled directions.

Contraindications and precautions

While warnings and precautions vary between countries and labeled statements must be observed, typical considerations that may apply are presented below.

- **Concurrent treatments.** Other insecticides and acaricides that could interact should be used carefully or avoided.
- **Sick and convalescing animals.** Use should be avoided or particular care taken.
- **Lactating animals.** Use should be avoided or particular care taken.
- **Pregnant animals.** Use should be avoided or particular care taken.
- **Young animals.** Use of organophosphates in animals less than 3–6 months is usually avoided.
- **Paralysis tick.** Where complete efficacy is necessary (e.g. with *Ixodes holocyclus* control) parasiticide treatment should be supplemented with thorough daily searching of the coat.
- **Human safety:**
  - Do not permit children access to pesticide formulations.
  - Keep away from food.
  - Wash hands thoroughly with soap and water after handling.
  - Protective clothing may be necessary.

Formulations and dose rates

While some dosage forms for external parasite control are available for oral administration or injection, most are administered externally. Some of the features of these formulations are described below.

Collars

A description of typically available collars is presented in Table 10.5.

Table 10.5 Ectoparasiticide dosage forms

Dosage form	Active constituent	Use rate	Species	Indication and typical duration of action			
				Ticks[1]	*Ix. holocyclus*	*Fleas*	*Other*
Collars		**g/kg collar**					
FORM	Amitraz	90	D	2 m	2 m		
OP	Chlorpyrifos	80/40	D/C	5/4 m		9/8 m	
SP	Deltamethrin	40	D	5–6 m		6 m	Ph 5–6 m
OP	Diazinon	150	D,C	5 m		9 m	
SP	Flumethrin	22.5	D	5 m	6 w	5 m	
CARB	+ propoxur	100					
OP	Naled	150/100	D/C	1 m		4 m	
BOT	Pennyroyal oil +	40	D,C			10 w	
BOT	eucalyptus oil	10					
SP	Permethrin	80	D,C	4 m		4 m	
CARB	Propoxur	100	D,C			5 m	
IGR	Pyriproxifen	5	C			13 m	
IGR	Pyriproxifen	2.5	D,C	5 m		5 m	
OP	+ diazinon	150					
IGR	S-methoprene	10/20	D/C			6 m	

Table 10.5 Ectoparasiticide dosage forms (*continued*)

Dosage form	Active constituent	Use rate	Species	Indication and typical duration of action			
				Ticks[1]	***Ix. holocyclus***	***Fleas***	***Other***
Spot-on		**mg/kg bwt**					
OP	Fenthion	10–20	D			2 w	
PP	Fipronil	6.7	D,C	4 w	2 w	4 w	L
PP	Fipronil	6.7	D	4 w	2w	4 w adult	L
GR	S-methoprene	6				8 w egg	
PP	Pyriprole	12.5	D	4 w		4 w	
NN	Imidacloprid	10	D,C			4 w	
NN	Imidacloprid	10	D			4 w	HW prevention
ML	Ivermectin	0.08					
NN	Imidacloprid	10/2.5	D			4 w	See Table 10.2
ML	Moxidectin	10/1	C				
NN	Imidacloprid	10	D	4 w		4 w	Ph 2–3 w, M 2–4 w, Stom
SP	Permethrin	50					
SP	Permethrin (55:45–40:60)	43–87	D	2–4 w	2 w	4 w	M
SP	Permethrin	45–100	D	3–5 w		3–5 w	M
IGR	+ pyriproxifen	0.5–0.75					
ML	Selamectin	6	D,C	2–4 w		4w	SOLN
SC	Metaflumizone	40	C			to 6 w	
SC	Metaflumizone	20	D	4 w		to 6 w	
FORM	Amitraz	20					
Dips/sprays		**mg/L dip**					
FORM	Amitraz (not chihuahuas)	250–500	D	7 d	7 d		SD
OP	Coumaphos	250	D				L
OP	Cypermethrin +	500	D	7 d	7 d	7 d	
SYN	PBO	500					
OP	Diazinon	500	D	3 w	7 d	3 w	
SPRAY: P	Dichorvos	2000	D,C			7–14 d	
OP	Fenitrothion	8000					
SPRAY: PP	Fipronil	7.5–15 mg/ kg bwt	D,C	4 w	2–3 w	12 w D 8 w C	
OP	Maldison	2.5–6000	D,C	7 d		7 d	SL
SPRAY		6000	D,C	7 d		7 d	
SYN	MGK326 +	3600					
SYN	PBO +	1800					
P	pyrethrins	2000					
IGR	methoprene						
SP	Permethrin (25:75)	1000	D			14 d	
P	Pyrethrins	100	D,C				
SPRAY P	Pyrethrins +	100–1000	D,C	1 d	1 d	1 d	L
SYN	PBO	180–5000					
Oral		**mg/kg bwt**					
IGR	Cyromazine	10	D			1 d	
OP	Cythioate	3	D	2 d	2 d	3–4 d	D
		1.5	C			3–4 d	
IGR	Lufenuron	10	D			4 w	
IGR	Methoprene	22	D			7 d	
NN	Nitenpyram	1	D,C			1 d	Ch
IGR	Pyriproxyfen	10	D,C			7 d	
Injection		**mg/kg bwt**					
IGR	Lufenuron	10	C			6 m	

Extra-label use of MLs has been reported in dogs and cats principally for *Otodectes*, *Demodex* and *Sarcoptes* control.
[1] Tick species against which a product is active is product specific and each product label should be read carefully.
ABBREVIATIONS: Species: D dog, C cat, D/C different dose rates in dog and cat; Ch *Cochliomyia hominovorax*, D *Demodex*, HW heartworm, L lice, M mosquito, S *Sarcoptes*, O *Otodectes*, N nematodes, Ph *Phlebotomus* spp., Stom *Stomoxys calcitrans*, IGR insect growth regulator, OP organophosphate, CARB carbamate, SYN synergist, FORM formamidine, P pyrethrin, PP phenylpyrazole, SP synthetic pyrethroid, ML macrocyclic lactone, BOT botanical, NN neonicotinoid, SC semicarbazone.

Collar technology has advanced significantly since the original vinyl matrices charged with the volatile organophosphate dichlorvos. More recent collars rely on alternative polymers that are hydrophobic and resist swelling and degradation when exposed to water. In addition to the active constituent, collars also may contain spreading agents such as silicone oils and fatty acids to assist dispersion over the coat of the host. Nonetheless, the release characteristics of the active constituent from collars are erratic and unpredictable and for this reason high levels of efficacy are seldom encountered. However, where subtotal parasite control is acceptable there is a valuable role for collars. Concerns have been expressed that the gradual decay in release rate over time may accelerate the likelihood of selection of parasite resistance. While this is plausible and strongly suspected, direct proof is unavailable.

After swimming or washing, re-establishment of pesticidal activity within the pelage may take 24–48 h. It is often recommended that collars be removed during these activities.

Particularly effective use of collars includes the use of deltamethrin collars for protection of dogs from the bites of sandflies and transmission of *Leishmania* spp and the protection of dogs from *Ixodes holocyclus* infection, given the usual preference of this tick to attach to the neck and head. However, there may be selection of ticks that prefer to attach at alternative sites.

The packaging of most collars should not be opened until ready to use, as the release of active agent is initiated by exposure to unsaturated conditions.

Precautions specific to collars include the following.

- **Skin irritation**. Regular inspection of neck recommended. Collar should be removed if irritation is observed.
- **Consumption**. While bioavailability varies from product to product, collars are nevertheless concentrated depots of pesticide. Measures should be instituted to ensure that animals do not chew or swallow collars.

Spot-ons

Topical high-concentration, low-volume preparations have been designed to increase both the convenience of treatment and compliance. Topical spot-on products are either absorbed systemically or distribute laterally and remain within the skin. Systemically active products include selamectin and fenthion. The products either rely on the lipid solubility of the drug or include permeation enhancers to ensure satisfactory transcutaneous passage. Once absorbed, the drugs are redistributed throughout the body and can be detected throughout the skin. The process of distribution throughout the skin of drugs that are not absorbed is poorly understood. However, imidacloprid, fipronil and permethrin are nevertheless active at skin locations remote from the site of application.

As has been described in other species, a decreasing drug concentration gradient would be expected between the site of application and remote skin locations, particularly with unabsorbed preparations. The impact that this may have on selection of resistant parasites is not known. Also unknown is the impact of skin lesions on drug distribution. Potential problems associated with spot-on products include toxicity from ingestion (either from close contact with treated animals or from self grooming which is particularly important in cats exposed to high-concentration permethrin products), skin lesions at the site of application, hair loss, change of hair color and, for products with flammable vehicles, temporary risk of ignition. The solvents in some products (e.g. imidacloprid spot-on) may be deleterious to domestic surfaces. Precautions should be taken at the time of administration by those applying products to ensure that human skin contact and inhalational exposure are minimized. The effect of wetting, by bathing, shampooing, swimming or rain, varies from product to product and labeled advice should be observed.

Dips and sprays

Products for use as immersion dips usually require dilution in water prior to use and are available as emusifiable concentrates (ECs) or wettable powders. ECs are formulated to provide a stable suspension of pesticide once diluted in water. It is preferable that, when applied, the pesticide preferentially binds to skin and hair, leaving the wash that runs away depleted of chemical. This ensures greater pesticide retention and higher concentrations in the coat. Sprays are generally ready-to-use solutions or suspensions of pesticide, requiring no dilution.

There is a higher likelihood of operator exposure during use of dips and sprays and particular attention should be paid to protective clothing and ventilation. With sprays particularly, care with flammable products is necessary. Storage and disposal of dips should be guided by labeled instructions. Some dip concentrates (especially certain diazinon products) can become highly toxic if stored inappropriately. The solvents in some products (e.g. fipronil spray) may be deleterious to domestic surfaces.

Resistance

Parasite resistance can be expected to arise wherever parasiticide application is most intense. At present, resistance of the cat flea, *Ctenocephalides felis*, has been described to the SPs, OPs and fipronil in field isolates and to imidacloprid and lufenuron in laboratory strains and can be predicted to eventually include all available products unless more judicious use practices are instituted.

Mechanisms of resistance that have been described include drug target site insensitivity, increased drug efflux and accelerated drug detoxification. Each mechanism requires a unique management strategy. For example, unlike the situation with increased drug degradation, with site insensitivity, increased dose rates cannot be expected to restore efficacy. Resistance has appeared in ticks, lice and flies affecting ruminants. Many of the tick and fly species selected by treatment of ruminants can potentially infect dogs and cats that are in close proximity. The response to treatment should always be closely monitored and lower than expected efficacy should be investigated.

There are many causes of apparent lack of efficacy, including misdiagnosis, incorrect dose rate, poor application, inappropriate retreatment interval and (very commonly) high and sustained challenge. Resistance is just one additional possible cause and should be confirmed, as its presence will require a change in treatment strategy.

FORMAMIDINES

Amitraz

N'-(2,4-dimethylphenyl)-*N*-[[(2,4-dimethylphenyl) imino]methyl]-*N*-methylmethanimidamide.

Clinical applications

Amitraz is applied externally and has broad-spectrum activity against all mites and ticks, with no significant activity against insect parasites of dogs and cats. Amitraz collars have been shown experimentally to reduce or prevent transmission of *Borrelia burgdorferi* by adult *Ixodes scapularis*.

Mechanism of action

Amitraz elicits a variety of behavioral changes in both argasid and ixodid ticks, often manifested as hyperactivity, leg waving and detaching behavior. It is thought that behavioral effects are secondary to the actions of amitraz on tick octopaminergic G protein-coupled receptors (GPCR). Indeed, sublethal and behavioral effects are considered more important in the mode of action than lethality. Other effects include diminished fecundity, inhibition of oviposition and reduced egg hatchability.

Although amitraz inhibits tick monoamine oxidase, the lethal biochemical lesion appears to be due to inhibition of mixed function oxidases.

Despite precautions against the use of amitraz with monoamine oxidase inhibitors (MAOIs) in mammals, MAOI inhibition by amitraz has only been demonstrated in vitro and not confirmed in vivo. However, amitraz has been shown to be an α_2-agonist and intoxication of dogs and cats can be controlled by use of α_2-antagonists such as yohimbine and atipamezole.

Pharmacokinetics

Orally administered amitraz is rapidly absorbed by dogs, with a T_{max} at 5 h, followed by hepatic biotransformation, with cumulative 96 h excretion of 57% in urine and 24% in feces. The elimination half-life is approximately 23 h. After dermal treatment with 1 mg amitraz/cm^2, peak blood concentrations occurred within 24–72 h and only 25–40% was recovered in urine and feces over a 10-day collection period, demonstrating the poor dermal absorption of amitraz. Similarly there was little absorption after dermal application of a spot-on formulation of amitraz (in combination with metaflumizone). However, amitraz distributed throughout the hair coat, reaching maximum concentration in 7–14 days, and quantifiable levels were present for 56 days.

Formulations and dose rates

General use recommendations are to charge dip washes at 250–500 mg/L. Efficacy is most unpredictable against *Demodex* spp. For generalized demodicosis, an increasing use rate has been recommended (extra-label) for increasingly refractory cases, as follows:

250 mg/L Initial use rate for mites and ticks, repeated every 2 weeks
250 mg/L Repeated weekly
500 mg/L Repeated weekly
1000 mg/L Repeated weekly
1250 mg/L Applied to one side of dog on rotating basis daily.

Some cases of demodicosis may be insensitive to amitraz and alternative approaches (e.g. use of MLs) may be warranted.

In cases of feline demodicosis that failed to respond to repeated lime sulfur treatments, weekly amitraz at 125 mg/L has been successful. However, transient sedation, salivation and behavioral changes were observed initially and use should be avoided in diabetic cats.

Amitraz is available as a spot-on formulation in combination with the insecticide metaflumizone with both actives applied to dogs to provide at least 20 mg/kg bodyweight of each compound.

Adverse effects

- No overt clinical signs of toxicity were observed in dogs receiving 0.25 mg/kg PO per day. CNS depression, bradycardia and hypothermia were present at 1.0 mg/kg PO per day.
- Amitraz may cause a transient sedative effect for 12–24 h after first and subsequent treatments.
- Some dogs may become pruritic after treatment.
- At high exposures (e.g. following accidental ingestion of an amitraz collar) the following adverse effects may occur:

- Severe signs of depression and reluctance to move
- Increased glucose concentrations (insulin concentration unchanged)
- Polyuria
- Bradycardia.

Treatment of intoxication

The adverse consequences of intoxication appear to be principally mediated by the α_2-agonist actions of amitraz. A specific α_2-antagonist, atipamezole (0.05 mg/kg IM), has been shown to control all toxic effects of amitraz within 20 min. Because of the short half-life of atipamezole and the considerably longer half-life of amitraz, initial antidotal treatment should be followed by oral yohimbine, 0.1 mg/kg every 6 h as needed.

INSECT GROWTH REGULATORS AND INSECT DEVELOPMENT INHIBITORS

In contrast to traditional adulticidal products for flea control, the insect growth regulators (IGRs) and insect development inhibitors (IDIs) have no significant direct adulticidal activity. They are, however, very effective at interrupting the environmental stages of the flea lifecycle. Because of the absence of adulticidal activity, they are usually combined with an adulticide if used in the face of pre-existing, symptomatic flea burdens. If flea populations are seasonal, use of IGRs and IDIs in anticipation of the onset of conditions conducive to flea infections can delay the onset of infection significantly. Used appropriately as a component of integrated flea control programs, these agents can provide long-lasting prevention of infection.

Cyromazine

N-cyclopropyl-1,3,5-triazine-2,4,6-triamine.

Clinical applications

Cyromazine is a triazine IGR with applications in sheep for the prevention of cutaneous myiasis and as a poultry feed-through agent for fly control in chicken feces. Because of its novel and specific mode of action, the mammalian toxicity is of a very low order.

Cyromazine has been shown in in vitro bio-assays to inhibit larval and pupal development in *Ctenocephalides canis* by disrupting cuticle turnover during ecdysis. This effect is also observed in the offspring of fleas feeding on dogs administered cyromazine orally.

Pharmacokinetics

Cyromazine is rapidly absorbed following oral administration, with most of the dose excreted in urine within 3 d. At low doses, coadministration with food results in loss of efficacy. However, at higher doses this effect is less clinically relevant.

Adverse effects

Despite an apparently high margin of safety for cyromazine, when combined with DEC for daily administration, serious and life-threatening adverse effects have been encountered, although the mechanism of these effects is unclear.

Fenoxycarb

Ethyl (2-(4-phenoxyphenoxy)ethyl)carbamate.

Clinical applications and mechanism of action

Fenoxycarb is a nonneurotoxic carbamate with potent insect juvenile hormone activity. The acute oral toxicity of fenoxycarb is remarkably low (oral LD_{50} in rat of more than 16,800 mg/kg). However, concerns about the potential chronic toxicity of fenoxycarb to mammals, particularly humans, are limiting its availability.

Fenoxycarb has been shown to directly effect oogenesis, embryogenesis, metamorphosis, fecundity and fertility of exposed *Ctenocephalides felis*. Indeed, unlike methoprene, which does not affect 24-h-old flea eggs, fenoxycarb is active throughout all stages of embryogenesis. The mode of action includes disruption of the midgut as well as inhibition of larval molting.

S-methoprene

Isopropyl(*E*,*E*)-(S)-11-methoxy-3,7,11-trimethyl-dodeca-2,4-dienoate.

Clinical applications and mechanism of action

S-methoprene is a terpenoid insect juvenile hormone mimetic that interferes with the metamorphosis and development of susceptible insects, resulting in ovicidal, embryocidal and larvicidal activity. These effects are produced by either direct exposure of eggs to methoprene or exposure of egg-laying adult female fleas.

Products containing methoprene include oral capsules, collars, topical spot-ons (in combination with fipronil) and sprays.

Pharmacokinetics

Methoprene is rapidly metabolized in mammals to acetates. Some parent compound is excreted in feces of host and flea, often sufficient for continuing effects on insect development. Methoprene is considered of low mammalian toxicity, with an acute oral LD_{50} in the dog of greater than 5000 mg/kg. It degrades quickly in aqueous environments and is unstable in the presence of ultraviolet light and therefore unsuitable for use in exposed situations.

Lufenuron

(*R,S*)-1-[2,5-dichloro-4-(1,1,2,3,3,3-hexafluoropropoxy)phenyl]-3-(2,6-difluorobenzoyl)urea.

Mechanism of action

The precise mechanism of action of lufenuron, a member of the benzoylphenylurea (BPU) class, is not known. However, while it does not directly inhibit chitin synthase, there is evidence that it inhibits the γ-S-GTP stimulated uptake of Ca^{2+} by chitin microfiber-containing excretory vesicles, disrupting vesicle fusion with the outer cell membrane and cuticle formation in exposed insects. Lufenuron is both ovicidal and larvicidal. The ovicidal action is most notable with higher concentrations of lufenuron. As concentrations deplete, eggs will hatch; however, the larvae are reduced in size and further development to pupae is inhibited. Excretion of lufenuron in flea feces provides a source of exposure to flea larvae, whose continued development is then impaired. In vitro studies of adult fleas have shown that sustained lufenuron exposure can be adulticidal. This activity is not encountered in vivo, as the concentrations of lufenuron in host blood are inadequate to disrupt adult flea chitin synthesis.

Although chitin occurs in most invertebrate phyla (the chitin content of the cuticle of larval insects is 30–60% while the weight of chitin in the cuticle of ticks is around 3%), it is absent among vertebrates, accounting for the high margin of mammalian safety associated with lufenuron.

Pharmacokinetics

The absorption of lufenuron following oral administration is improved in both rate and extent by the presence of food, with maximum concentrations achieved in around 6 h. Systemic bioavailability, at least in cats, may not be high, in view of an oral dose of 30 mg/kg providing efficacy for 1 month in comparison with parenteral administration of 10 mg/kg providing greater than 90% effect on flea development for 6 months. Lufenuron is highly lipophilic and accumulates in adipose tissue, forming a depot from where it slowly dissipates, extending the period of flea exposure following a single dose. Lufenuron is excreted unchanged in bile.

Formulations and dose rates

Applications and use rates are summarized in Table 10.5.

Pyriproxyfen

4-phenoxyphenyl (*R,S*)-2-(2-pyridyloxy)propyl ether.

Mechanism of action

Although a carbamate, pyriproxyfen has no cholinesterase activity but is a potent insect juvenile hormone mimetic. It is ovicidal and larvicidal when applied either directly to ova, via ingestion of fecal blood excreted by treated fleas, or indirectly via exposure of adults (both male and female fleas). It is photostable with extended residual activity in the environment. When young pupae are exposed pyriproxyfen diffuses across the pupal case, resulting in accelerated emergence and increased mortality of emerging adults, although the fecundity of surviving females is unaffected.

Pharmacokinetics

Pyriproxyfen is photostable and is available in a variety of formulations that permit persistence in the coats of treated dogs and cats. An analytical study of pyriproxyfen administered orally to cats at doses up to 50 mg/kg was unable to detect any drug in samples of hair. However, dogs and cats treated topically on the dorsal midline of the neck with 0.04 and 0.1 mg/kg as a 1% solution of pyriproxyfen had sustained levels of pyriproxyfen in their hair at concentrations above 0.02 mg/kg for more than 48 d. Not unexpectedly, there was a clear concentration gradient from the site of application to the hair of the hindquarters and considerable inter-animal variation in hair concentration. The minimum concentration causing inhibition of development of flea eggs has been shown to be 0.0001 mg/kg in hair.

MISCELLANEOUS EXTERNAL PARASITICIDES

Benzyl benzoate

Benzoic acid phenylmethyl ester.

Clinical applications

Benzyl benzoate is used as a pediculicide and scabicide in dogs, although its principal use in humans is as a repellent of ticks, chiggers and mosquitoes. It is generally applied as a spot treatment.

Pharmacokinetics

Benzyl benzoate is rapidly absorbed and is hydrolyzed to benzoic acid and benzyl alcohol, conjugated with glycine or glucuronide and eliminated in urine.

Adverse effects

- While generally considered of low toxicity, cats are about 10 times more sensitive than dogs (acute oral LD_{50} in cats is 2240 and in dogs 22,440 mg/kg) and its use in this species is contraindicated in some countries.

- Signs of poisoning include salivation, twitching of treated areas, generalized tremors, convulsions, respiratory failure and death.
- Treatment is symptomatic and supportive.

D-limonene

1-methyl-4-(1-methylethenyl)cyclohexene.

Clinical applications

D-limonene is a citrus fruit extract, available as an insecticidal dip for flea control. It has been shown to be neurotoxic to adult fleas, resulting in rapid immobilization. Vapors as well as direct exposure result in toxicity to fleas and toxicity is synergized by piperonyl butoxide.

Adverse effects

- D-limonene has been considered to be of little toxic concern, as the acute oral LD_{50} in rats is more than 5000 mg/kg.
- However, errors in dilution have led to exposure of cats to elevated dose rates 5–15 times the recommended use rate, inducing a toxic syndrome of salivation, muscle tremors, ataxia and hyperthermia.
- Treatment is supportive and symptomatic, with particular attention to both decontamination and body temperature control.
- A similar toxic syndrome has been reported in a dog, who developed erythema multiforme major and disseminated intravascular coagulation.

Lime sulfur

Solution of calcium polysulfides and thiosulfate.

Clinical applications

Lime sulfur is a traditional pesticide that has been popular in cats for control of *Notoedres, Sarcoptes, Demodex, Cheyletiella, Lynxacarus*, chiggers and lice infections. Lime sulfur is fungicidal, bactericidal, keratolytic and antipruritic. Concentrated suspensions are diluted to 2% prior to use.

Adverse effects

- If inadequately diluted, skin irritation and scalding may be observed.
- Lime sulfur preparations have an unpleasant odor.
- Lime sulfur can stain light-colored coats and tarnish silver jewelry.
- To prevent possible oral ingestion and toxicity, cats should not be allowed to groom until the coat has dried after treatment.

Linalool oil

3,7-dimethyl-1,6-octadien-3-ol.

Linalool oil occurs naturally in a large variety of plants and is a constituent of citrus peel and has found applications in perfumes and flavors.

Clinical applications

Linalool oil has been shown to kill the eggs, larvae and pupae of the cat flea (*Ctenocephalides felis*) and to eliminate adult fleas rapidly from cats immersed in a dip charged with 10,000 mg/L linalool or 5000 mg/L linalool plus MGK 264. Apart from the disagreeable odor and temporary oiliness of the coat, the low vertebrate toxicity and broad-spectrum flea activity make linalool a possible candidate for use.

Rotenone

(2*R*,6as,12aS)-1,2,6,6*a*,12,12*a*-hexahydro-2-isopropenyl-8,9-dimethoxychromeno[3,4-*b*]furol-[2,3-*h*]chromen-6-one.

Clinical applications

Rotenoid-containing plants have been used as fish poisons for many centuries, if not millennia, but it was not until 1892 that the active moiety was isolated, being named rotenone in 1902. Rotenone is most widely sourced from *Derris elliptica* and *D. malaccensis* in Asia and from *Lonchocarpus utilis* and *L. urucu* in South America. Plant extracts contain six rotenoids, of which rotenone is the most active and abundant. Rotenone solutions decompose on exposure to light or air.

Principal applications are in combination with synergists and pyrethrins for flea and ear mite control.

Mechanism of action

Rotenone toxicity to insects results in inactivity, locomotor instability and refusal to eat, followed by knockdown, paralysis and slow death by respiratory failure. Biochemically, rotenone is one of the most potent inhibitors of the NADH dehydrogenase system, acting on Fe-S proteins to inhibit electron transport between NADH and ubiquinone (coenzyme Q) in both insects and vertebrates.

Pharmacokinetics

Rotenone is sparingly soluble in water but readily soluble in many organic solvents and oils. Around 20–30% of an oral dose is absorbed, but this amount is increased if administered in oil. Rotenone is rapidly metabolized in the liver and excreted in both feces and urine.

Adverse effects

- Rotenone is considered relatively safe at normal use rates in dogs and cats.
- Early signs of intoxication include vomiting, which would serve to limit further exposure.

NEONICOTINOIDS

The neonicotinoids act selectively on the insect nicotinic acetylcholine receptor (nAChR), initially stimulating postsynaptic receptors, increasing Na^+ ingress and K^+ egress and then paralyzing nerve conduction, resulting in rapid death. Because of important structural differences between vertebrate and insect nAChR, the neonicotinoids have a high order of vertebrate safety, with a selectivity ratio (IC_{50} vertebrate nAChR to IC_{50} insect nAChR) in the order of 565. At physiological pH in mammals, 90% of nicotine (pKa = 7.9) is protonated, an important component of interaction with the mammalian nAChR. By contrast, the neonicotinoids are unprotonated at this pH. Furthermore, they have a negatively charged nitro or cyano group that interacts with cationic amino acids such as lysine, arginine or histidine in the insect nAChR-binding region. The neonicotinoids as a class have low hydrophobicity, systemic activity, act more by insect ingestion than contact, are ovicidal, show no cross-resistance to fipronil, OPs, SPs and carbamates, and have low mammalian and fish toxicity. They are subject to extensive detoxification by oxidative metabolism in mammals and quickly excreted.

Nitenpyram

N-[(6-chloro-3-pyridinyl)methyl]-*N*-ethyl-*N*′-methyl-2-nitro-1,1-ethenediamine.

Pharmacokinetics

Nitenpyram is administered orally to dogs and cats, is rapidly absorbed, with an elimination half-life of 2 and 16 h in dogs and cats respectively. The principal route of excretion is the kidney. While virtually 100% activity against adult fleas is observed for the 24-h period after treatment, greater than 95% activity was present between 24 and 48 h, with no significant activity thereafter.

Adverse effects

- Acute and repeated dose toxicity studies have demonstrated that nitenpyram has a high margin of safety in dogs and cats and appears safe to use in reproducing males and females.
- The toxic syndrome is not elicited until more than 100 mg/kg (100 times higher than the recommended use rate) is administered to either dogs or cats and is manifested by transient and spontaneously resolving salivation, vomiting, lethargy, tachypnea, soft stools and tremors.

Imidacloprid

1-[(6-chloro-3-pyridinyl)methyl]-*N*-nitro-2-imidazolidinimine.

Clinical applications

Imidacloprid was developed initially and principally for the control of agricultural pests but has been demonstrated to be a very effective pediculicide in dogs and cats.

Pharmacokinetics

In contrast to nitenpyram, which is administered orally and has a short duration of activity, imidacloprid is formulated for topical spot-on application in both cats and dogs, with adulticidal activity of at least 95% against fleas for up to 4 weeks. In addition, debris falling from treated animals has been shown to be larvicidal to fleas in direct contact in the environment.

Adverse effects

- Imidacloprid has a low order of mammalian toxicity, with an acute oral LD_{50} in rats of 450 mg/kg and in mice of 150 mg/kg, acute dermal LD_{50} in rat of more than 5000 mg/kg and a no observable effect level (NOEL) in a 52-week study in the dog of 500 ppm of diet.
- It has a very acceptable safety profile in dogs and cats, with a therapeutic margin of at least 20-fold with a single treatment and more than fivefold with repeated weekly treatments.
- In addition, no adverse effects were observed when administered during pregnancy and lactation.

PHENYL PYRAZOLES

Fipronil

5-amino-1-[2,6-dichloro-4-(trifluoromethyl) phenyl]-4-[(trifluoromethyl)sulfinyl]-1H-pyrazole-3-carbonitrile.

Clinical applications

Fipronil was discovered in 1987 and was developed initially for use in pest control in agriculture and public health. In dogs and cats, fipronil is available as a high-volume spray or a low-volume spot-on, with activity against ticks, fleas and ear mites. Hair shed from dogs for up to 2 weeks after topical treatment retains sufficient fipronil to kill dust mites (*Dermatophagoides* spp) coming in contact. There is also some evidence that the speed of kill of ticks may be sufficient to reduce or prevent the transmission of a number of disease agents, including *Ehrlichia canis, Borrelia burgdorferi* and *Anaplasma phagocytophilum*.

Mechanism of action

Recent investigations suggest that the mechanism of action of fipronil is complex, involving multiple interactions of both parent fipronil and its oxidation product, fipronil sulfone, on GABA-gated and glutamate-gated chloride channels in the insect nervous system. Both fipronil and fipronil sulfone inhibit GABA receptors as well as desensitizing and nondesensitizing GluCls, though the activity of fipronil sulfone is much higher than fipronil for desensitizing GluCls. The net result of insect exposure to fipronil is blockade of inhibitory nerve transmission, resulting in hyperexcitability and death of susceptible parasites. GluCls have been observed only in invertebrates The binding affinities of fipronil and fipronil sulfone to mammalian $GABA_A$ receptors are much less than in arthropods ($GABA_A$ receptor binding IC_{50} human:insect of 135 and 17 respectively) with no binding to other types of mammalian GABA receptor, accounting (in combination with the low systemic bioavailability after dermal administration) for the selectivity of action. However, fipronil and its metabolites and degradation products are highly toxic to some species of fish.

Pharmacokinetics

Fipronil is not thought to be significantly absorbed from topical sites of application but to translocate dermally, being confined to the lipids of hair follicles and sebaceous glands. From this reservoir, drug is released for many weeks, accounting for the sustained activity against fleas and ticks. On the basis of studies in humans, inadvertently ingested fipronil appears to be rapidly and well absorbed from the gastrointestinal tract, extensively metabolized to the sulfone and subject to significant enterohepatic recirculation. The elimination half-life is 7–8 h for fipronil but 7–8 d for fipronil sulfone.

Known drug interactions

- It has been suggested, on the basis of a review of mechanisms of action, that prior exposure of arthropods to the organochlorine class of pesticides may predispose to resistance to fipronil. This hypothesis has not yet been tested, but resistance of fleas to fipronil has already been reported.
- Piperonyl butoxide (by blocking oxidation of fipronil to its sulfone) appears to antagonize the antiparasitic action of fipronil.

Pyriprole

1-[2,6-dichloro-4-(trifluoromethyl) phenyl]-4-[(difluoromethyl)thio]-5-[(2-pyridinylmethyl)amino]-1H-pyrazole-3-carbonitrile.

Clinical applications and dose rates

Pyriprole is formulated as a high-concentration solution in diethylene glycol monoethyl ether for topical application to dogs at a dose rate of at least 12.5 mg/kg bodyweight. Efficacy has been established for the treatment and prevention of flea infestation (*Ctenocephalides canis* and *C. felis*) in dogs, with efficacy persisting for a minimum of 4 weeks. Pyriprole kills fleas within 24 h of exposure and may be used as part of a treatment strategy for the control of flea allergy dermatitis (FAD). Efficacy has also been demonstrated for the treatment and prevention of tick infestation (*Ixodes ricinus*, the least sensitive of the tick species tested, *Rhipicephalus sanguineus, Ixodes scapularis, Dermacentor reticulatus, Dermacentor variabilis, Amblyomma americanum*) in dogs with sustained acaricidal efficacy for around 4 weeks. Pyriprole kills ticks within 48 h of exposure but some ticks may remain attached.

Mechanism of action

Pyriprole is an analog of fipronil and is expected to share its mechanism of action. Susceptible parasites are killed after contact with pyriprole rather than by systemic exposure.

Pharmacokinetics

Following topical application pyriprole is rapidly (within 24 h) and widely distributed in the hair coat and stored in sebaceous glands from which it is slowly released. There is little metabolism or pyriprole in the skin. About 50% of a topical dose is absorbed ($t_{1/2}$ absorption about 21 d) with rapid hepatic clearance and excretion principally in feces (60%) with lesser amounts in urine (20%). Because of the slow absorption and rapid hepatic metabolism, parent drug is generally not detectable in plasma, though the oxidation products (sulfoxide and sulfone) are.

Adverse effects

Local reactions at the application site may include fur discoloration, local alopecia or pruritus. A greasy appearance or clumpiness of hair is common at the site of application. Most signs disappear within 48 h of the application. Transient hypersalivation may occur if the dog licks the application site immediately after treatment.

At a dose rate of 37.5 mg/kg, transient and mild neurological signs (slight inco-ordination and unsteadiness) were observed in some animals for up to 3 h. At

62.5 mg/kg, transient tremors, ataxia, panting and convulsions were noted but disappeared within 18 h. At 125 mg/kg, vomiting, anorexia, reduced bodyweight, muscle tremors, seizures, unsteadiness and labored breathing were present but resolved within 48 h. However, loss of appetite persisted in some cases.

Contraindications and precautions

Dogs should not be bathed or shampooed in the 48 h before treatment. Immersion of dogs in water or shampooing within 24 h after treatment may reduce efficacy, but weekly immersion in water did not affect efficacy against fleas and ticks.

Safety has not been established during pregnancy and lactation, nor in breeding animals, although in laboratory animal studies no indications of relevant effects on reproduction or fetal development were observed.

Do not use in dogs less than 8 weeks of age or less than 2 kg bodyweight. Do not use in cases of known hypersensitivity or on sick or convalescing dogs. Do not use on cats or rabbits.

SEMICARBAZONE

Metaflumizone

2-[2-(4-cyanophenyl)-1-[3-(trifluoromethyl)phenyl] ethylidene]-*N*-[4-(trifluoromethoxy)-phenyl] hydrazinecarboxamide.

Clinical applications and dose rates

Metaflumizone is formulated for use in the cat as a high-concentration solution in dimethyl sulfoxide, γ-hexalactone and a surfactant. The minimum topical dose rate is 40 mg/kg and efficacy has been confirmed for the treatment and prevention of flea infestation (*Ctenocephalides canis* and *C. felis*) when used every 4–6 weeks. It acts slowly, with flea deaths accumulating over 2–4 d, but it may be used as part of a treatment strategy for the control of flea allergy dermatitis (FAD).

Metaflumizone is also formulated in combination with the acaricide amitraz for topical use in dogs at a minimum dose rate of 20 mg/kg of each of the active constituents. Prevention of flea infestation for up to 6 weeks is claimed, though it was noted in a multicenter field trial that at the conclusion of the study more dogs in the metaflumizone-amitraz group had low flea burdens than a positive control group, though efficacy was still above 90%. The amitraz component of the combination product provides efficacy against ticks for up to 4 weeks.

Mechanism of action

Metaflumizone is a sodium channel blocker and is chemically a semicarbazone, closely related to the dihydropyrazoles of which indoxacarb is the characteristic agent. The voltage-dependent sodium channel is a complex multimeric protein and the precise location at which metaflumizone binds has not yet been described. It does appear to bind slowly in a manner not dissimilar to that of the local anesthetics. At concentrations as low as 100 nM, metaflumizone blocked sodium flux under depolarizing conditions, leading to paralysis and death of exposed insects. The insecticidal activity of metaflumizone occurs mainly following ingestion rather than via contact. Activity at the molecular level is often stereospecific. For example, the S enantiomer of the dihydropyrazles can be 10–100 times more insecticidally active than the R counterpart. Which of the isomers of metaflumazone is most active has not been reported, though the formulation contains E and Z isomers in a ratio of 9:1.

Pharmacokinetics

After topical application metaflumizone is distributed throughout the pelage within 1–2 d in cats and 7–14 d in dogs and concentrations slowly deplete over 56 d. There is considerable variation between animals and between skin sites in concentration and depletion rate. Dermal absorption and systemic bioavailability appear to be very low in both dogs and cats, though plasma levels were detectable in some male dogs.

Adverse effects

Transient salivation is reported, possibly following auto- or allo-grooming. However, metaflumizone appears to induce ingestion avoidance behavior in both dogs and cats which should limit the likelihood of significant oral exposure.

Local reactions at the application site include temporary oily appearance and clumping or spiking of the coat and color change of fur.

Contraindications and precautions

- Do not administer to cats or dogs less than 8 weeks of age.
- The safe use of metaflumizone in pregnant or lactating animals has not been established.
- Avoid prolonged intense exposure to water, especially in 24-h period after application.
- Do not use in cases of known hypersensitivity or on sick or debilitated animals.

REPELLENTS

The ideal repellent has been described as one that is active against multiple species of arthropods, effective for more than 8 h, has no irritant properties to skin or mucosae, no systemic toxicity, resistant to being rubbed or washed off, odorless and nongreasy. While the perfect repellent has not yet been identified, a number of significant advances have recently been made, especially by military entomologists seeking to protect soldiers from arthropod-borne diseases as well as the painful bites and allergic reactions associated with arthropods.

It should be noted that the term repellent is usually applied to a host of behavioral responses by arthropods with a common feature of interruption of contact with the host. However, there are a number of quite distinct responses that are likely mediated by quite separate mechanisms. For example, amitraz acts via octopamine receptors to elicit detaching activity. The pyrethrins at sublethal doses act via sodium channel excitation to prevent oviposition and to repel, while the action of DEET is unknown.

Repellents have been defined as chemicals that cause insects to make oriented movements away from the repellent while deterrence is defined as inhibition of feeding or oviposition. Approaches to the discovery of novel repellents include random screening of chemical libraries, screening of extracts based on ethnobotanical studies and more recently the application of QSAR (quantitative structure-activity relationship) modeling. The well-established pyrethrins, synthetic pyrethroids, garlic (recently demonstrated to be an effective tick repellent in studies with Swedish marines), dimethyl phthalate, ethohexadiol (Rutgers 6–12) and benzyl benzoate all continue to have roles as repellents. However, the most widely used repellents in veterinary practice are DEET, MGK 326 and a variety of natural volatile oils, described below. Oral thiamine has been shown to have no repellency activity against fleas (*Ctenocephalides felis*).

Recently developed repellents that have demonstrated greatest activity against a variety of insects and ticks that may be expected to find important roles in protecting dogs and cats include:

- 2% soybean oil (refined extracts from *Glycine max*, principally glycerides of linoleic and oleic acids) which had activity against black flies and mosquitoes greater than that provided by 25% DEET
- 19.2% icaridin (previously KBR 3023 or picaridin) (RS-sec-butyl 2-(2-hydroxy ethyl) piperidine-1-carboxylic acid) shown by military tests in the tropics to provide protection equivalent to that of 35% DEET but to be less irritating
- 10–20% p-menthane-3,8-diol (PMD) (a monoterpene obtained from the distillation of the leaves of the lemon-scented gum or *Corymbia citriodora* ssp *citriodora*) which provides protection against ticks, flies and mosquitoes
- natural citronella oil (obtained from steam distillation of the grasses *Cymbopogon nardus* and *C. winteranus* and containing a large number of terpenes, alcohols and aldehydes such as d-limonene, linalool, eugenol, citronellal and pinene) which provides short-term efficacy against mosquitoes and blackflies.

The period of protection provided by repellents is subject to a number of sources of variation, including pest factors (species, density, parity, nutritional status, season), host factors (age, sex, level of activity, intrinsic attractiveness) and environmental factors (ambient light, temperature, humidity, wind speed, rain). The mechanism by which repellents exert their effect is not certain, but there do appear to be certain chemical structural features that are associated with repellent activity. Chemoreceptors in the antennae of insects are important in host finding and are an obvious target of repellents. Ticks do not have antennae, but electrophysiological studies of chemoreceptor cells in the sensilla of the tarsus of *Ixodes ricinus* have shown that they respond to repellent exposure.

DEET

N,N-diethyl-*m*-toluamide (now termed N,N-diethyl-3-methylbenzamide).

Technical DEET usually contains 95% *m* isomer, with lesser amounts of the *o* and *p* isomers, which are less effective repellents. DEET is usually diluted in isopropyl or ethyl alcohol for use as a spray at a concentration of 2–60%. Studies in humans have demonstrated that the period of complete protection time or CPT (defined as the time from application to first bite) is related to the logarithm of the DEET concentration with a plateau at around 50%. Recently it has been shown that avoidance activity by ticks when exposed to DEET does not require direct contact, indicating that the vapor phase of DEET was sufficient. However, rising ambient temperature is associated with decreasing DEET efficacy.

Clinical applications

DEET has activity against mosquitoes, blackflies, midges, chiggers, ticks, fleas and leeches.

Pharmacokinetics

About 8–13% of topically applied DEET is absorbed in dogs from intact skin, with maximum blood concentrations attained within 1 h. DEET is then cleared quickly, with hepatic biotransformation and urinary excretion. Accumulation and persistence of DEET in skin have been observed. Topical DEET has been shown to increase the transdermal flux of concurrently administered products.

Adverse effects

- DEET is usually well tolerated by dogs and cats, although repeated applications of concentrated products have been associated with vomiting, tremors and hyperactivity.
- Treatment is directed at reducing exposure and symptoms and is usually successful.
- A rare syndrome of toxic encephalopathy described in children does not appear to have a counterpart in dogs and cats.

Di-*N*-propylisocinchomeronate (MGK 326)

Dipropyl 2,5-pyridinedicarboxylate.

MGK 326 is widely used as a component of companion animal external parasiticides. It is considered very safe, with an acute oral LD_{50} in the rat of more than 5200 mg/kg. There is little published material describing objective assessments of efficacy. A recent review of the efficacy of MGK 326 by the Pest Management Regulatory Agency in Canada concluded that there was insufficient evidence in support of a repellent effect.

SYNERGISTS

The discovery in 1940 that sesame oil potentiates the insecticidal activity of pyrethrins stimulated a search for synergistic compounds and resulted in the characterization of the methylene-dioxyphenyls. The synergists most widely incorporated into veterinary insecticides include piperonyl butoxide and MGK 264, described below. These products act as competitive inhibitors of mixed-function oxidases in both insects and mammals. Selectivity for insects is assured by poor absorption in mammals and rapid metabolism. However, exposure of mammals to sustained high concentrations has been associated with hepatic enzyme induction and increased liver weight. By inhibiting insect detoxification pathways, synergists increase the available concentration of insecticide, increasing effectiveness. Synergists thus allow a reduction in the content of the insecticide with retention of efficacy.

It should be noted that the use of inhibitors of mixed-function oxidases will not invariably lead to synergy. For those compounds that are activated by oxidative pathways, a reduction in insecticidal activity will be observed. This is the case with fipronil and the phosphoro(di)thioates (see Organophosphates), which require oxidative desulfuration for activation. Another consideration is the effect of temperature on synergy. In a study of the interaction of imidacloprid and piperonyl butoxide, it was observed that 16-fold synergy was observed against adult fleas at 26°C but no effect at a temperature (35°C) likely to be encountered in the coat of dogs and cats. It should be emphasized that synergy will not be present if resistance is due to target site insensitivity and synergy will be reduced or absent if resistance arises because of accelerated drug efflux.

Piperonyl butoxide

5-[2-(2-butoxyethoxy)ethoxymethyl]-6-propyl-1,3-benzodioxole.

Piperonyl butoxide (PBO) was first developed in 1947 and is still widely used. It is usually combined with pyrethrin or rotenone preparations in ratios of 5–20:1 by weight. PBO appears very safe in companion animals, with an acute oral LD_{50} in the cat and dog of more than 7500 mg/kg. Rarely, cats have been reported to develop central nervous system signs. PBO is poorly absorbed from the gastrointestinal tract of dogs, with more than 80% recovered in feces. The absorbed fraction is rapidly excreted in urine.

N-octyl bicycloheptene dicarboximide (MGK 264)

2-(ethylhexyl)-3a,4,7,7a-tetrahydro-4,7-methano-1 *H*-isoindole-1,3(2*H*)-dione.

MGK 264 is widely used as a component of products for cats and dogs containing pyrethrins and synthetic pyrethroids. The acute oral LD_{50} in rats is reported to be 4980 mg/kg. Although there are no reports of inefficacy or adverse effects, there is little objective assessment of its efficacy and safety in the literature. A recent review of the efficacy of MGK 264 by the Pest Management Regulatory Agency in Canada concluded that there was insufficient evidence in support of any synergism.

ANTICHOLINESTERASE PARASITICIDES

Organophosphates

Examples of available organophosphate preparations are presented in Table 10.5.

Pharmacokinetics

All commercially available organophosphate (OP) pesticides are very lipid soluble, with rapid absorption expected from most routes of exposure. In healthy animals, the OPs are metabolized by a variety of oxidative processes both in tissues and blood (especially by esterases) and in the liver, and conjugated with glucuronide, sulfate and glycine. Excretion is mainly in the urine. Many OPs may form slow-release depots in fat.

Inhibition of cholinesterase (both pseudocholinesterase in plasma and acetylcholinesterase) is essentially irreversible and return of activity necessitates synthesis of new enzymes. While regeneration can be rapid in nerve cells and liver, renewed erythrocyte enzyme, given the absence of a nucleus, requires production of new erythrocytes. Therefore, the duration of depression of erythrocyte cholinesterase activity following exposure is related to the life-span of these cells and may be more a measure of exposure than of current clinical condition.

A number of organophosphates must first be oxidized in order to produce an active form. Examples include diazinon and malathion, which are desulfurated to diazoxon and malaoxon respectively, and trichlorphon, which is activated to dichlorvos.

Adverse effects

- Cats are more sensitive to the toxic effects of OPs than dogs and only malathion is commonly used.
- In addition to the classic syndrome of increased muscarinic and nicotinic activity, certain nonanticholinesterase effects have been described, the most infamous of which is organophosphate-induced delayed neuropathy (OPIDN), a delayed (2–4 weeks after exposure) sensorimotor polyneuropathy affecting predominantly the hindlimbs. OPIDN follows phosphorylation and aging of a protein in neurones called neuropathy target esterase (NTE). The affinity of clinically useful OPs for NTE is orders of magnitude lower than for acetylcholinesterase and consequently OPIDN has rarely been encountered in dogs and cats. In those OPs capable of interacting with NTE (trichlorphon and chlorpyrifos), because of differential affinities, a significant acute cholinergic syndrome would be expected to precede the onset of delayed neuropathy. However, cats appear to be particularly susceptible to chlorpyrifos toxicity and delayed neuropathy has been described.
- The effect of chronic exposure to low doses of OPs has been the subject of much investigation. While cognitive enhancement has been observed (and led to the use of specific OPs for the treatment of Alzheimer's disease), concerns have been raised about possible adverse neurobehavioral effects. Available data, which include a number of epidemiological surveys, suggest that these concerns may be unwarranted.

Toxicity of specific organophosphates

- In comparison with other species, cats appear particularly sensitive to **chlorpyrifos**. The onset of signs of intoxication may be delayed for several days following topical exposure. Usual treatment protocols are appropriate but, in contrast with dogs, recovery may take significantly longer.
- Under conditions that may be found in emulsifiable concentrates (EC) contaminated with trace quantities of water, **diazinon** breaks down to highly toxic tetra ethyl pyrophosphates (TEPPs), especially *O*,*O*-TEPP (monotepp) and *O*,S-TEPP (sulfotepp), which are 300 and 2500 times more toxic, respectively, than diazinon. Outdated products and inadequate storage conditions can increase the likelihood of toxicity. Deaths of dogs have been recorded in a number of countries and EC formulations are expected to be withdrawn.
- **Fenthion** should not be used on chihuahuas.
- Incorrect storage of **malathion** (e.g. at 40°C for protracted periods) can lead to the formation of degradation products that can increase the toxicity of malathion preparations. Despite these potential limitations, malathion remains one of the least toxic organophosphates for use in both dogs and cats.

Treatment of organophosphate toxicity

Having obtained a history and secured the diagnosis, the essential principles of treatment of poisoning should be applied: stabilize vital signs, prevent continued exposure to or absorption of poison, administer antidotes, accelerate metabolism and excretion of absorbed poisons, and provide supportive and symptomatic therapy. Specific antidotal treatments are described below.

Oximes

Oximes were developed purposefully and specifically in the mid-1950s, on the basis of pharmacological theory, to restore the activity of acetylcholinesterase inhibited by combination with organophosphates. Organophosphates interact with the serine hydroxyl group within the active site of acetylcholinesterase to form a stable phosphorylated and inactive enzyme. Enzyme activity is returned very slowly by hydrolysis but, in the face of significant exposure to organophosphates, natural reactivation is insufficient to restore function. Oximes accelerate the reactivation of inhibited enzyme by nucleophilic attack, leading to dephosphorylation and restitution of the catalytic site of the enzyme. Simultaneously, the oxime, with a greater affinity for phosphorus, is sacrificed by phosphorylation. The phosphorylated oxime is also a potent anticholinesterase but fortunately is quickly hydrolyzed and inactivated.

While oximes can lead to dramatic improvements in clinical recovery if used soon after intoxication, with time (at a rate and extent dependent on the characteristics of the organophosphate) the phosphorylated enzyme is dealkylated, resulting in irreversible phosphorylation, unavailable to nucleophilic attack and restoration of activity. Nevertheless, in human poisonings, it is recommended, on the basis of successful interventions, that oxime therapy be continued for several days.

The value of oximes in the management of intoxication with diethoxy (chlorpyriphos, coumaphos and diazinon) and dimethoxy (cythioate, dichlorvos, fenitrothion, fenthion, malathion, naled, phosmet and trichlorphon) organophosphates has been well demonstrated, but less well described is their role in the treatment of poisoning by other types of organophosphate. Fortunately, most clinically useful organophosphates fall within these two categories; however, toxic exposure to certain other organophosphates used in agriculture and warfare may be less responsive to treatment.

The predominant oxime in clinical use is 2-PAM chloride (pralidoxime), a quaternary ammonium oxime. It is subject to enteric and hepatic metabolism and is therefore seldom administered orally. Usually, it is initially given by slow intravenous injection, followed by subcutaneous or intramuscular injection as necessary. The drug is cleared rapidly in dogs by renal excretion, the rate of which is increased by acidosis. Repeated dose regimens may need adjustment in the face of significant renal dysfunction.

The usual dose regimen is 10–20 mg/kg by slow intravenous injection, repeated IM or SC as necessary on the basis of clinical response. It should be noted that oximes have atropine-like activity and are also cholinesterase inhibitors, most manifest at high doses. Thus increasing the dose rate above 20 mg/kg is unlikely to be beneficial. In addition, they can depolarize neuromuscular junctions and potentiate the effect of succinylcholine.

Atropine

While organophosphate intoxication leads to both muscarinic and nicotinic affects, muscarinic signs (DUMBELS – diarrhea, urination, miosis, bronchoconstriction, emesis, lacrimation, salivation) can be attenuated by the use of atropine (racemic dl-hyoscyamine), available as atropine sulfate. Atropine is administered to effect (atropinization, as judged by pupil size), usually commencing with 0.2–0.5 mg/kg, one-quarter of the dose given IV and the balance IM or SC. A further dose may be administered in 15–30 min, as indicated by patient response, and additional doses at 3–6 h intervals for several days.

Known drug interactions

- The literature warns against the concurrent use of phenothiazine derivatives and organophosphates which appears to be based on an early (1962) case report of accidental but lethal poisoning in a mentally disturbed human patient concurrently administered promazine. Subsequent attempts to reproduce the interaction have not been uniformly successful. However, in the interests of prudence, it is generally recommended that, when tranquilization is required, drugs other than phenothiazines (e.g. diazepam) should form the first line of use.
- Succinylcholine activity is greatly potentiated by inhibition of the esterases that usually inactivate it. Therefore, if use remains indicated, great care in selection of the dose regimen will be necessary.
- Levamisole and pyrantel are theoretically expected to interact but clinical experience does not support this.
- Other drugs that act as cholinesterase inhibitors, such as morphine, neostigmine, physostigmine, pyridostigmine and the aromatic diamidines (e.g. imidocarb and pentamidine), should be avoided.

Carbamates

Carbamates such as carbaryl, methiocarb and propoxur are widely used in both dogs and cats. Unlike OPs, the dose resulting in the first signs of toxicity is widely separated from the lethal dose.

Examples of available carbamate preparations are presented in Table 10.5.

Treatment of carbamate poisoning

Atropine administration (as described for OP poisoning above) alone is the mainstay of antidotal treatment. Oximes have been found to enhance intoxication with carbaryl, as they do not interact with carbamylated cholinesterase but do act to inhibit cholinesterase. Recovery from carbamate poisoning is usually rapid, with carbamylated enzyme being spontaneously reactivated at a rate similar to oxime reactivation of phosphorylated enzyme.

PYRETHRINS AND SYNTHETIC PYRETHROIDS

The insecticidal properties of pyrethrum flowers have been recognized for more than a century. Isolation and identification of the active moieties revealed a set of six pyrethrins. High demand for use, combined with high cost of production and the light-instability of the naturally derived pyrethrins, motivated the search for more stable and more active synthetic analogs, resulting in the development of a host of synthetic pyrethroids (SPs).

While the pyrethrins are principally insecticidal, with the development of the synthetic pyrethroids, more recent compounds (especially cypermethrin, deltamethrin and flumethrin) also have significant activity against ticks. The synthetic pyrethroids have greater photostability than their pyrethrin predecessors and have greater persistence as topical preparations on animals.

Generally, these compounds are metabolized quickly and efficiently by mammals. Factors influencing the rate of metabolism include the *cis* isomer content, which is metabolized more slowly than *trans* isomers, and the presence of an α-cyano function, which also slows metabolism.

While these compounds have a high order of safety in mammals, some individual cats appear sensitive to the more recent SPs. The nature of the increased sensitivity is not known, but it is known from studies in laboratory mammals that single amino acid substitutions in the sodium ion channel pyrethroid-binding site can change sensitivity dramatically. It is possible that cats may be a pharmacogenomically distinct species in this respect, but this awaits investigation.

Two syndromes of toxicity in mammals have been described.

- **Type I.** Associated with pyrethrins and non-α-cyano SPs (resmethrin, permethrin).
  - Progressive development of whole-body tremor (which can lead to hyperthermia), exaggerated startle reflex, muscle twitching.
  - Treatment is described in the permethrin entry below.
- **Type II.** Associated with α-cyano SPs (cypermethrin, deltamethrin, flumethrin). In addition to inhibition of sodium channels, type II pyrethroids may also block voltage-gated chloride channels and this effect may be attenuated by use of ivermectin or phenobarbital.
  - Salivation, increased extensor tone, incoordination, writhing spasms, seizures, apnea, death.
  - In addition to actions on sodium channels, type II SPs act as antagonists to GABA receptors in mammals.

Pyrethrins

EXAMPLES

Pyrethrin I, II, cinerin I, II, jasmolin I, II.

Pyrethrum extract is obtained from the flower heads of *Chrysanthemum cinerariaefolium* and consists of a mixture of esters. The esters are unstable in the presence of ultraviolet light and are rapidly metabolized and inactivated by both insects and mammals. The inclusion of mixed-function oxidase inhibitors (such as PBO) in pyrethrin formulations enhances their longevity and insecticidal efficacy.

Although the selective toxicity of the pyrethroids has traditionally been attributed to differences in metabolism between arthropods and mammals, experimental evidence suggests that mammalian nerves have reduced sensitivity of around 250-fold (lower intrinsic sensitivity (10×) and lower sensitivity at mammalian body temperature (5×) combined with faster recovery time (5×)) which must be multiplied by a more rapid detoxification (9×) (related to enzyme activity and body size differences) for a total differential sensitivity of approximately 2000 times.

Mechanism of action

Pyrethrins have rapid knockdown activity against susceptible flying insects and fleas and a separate delayed lethal effect. Knockdown effects are almost immediate and thought to be due to excessive sensory hyperactivity of the peripheral nervous system. Resistance to this action is due to selection of a target site with altered amino acid sequence and insensitive to pyrethrin binding. The pyrethroids slow the kinetics of both opening and closing of individual sodium channels, resulting in delayed and prolonged ion channel opening. This causes prolongation of the whole-cell sodium current during a depolarizing pulse and marked slowing of the tail sodium current upon repolarization. Pyrethroids also cause a shift of the activation voltage in the direction of hyperpolarization. These changes in sodium channel kinetics lead to membrane depolarization and an increase in depolarizing after-potential. The latter reaches the threshold for excitation, causing repetitive after-discharges. The membrane depolarization of sensory neurones increases discharge frequency and that of nerve terminals increases the release of transmitter and the frequency of spontaneous miniature postsynaptic potentials.

Synthetic pyrethroids

Resmethrin

5-benzyl-3-furylmethyl (1*RS*,3*RS*;1*RS*,3*SR*)-2,2-dimethyl-3-(2-methylprop-1-enyl) cyclopropanecarboxylate.

Resmethrin (named after Rothamstead Experimental Station where it was developed in 1967) is considerably more active than natural pyrethrins and has lower mammalian toxicity but is unstable in UV light. It is available for use as an insecticidal shampoo.

Permethrin

3-phenoxybenzyl (1*RS*,3*RS*;1*RS*,3*SR*)-3-(2,2-dichlorovinyl)-2,2-dimethylcyclopropanecarboxylate.

Permethrin was first described in 1973 as a synthetic pyrethroid with improved heat- and photostability. It is widely used in agriculture and both veterinary and human medicine. The active constituent is available in various *cis* : *trans* ratios varying from 40 : 60 to 25 : 75.

The antiparasitic activity and mammalian toxicity are directly related to the *cis* content.

Toxicology
Permethrin can be classified as having a low potential for mammalian toxicology with an oral LD_{50} in rats ranging from 430 mg/kg to 4000–6000 mg/kg as the *cis* : *trans* ratio changes from 40 : 60 to 20 : 80. Apart from the isomeric composition, other important factors that influence the degree of toxicity include the vehicle, test species, gender, age and fasting status. The acute percutaneous LD_{50} is greater than 200 mg/kg in both rats and rabbits. As with many of the synthetic pyrethroids, permethrin is a mild eye and skin irritant. No mutagenic, teratogenic or carcinogenic activity has been observed in specific studies. It should be noted that, in contrast to low potential for toxicity in most mammals, fish, bees, aquatic invertebrates and cats are very sensitive to permethrin and care should be taken to dispose of surplus product according to label or local regulatory requirements.

Adverse effects
- Permethrin intoxication in cats is manifested principally by hyperexcitability, tremors and seizures.
- While these signs may frequently be unresponsive to diazepam (which is more effective in control of toxicity due to Type II GABA-ergic pyrethroids), intravenously administered methocarbamol at a dose rate of 55–220 mg/kg (one-third as a bolus followed by the remainder to effect based on response to the bolus) has been successful. The elimination half-life of methocarbamol in the cat is not known, but in the dog is approximately 0.6 h.
- In refractory or recurrent cases, further methocarbamol may be administered to a total daily dose of 330 mg/kg and use of pentobarbital, phenobarbital or general anesthesia with isoflurane may need to be considered. After administration of appropriate supportive treatment, most cases recover without permanent adverse effects in 1–3 d.
- However, cats exposed to high-concentration permethrin products with delayed initiation of treatment are at increased risk of death.

Cypermethrin
(*RS*)-α-cyano-3-phenoxybenzyl (1*RS*,3*RS*;1*RS*, 3*SR*)-3-(2,2-dichlorovinyl)-2,2-dimethylcyclopropanecarboxylate.

Cypermethrin, first described in 1975, is the α-*cy*ano derivative of *permethrin* (giving rise to its name), with three centers of optical activity and consequently four enantiomeric pairs for a total of eight isomers. The inclusion of the α-cyano function increases the biological activity (including mammalian toxicity) substantially, with retention of favorable heat- and photostability. In addition, the *cis* isomers are more active than their *trans* counterparts, although the preparations available for companion animals rely only upon racemic mixtures.

Cypermethrin is available as a PBO-synergized insecticidal shampoo for dogs and cats.

Deltamethrin
(*S*)-α-cyano-3-phenoxybenzyl (1*R*,3*R*)-3-(2,2-dibromovinyl)-2,2-dimethyl cyclopropane carboxylate.

Deltamethrin is an optically resolved single isomer first described in 1974. It is among the most potent of the SPs, with broad-spectrum insecticidal and acaricidal activity. It is available in some countries as a collar with significant repellent activity against sandflies (*Phlebotomus* and *Lutzomyia* spp), as well as providing sustained control of fleas and ticks (including *Ixodes ricinus* and *Rhipicephalus sanguineus*). Some useful activity in reduction of feeding success of *Triatoma infestans* (vector of Chagas disease) has been observed.

Flumethrin
(*RS*)-α-cyano-4-fluoro-3-phenoxybenzyl (1*RS*, 3*RS*; 1*RS*,3*SR*)-3-(β,4-dichlorostyryl)-2,2-dimethylcyclopropane carboxylate.

Flumethrin has high activity against cattle ticks (*Boophilus* spp) and has been developed as a collar combined with propoxur for the control of ticks and fleas in dogs.

ANTIPROTOZOAL DRUGS

Reflecting the diversity and specialization of the protozoa, there is no drug that could be stated to have broad-spectrum activity. Rather, a large and complex collection of antiprotozoal drugs with a variety of mechanisms of action, many yet still to be elucidated, has been developed to assist the management of the often severe protozoal diseases of humans, livestock and companion animals.

The name, class and dose rate of drugs used to treat protozoal infections are detailed in Table 10.6. Those drugs which are not covered elsewhere in the chapter or book are described in more detail below.

Allopurinol

1,5-dihydro-4 *H*-pyrazolo[3,4-d]pyrimidin-4-one.

Clinical applications
Allopurinol, a purine analog, was developed originally as a xanthine oxidase inhibitor with clinical application for the reduction in uric acid formation (e.g. in manage-

Table 10.6 Clinical applications and dose rates of antiprotozoal drugs in dogs and cats

Class/Drug/Indications/Dose regimen/Comments

8-AMINOQUINOLINE

Act by generating reactive oxygen species or by interfering with electron transport.

Primaquine phosphate

Babesia felis 0.5 mg/kg PO on three occasions at intervals of 3 days

Identified during WWII in a systematic synthetic chemistry study to find safer 8-AQ antimalarial drugs. Low margin of safety in cats (has caused death at 1 mg/kg). Clinical cure achieved but not sterilization of infection. Repeated or chronic therapy may be required. Little PK information in dogs and cats, but in other species is well absorbed after oral administration with peak concentrations in 2–3 h, volume of distribution greater than body water, extensive metabolism, elimination half-life of parent drug of 6 h and excretion of metabolites in urine. Toxic effects include methemoglobinemia and hemolysis in face of G6PD deficiency.

AMINOACRIDINE

Aminoacridines intercalate readily with giardial DNA leading to inhibition of nucleic acid synthesis. However, differing relative drug uptake rates between mammalian and giardial cells may account for selective toxicity.

Quinacrine (mepacrine) hydrochloride

Giardiosis 6.6 mg/kg PO q.12 h for 3–5 days

Bitter tasting. Absorbed rapidly from gastrointestinal tract, distributed widely, concentrates in liver, spleen, lungs and adrenal glands. Peak concentrations within 8–12 h, elimination half-life up to 14 days with excretion principally in urine. Adverse effects include anemia, vomiting and diarrhea. Nonclinically important yellow discoloration of skin and urine common. Lowest adverse intravenous dose in cat reported as 10 mg/kg.

AROMATIC DIAMIDINE

The specific mode of action of the aromatic diamidines is unclear. However, transmembrane transport proteins (especially the high affinity purine 2 (P2) transporter) actively accumulate aromatic diamidines within susceptible protozoa. As di-cations (and therefore poorly absorbed after oral administration), aromatic diamines also interact electrostatically with cellular polyanions, in particular with AT-rich regions of RNA and DNA acid duplexes via intercalation and minor-groove binding, leading to structural disorganization (especially unwinding) of kinetoplast supercoiled DNA and inhibition of replication, RNA polymerization and protein synthesis. Other potentially toxic effects arise from action on multiple cellular targets including inhibition of synthesis of trypanothione, a vital cofactor in kinetoplast function, reduction in mitochondrial membrane potential and selective inhibition of plasma membrane Ca^{2+}-ATPase. Reducing inositol uptake by host erythrocytes may lead to energy deprivation and death of parasitic *Babesia*.

Diminazene diaceturate

(preparations often contain 55% antipyrine to stabilize 45% diminazine in aqueous environment)

Babesia canis/gibsoni 3.5–4.2 mg/kg IM

Trypanosoma brucei/congolense 3.5–7 mg/kg IM q.14 days

Hepatozoon canis 3.5 mg/kg IM

Cytauxzoon felis 2 mg/kg IM twice at interval of 7 days

The pharmacokinetics of diminazene following IM injection in the dog show marked interanimal variability. Absorption is rapid with T_{max} at 20 min. There is rapid distribution and concentration in the liver from where slow redistribution to tissues takes place. After IV administration, the elimination half-life was up to 60 h. Adverse effects in dogs include nervous signs, anaphylaxis and vomiting. Cats appear to be more sensitive than dogs to diminazene.

Imidocarb dipropionate

Babesia canis/gibsoni 2–6.6 mg/kg SC or IM twice at interval of 14 days (may also protect from reinfection for 2–6 weeks)

Hepatozoon canis 5 mg/kg SC once; or imidocarb 5 mg/kg SC q.14 days + doxycycline 10 mg/kg PO q.24 h 14 days

The pharmacokinetics after IV administration were biphasic with a large volume of distribution. The mean terminal half-life was 207 min. The margin of safety is low, with doses of 9.9 mg/kg. Pain on injection, local reactions, salivation, vomiting and anaphylaxis are most frequently reported adverse signs. Atropine preadministration can limit cholinergic signs. At lower dose rates clinical cure is more likely than parasitological cure and relapse is possible. In endemic areas, parasitological cure is not recommended. In the presence of endotoxin-induced fever in dogs, the volume of distribution and clearance are decreased with no change in elimination half-life. Imidocarb has been shown to block LPS-induced TNF-α production and to increase serum IL-10 levels, novel anti-inflammatory actions that may contribute to its antiprotozoal activity.

Pentamidine

Pneumocystis carinii (*jiroveci*) 4 mg/kg IM q.24 h 3 weeks

Babesia gibsoni/canis 16.5 mg/kg IM q.24 h 2 days

Leishmaniosis 4 mg/kg IM q.48 h 30–40 days

Pentamidine is well absorbed after IM administration concentrating in a variety of tissues, particularly the liver, kidney and spleen, from where the drug dissipates slowly over a period of many weeks. Adverse effects associated with treatment include pain at the injection site, hyoptension, vomiting, diarrhea, hypoglycemia, diabetes mellitus, hypocalcemia and renal failure.

Phenamidine isethionate

Alternative to pentamidine for treatment of *Babesia gibsoni* 7.5–15 mg/kg IM, SC q.24 h 1–2 days

Usually well tolerated but some dogs may have a temporary hypersensitivity reaction with salivation, vomiting and diarrhea, and facial swelling. Concurrent use of cholinesterase inhibitors is contraindicated.

AZO DYE

Mode of action may involve DNA intercalation and inhibition of protein synthesis and cell replication.

Table 10.6 Clinical applications and dose rates of antiprotozoal drugs in dogs and cats (*continued*)

Trypan blue
Babesia canis 10 mg/kg IV (slow) as a 1% solution
Adverse effects include shock if administered quickly and periphlebitis.

AZOLE
Ergosterol is principal sterol in plasma membrane of certain protozoa. Azoles inhibit cytochrome P450-dependent C-14α demethylation of lanosterol, depriving cells of ergosterol and impairing normal cell membrane function. See Chapter 9 Antifungal Drugs
Ketoconazole *Leishmania* spp, *Acanthamoeba* spp.
Albaconazole (experimental) *Trypanosoma cruzi*

BENZIMIDAZOLE/PRO-BENZIMIDAZOLE
See entry under Internal Parasiticides
Albendazole
Giardia infection in both cats and dogs 25 mg/kg q.12 h for 2–5 days
Febantel
Bioactivated enzymatically by the host to fenbendazole and oxfendazole. Active (as fenbendazole) against giardiosis.
Fenbendazole
Giardia infection in both cats and dogs 25 mg/kg PO q.12 h for 5 days

HYDROXYNAPHTHOQUINONE
Hydroxynaphthoquinones selectively block mitochondrial electron transport thereby inhibiting ATP and pyrimidine biosynthesis in susceptible protozoa.
Atovaquone
Pneumocystis and (uniquely) *Toxoplasma* tissue cysts (bradyzoites) 15 mg/kg PO q.24 h for 3 weeks
Babesia gibsoni (Asian genotype) atovaquone 13.3 mg/kg PO q.8 h (with fatty meal) + azithromycin 10 mg/kg PO q.24 h, for 10 days. Intestinal absorption increased with fatty meal. Lipid soluble. Little metabolism. Enterohepatic cycling. Can be used in combination with azithromycin for *Babesia* control. Adverse effects include nausea, vomiting, diarrhea, hypoglycemia, anemia, neutropenia. Other members of the class (parvaquone and buparvaquone) do not appear as effective in dogs and cats.

HYDROXYQUINOLINE
Potent inhibitors of mitochondrial respiration in susceptible protozoal species, acting at a site near cyctochrome *b*.
Decoquinate
Hepatozoon americanum 10–20 mg/kg PO q.12 h indefinitely. Used as adjunct to primary treatment with trimethoprim, sulphonamide, clindamycin and pyrimethamine.

NITROFURAN
Nitrofurans inhibit oxidative reactions, including decarboxylation of pyruvate to acetyl coenzyme A (catalyzed by pyruvate:ferredoxin oxidoreductase or PFOR) reducing the available energy for vital cellular functions. In addition, reductive metabolism of the nitro group generates reactive metabolites that bind covalently with DNA, inhibiting replication and transcription.
Furazolidone
Giardia 4.4 mg/kg PO q.12 h 5–7 days
Cystoisospora 8–20 mg/kg PO q.24 h 7 days
Entamoeba 2.2 mg/kg PO q.8 h 7 days
Experimental studies have revealed no adverse effects associated with daily oral administration for two years with doses up to 2.5 mpk. Long term dosing with higher doses led to a variety of effects including cataracts decreased sperm motility and abnormal sperm and neurological signs. Studies of reproductive toxicity, embryotoxicity and teratogenicity revealed no adverse effects.
Nifurtimox
Trypanosoma cruzi 2–7 mg/kg PO q.6 h for 3–5 months
Nifurtimox requires one electron reductions to form nitro ion radicala that reduce molecular oxygen to form superoxide anion, regenerating the parent nitro compound through redox cycling. Overproduction of superoxide anion overwhelms cell pathways to remove it, and other reactive oxygen species (H_2O_2 and OH•) are formed, resulting in lipid peroxidation and damage to membranes, proteins, and DNA. LD50 greater than 4,000 mg/kg in both cat and dog. Daily dosing of dogs for 52 weeks was without adverse effects at a dose rate of 30 mg/kg.

NITROIMIDAZOLE
Nitroimidazoles are prodrugs that require reductive activation of the nitro group by susceptible organisms. Selective toxicity toward anaerobic and microaerophilic pathogens such as the amitochondriate protozoa (*Pentatrichomonas, Entamoeba* and *Giardia*) reflects differences in energy metabolism, where electron transport includes ferredoxins, small Fe-S proteins that have a sufficiently negative redox potential to donate electrons to nitroimidazoles. Single electron transfer forms highly reactive nitro radical anions that kill susceptible organisms by radical-mediated mechanisms that target DNA and possibly other vital biomolecules. Nitroimidazoles are catalytically recycled; loss of electrons from the active metabolite regenerates the parent nitroimidazole. Increasing levels of O_2 inhibit nitroimidazole-induced cytotoxicity as O_2 competes for electrons generated by energy metabolism.
Metronidazole (classified as a 5-nitroimidazole)
Balantidium coli 15–30 mg/kg PO q.12–24 h 5–7 days
Entamoeba histolytica 25 mg/kg PO q.12 h 5–7 days
Giardia duodenalis 25 mg/kg PO q.12 h 5–7 days
Metronidazole is well absorbed and widely distributed, subject to hepatic metabolism with an elimination half life of 3–13 h Adverse effects include vomiting, hepatotoxicity, neutropenia and neurological signs. Diazepam (IV bolus followed by PO q.8 h for 3 d) has been reported to significantly accelerate recovery from neurological toxicity. Other members of the class include **ipronidazole, ronidazole** (more active against *Tritrichomonas fetus* than metronidazole), and **tinidazole**.

Table 10.6 Clinical applications and dose rates of antiprotozoal drugs in dogs and cats (*continued*)

Benznidazole (classified as a 2-nitroimidazole)
Trypanosoma cruzi 5–7 mpk PO q.24 h 2 months
After oral administration to dogs, rapid and complete absorption has been observed with T_{max} at 1–5 h. The drug is widely distributed, concentrating 4–7-fold in a variety of tissues, including lung, kidney, liver and brain. Elimination half-life is 6–10 h. Reported to have fewer side effects than nifurimox.

PENTAVALENT ANTIMONIALS
Available drugs are prepared by reacting gluconic acid (sodium stibogluconate) or meglumine (*N*-methyl-d-glucamine; meglumine antimonate) with pentavalent antimony. The reaction mixture is allowed to age and a complex mixture of antimony-sugar polymeric compounds is isolated. The dose rate of either compound is designed to deliver equal Sb^{V} doses.

Meglumine antimonate
Leishmaniasis 50–75 mg/kg IM or SC q.12 h for 10 days. Best activity associated with combined use with allopurinol.

Sodium stibogluconate (antimony sodium gluconate)
Leishmaniasis 30–50 mg/kg q.24 h SC, IV 20–30 days

POLYENE ANTIFUNGAL
See Chapter 9, Systemic Antifungal Therapy

Amphotericin B
Leishmaniasis Dose rates are 1–2 times higher than those recommended for the treatment of systemic mycoses in dogs.

PURINE ANALOG
Allopurinol
Leishmaniasis 15 mg/kg q.12 h PO 3–6 months; 6–10 mg/kg q.8 h PO 3–24 months; maintenance treatment 20 mg/kg q.24 h, 1 week per month.

THIAMINE INHIBITOR
Amprolium
Cystoisospora infections in dogs and cats 300–400 mg/kg PO q.24 h 5 days

TRIAZINES/BENZENE ACETONITRILES
Triazines interfere with normal apicomplexan parasite division, leading to the presence of multinucleate schizonts, within which large vacuoles develop before they eventually degenerate. This class (originally developed as herbicides) may act on enzyme pathways (respiratory chain and pyrimidine synthesis) within apicoplasts and mitochondria.

Toltrazuril
Cystoisospora 5–10 mg/kg PO (single dose)
Hepatozoon canis (and possibily *Neospora caninum*) 5–10 mg/kg PO q.24 h for 2–6 days
Toltrazuril is a broad-spectrum antiprotozoal drug widely used for coccidiosis control in poultry and pigs. The drug is slowly absorbed after oral administration and has prolonged elimination with a half-life of several days. It has been observed that the outcome of treatment of neosporosis is improved if T cell function is normal. Other members of the class include diclazuril and the active toltrazuril metabolite ponazuril.

ANTIBACTERIAL DRUGS WITH ANTIPROTOZOAL ACTIVITY
The recent finding of a remnant chloroplast (the plastid or apicoplast) in most apicomplexan protozoa helps to explain the presence of many (but not all) antibacterial prokaryotic drug targets in eucaryotic protozoa. Further details of pharmacology are presented in Chapter 8.

Aminoglycoside
Paromomycin
Cryptosporidiosis 125–165 mg/kg PO q.12 h 5 days
Absorption from gastrointestinal tract usually poor. However, acute renal failure has been described in cats. Used topically and parenterally in humans to treat cutaneous and visceral leishmaniasis respectively.

Dihydrofolate reductase inhibitor (diamino pyrimidine)
Ormetoprim
Cystoisospora spp 66 mg/kg q.24 h 7–23 days
Combined with sulfadimethoxine in a ratio of 1 : 5 in tablets for dogs.

Pyrimethamine
Cats appear particularly sensitive to bone marrow suppression by pyrimethamine, and toxicity may be prevented or reduced by administration of folic acid or yeast supplements.
Toxoplasma gondii Pyrimethamine 0.25–1 mg/kg PO q.24 h + trimethoprim/sulfonamide 15–30 mg/kg PO q.12 h 2–4 weeks
Hepatozoon americanum Pyrimethamine 0.25 mg/kg q.24 h + trimethoprim/sulfadiazine 15 mg/kg PO q.12 h + clindamycin 10 mg/kg PO q.8 h 14 days (relapses noted within 3–4 months) (+ decoquinate)
Neospora caninum Pyrimethamine 1 mg/kg PO q.24 h + trimethoprim/sulfadiazine 15–30 mg/kg PO q.12 h 2–4 weeks

Trimethoprim
Acanthamoeba, Pneumocystis, Cystoisospora, Neospora and *Toxoplasma* (CNS and enteric forms) 15–30 mg/kg PO q.12 h 10–30 days in combination with a sulfonamide (usually sulfadiazine)

Table 10.6 Clinical applications and dose rates of antiprotozoal drugs in dogs and cats (*continued*)
Fluoroquinolone **Enrofloxacin** May have a role in the treatment of *Cytauxzoon felis* infection: 5 mg/kg PO or SC q.12 h 7–10 days In an experimental study of dogs with *Leishmania* infection, enrofloxacin (20 mg/kg PO q.24 h 30 d) had no direct antiprotozoal activity but proved capable of stimulating macrophage killing in the cells infected by the parasite and may be a useful adjunct to specific antileishmanial treatment.
Lincosamide **Clindamycin** *Neospora caninum* 10 mg/kg PO q.8 h 4–8 weeks *Toxoplasma* (CNS and enteric) 12.5 mg/kg PO, SC, IM q.12 h 4 weeks *Toxoplasma* (oocyst shedding) 25–50 mg/kg PO q.24 h *Toxoplasma* uveitis 12.5 mg/kg SC, PO q.12 h 14–28 days
Macrolide **Azithromycin** *Toxoplasma, Cryptosporidium* and *Pneumocystis* 5–10 (dog) or 7–15 (cat) mg/kg PO q.12 h 5–7 days
Sulfonamide **Sulfadimethoxine** *Cystoisospora* 50 mg/kg PO followed in 12 h by 25 mg/kg q.12 h 4–9 days
Tetracyclines **Doxycycline** *Entamoeba, Balantidium coli, Cystoisospora, Toxoplasma* 5–10 mg/kg PO q.24 h 14–28 days **Tetracycline** *Balantidium coli* 22 mg/kg PO q.8 h for 7–10 days

ment of dalmatian bronzing syndrome). Extensions of use have included protection of hypoxic tissues from reperfusion oxidative injury and have recently been extended to the treatment of leishmaniasis and *Trypanosoma cruzi* infections.

Mechanism of action

The mode of action of allopurinol against protozoan parasites is unrelated to its ability to inhibit xanthine oxidase, which enzyme is not present in *Leishmania* or *Trypanosoma* spp. Allopurinol is activated by susceptible protozoa to allopurinol ribonucleoside, which inhibits succinyl AMP-synthase, blocking the formation of AMP. GMP reductase is also inhibited, preventing the conversion of GMP to AMP. The net affect of allopurinol is to completely inhibit purine biosynthesis. Allopurinol ribonucleoside is converted to an AMP analog, which is then phosphorylated to the ATP analog. The resulting aminopyrazolopyrimidine nucleotide is incorporated into parasite RNA, causing the breakdown of mRNA, inhibition of protein synthesis and parasite death. While allopurinol is a successful antimetabolite for susceptible protozoa, oxypurinol, the major metabolite in dogs, is not.

Formulations and dose rates

See Table 10.6.

Combination treatment of leishmaniasis involves use of meglumine antimonate (see below) plus allopurinol.

Pharmacokinetics

Following oral administration to dogs, allopurinol is rapidly absorbed, reaching peak concentrations in less than 2 h. The elimination half-life of allopurinol is less than 2 h. There is significant and rapid conversion to oxypurinol.

The pharmacokinetic characteristics in dogs are not favorable for activity against protozoa. Methods to block xanthine oxidase and the conversion of allopurinol to oxypurinol may allow greater persistence of allopurinol and greater efficacy.

Adverse effects

- Xanthine urolith formation
- Vomiting
- Diarrhea
- Myelosuppression
- Dermatological eruption

Known drug interactions

Urinary acidification increases likelihood of xanthine uroliths.

Amprolium

1-[(4-amino-2-propyl-5-pyrimidinyl)methyl]-2-methylpyridinium hydrochloride.

Amprolium is a structural analog of thiamine, with which it competes for transport and uptake by *Cystoisospora* spp and other coccidia. Parasite thiamine transport systems are much more sensitive to amprolium than those of the host, accounting for the species selectivity. However, prolonged high doses can cause thiamine deficiency, particularly in young animals.

The recommended dose regimen for control of *Cystoisospora* infections in dogs and cats is 300–400 mg/kg PO q.24 h for 5 days.

Antimonials

Antimony belongs to the same periodic group as arsenic, with which it shares a similar disposition and metabolism. Two pentavalent antimonial compounds (Sb^{V+}), meglumine antimonate and sodium stibogluconate (antimony sodium gluconate), have been and remain important in the management of human and animal infections with *Leishmania* species. Trivalent forms of antimony (Sb^{III+}), formed in vivo from the reduction of pentavalent antimony, are less effective and more toxic in dogs, although they have been used successfully in the treatment of human schistosomiasis. Dose rates are based on quantity of [Sb^{V+}].

Mechanism of action

A key mode of action of organic antimonials appears to be the inhibition of the action of phosphofructokinase, thereby preventing the phosphorylation of fructose-6-phosphate to fructose-1,6-diphosphate. The fall in concentration of fructose-1,6-diphosphate decreases parasite aldolase activity, depressing glycolysis and depleting the anaerobic parasite of energy, resulting in death. Fortunately, mammalian phosphofructokinase is not inhibited as readily by antimonial drugs as is that of *Leishmania* species. Sodium stibogluconate has also been demonstrated to specifically inhibit the relaxation of supercoiled plasmid pBR322 catalyzed by DNA topoisomerase I of *Leishmania donovani*, suggesting another possible mode of action. A recent study has also found that pentavalent (but not trivalent) antimonials also induce generation of parasite-killing waves of reactive oxygen species and nitric oxide via activation of extracellular signal-regulated kinase phosphorylation.

Resistance

Although the mechanism has not been elucidated, *Leishmania* resistant to pentavalent antimonial drugs have been isolated from dogs unresponsive to treatment. There is concern that resistant organisms could be transmitted to humans via the sandfly vector, thereby limiting therapeutic options. Of course, transmission of resistant *Leishmania* is likely to be bilateral and could originate in either host. Nonetheless, consideration of public health implications of drug use is an important part of drug selection.

Adverse effects

Adverse drug reactions are not commonly experienced when recommended dosage regimens are followed. However, in dogs with renal dysfunction, extra care should be taken as antimonials may contribute additional nephrotoxicity.

Meglumine antimonate

1-deoxy-1-(methylamino)-D-glucitol antimonate – 33.3% Sb.

Meglumine antimonate is a pentavalent form of antimony (*stibium*) that has been widely used parenterally in both human and veterinary treatment of leishmaniasis. While currently available as a solution for injection, liposomal formulations are being developed in order to target the drug to infected macrophages and thereby minimize adverse effects and increase efficacy. Recent studies have revealed that meglumine antimonate exists as a series of oligomers, with the major moiety being NMG-Sb-NMG, where NMG represents *N*-methyl-D-glucamine. The significance of this finding is that the degree of polymerization may vary from batch to batch and with time and may impact on Sb bioavailability, safety and efficacy.

Formulations and dose rates

See Table 10.6.

Although the most commonly recommended dose regimen is 100 mg/kg q.24 h SC for at least 20 days, it is likely, on the basis of the pharmacokinetic findings described below, that an improved dose regimen may be a reduced dose administered q.12 h or q.8 h. However, this approach has not yet been clinically evaluated, though from a combined pharmacokinetic and pharmacodynamic perspective it appears favorable.

Intralesional administration of meglumine antimonate (85 mg Sb^{5+} per lesion) has been reported to successfully resolve cutaneous lesions of leishmaniasis.

Pharmacokinetics

The pharmacokinetic profile of meglumine antimonate has only recently been described in the dog. After administration of 27.2 mg antimony (as meglumine antimonate) per kilogram, the mean terminal elimination half-life was approximately 10, 10 and 14 h for IV, IM and SC routes respectively. A C_{max} of around 25 µg/mL was observed at 60–90 min for both IM and SC routes, with bioavailability in excess of 90%. Clearance was 0.25 L/h/kg and volume of distribution 0.25 L/kg. Urinary excretion was the major route of elimination, with more than 80% of antimony recovered within 6 h of intravenous administration.

In another study, dogs were experimentally infected with *Leishmania* spp and treated with meglumine antimonate at 75 mg/kg SC q.12 h for 10 days. Peak plasma concentrations of 31 μg/mL were observed and antimony concentrations above 1 μg/mL were detected throughout the study.

It is hypothesized on the basis of mechanism of action that the most efficacious dose regimen is likely to be one that ensures that antimony concentrations in blood and at the site of action are maintained for as long as possible above a yet to be confirmed minimum concentration. Divided doses given repeatedly are likely to yield better outcomes in terms of efficacy and safety than the same total dose given less frequently.

In cases of antimony toxicity, the use of the chelating agent DMSA (2,3,dimercapto-succinic acid) has been proposed but not evaluated in dogs.

Adverse effects

- Relapses are the rule and it is to be expected that multiple treatment courses will be necessary.
- Infrequently, intravenous administration is associated with thrombophlebitis, intramuscular administration with severe muscle fibrosis and lameness, and subcutaneous administration with painful local swelling.
- The least significant reactions favor the adoption of subcutaneous administration.

Atovaquone

2-[*trans*-4-(4-chlorophenyl)cyclohexyl]-3-hydroxy-1,4-naphthoquinone.

Atovaquone, a hydroxynaphthoquinone, is highly lipophilic with structural similarity to ubiquinone, whose activity it has been shown to inhibit. Atovaquone selectively blocks mitochondrial electron transport and ATP and pyrimidine biosynthesis in susceptible protozoa. It is administered orally but has poor bioavailability unless coadministered with a fatty meal, which increases the fraction absorbed threefold. The drug is highly protein bound, does not appear to be metabolized and has an elimination half-life of 2–3 days in humans. It is administered to dogs at 15 mg/kg PO q.12 h for 3 weeks and is active against *Pneumocystis* and (uniquely) *Toxoplasma* tissue cysts (bradyzoites). The activity of atovaquone in a mouse model of toxoplasmosis was significantly improved by coadministration of sulfadiazine or pyrimethamine. Recently, liposome-encapsulated atovaquone has been shown to be active in the experimental treatment of visceral leishmaniasis.

Parvaquone and buparvaquone, the butyl analog of parvaquone, have not been found to be effective antiprotozoal drugs in dogs or cats.

Benznidazole

N-benzyl-2-(2-nitroimidazole-1-yl)acetamide.

Benznidazole, a 2-nitroimidazole and analog of the more familiar 5-nitroimidazole metronidazole, acts by interfering with polymerases and DNA templates of susceptible protozoa, inhibiting RNA and protein synthesis. The nitro group is reduced by parasite metabolic pathways, resulting in the formation of reactive anion species, toxic to a parasite that is deficient in catalase and peroxidase activity.

Following oral administration, benznidazole is absorbed rapidly and completely, with peak plasma concentrations achieved in 3–4 h. Benznidazole appears to be extensively metabolized, with only 5% of unchanged drug excreted in urine. The elimination half-life is approximately 12 h.

Benznidazole is indicated for the treatment of infection with *Trypanosoma cruzi*. In humans it is administered orally at 2–4 mg/kg q.12 h for 30–60 days. The dose regimen in dogs has not been clearly defined. Relapses are frequent and parasitological cure is not reliably achieved. Best results are associated with treatment of early infections.

Adverse effects include vomiting, skin reactions and encephalopathy, frequently leading to cessation of treatment.

Decoquinate

Ethyl 6-(*n*-decycloxy)-7-ethoxy-4-hydroxyquinoline-3-carboxylate.

Decoquinate, used currently as an anticoccidial agent in cattle and formerly in poultry (before resistant *Eimeria* were rapidly selected, rendering efficacy insufficient), has recently been evaluated for a possible role in the management of a variety of protozoal infections, including hepatozoonosis.

Decoquinate is a potent inhibitor of mitochondrial respiration in susceptible protozoal species, acting at a site near cyctochrome *b*. However, alternative respiratory pathways appear to be selected rapidly, consistent with field experience of the early emergence of decoquinate-resistant *Eimeria* in poultry and experimental selection of resistant *Toxoplasma*. In poultry *Eimeria*, the species most studied, decoquinate has various effects according to the stage of the protozoal life-cycle, including a static effect on sporozoites, a lethal effect on schizonts and an inhibitory effect on oocyst sporulation.

The pharmacokinetic profile of decoquinate has not yet been described in the dog. However, aqueous solubility of decoquinate is very low and gastrointestinal absorption is therefore expected to be very low, but influenced by feeding regimen. In poultry, parenteral decoquinate is cleared rapidly (96% eliminated from blood within 1 h). Rapid clearance after oral administration is supported by studies in poultry and ruminants that demonstrate that efficacy against coccidia is lost if continuous daily administration is interrupted. Poor absorption and rapid clearance may explain the high margin of safety for the host.

In dogs, prolongation of remission from the signs of infection with *Hepatozoon americanum* has been produced by oral administration of decoquinate at 10–20 mg/kg q.12 h in food, indefinitely. It is thought that decoquinate inhibits the development of early asexual stages. Discontinuation of treatment is associated with relapse. It should be noted that treatment of acute disease requires a combination of trimethoprim-sulfadiazine, clindamycin and pyrimethamine.

Furazolidone

3-[(5-nitro-2-furanyl)methylene]amino)-2-oxazolidinone.

The mode of action of furazolidone in bacteria and susceptible protozoa (including *Giardia* and trichomonads) has not been definitively determined but appears to include inhibition of oxidative reactions, including the decarboxylation of pyruvate to acetyl coenzyme A, thereby reducing the available energy for vital cellular functions. In addition, it is likely that intracellular reductive metabolism of the nitro group of furazolidone generates reactive metabolites that bind to parasite DNA, blocking replication and transcription. On the basis of studies in pigs and humans, furazolidone is likely to be well absorbed from the gut of dogs and cats. Peak concentrations are observed within 3 h and the elimination half-life is around 5 h. Furazolidone is widely distributed and metabolized extensively, with renal excretion predominating, with little parent drug present. An orange metabolite contains an intact 5-nitro-2-furfural moiety and is the most abundant single furazolidone-related metabolite found in pig urine. Twenty-four hours after administration to rats MAO activity in liver and brain was inhibited by 95% (probably due to a metabolite of furazolidone that contains a free hydrazine group), slowly returning to normal over 21 days. Caution may be necessary with concurrent feeding of tyramine-rich foods such as cheese. See Table 10.6 for clinical applications and dose rates.

Nifurtimox

4-[(5-nitrofurfurylidene)amino]-3-methylthiomorpholine-1,1-dioxide.

Nifurtimox is a nitrofuran active against the amastigotes and trypomastigotes of *Trypanosoma cruzi*, the agent of Chagas' disease. Nifurtimox is well absorbed following oral administration, reaching maximum concentrations in 3–4 h and with an elimination half-life of only 3 h.

In common with other nitrofurans, the mode of action of nifurtimox involves various reduction and oxidation reactions of its nitro constituent, leading to the production by parasite enzymes of a variety of reactive oxygen species that react with cellular macromolecules and are lethal to the parasite. In addition, nifurtimox leads to the inactivation of the critical trypanosomatid enzyme, trypanothione reductase.

Nifurtimox is most active against acute stages of infection with *T. cruzi* and relapses are common. The recommended regimen is 2–7 mg/kg PO q.6 h for 3–5 months.

Pentamidine isetionate

4,4′-(pentamethylenedioxy)dibenzamidine bis(2-hydroxyethanesulfonate).

The mode of action of pentamidine and other aromatic diamidines is not well understood but a number of possible mechanisms have been identified. The aromatic diamidines have a high binding affinity for kinetoplast DNA, causing kinetoplast replication and function to be depressed. The synthesis of trypanothione, a vital cofactor in kinetoplast function, is inhibited by pentamidine at the level of conversion of *S*-adenosylmethionine to decarboxyl-*S*-adenosylmethionine. In addition, pentamidine appears to be a type II topoisomerase inhibitor, promoting linearization of trypanosome kinetoplast DNA.

Pentamidine is well absorbed after IM administration, concentrating in a variety of tissues, particularly the liver, kidney and spleen, from where the drug dissipates slowly over a period of many weeks.

Adverse effects associated with treatment include pain at the injection site, hypotension, vomiting, diarrhea, hypoglycemia, diabetes mellitus, hypocalcemia and renal failure. Other aromatic diamidines include diminazene diaceturate, phenamidine and imidocarb. All may produce cholinergic signs which can be relieved by atropine and with all, concurrent use of drugs with anticholinesterase activity must be undertaken with great care.

See Table 10.6 for applications and dose rates.

Primaquine phosphate

N^4-(6-methoxy-8-quinolinyl)-1,4-pentanediamine diphosphate.

The mode of action of primaquine, an 8-aminoquinoline, is not understood but two potential mechanisms have been described. The 8-aminoquinolines inhibit the function of DNA in a way distinct from that associated with the 4-aminoquinolines. Primaquine appears also to act via a quinoline-quinone metabolite to inhibit the function of ubiquinone or coenzyme Q, blocking cellular energy production.

Related to the mechanism of action is the likelihood of hemolytic anemia in animals with glucose-6-phosphate dehydrogenase deficiency. Primaquine can cause marked hypotension if administered parenterally. After oral treatment, primaquine is nearly completely absorbed, with a large volume of distribution. There is extensive hepatic metabolism and slow elimination.

The principal clinical application of primaquine phosphate is in the treatment of infection with *Babesia felis* at a dose regimen of 0.5 mg/kg PO on three occasions at an interval of 3 d. Reductions in parasitemia are dramatic and quick. Primaquine use in cats is frequently associated with vomiting after oral administration and mortality if doses exceed 1 mg/kg. In addition, infections are not sterilized, which could lead to recurrence.

Quinacrine hydrochloride

Quinacrine hydrochloride (mepacrine hydrochloride) is a yellow dye with a bitter taste that is administered orally for the treatment of *Giardia* infection and cutaneous leishmaniasis. It is well absorbed and widely distributed, with concentration in the liver and sustained release for up to 2 months following a single dose. It may cause skin and sclera to develop a yellowish tinge. It is administered at 6.6 mg/kg PO q.12 h for 3–5 d. For cutaneous leishmaniasis, quinacrine has been administered by intralesional injection or infiltration of a 5% solution three times at intervals of 3–5 d.

Trypan blue

3,3′-[(3,3′-dimethyl(1,1′-biphenyl)-4,4′-diyl)bis(azo)] bis(5-amino-4-hydroxy-2,7-naphthalenedisulfonic acid) tetrasodium salt.

Trypan blue is an antiprotozoal drug first used to treat *Babesia* infection in 1909 and still commonly used to treat *Babesia canis*. The complex chemical structure has been progressively simplified, yielding such other widely used drugs as imidocarb. Trypan blue is administered IV at a rate of 10 mg/kg as a 1% solution. Babesia are cleared from the blood within 24–48 h, corresponding to noticeable signs of recovery in dogs with uncomplicated cases. Trypan blue can cause blue discoloration of mucous membranes and plasma following administration and there is a potential for relapse of babesiosis.

FURTHER READING

Books

Campbell WC, Rew RS (eds) 1986 Chemotherapy of parasitic diseases. Plenum Press, New York

Greene CE 2006 Infectious diseases of the dog and cat, 3rd edn. Saunders Elsevier, St Louis, MO

Hayes WJ, Laws ER (ed.) 1991 Handbook of pesticide toxicology. Academic Press, San Diego, CA

Plumb DC 2005 Veterinary drug handbook, 5th edn. Blackwell Publishing Professional, Ames, IA

Quinn PJ, Donnelly WJC, Carter ME et al 1997 Microbial and parasitic diseases of the dog and cat. WB Saunders, London

Vercruysse J, Rew RS (eds) 2002 Macrocyclic lactones in antiparasitic therapy. CABI Publishing, Wallingford, UK

Journals

In additional to the major veterinary clinical journals, the following journals frequently contain reviews of parasiticide pharmacology.

Advances in Parasitology
Annual Reviews of Entomology
International Journal for Parasitology
Journal of Veterinary Pharmacology and Therapeutics
Medical and Veterinary Entomology
Parasitology Research
Trends in Parasitology
Veterinary Parasitology

Websites

Websites referred to in Chapters 1 and 3 contain information relevant to antiparasitic drugs. Safety and toxicology summaries are available for many antiparasitic drugs at: www.inchem.org/ (Chemical Safety Information from Intergovernmental Organizations). Latest review of agents used in the prevention and treatment of heartworm available at the website of the American Heartworm Society: www.heartwormsociety.org/heart.htm.

APPENDIX: PARASITES OF DOGS AND CATS

Parasite*	Potential sources of infection	Public health significance	Treatment options in dogs and cats	Comments
Esophagus				
Spirocerca lupi (nem) (d)	IH (dung beetles), PH (lizards, chickens, mice, snakes)	Signal (infection rare in humans)	Surgery, ivermectin, doramectin, benzimidazoles	Can cause stomach nodules, esophageal tumors, pulmonary metastasis, hypertrophic pulmonary osteoarthropathy, and aortic aneurysm
Stomach				
Aonchotheca (Capillaria) putori (nem) (c)	FO	None	Levamisole, ivermectin	Cause of gastric pain
Cyathospirura dasyuridis (nem) (d)	Dingo and dasyurid habitats	None	(Fenbendazole)	Prominent tumor around coiled parasites in stomach
Gnathostoma spinigerum (nem) (d,c)	IH (Snakes, frogs, freshwater fish)	Signal (VLM, eosinophilic meningitis)	(Albendazole, fenbendazole, ivermectin)	Gastric tumors in cats can rupture and cause death. Prolonged visceral migration to reach stomach
Ollulanus tricuspis (nem) (c)	L3 in vomitus, FO, hyperinfection	None	Fenbendazole	
Physaloptera spp *(praeputialis, rara)* (nem) (d)	IH (beetle, cockroach, cricket)	Signal	Mebendazole, pyrantel	Cause of recurrent and intractable vomiting
Spirocerca lupi (nem) (d)				See 'Esophagus'
Spirura ritypleurites (nem) (d,c)	IH (cockroach), PH (reptiles, mammals)	None	(Fenbendazole, ivermectin)	Low pathogenicity
Small intestine				
Ancylostoma caninum (nem) (d)	FO, SP, TM, PH (coprophagic insects)	CLM, myositis, eosinophilic enteritis	Pyrantel, BZs, ivermectin, milbemycin oxime, nitroscanate	Intestinal and muscle hypobiosis may interfere with successful treatment. Blood loss up to 0.2ml/worm/day
A. tubaeforme (nem) (c)	FO, SP, PH (coprophagic insects, small mammals, birds)	None	As above + emodepside	
A.braziliense (nem) (c)	FO, SP	CLM	As above	Causes classic creeping eruption in humans
A.ceylanicum (nem) (d,c)	FO, SP	CLM, intestinal helminthosis	As above	
Uncinaria stenocephala (nem) (d)	FO, SP	CLM	As above	Not hematophagous
Toxocara canis (nem) (d)	FO, TP, TM, PH (invertebrates, birds, small mammals)	VLM, OLM, CT	BZs, pyrantel, nitroscanate, milbemycin oxime, ivermectin, selamectin, DEC, piperazine	Larval reservoirs in tissues of bitch. Adult *T. canis* extremely fecund. Environmentally resistant eggs. Male dogs have patent infections

Parasite*	Potential sources of infection	Public health significance	Treatment options in dogs and cats	Comments
T.cati (nem) (d,c)	FO, TM, PH (rodents, birds)	Possible VLM Negligible importance compared with *T canis*	As above + emodepside	Rare in dogs. No liver-lung migration when infection acquired by TM or PH routes.
Toxascaris leonina (nem) (d,c)	FO, IH (mouse)	None	BZs, pyrantel, nitroscanate, milbemycin oxime, DEC, piperazine, emodepside	Nonmigratory in definitive host. Dose limiting for many MLs
Baylisascaris procyonis (nem) (d)	FO, raccoon feces, PH (rodents, birds)	Signal VLM, OLM, cerebral nematodiasis	Piperazine, pyrantel, fenbendazole, mebendazole, milbemycin oxime	Primary definitive host is the raccoon. Potentially serious disease in humans
Strongyloides felis (nem) (c)	SP	CLM possible	Thiabendazole	Pulmotracheal migration
Strongyloides stercoralis (nem) (d)	SP, autoinfection	CLM (*larva currens* – racing larva, 5–10 cm/h), intestinal helminthosis Immunocompromised at particular risk	Ivermectin, fenbendazole, mebendazole, DEC	Pulmotracheal migration. Infective larvae amplified by free-living cycles (heterogonic development)
Trichinella spiralis (nem) (d,c)	Ingestion of infective larvae in muscle of infected animal (any homeotherm, esp pig, rodent)	Signal	(BZs)	Adults short-lived in intestine, but source of muscle invasion
Anoplotaenia dasyuri (cest) (d)	IH (macropod)	None	(Praziquantel)	Tasmanian devil tapeworm
Diphyllobothrium latum (cest) (d,c)	IH (freshwater fish – muscle, roe, especially pike)	Signal (of presence of IH)	Praziquantel	Human is primary final host. Depletes host of vitamin B12
Diplopylidium spp (cest) (d,c)	IH (reptiles)	None	(Praziquantel, epsiprantel)	Common in Middle East
Dipylidium caninum (cest) (d,c)	IH (metacestode in fleas – *C. felis* (rarely *C. canis*), *Pulex irritans*, biting lice –*Trichodectes canis*)	Signal (of presence of IH)	Praziquantel, epsiprantel	Most common tapeworm of dogs and cats. Can be eliminated with effective flea control
Echinococcus granulosus (cest) (d)	IH (metacestode in liver and lungs of sheep, cattle, macropod, deer, etc.)	FO Infective eggs in dog feces. Cystic echinococcosis (CE)	Praziquantel, epsiprantel	Nonpathogenic to dog. Huge biotic potential: massive worm infections not unusual. Prolific egg production. Calliphorid flies readily transport eggs from feces to food. Asexual reproduction amplifies infective load in IH
E. multilocularis (cest) (d,c)	IH (metacestode in organs of voles and other rodents)	Signal and direct (infective eggs in dog or cat feces). Alveolar echinococcosis (AE)	Praziquantel, epsiprantel	Sylvatic interface of urban areas brings humans, dogs and cats into contact with foxes (primary final host). AE rarely found in liver of dog
E. oligarthrus (cest) (c)	IH (caviomorph rodents)	Signal and direct *E. oligarthrus* echinococcosis	(Praziquantel, epsiprantel)	Principal final host is *Felis concolor* (cougar)

Parasite*	Potential sources of infection	Public health significance	Treatment options in dogs and cats	Comments
E. vogeli (cest) (d)	IH (caviomorph rodents)	Signal and direct *E. vogeli* echinococcosis	(Praziquantel, epsiprantel)	Principal final host is bush dog (*Speothos venaticus*)
Hymenolepis diminuta (cest) (d)	IH (*Cten. felis*, grain beetles)	Signal	Praziquantel	Usual definitive hosts are rodents
Joyeuxiella spp (cest) (d,c)	IH (reptiles)	None	(Praziquantel, epsiprantel)	Common in Middle East
Mesocestoides spp (cest) (d,c)	IH (metacestode in any vertebrate)	Signal	Adulticide: praziquantel	Multiply asexually in small intestine. Tetrathyridia can invade and establish in peritoneal cavity. See also 'Serous cavities'
Spirometra spp (cest) (d,c) *mansonoides* (c) *mansoni* (d,c) *erinacei* (d,c)	IH (pig, snake, lizard, frog, tadpole, mouse, rat, etc.)	Signal (sparganosis)	Praziquantel, epsiprantel, mebendazole, niclosamide, nitroscanate	Adult parasites are prolific egg layers. Metacestode called a spargana. Proliferative sparganosis reported in dogs
Taenia hydatigena (cest) (d)	IH (metacestode in peritoneum of ruminant, pig)	None	Praziquantel, epsiprantel, niclosamide, BZs	Most adult taeniids are nonpathogenic. Prolific egg production. Prolonged egg survival in favorable environment. Tabanid flies readily transport eggs from feces to food
T. krabbei (cest) (d)	IH (metacestode in muscle of reindeer)	None	Praziquantel, epsiprantel, niclosamide, BZs	May be a subspecies of *T. ovis*
T. multiceps (cest) (d)	IH (metacestode in CNS of sheep)	FO Infective eggs in dog feces	Praziquantel, epsiprantel, niclosamide, BZs	Metacestodes can cause neurocoenurosis in humans
T. ovis (cest) (d)	IH (metacestode in muscle of sheep)	None	Praziquantel, epsiprantel, niclosamide, BZs	*T. ovis* live for many years, producing 250,000 eggs/d. Infection of sheep major cause of condemnation
T. pisiformis (cest) (d)	IH (metacestode in peritoneum of rabbit)	None	Praziquantel, epsiprantel, niclosamide, BZs	Adults grow to 2 m in length
T. serialis (cest) (d)	IH (metacestode in connective tissue of rabbit)	FO Infective eggs in dog feces	Praziquantel, epsiprantel, niclosamide, BZs	Adults grow to length of 80 cm
T. taeniaeformis (cest) (c)	IH (metacestode in liver of rodent)	None	Praziquantel, epsiprantel, niclosamide, BZs	May cause enteric signs in infected cats
Alaria alata/canis (trem) (d,c)	IH (amphibian), PH (reptile, bird, mammal), TM	None	(Praziquantel)	Migration through abdominal and thoracic cavities
Apophallus venustis (trem) (d,c)	IH (metacercariae in raw fish)	Signal	(Praziquantel, albendazole)	Heterophyid fluke
Cryptocotyle lingua (trem) (d,c)	IH (sea fish)	Signal	(Praziquantel, albendazole)	Metacercariae in skin of sea fish. Occasional cause of diarrhoea.
Echinochasmus perfoliatus (trem) (d,c)	IH (freshwater molluscs, fish, tadpoles)	Signal	(Praziquantel)	Echinostomatid fluke
Euparyphium ilocanum (trem) (d,c)	IH (freshwater molluscs, fish, tadpoles)	Signal	(Praziquantel)	Echinostomatid fluke

Parasite*	Potential sources of infection	Public health significance	Treatment options in dogs and cats	Comments
Heterophyes heterophyes (trem) (d,c)	IH (metacercariae in raw fish)	Signal	Praziquantel	
Metagonimus yokogawai (trem) (d,c)	IH (metacercariae in raw fish, esp cyprinids, trout)	Signal	(Praziquantel, albendazole)	Heterophyid fluke
Nanophyetus salmincola (trem) (d,c)	IH (metacercariae in raw fish)	Signal	Praziquantel	Vector of *Neorickettsia helminthoeca* (agent of salmon poisoning)
Phagicola longa (trem) (d,c)	IH (metacercariae in raw fish)	Signal	(Praziquantel, albendazole)	Heterophyid fluke
Pharyngostomum cordatum (trem) (c)	IH (tadpole), PH (toads, snakes)	None	(Praziquantel)	High doses of praziquantel (30 mg/kg SC) necessary
Pygidiopsis genata (trem) (d,c)	IH (metacercariae in raw fish)	Signal	(Praziquantel, albendazole)	Heterophyid fluke
Oncicola canis (acanth) (d,c)	PH (armadillo)	None	(Niclosamide, pyrantel)	More frequent in nonurban areas
Besnoitia spp (prot) (c)	IH (rodents, opossum)	None	Treatment generally not indicated	Usually nonpathogenic. Oocysts indistinguishable from those of Toxoplasma
Cryptosporidium parvum (prot) (d,c)	FO, water borne	Direct transmission (FO) (serious disease in the immunocompromised)	Paromomycin, azithromycin	No ideal specific treatment regimen described. Prolonged excretion of oocysts common. Infective dose of oocysts low. Excreted cysts immediately infective
Giardia duodenalis (prot) (d,c)	FO, water borne	Possible direct (FO)	Metronidazole, furazolidone, albendazole, fenbendazole, vaccination	Strain variations may lead to differences in host specificity and zoonotic potential. Excreted cysts immediately infective
Hammondia spp (prot) (d,c)	IH (goat, rat)	None	Treatment generally not indicated	Usually nonpathogenic. Oocysts indistinguishable from those of Toxoplasma
Cystoisospora (Isospora) spp (prot) (*canis, ohioensis, neorivolta, burrowsi* (d) *felis, rivolta* (c))	FO, IH (mammal)	None	Sulfonamides ± trimethoprim, toltrazuril, amprolium, furazolidone	Tissue cysts in lymphoid tissue. Often sign of underlying comorbidity or immunosuppression
Enteric *Sarcocystis* spp (prot) (d,c)	IH (herbivore)	None	Treatment generally not indicated (maduramicin)	Enteric species nonpathogenic for dog and cat, but species infecting dogs may be pathogenic for ruminants and pigs
Large intestine/cecum				
Strongyloides tumefaciens (nem) (c)	FO	None	(Thiabendazole)	Found in adenomatous nodules in the colon
Trichuris spp (nem) *vulpis* (d) *campanula* (c) *serrata* (c)	FO	Oral infection possible but unusual	Oxantel, BZs, milbemycin oxime, febantel + pyrantel	Possible coinfection in dog with *Giardia* or *Balantidium*. Prolonged egg survival containing infective larvae

Parasite*	Potential sources of infection	Public health significance	Treatment options in dogs and cats	Comments
Balantidium coli (prot) (d)	FO	Direct FO	Metronidazole	Pig is primary host and of greatest public health significance
Entamoeba histolytica (prot) (d,c)	FO	Signal (Humans usually source of infection in dogs and cats)	Intestinal: paromomycin, Extraintestinal: metronidazole	Extraintestinal forms of infection not commonly encountered in animals
Pentatrichomonas hominis (prot) (d,c)	FO	Direct FO	Metronidazole, paromomycin	Rarely associated with clinical signs
Tritrichomonas foetus (prot) (d,c)	FO	Direct FO	(Ronidazole)	Opportunistic pathogen. Treatment often difficult
Liver/pancreas				
Caldodium hepaticum (Capillaria hepatica) (nem) (d,c)	Ingestion of infective larvae in food or water contaminated with rodent feces	Signal (eggs not usually passed by dogs and cats)	(BZs)	Primarily a parasite of rodents. Infection in dogs and cats usually asymptomatic and never patent
Echinococcus multilocularis (ces) (d)	(See Small intestine)	Signal	Surgery (albendazole)	Adults infect small intestine. Alveolar echinococcosis or metacestodosis of liver
Amphimerus felineus (trem) (d,c)	IH (freshwater fish, esp. common sucker fish)	Signal	(Praziquantel)	
Clonorchis sinensis (trem) (d,c)	IH (freshwater fish esp. cyprinids)	Signal	Praziquantel	Human is primary final host
Dicrocoelium dendriticum (trem) (d,c)	IH (ants)	Signal	Albendazole	Primary final hosts are ruminants
Eurytrema procyonis (trem) (c)	IH (grasshopper)	None	(Praziquantel)	Pancreatic fluke
Metorchis spp (trem) (d,c)	IH (freshwater fish esp. silver bream and common sucker)	Signal	(Praziquantel)	Reported in Canadian sledge dogs
Opisthorchis spp (trem) (d,c)	IH (freshwater fish esp. cyprinids)	Signal	Praziquantel	Human is primary final host for *O. viverrini* and cat for *O. felineus*
Platynosomum spp *(fastosum, concinnum)* (trem) (c)	IH (lizards, frogs)	None	Praziquantel	Infection can be fatal in cats in endemic areas
Pseudamphistomum truncatum (trem) (d,c)	IH (freshwater fish)	Signal	(Praziquantel)	Opisthorchiid fluke
Respiratory system				
Aelurostrongylus abstrusus (nem) (c)	IH (snails, slugs), PH (rodents, birds, frogs, reptiles)	None	Fenbendazole, ivermectin, selamectin, levamisole	Spontaneous clearance of infection possible after 3–4 months
Anafilaroides rostratus (nem) (c)	IH (terrestrial gastropod)	None	(Albendazole, fenbendazole, ivermectin)	Cause of tracheobronchitis in cats in Sri Lanka
Angiostrongylus vasorum (nem) (d)	IH (many species of terrestrial and aquatic snails)	None		Granulomas in lungs, peribronchial lymph node hyperplasia. See Cardiovascular system
Crenosoma vulpis (nem) (d)	IH (snail)	None	Levamisole, milbemycin oxime	Parasite of canids, especially the fox

Parasite*	Potential sources of infection	Public health significance	Treatment options in dogs and cats	Comments
Eucoleus (Capillaria) aerophila (nem) (d,c)	FO, PH (earthworm, rodent)	Signal	Levamisole, fenbendazole, ivermectin	Can lead to fatal bronchopneumonia in young animals
Eucoleus (Capillaria) boehmi (nem) (d)	FO	None	Ivermectin	Lives in nasal cavity. Eggs passed in nasal secretions and feces
Filaroides hirthi (nem) (d)	Transmission in saliva, vomit. Autoinfection		Albendazole, fenbendazole, ivermectin	Parenchyma of lung. First larval stage is infective allowing autoinfection
Mammomonogamus ieri (nem) (c)	IH (lizard)	Signal	(Ivermectin)	Attaches to mucosa of nares causing nasal discharge
Oslerus (Filaroides) osleri (nem) (d)	Oral transmission to pups in saliva of bitch, FO	None	Ivermectin, fenbendazole, levamisole	Nodules near tracheal bifurcation. Treatment frequently unsuccessful
Paragonimus westermani (trem) (d,c)	IH (crab)	Signal	Fenbendazole, albendazole, praziquantel/febantel	Human is primary final host. Aberrant migration to CNS and elsewhere possible
P.ohirai (trem) (d,c)	IH (crab)	Signal	Fenbendazole, albendazole, praziquantel/febantel	
P.kellicotti (trem) (d,c)	IH (crayfish)	Signal	Fenbendazole, albendazole, praziquantel/febantel	New cases often follow introduction of IH
Linguatula serrata (pent) (d)	IH (viscera of infected ruminants or rats)	Signal, direct (nasal discharge of dogs)	(Ivermectin); avoid ingestion of uncooked ruminant or rat viscera	Infective larvae discharged in nasal secretions.
Annelida (leeches)	Direct exposure to terrestrial and aquatic species	Signal	Physical removal (can immobilize leech with chloroform, possibly halothane and other anesthetic gases). Repellents (esp. DEET)	May cause stridor and suffocation when attached to and obstructing URT. See Skin
Pneumonyssoides caninum (mite) (d)	Direct contact with nares of infected canid	None	Ivermectin, milbemycin oxime, selamectin	Frequent cause of sneezing in endemic areas
Cuterebra spp (fly) (d,c)	Direct exposure to gravid female fly	None	Physical removal (ML)	Larvae have been found in trachea of cat with dyspnoea. See Skin
Pneumocystis carinii (jiroveci) (prot) (d,c)	Air-borne droplets from infected animal	Direct Possible infection if close contact with immunocompromised human	Trimethoprim/ sulfonamide, pentamidine, albendazole	Disease usually accompanies immunodeficiency
Cardiovascular system				
Heart and pulmonary artery				
Angiostrongylus vasorum (nem) (d,c)	IH (land molluscs), PH (frogs)	None	Ivermectin, milbemycin oxime, fenbendazole, levamisole	Found in pulmonary artery, right ventricle
Dirofilaria immitis (nem) (d,c)	Mosquito borne	Signal Human pulmonary dirofilarial lesions often mistaken for lung tumor	Prophylaxis: MLs, DEC Macrofilaricides: arsenicals, MLs Microfilaricides: MLs, levamisole	See www.heartwormsociety.org for latest management guidelines. Cat infection can be severe, but rarely patent

Parasite*	Potential sources of infection	Public health significance	Treatment options in dogs and cats	Comments
Hepatozoon americanum (prot) (d)				See Muscular system
Trypanosoma cruzi (prot) (d)	Vector borne (Reduviids – *Triatomae* spp – kissing bugs). Blood transfusion	Signal	Nifurtimox, benznidazole (trifluralin, albaconazole)	American trypanosomiasis, Chagas' disease
Aorta				
Spirocerca lupi (nem) (d)				See Esophagus
Veins				
Heterobilharzia americana (trem) (d)	IH (freshwater snails) Infection via skin penetration of cercariae	None	Fenbendazole, praziquantel	Adults present in mesenteric veins. Eggs enter intestine and passed in feces
Schistosoma spp (esp *japonica*) (trem) (d,c)	IH (freshwater snails) Infection via skin penetration of cercariae	Signal Can cause serious disease in humans	(Fenbendazole, praziquantel)	Adults present in mesenteric veins. Eggs enter intestine and passed in feces
Blood				
Dirofilaria immitis (nem) (d,c)				Microfilaria. See Heart and pulmonary artery
D. repens (nem) (d)			(Doramectin)	Microfilaria. See Skin and subcutis
Acanthocheilonema (Dipetalonema) reconditum (nem) (d)				Microfilaria See Skin and subcutis
Brugia spp (esp. *malayi, pahangi, patei*) (nem) (d,c)			(Diethylcarbamazine)	Microfilaria in blood. See adults in Lymphatics
Babesia canis (3 subspecies: *canis, vogeli* and *rossi*) (prot) (d)	Tick borne (*Rhipicephalus sanguineus, Dermacentor* spp)	Signal (of vector ticks. Canine babesias not yet described in man)	Imidocarb, diminazene, phenamidine, pentamidine, trypan blue, quinuronium, (clindamycin)	Supportive treatment important, many dogs recover without specific treatment. Coinfection with *Ehrlichia canis* not uncommon.
Babesia gibsoni (2 subspecies: North American and Asian) (prot) (d)	Tick borne (*Haemaphysalis bispinosa, Rhipicephalus sanguineus*)	Signal (of vector ticks. Canine babesias not yet described in man)	Diminazene, phenamidine, pentamidine (clindamycin), atovaquone + azithromycin	Supportive treatment important, generally more pathogenic than *B. canis*
Babesia felis (prot) (c)	Vectors not known	None	primaquine	Highly pathogenic species
Cytauxzoon (Theileria) felis (prot) (c)	Tick borne (*Dermacentor variabilis, Amblyomma americanum*)	None	(Diminazene), (imidocarb), (enrofloxacin)	Treatment protocols have had poor success, with mortality often in excess of 50%
Hepatozoon canis (prot) (d)	Tick borne (tick must be ingested by final host) (*Rhipicephalus sanguineus, Dermacentor* spp), TP	Rare (one possible case report in human)	Imidocarb, doxycycline	Usually disease is mild. Target organs include spleen, bone marrow and lymph nodes.
Trypanosoma brucei (prot) (d)	Vector borne (Tsetse flies – *Glossina* spp)	Signal	Diminazene	African trypanosomiasis
Trypanosoma congolense (prot) (d,c)	Vector borne (Tsetse flies – *Glossina* spp)	None	Diminazene	Cause of nagana in cattle
Trypanosoma cruzi (prot) (d)				Cause of acute myocarditis. See Heart
Trypanosoma evansi (prot) (d,c)	Mechanically transmitted by biting flies (Tabanus, Stomoxys spp)	None	Diminazene	Classic disease is surra in horses

Parasite*	Potential sources of infection	Public health significance	Treatment options in dogs and cats	Comments
Lymphatics				
Brugia spp (esp. *malayi, pahangi, patei*) (nem) (d,c)	Mosquito borne	Signal	(DEC)	Adults in lymphatics, microfilaria in blood
Urogenital system				
Pearsonema (Capillaria) spp (esp. *plica* and *feliscati*)(nem) (d,c)	IH (earthworm)	None	Ivermectin	Usually asymptomatic
Dioctophyma renale (nem) (d)	IH (annelid, attached to crayfish), PH (freshwater fish)	Signal	Surgery (ivermectin)	Adult resides in and destroys the right kidney. Female can be 100 cm length and 1 cm diameter – largest known nematode
Encephalitozoon cuniculi (prot) (d,c)	IH (spores in urine and feces of mice, rabbits), TP	Signal Possible direct FO, urine–oral	Albendazole (humans), trimethoprim/ sulfonamide/ pyrimethamine ± albendazole	Spores shed in urine of infected dogs and cats. Different strains have distinct species preferences: III for dogs, I for cats
Muscular system				
Ancylostoma caninum (nem) (d)				Hypobiotic larvae in skeletal muscle. See Small intestine
Toxocara canis, cati (nem) (d,c)			Fenbendazole, albendazole	Hypobiotic larvae in skeletal muscle. See Small intestine
Trichinella spiralis (nem) (d,c)		Signal	Albendazole, fenbendazole	Infective larvae encapsulated in striated muscle. See Small intestine
Hepatozoon americanum (prot) (d)	Tick borne (tick must be ingested by final host) (*Amblyomma maculatum, A. cajennense*), TP	Rare	Trimethoprim/ sulfonamide, clindamycin, pyrimethamine (TCP) + decoquinate	Often fatal disease. No ideal treatment regimen identified. Relapses common. Targets skeletal muscle and myocardium. Periosteal proliferation
Neospora caninum (prot) (d)				Bradyzoites. See Polysystemic
Toxoplasma gondii (prot) (d,c)				Bradyzoites. See Polysystemic
Skin, subcutis, connective tissue				
Acanthocheilonema (Dipetalonema) reconditum (nem) (d)		None	Levamisole	Microfilaria in blood, adults in connective tissue
A. dracunculoides (nem) (d)		None	(Levamisole, MLs)	Microfilaria in skin, adults in peritoneal cavity
Cercopithifilaria(Dipetalonema) grassi (nem) (d)		None	(Levamisole, MLs)	Microfilaria in skin, adults in subcutis
Dirofilaria immitis (nem) (d,c)				Fourth and fifth larval stages in connective tissue prior to migration to heart. Microfilarial dermatitis described. See Blood

Parasite*	Potential sources of infection	Public health significance	Treatment options in dogs and cats	Comments
Dirofilaria repens (nem) (d,c)	Mosquito borne	Signal	Doramectin, levamisole, melarsomine	Adults in subcutaneous nodules. Microfilaria in blood
Dracunculus medinensis (nem) (d)	IH (*Cyclops* spp)	Signal (of presence of IH)	Surgical removal (DEC, ivermectin, albendazole ineffective)	Larvae directly deposited onto skin. Human is primary final host of the 'Guinea worm'
D. insignis (nem) (d)	IH (*Cyclops* spp)	Signal Human infection rare	As above	North American form of *D. medinensis*
Pelodera (Rhabditis) strongyloides (nem) (d) Other nematodes associated with dermatitis include *Ancylostoma* spp, *Uncinaria stenocephala*, *Strongyloides* spp	Direct contact with infected organic matter	Signal	OPs	Dermatitis and pruritus
Taenia crassiceps (cest) (d)	FO (esp. fox feces), ingestion of infected rodents	Signal	No defined regimen (surgery and albendazole)	Metacestode infection (cysticercosis) of skin and peritoneal and thoracic cavities
Annelida, sublcass *Hirudinea* (leeches – many genera)	Direct exposure to terrestrial and aquatic species	Signal	Physical removal (ivermectin, levamisole)	Signs include anemia from bloodsucking, upper respiratory or urinary tract obstruction. Leeches may act as vectors of a number of blood-borne diseases
Ctenocephalides felis felis (flea) (d,c) (also *C. felis strongylus*, *C. canis*, *C. orientis*)	Direct contact with adults in environment or infected host (including dog, cat, fox, ferret, rodent, etc.)	Signal Transient infection only in humans. Also possible vector of plague, typhus and Lyme disease	Adulticides: selamectin, fipronil, pyriprole, meflumizone, imidacloprid, pyrethrins, SPs, OPs, carbamates Preventatives: IGRs	Hematophagus – a female can consume 13.6 µl daily. IH of *Dipylidium caninum*, *Acanthocheilonema reconditum*, *Hymenolepsis* spp. Vector of *Bartonella hensalae*, *Rickettsia prowazekii* and less commonly *Yersinia pestis*, *Borrelia burgdorferi*. Flea allergy dermatitis
Pulex spp *(simulans* and *irritans)* (flea) (d,c)	Humans	Signal Direct infection	Adulticides as for *C. felis*	IH of *Dipylidium caninum*, *Hymenolepis diminuata*
Echidnophaga gallinacea (flea) (d,c)	Poultry	Signal Direct infection	Adulticides as for *C. felis*	Stickfast flea. Can transmit plague and murine typhus
Tunga penetrans (flea) (d,c)	Humans, pigs, armadillo	Signal Direct infection	Physical removal; prevention: topical imidacloprid + permethrin	Sand flea or chigoe. Burrows into and feeds within skin

Parasite*	Potential sources of infection	Public health significance	Treatment options in dogs and cats	Comments
Transitory flea infestations: *Archaeopsylla erinacei* (European hedgehog flea) *Spilopsyllus cuniculi* (European rabbit flea) *Cediopsylla simplex* (American rabbit flea) *Hoplopsyllus anomalus* (wild rodent flea) *Chaetopsylla* spp (parasitic on canid, hyaenid, ursid and mustelid carnivorans) *Xenopsylla cheopis* (rat flea)	Direct contact with principal host or infected environment	Signal *Xenopsylla cheopis* can transmit *Yersinia pestis* and the agent of murine typhus, *Rickettsia mooseri*	Adulticides as for *C. felis*	Most commonly encountered in hunting and roaming cats and dogs where transient exposure may allow transmission of a number of important diseases
Linognathus setosus (phth) (d)	Direct contact	None	Adulticides as for *C. felis*	Sucking louse
Trichodectes canis (phth) (d)	Direct contact	None	Adulticides as for *C. felis*	Biting louse. IH of *Dipylidium caninum*
Heterodoxus spiniger (phth) (d)	Direct contact	None	Adulticides as for *C. felis*	Biting louse. IH of *Acanthocheilonema reconditum*
Felicola subrostrata (phth) (c)	Direct contact	None	Adulticides as for *C. felis*	Biting louse
Transitory lice infestations: *Pediculus capitus* (human head louse) *Phthirus pubis* (human crab louse)	Human	Signal Direct infection	Adulticides as for *C. felis*	Control necessitates treatment of human source of infection. No significant environmental reservoir
Cuterebra spp (esp. *fontinella*) (fly) (d,c)	First stage larvae in environment	Signal	Physical removal, ivermectin	Larvae migrate in fascial planes and third stage larvae usually in subcutis of neck
Dermatobia hominis (fly) (d,c)	Transport hosts (hematophagous insects) deposit larvae on skin	Signal	Physical removal, ivermectin	Larvae develop in furuncle in subcutis
Cordylobia anthropophaga (fly) (d)	First stage larvae in environment	Signal	Physical removal	Tumbu fly. Larvae penetrate and develop within skin
Wohlfahrtia spp (*vigil, opaca*) (fly) (d,c)	Adult fly larviposits on skin	Signal	Ivermectin, other MLs, OPs (nitenpyram)	New World flesh fly. Cause of furuncular myiasis
Wohlfahrtia magnifica (fly) (d,c)	Adult fly deposits larvae directly into wounds or body openings	Signal	Ivermectin, other MLs, OPs (nitenpyram)	Old World flesh fly. Larvae cause massive tissue destruction as they develop
Cochliomyia hominovorax (fly) (d,c)	Adult fly oviposits adjacent to wound	Signal	Ivermectin, other MLs, OPs nitenpyram	New World screwworm. Larvae develop only in living tissue
Chrysomya bezziana (fly) (d,c)	Adult fly oviposits adjacent to wound	Signal	Ivermectin, other MLs, OPs (nitenpyram)	Old World screwworm. Larvae develop only in living tissue
Other wound myiasis flies: *Sarcophaga* spp, *Musca* spp, *Calliphora* spp	Adult flies oviposit in wounds	None	Debridement, ivermectin, other MLs, OPs (nitenpyram)	Attracted to infected, soiled wounds, especially if myiasis already established

Parasite*	Potential sources of infection	Public health significance	Treatment options in dogs and cats	Comments
Culicidae (mosquitoes and gnats) (d,c)	Direct	Signal Vectors of many agents	Repellents, avoidance, habitat control	Various species are vectors of *Dirofilaria immitis, D. repens, Brugia* spp
Simuliidae (black flies) (d,c)	Direct	Signal	Repellents, avoidance, habitat control	Impart painful bite. Attack ears. May induce hypersensitivity reactions
Ceratopogonidae (Culicoides midges) (d,c)	Direct	Signal	Repellents, avoidance, habitat control	Impart painful bite
Psychodidae (sand flies) (d,c)				
Phlebotomus spp	Direct	Signal Dominant vector of Leishmania	Repellents, avoidance, habitat control, deltamethrin collar, imidacloprid + permethrin	Old World vector of leishmaniasis
Lutzomyia spp	Direct	Signal Dominant vector of Leishmania	As for Phlebotomus	New World vector of leishmaniasis
Tabanidae (horse flies) (d,c)	Direct	Signal Can mechanically transfer *Echinococcus* eggs to human food	Repellents, avoidance, habitat control	Painful bites. Physical transfer of taeniid eggs (incl. *Echinococcus*) from feces to food
Anthomyidae (flies) (d,c) *Stomoxys calcitrans*	Direct	Signal	Repellents, avoidance, habitat control	Stable fly. Painful bite with predilection for dog ears
Musca spp (esp *vetustissima*)	Direct	Signal	Repellents, avoidance, habitat control	Bush flies. Cannot bite, but mouth parts well developed for lapping up fluids. IH of *Thelazia* spp
Glossina spp	Direct	Signal Vector of trypanosomes	Repellents, avoidance, habitat control	Tsetse flies
Hippoboscidae (flies) (d)	Direct	Signal	Repellents, OPs	Bite in clusters. Vector of *Acanthocheilonema dracunculoides*
Amblyomma americanum (ix) (d,c)	3 host tick Indiscriminate in host selection	Signal Vector of Q fever, RMSF and tularemia	Physical removal, amitraz, fipronil, pyriprole, OPs, SPs	Lone star tick. Vector of *Coxiella burnetii, Francisella tularensis, Cytauxzoon felis, Rickettsia rickettsii*
A. cajennense (ix) (d,c)	3 host tick	Signal Vector of Q fever and RMSF	Physical removal, amitraz, fipronil, OPs, SPs	Cayenne tick. Vector of *Coxiella burnetii, Rickettsia rickettsii*
A. hebraeum (ix) (d,c)	3 host tick	Signal Vector of African tick-bite fever (*Rickettsia africae*)	Physical removal, amitraz, fipronil, OPs, SPs	Bont tick. Preference for perineal region. Long mouthparts can inflict serious wound. Difficult to dislodge with acaricides
A. maculatum (ix) (d,c)	3 host tick	Signal Vector of RMSF	Physical removal, amitraz, fipronil, OPs, SPs	Gulf coast tick
A. variegatum (ix) (d,c)	3 host tick	Signal Vector of yellow fever virus and *Rickettsia africae*	Physical removal, amitraz, fipronil, OPs, SPs	Variegated tick of Africa

Parasite*	Potential sources of infection	Public health significance	Treatment options in dogs and cats	Comments
Dermacentor andersoni (ix) (d,c)	3 host tick	Signal Humans susceptible to paralysis. Vector of tularemia, Q fever and RMSF	Physical removal, amitraz, fipronil, OPs, SPs	Rocky Mountain wood tick. Cause of tick paralysis (cats appear resistant). Vector of *Francisella tularensis, Coxiella burnetii, Rickettsia rickettsii*
D. occidentalis (ix) (d,c)	3 host tick	Sign. Vector of Q fever, tularemia	Physical removal, amitraz, fipronil, OPs, SPs	Pacific coast tick. Vector of *Francisella tularensis, Coxiella burnetii, Francisella tularensis*
D. reticulatus (ix) (d)	3 host tick	Signal	Physical removal, amitraz, fipronil, pyriprole, OPs, SPs	Marsh tick. Vector of *Babesia canis*
D. variabilis (ix) (d)	3 host tick Only adult ticks feed on dogs	Signal Humans susceptible to paralysis. Vector of Q fever, tularemia and RMSF	Physical removal, amitraz, fipronil, pyriprole, OPs, SPs selamectin	American dog tick. Cause of tick paralysis (cats appear resistant). Vector of *Francisella tularensis, Cytauxzoon felis, Rickettsia rickettsii*
Haemaphysalis spp (incl. *leachi, longicornis*) (ix) (d,c)	3 host ticks	Sign Vector of Q fever	Physical removal, amitraz, fipronil, OPs, SPs	Vector of *Coxiella burnetii, Babesia canis*
Ixodes canisuga (ix) (d)	3 host tick	None	Physical removal, amitraz, fipronil, OPs, SPs	British dog tick. Carrier but not transmitter of *Borrelia burgdorferi*
I. dammini (ix) (d,c)	3 host tick White tailed deer is principal final host	Signal Vector of agent of Lyme disease	Physical removal, amitraz, fipronil, OPs, SPs	Deer tick. Vector of *Babesia microti*, HE agent
I. hexagonas (ix) (d)	3 host tick	Signal Possible vector of *Borrelia burgdorferi*	Physical removal, amitraz, fipronil, OPs, SPs	Hedgehog tick
I. holocyclus (ix) (d,c)	3 host tick Bandicoot is principal final host	Signal Vector of Q fever and *Rickettsia australis*. Humans susceptible to paralysis	Physical removal, amitraz, fipronil, OPs, SPs	Holocyclotoxin causes ascending paralysis. Vector of *Coxiella burnetii*
I. pacificus (ix) (d,c)	3 host tick	Signal Vector of agent of Lyme disease	Physical removal, amitraz, fipronil, OPs, SPs	California black legged tick. Vector of *Borrelia burgdorferi*
I. ricinus (ix) (d,c)	3 host tick Infects many mammalian species	Signal Vector of *Borrelia burgdorferi, Babesia divergens, Coxiella burnetii*	Physical removal, amitraz, fipronil, pyriprole, OPs, SPs	Castor bean tick. Vector of *Borrelia burgdorferi*
I. scapularis (ix) (d,c)	3 host tick	Signal Vector of agent of Lyme disease	Physical removal, amitraz, fipronil, pyriprole, OPs, SPs	Black legged tick. Vector of *Borrelia burgdorferi*
Rhipicephalus sanguineus (ix)(d,c)	3 host tick Each stage prefers dog Survives well indoors	Signal Vector of Mediterranean spotted fever and RMSF	Physical removal, amitraz, fipronil, pyriprole, OPs, SPs	Brown dog tick. Vector of *Acanthocheilonema* spp, *Babesia* spp, *Hepatozoon canis, Mycoplasma (Haemobartonella), Ehrlichia canis, Rickettsia conorii* and *R. rickettsii*

Parasite*	Potential sources of infection	Public health significance	Treatment options in dogs and cats	Comments
Other Ixodid tick species *Hyalomma, Boophilus, Rhipicentor*	Contact with infested areas. 2 host, 1 host and 3 host respectively	Signal	Physical removal, amitraz, fipronil, OPs, SPs	Dog and cat are not preferred hosts
Otobius megnini (argasid or soft tick) (d)	Infected environment Wild ungulates are principal host	None	Physical removal	Spinose ear tick. Only larvae and nymphs found in ear. Adults do not feed
Cheyletiella spp (esp. *yasguri* and *blakei*) (mite) (d,c)	Direct contact	Direct contact Transient infection	Lime sulfur, ivermectin, amitraz, pyrethrins, carbaryl, malathion	'Walking dandruff' observed as active mites dislodge epidermal debris
Demodex canis (mite)(d)	Direct contact. Especially from bitch to neonate	None	Amitraz, ivermectin, milbemycin oxime, doramectin	Localized and generalized forms, the former usually healing spontaneously
Demodex cati, gatoi (mite) (c)	Direct contact	None	Lime sulfur, carbaryl, malathion, rotenone	Localized and generalized, usually less severe than canine form
Dermanyssus gallinae (mite) (d,c)	Direct contact	Signal	Lime sulfur, ivermectin, pyrethrins, carbaryl, malathion	Red mite of poultry
Lynxacarus radovsky (mite) (c)	Direct contact	Direct contact Transient infection	Ivermectin, OPs, SPs	Cat fur mite
Notoedres cati (mite) (d,c)	Direct contact	Direct contact Transient infection	Selamectin, ivermectin, milbemycin oxime, amitraz, lime sulfur	Rarely infects dogs
Otodectes cynotis (mite) (d,c)	Direct contact	Direct contact Infection rare	Selamectin, ivermectin, rotenone, pyrethrins, carbaryl, thiabendazole	Ear mite. Ectopic skin populations provide source of reinfection if treatment is solely intra-aural
Sarcoptes scabiei (mite) (d,c)	Direct contact	Direct contact Transient infection	Selamectin, ivermectin, milbemycin oxime, amitraz, lime sulfur	Highly contagious. Under most favorable conditions nymphs can survive up to 21 days in environment
Trombiculidae (mite) (d,c)	Contact with infected environments (woods and fields)	Sign Some species are vector of scrub typhus	Amitraz, OPs, repellants	Harvest (chigger) mites. Only the six-legged larvae parasitize mammals
Neospora caninum *(prot) (d)*				Infection may present as nodular dermatitis. See Polysystemic
Leishmania spp (prot) (d)				See Polysystemic
Eye				
Angiostrongylus vasorum (nem) (d)				Adult found in anterior chamber of eye of infected dog. See Cardiovascular system

Parasite*	Potential sources of infection	Public health significance	Treatment options in dogs and cats	Comments
Dirofilaria immitis (nem) (d)				Aberrant migration can cause severe intraocular inflammation. See Heart and pulmonary artery
Thelazia callipaeda (nem) (d,c)	IH (muscids)	Signal	Ivermectin, moxidectin (as topical treatment)	Physical removal of worms is also possible
T.californiensis (nem) (d,c)	IH (muscids)	Signal	Ivermectin	Physical removal of worms is also possible
Toxocara canis (nem) (d)				Aberrant migration. See Small intestine
Toxoplasma gondii (prot) (c)			Clindamycin (atovaquone)	Chorioretinitis and anterior uveitis. See Polysystemic
Central nervous system				
Angiostrongylus cantonensis (nem) (d)	IH (snails – including giant African snail, slugs), PH (frogs, toads, freshwater prawn, crabs)	Signal (Infection esp. via consumption of raw snails)	Anthelmintic treatment may increase host death rate.	Primary definitive hosts are *Rattus* spp. Cause of ascending paresis and lumbar hyperalgesia in dogs
Baylisascaris procyonis (nem) (d)				Aberrant larval migration See Small intestine
D. immitis (nem) (d)				Aberrant larval migration. See Blood
Toxocara canis (nem) (d)				Aberrant migration. See Small intestine
Acanthamoeba spp (prot) (d)	Water and soil borne (ingestion and inhalation)	Signal	Amphotericin B, ketoconazole, sulfonamide + trimethoprim	Cause cutaneous, pulmonary and CNS disease
Encephalitozoon cuniculi (prot) (d,c)				See Urogenital system
Neospora caninum (prot) (d)				See Polysystemic
Visceral *Sarcocystis* spp (prot) (d,c)	Unknown	Unknown		Reported in rare cases of CNS disease. See Small intestine
Toxoplasma gondii (prot) (d,c)				See Polysystemic
Trypanosoma *spp (prot) (d,c)*				See Blood
Cuterebra spp (esp. *fontinella*) (fly) (d,c)				Aberrant migration in CNS, commonly in olfactory bulbs, optic nerves and cribriform plate. See Skin

Parasite*	Potential sources of infection	Public health significance	Treatment options in dogs and cats	Comments
Polysystemic				
Leishmania braziliense (prot) (d)	Vector borne (sandflies: *Lutzomyia* spp)	Signal (mucocutaneous leishmaniasis)	Pentavalent antimonials, allopurinol, amphotericin B, paromomycin	New World leishmaniasis. Recurrence of infection after treatment usual
Leishmania chagasi (prot) (d)	Vector borne (sandflies: *Lutzomyia* spp)	Signal Dog is reservoir host (visceral leishmaniasis)	Pentavalent antimonials, allopurinol, amphotericin B, paromomycin	New World leishmaniasis. Recurrence of infection after treatment usual
Leishmania infantum (prot) (d)	Vector borne (sandflies: *Phlebotomus* spp)	Signal Dog is reservoir host (infantile visceral leishmaniasis, adult infection in the immunocompromised)	Pentavalent antimonials, allopurinol, amphotericin B, paromomycin	Old World leishmaniasis. Recurrence of infection after treatment usual
Neospora caninum (prot) (d)	IH (herbivore), TP	Unknown	No rigorous study, but expect *T. gondii* regimens to be similarly effective	Significant cause of abortion in cattle
Sarcocystis spp (prot) (d,c)				See Small intestine
Toxoplasma gondii (prot) (c)	IH (bradyzoites in tissues of mammals, birds) TP, TM (tachyzoites) FO (sporozoites), PH (e.g. cockroaches)	Food borne, water borne Ingestion of sporozoites from cat feces. Main risk factor in pregnancy: inadequately cooked or cured meat	Systemic: clindamycin, doxycycline, sulfonamide + trimethoprim or pyrimethamine Enteric: above, toltrazuril, monensin	Cat is only definitive host. No correlation between cat ownership and human infection. Excreted oocysts not infective for 24 h and very resistant to environmental conditions
Toxoplasma gondii (prot) (d)	IH, FO, TP	Signal (no direct transmission, unless dog consumed by human)	Clindamycin, doxycycline, sulfonamide + trimethoprim or pyrimethamine	Extraintestinal infection only
Serous cavities				
Dioctophyma renale (nem) (d)				Rarely, adults found free in peritoneal cavity. See Urogenital system
Acanthocheilonema (Dipetalonema) dracunculoides (nem) (d)				Adults in peritoneal cavity. For microfilaria, see Skin
Mesocestoides spp (cest) (d,c)	IH (metacestode in any vertebrate)	Signal	Metacestocide: fenbendazole	Metacestodes can populate peritoneal cavity and multiply asexually to enormous numbers. See also Small intestine
Spirometra spp (cest) (d,c)			Praziquantel + mebendazole	Proliferative sparganosis within peritoneal cavity. See Small intestine
Taenia crassiceps (cest) (d)	FO (esp. fox feces), ingestion of infected rodents	Signal	(Praziquantel)	Metacestode infection (cysticercosis) of skin and peritoneal and thoracic cavities.

Parasite*	Potential sources of infection	Public health significance	Treatment options in dogs and cats
ABBREVIATIONS			
d dog	IH intermediate host	HGE human granulocytic ehrlichiosis	BZs benzimidazoles
c cat	PH paratenic host		OPs organophosphates
nem nematode	FO fecal–oral	VLM visceral larva migrans	SPs synthetic pyrethroids
cest cestode	TM transmammary	CLM cutaneous larva migrans	MLs macrocyclic lactones
trem trematode	TP transplacental	OLM ocular larva migrans	IGRs insect growth regulators
phth phthirapteran (louse)	SP skin penetration	CE cystic echinococcosis	DEC diethyl carbamezine
ix ixodid tick	L3 third stage larvae	AE alveolar echinococcosis	( ) suggestion only, drug not thoroughly tested for this indication
prot protozoan		RMSF Rocky Mountain spotted fever	

11

Glucocorticosteroids and antihistamines

Michael J Day

GLUCOCORTICOSTEROIDS

Relevant pathophysiology

Endogenous glucocorticosteroids are derived from the adrenal cortex and have pleotropic metabolic effects on numerous cells and tissues throughout the body. The pharmacological correlates of the endogenous glucocorticoids are among the most commonly used drugs in companion animal medicine. These agents are used chiefly for their anti-inflammatory and immunosuppressive effects; however, these properties are not selective and the corticosteroids will also affect other body systems, potentially giving rise to unwanted side effects. Therefore the most important consideration in administering glucocorticoid therapy is to achieve a balance between control of clinical disease and the potential induction of side effects.

The glucocorticoid hormones pass through the membrane of cells within the target tissue, where they bind to intracytoplasmic steroid receptors. The complex of steroid and receptor then passes to the nucleus and associates with DNA to alter gene transcription and ultimately the production of proteins that control a wide range of cellular processes (e.g. structure, enzyme synthesis and activity, membrane permeability).

Metabolic effects

The major metabolic effects of glucocorticoids are gluconeogenesis, protein catabolism and lipolysis. In addition to enhancing gluconeogenesis in extrahepatic tissues and increasing hepatic storage of glycogen, the glucocorticoids reduce the uptake and utilization of glucose by tissues and may decrease expression of the insulin receptor by these target cells. The ensuing hyperglycemia leads to increased release of insulin from pancreatic β-cells.

Glucocorticoids cause reduced tissue protein synthesis and increased protein catabolism, resulting in increased levels of protein within the liver and plasma, and associated muscle atrophy. The increased lipolysis mediated by glucocorticoids results in mobilization of fatty acids and redistribution of fat, particularly to the liver.

Other metabolic effects include:

- the antagonism of release or effect of antidiuretic hormone
- reduced intestinal absorption
- enhanced secretion of gastric acid
- reduced production and altered nature of gastric mucus
- cutaneous atrophy
- increased tissue mobilization of calcium that may lead to osteoporosis and soft tissue mineralization
- inhibition of chondrocyte growth.

Increased levels of glucocorticoids lead to reduced production of hypothalamic corticotropin-releasing hormone (CRH) and pituitary adrenocorticotropic hormone (ACTH) via the 'negative feedback loop' of the hypothalamic-pituitary axis (HPA), and may also influence thyroid hormone levels via depression of TSH production.

The production of other pituitary hormones (prolactin, luteinizing hormone, follicle-stimulating hormone) is also suppressed by glucocorticoids. Glucocorticoids may also have a range of mineralocorticoid effects, including mediating the retention of Na^+, Cl^- and water, and increasing the excretion of K^+ and H^+ by distal tubules.

Anti-inflammatory effects

The anti-inflammatory effects of glucocorticoids are numerous, and endogenous production is one means of downregulating the inflammatory response when no longer required, in order to prevent unwanted ('bystander') damage to normal tissue.

In this context, glucocorticoids are antagonistic to:

- capillary blood flow and vasodilation (and therefore edema formation, and loss of protein and leukocytes from the vasculature into inflamed tissue and subsequent migration of these cells)
- vasoproliferation
- platelet aggregation
- fibrin deposition
- fibroblast proliferation and formation of collagen.

Glucocorticoids suppress the inflammatory function of leukocytes (specifically granulocytes, mast cells and monocyte-macrophages) by stabilizing the membranes of these cells. This prevents release of inflammatory mediators such as histamine and arachidonic acid metabolites of both the cyclo-oxygenase and lipoxygenase pathways. They also inhibit particular metabolic pathways, e.g. production of proinflammatory cytokines such as IL-1, IL-6 and TNF-α.

Glucocorticoids downregulate expression of Fc receptors on macrophages, thereby decreasing phagocytosis of opsonized particles (e.g. antibody-coated erythrocytes or platelets). The effects of glucocorticoids on neutrophil function are controversial. These drugs are generally considered to induce impairment of chemotaxis, adhesiveness, bacterial killing and lysosomal enzyme secretion. However, a recent study of neutrophil function in dogs administered prednisolone (1 mg/kg) has shown elevated IgG- or C3b-mediated phagocytosis, increased chemotaxis and chemiluminescence, and reduced adherence to nylon wool. Glucocorticoids may induce the characteristic blood leukocyte profile (neutrophilia, lymphopenia, monocytosis and eosinopenia) known as the 'stress leukogram'.

Effect on immune mechanisms

Glucocorticoids may mediate immunosuppression by influencing several stages of the immune response. The downregulation of macrophage function may inhibit antigen processing and presentation, and glucocorticoids may be directly suppressive of T lymphocytes and the cell-mediated immune effects that they mediate. In experimental systems, there is some evidence that glucocorticoids may selectively enhance the function of specific T-lymphocyte subsets but this is not yet defined in companion animal species. Interestingly, when dexamethasone was incorporated into in vitro cultures of feline lymphocytes there was an increase (rather than the predicted decrease) in proliferative activity of both $CD4^+$ and $CD8^+$ T lymphocytes. However, a combination of dexamethasone and ciclosporin induced inhibition of proliferation greater than observed with ciclosporin alone.

By contrast, B lymphocytes are considered to be more resistant to the suppressive effects of glucocorticoids, so these hormones do not inhibit antibody production, other than indirectly by removing the 'help' that T cells provide for B-lymphocyte activation. Despite this, in a recent study, beagle dogs given a 14-day course of prednisolone (2 mg/kg PO) had significantly decreased serum IgG, IgM and IgA concentrations, in addition to reduced numbers of circulating $CD4^+$ and $CD8^+$ T lymphocytes and surface membrane immunoglobulin-expressing B lymphocytes.

A further effect of glucocorticoids on humoral immunity is that of reducing antibody affinity for cell membrane epitopes, causing elution of antibody from the surface of target cells (e.g. erythrocytes or platelets). Glucocorticoids are also inhibitory of complement pathways. They may impede the passage of immune complexes through basement membranes, although a 7-day course of glucocorticoid (prednisone 2.2 mg/kg) was unable to reduce canine serum C3 concentration.

Examples

There is a range of glucocorticoid drugs, which are most usefully categorized by their relative anti-inflammatory potency and duration of action. The names of these agents are summarized in Table 11.1.

The synthetic glucocorticoids may be formulated as esters, and the nature of this ester will determine the bioavailability of the glucocorticoid moiety. Esters of succinate, hemisuccinate or phosphate allow rapid release (minutes) of steroid, and include agents such as prednisolone sodium succinate, hydrocortisone sodium succinate and dexamethasone sodium phosphate.

Glucocorticoids bound to polyethylene glycol are available within minutes to hours of administration. Esters of acetate, diacetate, tebutate, phenylproprionate or isonicotinate are moderately insoluble, allowing steroid release over days to weeks, and include preparations such as isofluprednone acetate, methylprednisolone acetate, dexamethasone phenylproprionate and dexamethasone isonicotinate. Poorly soluble esters of acetonide, hexacetate, pivalate or diproprionate allow steroid release over a period of weeks to months (e.g. triamcinolone acetonide).

Budesonide is a locally active glucocorticosteroid that is used in asthma inhalers. An enteric-coated formulation of budesonide is now available. It is locally active in the gut following a pH-dependent release and is claimed to produce less HPA suppression than conventional glucocorticoids, as it is destroyed 90% on first pass through the liver. However, steroid hepatopathy has still been noted in dogs, and significant HPA suppression has been demonstrated. There are anecdotal reports of budesonide's efficacy in canine and feline inflammatory bowel disease (IBD). However, some early studies actually used the nonenteric-coated formulation from inhalers, and the appropriate dose of the enteric-

Table 11.1 Summary of the anti-inflammatory potency and duration of action of glucocorticoid drugs

Glucocorticoid	Anti-inflammatory potency	Duration of action
Cortisone	0.8	Short-acting
Hydrocortisone	1.0	Short-acting
Prednisolone/prednisone	4.0	Intermediate
Methylprednisolone	5.0	Intermediate
Triamcinolone	5.0	Intermediate*
Flumethasone	15.0	Long-acting
Dexamethasone	30.0	Long-acting
Betamethasone	35.0	Long-acting

Short-acting <12 h, intermediate-acting 12–36 h, long-acting >48 h.
* Triamcinolone may act for up to 48 h.

coated formulation is not yet determined. Further studies of budesonide are indicated before it can be recommended for use in dogs or cats. Fluticasone is a glucocorticoid that can be administered via the inhalational route for example to cats with allergic bronchial disease using a standard pediatric spacer with a cat face mask.

Topical cutaneous forms of glucocorticoid would include acetonide or valerate esters of hydrocortisone, prednisolone, betamethasone and dexamethasone. Topical ocular preparations of dexamethasone or prednisolone formulated as various esters are available. The absorption of these varies, and the agent selected will depend upon whether the disease process is intraocular, corneal or subconjunctival. Alcohol-based formulations are most readily absorbed, while acetate esters are more readily absorbed by cornea and conjunctiva than succinate or phosphate esters.

Clinical applications

The clinical indications for glucocorticoids are in the treatment of inflammatory, immune-mediated (autoimmune) or neoplastic (e.g. lymphoma, mast cell tumor) disease, for adjunct therapy in hypoadrenocorticism, and in the emergency management of acute anaphylaxis, shock, asthma, heat stroke or trauma of the central nervous system (controversial).

The major anti-inflammatory application of systemic glucocorticoid therapy in companion animals is for cutaneous hypersensitivity disease. A recent evidence-based review has suggested that there is a firm basis for the use of oral glucocorticoids in the management of canine atopic dermatitis. Immunosuppressive glucocorticoid therapy is still the mainstay of treatment for immune-mediated or autoimmune diseases in these species (e.g. immune-mediated hemolytic anemia (IMHA) and thrombocytopenia, immune-mediated polyarthritis, autoimmune skin diseases, IBD) and forms part of the multidrug protocols used for chemotherapy of round cell neoplasia. Topical corticosteroids are employed in the management of some immune-mediated or inflammatory ocular diseases.

Mechanism of action

The mechanism of action of the glucocorticoid drugs reflects the effects of endogenously produced glucocorticoid hormones described above, but synthetic glucocorticoids have greater glucocorticoid activity and less mineralocorticoid activity than endogenous cortisol. The only synthetic glucocorticoids with mineralocorticoid activity are hydrocortisone, cortisone and prednisolone, which have a relative mineralocorticoid potency of 1.0, 0.8 and 0.25 respectively.

Formulations and dose rates

Glucocorticoids may be administered topically, orally or by intravenous, intramuscular or intralesional (e.g. subconjunctival) injection. The main consideration in clinical administration of glucocorticoid drugs is to achieve an appropriate clinical response, without inducing the range of corticosteroid side effects.

An appropriately potent agent, with an appropriate duration of action, should be selected for any individual case. The dose rates for achieving an anti-inflammatory or immunosuppressive effect are well defined for the various disease indications but, for the most commonly administered agent (oral prednisolone), an anti-inflammatory dose is generally considered to be 0.25–0.5 mg/kg q.12 h or 0.5–1.0 mg/kg q.24 h for the dog, and 1–2 mg/kg q.12 h or 2 mg/kg q.24 h for the cat.

The initial anti-inflammatory dose would be administered for an 'induction period' of 5–7 days and then tapered to a maintenance dose. For example, a maintenance dose of 0.25–0.5 mg/kg q.12 h for 5–7 days may be used for the dog, followed by glucocorticoid administration for a withdrawal period at a dose of 0.5–1.0 mg/kg every other day. In some cases, alternate-day therapy may be extended to every third or fourth day.

The cat is considered more 'steroid resistant' (to the immunosuppressive rather than the adrenosuppressive effects of glucocorticoids) than the dog, which may reflect reduced expression of glucocorticoid (dexamethasone)-binding receptors in the tissues (skin and liver) of this species. A recommended immunosuppressive dose of prednisolone for the cat is therefore 2.2–6.6 mg/kg q.12 h, and for the dog 1.0–2.0 mg/kg q.12 h. Some authors recommend that these doses are given as a single daily dosage in the morning (dog) or evening (cat).

The duration of therapy will depend upon the individual patient and disease entity being treated but in order to avoid side effects, glucocorticoids should be administered for the shortest period possible. In some diseases, combination therapy with other agents may be possible and permit reduced doses of glucocorticoids to be used (e.g. concurrent administration of azathioprine and prednisolone in canine IMHA).

Following administration of an induction protocol (typically 10–28 days for an immunosuppressive regimen), the glucocorticoids should be gradually tapered towards an alternate-day maintenance regimen, but only when there is clear evidence of disease remission. For example, in a dog given an induction dose of 1.0 mg/kg of prednisolone q.12 h (for 10–28 days), a tapering protocol might consist of stepwise dose reduction to 0.75 mg/kg q.12 h (10–28 days), to 0.5 mg/kg q.12 h (10–28 days), to 0.25 mg/kg q.12 h (10–28 days) to 0.25 mg/kg q.24 h (10–28 days). This may be followed by a withdrawal regime of 0.25–0.5 mg/kg every other day for a period of at least 21 days, and subsequently dosing every third day may be attempted.

Treatment should never be ceased abruptly, as there is a risk of inducing signs of hypoadrenocorticism. Should disease relapse occur during the tapering period, the glucocorticoid dose should be increased to one equivalent to, or greater than, the initial dose used in the induction regimen. In many instances, glucocorticoid therapy may eventually be withdrawn entirely but in some individuals with particular diseases, a life-long maintenance dose may be required.

In adjunct therapy for systemic anaphylaxis, administration of glucocorticoids such as dexamethasone sodium phosphate (1–4 mg/kg IV) or prednisolone sodium succinate (10–25 mg/kg IV) has been reported following appropriate management of circulatory collapse. Similarly, for management of acute spinal cord injury, high-dose glucocorticoid (e.g. methylprednisolone sodium succinate, 30 mg/kg IV) within 8 h of injury is recommended by some authors.

For inhalational therapy, in cats with allergic bronchial disease, most clinicians recommend using both a β-blocker (such as albuterol – see Chapter 18) and topical glucocorticoids such as fluticasone. The drugs can be administered using a standard pediatric spacer equipped with a cat face mask on the 'patient' end. The dose of albuterol is two 'puffs' from a generic inhaler and is combined with a standard dose of inhaled fluticasone of 220 μg. Both are vaporized in the spacer, the face mask placed over the cat's face and it is allowed to breath through the mask for seven to ten seconds.

The inhalation procedure is usually given every 12 hours and is started in addition to oral prednisolone if the cat is symptomatic at the time. Usually the prednisolone can be stopped after five to ten days and the inhalation continued for at least a further month. Assuming adequate control, the dose of fluticasone can then be reduced to 110 μg every 12 hours for another month and then stopped. Whether or not the albuterol is required throughout this period is debatable. Some clinicians do not use albuterol except at times when cats are symptomatic.

Pharmacokinetics

Synthetic glucocorticoids are readily absorbed from any site of administration and bind with less avidity to serum proteins than endogenous cortisol, thereby diffusing more readily into the tissues. The synthetic molecules have greater affinity for the cytoplasmic steroid receptor and are less rapidly degraded, both effects contributing to a prolonged duration of action. Prednisone and cortisone require activation in the liver to prednisolone and cortisol respectively, so the use of these agents topically or with end-stage liver disease is generally considered to be contraindicated.

Adverse effects

The adverse effects of glucocorticoids are largely attributable to an enhancement of the range of metabolic changes induced by these agents at the physiological level, with the resultant syndrome of 'iatrogenic hyperadrenocorticism' (Cushing's disease) and associated atrophy of the adrenal cortices due to suppression of the HPA. Individuals vary greatly in their sensitivity to the adverse effects of glucocorticosteroids.

- Adrenal atrophy is slowly reversible following cessation of glucocorticoid therapy, but hypoadrenocorticism can occur if glucocorticoids are withdrawn suddenly or if the animal is subject to a stressful event and cannot make an appropriate physiological response.
- Excess gluconeogenic, protein catabolic and lipolytic effects (confounded by antagonism of insulin and antidiuretic hormone) may lead to the development of hepatomegaly ('steroid hepatopathy' – dogs are exquisitely sensitive), hyperglycemia (with secondary diabetes mellitus) and clinical signs such as polyuria/polydipsia, polyphagia and weight gain.
- Cats are particularly susceptible to the hyperglycemic effects of glucocorticosteroids (stress hyperglycemia).
- Dogs are particularly susceptible to steroid-induced polyuria and polydipsia, which is an almost inevitable consequence of glucocorticosteroid treatment at pharmacological doses sufficient to induce remission of inflammation in the dog.
- Glucocorticosteroids induce synthesis of alkaline phosphatase in the dog but not the cat. This has recently been shown to relate to activation of the corticosteroid-induced alkaline phosphatase gene within canine hepatocytes. This does not have any pathological consequences but may create a diagnostic dilemma when the clinician is attempting to screen for hepatic pathology.
- Long term administration of corticosteroids has been shown to induce proteinuria and glomerular pathology in the dog.
- Chronic high-dose glucocorticosteroid treatment can cause cutaneous protein catabolism, which may result in an atrophic dermatopathy characterized by thin, alopecic skin that occasionally has evidence of calcinosis cutis.
- Suppression of the immune and inflammatory systems may potentiate viremia (e.g. in cats that are carriers of feline herpes virus or calicivirus) or result in increased susceptibility to secondary infection (e.g. urinary tract infection).

- Other potential adverse effects include:
  - hypertension
  - Na^+ and water retention (insignificant with most synthetic glucocorticosteroids)
  - peripheral edema (rare)
  - gastric ulceration and hemorrhage (usually only when there is another concurrent ulcerogenic stimulus such as NSAID administration, altered gut blood flow)
  - pancreatitis (degree to which glucocorticosteroids used at anti-inflammatory doses are a risk factor in pancreatitis is controversial)
  - osteoporosis (more an issue in humans than dogs and cats)
  - myopathy (rare)
  - behavioral changes
  - neuropathy (rare)
  - cataract
  - glaucoma.
- Adverse effects are less common in cats than dogs given chronic glucocorticoid therapy and are usually restricted to the development of polydipsia, polyuria (although usually not to the degree experienced by dogs), polyphagia and weight gain.

Contraindications and precautions

- There is a range of contraindications for glucocorticoid administration, which are largely situations in which the immunomodulatory or metabolic effects of these drugs would amplify an existing pathology in an individual patient, for example those with:
  - infectious disease (particularly bacterial, viral or fungal)
  - diabetes mellitus
  - liver disease (unless specifically indicated to treat the pathology present)
  - protein-losing nephropathy (unless specifically indicated to treat the pathology present; however, there is no good evidence that glucocorticosteroid treatment reduces protein loss in immune-mediated glomerulonephropathy).
- Corticosteroids may induce abortion or congenital defects if administered during pregnancy.
- Corticosteroids may inhibit growth if given to immature animals.
- Wound or fracture healing may be inhibited by glucocorticoids.
- Topical ophthalmic corticosteroid should not be instilled into an eye with infection, glaucoma or corneal ulceration because of the risk of inducing corneal perforation and delaying repair, and the possibility of secondary infection.
- Owners should be advised to wear gloves when applying topical corticosteroids.

Known drug interactions

A range of drug interactions is reported for glucocorticoids.

- Increased insulin requirements with concurrent glucocorticoid therapy.
- Increased metabolism of glucocorticoids by phenytoin, phenobarbital, rifampicin (rifampin).
- Reduced blood levels of salicylates with glucocorticoid therapy.
- Hypokalemia when glucocorticoids are given concurrently with amphotericin B or potassium-depleting diuretics (e.g. furosemide); when these agents are used together with digitalis therapy, there is an increased risk of digitalis toxicity in the presence of hypokalemia.
- Concurrent administration of glucocorticoids and ciclosporin leads to reduced hepatic metabolism of each drug, with elevated blood levels of both agents.
- Glucocorticoids reduce hepatic metabolism of cyclophosphamide.
- Erythromycin reduces hepatic metabolism of methylprednisolone.
- Concurrent administration of drugs known to induce gastrointestinal ulceration (e.g. nonsteroidal anti-inflammatories) with glucocorticoids increases the risk of such ulceration, which may also occur more readily in animals given corticosteroids for spinal cord trauma.
- Estrogens may potentiate the effects of glucocorticoids.
- Glucocorticoids at immunosuppressive doses should be administered with care to myasthenic animals as they may lead to an exacerbation of weakness, the mechanism of which has been poorly defined. Myasthenic dogs should initially be given glucocorticoids at anti-inflammatory doses, and these may be increased to immunosuppressive levels over a 1–2 week period. Patients should be carefully monitored over this time. As a general rule, the more severe the weakness, the lower the dose of glucocorticoids that should be used.
- Animals receiving immunosuppressive doses of glucocorticoids may make a diminished response to vaccines and should not be given live viral vaccines. However, one early study of dogs administered distemper virus vaccine after a 21-day course of prednisolone (1 mg/kg or 10 mg/kg PO) revealed adequate serum neutralizing antibody and protection from challenge with virulent virus.

ANTIHISTAMINES

Relevant pathophysiology

In a clinical setting, the major use of the antihistamines is to counteract the effects of the histamine release that follows mast cell degranulation in hypersensitivity disease. The most significant means of causing such degranulation is via the interaction of allergen with mast cell-bound IgE molecules. A 'sensitized' mast cell is coated by allergen-specific IgE that affixes to the cell surface through interaction with the high-affinity Fcε receptor (FcεR type 1). The allergen must 'cross-link' two adjacent IgE molecules by interacting with at least one of the antigen-binding sites of each IgE molecule.

The intracellular signaling pathways that are rapidly activated following these interactions are complex and beyond the scope of this discussion. However, the major effects involve aggregation of the Fcε receptors, physical movement of membrane phospholipids, elevation of cAMP and intracellular Ca^{2+} influx. Alternative means of initiating mast cell degranulation involve allergen cross-linking IgG molecules bound to mast cell membrane FcγRIII molecules, the binding of the biologically active complement fragments C3a or C5a to specific receptor molecules, the binding of a range of drugs or lectins to carbohydrate residues on the FcεR or the effects of physical stimuli (cold, trauma), neuropeptides or cytokines.

Mast cell granules contain a potent cocktail of preformed inflammatory mediators, including histamine, heparin, serotonin, kininogenase, tryptase, chymase, exoglycosidases, eosinophil and neutrophil chemotactic factors and platelet-activating factor. In addition, there is a range of synthesized mediators, the most significant of which are derived from the precursor molecule arachidonic acid, which in turn is a cleavage product of membrane phospholipids. Arachidonic acid is modified by two distinct pathways that give rise to prostaglandins, thromboxanes (cyclo-oxygenase pathway) and leukotrienes (lipoxygenase pathway).

Mast cells also produce a wide range of proinflammatory and immunoregulatory cytokines, including IL-1, IL-3, IL-4, IL-5, IL-6, IL-8, IL-9, IL-13, TNF-α, TGF-β and GM-CSF. The release of preformed mediators and arachidonic acid metabolites occurs rapidly (seconds to minutes) after mast cell activation, whereas cytokine release occurs several hours later.

The end-effects of mast cell degranulation include:

- vasodilation with tissue edema, leakage of serum proteins and extravasation of leukocytes, contributing to the local inflammatory response
- smooth muscle contraction (bronchoconstriction)
- pruritus.

The effects of mast cell degranulation may be localized (skin, respiratory tract) or it is possible for systemically administered antigen (e.g. drugs) to activate connective tissue mast cells throughout the body, causing anaphylactic shock due to generalized vasodilation (and reduced blood pressure) and localized edema. Many of these effects are a sequel to the binding of histamine to specific H_1-receptors, and the major effect of one class of antihistamine drugs is blockade of this interaction (H_1-receptor competitive antagonism). H_1-receptors are distributed on blood vessels, airway and gastrointestinal smooth muscle cells, cardiac and central nervous system cells.

Although the major veterinary clinical application of H_1-blockers is in the management of allergic skin disease, certain of these agents have a range of other properties, including anticholinergic and antiserotonin effects, stabilization of mast cells, basophils and eosinophils, local anesthetic, antiemetic and behavior-modifying effects.

Histamine may also bind to a second class of receptor molecules (H_2-receptors) that are particularly expressed by gastric parietal cells (also cells of the uterus, heart and central nervous system). Occupation of the H_2-receptor by histamine mediates a range of effects, including enhanced secretion of gastric acid (which also requires activation through gastrin and acetylcholine receptors), stimulation of other exocrine secretions, some instances of inhibition of smooth muscle contraction, enhanced cardiac function and some effect on enhanced capillary vasodilation. H_2-blocking drugs have also been identified and have greatest clinical application in control of overproduction of gastric acid, e.g. in duodenal ulceration. These drugs are discussed in Chapter 18.

Examples

Antihistamines have a similar basic chemical structure to histamine. The H_1-blockers are conveniently grouped on the basis of this chemical structure.

- Ethanolamine derivatives (clemastine, dimenhydrinate, diphenhydramine, doxylamine)
- Ethylenediamine derivatives (pyrilamine, tripelennamine)
- Phenothiazine derivatives (promethazine, alimemazine (trimeprazine))
- Piperazine derivatives (cetirizine, hydroxyzine)
- Propylamine derivatives (bromopheniramine, chlorphenamine (chlorpheniramine))
- Others (astemizole, azatadine, cyproheptadine, loratadine, oxatomide, terfenadine)

The behavior-modifying tricyclic antidepressants (amitriptyline, clomipramine, doxepin) are also H_1-receptor antagonists and have been used in the management of pruritic dogs and cats.

Clinical applications

In veterinary medicine, H_1-blockers are used most frequently in the management of allergic pruritus in the dog and cat. Despite this, a recent evidence-based review has concluded that there is currently insufficient evidence to recommend the use of this range of drugs in the management of canine atopic dermatitis. H_1-blockers may also be used as adjunct therapy for the management of systemic anaphylaxis, to control ongoing mediator release following the acute therapy of circulatory collapse (e.g. with adrenaline (epinephrine), fluids).

Formulations and dose rates

Suggested dosage regimens for the use of H_1-blockers in the management of pruritus have been reviewed in an excellent paper by Scott & Miller (1999), and these data are reproduced here (Tables 11.2 and 11.3). Effective antihistamine therapy is problematic in the dog and cat, and the owner and veterinary surgeon must be prepared to invest some time in optimizing a regimen for any individual patient.

Table 11.2 Antihistamine dosage for the pruritic dog (from Scott & Miller 1999)

Antihistamine	Dose (mg/kg)	Frequency of administration
Amitriptyline	1–2	q.12 h
Astemizole	1	q.12–24 h
Azatadine	1 mg/dog	q.24 h
Brompheniramine	0.5–2	q.12 h
Cetirizine	0.5–1	q.24 h
Chlorphenamine (chlorpheniramine)	0.2–2	q.8–12 h
Clemastine	0.05–1.5	q.12 h
Clomipramine	1–3	q.24 h
Cyproheptadine	0.1–2	q.8–12 h
Dimenhydrinate	8	q.8 h
Diphenhydramine	1–4	q.8 h
Doxepin	0.5–1	q.8–12 h
Doxylamine	1–2	q.8 h
Hydroxyzine	2–7	q.8 h
Ketotifen	2–4 mg/dog	q.12 h
Loratadine	0.5	q.24 h
Oxatomide	0.5–2	q.12 h
Promethazine	1–2.5	q.12 h
Pyrilamine	1–2	q.8–12 h
Terfenadine	0.25–10	q.12–24 h
Trimeprazine	0.5–5	q.8–12 h
Tripelennamine	1	q.12 h

Table 11.3 Antihistamine dosage for the pruritic cat (from Scott & Miller 1999)

Antihistamine	Dose (mg/kg)	Frequency of administration
Amitriptyline	5–10	q.12–24 h
Chlorphenamine (chlorpheniramine)	2–4	q.12–24 h
Clemastine	0.68	q.12 h
Cyproheptadine	2	q.12 h
Diphenhydramine	2–4	q.12 h
Hydroxyzine	5–10	q.8–12 h
Oxatomide	15–30	q.12 h
Promethazine	5	q.24 h

Not every antihistamine will be effective in any one patient, so several agents and dosage regimens may need to be tested in order to achieve control of pruritus. This may involve the testing of a number of different antihistamine drugs in sequence, with each agent being evaluated for clinical effect over a 7–14 day period. Factors such as cost and frequency of dosing should be considered in selection of an appropriate antihistamine for any individual case.

The antihistamines that appear most efficacious in the dog include oxatomide, clemastine, cyproheptadine and amitriptyline (achieving control of pruritus in 16–33% of cases) and in the cat chlorphenamine (chlorpheniramine), oxatomide, clemastine and cyproheptadine are reported to be clinically effective in 40–73% of published cases. There are, however, few blinded, placebo-controlled trials of these agents upon which to base specific recommendations.

In the management of pruritus, antihistamines are generally given in conjunction with glucocorticoid, and when pruritus is controlled (generally within 5 days) the glucocorticoid is withdrawn and antihistamine therapy maintained to prevent recurrence of pruritus. There is some evidence that the effect of antihistamines may be enhanced by concurrent supplementation with essential fatty acids.

Scott & Miller (1999) have recommended an initial 14-day trial of antihistamine, followed by withdrawal of the drug to allow clinical relapse. When relapse occurs, the antihistamine therapy is started again and is continued for a 30-day period. There is no clinical benefit to be derived from using H_2-blockers in the therapy of canine atopic dermatitis, and there is no additive effect to be gained from administration of combined H_1- and H_2-blockers to such patients.

In adjunct therapy for systemic anaphylaxis, administration of diphenhydramine (0.5–1.0 mg/kg IV to a total dose of 50 mg) has been reported following appropriate management of circulatory collapse.

Pharmacokinetics

The pharmacokinetics of antihistamines in the dog and cat are largely unknown but following oral administration, these drugs are rapidly absorbed, achieving peak plasma levels within 1 h. Metabolism generally occurs in the liver and excretion is via the urine. Antihistamines may cross the placenta and be secreted in milk. A recent study has reported the pharmacokinetics of clemastine in the dog. After oral administration (0.5 mg/kg), the bioavailability was 3% and the drug was unable to inhibit wheal formation after intradermal injection of histamine. By contrast, intravenous administration (0.1 mg/kg) inhibited wheal formation for up to 7 h post injection. The results of this study suggest that oral clemastine administered at currently recommended dose rates (see above) is unlikely to be an effective therapy. Similar studies are required for other antihistamines used in companion animals.

Adverse effects

- H_1-blockers may induce a wide range of adverse effects, which vary with the drug used and the individual patient; however, these are generally mild and do not warrant discontinuation of therapy.
- Depending upon the drug used, some form of adverse effect was recorded in 0–25% of treated dogs in published studies.
- The most commonly recognized adverse effect is CNS depression (lethargy, depression, drowsiness, somnolence), which has been recorded in dogs given amitriptyline, chlorphenamine (chlorpheniramine), clemastine, diphenhydramine, hydroxyzine, terfenadine or alimemazine (trimeprazine). This depression may spontaneously resolve after 3–7 days, even in the face of continued antihistamine administration.
- Less common side effects include the following.
  - Excitement (restlessness, nervousness, tremors, hyperactivity), due to reduced seizure threshold, has been reported in dogs given cyproheptadine, doxepin, hydroxyzine or terfenadine.
  - Gastrointestinal effects (anorexia, vomiting, diarrhea, constipation) are recorded in dogs treated with amitriptyline, chlorphenamine (chlorpheniramine), clemastine, diphenhydramine, doxepin, hydroxyzine or terfenadine. These effects may sometimes be prevented if the drugs are given with food.
  - Anticholinergic effects (dry mouth, throat, nose and eyes; urinary retention or dysuria; intestinal atony) have been recorded in dogs given chlorphenamine (chlorpheniramine) or clemastine.
  - An increase in pruritus has occasionally been recognized in dogs treated with chlorphenamine (chlorpheniramine), diphenhydramine, hydroxyzine or terfenadine. This may occur more frequently with higher dosages of the drugs.
  - Cardiovascular effects (tachycardia, arrhythmia, hypertension) have been reported after overdosing with some antihistamines.
- Similar adverse effects have been recorded in 10–40% of cats treated with antipruritic doses of H_1-blockers. These include:
  - drowsiness (with chlorphenamine (chlorpheniramine))
  - diarrhea (with clemastine)
  - polyphagia, sedation, increased vocalization and vomiting (with cyproheptadine).

Known drug interactions

- H_1-blocking antihistamines are reported to act synergistically with products containing ω-6/ω-3 fatty acids in the control of pruritus in the dog and cat, and have also been administered concurrently with glucocorticoids, enabling a reduced dosage of glucocorticoid to be used.
- Contraindications include the concurrent administration of monoamine oxidase inhibitors (e.g. amitraz), which may potentiate the anticholinergic effects of these antihistamines, or coadministration of other CNS depressant agents (e.g. barbiturates, narcotics, anesthetics), which may cause additive CNS depression.
- Antihistamines may partially counteract the anticoagulative effects of histamine or warfarin.
- Astemizole or terfenadine should not be coadministered with ketoconazole, itraconazole, fluconazole, clarithromycin or erythromycin, as these drugs may increase the plasma levels of the antihistamine by inhibiting metabolism, and enhance the potential for the antihistamine to induce cardiac arrhythmia (reported in humans but not in dogs).
- The phenothiazine antihistamines should not be administered with quinidine, antidiarrheal mixtures (e.g. kaolin/pectin), antacids or adrenaline (epinephrine).
- Doxylamine, diphenhydramine or pyrilamine may also enhance the effects of adrenaline.

Contraindications and precautions

- Antihistamines are not recommended for animals with hepatic or cardiovascular disease, hypertension, glaucoma, hyperthyroidism or a history of seizures, urinary retention or intestinal atony.
- There is no information on the safety of administration during pregnancy or potential effects of transfer in the milk. Antihistamine therapy should be withdrawn before performing intradermal skin testing for allergy.

REFERENCE

Scott DW, Miller WH 1999 Antihistamines in the management of allergic pruritus in dogs and cats. J Small Anim Pract 40: 359-364

FURTHER READING

Aronson LR, Drobatz KJ, Hunter CA, Mason N 2005 Effects of CD28 blockade on subsets of naïve T cells in cats. Am J Vet Res 66: 483-492

Cohn LA 1991 The influence of corticosteroids on host defence mechanisms. J Vet Intern Med 5: 95-104

Cohn LA 1997 Glucocorticosteroids as immunosuppressive agents. Semin Vet Med Surg 12: 150-156

DeBoer DJ, Griffin CE 2001 The ACVD task force on canine atopic dermatitis (XXI): antihistamine pharmacotherapy. Vet Immunol Immunopathol 81: 323-329

Dunn J 1998 Therapy of immune-mediated disease in small animals. In Pract 20: 147-153

Hill PB, Martin RJ 1998 A review of mast cell biology. Vet Dermatol 9: 145-166

Hansson H, Bergvall K, Bondesson U et al 2004 Clinical pharmacology of clemastine in healthy dogs. Vet Dermatol 15: 152-158

Lucena R, Ginel PJ, Hernandez E, Novales M 1999 Effects of short courses of different doses of prednisone and dexamethasone on serum third component of complement (C3) levels in dogs. Vet Immunol Immunopathol 68: 187-192

Lyles KW, Jackson TW, Nesbitt T, Quarles LD 1993 Salmon calcitonin reduces vertebral bone loss in glucocorticoid-treated beagles. Am J Physiol 264: E938-E942

Miller E 1992 Immunosuppressive therapy in the treatment of immune-mediated disease. J Vet Intern Med 6: 206-213

Moore GE, Mahaffey EA, Hoenig M 1992 Hematologic and serum biochemical effects of long-term administration of anti-inflammatory doses of prednisolone in dogs. Am J Vet Res 53: 1033-1037

Nara PL, Krakowka S, Powers TE 1979 Effects of prednisolone on the development of immune responses to canine distemper virus in beagle pups. Am J Vet Res 40: 1742-1747

Olivry T, Mueller RS 2003 Evidence-based veterinary dermatology: a systematic review of the pharmacotherapy of canine atopic dermatitis. Vet Dermatol 14: 121-146

Olivry T, Sousa CA 2001 The ACVD task force on canine atopic dermatitis (XX): glucocorticoid pharmacotherapy. Vet Immunol Immunopathol 81: 317-322

Paterson S 1994 Use of antihistamines to control pruritus in atopic dogs. J Small Anim Pract 35: 415-419

Paterson S 1995 Additive effects of EFAs in dogs with atopic dermatitis after partial response to antihistamine therapy. J Small Anim Pract 36: 389-394

Rinkardt NE, Kruth SA, Kaushik A 1999 The effects of prednisone and azathioprine on circulating immunoglobulin levels and lymphocyte subpopulations in normal dogs. Can J Vet Res 63: 18-24

Rohrer CR, Hill RC, Fischer A et al 1999 Gastric hemorrhage in dogs given high doses of methylprednisolone sodium succinate. Am J Vet Res 60: 977-981

Solter PF, Hoffmann WE, Chambers MD, Schaeffer DJ, Kuhlenschmidt MS 1994 Hepatic total 3-alpha-hydroxy bile-acids concentration and enzyme-activities in prednisone-treated dogs. Am J Vet Res 55: 1086-1092

Trowald-Wigh G, Hakansson L, Johannisson A, Edqvist LE 1998 The effect of prednisolone on canine neutrophil function: in vivo and in vitro studies. Acta Vet Scand 39: 201-213

Van Den Broek AHM, Stafford WL 1992 Epidermal and hepatic glucocorticoid receptors in cats and dogs. Res Vet Sci 52: 312-315

Waters CB, Adams LG, Scott Moncrieff JC et al 1997 Effects of glucocorticoid therapy on urine protein-to-creatinine ratios and renal morphology in dogs. J Vet Intern Med 11: 172-177

Watson ADJ, Nicholson A, Church DB, Pearson MRB 1996 Use of anti-inflammatory and analgesic drugs in dogs and cats. Austr Vet J 74: 203-210

Wiedmyer CE, Solter PF, Hoffman WE 2002 Kinetics of mRNA expression of alkaline phosphatase isoenzymes in hepatic tissues from glucocorticoid-treated dogs. Am J Vet Res 63: 1089-1095

12

Immunomodulatory therapy

Michael J Day

INTRODUCTION

In clinical veterinary medicine there are numerous situations in which it would be advantageous to either enhance the immune system (immunostimulatory therapy) or downregulate it (immunosuppressive therapy).

The form of immunomodulatory therapy most commonly used in veterinary practice is immunosuppression and currently this is achieved through the use of glucocorticoids, given alone or in combination with a range of adjunct drugs. These agents cause 'blanket immunosuppression' of both deleterious and beneficial immune responses. Methods of inducing selective immunosuppression of a specific pathological immune response that leave general immunity intact are currently a major research focus.

By contrast, immunostimulation is at present difficult to achieve in the practice situation by pharmacological means. Although some agents are advocated for their immune-stimulatory properties, there have been few studies of the effects of these drugs on immunological parameters in companion animals.

This chapter will not address the application of the glucocorticoids (which are reviewed in Chapter 11) but will describe other agents with immunomodulatory capacity that are currently available to veterinary practitioners. Potential future developments in this important area will also be addressed.

Relevant pathophysiology

The rational use of immunomodulatory agents requires a working knowledge of the immune response. An overview of the complex interactions that make up any immune response is given in Figure 12.1. The key regulatory cell of the immune system is the $CD4^+$ T lymphocyte, which is activated following molecular interactions with an 'antigen-presenting cell' that has previously processed native antigen to a form that can be recognized by the antigen-specific T-cell receptor. The activated T cell in turn induces the specific immunological effector mechanisms that deal with the antigenic insult to the host.

There are several regulatory subsets of $CD4^+$ T cells that mediate different end-effects. The Th2 $CD4^+$ T cell induces B lymphocyte differentiation to antibody-secreting plasma cells (humoral or type 2 immunity). The Th1 $CD4^+$ T cell activates a range of cytotoxic cell populations, which can destroy neoplastic or infected target cells, or enable phagocytes to destroy intracellular pathogens (cell-mediated or type 1 immunity). By contrast, the effector function of Th3 or Treg $CD4^+$ T cells inhibits or 'suppresses' the immune response rather than amplifying it. All these regulatory functions are mediated by cytokines – soluble factors released from cells that initiate intracellular signaling pathways with resultant gene transcription in effector cells expressing appropriate cytokine receptors. There is intrinsic interconnection between the immune and inflammatory pathways and factors such as the complement cascade provide a bridge between the systems.

Immunomodulatory agents have the ability to act at different levels of these complex pathways. In some instances, a drug has a selective and specific action on one individual component (e.g. ciclosporin chiefly affects T lymphocytes) but this may have broad effects on other populations that are regulated by the target cell. By contrast, the mechanism and target of many other immunomodulatory agents are incompletely understood, despite the clinical effects observed.

DRUGS WITH IMMUNOSUPPRESSIVE EFFECTS

Azathioprine

Clinical applications

Although azathioprine is classified as a cytotoxic drug, it is used almost exclusively in small animal practice in the management of immune-mediated disease. Azathioprine has been used successfully in a large range of immune-mediated and inflammatory disorders in dogs and to a lesser extent in cats. This drug is often administered as an adjunct to immunomodulatory therapy with corticosteroids as this combination may have complementary immunological effects and concurrent azathioprine treatment usually permits lower doses of corticosteroids to be used in the maintenance phase of therapy.

Disorders in which azathioprine has been used include myasthenia gravis, immune-mediated hemolytic anemia,

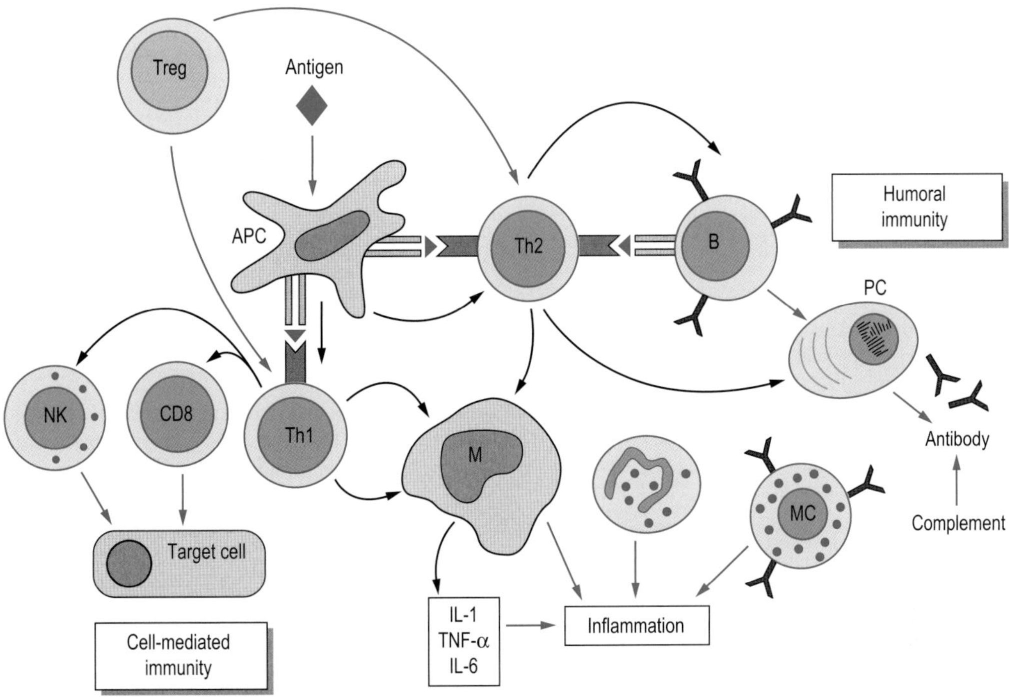

Fig. 12.1 **A summary of the cellular events leading to production of a humoral or cell-mediated immune response. Immunomodulatory agents may act at different points within these pathways. Black arrows represent cell signaling via cytokines. APC, antigen-presenting cell; B, B lymphocyte; IL-1, interleukin 1; IL-6, interleukin 6; M, macrophage; MC, mast cell; NK, natural killer cell; Th1, Th2, CD8, T lymphocytes; PC, plasma cell; TNF-α, tumor necrosis factor α.**

immune-mediated thrombocytopenia, autoimmune skin diseases such as erythema multiforme and pemphigus, inflammatory bowel disease, immune-mediated polyarthritis, anal furunculosis and uveodermatological syndrome. In addition, azathioprine has been used experimentally to prevent transplant rejection in dogs, most commonly as part of multicomponent treatment with ciclosporin, prednisone and antithymocyte serum. Use of azathioprine may not be indicated in acute antibody-mediated diseases as it does not decrease serum immunoglobulin except indirectly by inhibiting the function of T-helper cells. The onset of the immunosuppressive effects of azathioprine may be delayed (2–4 weeks) so this agent should be administered from the outset of any immunosuppressive protocol.

Mechanism of action

Azathioprine is an imidazole prodrug of 6-mercaptopurine, an established clinical agent for human leukemia. Azathioprine was developed to overcome the rapid inactivation of 6-mercaptopurine by a number of processes including enzymatic *S*-methylation, nonenzymatic oxidation or conversion to 6-thiourate by xanthine oxidase. 6-Mercaptopurine, an analog of the natural purine hypoxanthine, is converted to mercaptopurine-containing nucleotides. This leads to inhibition of purine synthesis or anabolism to thioinosine monophosphate (thio-IMP), a fraudulent nucleotide that interferes with the salvage pathway of purine synthesis. Thio-IMP is converted to thioguanosine monophosphate (thio-GMP) and further phosphorylated to thioguanosine triphosphate (thio-GTP), which causes DNA damage upon intercalation into the DNA backbone. Azathioprine may thus inhibit RNA and DNA synthesis and disrupt mitosis and cellular metabolism.

Azathioprine modulates cell-mediated immunity and T lymphocyte-dependent antibody synthesis. In a canine experimental study, azathioprine alone had no significant effect on serum immunoglobulin concentrations or the numbers of blood T or B lymphocytes although the drug was only administered for a 2-week period, reinforcing the need for longer term administration and observations.

Formulations and dose rates

Azathioprine is usually used as oral medication in dogs and cats, although it is available in some countries in parenteral formulations.

DOGS

- 2 mg/kg or 50 mg/m^2 PO q.24 h or q.48 h. This may be reduced after 2–4 weeks to 1 mg/kg once daily or every other day, although some clinicians prescribe 50 mg/m^2 dose every other day for extended periods

CATS

- Although azathioprine has been used successfully to treat immune-mediated disease in cats, serious bone marrow suppression has been reported in cats treated with doses used in dogs
- The recommended dose in cats is 1.5–3.125 mg/cat q.48 h. The tablets may be compounded into a suspension to assist oral dosing, but care is required to ensure that the intended dose is administered

Pharmacokinetics

Azathioprine is a prodrug that is well absorbed from the gut and cleaved in the presence of sulfhydryl compounds such as glutathione to 6-mercaptopurine. The enzymes xanthine oxidase and thiopurine methyltransferase (TPMT) catalyze the conversion of 6-mercaptopurine to inactive metabolites. In humans there is wide variation in the activity of TPMT which is subject to genetic polymorphism, with similar genetic variation in azathioprine metabolism also demonstrated in dogs and cats. Moreover, it is well documented that cats have significantly lower erythrocyte levels of TPMT than either dogs or humans, further underlining the potential safety issues in this species. Little parent azathioprine or 6-mercaptopurine is excreted as they are both extensively oxidized and methylated to metabolites that are excreted in urine.

Adverse effects

- Bone marrow suppression is more common in cats than in dogs and is believed to be more common in dogs on daily treatment than if treated every other day.
- In addition to dose-related marrow toxicity, idiosyncratic severe, irreversible, fatal leukopenia and thrombocytopenia have been reported in cats. As a result of this and the lower baseline activity of TPMT in this species, azathioprine is generally not recommended for use in cats. Chlorambucil is often used as an alternative in the management of immune-mediated disease in this species (see Chapter 15).
- Acute pancreatitis and hepatotoxicity have been associated with azathioprine use in dogs.
- Increased risk of infection may occur with prolonged azathioprine treatment.
- Azathioprine is mutagenic, carcinogenic and teratogenic and, as for all cytotoxic agents, the drug must be handled with appropriate care.

Known drug interactions

Concomitant administration of allopurinol, a xanthine oxidase inhibitor, and azathioprine increases the risk of azathioprine toxicity, as oxidation of mercaptopurine to inactive metabolites is greatly reduced by allopurinol. Dose adjustments may be necessary.

Ciclosporin

Clinical applications

Ciclosporin (ciclosporin A, ciclosporine, ciclosporine A) has traditionally been used as an immunosuppressant agent for transplantation surgery in humans, dogs and cats. In cats, the drug is administered concurrently with prednisolone for this purpose, whereas for canine renal transplantation a multiagent protocol is used with various combinations of ciclosporin (Sandimmun®, Novartis), antilymphocyte serum, donor bone marrow fractions, leflunomide, rapamycin and tacrolimus. A recent protocol reports the use of combination ciclosporin (Neoral®, Novartis), azathioprine and prednisolone for the prevention of acute renal allograft rejection in the dog.

Recently ciclosporin has found a wider range of therapeutic applications in veterinary medicine, including:

- medical therapy of canine anal furunculosis
- treatment of autoimmune diseases, including immune-mediated hemolytic anemia (IMHA), pure red cell aplasia, immune-mediated thrombocytopenia (IMTP) and systemic lupus erythematosus (SLE) in the dog and cat. There is still an insufficient evidence base for use of ciclosporin for these indications and recent reviews of the association between therapy and clinical outcome in canine IMHA have suggested that administration of concurrent oral prednisone and ciclosporin offers no benefit over prednisone monotherapy
- treatment of atopic dermatitis in the dog. This application is the only one for which the use of systemically administered ciclosporin is currently licensed in some markets for veterinary use and there are excellent supporting data which indicate the clinical efficacy of this drug in the management of this disease. Ciclosporin is also used to treat feline allergic skin disease (e.g. atopic dermatitis, eosinophilic granuloma complex).

The potential for systemic use of this drug in a range of other immune-mediated diseases is also being examined. For example, there are reports of successful application to the treatment of canine pemphigus foliaceus, epitheliotrophic lymphoma, reactive histiocytosis, sebaceous adenitis and inflammatory bowel disease. By contrast, ciclosporin appears not to be of clinical benefit in the treatment of canine immune-complex glomerulonephritis.

Topical ocular ciclosporin has immunosuppressive, anti-inflammatory and lacrimomimetic properties and is therefore indicated for immune-mediated diseases such as keratoconjunctivitis sicca (KCS, 'dry eye'), chronic superficial keratitis ('pannus') and nictitans plasmacytic conjunctivitis (plasmoma) in the dog. The efficacy of ciclosporin in KCS probably results from local (lacrimal gland) anti-inflammatory effects, although a direct stimulatory effect on glandular tissue by binding to lacrimal gland receptors has been proposed.

It has been shown that topical ciclosporin reduces apoptosis ('programmed cell death') by lacrimal epithelium and enhances apoptosis of infiltrating lymphocytes in canine KCS. The clinical effects of ciclosporin are greater in the early stages of KCS. Where the Schirmer tear test value is 0–1.0 mm/min, improved lacrimation may only occur in 50% of cases. In the cat, topical ciclosporin has been used for cases of eosinophilic keratoconjunctivitis, but variable efficacy is reported. The ocular application of ciclosporin is also discussed in Chapter 25.

Mechanism of action

Ciclosporin is a cyclic polypeptide containing 11 amino acids derived from a Norwegian soil fungus, *Tolypocladium inflatum*. The agent binds specifically to a cytoplasmic molecule (cyclophilin) that is expressed in high concentration in T lymphocytes. The complex of ciclosporin-cyclophilin in turn binds to and blocks another cytoplasmic molecule known as calcineurin. In a normal T cell, calcineurin is activated by the cytoplasmic influx of Ca^{2+} that follows T cell-receptor engagement by antigen presented by major histocompatibility molecules on the surface of an antigen-presenting cell. In turn, calcineurin activates the 'nuclear factor of activated T cells' (NF-AT), which migrates to the nucleus and binds the transcription factor AP-1. The complex of AP-1 with NF-AT induces the transcription of genes required for T-cell activation, particularly the gene encoding the cytokine interleukin 2 (IL-2).

The effects of ciclosporin on T lymphocytes include reduced production of IL-2, IL-3, IL-4, granulocyte colony-stimulating factor (G-CSF) and tumor necrosis factor (TNF-α), in addition to reduced clonal proliferation of the cell. This in turn results in reduced clonal proliferation of B lymphocytes and has indirect effects on a range of other cell types (granulocytes, macrophages, natural killer (NK) cells, eosinophils, mast cells). A recent in vitro study of the effects of ciclosporin on cultured feline lymphocytes has shown that this agent can potently suppress the proliferative response of both $CD4^+$ and $CD8^+$ T cells. Ciclosporin is also known to directly affect granulocyte function via reducing Ca^{2+}-dependent exocytosis of granule-associated serine esterases. In vitro studies of isolated canine skin mast cells have shown that ciclosporin is a potent inhibitor of histamine release induced by nonimmunological or immunological stimuli. Finally, the immunosuppression mediated by ciclosporin may reflect the induction of transforming growth factor β (TGF-β), a potent inhibitor of IL-2 stimulated T-cell proliferation.

Two further molecules have now been developed for such selective T-cell immunosuppression but are not yet used widely in veterinary medicine. The agent tacrolimus (formerly FK506) is derived from the bacterium *Streptomyces tsukabaensis* and the drug rapamycin (or sirolimus) is obtained from *Streptomyces hygroscopicus* (originally obtained from Rapa Nui or Easter Island). Tacrolimus selectively binds the T-cell cytoplasmic molecules known as FK-binding proteins (FKBP), while the complex of tacrolimus-FKBP also binds and inhibits calcineurin. FKBP and cyclophilin are both members of the family of intracellular immunophilin proteins. Tacrolimus blocks transcription of genes encoding IL-2 and IL-4. By contrast, rapamycin acts in a different fashion from ciclosporin or tacrolimus; it binds FKBP but the complex does not affect calcineurin, but blocks the complex signal transduction pathway triggered by binding of IL-2, IL-4 or IL-6 to their specific membrane receptors.

Formulations and dose rates

The licensed veterinary formulation of ciclosporin for systemic administration is Neoral® (Novartis). This is an orally administered, microemulsion formulation of ciclosporin, which has greater bioavailability and less variability in pharmacokinetics than the earlier human formulation that was used in companion animals (Sandimmun®, Novartis). The advantage of Neoral® is that it produces more stable blood concentrations, thus reducing the need for regular monitoring of this parameter. Neoral® is available as soft capsules containing either 10, 25, 50 or 100 mg of ciclosporin. Sandimmun® was used as either an oral capsule formulation or as a solution for intravenous injection.

For topical ophthalmic use, Optimmune® (Schering-Plough) is a 0.2% w/w ciclosporin ointment that is also a licensed veterinary formulation. A human formulation of tacrolimus ointment is currently being evaluated for topical cutaneous application in canine atopic dermatitis, anal furunculosis or deep pyoderma with localized sinus tract formation.

The recommended dose rate for Neoral® in the treatment of canine atopic dermatitis is 5 mg/kg q.24 h given at least 2 h before or after feeding. The aim of therapy is to achieve a blood trough concentration of 400–600 ng/mL of ciclosporin and appropriate assays for determination of blood concentration are generally accessible. Whilst such assays were routinely performed following administration of

Formulations and dose rates—cont'd

Sandimmun®, there is no such recommendation listed on the data sheet for Neoral® as this formulation has more predictable pharmacokinetics with a higher safety margin. Monitoring may be considered when ciclosporin is administered concurrently with ketoconazole (see below). The dose rate of ciclosporin should be gradually tapered as for other immunosuppressive medicines. For Neoral® administered for the control of chronic atopic dermatitis in dogs, the recommendation is for daily administration (as above) until there is clinical improvement. This will normally occur within 4 weeks of therapy and if there has been no response within 8 weeks, treatment should be stopped. Following control of clinical signs, Neoral® may be given every other day, then every 3–4 days and finally withdrawn. Recurrence of clinical signs following withdrawal of therapy requires reinstigation of daily dosing. This dosage regimen has now become reasonably standard for most applications of Neoral® but earlier literature on the use of ciclosporin A (often as Sandimmun®) may report a range of different dosage regimens for oral or intravenous administration.

Ciclosporin has been administered concurrently with prednisolone to achieve immunosuppression in diseases such as canine IMHA and in this instance should be gradually tapered in conjunction with reduction in the dosage of glucocorticoid. Current data sheet recommendations for Neoral® are, however, that this agent not be administered concurrently with other immunosuppressives.

In the medical management of canine anal furunculosis, reduced dosage of ciclosporin has been achieved by concurrent administration of ketoconazole (see below) which competitively inhibits enzymes involved in ciclosporin metabolism (e.g. cytochrome P450). Increased bioavailability occurs when grapefruit juice is administered concurrently with oral ciclosporin (Sandimmun®). However, as dogs and cats are unlikely to imbibe much, if any, grapefruit (or any other) juice, this is unlikely to be of clinical relevance in veterinary practice.

Optimmune® is administered to the conjunctival sac by applying a small quantity of ointment (0.5–1.0 cm) q.12 h. Lifelong therapy may be required for KCS and continuous therapy is required to stimulate tear production, which may not be evident for 2–6 weeks. Adjunct treatment (e.g. tear replacement) is also generally administered during the initial phases of treatment. In the treatment of pannus, intermittent therapy may be appropriate, with reduced frequency of application possible during periods of reduced exposure to UV light.

Tacrolimus is formulated as an ointment for topical application in the treatment of human atopic dermatitis (Protopic® 0.1% tacrolimus ointment; Fujisawa Healthcare). There is minimal systemic absorption and thus a low risk of adverse effects. Protopic® has been used to effectively treat dogs with atopic dermatitis, particularly cases with localized disease.

Pharmacokinetics

Pharmacokinetic studies of the original ciclosporin formulation, Sandimmun®, administered to dogs revealed that peak concentrations were generally achieved 2–4 h after oral administration, with only 20–25% of the dose absorbed and substantial variation between dogs. This low bioavailability may increase with longer duration of dosing. The bioavailability of Neoral® is higher, at approximately 35%, as a result of improved micellar formulation. While bile salts are required to emulsify Sandimmun® there is no effect of bile salts on Neoral® absorption. The absorption of Neoral® is impaired by ingestion of fatty meals within 30 min of administration, leading to the recommendation not to administer Neoral® within 2 h of feeding. Absorbed ciclosporin has high affinity for plasma lipoproteins, but up to 50% of absorbed drug is located within erythrocytes and leukocytes. Highest tissue concentrations occur in fat and the liver, with lower concentrations in pancreas, kidneys, skin and heart. Metabolism is extensive and carried out by the cytochrome P450 microsomal enzyme system. Metabolites are largely excreted in bile, with some minor (5%) urinary loss.

Adverse effects

- The immunosuppressive effects of ciclosporin have the potential to result in secondary infection or malignancy (particularly lymphoid). The dog and cat appear relatively tolerant of the drug but isolated cases of recrudescence of existing infection or development of primary infection have been recorded in both species. Ciclosporin should not be used in animals with pre-existing neoplastic disease.
- In the cat the major reported side effect is soft feces.
- In dogs a range of adverse effects has been recorded. The most common are vomiting, diarrhea or soft feces. These effects are mild and transient and do not warrant withdrawal of therapy. Other effects include: anorexia, gingival hyperplasia, papillomatosis, hirsutism, hair shedding, red and swollen ears, muscle weakness or muscle cramps. These signs rapidly resolve on withdrawal of the drug.
- Renal toxicity is rarely reported, except with high dose rates, which may also induce defective hepatic protein synthesis, inhibition of insulin release and peripheral insulin resistance. Ciclosporin should therefore be used with particular care in diabetic dogs and dogs with renal disease should be closely monitored (e.g. via serum biochemistry).
- Ciclosporin (or its excipients) may induce hypersensitivity and the drug should not be administered to animals that are sensitized. This particularly applies to the injectable products which contain Cremophor as a solubilizing agent.
- Ciclosporin should not be administered to pregnant or lactating animals as it may cross the placental barrier and pass into the milk. The safety of the drug has not been studied in breeding male dogs.
- Ciclosporin is not recommended for use in dogs under 6 months of age or those that weigh less than 2 kg.

- Optimmune® should not be administered where there is suspected ocular infection. If persistent mild ocular irritation is observed, the drug should be discontinued.
- Ciclosporin is concentrated within the cornea and is reported to have low systemic bioavailability. However, one published study has demonstrated a degree of systemic immunosuppression following local ophthalmic absorption of 2% ciclosporin applied for 1–3 months.

Known drug interactions

Much of the data on drug interactions with ciclosporin is derived from human medicine.

- Drugs that elevate human blood ciclosporin concentrations include: bromocriptine, danazol, diltiazem, doxycycline, erythromycin, fluconazole, itraconazole, ketoconazole, methylprednisolone, nicardipine and verapamil. In dogs ketoconazole and vitamin E are known to have this effect.
- Agents that can decrease human blood ciclosporin concentrations include: carbamazepine, phenobarbital, phenytoin, rifampicin (rifampin) and intravenous trimethoprim-sulfamethoxazole.
- Ciclosporin may potentially induce signs of CNS toxicity if coadministered with ivermectin or milbemycin.
- Ciclosporin may increase the nephrotoxicity of aminoglycoside antibiotics and trimethoprim and should not be coadministered with these agents.
- In the dog ketoconazole given at 5–10 mg/kg can increase the blood concentration of ciclosporin by up to fivefold and this agent may be used to reduce the required dose of ciclosporin. When ketoconazole is used in this fashion, the dose of Neoral® should be halved (i.e. 2.5 mg/kg q.24 h) or the treatment interval should be doubled (i.e. 5 mg/kg q.48 h). However, careful individualization of dose rates will be necessary due to interanimal variation in responses.
- Unlike the situation in humans, there is no interaction between concurrently administered methylprednisolone and ciclosporin in dogs.
- Animals treated with ciclosporin should not receive a live attenuated vaccine whilst being treated, or within 2 weeks before or after treatment.

Special considerations

Ciclosporin A remains a relatively expensive immunosuppressive drug. Owners should be instructed to administer the drug carefully to reduce their exposure. For example, Optimmune® should be applied using gloves and contact with the skin should be avoided.

Danazol

Clinical applications

In small animal medicine, danazol, a synthetic attenuated androgen, has been used as an adjunct therapy for canine immune-mediated hemolytic anemia (IMHA) and thrombocytopenia (IMTP). The use of danazol enables treatment with reduced doses of corticosteroid, thus decreasing the likelihood of glucocorticoid side effects in these patients. The use of danazol in this manner is contentious and there have been few controlled clinical trials demonstrating efficacy of the drug. In fact, recent studies in dogs with IMHA have suggested that danazol provides no benefit, above the immunosuppression achieved with prednisolone and azathioprine.

Mechanism of action

Use of danazol therapy in IMHA is based upon the following reported actions of the drug.

- Downregulation of Fc-receptor expression by macrophages, thereby decreasing extravascular hemolysis mediated by erythrocyte-bound antibody.
- Reduced number of immunoglobulin molecules coating erythrocytes.
- Alteration of T-lymphocyte immunoregulation.
- Incorporation of the drug into the erythrocyte membrane, stabilizing the membrane so the erythrocyte becomes less susceptible to hemolysis.

Formulations and dose rates

Danazol (Danocrine®; 50, 100 or 200 mg capsules; Winthrop Pharmaceuticals) is not a licensed veterinary product.

Danazol is reported to have a slow onset of action (2–3 weeks), so is administered at a dose of 3–5 mg/kg q.8 h PO, concurrently with prednisolone (and/or azathioprine). Following tapering of the prednisolone dose, danazol therapy is continued at 5 mg/kg q.24 h. Danazol may then be tapered after 2–3 months of normal hemograms.

Danazol therapy is suitable for dogs with chronic, stable IMHA but not those animals with acute-onset, severe hemolysis.

Pharmacokinetics

The pharmacokinetics of danazol in the dog are virtually unknown. By analogy with results from studies in experimental animals and humans, danazol is assumed to be largely metabolized in the liver of cats and dogs.

Adverse effects

- The most significant adverse effect reported in the dog is hepatotoxicity.
- Danazol is not currently recommended for use in the cat, as those few animals treated with the drug devel-

oped illness, with hyperbilirubinemia and elevated liver enzymes on serum biochemistry.

Known drug interactions

- Danazol should not be administered concurrently with anticoagulants, as the drug may decrease synthesis of procoagulant factors by the liver.
- Use in diabetic animals should be undertaken with care, as danazol may alter insulin requirements via an effect on carbohydrate metabolism.
- Similarly, care should be taken in patients with cardiac, renal or hepatic disease.
- Danazol is a teratogen that should not be administered during pregnancy.

Gold

Clinical applications

Administration of gold salts (chrysotherapy) has found greatest application in canine medicine in the treatment of autoimmune disorders, particularly autoimmune polyarthritis (e.g. rheumatoid arthritis, idiopathic polyarthritis) and the autoimmune skin diseases (e.g. pemphigus foliaceus, bullous pemphigoid). In the cat, gold salts have been used as therapy for pemphigus foliaceus, chronic gingivostomatitis, plasma cell pododermatitis and lesions of the eosinophilic granuloma complex. The majority of reported studies have been with aurothiomalate rather than auranofin as the latter drug is more expensive and reportedly less effective.

Mechanism of action

The mechanism of action of gold salts is very poorly understood, but they are reported to have anti-inflammatory, immunomodulatory, antirheumatic and antimicrobial effects. Effects on the immune system include:

- inhibition of lymphocyte proliferation (possibly T-helper cells)
- inhibition of immunoglobulin production
- inhibition of complement component C1
- inhibition of neutrophil and monocyte-macrophage function, particularly the release of lysosomal enzymes and prostaglandins
- inhibition of connective tissue enzymes (elastase, collagenase, hyaluronidase)
- protection from oxygen radicals.

Formulations and dose rates

Gold salts are available for oral administration as auranofin (Ridaura®; 3 mg tablets containing 29% gold) or in an injectable form as aurothiomalate (Myocristin®; 20, 40 or 100 mg/mL suspension containing 50% gold). These drugs are not currently licensed for companion animal use.

DOGS

- Auranofin has been administered to dogs at a dose of 0.05–0.2 mg/kg q.12 h PO, with a maximum daily dose of 9 mg/day
- Aurothiomalate is administered to dogs under 10 kg bodyweight by deep IM injection using a dosage regimen of 1 mg in week 1, 2 mg in week 2 and then 1 mg/kg every 7–28 days
- For a dog of over 10 kg bodyweight, the recommendation is 5 mg in week 1, 10 mg in week 2 (to a maximum of 1 mg/kg) and then 1 mg/kg every 7–28 days

CATS

- IM aurothiomalate is given, using the protocol described above for smaller dogs. The drug has a slow onset of action and administration for 6–12 weeks may be required before clinical benefit is observed. Because of this, many clinicians advocate the use of low-dose glucocorticoids (e.g. prednisolone 1–2 mg/kg q.12–48 h PO) during the initial phase of treatment
- Once disease remission is achieved, the dose or dosage interval should be reduced where possible

Pharmacokinetics

Following oral administration, gold is absorbed from the intestine (approximately 20–25% of the gold content of the drug) and binds plasma proteins with moderate affinity. Gold particularly concentrates within liver, kidney, spleen, lungs and adrenal glands. At the cellular level, gold also accumulates predominantly within macrophages. Approximately 60% of the absorbed dose is excreted in urine and unabsorbed gold is excreted in the feces.

After IM injection, gold is rapidly absorbed, with peak serum concentrations achieved in 4–6 h and up to 95% of the agent is bound to plasma proteins. The half-life in blood is approximately 6 d. The drug is predominantly concentrated in the synovium, with lower levels in liver, kidney, spleen, bone marrow, adrenals and lymph nodes. Approximately 70% of the absorbed dose is excreted in urine and the remainder is lost in the feces.

Adverse effects

- Gold salts are contraindicated in patients with SLE, diabetes mellitus or hematological, hepatic, renal or cardiac disease.
- Recorded adverse effects include diarrhea (more commonly with auranofin than aurothiomalate), blood dyscrasias (especially thrombocytopenia, hemolytic anemia, leukopenia), hemorrhage or ulceration of mucous membranes, mucocutaneous disease of the erythema multiforme–toxic epidermal necrolysis spectrum, encephalitis, neuritis, hepatotoxicity or renal disease (damage to proximal tubules).
- Nephrotoxic effects are particularly marked in cats and may lead to proteinuria.

Known drug interactions

- There are few data for veterinary patients, but in humans the potential for toxicity is elevated with concurrent administration of penicillamine or antimalarial drugs.
- Gold salts should not be administered concurrently with cytotoxic immunosuppressive drugs.

Special considerations

The use of gold salts should only be considered following unsuccessful trials of other less toxic and expensive immunosuppressive agents. Animals receiving chrysotherapy should have regular monitoring of hematological and renal (urinalysis) parameters at baseline, then every 2 weeks initially and then every 1–2 months. Gold salts are potentially teratogenic and their use is contraindicated in pregnancy.

Intravenous immunoglobulin

Clinical applications

Intravenous infusion of a preparation of intact human immunoglobulin (IVIG) precipitated from pooled plasma (Gamimune®, Miles Inc.) has been used in the treatment of canine nonregenerative IMHA or IMTP refractory to standard immunosuppressive therapy. IVIG has more recently found application in the treatment of some forms of immune-mediated skin disease (in particular those of the erythema multiforme–toxic epidermal necrolysis spectrum).

Mechanism of action

The mode of action of the immunoglobulin is probably via:

- saturation of Fc receptors on macrophages, preventing binding of cell-bound autoantibody. IVIG inhibits the binding of canine IgG to monocytes and inhibits phagocytosis of antibody-coated canine erythrocytes in vitro. This effect likely underlies the mode of action of IVIG in the treatment of IMHA and IMTP.
- modulation of T- and B-lymphocyte function via binding of immunoglobulin to molecules on the surface membrane of these cells. IVIG has been shown to bind to canine T ($CD4^+$ and $CD8^+$) and B lymphocytes in vitro. In humans, there is evidence that the immunoglobulin in IVIG blocks the interaction between the molecules Fas (CD95) and Fas-ligand (CD95R) which are involved in the induction of apoptosis in lymphocyte-mediated cytotoxic destruction of target cells. This effect likely underlies the mode of action of IVIG in the treatment of immune-mediated skin diseases such as erythema multiforme which involve lymphocyte-mediated killing of epidermal keratinocytes.

Formulations and dose rates

- The immunoglobulin is administered at a dose of 0.5–1.5 g/kg by IV infusion over a 6–12 h period and is generally given concurrently with other immunosuppressive therapy. In most cases only a single treatment is performed
- Following infusion, canine patients develop a rapid, transient elevation of hematocrit and evidence of reticulocytosis

Adverse effects

No adverse effects have been recorded in dogs transfused with IVIG; however, the half-life of human immunoglobulin in dogs (7–9 days) is shorter than in humans, which might suggest that the dog makes an endogenous antibody response to the human molecules. Repeated administration will likely sensitize a dog such that hypersensitivity reactions may occur on subsequent exposures.

Special considerations

The product is expensive and may have limited availability when demand is high for human patients.

Leflunomide

Clinical applications

Leflunomide, a synthetic isoxazole derivative and disease-modifying antirheumantic drug, has been shown to be a potent immunosuppressive agent in experimental models of immune-mediated disease and in the therapy of human autoimmune disease, particularly rheumatoid arthritis. In veterinary medicine, this agent has to date found widest application in experimental studies of transplantation in the dog, where it is used in combination with other immunosuppressive modalities.

One study has shown that leflunomide can also be effective in the treatment of canine immune-mediated diseases that are refractory to standard therapies, or where there are side effects from glucocorticoid administration. Leflunomide treatment has been reported as being of benefit for dogs with IMHA, IMTP, Evans' syndrome, multifocal nonsuppurative encephalitis/meningomyelitis, immune-mediated polymyositis and pemphigus foliaceus. The drug is particularly effective in the therapy of canine reactive histiocytosis. Combination therapy with leflunomide and methotrexate has recently been reported as efficacious in cats with immune-mediated polyarthritis.

Mechanism of action

The primary immunomodulation mechanism of action of leflunomide is selective inhibition of dihydro-orotate dehydrogenase, a mitochondrial enzyme essential for de novo pyrimidine biosynthesis, which particularly affects

T and B lymphocytes that lack a pyrimidine salvage pathway.

Formulations and dose rates

In the studies cited above, leflunomide was initially administered in conjunction with other immunosuppressive therapy (with progression to leflunomide monotherapy) at a dose of 4 mg/kg q.24 h PO, with the plasma trough level adjusted to 20 μg/mL. Leflunomide is not a licensed veterinary medicine.

Pharmacokinetics

Following oral administration, leflunomide is almost completely absorbed and immediately subject to nonenzymatic conversion in the intestinal mucosa, portal circulation and liver to the active metabolite A77 1726 (3 cyano-3-hydroxy-N-[4-trifluoromethylphenyl] crotonamide or M1). Little leflunomide is detectable in plasma, indicative of the extensive metabolism. M1 is further biotransformed in the liver and excreted by both biliary and renal routes. Reabsorption from the small intestine after biliary excretion leads to enterohepatic recycling, contributing to the long elimination half-life of M1 of more than 7 d.

Megestrol acetate

Clinical applications

Megestrol acetate is an oral progestin most commonly used for prevention or postponement of estrus in the bitch or queen and a range of canine reproductive and behavioral problems (see Chapters 7 and 23). The drug is also used in the management of feline miliary dermatitis and the eosinophilic granuloma complex, both of which are manifestations of cutaneous hypersensitivity in the cat. However, because of the high incidence of adverse effects, the drug is not recommended for management of these disorders unless there is no alternative.

Mechanism of action

The mechanism of action of megestrol acetate in these disorders is not completely understood. The drug has more potent anti-inflammatory and adrenal-suppressive effects than corticosteroids, but the additional possibility of immunosuppressive properties has been discussed by some authors.

Formulations and dose rates

CATS

- The dosage regimen for feline cutaneous hypersensitivity disease is 2.5–5 mg/cat q.48–72 h PO until a response is observed and then the dose is reduced to 2.5–5 mg/cat q.7 d
- A maintenance dose of 2.5 mg/cat q.7–14 d may be required to prevent recurrence, or repeated courses of treatment may be given

Adverse effects

Multiple side effects have been reported and include:

- increased appetite
- weight gain
- depression/lethargy
- mammary gland hyperplasia and carcinoma
- diabetes mellitus (transient and permanent)
- bone marrow suppression
- endometrial hyperplasia
- pyometra
- adrenocortical suppression
- thinning and increased fragility of the skin.

Contraindications and precautions

- Progestins should not be used in intact females, breeding animals and in animals with diabetes mellitus (increases insulin resistance)
- Concurrent corticosteroid use is contraindicated.

Pentoxifylline

Clinical applications

Pentoxifylline (Trental®, Hoechst) has found application in the therapy of a range of canine skin diseases, including vasculitis, rabies vaccine-induced ischemic dermatitis, dermatomyositis, ulcerative dermatosis of shelties and collies, and contact allergy. There is some evidence that the drug has a useful adjunct role in the therapy of atopic dermatitis.

Mechanism of action

Pentoxifylline is a methylxanthine derivative and nonselective inhibitor of the cyclic nucleotide phosphodiesterases that increase the rate of breakdown of cAMP and cGMP. The drug has two major clinical effects:

- increasing microvascular blood flow, thereby enhancing oxygenation of ischemic tissue. This effect is attributed to increased erythrocyte membrane deformability, vasodilation, reduced erythrocyte and platelet aggregation and enhanced fibrinolysis
- immunomodulation, particularly by suppressing synthesis of proinflammatory cytokines (IL-1, IL-6, IL-12, TNF-α) by lymphocytes and keratinocytes and inhibiting adhesion between leukocytes and endothelial or epithelial cells. There may also be inhibitory effects on neutrophil, T and B lymphocytes and NK cell activity.

Formulations and dose rates

- A range of dose rates is reported and long-term therapy is generally indicated with a trial period of 2–3 months
- Pentoxifylline has been administered to dogs with dermatomyositis or ulcerative dermatosis at 400 mg/dog q.12 h (or for small dogs 200 mg/dog q.12 h) and to dogs with contact dermatitis or

atopic dermatitis at 10 mg/kg q.12 h PO. Combination prednisone and pentoxifylline therapy is reported for the management of cutaneous rabies vaccine-induced vasculitis in dogs. Pentoxifylline is not a licensed veterinary medicine

Pharmacokinetics
One study has examined the pharmacokinetics of pentoxifylline in the dog following oral administration at 15 mg/kg q.8 h for a 5-d period. The drug was rapidly absorbed and eliminated within hours of absorption, with lower plasma concentrations achieved on day 5 than day 0.

Adverse effects
Anorexia and vomiting.

Tetracycline and niacinamide

Clinical applications
The combination of niacinamide and tetracycline has been used to treat a range of immune-mediated dermatopathies of the dog, particularly discoid lupus erythematosus and the cutaneous manifestations of SLE.

Mechanism of action
Niacinamide has been shown to block mast cell degranulation and inhibit protease release from leukocytes, whereas tetracycline is able to suppress complement activation, antibody production, leukocyte chemotaxis, prostaglandin synthesis and the production of lipases and collagenases. The specific means by which these drugs downregulate aberrant immune responses in these disorders is not clearly understood. However, laboratory studies of the tetracycline group have shown that doxycycline and minocycline can inhibit nitric oxide synthase and augment cyclo-oxygenase-2 and PGE_2 production by macrophages. Additionally, these drugs can inhibit matrix metalloproteases and block angiogenesis.

Formulations and dose rates

- The recommended dosage regimen is 500 mg per dog (250 mg/dog if below 10–15 kg bodyweight; alternatively 5–12 mg/kg) of each drug, given q.8 h for at least a 3-month trial period. When a clinical response is recorded, the dosage is decreased to q.12 h for 2 months and then q.24 h. If there is no relapse on once-daily therapy, the niacinamide is withdrawn and tetracycline monotherapy continued
- In cases of more severe clinical disease, initial therapy may be combined with prednisolone (2 mg/kg q.24 h) with the aim of tapering the glucocorticoid and maintaining combination niacinamide/tetracycline. Up to 50% of dogs with DLE are successfully managed on this therapy, but it is less effective in the treatment of other immune-mediated skin diseases (e.g. pemphigus foliaceus, bullous pemphigoid, dermatomyositis)

Adverse effects
Reported adverse effects include: anorexia, vomiting, diarrhea, elevated liver enzymes, hyperexcitability, depression, lameness. These may be largely attributed to the niacinamide component of the regimen.

DRUGS WITH IMMUNOSTIMULATORY EFFECTS

Acemannan

Clinical applications
Acemannan has most often been used in veterinary medicine by intralesional injection into canine and feline cutaneous fibrosarcomas. The resultant tumor necrosis and encapsulation facilitates subsequent surgical excision.

The agent has also been used in animals with squamous cell carcinoma, histiocytoma, myxosarcoma, adenocarcinoma, lymphoma, mast cell tumor and infiltrative lipoma.

Acemannan has been administered to cats with FeLV or FIV infection and is suggested to improve both quality of life and survival time; however, these were not placebo-controlled studies.

Mechanism of action
Acemannan is a β-(1,4)-acetylated mannan-based polysaccharide derived from the plant aloe vera (*Barbadensis milleri*). The reported range of biological effects of acemannan includes:

- stimulation of the production of IL-1α, TNF-α, IL-6, nitric oxide and prostaglandin E_2 by macrophages
- enhanced macrophage phagocytosis
- antiviral activity
- induction of tumor cell apoptosis or necrosis.

Formulations and dose rates

Intralesional treatment of canine and feline cutaneous fibrosarcomas
- 2 mg intralesional q.7 d for 6 weeks given concurrently with intraperitoneal injection of 1 mg/kg q.7 d for 6 weeks

Adverse effects
- Pyrexia
- Anorexia
- Depression
- Diarrhea
- Syncope, transient bradycardia and disorientation
- Tachypnea and/or tachycardia
- Collapse and pain on injection

Immunoregulin

Clinical applications

Immunoregulin has been used in a range of clinical situations, including:

- FeLV or feline viral rhinotracheitis infection
- canine staphylococcal pyoderma
- canine oral melanoma, mast cell tumor.

Mechanism of action

Immunoregulin is a killed suspension of the bacterium *Propionibacterium acnes*, which is reported to have a range of immunostimulatory effects, including enhancement of antibody production, cell-mediated immunity, macrophage and NK cell function.

Formulations and dose rates

A range of dosage regimens is reported.

CATS

- Immunoregulin has been given at 0.25 (for a 2.5 kg cat) –0.5 mL (for a 5 kg cat) IV twice weekly for 2 weeks, then once weekly for 3 weeks and finally once monthly for 2 months

DOGS

- For dogs with staphylococcal pyoderma the drug is administered as an adjunct to standard therapy in chronic cases of the disease. The recommended dose rates depend upon bodyweight (0.25 mL for a dog under 7 kg, 0.5 mL for a dog 7–20 kg, 1.0 mL for a dog 21–34 kg, 2.0 mL for a dog over 34 kg) and the drug is given by IV injection twice weekly during weeks 1 and 2 of therapy, then by weekly injection during weeks 3–12. A response should be observed within 12 weeks, but some dogs may require a monthly injection to maintain remission

Adverse effects

- Mild anaphylactoid reactions characterized by vomiting, anorexia, pyrexia and lethargy.
- There may be localized inflammation if there is extravasation of the agent during injection.

Ivermectin

Clinical applications

Ivermectin is a broad-spectrum parasiticide that is widely used in veterinary medicine. The drug is currently unlicensed for use in the dog, with the exception of a specific formulation (Heartgard®) used as a heartworm preventive in many countries. A range of ectoparasitic infections of the dog have been treated using the 1% w/v bovine preparation (Ivomec®, Merial). The antiparasitic effects of ivermectin are discussed in Chapter 10.

Mechanism of action

On the basis of studies in other species, it has sometimes been proposed that ivermectin has an immunomodulatory, as well as antiparasitic, effect. In one reported study, administration of Ivomec® to healthy laboratory beagles had no effect on blood lymphocyte counts, CD4 : CD8 T-cell ratios or lymphocyte blastogenic responses in vitro. The authors suggest that ivermectin may act in a similar fashion to levamisole, being able to restore subnormal immune function, but not enhance immunity to supranormal levels (see below).

Formulations and dose rates

- A range of ectoparasitic infections of the dog has been treated using the 1% w/v bovine preparation (Ivomec®, Merial) given by subcutaneous injection at a dose of 0.2–0.3 mg/kg. Regimens of two such injections 2 weeks apart, or weekly injections for a 2-month period, have been described
- Ivomec® has also been administered orally over longer periods at 0.6 mg/kg q.24 h

Contraindications and precautions

At doses above those approved for heartworm prophylaxis, ivermectin must be used cautiously in collies, shelties or related breeds. Care must also be taken when using in dogs with circulating microfilaria of *Dirofilaria immitis*.

Levamisole

Clinical applications

Levamisole is an anthelmintic agent used principally for the treatment and control of a range of nematodes in domestic species and as a microfilaricide in dogs. In the context of this chapter, levamisole has often been advocated as an adjunctive immunostimulant drug in small animal medicine, with particular application to canine microbial disease with underlying immunodeficiency. The basis for this usage might lie in the fact that this agent has immunomodulatory properties and is sometimes used as a vaccine adjuvant in domestic livestock. Fundamentally, however, the immunomodulatory properties of levamisole in companion animals remain unproven, and use of this agent is associated with a range of potentially severe side effects. It is difficult to recommend its use given these circumstances.

The specific clinical applications to which levamisole have been applied include:

- chronic, recurrent cutaneous infection, particularly canine deep pyoderma
- aspergillosis or penicillosis
- immunodeficiency of Weimaraner dogs

- immunostimulation in neoplastic disease. Limited studies of levamisole used in this context have shown no significant benefit when used as an adjuvant to surgical management of mammary adenocarcinoma (cat and dog), or when given with combination chemotherapy for canine lymphoma.

In the dog, levamisole has also been used in combination with prednisolone for the treatment of SLE. The drug has occasionally been used as adjunct therapy in feline chronic gingivostomatitis or eosinophilic granuloma complex, but there appears to be little conclusive evidence for an effect in these conditions. The antiparasitic effects of levamisole are discussed in Chapter 10.

Mechanism of action

The mechanism by which levamisole causes immunomodulation is poorly understood and there have been very few studies of the effect of this drug on immune parameters in the dog and cat. Properties that have been attributed to this agent include:

- enhancement of T-lymphocyte number and function, but no direct effect on B lymphocytes or antibody production
- enhanced chemotaxis, phagocytosis and intracellular killing by granulocytes and monocytes.

Levamisole will not enhance immune function to 'supranormal' levels but may improve subnormal immunity. The drug may enhance the immune response to an antigenic stimulus (e.g. vaccine) given concurrently. It has been suggested that levamisole may affect the metabolism of cyclic nucleotides, by increasing cAMP breakdown and decreasing cGMP inactivation.

Early studies of dogs with generalized demodicosis demonstrated that levamisole therapy was able to restore the depressed blood lymphocyte mitogen responsiveness that accompanies this disease without altering cutaneous mite populations. In dogs with SLE, there is a peripheral blood lymphopenia with an alteration in the CD4 : CD8 T-lymphocyte ratio in circulating blood, due to a decrease in the number of $CD8^+$ T cells. Following successful levamisole therapy, there is elevation in $CD8^+$ T-cell number, but if therapy is clinically unsuccessful the number of $CD8^+$ cells remains low.

Formulations and dose rates

Levamisole is the levoenantiomer of the synthetic anthelmintic tetramisole and is most widely available as levamisole hydrochloride. As levamisole is not currently licensed for companion animal use, the forms of the drug most commonly administered to dogs and cats are those produced for large animal purposes – either an oral bolus, an oral solution or an injectable solution (e.g. Levadin®, Vetoquinol). The difficulty in accurately breaking the bolus makes this form more suitable for larger dogs, whereas for smaller companion animals oral administration of the injectable or oral solutions is the method of choice.

- A range of dosages is reported for the use of levamisole as an adjunct immunostimulant in the dog, but those most commonly quoted are 2.2 mg/kg PO every other day, or 0.5–2.0 mg/kg PO given three times per week. It has been suggested that dosage out of this range may cause immunosuppression rather than enhancement
- In the therapy of canine SLE, oral levamisole is administered at 2.0–5.0 mg/kg (to a maximum of 150 mg per dog) on alternate days, concurrently with prednisolone at 0.5–1.0 mg/kg q.12 h. The prednisolone is tapered and eliminated over 1–2 months, whereas levamisole is continued at the same dose for a 4-month period. If an animal undergoes disease relapse, treatment with levamisole alone for 4 months is recommended
- In the cat, the reported immunomodulatory dose of levamisole is again variable, but one regimen uses the drug at 25 mg/cat PO q.24 h for three doses only

Pharmacokinetics

Levamisole is rapidly absorbed from the gut and becomes widely distributed throughout the body, with peak plasma levels obtained in 1–2 h. The plasma elimination half-life in the dog is 2–4 h and the majority (95%) of the drug is metabolized in the liver and excreted in urine (primarily) and feces.

Adverse effects

- In the dog: lethargy, vomiting, diarrhea, panting, shaking, agitation, behavioral changes, hemolytic anemia, agranulocytosis, dyspnea, pulmonary edema and cutaneous drug eruption (particularly of the erythema multiforme–toxic epidermal necrolysis spectrum).
- In the cat: hypersalivation, excitement, mydriasis and vomiting.

Contraindications and precautions

- Levamisole should not be given to lactating animals or to animals that are debilitated or have marked impairment of renal or hepatic function.
- There is no information regarding the safety of the drug in pregnant companion animals. However, no embryotoxicity or teratogenicity was noted in continuous feeding studies of pregnant rats, rabbits or pigs.

Known drug interactions

The toxic effects may be enhanced by the use of concurrent cholinesterase inhibitors (e.g. neostigmine, organophosphates) or nicotine-like agents (e.g. diethylcarbamazine).

Muramyl tripeptide

Clinical applications

Muramyl tripeptide is a derivative of the cell wall of *Mycobacterium* spp that acts on monocyte-macrophages, causing enhanced release of proinflammatory cytokines and cytotoxic function of these cells. The agent has been incorporated into liposomes (muramyl tripeptide phosphatidyl-ethanolamine) and used in several studies to treat canine patients with osteosarcoma, hemangiosarcoma and malignant melanoma. In these studies muramyl tripeptide was used as an adjunct to surgery and chemotherapy and appeared to reduce the prevalence of metastasis and enhance survival time. By contrast, in studies of canine and feline mammary adenocarcinoma, administration of liposome-encapsulated muramyl tripeptide did not enhance survival time of affected animals.

Recombinant cytokines

Cytokines are a key regulatory component of the immune system that may be involved in the activation or suppression of an immune response (see Fig. 12.1). Those cytokines that positively influence immune effector mechanisms are logical candidates for therapeutic application in immunosuppressed patients. Knowledge of the molecular sequence of cytokine molecules enables preparation of commercial quantities of recombinant cytokines and such products are now routinely employed in human medicine.

Although sequence data for numerous canine and feline cytokines are published and some recombinant dog and cat cytokines have been produced, there is only one licensed product for companion animal use (Virbagen Omega®, see below). However, the close sequence homology between some human and companion animal cytokines has historically enabled the clinical use of recombinant human (rHu) cytokines in veterinary species.

Although profound effects are often reported following the administration of rHu cytokines, these molecules still bear a degree of antigenic dissimilarity to those of the dog or cat, permitting recipient animals to mount an anti-rHu cytokine antibody response. The onset of this antibody response not only neutralizes any therapeutically administered rHu cytokine, but the antibodies can also bind to and neutralize the activity of the corresponding endogenous cytokine. For this reason, administration of rHu cytokines to animals is generally only of short-term benefit, although regimens have been developed that minimize the onset of the anticytokine response. Such responses are not engendered when endogenous canine or feline recombinant cytokines are administered.

Granulocyte colony-stimulating factor (G-CSF)

The effect of G-CSF is to enhance bone marrow granulopoiesis, so this molecule has clinical application to animals with neutropenia induced by:

- infection (e.g. canine ehrlichiosis or parvovirus, FeLV, FIV)
- myelosuppressive drugs used in chemotherapy
- bone marrow lymphoid neoplasia or myeloproliferative disease
- bone marrow immune-mediated aplasia.

rHuG-CSF (Neupogen®, 300 μg/mL solution for injection) can induce neutrophilia in the dog and cat, which reaches a maximum level on days 10–14 of therapy. Neutralizing antibodies to the human molecule develop after 21 days (in normal dogs and cats, but probably not in those undergoing intensive chemotherapy), so treatment beyond this time is inadvisable as profound neutropenia may occur.

A range of dosage regimens is reported for treatment of neutropenia associated with chemotherapy, including 10–100 μg/kg q.24 h SC in the dog and 3–10 μg/kg q.12 h SC in the cat. There is some evidence that rHuG-CSF can modify neutrophil counts in puppies with parvovirus infection, but this cytokine did not elevate blood neutrophil levels in cats with panleukopenia.

There are a number of published studies that have investigated use of the recombinant canine molecule (rCaG-CSF). When administered to healthy dogs (5 μg/kg q.24 h SC for 4 weeks) there was rapid elevation of blood neutrophil count 24 h after the first injection and this peaked on day 19. There was an additional monocytosis, but leukocyte counts returned to normal levels 5 d after cessation of therapy. No toxicity was observed.

rCaG-CSF has been administered to dogs with cyclic hematopoiesis (up to 2.5 μg/kg q.12 h) and was shown to prevent neutropenia and the associated clinical signs in these patients, without totally eliminating the cycling of neutrophils.

rCaG-CSF (daily for 20 d) was able to prevent neutropenia in normal dogs given the myelosuppressive agent mitoxantrone (or mitozantrone – British Approved Name) and therefore has application in the prevention of neutropenia associated with chemotherapy. Canine G-CSF has also been administered to normal cats (5 μg/kg q.24 h SC for 42 d) with marked neutrophilia developing 24 h after the first injection and persisting for the duration of treatment. No adverse effects were recorded in these cats and no antibody was produced to the canine protein. Administration of rCaG-CSF to cats with Chédiak–Higashi syndrome enhanced neutrophil number and function.

Fewer investigations have been performed with recombinant granulocyte-macrophage colony-stimulating factor (GM-CSF). rHuGM-CSF induces neutrophilia, monocytosis, eosinophilia and thrombocytopenia in normal dogs and can ameliorate the effects of total body irradiation on bone marrow hematopoiesis. rCaGM-CSF has similar effects on leukocyte and platelet numbers in normal dogs but is less effective than the human product in counteracting the bone marrow effects of total body irradiation.

Interferon-α

A number of studies have examined the potential benefit of administration of rHuIFN-α (Roferon®) to cats. In one study of experimental FeLV infection, oral administration (generally given at 30 U/cat q.24 h on a 1-week-on, 1-week-off cycle) was shown to ameliorate the clinical course of disease (but not viremia) and there are anecdotal reports of efficacy in managing the clinical effects of spontaneously arising FeLV, FIV and FIP infections. It is presumed that the agent has a localized effect on oropharyngeal lymphoid tissue, as there is poor systemic absorption following oral administration.

rHuIFN-α has also been administered SC at high dose (10 U/kg q.24 h for 8 d, then alternate days for another 2–3 weeks) to cats experimentally infected with FIP virus. Treated cats had suppression of clinical signs and serum antibody levels, with a small increase in survival times. Similar beneficial effects were reported in FeLV-infected cats given combined rHuIFN-α and AZT.

As for other human recombinant products, neutralizing antibodies are induced after several weeks (with SC but not oral therapy) and the cats become refractory to therapy.

Interferon-ω

Interferon-ω is a type I interferon that is related to interferon-α. A recombinant version of feline interferon-ω has been produced commercially (Virbagen Omega®, Virbac Ltd) and is licensed in Europe for specific indications in the dog and cat.

Clinical applications

Virbagen Omega® is licensed for therapeutic use in dogs (over 1 month of age) with enteric parvovirus infection and is claimed to be able to reduce mortality and clinical signs in such cases. In the cat, Virbagen Omega® is licensed for the treatment of FeLV and FIV infections. When administered to cats during the symptomatic (but nonterminal phase) of these infections, the product claims to reduce the clinical signs and mortality associated with infection. Although not licensed for other applications, the use of Virbagen Omega® has been investigated in cats with upper respiratory tract calicivirus infection (and chronic gingivostomatitis), herpesvirus infection (and keratoconjunctivitis) or feline infectious peritonitis virus infection. The use of this product has also been examined in noninfectious disease (e.g. canine atopic dermatitis) but no clear benefits have been proven.

Mechanism of action

The precise mode of action of Virbagen Omega® is not described but in general, type I interferons bind to surface receptors expressed by a range of cells (both virally infected and noninfected) and trigger an intracellular signaling pathway resulting in gene transcription of host cell proteins that inhibit viral replication within infected cells, upregulate expression of molecules involved in antigen presentation (class I molecules of the major histocompatibility complex) and activate NK cells to destroy virally infected cells through cytotoxic mechanisms.

Formulations and dose rates

Virbagen Omega® comes as a vial containing 10 million units (MU) of lyophilized recombinant interferon-ω. Solvent for resuspension of the lyophilizate into a 1 mL volume is provided. For dogs with parvoviral enteritis, a dose of 2.5 MU/kg is injected intravenously each day for 3 d. For cats with retroviral infection, a dose of 1 MU/kg is injected subcutaneously once daily (starting on day 0) for d. This 5-d treatment is then repeated from day 14 and again from day 60.

Adverse effects

- Transient hyperthermia 3–6 h after injection.
- Vomiting.
- Mild leukopenia, thrombocytopenia and anemia that revert to normal within 1 week after the last injection.
- Mild elevation in alanine aminotransferase that reverts to normal within 1 week after the last injection.
- Soft feces to mild diarrhea in cats only.
- Transient fatigue during treatment in cats only.

Animals receiving Virbagen Omega® should not be vaccinated during or after therapy until the animal is clinically normal. The safety of the agent has not been established in pregnant or lactating animals. In humans treated with multiple doses of type I interferon, autoimmune diseases have occasionally been recognized. This has not yet been reported in animals but remains a consideration. If this product is administered intravenously to cats there is a greater frequency of adverse effects (including hyperthermia, soft feces, anorexia, decreased drinking and collapse).

Known drug interactions

There is no specific information available on drug interactions. Animals treated with this product are likely to receive a range of therapeutics (e.g. antibiotics, fluids, vitamins, nonsteroidal anti-inflammatory drugs) which should be used cautiously after appropriate risk : benefit analysis.

Special considerations

Special care should be taken by those administering this product. If accidentally self-injected, medical assistance should be sought immediately.

Interleukin-2

Recombinant human interleukin-2 (rHuIL-2) has been administered as adjunct therapy (with surgical resection and/or chemotherapy) to dogs with neoplastic disease in order to enhance the endogenous antitumor immune response. Patients with a range of tumors have been studied, but greatest promise came from sequential administration of rHuTNF and rHuIL-2 to dogs with oral melanoma or mast cell tumors. rHuIL-2 has been administered by IV or SC injection, or by nebulization of IL-2 or liposomes containing IL-2 in an attempt to reduce the formation of pulmonary metastases.

Recent studies have shown that injected cDNA encoding the IL-2 sequence localizes to the lung and transfects pulmonary cells that subsequently produce IL-2. rHuIL-2 has been coadministered with rHuIFN-α to cats with FeLV-induced disease, but the clinical response was disappointing.

Adverse effects of IV infusion of rHuIL-2 into dogs include vomiting, diarrhea and lethargy. Adjunct IL-2 gene therapy has been performed in the dog by intratumoral injection of an IL-2 gene transfected cell line, or adenoviral vector containing IL-2 cDNA. Although these procedures show clinical promise, there is a range of reported side effects.

MISCELLANEOUS AGENTS REPORTED TO HAVE IMMUNOSTIMULATORY ACTIVITY

Regressin-V

Regressin-V is a mixture of components derived from the cell wall of *Mycobacterium* that has been used as an adjunct immune stimulant (given before surgery) in bitches with mammary neoplasia. The suggested effects of this agent are to enhance T-cell activation and proinflammatory cytokine release from macrophages.

Serratia marcescens

An extract of *Serratia marcescens* has the ability to induce myelostimulation and to activate macrophages with release of proinflammatory cytokines. The agent has been shown to reduce the myelosuppression caused by administration of doxorubicin to dogs and to enhance the synthesis of endogenous G-CSF measured several hours after administration.

Staphage lysate

Clinical applications

Staphage lysate is a bacterin prepared by bacteriophage lysis of human-origin *Staphylococcus aureus*. Staphage lysate has been given as adjunct therapy to dogs with idiopathic recurrent superficial pyoderma but has not been extensively evaluated in cases of deep pyoderma. Treatment has been shown to be beneficial in up to 70% of cases of superficial pyoderma.

Mechanism of action

The objective of administration is to enhance the host immune response to *Staphylococcus* spp; however, repeated injection of staphage lysate does not lead to elevated levels of serum antibody specific for *S. intermedius* antigens in dogs with superficial pyoderma.

Formulations and dose rates

- One suggested dosage regimen is to administer staphage lysate, concurrently with appropriate antibiotics, at 0.5 mL twice weekly for 6 weeks by SC injection. Following cessation of antibiotics, staphage lysate monotherapy is continued for a further 4–8 weeks
- In order to maintain remission, intermittent administration of staphage lysate may be required thereafter

Adverse effects

- Local injection site reactions
- Pyrexia
- Lethargy
- Vomiting

Staphoid AB

Clinical applications

Staphoid AB is a bacterin preparation that contains a mixture of *Staphylococcus aureus* cell wall antigen, together with α- and β-toxins. This agent is marketed in some countries for the prevention of staphylococcal mastitis in cows and has been evaluated in canine pyoderma, but appears less efficacious than staphage lysate.

Formulations and dose rates

The suggested dosage regimen involves administration of increasing increments given by a combination of intradermal and SC injection over a 5-d period (total dose 0.25 mL on day 1, increasing to 1.25 mL on day 5), then weekly for 3 weeks (increasing from 1.5 to 2.0 mL) and monthly (2.0 mL doses) thereafter.

Adverse effects

- Injection site reactions
- Pyrexia
- Lethargy

FUTURE IMMUNOTHERAPY

The future of immunomodulatory therapy clearly lies in targeted immunotherapy, which will very specifically alter a single immunological parameter without blanket immunosuppression or other adverse effects that characterize administration of many of the pharmacological agents that are the mainstream of veterinary immunomodulation today. There are currently many experimental approaches that are starting to transfer into clinical practice in human medicine. These are too numerous to review in detail here, but selected examples might include the following.

- **Peptide immunotherapy for autoimmune or allergic disease.** In this instance a specific peptide derived from an autoantigen or allergen is delivered to the immune system via a novel route (e.g. by the oral or intranasal route, perhaps linked to a new-generation 'mucosal adjuvant'). By mechanisms that are not fully understood (but probably involve induction of specific regulatory T-cell populations), presentation of this peptide antigen is often able to selectively 'disarm' those autoreactive or allergen-specific T lymphocytes that are the cause of disease, yet leave intact those T cells that are involved in 'appropriate' immune responses to pathogens.
- **Cytokine gene therapy.** Examples of the use of gene therapy are already to be found within the veterinary literature. In this approach, genes encoding specific regulatory cytokines may be delivered to a specific site in the body, either as a 'naked' plasmid or incorporated into a cellular vector. The localized synthesis of cytokines that ensues can specifically direct the nature of the local immune response (e.g. to a tumor, within a site of inflammation such as the synovium of an arthritic animal or to a vaccine within regional draining lymphoid tissue).
- **Monoclonal antibody therapy,** using monoclonal antibodies that have been synthetically constructed to avoid immunogenicity in the host animal. Monoclonal antibodies may be used to selectively block or enhance molecular interactions between immune cells, to neutralize cytokine activity, or to act as 'delivery vehicles' for a range of toxins, cytokines or prodrugs to specific cells (e.g. neoplastic) expressing epitopes recognized by the antibodies.

FURTHER READING

Affolter VK, Moore PF 2000 Canine cutaneous and systemic histiocytosis: reactive histiocytosis of dermal dendritic cells. Am J Dermatopath 22: 40-48

Amatori FM, Meucci V, Giusiani M et al 2004 Effect of grapefruit juice on the pharmacokinetics of cyclosporine in dogs. Vet Rec 154: 180-181

Beale KM 1988 Azathioprine for treatment of immune-mediated diseases of dogs and cats. JAVMA 192: 1316-1318

Bernsteen L, Gregory CR, Kyles AE et al 2003 Microemulsified cyclosporine-based immunosuppression for the prevention of acute renal allograft rejection in unrelated dogs: preliminary experimental study. Vet Surg 32: 213-219

Day MJ 1999 Immunotherapy. In: Day MJ (ed.) Clinical immunology of the dog and cat. Manson Publishing, London, pp 266-277

Day MJ 2005 Immunotherapy. In: Hillier A, Foster AP, Kwochka KW (eds) Advances in veterinary dermatology, volume 5. Blackwell Publishing, Oxford, pp 107-122

DeMari K, Maynard L, Eun HM, Lebreux B 2003 Treatment of canine parvoviral enteritis with interferon omega in a placebo-controlled field trial. Vet Rec 152: 105-108

DeMari K, Maynard L, Sanquer A et al 2004 Therapeutic effects of recombinant feline interferon-omega on feline leukaemia virus (FeLV)-infected and FeLV/feline immunodeficiency virus (FIV)-coinfected symptomatic cats. J Vet Intern Med 18: 477-482

Foster AP 2004 Immunomodulation and immunodeficiency. Vet Dermatol 15: 115-126

Foster AP, Shaw SE, Duley JA, Shobowale-Bakre E-M, Harbour DA 2000 Demonstration of thiopurine methyltransferase activity in the erythrocytes of cats. J Vet Intern Med 14: 552-554

Gauguere E, Steffan J, Olivry T 2004 Cyclosporin A: a new drug in the field of canine dermatology. Vet Dermatol 15: 61-74

Gregory CR, Stewart A, Sturges B et al 1998 Leflunomide effectively treats naturally occurring immune-mediated and inflammatory diseases of dogs that are unresponsive to conventional therapy. Transplant Proc 30: 4143-4148

Grundy SA, Barton C 2001 Influence of drug treatment on survival of dogs with immune-mediated hemolytic anemia: 88 cases (1989–1999). JAVMA 218: 543-546

Kruth SA 1998 Biological response modifiers: interferons, interleukins, recombinant products, liposomal products. Vet Clin North Am Small Anim Pract 28: 269-295

Larche M, Wraith DC 2005 Peptide-based therapeutic vaccines for allergic and autoimmune diseases. Nature Med 11: S69-S76

Marsella R, Olivry T 2001 The ACVD task force on canine atopic dermatitis (XXII): nonsteroidal anti-inflammatory pharmacotherapy. Vet Immunol Immunopathol 81: 331-345

Marsella R, Nicklin CF, Saglio S, Lopez J 2004 Investigation on the clinical efficacy and safety of 0.1% tacrolimus ointment (Protopic®) in canine atopic dermatitis: a randomized, double-blinded, placebo-controlled, cross-over study. Vet Dermatol 15: 294-303

Mathews KA, Sukhiani HR 1997 Randomized controlled trial of cyclosporine for treatment of perianal fistulas in dogs. JAVMA 211: 1249-1253

Mathews KA, Holmberg DL, Miller CW 2000 Kidney transplantation in dogs with naturally occurring endstage renal disease. J Am Anim Health Assoc 36: 294-301

Mouatt JG 2002 Cyclosporin and ketoconazole interaction for treatment of perianal fistulas in the dog. Aust Vet J 80: 207-211

Nabel GJ 1999 A transformed view of cyclosporine. Nature 397: 471-472

Nichols PR, Morris DO, Beale KM 2001 A retrospective study of canine and feline cutaneous vasculitis. Vet Dermatol 12: 255-264

Olivry T, Rivierre C, Jackson HA et al 2002 Cyclosporine decreases skin lesions and pruritus in dogs with atopic dermatitis: a blinded randomized prednisolone-controlled trial. Vet Dermatol 13: 77-87

Radowicz SN, Power HT 2005 Long-term use of cyclosporine in the treatment of canine atopic dermatitis. Vet Dermatol 16: 81-86

Read RA 1995 Treatment of canine nictitans plasmacytic conjunctivitis with 0.2 per cent cyclosporin ointment. J Small Anim Pract 36: 50-56

Rinkhardt NE, Kruth SA, Kaushik A 1999 The effects of prednisone and azathioprine on circulating immunoglobulin levels and lymphocyte subpopulations in normal dogs. Can J Vet Res 63: 18-24

Rosenkrantz WS 2004 Pemphigus: current therapy. Vet Dermatol 15: 90-98

Salvaggione OE, Kidd L, Prondzinski JL et al 2002 Canine red blood cell thiopurine S-methyltransferase: companion animal pharmacogenetics. Pharmacogenetics 12: 713-724

Salvaggione OE, Yang C, Kidd LB et al 2004 Cat red blood cell thiopurine S-methyltransferase: companion animal pharmacogenetics. J Pharmacol Exp Therapeut 308: 617-626

Scott-Moncrieff JC, Reagan WJ, Synder PW, Glickman LT 1997 Intravenous administration of human immune globulin in dogs with immune-mediated hemolytic anemia. JAVMA 210: 1623-1627

Steffan J, Alexander D, Brovedani F, Fisch RD 2003 Comparison of cyclosporine A with methylprednisolone for treatment of canine atopic dermatitis: a parallel, blinded, randomized controlled trial. Vet Dermatol 14: 11-22

Nonsteroidal anti-inflammatory drugs and chondroprotective agents

Peter D Hanson and Jill E Maddison

Nonsteroidal anti-inflammatory drugs (NSAIDs) are nonnarcotic agents that have analgesic, anti-inflammatory and antipyretic activity. NSAIDs are classified by their chemical structure as well as by their specific inhibitory activity for enzymes associated with eicosanoid production (e.g. production of prostaglandins, prostacyclins, thromboxanes, leukotrienes, lipoxins, etc.). With greater understanding of the importance of managing pain in small animal practice, NSAID use has continued to increase. NSAIDs are widely prescribed for the control of pain and inflammation associated with osteoarthritis, trauma and surgery. They have advantages over narcotic analgesics in that they do not produce sedation or ataxia and allow more rapid recovery from anesthesia. In situations where greater analgesia is required (e.g. orthopedic surgery), NSAIDs may be combined with narcotic analgesics. Such a multimodal approach may allow reduction of the narcotic dose, thereby reducing the sedation observed with the narcotic alone.

The safety of NSAIDs is reasonably well understood. There is some variation in the side effect profiles for the various NSAIDs based on their specific mechanisms of action. As a class, the most common side effects are gastrointestinal, renal and hepatic. Additionally, some NSAIDs affect platelet activity and may prolong bleeding times. There is considerable species variation with NSAIDs regarding enzyme specificity, pharmacokinetics, metabolism and safety profile. Consequently, appropriate patient selection and monitoring must be considered when choosing a NSAID.

Clinical applications

Many NSAIDs are approved by regulatory agencies around the world for use in small animal practice. The majority are approved for use in dogs and only a few for use in cats. Oral and parenteral formulations are commonly available. Where an approved product exists for a given indication and species, it should be used preferentially over an unapproved product.

- The most common approved NSAID indications are for the management of noninfectious/nonallergic inflammatory disorders to control pain and inflammation associated with osteoarthritis, trauma and surgery.

A number of other uses of NSAIDs have also developed. Although these indications have not been subjected to regulatory review, they are based on the broad anti-inflammatory activity of NSAIDs use in other species and often supported by published literature for the target species.

- NSAIDs that inhibit cyclo-oxygenase-2 (COX-2) have activity against certain tumors that depend on COX-2 activity directly or indirectly. The original work involved piroxicam used alone or with platinoid therapy (e.g. cisplatin) to treat transitional cell carcinoma (TCC) of the urinary bladder in dogs. Subsequent work with TCC and other tumors (e.g. osteosarcoma, melanoma, squamous cell sarcoma) has included deracoxib, firocoxib and meloxicam.
- The ability of some NSAIDs to reduce platelet aggregation is exploited in canine medicine by the use of aspirin to reduce the potential for thromboembolus formation. Aspirin is also used in cats with hypertrophic cardiomyopathy to reduce the potential for thrombus formation and where a saddle thrombus of the aorta or iliac arteries has been diagnosed.
- NSAIDs are being used more frequently in ophthalmology for conditions such as keratitis and scleritis. Following topical application, they do not inhibit re-epithelialization of the cornea. Both flunixin and phenylbutazone have been used systemically in the management of nonulcerative kerato-uveitis and corneal ulceration in the horse and may have similar applications in the dog. Systemic use of firocoxib and meloxicam is being investigated by ophthalmologists in this area as well.
- Preoperative aspirin treatment may be of value in dogs undergoing intraocular surgery, as it may minimize the postoperative increase in protein content of the aqueous humor. Flunixin and dexamethasone have been reported to act synergistically in inhibiting postoperative aqueous humor protein increases. However, the potential adverse drug interaction that may occur should be carefully considered before using this drug combination.

- NSAIDs are used in the management of some immunological diseases such as systemic lupus and rheumatoid arthritis because of their anti-inflammatory effects. However, research indicates that NSAIDs may have a more direct effect in these diseases by stimulating T-suppressor cells in their action against T-helper cells and autoantibody-producing B cells.
- NSAIDs appear to have a role in the management of endotoxic shock, as plasma concentrations of prostaglandins, thromboxane and prostacyclin are increased and are thought to contribute to the decreased cardiac output, blood pressure, oxygen tension and acidosis that occurs. However, if therapy is to be effective it must be administered either prior to or immediately after the onset of endotoxemia in conjunction with other supportive therapy.
- NSAIDs are used as antipyretic agents in cattle and other species. Because of this, they are used in cats with high fevers and to a lesser extent in dogs.

Mechanism of action

The mechanism of action of NSAIDs includes inhibition of several mediators of inflammation in the arachidonic acid cascade (Fig. 13.1). Eicosanoids are formed from arachidonic acid by the action of COX and lipoxygenase (LOX). COX activity leads to production of prostaglandins, prostacyclins and thromboxanes, whereas LOX activity leads to production of leukotrienes and lipoxins.

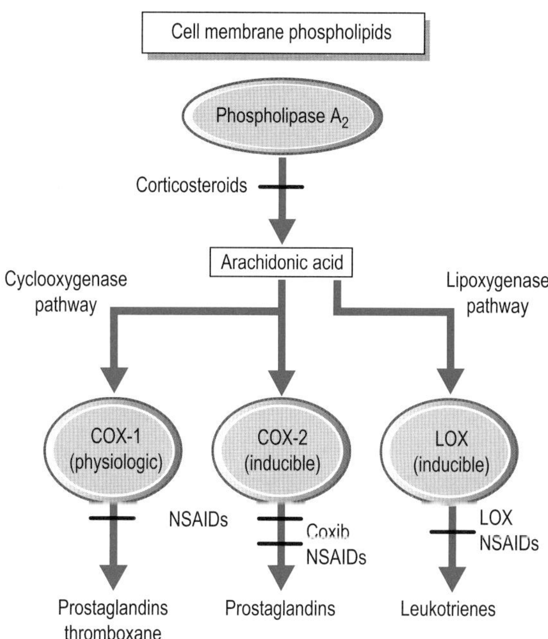

Fig. 13.1 Simplified illustration of the arachidonic acid cascade. Corticosteroids act by inhibiting the activity of phospholipase A_2, thereby preventing the formation of arachidonic acid. NSAIDs act by inhibiting components of the cyclo-oxygenase and lipoxygenase pathways. Within the cyclo-oxygenase pathway, activity may be selective or nonselective for COX-1 and COX-2.

It is currently understood that prostaglandin synthesis is catalyzed by at least two forms of cyclo-oxygenase: COX-1 and COX-2. COX is present in all cells except mature blood cells. However, the distribution of COX activity between and within tissues is very heterogenous. COX-1 is constitutively expressed and enzymatically active in a variety of tissues, including the stomach, intestine, kidneys and platelets. COX-1 activity is primarily physiological, including gastric mucosal protection, renal blood flow and vascular hemostasis. In some situations, COX-1 may have inflammatory activity, but this is not its predominant function. COX-2 expression is primarily induced by mediators such as serum growth factors, cytokines and mitogens. COX-2 activity is primarily associated with pathological processes (pain, inflammation and fever). COX-2 has some physiological activity related to maintenance of renal blood flow, reproduction and cell signaling, but its activity is most evident with inflammation.

Recently a third cyclo-oxygenase, COX-3, has been reported. Although COX-3 is described as the product of a splice variant of COX-1 and it may constitute the centrally mediated mechanism of action for paracetamol (acetaminophen), its exact role remains unclear. There is evidence that additional COX variants will be delineated in the future.

The other major products of arachidonic acid metabolism are the leukotriene series, the production of which is mediated by the enzyme LOX, found in lungs, platelets and white blood cells. It has been hypothesized that NSAIDs are less efficacious as anti-inflammatory agents than glucocorticosteroids because precursor mediators of inflammation are free to enter the lipoxygenase pathway and still produce inflammation. Although it is claimed that some NSAIDs, such as ketoprofen, also inhibit lipoxygenase in vitro, this effect tends to be species and tissue dependent and has not been demonstrated with clinical dose rates in vivo. Newer dual COX/LOX inhibitors have been studied for human application, with one, tepoxalin, entering the veterinary market. Still, there is no evidence to date that such drugs have greater clinical efficacy and safety than pure COX inhibitors.

Prostaglandins and inflammation

Prostaglandins and leukotrienes do not cause pain directly but both cause hyperalgesia. Hyperalgesia is a pain response to stimuli that are not normally painful, induced by the lowering of the nociceptor threshold level. Prostaglandins act as mediators of inflammation and amplify nociceptive input and transmission to the spinal cord via sensory afferents in the peripheral nerves. They also have a powerful effect on spinal nociceptive processing by facilitating firing of central neurones and augmenting neurotransmitter release from primary spinal sensory afferents.

Prostaglandins, in particular PGE_2, sensitize receptors on afferent nerve endings to agents that do cause pain, e.g. bradykinin, serotonin and histamine. PGE_2 is a potent pyretic agent, a potent dilator of vascular smooth muscle and its production is stimulated by interleukin-1 released in response to bacterial and viral infections.

Cyclo-oxygenase

COX catalyzes the first two steps in the biosynthesis of the prostaglandins from arachidonic acid to form PGG_2 which is then acted on by various enzymes to produce the prostanoids; prostacyclin synthetase produces prostacyclin (PGI_2), thromboxane synthetase produces thromboxane and prostaglandin isomerase produces PGE_2 and PGF_2 as well as other prostaglandins.

Arachidonic acid is a 20-carbon unsaturated fatty acid component of cell phospholipids and is synthesized from the essential dietary fatty acids linoleic and linolenic acid. When membranes are damaged, endogenous peptides called lipocortins are released, which activate phospholipase A_2. This release is initiated by stimuli that damage or distort the cell membrane, such as infection, trauma, fever or platelet aggregation. Arachidonic acid is released from membrane phospholipids through the action of phospholipase A_2 and C. When released, arachidonic acid enters the opening of the cyclo-oxygenase enzyme channel, where it is oxygenated and a free radical extracted. The result is the cyclic five-carbon structure that characterizes the prostaglandins.

As noted above, there are two main isoforms of cyclo-oxygenase: COX-1 and COX-2. Both isoforms of the enzyme consist of a long narrow channel with a hairpin bend at the end. In humans, COX-2 has a substitution of valine for an isoleucine present in COX-1. This creates a conformational change in the COX-2 enzyme channel, making it wider. NSAIDs that inhibit COX do so by blocking the enzyme channel and preventing the activation of arachidonic acid. Nonselective NSAIDs, those that inhibit both COX-1 and COX-2, have a narrower conformation, allowing them to occupy and block either enzyme channel. Those that are selective for COX-2 have a broader configuration, allowing them to readily block the COX-2 channel but less effectively enter the COX-1 channel.

There are notable differences in the kinetics of binding of NSAIDs to COX-1 and COX-2. COX-1 inhibition involves hydrogen bonding, is instantaneous and is generally competitively reversible. Even so, effects may be irreversible, such as with aspirin that induces an acetylation in the COX-1 binding channel and irreversibly inactivates platelet COX-1. COX-2 inhibition may involve covalent binding and may result in a conformational change. It is time dependent and is slowly to nonreversible.

Cyclo-oxygenase selectivity

With identification that cyclo-oxygenase consists of COX-1 and COX-2 and indication that the major activity of COX-1 is constitutive and that of COX-2 is inflammatory, considerable interest arose to identify compounds that were selective for the COX-2 isoenzyme. Starting with NSAIDs used in human medicine, the selectivity of the compounds for COX-1 and COX-2 was determined. This was followed by retrospective evaluation of the incidence of adverse effects, primarily gastrointestinal, associated with each compound. It was observed that NSAIDs with greater COX-1 selectivity had higher rates of gastrointestinal toxicity. Consequently, COX-1 selectivity became a surrogate marker for NSAID safety and the search centered on finding NSAIDs that had greater COX-2 selectivity, or less COX-1 activity, at therapeutic ranges. Although the correlative data for this are reasonably sound and serve as a starting point for compound selection, the safety and efficacy of a compound depend on many factors and can only be established through appropriately designed clinical studies with the compound in the target species.

The selectivity for inhibition of COX is the ratio of the effects of inhibition of COX-1 and COX-2 for a given NSAID. It is often calculated as the ratio of the amount of drug necessary to inhibit 50% (i.e. the inhibitory concentration 50 or IC_{50}) for each enzyme. A COX-1/COX-2 IC_{50} ratio that is less than one (<1) signifies a drug that is nonselective or selective for COX-1. Conversely, a COX-1/COX-2 IC_{50} ratio greater than one (>1) indicates a drug is selective for COX-2 (Table 13.1). (NB: some papers invert the ratio and express it as COX-2/COX-1. Then a ratio less than 1 is COX-2 selective and a ratio greater than 1 is COX-1 selective.) This has been further refined by some to define a nonspecific COX inhibitor as one with no meaningful or clinical differences in COX-1 or COX-2 inhibition. A preferential COX-2 inhibitor is 2–100-fold more selective for COX-2. Such a drug has analgesic and anti-inflammatory activity at doses that inhibit COX-2 but not COX-1. However, some COX-1 inhibition is possible at elevated or therapeutic dosages. A specific COX-2 inhibitor is more than 100-fold selective for COX-2 and has no COX-1 activity across a wide dosage range. A point that is frequently confused is that a specific COX-2 inhibitor does not necessarily inhibit COX-2 any more than a nonspecific COX inhibitor. Rather, it inhibits COX-2 at high levels while not inhibiting COX-1.

Table 13.1 COX selectivity for approved[a] veterinary NSAIDs listed in approximate order of increasing selectivity for COX-2. Data are based on the ratio of IC_{50} values for inhibition of COX-1/COX-2

NSAID	Trade name	Canine whole-blood assay	Cell line assay (various sources)
Dipyrone	Generic	No data	No data
Ketoprofen	Ketofen® and generic	0.2	0.06–0.15
Vedaprofen	Quadrisol®	0.26	No data
Tepoxalin	Zubrin®	No data	0.1–1.0
Phenylbutazone	Generic	0.6	2.6
Tolfenamic acid	Generic	No data	15.0
Meclofenamic acid	Arquel®	No data	15.4
Flunixin meglumine	Banamine® and generic	1.5	0.64
Indometacin	Generic	4.0	No data
Etodolac	Etogesic®	4.2	0.5–3.4
Meloxicam	Metacam®	2.1–10	2.9
Carprofen	Rimadyl® and generic	6.5–15	65–129
Deracoxib	Deramaxx®	12–36.5	1275
Firocoxib	Previcox®	380	1938

[a] NSAIDs listed are approved in various markets and may not be available in all countries.
Data from Brideau et al (AJVR 2001;62:1755-1760); Haven et al (Proc ACVIM 1998); Li et al (Bioorg Med Chem Lett 2004;14:95-98); McCann et al (AJVR 2004;65:503-512); Ricketts et al (AJVR 1998;59:1441-1446); Schering-Plough monograph.

Although simple in concept, interpretation of selectivity data is complicated by biology. The results of studies of the relative selectivity of different NSAIDs for COX-1 and COX-2 vary markedly depending on the tissue used in the assay system, the assay method itself and the species from which the test cells were derived. Results from in vitro assays often use cell lines that overexpress the enzymes. These may be tumor cells, cloned cells or cells from other species, etc. Such assay systems are most useful for screening 'relative' selectivity of a drug for the enzymes, but they may not be physiologically relevant.

Use of the whole-blood assay for the target species has become the gold standard for COX selectivity. In this approach, drug at varying concentrations is incubated with whole blood from the target species. The blood is allowed to clot and the inhibitory effects on production of thromboxane, TxB_2, are used to assess COX-1 activity. A similar set of samples is incubated with lipopolysaccharide and the inhibitory effects on production of PGE_2 are used to assess COX-2 activity (Fig. 13.2). COX activity may still vary within a species in different tissues (e.g. whole blood vs gastrointestinal vs synovial). Still, the whole blood assay is a more physiological model than most cell lines and retains utility as the gold standard for comparing NSAID activity.

Another point of discussion regarding selectivity is whether the COX-1/COX-2 ratios are based on the IC_{50} values, IC_{80} values or a combination of the COX-1 IC_{20} value relative to the COX-2 IC_{80} value. Recall that the IC_{50} values indicate a drug's ability to inhibit 50% of the enzyme. Use of IC_{50} values is a standard approach for assessing enzyme activity. However, reports suggest that peak analgesic and anti-inflammatory activity occur when COX-2 is inhibited by more than 80% (i.e. the IC_{80}). Similarly, there is suggestion that gastrointestinal side effects are more frequent when COX-1 is inhibited by more than 10–20% (i.e. the IC_{10} or IC_{20}). A further complication associated with COX inhibition data is that not all compounds have similar slopes to the inhibition curves. Point data, such as the IC_{50} ratio or IC_{80} ratio, do not give an indication of this slope. A compound with a steep slope would have a narrow concentration range to go from no enzyme inhibition to maximal inhibition. Conversely, a flatter slope would indicate that a change in enzyme inhibition requires a relatively greater change in drug concentration. This slope information has potential utility in understanding the therapeutic range associated with efficacy and safety of a compound.

To summarize the use of COX selectivity assays, a few key points may be made.

- The current standard for comparing drugs and their COX selectivity is the whole-blood assay using blood from the species of interest.
- Only compare drugs based on assessment with the same assay method, regardless of which method was used.
- Do not extrapolate results for one species to another. They may be similar but they may also be quite different.
- Consider efficacy and safety data from clinical studies in addition to COX selectivity data.

Although preferential COX-2 inhibition appears to be an important factor in improving the safety of NSAIDs, this is not the only consideration. Other factors that

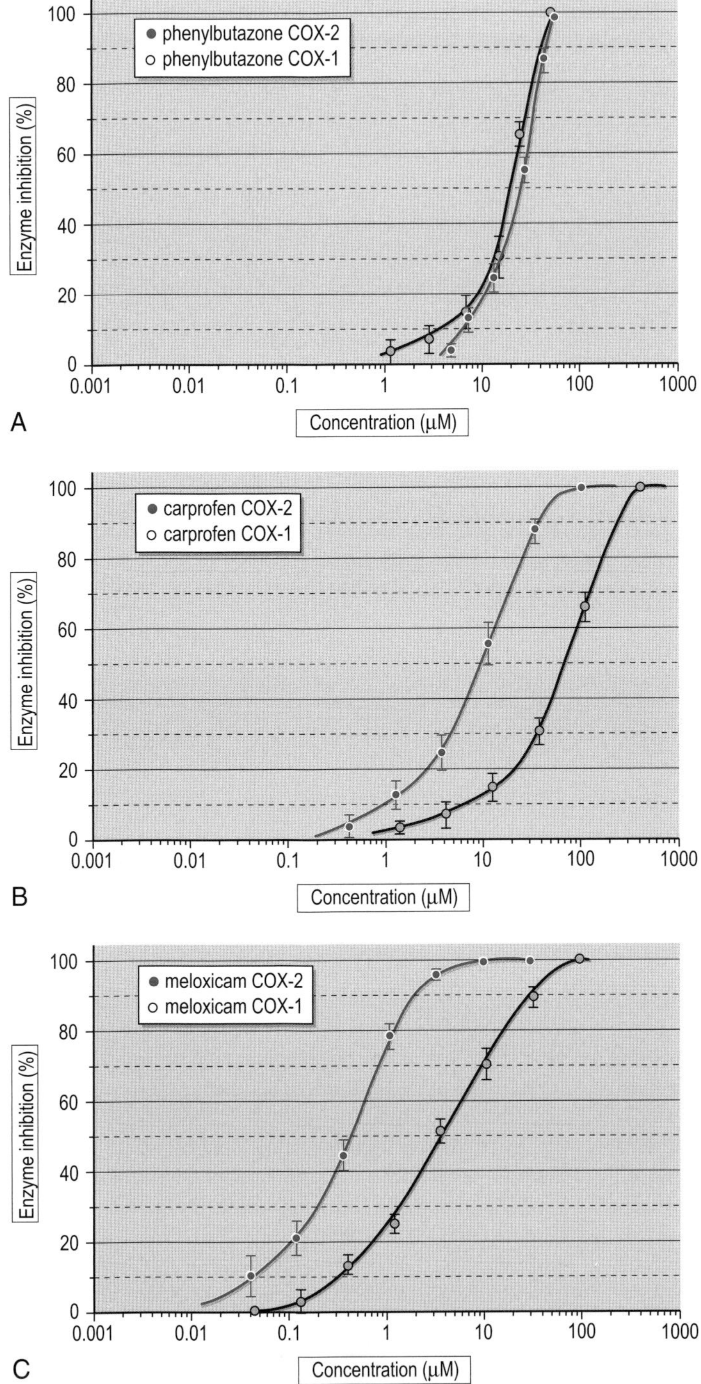

Fig. 13.2 **Whole-blood assay inhibitory concentration curves to assess COX selectivity in dogs. Points and curves represent the inhibition of TxB_2 (COX-1 activity) and PGE_2 (COX-2 activity) over a range of drug concentrations. (A) An example of a nonspecific COX inhibitor – phenylbutazone. (B–D) Examples of preferentially specific COX-2 inhibitors – carprofen, meloxicam and deracoxib, respectively. (E) An example of a specific COX-2 inhibitor – firocoxib. (Based on data presented in Brideau et al 2001, McCann et al 2004 and personal communication.)**

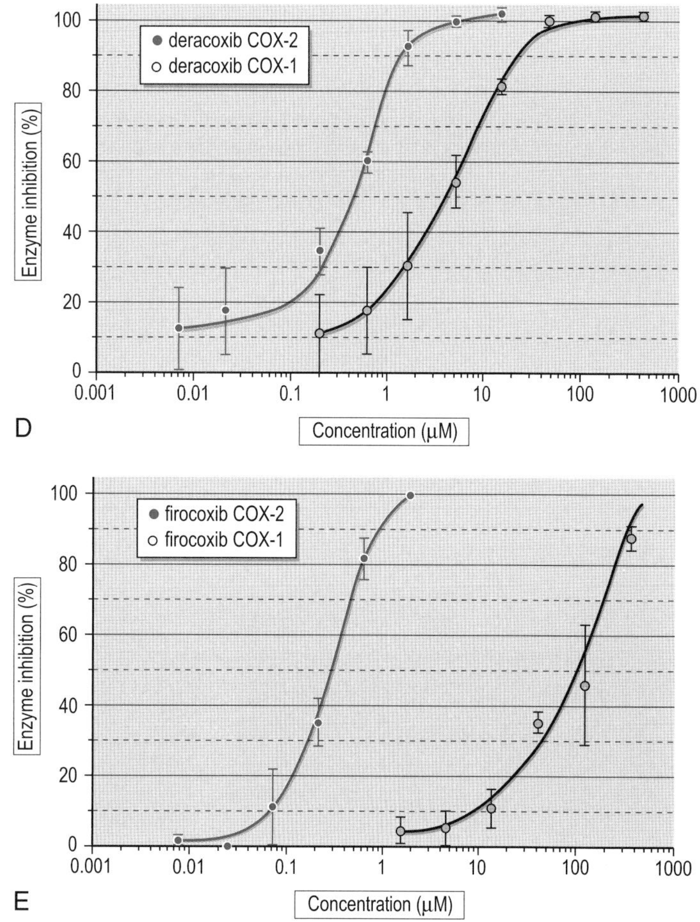

Fig. 13.2, cont'd

may influence the degree of safety of NSAIDs include the degree of acidity of any prodrug, the plasma half-life, the degree of enterohepatic recycling and the potential for polymorphism in metabolism. One example of this is found with the human drug celecoxib when used in dogs. It has been shown that beagle dogs exhibit polymorphism in the cytochrome P450 system that leads to some dogs metabolizing celecoxib rapidly and others slowly. Another example relates to gastrointestinal ulcers and ulcer healing. Inhibition of COX-1 is associated with a greater propensity for ulcer formation, suggesting that COX-2 selective drugs reduce the risk of ulcer formation. However, existing ulcers have increased COX-2 in the ulcer margin and model studies have demonstrated that COX-2 inhibition delays healing of these ulcers. Most of these studies have included complete inhibition of the COX-2 enzyme, so more work remains to understand if thresholds or time courses for the level of inhibition and delayed healing exist.

Non-COX-related mechanisms of action

A relatively new approach in small animal practice is the use of dual COX/LOX inhibitors. This target has been active for a while in human medicine; however, no compounds have come to market yet. The concept is to inhibit lipoxygenase and the formation of leukotrienes. Leukotrienes are inflammatory, active in a number of tissues and have a negative effect on the microcirculation of gastrointestinal mucosa, leading to a loss of the protective mucosal barrier. It is thought that inhibition of LOX helps preserve mucosal integrity, is anti-inflammatory and, in conjunction with inhibition of COX, provides analgesia comparable to other NSAIDs.

Inhibition of prostaglandin synthesis may only partially explain the therapeutic effects of NSAIDs. As well as their peripheral anti-inflammatory actions, some NSAIDs may also have a central component to pain relief and even have centrally mediated anti-inflammatory actions. Most NSAIDs, however, cross the blood–brain barrier poorly. Paracetamol (acetaminophen) does cross this barrier and appears to exert its main antipyretic and analgesic effects in the CNS. Similarly, there is evidence to suggest that coxibs also cross this barrier and may exert a central effect in addition to their peripheral effects.

It is not always possible to distinguish between the anti-inflammatory and analgesic effects of NSAIDs. Clinical analgesic efficacy does not necessarily correlate with anti-inflammatory effects and the analgesic action of some compounds such as paracetamol occurs in the absence of anti-inflammatory activity.

Some NSAIDs inhibit phosphodiesterase, which elevates the intracellular concentrations of cyclic AMP. Cyclic AMP has been shown to stabilize membranes, including lysosomal membranes in polymorphonuclear neutrophils, thereby reducing the release of enzymes, such as β-glucuronidase, that play an important role in the inflammatory process.

Other postulated mechanisms of actions of NSAIDs include acting as antagonists at prostaglandin-binding sites and as antioxidants, scavengers of free radicals and/or inhibitors of the formation of other cytotoxic chemicals.

General pharmacokinetics and pharmacodynamics

Chemical structure

Many NSAIDs are chiral molecules and available as racemates – a balanced combination of optical isomers. This is particularly true for the 2-aryl propionic acid group (except naproxen), which includes the profens carprofen, ketoprofen and vedoprofen. The S-enantiomers are generally more active than the R-enantiomers, although studies have demonstrated that R-enantiomers of some NSAIDs can have activity. The effectiveness of an individual drug could be dependent on the differential distribution and elimination of each enantiomer combined with its intrinsic activity. Several profens undergo metabolic chiral inversion, which can take place in several organs but predominantly the liver. Usually the R-enantiomer is converted to the active S-enantiomer, although the reverse can occur (e.g. with carprofen in the horse). However, it has been demonstrated that there is negligible chiral conversion in the dog.

A few NSAIDs are nonchiral and remain as the parent compound or a metabolite. In these cases, depending on any activity of metabolites, it is easier to estimate potential exposure to the drug and its effects.

Absorption

Orally administered NSAIDs are well absorbed from the upper gastrointestinal tract, although the rate and extent of absorption can be influenced by species, intragastric pH, presence of food, gastrointestinal motility and lesions and drug concentration. Most NSAIDs are weak acids and therefore absorption from the canine and feline stomach is facilitated by the low pH of gastric fluid. Efficient absorption also occurs in the small intestine, despite the less acidic environment, because of the large surface area and the fact that nonionized forms of most NSAIDs are lipophilic.

Many NSAIDs are formulated for parenteral administration and are well absorbed from intramuscular or subcutaneous sites. NSAIDs have also been formulated for topical use. Topical administration can result in measurable drug levels in tissues and synovial fluids comparable to that observed after oral administration.

Distribution

The NSAIDs are generally distributed extracellularly, with a small volume of distribution. One reason for this is that most NSAIDs have an ionic charge. However, because most are weak acids they readily penetrate inflamed tissues. As a result, the duration of effect of NSAIDs may exceed their apparent systemic half-life. This is thought to be due to the concentration of NSAIDs in locations where the pH of extracellular fluid is decreased, such as at sites of inflammation. A few NSAIDs, including firocoxib, lack ionic moieties and have an inherently high volume of distribution and broad tissue penetration.

Protein binding

All NSAIDs are highly protein bound (>90%), with the exception of salicylate (50% protein bound). This is believed to be another factor in the accumulation of drug in protein-rich inflammatory exudate. As a result of being highly protein bound, NSAIDs can be involved in drug interactions via protein displacement. They can sometimes be displaced from protein-binding sites (resulting in increased biologically active drug) but more commonly displace other less avidly bound drugs such as anticoagulants, hydantoins, glucocorticoids and sulfonamides. This may result in acute potentiation of the effect of other drugs. However, in general, the clinical significance of simple protein displacement interactions is believed to be minimal, as the acute increase in free drug concentration is immediately available for redistribution, metabolism and excretion. Most NSAIDs only bind to albumin and once binding sites are saturated, the concentration of free drug rapidly increases.

Metabolism and elimination

Metabolism of NSAIDs is usually mediated by hepatic mixed-function oxidases. A variety of conjugation reactions is commonly involved in NSAID metabolism and there are major species differences. Although hepatic biotransformation of most NSAIDs results in inactive or less active metabolites, there are some exceptions. For example, aspirin and phenylbutazone are converted to active metabolites (salicylate and oxyphenbutazone respectively). As noted previously, polymorphism of cytochrome P450 and other metabolic enzymes may also impact elimination in a drug-dependent manner.

The high level of protein binding and the relative acidity of dog and cat urine results in only a small fraction of the administered dose of most NSAIDs being excreted unchanged in the urine. Excretion is predominantly renal by glomerular filtration and tubular excretion, but some biliary elimination of conjugates occurs, which are available for enterohepatic recycling. The rate of renal excretion is frequently pH dependent and may be inhibited competitively by other weak acids. NSAIDs are excreted at varying rates depending on the metabolic pathway and extent of enterohepatic circulation. The elimination half-life therefore varies considerably between drugs and species. A corollary of this is that toxicity and pharmacokinetic data on NSAIDs generated in one species can never be transposed to another.

Side effects

Gastric ulceration

Prostaglandin inhibition

The ability of NSAIDs to reduce the production of prostaglandins and thromboxane and thus reduce inflammation is believed to be important for the potential toxicity of many members of this drug class. Prostaglandins play an important role in a wide variety of body functions. Of particular relevance to NSAID gastrointestinal toxicity is the role of PGI_2 (prostacyclin) and PGE_2 in maintaining the integrity of the protective barrier that prevents gastric mucosa from damage by gastric acid.

The PGE series and PGI_2 play an essential role in protecting the gastric mucosa. They are largely COX-1 dependent in this role. They:

- decrease the volume, acidity and pepsin content of gastric secretions
- stimulate bicarbonate secretion by epithelial cells
- produce vasodilation in gastric mucosa
- increase gastric and small intestinal mucus production
- stimulate turnover and repair of gastrointestinal epithelial cells
- increase the movement of water and electrolytes in the small intestine.

Other mechanisms

It is of interest that there is little correlation between the ulcerogenicity of NSAIDs and their anti-inflammatory activity. Some have hypothesized that this relates to anti-inflammatory activity resulting from COX-2 inhibition and ulcerogenicity relating to COX-1 inhibition. However, this is not the full explanation because some NSAIDs that inhibit gastric mucosal prostaglandin production or concentration are not overly ulcerogenic. The propensity of a NSAID to induce gastrointestinal damage depends in part on the relative rate of gastric absorption and systemic availability of the drug via the circulation to the mucosa.

Direct chemical damage to the gastric mucosa is believed to be important as well as reduced prostaglandin synthesis. For example, aspirin is not very soluble in acid solutions and therefore precipitates in gastric fluid, which may be an important factor causing gastric ulceration. However, gastric ulceration is also associated with systemic administration of NSAIDs.

NSAID-induced gastric damage is also believed to involve increased neutrophil adherence, which may result in increased release of oxygen-derived free radicals and proteases or capillary obstruction. The evidence for this is based on the observation that NSAID administration increases the number of leukocytes, mainly neutrophils, adhering to the local vascular endothelium and NSAID-induced gastropathy is reduced in neutropenic animals or if monoclonal antibodies are used to prevent leukocyte adhesion.

In addition, NSAIDs reduce the rate of mitosis at the edge of ulcer sites, creating a cycle that may delay or prevent ulcer healing. Inhibition of COX by NSAIDs may also lead to diversion of arachidonic acid into the lipoxygenase pathway, yielding leukotrienes, hydroperoxyeicosatetraenoic acids and active oxygen radicals, which adversely affect mucosal integrity. Although theoretically possible, this shunting has not been established as a clinical concern and gastrointestinal adverse event reporting has been similar between COX/LOX inhibitors and more traditional COX inhibitors.

An examination of the relative COX-1/COX-2 ratios for various drugs used in veterinary medicine (see Table 13.1) is illuminating and supports the contention that gastrointestinal toxicity is not entirely due to inhibition of physiologically important prostaglandins. Until recently, the drugs most selective for COX 2 based on the canine whole-blood assay had similar selectivity for COX-2 of approximately 10–30-fold greater than that for COX-1. Even so, carprofen, deracoxib and meloxicam have reported adverse event rates that are not greatly different from each other or less selective NSAIDs. These results may be influenced by the fact that fewer dogs are dosed with the nonselective NSAIDs and the duration of use for these is typically less. A new entry for dogs, firocoxib, has COX-2 selectivity that is more than 350-fold greater than that for COX-1. Although the registration study data were promising, it remains to be seen whether a meaningful difference in adverse events will be associated with the greater COX-2 selectivity. Appropriate case selection and monitoring remain a requirement for use of any NSAID.

Enterohepatic recycling

One of the problems in small animal practice is that dogs and particularly cats appear more sensitive to the gastrointestinal side effects of some NSAIDs than other species. For dogs, this may in part be a result of increased enterohepatic recycling and therefore longer half-lives of many NSAIDs. In cats, it may result from decreased ability to glucuronidate and metabolize the NSAIDs, again resulting in longer half-lives. Increased enterohepatic recycling causes the duodenum to be repeatedly exposed to high concentrations of a NSAID as well as increasing systemic residence time.

The degree of recycling may in part be correlated with the risk of gastrointestinal ulceration, particularly with drugs that inhibit COX-1 as part of their mechanism. Studies in rats suggest that enterohepatic recycling is the main factor contributing to the ability of a NSAID to cause enteropathy. Drugs that do not undergo enterohepatic recycling (i.e. have low or no biliary excretion) may have less impact on the gastrointestinal tract. For example, in humans, nabumetone has an improved gastrointestinal safety profile comparable to that of coxibs. It was initially believed that its safety was due to preferential COX-2 inhibition but this was not supported by several studies. It is now believed that its safety is based on two factors: (1) it is nonacidic and therefore does not have a direct toxic effect on gastric mucosa and (2) it is metabolized by first-pass metabolism and its metabolites do not undergo enterohepatic recycling.

NSAIDs suspected of undergoing various degrees of enterohepatic recycling in dogs include naproxen, piroxicam, indometacin, flunixin, etodolac, tolfenamic acid, deracoxib, firocoxib and carprofen, to a limited extent. However, it is clear that there is no one factor responsible for gastrointestinal toxicity, as preferential and highly selective COX-2 inhibitors appear to have reduced gastrointestinal toxicity overall but do on occasion have ulcers reported as an adverse effect.

Plasma half-life

Prolonged plasma half-lives are believed to contribute to the potential for NSAIDs to cause adverse effects in humans. Although ideally a longer half-life is desirable so that dosing may be maintained at convenient intervals, a longer half-life has been associated with increased risk of renal impairment and gastrointestinal complications in humans.

Half-life also plays a role when switching from one NSAID to another and may be a contributor to reported adverse events. It takes 5–7 half-lives to clear 97–99% of a drug from the body. In dogs, the approved NSAIDs have half-lives that range from approximately 2 to 24 h. This would suggest, depending on the drug, that a wash-out of 10 h to 7 d is appropriate to allow elimination of one NSAID before starting another. Because of this variability and the potential for subclinical toxicity to be exacerbated by the new NSAID, it is often recommended to wait at least 5–7 d as a wash-out when switching NSAIDs.

Gastric adaptation

The incidence of side effects may be less than expected in patients on chronic NSAID therapy because of the phenomenon of gastric adaptation. Gastric adaptation has been demonstrated in dogs, humans and rats after about 14 d of continuous aspirin therapy. It involves increased gastric blood flow, reduced inflammatory infiltrate and increased mucosal cell regeneration and mucosal content of epidermal growth factor. Whether such adaptation also applies to the small intestine is still debated. There is suggestion that long-term usage of NSAIDs, including COX-2 selective NSAIDs, increases the incidence of duodenal ulcers.

Exacerbating factors

The ulcerogenic potential of NSAIDs is increased by:

- concurrent corticosteroids
- dehydration
- hypovolemic shock
- disruption to normal gut blood flow.

The potential for gastric ulceration to occur with NSAID use is substantially magnified if the drugs are given concurrently with corticosteroids. There is debate whether corticosteroids alone cause gastric ulceration. They do not inhibit COX-1 directly, but rather diminish the generation of arachidonic acid that may be acted on by COX and LOX. There is no doubt that their ulcerogenic potential is enhanced in certain clinical situations, for example after spinal surgery, in hypovolemic states and, most importantly, when administered concurrently with NSAIDs. There is also debate whether a single concomitant administration of a NSAID and corticosteroid increases this risk. The prudent choice is to avoid combining the treatments if possible. If not, then coadministration of a protective agent, such as misoprostol, should be considered and the patient monitored closely.

Similarly, the use of NSAIDs in clinical situations where gastrointestinal blood flow may be reduced (e.g. dehydration, hypovolemic shock), thus enhancing the drug's ulcerogenic potential, has little merit. The use of NSAIDs in the management of a patient with hypovolemic shock secondary to trauma has no rational basis and is clinically insupportable, particularly when such drugs are used concurrently with corticosteroids.

There continues to be debate regarding the possible beneficial role that NSAID use may have in treatment of septic and endotoxic shock. The efficacy of some NSAIDs, especially flunixin, in endotoxic shock in horses and dogs has been demonstrated but the drug must be administered prior to or immediately after the onset of endotoxemia.

Renal toxicity

A second potential side effect of NSAIDs is renal toxicity following reduced renal blood flow and glomerular filtration rate secondary to inhibition of renal prostaglandin synthesis. Immunohistochemical staining of kidney tissue has revealed the presence of both COX-1 and COX-2. Renal prostaglandins are involved in maintaining renal blood flow via their vasodilatory actions. In a healthy, well-hydrated animal, reduced renal prostaglandin production is of little consequence. However, significant renal toxicity can result if an animal is volume depleted, is avidly retaining sodium (e.g. in congestive heart failure or hepatic cirrhosis) or has pre-existing renal insufficiency. Renal toxicity with NSAIDs has been described in humans and horses but has not been well documented in dogs and cats. However, a recent study demonstrated that creatinine clearance was significantly lower in dogs given carprofen or ketoprofen at induction of anesthesia compared to controls given saline.

When the sympathetic and renin-angiotensin systems are activated by sodium depletion, volume depletion or systemic hypotension, noradrenaline (norepinephrine) and angiotensin II act as potent vasoconstrictors, which may reduce renal blood flow, especially in the medulla. PGI_2 in the glomerulus and PGE_2 in the medulla counteract the vasoconstrictor actions of noradrenaline (norepinephrine) and angiotensin II and therefore protect the kidney from ischemic damage. Production of PGI_2 and PGE_2 is stimulated by vasoconstrictive substances. If the production of these protective prostaglandins is blocked by NSAID administration, renal failure may result.

The potential for renal toxicity to occur in a volume depleted dog is a further potent reason why NSAIDs should not be administered to any animal in shock post-traumatically or to any animal that may have significant gastrointestinal disease resulting in dehydration and volume depletion. As discussed above, selective COX-2 inhibitors may not prove to be safer than nonselective NSAIDs in the volume-depleted dog.

Hepatotoxicity

Hepatic toxicity is uncommon in animals receiving NSAIDs; however, there have been recent reports of idiosyncratic hepatotoxicity associated with carprofen use in dogs. Idiosyncratic hepatic toxicity, although rare, has been associated with the use of most classes of NSAIDs in humans. Hepatic toxicity has been associated with the use of phenylbutazone in aged horses but has not been reported in dogs. Paracetamol (acetaminophen) overdose can cause serious hepatocellular damage in dogs and adult humans but, interestingly and inexplicably, this occurs less often in cats and human infants. However, the therapeutic margin of paracetamol is low in cats where it causes methemoglobinemia, anemia and other signs.

Adverse effects on hematology and hemostasis

Prolongation of bleeding times due to inhibition of platelet thromboxane production can potentially occur after administration of NSAIDs, although at dose rates used clinically most NSAIDs do not impair hemostasis. This may be due to the fact that COX-1 blockade of thromboxane production is balanced by COX-2 inhibition in endothelial cells, resulting in reduced release of PGI_2 which normally causes vasodilation and reduced platelet aggregation. However, bleeding may occur with the use of drugs that irreversibly bind to COX-1, such as aspirin and phenylbutazone, as the effect persists for the life of the platelet (which is unable to synthesize additional thromboxane as it lacks a nucleus). Studies with more COX-2 selective drugs, such as carprofen, deracoxib and firocoxib, have not shown prolongation of bleeding time, in some cases even at high dosages.

Thromboxane is a potent vasoconstrictor and stimulus for platelet aggregation and the reduced vasoconstriction and platelet aggregation that occur may be significant in patients with bleeding tendencies or may complicate surgical procedures. NSAIDs should be used with extreme care in breeds, such as dobermans and Scottish terriers, that have a high incidence of von Willebrand's disease.

Myelotoxicity (agranulocytosis) occurs relatively commonly in humans but is rare in dogs. Blood dyscrasias have been reported occasionally in association with the use of phenylbutazone in dogs.

Human use of coxibs and even some nonselective NSAIDs has been associated with an increased risk of cardiovascular events, particularly stroke and heart attack. Several theories have been proposed to explain this potential. These include a drug-related increase in blood pressure, unbalanced inhibition of prostacyclin and thromboxane and drug-dependent oxidative damage to low-density lipid which causes vascular inflammation. Although still under investigation, the strongest theory relates to coxibs not being platelet inhibitors. In this manner, they do not inhibit thromboxane and the propensity for clot formation is increased. At the same time, they inhibit prostacyclin which plays a role in modulating the effects of thromboxane. In a large-scale human trial of long-term treatment administration with rofecoxib, there was an overall risk of 1.96 compared with placebo for the development of confirmed thrombotic cardiovascular serious events.

Fortunately for veterinary medicine, the pathogenesis of cardiovascular disease in humans and animals is different. Animals do not have the same risk factors as humans, are not generally prone to atherosclerosis and have much lower rates of serious thrombotic cardiovascular events. Reviews by regulatory authorities in the United States and Europe found no evidence for increased cardiovascular events with NSAIDs, including coxibs, in dogs.

Injury to articular cartilage

Chronic NSAID therapy may worsen cartilage degeneration in animals with osteoarthritis through impaired proteoglycan synthesis. It is not clear whether this effect occurs at standard clinically recommended dose rates. Aspirin, indometacin, ibuprofen and naproxen caused increased degeneration in arthritic joints in experimental murine and canine models whereas ketoprofen and diclofenac did not. Meloxicam also does not appear to adversely affect synthesis of cartilage proteoglycans in vitro. Carprofen may adversely affect chondrocyte metabolism but only if present in synovial fluid at high concentrations that do not appear to be reached in vivo. The clinical relevance of these findings has not been determined.

Known drug interactions

NSAIDs should not be administered with corticosteroids or other NSAIDs. The combination of two NSAIDs or a NSAID and a corticosteroid in the same commercial product is difficult to defend on toxicological grounds.

In humans there is an increased risk of convulsions if NSAIDs are administered with fluoroquinolones; this has not been reported to date in animals.

NSAIDs may antagonize the hypotensive effects of antihypertensives such as β-blockers.

NSAIDs may decrease the action of furosemide and angiotensin-converting enzyme (ACE) inhibitors. Furosemide and ACE inhibitors stimulate prostaglandin synthesis to increase renal blood flow, produce vasodilation and cause natriuresis. However, the clinical relevance of this interaction is unknown.

Because of avid protein binding, NSAIDs may displace other drugs from protein-binding sites, e.g. oral anticoagulants, glucocorticoids, sulfonamides, methotrexate, valproic acid and phenytoin. However, redistribution of free displaced drug, combined with metabolism and excretion, usually minimizes any potential adverse consequences.

APPROVED NSAIDS FOR SMALL ANIMAL PRACTICE (ORDERED ALPHABETICALLY)

Carprofen

(Rimadyl® and generic)

Carprofen is available throughout the world.

Clinical applications

Carprofen is indicated for perioperative analgesia and management of acute pain and chronic pain, including osteoarthritis, in dogs and cats. Studies of its comparative efficacy in relation to opioid analgesics for postoperative analgesia in both dogs and cats suggest that it is as efficacious or more so and longer lasting than drugs such as pethidine (meperidine) and butorphanol. The timing of administration appears to be important; one study suggested that preoperative administration of carprofen had a greater analgesic effect than administration in the early postoperative period.

Formulations and dose rates

Carprofen is available in oral and injectable formulations.

DOGS (DOSAGE VARIES BY MARKET)

Surgical pain

- 4.0 mg/kg IV, SC or IM. Repeat in 12 h if needed
- 4.4 mg/kg PO q.24 h or divided (2.2 mg/kg) and administered q.12 h. For the control of postoperative pain, administer approximately 2 h before the procedure

Chronic pain

- 2.0–4.0 mg/kg either q.24 h or divided and administered q.12 h PO for 7 d then titrated to the lowest effective dose, or 2 mg/kg q.24 h
- 4.0–4.4 mg/kg either q.24 h or divided (2.0–2.2 mg/kg) and administered q.12 h PO

CATS

Pharmacokinetic studies and clinical experience in Europe suggest that acute administration of a single dose of 2.0–4.0 mg/kg IV, SC or IM appears safe in cats; however, recommendations for safe dosing schedules for longer term treatment have not been made and repeated administration is not recommended.

Mechanism of action – additional information

Carprofen is a member of the propionic acid class of NSAIDs. Although the therapeutic effects of carprofen are not believed to be principally dependent on inhibition of prostaglandin synthesis, it is a moderately potent inhibitor of phospholipase A_2 and a weak and reversible inhibitor of COX with a preferential activity for COX-2.

Relevant pharmacokinetic data

The mean half-life of elimination is approximately 8 h after single oral administration in dogs and approximately 20 h in cats. Carprofen is eliminated in dogs primarily by means of biotransformation in the liver, followed by rapid excretion of the resulting metabolites in feces (70–80%) and urine (10–20%). Some enterohepatic circulation has been detected.

Adverse effects

- The majority of adverse events reported are those typical for the NSAID class.
- Idiosyncratic hepatotoxicity has been reported in dogs treated with carprofen. Labrador retrievers may be overrepresented. The mechanism of the hepatotoxicity is not known but it has been speculated that glucuronide metabolites may react with plasma and hepatocellular proteins, resulting in the formation of antigenic NSAID-altered proteins that cause immune-mediated hepatic toxicosis. Drug withdrawal is usually associated with recovery, but some cases have been fatal.
- The safety of chronic carprofen use in cats has not been determined. Duodenal perforation has been reported in a cat treated with carprofen at a dose of 2.2 mg/kg q.12 h for 7 d. The considerably longer half-life in cats compared to dogs indicates that chronic dosage recommendations for dogs cannot be extrapolated to cats.

Deracoxib

(Deramaxx®)

Deracoxib is available in the United States, Europe and Australia. Structurally it is closely related to celecoxib, a coxib for humans. However, deracoxib is indicated only for use in dogs.

Clinical applications

Deracoxib is indicated for management of pain and inflammation associated with osteoarthritis and for postoperative pain following orthopedic surgery. Additional reports indicate it has been used in the treatment of osteosarcoma.

Formulations and dose rates

Deracoxib is available as an oral chewable tablet.

DOGS

Orthopedic surgery

- 3–4 mg/kg PO q.24 h as needed for 7 d

Osteoarthritis

- 1–2 mg/kg PO q.24 h

Mechanism of action – additional information

Deracoxib is a member of the coxib class of NSAIDs. Data indicate that it inhibits the production of PGE_1 and 6-keto PGF_1 by its inhibitory effects on prostaglandin biosynthesis. Deracoxib inhibited COX-2 mediated PGE_2 production in LPS-stimulated human and dog whole blood. At doses of 2–4 mg/kg/d, deracoxib does not inhibit COX-1 based on in vitro studies using cloned canine cyclo-oxygenase.

Relevant pharmacokinetic data

Deracoxib has a half-life of approximately 3 h, although a longer duration of effectiveness is observed. Nonlinear elimination kinetics are exhibited at doses above 8 mg/kg/d, at which competitive inhibition of constitutive COX-1 may occur. At doses of 20 mg/kg, the half-life increases to 19 h.

Adverse effects

Adverse events reported are those typical for the NSAID class.

Dipyrone

(Generic)

Clinical applications

Dipyrone is approved for use in dogs and cats in Europe and Canada, although its use in cats is strongly discouraged as safety trials in this species are lacking. Even in dogs, with the availability of newer, safer NSAIDs, there is little reason to consider the use of dipyrone today. It is a member of the pyrazolone class of NSAIDs. It has been primarily used as an antipyretic agent, as the analgesia produced is inadequate for moderate-to-severe postoperative pain. However, it can control mild-to-moderate visceral pain. The role of dipyrone in veterinary medicine is very limited, particularly with the development of newer, more effective and safer NSAIDs. Its use in food-producing species is prohibited because of its potential for causing blood dyscrasias in humans.

The most common formulation in which dipyrone is used clinically is in combination with hyoscine (e.g. Buscopan®, Spasmogesic®) for the management of abdominal pain in dogs and horses.

Formulations and dose rates

DOGS AND CATS

Dipyrone is available as a solution for injection and tablets.

- The dose is approximately 25 mg/kg PO or IV q.12 h or q8 h
- The injectable solution should preferably be used IV as IM or SC injection causes tissue irritation

Relevant pharmacokinetic data

Dipyrone is rapidly and well absorbed following oral administration in the dog, with an elimination half-life of 5–6 h. It is largely excreted in the urine.

Adverse effects

There is little published information on the toxicity profile of dipyrone in dogs and cats. However, it has been associated with toxic effects in humans, including bone marrow toxicosis and teratogenicity, and it is believed that similar adverse effects may occur in dogs and cats. Concern that dipyrone may not be safe is supported by the fact that extra-label use of dipyrone in food animals is specifically prohibited by the Food and Drug Administration's Committee of Veterinary Medicine in the USA for several reasons, including lack of data indicating that dipyrone is safe and effective.

Cyanosis and extreme dyspnea have been reported to occur with use of hyoscine-dipyrone combination in cats in Australia. This adverse reaction was fatal in the three cats reported and was believed by the manufacturer to be due to a hypersensitivity reaction to the product. It is well documented that dipyrone can elicit hypersensitivity reactions in humans. Following this, the product was not recommended for use in cats.

Additional known or suspected drug interactions

There have been questionable interactions reported between dipyrone and phenothiazine tranquilizers whereby animals apparently lose their ability to thermoregulate.

Etodolac

(Etogesic®)

Clinical applications

Etodolac is indicated for the management of chronic osteoarthritis in dogs.

Formulations and dose rates

Etodolac is available in tablet form.

DOGS

- 10–15 mg/kg PO q.24 h

Mechanism of action – additional information

Etodolac is a member of the pyranocarboxylic acid class of NSAIDs. Results of in vitro studies indicate that etodolac preferentially inhibits COX-2, although therapeutic dosages likely also inhibit COX-1.

Relevant pharmacokinetic data

Etodolac is well absorbed when administered orally in dogs and has a large volume of distribution. It undergoes extensive enterohepatic recycling and has a serum half-life of 9.7–14.4 h.

Adverse effects

- Gastric tolerance was demonstrated in a study of dogs treated for 28 d at a mean dose of 12.8 mg/kg daily. In that study, gastrointestinal lesion scores were not different in dogs treated with etodolac, carprofen or placebo and significantly less than in dogs treated with buffered aspirin. However, in safety studies at approximately three times the maximum recommended dose level, gastrointestinal toxicity was observed.
- Transient decreases in serum proteins have been reported in chronically treated dogs. Excessive hemorrhage was reported with use of etodolac in five of six dogs undergoing stifle surgery compared with two of six control dogs.

Firocoxib

(Previcox®)

Firocoxib is available throughout the world.

Clinical applications

Firocoxib is indicated for management of pain and inflammation associated with osteoarthritis. In Australia/New Zealand, claims also include other musculoskeletal disorders and soft tissue surgery. Additional reports indicate it has been used in the treatment of transitional cell carcinoma, but there is no claim for this indication.

Formulations and dose rates

Firocoxib is available as an oral chewable tablet for dogs and an oral paste for horses.

DOGS

- 5 mg/kg PO q.24 h

HORSES

- 0.1 mg/kg PO q.24 h

CATS

- Firocoxib is not approved for use in cats. However, one paper reports efficacy in a fever model at dose levels of 0.75–3.0 mg/kg PO q.24 h

Mechanism of action – additional information

Firocoxib is a member of the coxib class of NSAIDs with anti-inflammatory and analgesic properties. It is not used in humans and was developed specifically for animal species. Results from in vitro studies showed firocoxib to be highly selective for the COX-2 enzyme when canine blood was exposed to drug concentrations comparable to those observed following a once-daily 5 mg/kg oral dose in dogs.

Relevant pharmacokinetic data

Firocoxib has a half-life in dogs of approximately 7.8 h. In horses, it averages 30–40 h. Steady-state concentrations are achieved in horses beyond 6–8 daily oral doses. In cats, the half-life is reported to range from approximately 9 to 12 h.

Adverse effects

Adverse events reported are those typical for the NSAID class.

Flunixin meglumine

(Banamine® and generic)

Clinical applications

Flunixin is one of the most potent inhibitors of COX. It is registered for use in dogs in some countries but not in the United States, where it is only approved for use in horses and cattle. It has been shown to provide good analgesia for acute and surgical pain (better, for example, than butorphanol) but the potential for side effects is of major concern. It has been used as a postoperative analgesic (single dose only) in cats, although it is not approved for use in this species.

Flunixin has been shown to have similar efficacy to phenylbutazone in the management of acute flare-ups of musculoskeletal disorders in dogs. This is in contrast to horses, where flunixin is a better anti-inflammatory and analgesic than phenylbutazone. The development of equally or more efficacious and safer NSAIDs that can be given by parenteral as well as oral routes means that there are now few indications for the use of flunixin in the safe management of acute or chronic pain in dogs or cats.

Flunixin is effective in the management of a variety of inflammatory ocular conditions, particularly if given prophylactically. It is also used as an adjunct in the treatment of endotoxic shock and has been demonstrated to increase survival in dogs with experimental septic peritonitis and after injection with *Escherichia coli* endotoxin. In dogs with experimental gastric dilation and torsion, flunixin did not alter cardiac indices or blood flows significantly but did reduce prostacyclin levels, suggesting that it may attenuate or inhibit the continued effects of endotoxic damage. Other NSAIDs may have similar beneficial effects in endotoxemia.

Formulations and dose rates

Flunixin is available in oral and injectable formulations.

DOGS

Surgical pain
- 1.1 mg/kg IV, SC or IM q.24 h, maximum of 3 doses (1 dose preferred)

Pyrexia
- 0.25 mg/kg IV, SC or IM q.24 h or q.12 h PRN for 1–2 treatments

Ophthalmological procedures
- 0.25–1.0 mg/kg q.24 h or q.12 h PRN for 1–2 treatments

CATS

Surgical pain
- 0.25–1.0 mg/kg IV, SC or IM q.24 h, maximum of 3 doses (1 dose preferred)

Pyrexia
- 0.25 mg/kg IV, SC or IM q.24 h or q.12 h PRN for 1–2 treatments

Mechanism of action – additional information

Flunixin is an aminonicotinic acid NSAID.

Relevant pharmacokinetic data

Flunixin has a short half-life in dogs of 2.4–3.7 h but sequesters in inflamed tissues, resulting in a duration of action of approximately 24 h. Mean elimination half-life in cats has been reported to be 0.7–1.5 h.

Adverse effects

Significant gastrointestinal toxicity occurs in dogs with chronic use; therefore, acute and preferably single dose use only is advisable.

Additional known or suspected drug interactions

Significant renal dysfunction has been documented in dogs anesthetized with methoxyflurane and given a single dose of flunixin (1.0 mg/kg).

Indometacin and copper indometacin

(Cu-Algesic®)

Indometacin is commonly used in humans. It is an acetic acid derivative and a member of the indoline class. Despite its short half-life in dogs (0.3 h), indometacin is highly ulcerogenic at doses of 1 mg/kg, 5% of the toxic dose in humans.

Indometacin is marketed in Australia in combination with copper for use in dogs and horses. Copper is reported to have anti-inflammatory and antioxidant effects. Copper-complexed NSAIDs are reported to be more potent anti-inflammatory agents than NSAIDs alone in laboratory animals. The copper–NSAID formulation is said to alter the pharmacokinetics of the compound sufficiently (reduced enterohepatic recycling) to result in reduced potential for gastrointestinal toxicity.

To date, controlled clinical trials have not been conducted to prove or disprove the compound's efficacy in the management of inflammatory disorders in dogs and horses. However, uncontrolled clinical trials support the relative lack of gastrointestinal toxicity when the drug is used in dogs compared with the use of indometacin alone. Anecdotal reports suggest that its efficacy is similar to or slightly better than aspirin or phenylbutazone in the management of osteoarthritis in dogs.

Formulation and doses

Copper-indometacin is available as an oral tablet.

DOGS

Surgical pain

- 0.2 mg/kg PO for short-term use and 0.1 mg/kg PO for long-term use to treat musculoskeletal/locomotor inflammatory conditions

Ketoprofen

(Ketofen®, Romefen®)

Clinical applications

Ketoprofen is registered for management of acute mild-to-moderate pain and at a lower dosage for osteoarthritis. It can be used in both dogs and cats. Several studies indicate that, except perhaps in the first postoperative hour, ketoprofen provides more effective, longer-lasting analgesia after soft tissue and orthopedic surgery than the synthetic opioids such as pethidine (meperidine), oxymorphone, buprenorphine and butorphanol.

Ketoprofen has been demonstrated to be an effective antipyretic agent in cats.

Formulations and dose rates

Ketoprofen is available in oral and injectable formulations.

DOGS

- 1 mg/kg IV, SC, IM or PO q.24 h for up to 5 d for acute pain and inflammation
- 0.25 mg/kg PO q.24 h for chronic pain, such as with osteoarthritis

CATS

- 1 mg/kg SC or PO q.24 h for 3–5 d

Mechanism of action – additional information

Ketoprofen is a member of the propionic acid class of NSAIDs. Depending on the species, tissue and assay system used, ketoprofen may inhibit lipoxygenase as well as COX. For example, it inhibits lipoxygenase in human lung tissue and rabbit leukocytes but not in guinea-pig lung. However, lipoxygenase inhibition by ketoprofen has not been demonstrated in vivo to date in domestic animals.

Ketoprofen is well absorbed orally but the presence of food or milk decreases oral absorption. The elimination half-life in cats and dogs is 3–5 h.

Adverse effects

- Ketoprofen appears to have a relatively good safety profile, although it is principally used for short courses only.
- The most common adverse effect is vomiting.
- Endoscopic studies suggest that ketoprofen is less ulcerogenic than aspirin but may be more likely to cause ulceration than carprofen.

Meclofenamic acid

(Arquel®)

Meclofenamic acid is approved for use in dogs and is commonly used in equine medicine. It is an anthranilic acid or fenamate NSAID. Its use in dogs is limited because of the potential for gastrointestinal side effects. The dose is 1.1 mg/kg PO q.24 h or q.48 h for 5–7 d only. The drug has been incriminated in one reported case of aplastic anemia in a dog.

Meloxicam

(Metacam®)

Meloxicam is available throughout the world.

Clinical applications

Meloxicam is indicated for management of chronic soft tissue or musculoskeletal pain, including osteoarthritis in dogs. It is effective also for the management of perioperative pain in dogs undergoing orthopedic or soft tissue surgery.

Meloxicam was recently registered in some markets for use in cats for short-term (1 d) treatment. It appears to have similar efficacy to ketoprofen.

Meloxicam is approved in Europe for use in horses for alleviation of inflammation and relief of pain in both acute and chronic musculoskeletal disorders.

Formulations and dose rates

Meloxicam is available as an injectable preparation, an oral suspension and a chewable tablet.

DOGS

- An initial dose of 0.2 mg/kg SC or PO followed by 0.1 mg/kg PO q.24 h

CATS

- A single dose of 0.3 mg/kg SC. Longer term use at this dose has been associated with significant adverse effects. Anecdotal reports suggest that a reduced dose of approximately 0.025 mg/kg q.24 h may be tolerated for up to 7 d

HORSES

- 0.6 mg/kg PO q.24 h for up to 14 d

Mechanism of action – additional information

Meloxicam is a member of the oxicam class of NSAIDs. It has been shown in several studies to be a preferential

COX-2 inhibitor, although there are other studies that suggest it has equipotent COX-1 and COX-2 activity.

Relevant pharmacokinetic data

Meloxicam has a half-life of approximately 24 h in dogs. There is some evidence of enhanced drug accumulation and terminal elimination half-life prolongation when dogs are dosed for 45 d or longer. The half-life in cats is approximately 21 h. In horses, it is approximately 8 h.

Adverse effects

Adverse events reported are those typical for the NSAID class.

Phenylbutazone

(Generic)

Phenylbutazone was one of the first NSAIDs used in canine medicine and has been available since the 1950s. It is a member of the pyrazolone class of NSAIDs and has similar anti-inflammatory activity to the salicylates.

Clinical applications

Phenylbutazone is primarily used in dogs in the management of chronic osteoarthritis. In contrast to equine medicine, where phenylbutazone is commonly used postoperatively to reduce inflammation and swelling, postoperative use of phenylbutazone is not recommended in the dog because of potential toxicity. This is particularly so now that safer and more effective NSAIDs are available for postoperative use. In canine medicine, it has few advantages over newer NSAIDS in the management of inflammatory conditions such as osteoarthritis.

Formulations and dose rates

DOGS

- Phenylbutazone is usually administered to dogs orally but is available as a parenteral formulation for intravascular use in some countries
- Topical formulations are also available in some countries
- 2–20 mg/kg PO q.24 h or in divided doses for up to 7 d, then reduce to lowest effective dose

Adverse effects

Although direct teratogenic effects have not been confirmed, rodent studies have demonstrated reduced litter sizes, increased neonatal mortality and increased stillbirths. Therefore, its use in pregnancy should be avoided unless the potential benefit outweighs the risk.

Additional known or suspected drug interactions

- Phenylbutazone and oxyphenbutazone can induce microsomal enzymes and increase the metabolism of drugs affected by this system, e.g. digitoxin, phenytoin.
- Conversely, other microsomal enzyme inducers, e.g. barbiturates, rifampicin (rifampin), corticosteroids, chlorphenamine (chlorpheniramine), diphenhydramine, may decrease the plasma half-life of phenylbutazone.
- Phenylbutazone may increase the chances of hepatotoxicity developing if administered concurrently with potentially hepatotoxic drugs.
- May cause falsely low T_3 and T_4 values (but does not cause clinical hypothyroidism).

Tepoxalin

(Zubrin®)

Tepoxalin is available in Australasia, Europe and the United States. It was originally a candidate for use in humans but was subsequently developed only for dogs.

Clinical applications

Tepoxalin is indicated for management of pain and inflammation associated with osteoarthritis.

Formulations and dose rates

Tepoxalin is available as an oral fast-melt tablet for dogs.

DOGS

- 10 mg/kg or 20 mg/kg PO on the initial day of treatment, followed by a daily maintenance dose of 10 mg/kg PO q.24 h. Tepoxalin should be administered with food or within 1–2 h after feeding

Mechanism of action – additional information

The mechanism of action of tepoxalin, like other NSAIDs, is believed to be associated with the inhibition of cyclo-oxygenase activity. Additionally, tepoxalin has been shown to be an inhibitor of lipoxygenase and is thus classified as a dual inhibitor of arachidonic acid metabolism (i.e. a COX/LOX inhibitor).

Relevant pharmacokinetic data

The half-life of tepoxalin in plasma is short, approximately 2 h, due to conversion to an active carboxylic acid metabolite. The active metabolite has a long half-life, approximately 12–14 h, which justifies once-daily dosing.

Adverse effects

Adverse events reported are those typical for the NSAID class.

Tolfenamic acid

(Tolfedine®)

Tolfenamic acid is approved for use in dogs and cats in Europe and Australasia but not the United States. It is an anthranilic acid NSAID. There is little information available as to its efficacy and potential for side effects in these species. In one study in beagles, good gastric tolerance (assessed endoscopically) was demonstrated at an oral dose of 4 mg/kg q.24 h for 5 weeks. Tolfenamic acid has an elimination half-life of 6.5 h after IV or SC administration and undergoes marked enterohepatic recycling.

Vedaprofen

(Quadrisol®)

Clinical applications

Vedaprofen is approved for use in dogs and horses. It is indicated for the reduction of inflammation and relief of pain associated with musculoskeletal disorders and trauma.

Formulations and dose rates

Vedaprofen is available as an oral gel (dogs and horses) and injectable formulation (horses).

DOGS

Musculoskeletal disorders and trauma

- 0.5 mg/kg PO q.24 h for up to 1 month

HORSES

Musculoskeletal disorders and trauma

- 2.0 mg/kg PO initial dose followed by 1.0 mg/kg PO q.12 h for up to 14 d

Colic

- 2.0 mg/kg IV once

Mechanism of action – additional information

Vedaprofen is a member of the propionic acid class of NSAIDs. It is reported to have preferential activity for COX-2 relative to COX-1. However, in the canine whole-blood assay, it is selective for COX-1 similar to ketoprofen.

Relevant pharmacokinetic data

Vedaprofen is a racemic mixture. The half-life is approximately 13 h in dogs and 6–8 h in horses.

Adverse effects

Adverse events reported are those typical for the NSAID class. Vedaprofen is reported to have a narrow therapeutic index, with gastrointestinal effects making up the primary toxicity.

UNAPPROVED NSAIDS USED IN SMALL ANIMAL PRACTICE

Aspirin (acetylsalicylic acid)

(Generic)

Clinical applications

Aspirin is approved for use in dogs and cats in some markets but the available data supporting its safety and efficacy are scarce and not of the same standard as for more recently approved NSAIDs. Still, it is widely used because it is inexpensive, available as an over-the-counter preparation and can be clinically efficacious in many dogs with chronic osteoarthritis. It is a member of the salicylate class of NSAIDs. Clinical reports of aspirin-induced toxicosis are infrequent despite the widespread use of the drug and its theoretical potential for toxicity. The pharmacokinetics of the drug are well known in dogs and cats and steps can be taken to minimize the potential toxic effects. However, subclinical gastrointestinal bleeding has been documented after even a single dose of aspirin, possibly due to local acidity.

In addition to its use in canine (and sometimes feline) osteoarthritis, aspirin is used for the prevention of thromboemboli in dogs being treated for heartworm disease and in cats with hypertrophic cardiomyopathy and aortic saddle thrombus.

Formulations and dose rates

Aspirin is administered orally and is available in plain, buffered or enteric-coated formulations. Plain aspirin is associated most commonly with gastrointestinal irritation but the bioavailability of enteric-coated products can be very variable and buffered aspirin can be difficult to obtain. Enteric-coated tablets are not recommended for dogs because of the erratic and incomplete absorption. Buffering hastens stomach emptying of aspirin, thus decreasing the contact time of aspirin with the gastric mucosa and decreasing gastric absorption. Aspirin should be given with food to reduce gastrointestinal irritation.

DOGS

Analgesia, anti-inflammatory

- 10–25 mg/kg PO q.12 h

Antipyretic

- 10 mg/kg PO q.12 h

In association with adulticide heartworm therapy

- 5–10 mg/kg PO q.24 h

Antithrombosis

- 0.5 mg/kg PO q.24 h

Disseminated intravascular coagulation

- 7.5–15 mg/kg PO q.24 h or q.48 h for 10 d

CATS

Analgesia, anti-inflammatory, antithrombotic

- 10–20 mg/kg PO q.48–72 h

Mechanism of action – additional information

Aspirin is deacetylated to form salicylate and the parent compound has a very short half-life. It is believed that salicylate accounts for most of the analgesic and anti-inflammatory properties of aspirin whereas aspirin itself provides the antithrombotic activity. Aspirin induces an irreversible inhibition of COX; thus the pharmacological effect persists until new enzyme is synthesized. Platelets have no ability to synthesize new proteins as they are anuclear; therefore, inhibition of thromboxane synthesis will last the life of the platelet, resulting in impaired primary hemostasis. With other NSAIDs, COX inhibition only lasts while the drug is present.

Relevant pharmacokinetic data

There are major species differences in the metabolism of aspirin.

- The half-life of salicylate is 37.5 h in cats and 8.5 h in dogs. Cats are relatively deficient in glucuronyl transferase, which is responsible for conjugating salicylate with glucuronic acid. Thus hepatic clearance in the cat is very prolonged.
- Newborn animals are also deficient in microsomal enzymes required for biotransformation and have limited ability to excrete aspirin in urine.
- In contrast to dogs and cats, aspirin has a very short half-life in horses and is therefore not a useful anti-inflammatory/analgesic in this species. However, aspirin has a profound effect on platelet function in horses – a single dose of 17 mg/kg inhibits platelet function and prolongs bleeding times for at least 48 h.
- Salicylate is excreted into milk but levels appear very low. It will cross the placenta and fetal levels may exceed those in the mother.
- Salicylate and its metabolites are rapidly excreted by the kidneys by both filtration and renal tubular excretion. Substantial tubular reabsorption occurs and is highly pH dependent. Excretion can be significantly enhanced by increasing urine pH.

Adverse effects

In addition to the expected side effects of NSAIDs discussed previously, aspirin may cause the following adverse effects.

- Hypersensitivity reactions have been reported in dogs, although they are rare.
- Salicylates are possible teratogens, so use in pregnancy should be avoided. In addition, aspirin has been shown to delay parturition.
- Overdosage initially results in respiratory alkalosis with a compensatory hyperventilatory response. Profound metabolic acidosis follows.

Additional known or suspected drug interactions

- In cats, concurrent treatment with furosemide and aspirin substantially alters digoxin pharmacokinetics and digoxin dosage should be reduced by approximately 30%. In dogs aspirin has been demonstrated to decrease clearance of digoxin and therefore increase plasma levels.
- Furosemide may compete with the renal excretion of aspirin and delay its excretion.
- The extrarenal venodilatory effects of furosemide are prostaglandin mediated and abolished by prior treatment with aspirin. Therefore the clinical efficacy of furosemide may be reduced in animals with congestive heart failure if aspirin is administered concurrently.
- Phenobarbital may increase the rate of aspirin metabolism through hepatic enzyme induction.
- Aspirin may also inhibit the diuretic activity of spironolactone.
- Aspirin should not be administered with any other nonsteroidal drug and virtually never administered concurrently with corticosteroids (although the manufacturer's recommendation to use both aspirin and prednisolone in relation to treatment of heartworm disease with melarsomine appears to be an exception).
- Buffered aspirin may chelate tetracycline products if given simultaneously – space doses by at least 1 h.
- It is possible, but has not been proved, that concurrent administration of aspirin and aminoglycoside antimicrobial drugs may increase the risk of nephrotoxicity.

Special considerations

Aspirin is stable in dry air but readily hydrolyzes to acetate and salicylate when exposed to water or moist air; it will then exude a strong, vinegar-like odor. Accordingly, aspirin tablets should be stored in tight, moisture-resistant containers, not used if the bottle smells of vinegar and not used past their expiry date.

Ibuprofen

(Generic)

Ibuprofen is a popular over-the-counter NSAID for people but it is not approved for use in animals. Ibuprofen is a member of the propionic acid class of NSAIDs.

There are numerous reports in the literature of serious gastrointestinal and renal toxicity in dogs treated with ibuprofen at doses that are insufficient to have anti-inflammatory efficacy. Ibuprofen toxicity occurs relatively frequently in dogs as a result of accidental exposure or owner administration of the drug in the absence of veterinary advice.

Ketorolac

(Toradol®)

Ketorolac is a cyclized propionic acid NSAID that is used in humans mainly as a postsurgical analgesic rather than as an anti-inflammatory. It is not approved for use in dogs. It is reported to be as effective as morphine for mild-to-moderate postoperative pain. It is most often given parenterally, although oral formulations are available. Longer-term use in humans is associated with a significant incidence of peptic ulceration and renal compromise. In veterinary medicine, ketorolac has been used to control postoperative pain in dogs; it is as effective as flunixin and more effective than butorphanol or a low dose of oxymorphone. Its use in dogs has been associated with significant gastrointestinal toxicity.

Naproxen

(Naprosyn®, Aleve®)

Clinical applications

Naproxen is widely used in humans and has been used for the management of chronic musculoskeletal pain in dogs although it is not approved for dogs. However, the incidence of adverse effects is relatively high with its use and there would appear to be little therapeutic benefit in using this drug in comparison to other more effective and safer NSAIDs.

Formulations and dose rates

Naproxen is available in tablet formulation.

DOGS

- Naproxen has been administered chronically to dogs at doses starting at 5 mg/kg PO on the first day and 2 mg/kg PO q.24 h or q.48 h thereafter

Mechanism of action – additional information

Naproxen is a member of the propionic acid class of NSAIDs.

Relevant pharmacokinetic data

Naproxen undergoes extensive enterohepatic recycling in the dog, resulting in prolonged elimination. The half-life in dogs is as long as 92 h, in comparison to 8.3 h for horses and 14–24 h for humans.

Paracetamol (acetaminophen)

(Crocin®, Panadol®, Tylenol®, Calpol®, etc. and generics)

Clinical applications

Paracetamol (acetaminophen) is not approved for use in dogs and cats. It is a para-aminophenol derivative. It has analgesic and antipyretic actions through presumed central COX inhibition. Recent reports have suggested that paracetamol may act by inhibition of 5-HT_3 receptors and COX-3, the product of a splice variant of COX-1. It does not inhibit peripheral COX. Although paracetamol is believed to have no significant anti-inflammatory activity, it has been reported to be as effective as aspirin in the treatment of musculoskeletal pain in dogs.

Adverse effects

Adverse effects in dogs are reported to be few because of the lack of peripheral COX inhibition. Cats, however, are very sensitive to paracetamol and as little as 46 mg/kg (e.g. half a 500 mg tablet) can cause toxic signs. The clinical signs of paracetamol toxicity in cats are edema of the face (mechanism unknown), cyanosis and methemoglobinemia, anemia, hemoglobinuria and icterus.

Methemoglobinuria occurs as a result of oxidation of heme, which allows methemoglobin, which is not capable of binding oxygen, to accumulate. Oxidized heme also shifts the oxydissociation curve to the left, which impairs the unloading of oxygen in tissues, exacerbating the tissue anoxia. The sulfhydryl-containing tripeptide, reduced glutathione, is thought to be important in methemoglobin production. Cat hemoglobin has at least eight sulfhydryl groups per molecule, more than are found in other species, which may render it particularly sensitive to oxidation when glutathione levels fall.

Intravascular or extravascular hemolysis occurs because of Heinz body anemia. Heinz bodies are microscopic, round, refractile structures on the internal aspect of the erythrocyte membrane. They represent sites of hemoglobin denaturation due to oxidant injury. Clinical reports of paracetamol toxicosis in cats suggest that erythrocyte destruction can occur for up to 3 weeks. In one cat, hemoglobin casts caused urethral obstruction, an unusual but potentially fatal sequela.

Icterus in cats with paracetamol toxicity is probably more likely to result from hemolysis than hepatocellular necrosis. In contrast to humans and dogs, hepatocellular necrosis is reported to be of less significance in cats with paracetamol toxicosis.

It is not understood why hepatic necrosis is less important in cats than in other species, as high concentrations of the drug remain in the blood for a long time and a greater proportion is oxidized. Another anomaly occurs in humans, where doses high enough to cause hepatic necrosis in adults cause very little damage in children.

Paracetamol in all species is metabolized by three pathways: glucuronidation, sulfation and cytochrome P450-mediated oxidation. The metabolites of glucuronidation and sulfation are not toxic but the oxidation pathway yields a reactive toxic metabolite (thought to be *N*-acetyl-*p*-benzoquinoneimine). This metabolite is normally conjugated with glutathione but when hepatic glutathione is depleted the metabolite binds covalently to amino acid residues of protein in the liver, resulting in centrilobular hepatic necrosis.

Glucuronidation is the major metabolic pathway in most species but cats have a low concentration of glucuronyl transferase, which catalyzes the final step, so metabolism via this pathway is insignificant. Sulfation is the major metabolic pathway in the cat but it is capacity limited – as the dose is increased, a greater percentage of the drug is oxidized.

Therapy of toxicosis

Treatment of paracetamol toxicity involves supportive therapy (intravenous fluids, typed blood transfusion if required) as well as more specific therapy.

N-acetylcysteine (140 mg/kg PO followed by 70 mg/kg PO every 6 h) is efficacious in the treatment of paracetamol toxicity in humans and dogs if given within a few hours following drug administration. In cats, paracetamol is slowly eliminated so *N*-acetylcysteine should be given if clinical signs are present regardless of the time elapsed since drug administration.

There are several mechanisms by which *N*-acetylcysteine is thought to act. It is rapidly hydrolyzed to cysteine and therefore can provide a substrate for glutathione in erythrocytes and the liver. It has also been shown to react directly with the reactive metabolite of paracetamol to form an acetylcysteine conjugate. It has also been shown to increase sulfate conjugation.

Other glutathione and sulfate precursors such as methionine (70 mg/kg q.8 h) have also been used successfully. The use of ascorbate to reduce methemoglobin has been recommended but has been shown not to be effective in dogs and has not been evaluated in cats.

It has been suggested that cimetidine may be useful for treatment of paracetamol toxicity as it is a potent inhibitor of cytochrome P450-mediated drug metabolism. In rats it is as efficacious as *N*-acetylcysteine in protecting against paracetamol-induced hepatic necrosis. However, its use in cats has not been evaluated and the potential benefit may be less in this species because hepatocellular damage is not as extensive as in other species.

Piroxicam

(Feldene®)

Clinical applications

Piroxicam is not approved for use in dogs. It has been used in the management of canine transitional cell carcinoma of the bladder. It is believed that its antitumor effect is by inhibition of COX-2, although piroxicam has not been shown to have cytotoxic activity in vitro. A small number of dogs (approximately 20%) may achieve partial or complete remission with piroxicam therapy. It has been reported that combination therapy with cisplatin (50–60 mg/m^2 intravenously, once every 21 d) increases the partial or complete remission rate to as high as 70%. It is also reported to be useful in the symptomatic relief of stranguria associated with cystitis, urethritis or transitional cell carcinomas. Because of its side effects, piroxicam is not recommended for musculoskeletal pain as there are other more effective and safer NSAIDs available.

Formulations and dose rates

Piroxicam is available in tablet form.

DOGS
- 0.3 mg/kg PO q.24 h

Mechanism of action – additional information

Piroxicam is a member of the oxicam class of NSAIDs.

Adverse effects

- The incidence of gastrointestinal and renal side effects in dogs treated with piroxicam is relatively high.
- The synthetic prostaglandin E analog misoprostol may be administered concurrently to reduce the likelihood of gastric ulceration occurring.

CHONDROPROTECTIVE AGENTS FOR SMALL ANIMAL PRACTICE

The use of chondroprotective agents in veterinary medicine started with equine medicine. Application in dogs followed but there is currently little use in cats. Therapeutic approaches may be divided into at least three broad categories:
- component building blocks necessary for cartilage function and regeneration, such as polysulfated glycosaminoglycans (PSGAGs)
- boundary lubricants to reduce joint trauma and improve joint motion, such as hyaluronan (HA)
- nutraceutical supplements to supply essential nutrients to joint function, such as chondroitin sulfate and glucosamine.

PSGAGs and other polysulfated polysaccharides are similar to the glycosaminoglycans present in articular cartilage. These agents are synthetic heparinoids and have affinity for proteoglycans and noncollagenous proteins in cartilage. Studies have documented a stimulatory role in the production of HA and glycosaminoglycan synthesis. It is believed that long-term use of these agents helps cartilage regeneration and/or repair. Additionally, activity has been attributed to PSGAGs for the inhibition of cartilage degradative enzymes and even as an anti-inflammtory with inhibition of PGE_2. Initial formulations were for intra-articular administration. However, at least in horses, there was occasional joint infection associated with treatment. Subsequently, intramuscular and oral formulations have been developed that apparently still give good joint penetration of the active ingredients. Potential adverse events, in addition to the iatrogenic infection described above, primarily include hemorrhage. Since these agents are heparinoids, they can interfere with normal clotting activity. Elevations in activated partial thromboplastin time, prothrombin time and activated clotting time have been reported. Clinically these effects may manifest as hemarthrosis, local hematoma and thrombocytopenia.

Boundary lubricants have been used primarily in equine medicine. Most of the products available vary based on molecular weight of the HA and any additional cross-linking or polymerization between HA chains. HA itself is a component of both synovial fluid and cartilage. In synovial fluid, its viscoelastic properties confer boundary lubrication. In cartilage, HA may not be the primary lubricant but may be involved in what is called boosted lubrication. In this case, as the opposing cartilage surfaces come together, water is driven into the cartilage and a concentrated pool of HA remains. Additionally, HA has been shown to have anti-inflammatory properties, particularly in terms of inhibiting chemotaxis of leukocytes. HA products for horses are available for intra-articular or intravenous administration.

Nutraceutical supplements are defined variously around the world. One definition, from Health Canada, is 'a product isolated or purified from foods and generally sold in medicinal forms not usually associated with food and demonstrated to have a physiological benefit or provide protection against chronic disease'. Nutraceuticals are not generally regulated as drugs, but rather as foodstuffs or nutritional supplements. As such, most nutraceuticals have not undergone the safety and efficacy testing, nor the manufacturing rigor, required of pharmaceuticals. In the area of joint disease, the most commonly used nutraceuticals include chondroitin sulfate and glucosamine, generally in association with ascorbic acid (vitamin C) and manganese. Additionally, some preparations include special fatty acids, such as omega-3, coenzyme Q10 (ubiquinone), various other antioxidants and various other free radical-scavenging agents. These products may be available as powders, in gelatin capsules, as liquids or in pet foods. Because these products are less regulated and there literally are hundreds of offerings, it is important to purchase them from reputable companies that guarantee their content and have study data to support their use.

The most extensively studied nutraceuticals in small animal practice are chondroitin sulfate and glucosamine. Chondroitin sulfate is a normal component of cartilage and is part of the proteoglycan molecule. In joint disease, proteoglycans and their synthesis are diminished. Chondroitin sulfate is believed to stimulate production of glycosaminoglycans and cartilage matrix production. The mechanism of action for glucosamine is not fully determined, although it is believed to influence synthesis of HA and glycosaminoglycans. Glucosamine appears to be synergistic with chondroitin sulfate and the combination of the two may also inhibit proteolytic enzymes to further retard joint damage. These effects are slow acting and may take 4–6 weeks of supplementation for improvement to be seen.

APPROVED CHONDROPROTECTIVE DRUGS FOR SMALL ANIMAL PRACTICE

Pentosan polysulfate

(Cartrophen Vet®, Elmiron®)

Clinical applications

Pentosan polysulfate is approved for use in dogs in Europe and Australasia. It is indicated for the treatment of primary and secondary osteoarthritis. Clinical efficacy has been demonstrated in dogs with chronic osteoarthritis. Anecdotal reports suggest that pentosan has value in assisting healing after surgical procedures such as cranial cruciate repair and luxating patella fixation.

Pentosan has also been used in the management of refractory cases of feline lower urinary tract disease or recurrent urinary tract infection in dogs.

Formulations and dose rates

Available in injectable (SC) or oral formulations. Intra-articular administration has been shown to predispose to the development of septic arthritis.

CATS AND DOGS

- 3 mg/kg PO or SC once weekly for four treatments

Mechanism of action

Pentosan polysulfate is a polysulfated polysaccharide drug that acts as a chondroprotective agent. It can:

- retard the degradation of articular cartilage in osteoarthritis through inhibition of many enzymes that are implicated in the degradation of cartilage
- in some circumstances have a positive effect on chondrocyte metabolism, which may encourage repair of articular cartilage

- stimulate the synthesis of HA (the major nonproteinaceous component of synovial fluid). The quantity and molecular weight of HA are often reduced in arthritic joints. HA is important for the maintenance of viscosity, soft tissue boundary lubrication and protection of articular cartilage from mechanical damage
- improve circulation to subchondral bone.

Adverse effects

Polysulfated polysaccharides have anticoagulant activity, although when administered as recommended they should not prolong bleeding time. However, care should be exercised when giving these drugs to animals with known clotting disorders. Administration should be delayed for 1–3 d postoperatively.

Polysulfated glycosaminoglycan

(Adequan®)

Clinical applications

Polysulfated glycosaminoglycan (PSGAG) is approved for use in dogs in Europe, Canada and the USA. Indications are the prevention and modification of progression of secondary osteoarthritis. Young dogs predisposed to development of hip dysplasia that were given PSGAG by intramuscular injection twice weekly had better radiographic scores for subluxation at 8 months of age than control dogs but there were no significant treatment effects on the gross lesions or cartilage biochemistry. In another study of beagles, prophylactic administration of PSGAG provided partial protection against articular cartilage degeneration induced by medial meniscectomy. However, a multicenter, dose–response, clinical study in dogs with osteoarthritis failed to find a significant beneficial effect of PSGAG treatment.

Mechanism of action

PSGAG is derived from bovine trachea and lung and it is a mixture of highly sulfated glycosaminoglycans, mainly composed of chondroitin sulfates. Some in vitro studies demonstrated an anabolic effect of PSGAG on articular cartilage, with increased matrix synthesis by chondrocytes. Also, PSGAG inhibited the degradative actions of some inflammatory mediators and enzymes in vitro and reduced concentrations of collagenases in articular cartilage in dogs with induced osteoarthritis.

Formulations and dose rates

Available in an injectable formulation for intramuscular administration.

DOGS

- 4.4 mg/kg IM, twice weekly for up to 4 weeks (maximum of 8 injections) (from packet insert)

Pharmacokinetics

Studies in rabbits and horses have shown that PSGAG is incorporated into articular cartilage, meniscus and synovial fluid following intramuscular and intra-articular injection.

Adverse effects

PSGAG is a synthetic heparinoid and increases bleeding times in dogs and cats. Do not use it in dogs in shock or with suspected bleeding disorders.

FURTHER READING

Bergh MS, Budsberg SC 2005 The coxib NSAIDs: potential clinical and pharmacological importance in veterinary medicine. J Vet Intern Med 19: 633-643

Brideau C, Van Staden C, Chan CC 2001 In vitro effects of cyclooxygenase inhibitors in whole blood of horses, dogs and cats. Am J Vet Res 62: 1755-1760

Brooks P, Emery P, Evans JF et al 1999 Interpreting the clinical significance of the differential inhibition of cyclooxygenase-1 and cyclooxygenase-2. Rheumatology 38: 779-788

Chandrasekharan NV, Dai H, Roos KLT et al 2002 COX-3, a cyclooxygenase-1 variant inhibited by acetaminophen and other analgesic/antipyretic drugs: cloning, structure and expression. PNAS 99: 13926-13931

Forsyth SF, Guilford WG, Pfeiffer DU 2000 Effect of NSAID administration on creatinine clearance in healthy dogs undergoing anaesthesia and surgery. J Small Animal Pract 41: 547-550

Johnson SA, Fox SM 1997 Mechanisms of action of anti-inflammatory medications used for the treatment of osteoarthritis. JAVMA 210: 1486-1492

Lees P, Landoni MF, Giraudel J, Toutain PL 2004 Pharmacodynamics and pharmacokinetics of nonsteroidal anti-inflammatory drugs in species of veterinary interest. J Vet Pharm Therap 27: 479-490

Lees P, Giraudel J, Landoni MF, Toutain PL 2004 PK-PD integration and PK-PD modeling of nonsteroidal anti-inflammatory drugs: principles and applications in veterinary pharmacology. J Vet Pharm Therap 27: 490-502

Mathews KA 1996 Nonsteroidal anti-inflammatory analgesics in pain management in dogs and cats. Can Vet J 37: 539-545

McCann ME, Andersen DR, Zhang D et al 2004 In vitro effects and in vivo efficacy of a novel cyclooxygenase-2 inhibitor in dogs with experimentally induced synovitis. Am J Vet Res 65: 503-512

Papich MG 1997 Principles of analgesic drug therapy. Semin Vet Med Surg 12: 80-93

Warner TD, Giuliano F, Vojnovic I, Bukasa A, Mitchel JA, Vane JR 1999 Nonsteroid drug selectivities for cyclo-oxygenase 1 rather than cyclo-oxygenase-2 are associated with human gastrointestinal toxicity: a full in vitro analysis. Proc Natl Acad Sci USA 96: 7563-7568

Wilson JE, Chandrasekharan NV, Westover KD, Eager KB, Simmons DL 2004 Determination of expression of cyclooxygenase-1 and -2 isozymes in canine tissues and their differential sensitivity to nonsteroidal anti-inflammatory drugs. Am J Vet Res 65: 810-818

Opioid analgesics

Richard Hammond, Macdonald Christie and Anthony Nicholson

INTRODUCTION

Pain

Recognition of pain in animals and its management

Most clinicians now accept that 'beneficial' effects of pain are limited (minimizing the extent of an injury, encouraging rest, learning of avoidance behavior). In animals under direct veterinary care, these responses are maladaptive and deleterious. Ongoing or severe pain confers no useful function in the clinical setting and is associated with a well-established, evidence-based list of negative aspects. These include: the shift to a catabolic state, reduced voluntary food intake, impaired respiratory function and delayed recovery from anesthesia, delayed wound healing, central/peripheral hypersensitization and chronic hyperalgesic states, and an increased development of metastatic disease following tumor removal. These aspects are in addition to the ethical considerations of alleviating suffering of patients under our care.

Despite this acceptance, many clinicians are unwilling to provide the plane of analgesia adequate for the preexisting level of pain or the proposed surgical intervention. Common (but not excusable) reasons for neglect of analgesia in small animals primarily are based upon misconceptions as to opioid safety or unwanted effects and inability to adequately recognize pain. Indeed, it has been hypothesized that evolutionary processes have contributed to making recognition of pain in animals difficult. Animals showing weakness, distress or pain become targets for predators. Therefore, the laws of survival require that abnormal behavior be avoided at all costs. Thus, just because an animal does not exhibit what the clinician thinks are typical signs of pain (e.g. vocalizing) does not mean that it is not in pain.

The indicators of pain in animals are often nonspecific and may be confused with disease (anorexia), hypovolemia (tachycardia), pulmonary disease (tachypnea) or reaction to being in a strange environment (altered behavior). In most cases there are few contraindications for giving the animal 'the benefit of the doubt' and using the administration of an analgesic as both diagnostic and therapeutic tool, an improvement of the animal on administration of the analgesic confirming and treating the presence of pain.

It is also important to recognize that pain is only one of many internal and environmental stressors placed on critically ill or postsurgical animals. Fear and anxiety can intensify the distress associated with pain. Therefore, sedation is often desirable in these patients and the combination of analgesics and anxiolytics (e.g. acepromazine, midazolam, medetomidine) may be very beneficial. Much can also be done to provide relief from pain and distress other than using drugs. Other strategies include:

- **wound care**: careful dressing and stabilization will limit movement and self-trauma; dressings/splints
- **nutrition**: important in wound healing and a useful diversionary activity
- **physiotherapy**: assists early mobilization and reduces inflammation
- **environment**: providing comfort and padding.

The importance of pre-emptive analgesia

A painful stimulus associated with tissue damage is detected by tissue nociceptors. The stimulus is transmitted via primary afferent neurones to the spinal cord or cranial nerve nuclei. Two main types of neurones are involved: C-fibers (slow, dull pain) and Aδ fibers (fast, sharp pain). These fibers enter the spinal cord via the dorsal horn and interact with other spinal nociceptive neurones and neurotransmitters to achieve perception of the stimulus in the higher centers in the brain. This system is highly malleable and can change over time according to input.

Both types of clinically important pain (inflammatory and neuropathic) are associated with a generalized increase in sensitivity of the whole nociceptive processing system. This leads to nonpainful stimuli being perceived as painful (allodynia) and an exaggeration of pain responses (hyperalgesia). The latter can occur at the site of injury (primary) or at distant tissues (secondary). Such sensitization is initiated almost immediately following a painful stimulus, both centrally within the nervous system as well as in the peripheral tissues. Peripheral sensitization occurs largely because of an increase in sensitivity of peripheral nociceptors to inflammatory and 'nociceptive' mediators released following tissue injury. This causes afferent neurones to fire more frequently. It also allows low-intensity signals to stimulate spinal cord neurones. Central sensitization occurs due to changes within the spinal cord. Nerve fibers in the dorsal horn of the spinal cord increase their excitability and afferent information is 'overinterpreted' by the spinal afferent system. The clinical significance of these mechanisms is that any pain perceived by the animal is more severe once tissue damage has occurred, and analgesics may be less effective.

This has given rise to the concept of pre-emptive analgesia: giving analgesics before tissue damage occurs. Postoperative pain may be more easily controlled when it is pre-empted by administration of analgesic therapy instituted before the patient is exposed to noxious stimuli, whether or not the patient is conscious. The reasons for this are not entirely understood but appear to be related to the fact that the organization and function of the nervous system change following painful stimuli. The significance of this hypersensitivity remains controversial in humans but it is important in several species of experimental animals. It may therefore be much easier to prevent pain produced by surgery than to suppress it once it is already present. In human patients, it has been clearly shown that fixed-interval administration of analgesics (a regular dose at a regular time) is more effective in achieving pain relief and requires lower overall doses of opioids than dosing on demand. It is therefore more effective (and humane) and safer to administer opioids to control pain likely to result from a procedure than attempt to reduce pain after severe signs have emerged.

Drugs

EXAMPLES

Morphine and its analogs (e.g. oxymorphone), pethidine (meperidine), methadone, codeine, fentanyl and its analogs (alfentanil and remifentanil), buprenorphine, butorphanol, pentazocine and tramadol.

The opioid analgesics remain the most potent and efficacious analgesic drugs in veterinary medicine. The prototype drug is morphine, named after the Greek god of dreams, Morpheus. It is derived from the dry residue of the exudate from the unripe seed capsule of the poppy *Papaver somniferum*. This residue is opium, which contains a mixture of alkaloids, of which there are two main types. These are the phenanthrene alkaloids, which include morphine and codeine, and the benzylisoquinoline alkaloids, of which papaverine is the main example, which have smooth muscle relaxant effects but no analgesic properties.

Drugs derived directly from the opium poppy are known as opiates while any substances that interact specifically with opioid receptors (see below), including endogenous peptides and opiates, are known as opioids.

Clinical applications

Opioids are effective for treatment of moderate-to-severe pain, particularly acute pain due to trauma and surgical procedures. Although these drugs can have significant side effects, these are significantly reduced in the face of pre-existing pain and for most animals are usually not of sufficient concern to prevent use of opioid drugs at clinical dose rates.

Chemical structure

Morphine has a five-ring structure that is the core for many of the semisynthetic opioids, including heroin (diacetyl morphine), oxymorphone, pentazocine, butorphanol, buprenorphine and naloxone.

Synthetic opioids have fewer rings and form either piperidines such as pethidine (meperidine) or the phenylpiperidines, which include fentanyl, sufentanil and alfentanil.

Remifentanil is also a phenylpiperidine, but as a 4-anilidopiperidine derivative of fentanyl, has an ester linkage in the piperidine ring, making it susceptible to metabolism by plasma esterases.

Methadone has a structure very different from that of morphine but retains the active moieties of morphine. Opioid antagonists, including naloxone, naltrexone and nalbuphine, structurally resemble agonists but generally have bulky unsaturated N-linked substitutions.

Opioid receptors and drug/effector mechanisms

Classes of opioid receptor

The opioid receptors are pharmacologically distinct, closely related membrane proteins that share common characteristics because they have evolved from a common ancestral G protein coupled receptor. Three types of opioid receptor have been identified in mammals. These are termed mu (μ, the Greek letter m, for 'morphine receptor', also MOP using standard nomenclature), kappa (κ, the Greek letter k, for ketocyclazocine, the first class of drug used to define the receptor functionally, also KOP using standard nomenclature) and delta (δ, the Greek letter d for deferens, because the mouse vas deferens was the first tissue used to define the receptor functionally, also DOP using standard nomenclature). Each of the three receptor proteins is encoded by an independent gene. A fourth closely related gene encodes an opioid-like receptor (NOP using standard nomenclature, also known as ORL-1) that interacts with some opioid-like peptides orphanin-FQ or nociceptin but not the classic opioid drugs. The potential role of this receptor in pain control is still being investigated.

Other types and subtypes of opioid receptor have been suggested on the basis of indirect pharmacological evidence but their existence has either been ruled out or they have not yet been clearly established. The sigma (σ) receptor is no longer considered to be an opioid receptor.

The epsilon (ε) receptor is not a distinct opioid receptor, being best explained by the presence of a very low density of μ receptors in some tissues. The suggestion that a subtype of μ-receptor is the target of the major active metabolite of morphine, morphine-6-glucuronide, has little or no experimental support. Further receptor subclassifications such as μ1 and μ2, δ1 and δ2 and κ1 and κ2 are controversial. It remains possible but not established that some subtypes arise from alternatively spliced mRNA products of transcripts of the three major receptors, or from hetero-oligomerization among the three major receptor types. The κ3 subtype is no longer accepted.

Effector mechanisms

Opioid drugs mimic the actions of endogenous opioids (endorphins), which are peptides produced in the nervous and endocrine systems that stimulate opioid receptors. A number of opioid peptides ranging in size from five to over 30 amino acids are synthesized from the three large precursors: pro-opioimelanocortin, pro-enkephalin and prodynorphin. Endogenous opioid systems appear to usually have only weak tonic activity but become highly active under certain environmental conditions, e.g. during extreme stress and pain. The analgesic activity of some opioid drugs (e.g. tramadol) is due to interaction with opioid receptors as well as other neurotransmitter systems.

Different opioid drugs bind to distinct opioid receptors with varying degrees of affinity and have differing durations of action, which result in different pharmacological profiles. To complicate matters, a given opioid drug may act as an agonist, a partial agonist or an antagonist at each type of receptor (Fig. 14.1). Selection of an opioid for a particular use depends on these properties as well as its absorption, distribution and metabolism.

All the cloned opioid receptor types belong to the Gi/Go-coupled superfamily of receptors. Under normal circumstances opioid receptors do not couple directly with Gs or Gq and none of the cloned receptors forms a ligand-gated ion channel. All three classic receptor types (μ, δ and κ) and the NOP-receptor couple through Gi/Go proteins generally share common effector mechanisms, e.g. they can all activate inwardly rectifying potassium conductance and inhibit voltage-operated calcium conductances in cell membranes to produce inhibition of excitability. However, different responses can be evoked in different cell types in response to activation of different opioid receptors. These are likely to reflect changes in the expression of G proteins and effector systems between cell types rather than any inherent differences in the properties of the receptors themselves.

Opioid receptor activation produces a wide array of cellular responses, the net result of which depends upon the location of each receptor type in the nervous system and on the specific biochemical cascades activated in different types of cell. For example, μ-opioid receptors are located throughout neural systems responsible for pain sensation, from the spinal cord to the brain. The inhibition of pain transmission produced by μ-opioid agonists is highly selective and other sensory modalities are not disrupted. μ-Receptors also occur on nerve cells responsible for generating respiratory rhythms in the brainstem and thus depress respiration when stimulated. Receptor selectivity, distribution and pharmacological responses produced by opioid agonists are summarized in Table 14.1.

All opioid receptors appear to function primarily by exerting inhibitory modulation of synaptic transmission in both the CNS and various peripheral nerve cells, including the myenteric plexus. Receptors are often found on presynaptic nerve terminals, where their action results in decreased release of neurotransmitters, or on nerve cell bodies, where they inhibit the generation of action potentials. In some parts of the nervous system opioid receptors inhibit excitatory neurotransmission and in others release of inhibitory neurotransmitters is impaired, leading to disinhibition or a net excitatory effect.

Known drug interactions with opioid receptors

Some opioids act with high efficacy and potency at one receptor type and with much lower potency and lower efficacy at other receptors; these are called full agonists, e.g. morphine at μ-receptors. Some opioids are partial agonists at one receptor type, e.g. buprenorphine is a partial μ-receptor agonist with little activity at other types. Others are mixed agonist-antagonists, having agonist actions at one receptor type and antagonist activity at others (e.g. nalbuphine is a μ-antagonist as well as a κ-agonist).

Endogenous opioid peptides display some selectivity for different receptor types. Enkephalins and β-endorphin interact selectively with both μ- and δ-receptors. Dynorphins are selective for κ-receptors and endomorphins are selective for μ-receptors; however, the existence of endomorphins will remain tentative

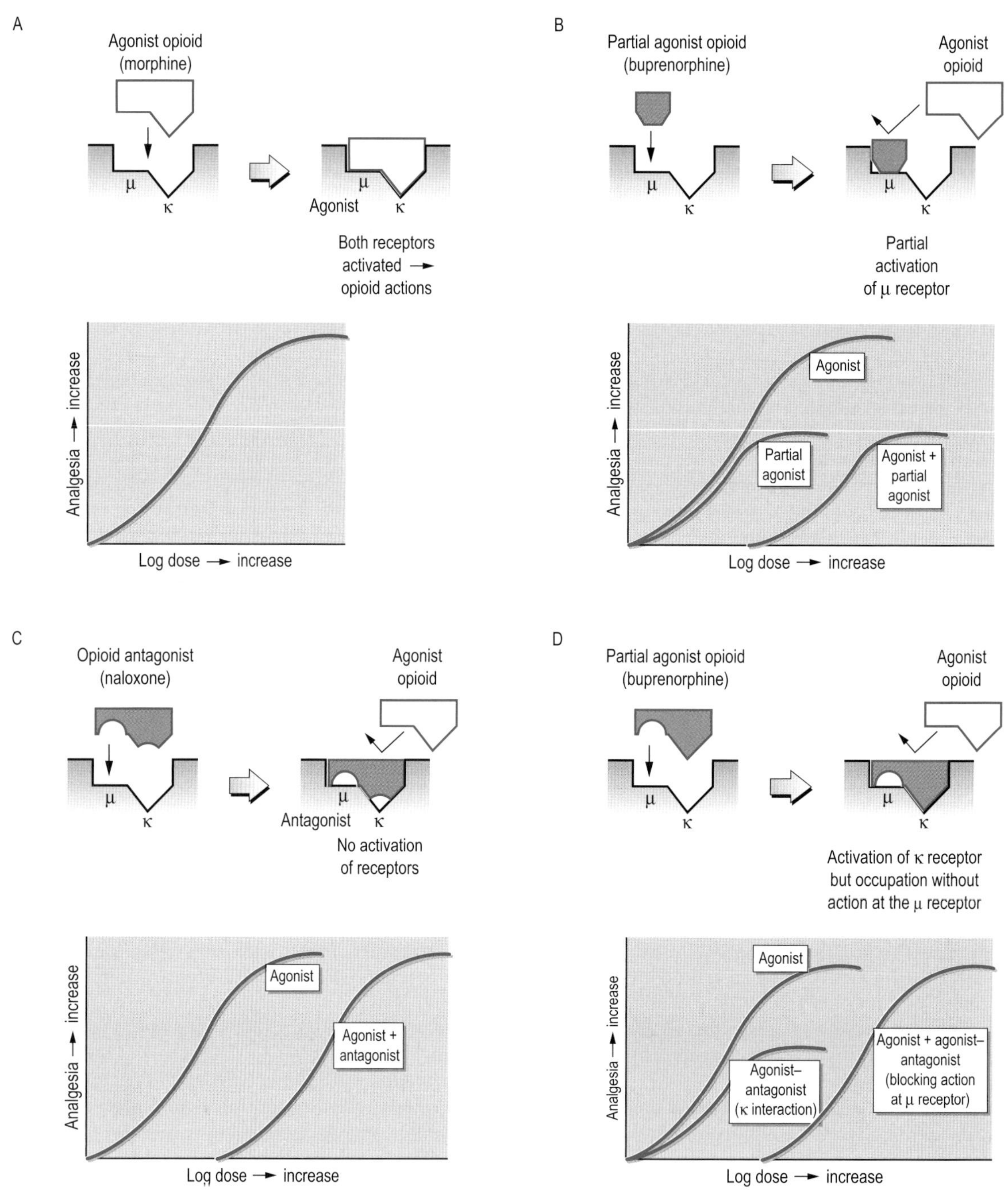

Fig. 14.1 **Opioid receptor interactions. A lock-and-key analogy is used to illustrate different drug interactions at mu (μ) and kappa (κ) receptors, below which is a relative dose–response curve for analgesic potency. (A) An opioid agonist stimulates both receptor types, which results in increased analgesic effect with increased dose. (B) A partial agonist weakly stimulates the μ-receptor to achieve a reduced maximum analgesic effect compared with a full agonist. A large dose of a partial agonist will block the receptor actions of the full agonist and so move its dose–response curve to the right and depress the maximal analgesic response. Buprenorphine, a commonly used partial agonist, has very strong receptor binding so that even with very large doses of an agonist, the limited analgesic effect of buprenorphine predominates. (C) Complete opioid antagonists possess no intrinsic activity but block the μ- and κ-receptors. Because of the competitive nature of the binding at the receptors, more agonist is required in the presence of antagonist to produce its full analgesic effect. (D) Agonist-antagonists have mixed activity at the two receptor types. Most, such as nalbuphine, have agonist activity at κ-receptors and antagonist activity at μ-receptors. In the presence of a full μ-agonist, these opioids tend to act as antagonists and increase the dose of full agonist required to achieve maximum analgesic effect.**

Table 14.1 Features of different opioid receptor types

Receptor type	Mu (μ)	Kappa (κ)	Delta (δ)
Some selective drugs used clinically	Fentanyl Morphine Methadone Oxycodone Pethidine (and most other opioid analgesics in use)	Butorphanol (also a partial μ-agonist) Pentazocine (also a partial μ-agonist) Nalbuphine (also a weak partial μ-agonist)	None available but some are in development
Location of receptors relevant for clinical effects	**Brain:** All pain sensation and modulation pathways Chemoreceptor trigger zone Respiratory centers Baroreflex centers Basal ganglia (motor effects) Limbic centers (emotional responses) Cortex and thalamus (sensory processing) **Spinal cord:** dorsal horn (pain sensation) **Myenteric plexus** (gut motility)	**Brain:** Basal ganglia Limbic centers Cortex and thalamus **Spinal cord:** dorsal horn **Kidney** **Myenteric plexus** (gut motility)	**Brain:** Basal ganglia Cortex and thalamus **Spinal cord:** dorsal horn
Selective actions	Analgesia (strong) Cough suppression Constipation Hypotension Sedation Motor excitation (some species) Respiratory depression – cause of overdose death Tolerance and dependence Vomiting	Analgesia (moderate from spinal cord) Diuresis Sedation Dysphoria Hallucinosis	Analgesia (mild–moderate from spinal cord) Motor excitation

until an endogenous mechanism for their synthesis is found. Most of the analgesic actions as well as side effects of the opioids used clinically are due to their interactions with μ-receptors and, to a lesser extent, κ-receptors in the CNS.

Most of the analgesic actions as well as unwanted effects of opioids have been ascribed to interactions with opioid receptors in the CNS. Opioid receptors are expressed preferentially on the CNS terminations of nociceptive primary afferent neurones and thence throughout ascending systems involved in the sensation and emotional appreciation of pain. Opioid receptors are also expressed on descending pain modulation systems. Throughout these neural pathways μ-opioid receptors dominate but κ- and δ-receptors are also present in some places, e.g. the dorsal horn of the spinal cord.

More recently, interest has developed in the modification of peripheral opioid receptors. Opioid receptors are also present on peripheral terminations of nociceptive nerve fibers. The cell bodies of these neurones in dorsal root ganglia express mRNAs for all three classic receptor types and receptor proteins. Opioid receptors are intra-axonally transported into the neuronal processes, where opioids are thought to inhibit nerve cell activity and produce pain relief only in circumstances where sensory nerves are sensitized to all stimuli, e.g. during inflammation. This forms the rationale for direct intra-articular instillation of opioids during joint surgery.

Adverse effects in relation to receptor class

The major effects of concern are respiratory depression, hypotension and bradycardia. These effects usually result from the CNS location of opioid receptors. Respiratory depression occurs primarily because μ-opioid receptor stimulation inhibits the activity of neurones in the ventral medulla that respond to hypercapnia (elevated P_aCO_2). Nausea and vomiting, motor excitation and bradycardia are also mediated by the actions of opioids on CNS opioid receptors. Some effects, such as reduced gastrointestinal motility, are due to the presence of opioid receptors throughout the myenteric plexus that control the tone and peristaltic rhythms of the gastrointestinal tract and its sphincters. Histamine release presumably results from an opioid receptor-independent action of some opioids on circulating mast cells.

Pharmacokinetics

Absorption

Most opioids are absorbed well from oral, intramuscular, subcutaneous and intravenous routes. Unwanted effects such as histamine release during intravenous administration of some agents (primarily pethidine) can make the intravenous route unsuitable.

While most opioids are readily absorbed after oral administration, extensive first-pass metabolism makes this route unsuitable in many cases. Rectal administration, e.g. suppositories, may sometimes partly overcome this limitation. Special routes of administration, such as intrathecal, can be used under some circumstances to achieve a high concentration of opioids at a principal site of analgesic action, the dorsal horn of the spinal cord, while minimizing side effects arising from sites higher in the neuraxis (see below).

Distribution and protein binding

Distribution and protein binding of different opioids vary greatly and are discussed under individual subheadings.

Metabolism and elimination

Rates of metabolism and routes of elimination also vary among opioids and are discussed under individual subheadings. Active metabolites are important in some circumstances. For example, the active metabolite of morphine, morphine-6-glucuronide, is approximately five times as potent as morphine. In most species this is a minor metabolite of little consequence but in patients with renal failure, it accumulates to significantly enhance therapeutic actions as well as side effects.

Adverse effects

Most opioids that act on μ-receptors produce a similar spectrum of unwanted effects, although there are individual differences as discussed for specific agents below.

Respiratory depression

Respiratory depression is the most serious unwanted effect of opioid agonists and is the primary cause of mortality due to overdose All aspects of respiratory activity are depressed but responsiveness to hypercapnia is most affected. Respiratory depression occurs as a result of actions on respiratory control nerve networks located in the ventral medulla. Respiratory reflexes, including the cough reflex, are also profoundly depressed and many weak opioid agonists (especially butorphanol) are useful cough suppressants. If P_aCO_2 is allowed to increase after opioid agonist administration then cerebral vasodilation may result in increased intracranial pressure. This may be detrimental in cases of closed head injury. In ventilated patients, however, where normocapnia is maintained, opioids will reduce intracranial pressure and cerebral metabolic oxygen demand.

Partial μ-receptor agonists tend to produce less respiratory depression than full agonists. In many species partial μ-agonists such as buprenorphine and mixed agonist-antagonists with weak partial μ-receptor activity, e.g. pentazocine and butorphanol, reach a ceiling effect beyond which no further respiratory depression can be produced despite increased analgesic effects from increasing doses. These opioids are therefore safer than full agonists which may be beneficial in some circumstances. However, it should be noted that partial μ-receptor agonists can produce severe respiratory depression when used in combination with sedatives that also depress respiration. It should also be noted that there is a ceiling effect associated with use of partial μ-agonists for pain relief, particularly after continuous administration for several days (see Tolerance and physical dependence). Opioids with some agonist activity at κ-receptors, such as butorphanol, also tend to produce less respiratory depression than pure μ-receptor agonists.

Nausea and vomiting

Nausea and vomiting are due to direct actions on opioid receptors located on dorsal medullary neurones in and around the area postrema. This brain region, which lacks a fully developed blood–brain barrier, is also known as the chemoreceptor trigger zone. While some opioids, such as morphine and oxymorphone, may induce more vomiting than others, all can potentially do so.

Bradycardia

Opioids may produce a dose-related bradycardia, although this tends to be more pronounced with fentanyl and its analogs. This action is caused by depression of brainstem cardiovascular control centers, resulting in an increased parasympathetic nervous tone. In all cases, this may be prevented or treated by use of a parasympatholytic such as atropine or glycopyrrolate. Pethidine has a structure similar to atropine and as a result does not reduce heart rate at normal clinical doses.

Myocardial contractility and vascular tone are well preserved when opioids are administered at clinical doses. As a result, the bradycardia produced by the clinical use of an opioid, especially in the presence of pre-existing pain, does not normally result in significant hypotension. Indeed, the dose-sparing effect of an opioid when used concurrently with an anesthetic often results in more favorable cardiovascular parameters.

Constipation

The use of opium for relief of diarrhea and dysentery predates its use for pain therapy. Synthetic opioids, particularly those that poorly penetrate the CNS (e.g. loperamide), are currently used to manage diarrhea (see Chapter 19). Constipation is not usually of concern during short-term opioid use for acute pain relief but management using stool softeners and other adjuncts may prove necessary during prolonged opioid therapy.

Constipation results primarily from inhibitory actions of opioids on neurones of the myenteric plexus, although the CNS is also involved to a minor extent. Both μ- and κ-opioid agonists (relative actions depend on species) markedly inhibit the propulsive contractions of peristalsis, slowing gastrointestinal transit and thereby increasing water resorption. Biliary and pancreatic secretion is inhibited and sphincter tone is increased, contributing to constipation.

Urinary retention

Urinary retention is a minor and variable side effect of opioids in most species, resulting from increased sphincter tone. Where high concentrations are administered intrathecally or into the extradural space, retention may be significant, for a period of some hours, and regular monitoring of urinary bladder tone should be performed. Opioids with agonist activity at κ-receptors produce diuresis, thus increasing urine flow.

Histamine release

Opioids are secretagogues and histamine release results from a nonopioid receptor-mediated action on circulating mast cells. Pethidine and to a lesser extent morphine may produce significant histamine release on intravenous administration of clinical doses. Intravenous use of pethidine should be avoided. In contrast, fentanyl produces little or no histamine release. Pruritus is a relatively common sequel to extradural administration of morphine (pethidine is not used via this route) and has been reported in many species including man, the horse and the dog. This is a receptor-mediated action (it is reversed by opioid antagonists such as naloxone) but has a poorly understood mechanism (it may be treated by subanesthetic concentrations of the sedative-anesthetic propofol, a drug with no known opioid receptor antagonism).

Excitatory motor effects

Motor excitation, muscular rigidity and explosive motor behavior can occur with μ-opioid receptor agonists at high doses in some species. These actions are dose related and mediated by the CNS. They are thought to arise from disinhibition of basal ganglia neural systems and possibly midbrain emotional motor systems. Cats, horses, pigs and ruminants are particularly susceptible to excitatory motor effects. Opioids are routinely and effectively used in these species and these effects are not normally seen at even high-end clinical doses.

Tolerance and physical dependence

Repeated or continuous use of opioids results in development of tolerance, or a need to administer an increased dose to produce the same effect, and physical dependence characterized by a withdrawal syndrome on cessation of use.

Tolerance can usually be overcome by increasing the dose of opioid used but this carries the risk of increasing physical dependence. The maximum analgesic effect achievable may be blunted in tolerant patients for partial agonists such as buprenorphine, pentazocine and butorphanol, regardless of dose. Tolerance and dependence do not develop appreciably after a single opioid dose but are of concern if therapy is continued for more than several days. Both phenomena are dose related and develop in parallel. Therefore, if there is need to escalate doses of opioids over a period of days to produce adequate control of pain then the likelihood increases that a withdrawal syndrome will be manifested on cessation of use.

Opioid withdrawal is intensely dysphoric if severe and can be minimized by use of gradually diminishing opioid doses. The syndrome differs somewhat among species but can include agitation, violent escape attempts, ptosis, yawning, lacrimation, rhinorrhea, diarrhea, urination, ejaculation and piloerection.

Indications and techniques of opioid use in small animals

Animals presenting in pain

Veterinary surgeons may be presented with an animal in pain, most frequently following trauma. In these cases moderate-to-high doses of opioid, often in combination with sedation and a second mode of analgesia (multimodal analgesia), are needed to overcome the preexisting nociception. However, the most frequent indication for opioid administration in veterinary practice is perioperatively. This may be preoperative, intraoperative, postoperative or a combination of any or all of these.

Preoperative analgesia

Preoperative opioids regularly form part of the premedication protocol, usually in combination with a sedative or tranquilizer. Premedicants commonly used in companion animal practice include acepromazine (ACP), medetomidine and the benzodiazepines diazepam and midazolam. All three agents have a synergistic effect with most opioids in current usage. With α_2-agonists this may be explained by a co-localization of receptor activity. Analgesic effects of medetomidine are principally (but not exclusively) due to spinal antinociception via binding to nonnoradrenergic receptors located on the dorsal horn. There is also some evidence of supraspinal analgesic mechanisms in the locus ceruleus.

In severely compromised animals in whom only low-level sedation is required, a low dose of an opioid alone may achieve the desired effect, although in general the level of sedation produced by standard clinical doses is poor for most opioids when used as the sole agent. Apart from providing increased sedation when used in combination with a sedative or tranquilizer, opioids as part of a premedication protocol can act in a pre-emptive fashion, reducing both the intraoperative and postoperative analgesic requirements. Controlling surgical pain in animals before they fully recover from general anesthesia is easier and requires less total drug to be administered than waiting for the animals to show obvious signs of pain and then administering an analgesic.

Opioids and anesthesia induction

Another preoperative application for some of the full opioid agonists is as a component of the protocol for induction of anesthesia. Selected opioid agents have been used for anesthetic induction in a number of situations because of the marked cardiovascular stability they provide, aside from bradycardia. This technique is most often reserved for very ill and moribund animals, the very elderly or those with a pronounced degree of cardiovascular compromise. In such cases, higher doses of ultra-fast acting pure agonist μ-receptor opioids (fentanyl, alfentanil) may be administered as part of a coinduction (immediately prior to the induction agent). As a result, the dose of induction agent will be significantly reduced but other unwanted effects such as ventilatory depression are minimized or, where seen, can be quickly managed in the anesthetized patient with a controlled airway. It is also recommended that where possible, without stressing the patient, animals be preoxygenated via facemask or oxygen chamber, prior to induction of anesthesia.

The onset of anesthesia during an opioid induction is much slower than that achieved with other intravenous agents such as thiopental and propofol. Delay in onset during induction relates to those factors that influence the transfer across the blood–brain barrier: lipid solubility, ionization and protein binding. Some opioids, fentanyl in particular, make animals hyperresponsive to sudden, loud sounds, which should therefore be avoided during induction.

Intraoperative use of opioids

Many studies have demonstrated a reduced requirement for inhalant anesthetic agents (reduction in the minimum alveolar concentration – MAC) in animals that have received opioid analgesics. This effect is dose dependent; however, even at extremely high dose rates the MAC reduction is still not 100%, which further indicates the inability of opioids to act as true anesthetic agents. Therefore opioid analgesics can be used to supplement the main anesthetic agent, whether it be infused or inhaled, and at the same time provide analgesia; this combination of drugs is often referred to as 'balanced anesthesia'.

There are two commonly used approaches to the delivery of intraoperative opioids: intermittent bolus and continuous infusion.

Intermittent boluses

All μ-agonists, with the exception of the ultra-short acting agent remifentanil, can be administered by intermittent intravenous bolus, the important difference between them being the dosing intervals, which need to be greater for the longer-acting drugs. If such administration is continued for a long surgical procedure, then the dosing interval will often need to be increased as the case progresses to avoid accumulation, which may only become apparent during recovery. Signs of accumulation observed during recovery include prolongation of recovery, in particular delayed extubation, respiratory depression and possibly excitatory behavior, including thrashing and vocalization, which can be difficult to distinguish from insufficient analgesia and an extreme response to pain.

Continuous infusion

Shorter-acting μ-agonists are well suited to this technique and more recently have been developed for this purpose. As well as acting as supplements to inhalational anesthesia, these drugs may also be used as part of a total intravenous anesthesia (TIVA) protocol in conjunction with a hypnotic agent such as propofol and muscle relaxants. In some instances, all three classes of drug may be administered as continuous infusions. By selection of the appropriate agents and infusion rates, this technique can provide precise control of anesthetic depth and hence reduce recovery times. Fentanyl has traditionally been the agent of choice for this indication in veterinary anesthetic practice. The cumulative nature of fentanyl when infused for more than 90 min and the introduction of remifentanil means that fentanyl is no longer the infusion opioid of choice in most circumstances.

Extradural and intrathecal administration of opioids

Other techniques for opioid administration perioperatively are extradural (epidural) and intrathecal (subarachnoid, spinal) placement of opioids alone or in combination with local anesthetic agents. These techniques can be used to supplement general anesthesia or heavy sedation and provide highly effective analgesia with MAC reduction of 30–60% and good cardiovascular stability. Patient and procedure selection are very important if these techniques are to be used without general anesthesia but they can be extremely successful in the right circumstances, such as a tail amputation in well-sedated dogs.

In conjunction analgesia lasts 12–24 h following a single dose of morphine with an onset time of 30–60 min, especially when used in combination with a local analgesic.

When administered into the extradural space or directly into the cerebrospinal fluid (subarachnoid space), opioids provide very profound analgesia by acting on the μ-receptors within the substantia gelatinosa of the spinal cord. The lower lipid solubility, and hence slower uptake into the cord, of morphine increases spread of the drug within the extradural space. This increases the number of dermatomes over which analgesia is produced and is considered beneficial in veterinary species. In humans the cranial spread of morphine is associated with a biphasic and often delayed respiratory depression. It is for this reason that morphine is rarely used for human extradural or spinal anesthesia. Highly lipid-soluble opioids such as fentanyl and butorphanol are best delivered via an epidural catheter so that repeated doses may be administered. This particular technique is not often used in veterinary medicine because of the technical skill involved in catheter placement and the subsequent patient monitoring required to avoid complications or inadvertent catheter removal.

In cats and dogs a spinal needle is usually inserted at the lumbosacral space, which especially in the dog generally ensures epidural rather than spinal drug delivery. Several recommendations have been made as regards these techniques to avoid complications. First, in large dogs it is recommended by some that no more than 6 mL of drug and diluent be injected into the epidural space of any size of animal and if cerebrospinal fluid flows back through the needle, indicating spinal placement, then only 25% of the calculated volume should be administered. It is also important to use sterile and preservative-free drugs to avoid problems with neurotoxicity, which may be more apparent with spinal administration than epidural.

Delayed respiratory depression is the most common and significant side effect of epidural or spinal opioid administration observed in small animals. Others observed in humans but not well documented in small animals include urinary retention, pruritus, nausea and vomiting. Animals may become sedated after epidural morphine due to its cephalad spread in the cerebrospinal fluid, but in general the sedation is no more than that seen with other routes of administration.

In many situations opioids are not the sole agent delivered by these techniques but are combined with other drugs, most commonly a local anesthetic but also analgesics of a different modality such as ketamine. Local anesthetic agents act at both the sensory and motor neurones, thus providing further analgesia and muscle relaxation, which is particularly useful for orthopedic procedures of the hindlimbs. However, sympathetic blockade may also occur, causing peripheral vasodilation and consequent hypotension and hypothermia, which in part can be ameliorated by ensuring an adequate hydration status and appropriate intravenous fluid administration during the procedure. Lidocaine (lignocaine) is frequently used for its rapid onset of action to provide early surgical analgesia while bupivacaine, ropivacaine and levo-bupivacaine tend to be used for their longer duration of action and relative selectivity for sensory over motor blockade.

Analgesia provided by neuraxial placement of opioids is useful for procedures of the hindlimbs particularly and also for forelimb procedures, thoracotomies and major intra-abdominal surgery.

Alternative routes of therapy

Other routes that have been used more recently for postoperative analgesia include intra-articular instillation of an opioid prior to joint closure, instillation into the interpleural space following intrathoracic surgery, and transdermal delivery of fentanyl.

Intra-articular

Intra-articular morphine has been shown to be an effective means of providing analgesia in multiple species including the horse and dog, especially where a joint is inflamed. Analgesia has been successfully provided to dogs following median sternotomy by the instillation of morphine into the interpleural space, a technique previously reserved for local anesthetics, bupivacaine in particular.

Fentanyl patches

Fentanyl patches have been developed for use in humans, as a means of providing analgesia for prolonged periods. Although formulated to provide appropriate fentanyl release rates for absorption through human skin, it has been shown that effective plasma levels can also be attained in dogs and cats.

It is important to note that in animals, the plasma concentrations of fentanyl vary considerably between individuals and in some animals it is unlikely that significant analgesia will be produced. It is therefore particularly important to carry out regular assessments of the adequacy of pain relief in animals treated with patches and to be prepared to provide additional analgesia when required.

Onset of analgesia is slow (up to 12 h) but the patches can provide effective pain relief for up to 72 h. All regulations relating to controlled substances still apply.

Small dogs and cats may be dosed with half a patch, but the patch should not be cut in half. Cover half the gel membrane with tape. 'Half-patch dosing' is suggested for pediatric, geriatric and systemically ill cats and small dogs.

The patch may be placed either on the dorsal or lateral cervical area or the lateral thorax. If the neck is used, collars/leashes cannot be placed over the patch. The thorax is easily used and contact maximized (especially in cats), but can be difficult to bandage. The site must be clean and dry at the time of application. The patch should not be placed where a heating pad may come into contact as this may increase release of drug from the patch. All patients wearing patches should have heart and respiratory rates monitored regularly.

CLINICAL PHARMACOLOGY OF INDIVIDUAL OPIOID AGONISTS

Choice of the most appropriate opioid analgesic, as well as its dose and route of administration in a given clinical situation, is dictated by the pharmacodynamic and pharmacokinetic factors discussed above. Table 14.2 summarizes important pharmacodynamic features of the available opioids discussed below and Table 14.3 lists appropriate doses and routes of administration in different species.

Morphine

Morphine is the opioid analgesic against which others are compared.

Table 14.2 Relative activities of opioid agonists and antagonists at μ- and κ-receptors

Drug	Receptor activity	Mu (μ)	Kappa (κ)	Analgesic efficacy
Morphine	Agonist	++	0	Strong
Pethidine (meperidine)	Agonist	+	+	Moderate-strong
Methadone	Agonist	++	0	Strong
Oxymorphone	Agonist	++	0	Very strong
Fentanyl	Agonist	++	+	Very strong
Alfentanil	Agonist	++	+	Very strong
Codeine*	Agonist	+	0	Weak
Tramadol**	Agonist	+	0	Moderate
Buprenorphine	Partial agonist	P+	P+?	Moderate
Butorphanol	Agonist–antagonist	P+	+	Moderate-weak
Pentazocine	Agonist–antagonist	P+	++	Moderate-weak
Nalbuphine	Agonist–antagonist	P+?	+	Moderate-weak
Naloxone	Antagonist	–	-	N/A
Nalorphine	Antagonist	–	P+	N/A
Nalmefene	Antagonist	–	-	N/A

++, Strong agonist activity; +, agonist activity; P+, partial agonist activity; 0, no activity; -, weak antagonist activity; – –, strong antagonist activity; N/A, not applicable,?, the action is very weak or absent.

* Opioid actions of codeine are due exclusively to its slow metabolic conversion to morphine.

** Tramadol is moderately analgesic because it is a dual μ-receptor agonist (its metabolites are more potent) and monoamine (noradrenaline and serotonin) transport inhibitor.

Table 14.3 Opioid dosages and duration of action

Drug	Route of administration	Dose rate (μg/kg)[†]		Duration of analgesic action (h)¶
		Dog	Cat[‡]	
Agonists				
Morphine	Intravenous	0.05–0.1	0.05	1–4[§]
	Intraoperative bolus	0.1	0.05	
	Intramuscular or subcutaneous	0.1–0.5	0.1–0.3	4–6
	Extradural	0.1–0.2	0.1–0.2	12–24
	Interpleural	0.5–1.0		8–12
	Intra-articular	0.1–1.0		8–12
	Oral	0.1–3.0	0.1–1.0	4–8
	Sustained release	1.5–3.0	N/A	8–12

Table 14.3 Opioid dosages and duration of action (*continued*)

Drug	Route of administration	Dose rate (μg/kg)[†]		Duration of analgesic action (h)¶
		Dog	Cat[‡]	
Pethidine (meperidine)	Intravenous	Contraindicated in small animals		
	Intramuscular or subcutaneous	2–10	2–10	1–2
Methadone	Intravenous	0.05–0.1	0.05–0.1	4–6[§]
	Intramuscular or subcutaneous	0.1–1.0	0.1–1.0	4–6
Oxymorphone	Intravenous	0.02–0.2	0.02–0.1	2–4[§]
	Intraoperative bolus	0.1	0.05	
	Intramuscular or subcutaneous	0.02–0.2	0.02–0.1	4–6
	Epidural	0.02–0.1	0.02–0.1	8–12
Fentanyl	Intraoperative IV bolus	0.002–0.005	0.001–0.005	0.3–0.5
	Constant rate IV infusion:			
	Loading dose	0.01	0.005	
	Infusion rate	0.0025–0.010 mg/kg/h	0.0025–0.005 mg/kg/h	
	Anesthetic induction IV + diazepam (0.5 mg/kg) or midazolam (0.2 mg/kg)	0.01	N/A	
	Transdermal:	2–4 μg/kg/h	2–4 μg/kg/h	≥72
	Patch sizes: 25, 50, 75 and 100 mg/h			
	Intravenous induction	0.04 mL/kg	Contraindicated	
	Intramuscular or subcutaneous	0.02–0.04 mL/kg	0.5–1.0	
Alfentanil	Intravenous	0.01–0.025		
Remifentanil*	Intravenous	0.1–0.6 μg/kg/min	0.05–0.3 μg/kg/min	Half-life approximately 4 min irrespective of infusion duration
Codeine	Oral	0.5–2.0	0.5–2.0	4–6
	With paracetamol (acetaminophen)	0.5–2.0	Contraindicated	6–8
	Subcutaneous	0.5–2.0	0.5–2.0	
Buprenorphine	Intravenous	0.005–0.02	0.005–0.01	3–4
	Intramuscular or subcutaneous	0.005–0.04	0.005–0.04	4–12
	Epidural	0.005–0.02	0.005–0.01	12–18
Butorphanol	Intravenous	0.2–0.4	0.2–0.4	1–3 (dog) 4 (cat)
	Intramuscular or subcutaneous	0.2–0.4	0.2–0.4	2–6
	Antitussive dose	0.05–0.1		6–12
	Oral	0.2–1.0	0.2–1.0	6–8
Pentazocine	Intravenous	1–3	0.75–1.5	1–3
	Intramuscular or subcutaneous	1–3	0.75–1.5	2–3
	Oral	2–10		4–6
Antagonists				
Naloxone	Intravenous	0.01–0.04		20 min (0.3)
	Intramuscular or subcutaneous			
Nalorphine	Intravenous	10–20		2–3
	Intramuscular or subcutaneous	10–20		2–3
Nalbuphine	Intravenous	0.5–1.5		1–6
	Intramuscular or subcutaneous	0.5–2.0		4–8
Nalmefene	Intravenous	0.03		≥4

[†] Dose selected will depend on desired effect, whether for sedation and/or analgesia, and other drugs concurrently administered.
[‡] Where no dose rate is given for cats there are generally no recommendations available in the literature, rather than that drug being contraindicated for use in cats. A similar or lower dose may be used with caution.
¶ Duration of action will be affected by concurrent drug administration, desired effect and type of procedure performed and therefore act as a guide only. These variables will influence the repeat dosing schedule and hence each animal should be assessed for evidence of pain and response to therapy.
[§] Intravenous boluses can be 'titrated' to effect by administering a bolus from the lower end of the dose range and repeating every 5–10 min until the desired effect is achieved. At the same time, it is important not to overdose the patient.
* IPPV or support ventilation is mandatory at all but lower doses.

Clinical applications

Morphine is effective for treatment of visceral pain as well as somatic pain, unlike nonopioid analgesics. Morphine is appropriate in most situations where medium- to long-term analgesia is required. It is commonly used for trauma patients and perioperatively and is the most commonly used opioid for epidural administration.

Clinical studies have shown the analgesic effectiveness of morphine, IV or IM, for arthrotomy, lateral thoracotomy and median sternotomy. It has also been demonstrated to be effective intra-articularly following arthrotomy and interpleurally after sternotomy.

Morphine is suitable for use as a premedicant, generally in combination with a sedative. It is generally given intramuscularly or subcutaneously. Dogs will often salivate, vomit, defecate and pant, while cats may salivate and appear nauseous. These effects are markedly reduced by combination with acepromazine. Cats may not appear to be sedated by morphine but generally they become more tractable, so venous access is easier to achieve. In humans a relatively high dose of morphine at the time of induction has been shown to significantly reduce the postoperative morphine requirements compared with patients who first received morphine at the end of surgery.

Extradural morphine may be delivered prior to surgery after anesthetic induction or at the end of the surgical procedure. Prior administration will provide some intraoperative analgesia, depending on the duration of the procedure, as well as lowering the requirement for volatile anesthetic, which may have the added benefit of a shorter recovery period. Other routes for postoperative use of morphine include intra-articular and interpleural. More commonly, local anesthetics will be instilled in preference to morphine, although a combination may prove to be most efficacious.

Mechanism of action

Morphine is a μ-receptor selective opioid agonist, with very low affinity at κ-receptors and virtually no activity at δ-receptors. It produces profound analgesia and sedation in the dog.

Formulations and dose rates

DOGS AND CATS

- IV: 0.05–0.1 mg/kg
- IM, SC: 0.1–0.5 mg/kg
- Extradural: 0.1–0.2 mg/kg
- Interpleural: 0.5 mg/kg
- Intra-articular: 1.0 mg/kg
- PO: 0.1–1.0 mg/kg, 1.5–3.0 mg/kg sustained release (dog)

Doses from the lower end of the range should be used in cats. When used preoperatively in cats, coadministration of a sedative/anxiolytic reduces the likelihood of excitement. Interpleural and intra-articular routes have not been described in cats. A common postoperative protocol for morphine involves an initial dose at 0.1 mg/kg administered slowly IV then waiting 5–10 min before administering a second dose if considered necessary. Further doses may be required at 30–60 min intervals to maintain adequate analgesia. Low-dose ACP can be a very useful adjunct in these situations.

Pharmacokinetics

Although morphine is well absorbed when administered orally, extensive first-pass metabolism occurs, as with most other opioids. It is therefore usually administered parenterally (SC, IM, IV). Peak analgesic action is seen about 10 min after IV injection and 45 min after SC injection. Analgesia may only last for 1–2 h after IV administration. However, the duration of analgesia is increased to up to 6 h following SC or IM administration. Extradurally administered morphine may provide analgesia for 24 h after an onset time to peak analgesia of 30–60 min.

Following IV administration, plasma morphine concentrations correlate poorly with pharmacological activity, in part because of delayed entry into the cerebrospinal fluid through the blood–brain barrier. Similarly, the analgesia and other effects continue despite decreasing plasma concentrations. It has been estimated that less than 0.1% of an intravenously administered dose of morphine has reached the central nervous system at the time of peak plasma concentration. This is because of low lipid solubility, a high degree of ionization at physiological pH (about 75%), protein binding (30–35%) and rapid conjugation to glucuronic acid.

Morphine is predominantly metabolized in the liver and kidney by conjugation with glucuronic acid to form morphine-3-glucuronide (75–85%) and morphine-6-glucuronide (5–10%). These metabolites are predominantly excreted in urine and so may accumulate in patients with renal failure. Morphine-6-glucuronide acts at μ-receptors to produce analgesia and respiratory depression while morphine-3-glucuronide has no pharmacological action. The actions of morphine-6-glucuronide may account for a significant part of the clinical efficacy of morphine. It may also be for this reason that morphine appears to be a less effective analgesic in cats who, as a species, are less able to perform conjugation.

Adverse effects

Central nervous system

CNS depression in the form of sedation and drowsiness is common following morphine administration in dogs, humans and nonhuman primates. In some circumstances this CNS depression may be viewed as a benefit rather than a side effect. Other species, cats, horses and swine in particular, display CNS stimulation, which manifests as motor excitement and mania. It may be that in these species the doses administered are in excess of those required to produce effective analgesia. Another unwanted effect associated with the administration of morphine is dysphoria (disquieted state accompanied by restlessness and a feeling of malaise), particularly when administered intravenously too quickly.

Stimulation of the Edinger–Westphal nucleus of the third cranial nerve results in miosis in dogs, rats, rabbits and humans. However, in the cat, horse, sheep and monkey the pupils dilate after morphine administration.

Respiratory system

Dose-related respiratory depression is common to all pure μ-agonists. The principal effect is a reduction in the sensitivity of the respiratory center to carbon dioxide, which is associated with increased irregularity in breathing pattern. Although dose-related respiratory depression is the most life-threatening side effect of morphine, most postoperative patients can tolerate the mild-to-moderate depression that occurs with therapeutic doses. Clinically significant hypoventilation is rarely a problem unless high doses (>1 mg/kg) are used. In many cases of animals with pre-existing pain, morphine may improve ventilatory parameters by slowing ventilation and increasing tidal volume. In stressed, painful animals, tachypnea and hypopnea are not infrequent.

In conscious dogs, following morphine administration, there is an initial rise in body temperature, which stimulates the respiratory center and results in panting. With time the body temperature declines and CNS depression ensues, leading to the more common respiratory depression.

Histamine release

Intravenous administration can cause histamine release if the drug is given too rapidly. Histamine release causes systemic hypotension, which can worsen circulatory shock, and IV morphine administration should therefore be avoided or used with great caution in such patients.

Cardiovascular system

Morphine has no, or very little, direct effect on the heart, causing no direct myocardial depression or predisposition to arrhythmias. However, bradycardia may occur with all opioids except pethidine (meperidine) and is commonly observed in anesthetized animals. This results from increased vagal activity due to medullary stimulation. Serious bradycardia is uncommon and can usually be managed by treatment with atropine. Although bradycardia is more profound in anesthetized human patients compared with conscious ones, slow IV administration to anesthetized small animal patients will generally ameliorate this effect.

Nausea and vomiting

Opioids directly stimulate the chemoreceptor trigger zone in the fourth ventricle of the brain, which in turn initiates the vomiting reflex. Dogs are more susceptible to this than cats, although both species will salivate and show signs of nausea. Dogs are more likely to vomit if their stomach is not properly emptied following at least 6 h fasting prior to anesthesia. In humans, vomiting is more likely to occur in ambulatory patients than those lying down, suggesting a vestibular component, which may in part explain its greater frequency in dogs. It is not uncommon for dogs also to defecate following vomiting. Morphine is more likely than other commonly used opioids to induce nausea, vomition and salivation in healthy animals when used as a premedicant. Signs of nausea and vomiting are rarely observed in anesthetized animals or in those recovering from surgery.

Gastrointestinal system

Opioids increase smooth muscle tone along the whole gastrointestinal tract, together with a decrease in propulsive peristalsis. These effects cause a delay in gastric emptying and constipation. There is also an increase of muscle tone in the biliary tract, with a decrease in bile formation and flow. Normal clinical use of morphine infrequently results in significant clinical signs attributable to these effects.

Musculoskeletal system

Muscle rigidity has been observed in humans given large doses of μ-agonist opioids rapidly IV during induction of anesthesia. This particularly affects the muscles of the chest wall and so limits ventilatory efforts. This phenomenon has not been reported to occur in small animals.

Epidural-specific side effects

Delayed respiratory depression, pruritus, urinary retention, nausea and vomiting are well recognized in humans given extra or subdural opioids. Respiratory depression is also the most common to occur in small animals, although its prevalence is low. If suspected, respiratory depression should be treated initially with buprenorphine or low-dose naloxone intravenously where there is need for an immediate reversal. The other unwanted effects are not generally seen in small animals, although urinary retention may occur, in which case expression of the bladder may be required.

Contraindications and precautions

- Caution should be exercised when administering morphine to animals with head trauma. It is important to ensure that ventilation is adequate to avoid problems associated with increased arterial CO_2.
- Rapid intravenous administration of large doses should be avoided in hypovolemic animals because of the risk of histamine release and a further decrease in arterial blood pressure.
- Epidural administration of any drug is best avoided during sepsis and in the presence of clotting abnormalities or localized skin infections.

Known drug interactions

- As with other opioids, morphine has a synergistic action with ACP, the most commonly used sedative in small animal practice. Because of the additive effect of this and similar combinations, caution would suggest that the individual dose of each drug be reduced from that given alone. This will of course be tempered by the animal's temperament and the desired effect. Of particular concern when using such combinations is the exacerbation of ventilatory depression.
- Similarly, morphine has at least additive actions on respiratory depression when used with other sedatives such as benzodiazepines and barbiturates.
- Verapamil augments the analgesia produced by morphine.

Pethidine (meperidine)

Clinical applications

Pethidine has only very mild sedative effects when given alone to healthy animals but is unlikely to induce bradycardia, unlike other opioids. Because of its short duration of action (1–2 h at the most), pethidine is of more practical use as a preanesthetic medication than as a postoperative analgesic. Vomiting is less common than with morphine when used as a premedicant.

Mechanism of action

Pethidine has a similar receptor selectivity profile to morphine, is slightly less efficacious and has lower potency. It has an extremely fast onset, even when given by the subcutaneous route (less than 5 min).

Formulations and dose rates

DOGS AND CATS

- 2–10 mg/kg IM, SC

Although absorption of pethidine can be variable after IM administration, this route is preferred to SC because of the local irritation and pain that may be produced. Pethidine is not to be administered IV in small animals because of marked histamine release.

Pharmacokinetics

Pethidine is moderately lipid soluble and has an onset of action shorter than that of morphine following IM injection. About 70% is protein bound to albumin, lipoprotein and α_1-acid glycoprotein.

Most pethidine is metabolized in the liver to norpethidine, pethidinic acid and norpethidinic acid, which are then excreted via the kidneys. Norpethidine can accumulate in renal failure and has about half the analgesic potency of pethidine. Norpethidine also causes CNS stimulation and may result in myoclonus and seizures, a situation more common with prolonged administration in the presence of renal impairment.

Adverse effects

- In equianalgesic doses, pethidine's respiratory depressant effects are comparable to morphine.
- Pethidine should not be given IV as it significantly depresses myocardial contractility and causes histamine release.
- Vomiting is rarely seen after administration and it does not cause excitement in cats or horses.
- Bradycardia is rarely seen due to pethidine's atropine-like structure which may cause tachycardia.
- Large doses of pethidine, greater than 20 mg/kg, will induce excitement and seizures in cats.

Known drug interactions

Pethidine should be used cautiously in conjunction with monoamine oxidase inhibitors such as selegiline (see Chapter 7). Use with monoamine oxidase inhibitors leads to excessive metabolism to norpethidine, with greatly increased risk of myoclonus and seizures.

Methadone

Methadone is a synthetic opioid with a pharmacological profile similar to morphine.

Clinical applications

Similar use to morphine, although not for epidural use as it is not available in preservative free formulation.

Mechanism of action

The potency and efficacy of methadone are similar to morphine and it is more selective for μ-receptors. Its analgesic efficacy is similar to morphine after a single dose but is several times greater after repeated administration. This may result from its very long plasma half-life, which in humans is on average 24 h; however, this does not appear to be the case in animals.

Formulations and dose rates

DOGS
- 0.05–0.1 mg/kg IV
- 0.1–1.0 mg/kg IM, SC

CATS
As with morphine, lower dose rates are recommended for use in cats, as is the concurrent use of a sedative/tranquilizer to avoid excitement.

Pharmacokinetics

The duration of action of methadone in dogs is 3–5 h. It has a more rapid onset of action than morphine, 15–20 min following IM or SC administration and 5–10 min after IV administration. Unlike morphine, methadone has a very high bioavailability following oral administration in humans (80–85%) but this may not be the case in dogs and cats.

Methadone has a long elimination half-life (24–35 h) in humans but the duration of action of a single dose is comparable to that of morphine. Similarly, in animals, the duration of action appears to be similar to morphine.

Adverse effects

- Methadone is less likely to cause nausea and vomiting than morphine when used as a premedicant.
- Sedation and dysphoria are less common following methadone administration, although cats may display excitement, as occurs with morphine. In one study, premedicant doses up to 0.5 mg/kg IM in cats did not produce any excitation or mania. Therefore, despite literature to the contrary, methadone would appear to be as safe and reliable an opioid to use in cats as morphine.
- Respiratory depression, bradycardia and cough suppression are associated with methadone administration, as occurs with morphine.
- Histamine release following IV administration would appear to be minimal, based on studies in which cardiovascular stability was maintained during administration of induction doses.

Contraindications and precautions

As for morphine.

Known drug interactions

As for morphine, although analgesia is not enhanced by verapamil.

Oxymorphone

Mechanism of action

Oxymorphone is not available in Europe or Australasia. It is a μ-agonist with approximately 10 times the potency of morphine.

Clinical applications

Oxymorphone is probably the opioid most widely used in veterinary practice in North America, where its indications are similar to those for morphine. Oxymorphone is useful at all perioperative stages, as well as for cases of trauma. It is much more effective as a premedicant when used in combination with a tranquilizer or sedative such as ACP or an α_2-agonist.

Formulations and dose rates

DOGS
- 0.02–0.2 mg/kg IM, SC, IV or epidural

CATS
- 0.02–0.1 mg/kg IM, SC or IV

Pharmacokinetics

The duration of action of oxymorphone is 2-6 h with shorter times resulting from IV administration.

Adverse effects

- Oxymorphone tends to have the same side effects as morphine, although there is less respiratory depression and nausea and vomiting.
- It causes pronounced auditory hypersensitivity.
- Panting occurs because of lowering of the temperature equilibrium point of the hypothalamic thermoregulatory center.
- Oxymorphone delivered intravenously does not induce histamine release, in contrast to morphine.

Contraindications and precautions

As for morphine.

Known drug interactions

As for morphine.

Fentanyl

Clinical applications

Because of its relatively short duration of action (30–60 min), fentanyl is often used as a continuous-rate infusion to maintain general anesthesia, in combination with other drugs, or as part of an induction protocol for seriously ill patients. Intraoperatively it may be used as an intermittent bolus prior to a noxious stimulus to provide analgesia and to blunt the hemodynamic response to the stimulus. Fentanyl has been demonstrated to be effective at reducing the MAC of inhaled volatile anesthetic agents, both clinically and in the laboratory. However, caution must be exercised in regard to maintenance of both adequate ventilation to prevent hypercapnia and an adequate heart rate to minimize or eliminate hypotension.

Fentanyl is also available in combination with a number of butyrophenone tranquilizers, e.g. droperidol (Leptan® or Innovar-Vet®) and fluanisone (Hypnorm®), in which combinations it is used to produce profound neuroleptanalgesia. These combination premixes are highly popular despite the fixed concentrations of the two drugs and the pharmacokinetic mismatch between the durations of the different agents.

Fentanyl is the opioid most often used as part of the protocol for induction of anesthesia in veterinary patients. This may then be followed by either short-term fentanyl infusion as part of balanced anesthesia or use of one of the fentanyl analogs with shorter elimination times. Fentanyl has also been administered to small animals via transdermal patches (see above). This property is by virtue of the very high lipid solubility of fentanyl which increases absorption into dermal lipid.

Fentanyl can be administered into the epidural space with a very rapid onset of action but an equally short duration of action because of its high lipid solubility. For best effect it should be administered as intermittent boluses through an epidural catheter. This is not a technique often attempted in veterinary practice. The effectiveness of epidural fentanyl is enhanced by combining it with a local anesthetic, particularly longer acting agents such as ropivacaine or bupivacaine. Combinations of these two drugs are available commercially for this use in humans.

Mechanism of action

Fentanyl is a potent selective μ-opioid agonist with an affinity at μ-receptors approximately 50–100 times that of morphine. It is highly effective and short acting.

Formulations and dose rates

Fentanyl is available as an injectable solution and in transdermal patches. Patch sizes available deliver 25, 50, 75 and 100 mg/h.

DOGS

Intraoperative IV bolus

- 2–5 μg/kg

Constant rate infusion – IV

- Loading dose: 10 μg/kg
- Infusion rate: 0.0025–0.010 μg/kg/min

Anesthetic induction

- 10 μg/kg fentanyl with diazepam (0.5 mg/kg) or midazolam (0.2 mg/kg) IV

Transdermal patches

- 2–4 μg/kg/h

CATS

Intraoperative IV bolus

- 1–5 μg/kg

Constant rate infusion – IV

- Loading dose: 5 μg/kg
- Infusion rate: 0.0025–0.005 μg/kg/min

Transdermal patches

- 2–4 μg/kg/h

Pharmacokinetics

Fentanyl is highly protein bound and lipid soluble, with wide redistribution to peripheral tissues.

Adverse effects

- Apart from being a potent analgesic, fentanyl causes profound sedation and respiratory depression.
- Auditory sensitization and altered thermoregulation (resulting in panting) may occur.
- Large intravenous doses will cause bradycardia, particularly when administered rapidly. This effect appears to be more profound during general anesthesia.

Contraindications and precautions

High doses of fentanyl during anesthesia may cause short-term ventilatory depression requiring assisted ventilation. This is rarely seen on anesthesia induction, with lower doses during anesthesia or on repeat bolusing.

Known drug interactions

- When combined with other central-depressant drugs, the side effects associated with fentanyl tend to be more pronounced.
- α_2-Agonists increase the degree of bradycardia while all central depressants tend to worsen respiratory depression.

Special considerations

Care must be taken when using transdermal patches to prevent ingestion by animals or young children. As fentanyl is a controlled substance, close monitoring of patch use and disposal is legally important.

Alfentanil, sufentanil

These short-acting opioid agents were developed as analogs of fentanyl in an attempt to produce a shorter acting, less cumulative alternative. As such, they have been largely replaced by remifentanil. At the time of writing they do, however, retain some clinical use and they retain the advantage over fentanyl of a shorter duration of action, particularly following a prolonged continuous infusion. Studies, both clinical and experimental, have been undertaken using alfentanil in dogs and cats. The results of these indicate that the actions and side effects of alfentanil in these species are very similar to those of fentanyl, in particular good analgesia, MAC reduction of inhaled agents, bradycardia and respiratory depression. Alfentanil is less potent than fentanyl while sufentanil is 5–10 times more potent. Both are full μ-agonists and more lipid soluble than fentanyl.

Remifentanil

Clinical applications

Remifentanil is a 4-anilidopiperidine derivative of fentanyl containing an ester linkage to propanoic acid, making it susceptible to esterase metabolism. The primary metabolite, remifentanil acid, has negligible activity compared with remifentanil. It is ultra-short acting and displays analgesic effects, consistent with its agonist activity at the μ-receptor. The effect of remifentanil on hemodynamics is typical of opioids (e.g. decreased blood pressure and heart rate). The reduced blood pressure is by virtue of the bradycardia and may be prevented or reversed by use of an anticholinergic. Remifentanil is proving to be a highly effective analgesic when used as part of balanced anesthesia in the dog. Infusion rates of between 0.05 and 0.6 μg/kg/min produce profound analgesia and MAC sparing effects. Where heart rate is supported, blood pressure is well maintained due to the reduction of inhaled volatile agent.

Remifentanil has also been shown to be effective alongside infused propofol as part of a total intravenous anesthetic technique. Because metabolism is independent of hepatic function, remifentanil is useful as part of anesthetic protocol for dogs with reduced hepatic function. There are two main unwanted effects. Unlike in humans, in whom ventilation is often well maintained, dogs require assisted ventilation even at low doses of infused remifentanil. Second, without the use of an anticholinergic, bradycardia may be profound. This is rapidly reversed on termination of the infusion. In addition, it should be recognized that as the analgesic effects wear off rapidly, analgesia should be pre-emptively provided by a different opioid (e.g. morphine) before terminating the remifentanil.

Mechanism of action

Remifentanil is a potent selective μ-opioid agonist.

Formulations and dose rates

Remifentanil is marketed as a sterile lyophilised powder for reconstitution with sterile water.

DOGS AND CATS

Constant rate infusion – IV

- Loading dose: not needed
- Infusion rate: 0.05–0.6 μg/kg/min

Pharmacokinetics

Remifentanil has a rapid onset of action (<1 min) and a rapid offset of action following discontinuation (<3–10 min). The time to offset of action is not prolonged to a clinically significant extent by renal impairment or prolonged infusion, i.e. it has no context-sensitive half-life. Remifentanil is rapidly distributed throughout the body and undergoes widespread vascular and extravascular metabolism, via nonspecific blood and tissue esterases, to remifentanil acid. The rapid, complete metabolism results in zero accumulation of the drug and therefore infusion rates remain constant. There is no need for adjustment of targeting to maintain plasma concentrations.

Adverse effects

- Remifentanil causes profound sedation and respiratory depression.
- Bradycardia is marked with clinical doses and may require anticholinergic intervention.

Contraindications and precautions

Remifentanil is formulated with glycine and should not therefore be instilled into the extradural space or administered intrathecally.

Codeine

Codeine (methylmorphine) occurs naturally in the opium poppy. It has similar actions to morphine but with only a quarter of its efficacy.

Clinical applications

Used for mild-to-moderate pain in humans and dogs, commonly in combination with paracetamol (acetaminophen), or alone as a cough suppressant.

Mechanism of action

The analgesic activity of codeine is probably due to slow metabolic conversion (demethylation) to morphine.

Formulations and dose rates

DOGS AND CATS

- 0.5–2.0 mg/kg PO, SC q.12 h

Dosage is similar when combined with paracetamol (acetaminophen) but this combination is contraindicated in cats.

Adverse effects

- Respiratory depression is less pronounced with moderate doses of codeine.
- It does not usually cause vomiting.
- Constipation may occur with prolonged administration.

PARTIAL AGONISTS

Buprenorphine

Clinical applications

Buprenorphine is the prototypical drug in this class; it is relatively safe, producing few side effects and minimal sedation. Buprenorphine has a high affinity for the μ-receptors and will competitively inhibit pure μ-agonists from binding. This property makes it useful for 'reversing' the effects of morphine or fentanyl if adverse consequences arise, while still maintaining a level of analgesia. Buprenorphine's analgesic properties in animals were first described in 1977 and it has been used extensively in laboratory species as a means of managing acute postoperative pain. It also was used extensively for pain management in clinical practice, although the lack of veterinary product licensing restricted this. This analgesic is now licensed for use in dogs in some markets.

Although it is widely used, misconceptions arising from misinterpretation of early animal studies have hampered its use in clinical pain management. Early studies indicated that it exhibited a 'bell-shaped' dose–response curve, with high dose rates producing a paradoxical reduction in analgesic efficacy. These initial results in laboratory animals were uncritically translated into clinical opinion, that additional doses of buprenorphine would reduce the agent's analgesic effects. Although repeated dosing with buprenorphine may eventually reach a plateau in terms of analgesic efficacy, inspection of the available animal data shows that dose rates far in excess of those used clinically are required for 'self-reversal'. This ceiling effect makes buprenorphine less useful for severe pain and inadequate analgesia may be seen following moderate-to-major bone trauma and surgery. Doses of 30 μg/kg will provide relatively long periods (8–10 h) of analgesia and 40 μg/kg may produce as much as 12 h of pain control. The onset of action is slow (30 min when given IV).

Buprenorphine is not available as an oral preparation (significant first-pass effect renders it inactive), but its lipophilic nature lends itself to absorption across skin or mucous membranes. The alkaline salivary pH of cats allows for excellent transmucosal absorption when the injectable drug is given in the mouth (it should not be mixed with flavored syrups, as swallowing will inactivate it; the injectable form is tasteless and well tolerated by cats). No studies have been performed on transmucosal usage in dogs, though the pH of their saliva is closer to that of humans, where bioavailability after mucosal administration is only 30%.

Recent studies of the clinical use of buprenorphine patches in companion animals have found them to be entirely ineffective.

Mechanism of action

Buprenorphine is a potent synthetic opioid with partial agonist activity at and very high affinity for μ-receptors.

Formulations and dose rates

DOGS

- 5–40 μg/kg IM, SC, IV or epidural prn or q.8 h

CATS

- 5–40 μg/kg IM, SC, IV or epidural prn or q.8 h

Pharmacokinetics

Buprenorphine has a long duration of action (8–12 h) due to its slow dissociation from μ-receptors. Onset of analgesia is about 45 min after subcutaneous administration. If more rapid onset is required, half the dose can be given slowly intravenously.

Adverse effects

- Respiratory depression is less than with morphine (probably because it is a partial agonist).
- Vomiting and gastrointestinal side effects do not occur to any great extent.

Known drug interactions

There is an augmentation of sedation and bradycardia when administered in conjunction with other central depressant drugs.

AGONISTS–ANTAGONISTS

Butorphanol

Clinical applications

Butorphanol provides poor-to-moderate pain relief that is more effective for visceral than somatic pain. As a sole agent, butorphanol provides mild sedation in dogs and next to none in cats. For this reason it is best administered with a sedative or tranquilizer if it is to be used as a premedicant. Because butorphanol is a partial agonist at μ-receptors, the analgesic efficacy of morphine or other full agonists at μ-receptors can be reduced if butorphanol is given concurrently.

Mixed partial agonists like butorphanol are not considered useful in the management of chronic pain.

First-pass effect destroys some of the drug and the analgesia is considered to be relatively short-lived (1–2 h). Because these drugs are κ-agonists and μ-antagonists, the pain relief is often less than optimal for chronic discomfort. However, visceral nociception is considered to be more responsive to κ-agonism, leading some urologists to advocate butorphanol's use in chronic bladder pain.

Butorphanol is a potent antitussive. It may also be used to antagonize pure μ-agonists with residual analgesia and reduction in side effects.

Mechanism of action

Butorphanol is a synthetic opioid that is a partial agonist at μ-receptors as well as being a κ-agonist.

Formulations and dose rates

DOGS AND CATS
- 0.2–0.4 mg/kg IM, SC or IV prn or q.6–12 h
- 0.2–1.0 mg/kg PO q.6–12 h

Pharmacokinetics

Analgesia occurs 20 min after SC administration and lasts for about 4 h. Duration of analgesia appears to be longer (2–6 h) in cats than in dogs (1–2 h). Visceral analgesia is achieved at lower doses (0.1 mg/kg) than somatic analgesia in cats (up to 0.8 mg/kg).

Adverse effects

- Butorphanol produces less respiratory depression than morphine because of its 'ceiling effect'.
- At normal clinical doses, butorphanol produces mild, transient depression of the cardiovascular system, which is more profound when combined with other central depressant drugs.

Known drug interactions

Cardiopulmonary side effects are more pronounced in the presence of α_2-agonists and inhalational anesthetic agents.

Special considerations

In many but not all countries, butorphanol is not a controlled substance, unlike most of the other opioids, as there is little potential for human abuse of the drug.

Pentazocine

Clinical applications

Pentazocine provides moderate pain relief and is most appropriately used as part of a premedication protocol for anesthesia.

Mechanism of action

Pentazocine is a synthetic opioid that is a partial agonist at μ-receptors as well as being a κ-agonist. Its analgesic efficacy is 25–50% that of morphine.

Formulations and dose rates

DOGS
- 1–3 mg/kg IM, SC or IV
- 2–10 mg/kg PO repeated q.3–4 h prn

CATS
- 0.75–1.5 mg/kg IM, SC or IV
- 2–10 mg/kg PO

Pharmacokinetics

Analgesia occurs 20 min after SC administration and lasts for 2–4 h. Duration of analgesia is dose related, lasting 20–120 min in cats after 0.75 and 1.5 mg/kg, respectively.

Adverse effects

- Pentazocine produces less respiratory depression than morphine.
- Intravenous administration may cause a transient decrease in arterial blood pressure.
- Ataxia, inco-ordination and disorientation may occur in dogs.
- Pentazocine causes dysphoria in cats. Alternative analgesics are recommended.

Tramadol

Clinical applications

Tramadol provides moderate pain relief. Because of its dual actions as a μ-agonist and monoamine transport inhibitor, it produces less respiratory depression for a given analgesic effect.

Mechanism of action

Tramadol is a synthetic opioid that is a weak agonist at μ-receptors. Its major metabolites are more potent agonists at μ-receptors. Tramadol also inhibits monoamine transporters (principally noradrenaline and serotonin) which is thought to produce analgesia synergistically with μ-agonism.

Formulations and dose rates

DOGS
- 1–5 mg/kg PO q.8–12 h

CATS
- 1–2 mg/kg PO q.12 h

Pharmacokinetics

Duration of analgesia is dose related, lasting 4–8 h.

Adverse effects

- Tramadol produces less respiratory depression than morphine.
- Sedation.
- May decrease seizure threshold.

Known drug interactions

Tramadol is contraindicated in patients treated with monoamine oxidase inhibitors (MAOIs) or monoamine transport inhibitors including noradrenaline uptake inhibitors, specific serotonin reuptake inhibitors, deprenyl.

OPIOID ANTAGONISTS

There are infrequent indications for antagonists of opioid agonists in veterinary medicine; the most common use is to reverse an absolute or relative opioid agonist overdose. However, a partial agonist such as buprenorphine or an agonist-antagonist (butorphanol) may be a better choice, as analgesia can be maintained while reversing the unwanted side effects such as respiratory depression or excitement and agitation.

When using opioid antagonists, care must be taken not to overtreat, thereby exposing the animal to the full pain of the procedure it has just undergone. If this happens, the animal may become agitated and excitable, from which point adequate pain control will be more difficult to achieve.

Naloxone

Clinical applications

Indications for use of naloxone are rare because of its ability to nonselectively antagonize all the effects of the μ-agonists, both good and bad. It is used occasionally in the management of behavior disorders such as tail chasing (see Chapter 7).

Mechanism of action

Naloxone is a pure antagonist at all opioid receptors but has greatest affinity for μ-receptors.

Formulations and dose rates

DOGS AND CATS

- 0.01–0.04 mg/kg IM, SC or IV

Pharmacokinetics

The onset of action is very rapid following intravenous administration and its duration of action is correspondingly short. For this reason a similar dose may also be given intramuscularly or subcutaneously to prolong its action. Depending on the reason for administration and the agonist being reversed, further doses may be required. In dogs treated with oxymorphone, naloxone administered intravenously and intramuscularly reversed the cardiopulmonary and sedative effects for about 30 and 60 min respectively.

Adverse effects

- Observed side effects of naloxone administration generally result from sympathetic stimulation due to reversal of analgesia and sedation and include catecholamine release, arrhythmias, hypertension and death.
- The most pronounced effect of its administration is the reversal of analgesia. For this reason, if it is to be used in an animal that has respiratory depression from narcotic overdose, it is recommended that the naloxone be diluted and given slowly to titrate to the desired effect.
- There are reports in the human literature of pulmonary edema and sudden death in response to naloxone administration.

Known drug interactions

Naloxone may have difficulty reversing the effects of buprenorphine because of a similar binding affinity of the two drugs for the μ-receptor.

Nalorphine

Nalorphine was the first antagonist identified and used clinically, but has now fallen into disfavor because of its dysphoric effects and the existence of superior alternatives.

Nalbuphine

Clinical applications

Nalbuphine is primarily used to reverse the undesired effects of pure μ-agonists while tending to maintain some analgesia. It can also be solely used for its agonist analgesic effect.

Mechanism of action

Nalbuphine is a μ receptor antagonist (some studies suggest it is a weak partial μ-agonist) and a κ-agonist.

Formulations and dose rates

DOGS AND CATS

- 0.5–1.5 mg/kg IM, SC or IV

Pharmacokinetics

In humans the duration of action of nalbuphine is 2–6 h. It is thought to have a similar duration in small animals.

Adverse effects

- Respiratory depression is minimal with nalbuphine, with no clinical effect upon the cardiovascular system.
- It will produce some sedation.

Nalmefene

Nalmefene is a newer pure opioid antagonist that has a longer duration of action than naloxone. The effective duration is reported to be dependent on the dose administered. In one laboratory study in dogs, nalmefene (0.03 mg/kg IV) was found to still be effective against oxymorphone (4.5 mg IV) at 4 h. It has been demonstrated to be effective for up to 8 h in humans.

15

Cancer chemotherapy

Jane M Dobson, Ann E Hohenhaus and Anne E Peaston

INTRODUCTION

Cancer is an important cause of morbidity and mortality in pet cats and dogs and as awareness and diagnosis of this disease increase, so too does the demand for treatment. Surgery, radiation therapy and chemotherapy are conventionally the three main methods of cancer treatment. Surgery and radiation are used in management of localized solid tumors, e.g. mammary carcinoma and soft tissue sarcoma, whereas chemotherapy is primarily used for management of systemically disseminated or multifocal malignant tumors. However, these treatments are not mutually exclusive and the optimum treatment for a particular patient may be achieved through multimodal therapy combining, for example, surgical management of a primary tumor (amputation of a limb affected by osteosarcoma) with systemic chemotherapy to try to prevent or delay development of systemic microscopic metastases.

The prerequisite to treatment selection is a definitive tumor diagnosis, preferably by histopathology, and a thorough examination of the patient to determine the extent of the disease in terms of local invasion at the primary site, lymph node involvement and distant metastasis. A medical evaluation of the patient is also required to identify any concomitant health problems, e.g. renal or hepatic disease, which may compromise the patient's ability to tolerate treatment. The feasibility and likely success of treatment are determined by the type, grade and extent of the tumor. Clearly a cure, i.e. total eradication of all tumor stem cells, is the desirable outcome but even the most effective methods of treatment currently available cannot achieve this aim in every case.

Prolonged palliation in conditions such as lymphoma is an achievable and acceptable goal. The decision to treat an animal with cancer is one which must be made jointly by the veterinarian (bearing in mind the type of tumor, its extent, the facilities and experience available) and the owner. and all involved must be clear on the goals, whether the intention of treatment is curative or palliative.

GENERAL INDICATIONS FOR CHEMOTHERAPY

The general indications for chemotherapy in small animal practice are as follows.

- Primary treatment of chemosensitive local or systemic tumors with curative intent, e.g. transmissible venereal tumor.
- Palliative intent, e.g. hematological malignancies, lymphoma/sarcoma.
- Adjuvant treatment in cases of malignant solid tumors with a high risk of metastasis. In these cases chemotherapy is used after surgical removal/irradiation of the primary and is directed against microscopic metastatic disease. In animals this is usually with palliative intent in tumors such as canine osteosarcoma.
- Neo-adjuvant treatment is when chemotherapy is used prior to surgery/radiation of the primary tumor with the intention of reducing the size of the primary mass and thus enhancing the chance of successful surgical removal or facilitating radiotherapy. This approach is not common, but has been investigated in dogs with osteosarcoma. This application has the possible advantage of enabling the clinician to estimate tumor chemosensitivity. However, if the tumor is nonresponsive, a serious disadvantage is the delay in institution of effective therapy.

RELEVANT PATHOPHYSIOLOGY OF CANCER

The genetic changes which occur in the transformation of normal cells to neoplasia enable cancer cells to proliferate excessively without the need for external growth signals, to develop a limitless capacity to replicate, to evade apoptosis, to stimulate and sustain angiogenesis and to invade adjacent tissues and metastasize. Of all these features of malignancy, cellular growth and division are the main targets of conventional chemotherapeutic drugs. Novel agents targeting angiogenesis are in clinical development in human medicine. Some agents which target cell signaling pathways are already licensed for use in human medicine and many more are in development.

Cell cycle

Most cytotoxic drugs act on the processes of cell growth and division and thus it is important to understand these processes.

Both normal and neoplastic cells progress through the cell cycle which consists of five major stages (Fig. 15.1).

- **M**, the mitotic phase
- **G_0**, the resting phase
- **G_1**, the intermitotic phase (synthesis of cellular components for DNA synthesis)
- **S**, the DNA synthesis phase
- **G_2**, the premitotic interval (synthesis of cellular components for mitosis)

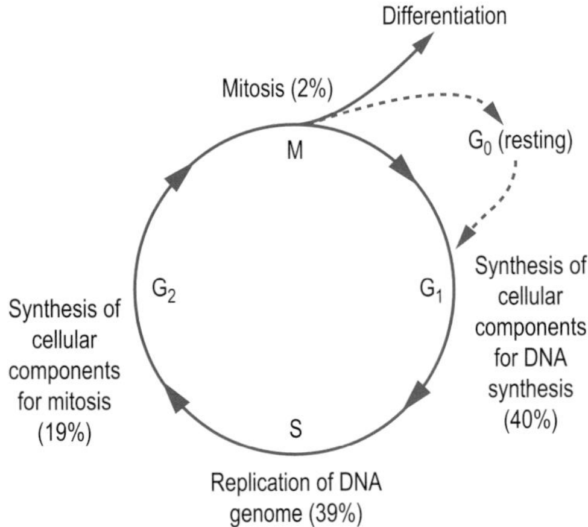

Fig. 15.1 The cell cycle.

Growth fraction

The growth fraction of a tumor is the proportion of tumor cells which are actively replicating, i.e. are within the cell replication cycle. The majority of chemotherapy drugs are most active against cells in the cell cycle as opposed to the G_0, resting cells (i.e. cell cycle dependent). These drugs will be most effective against tumors with a high growth fraction.

Most tumors initially grow in an exponential manner but reach a plateau by the time the mass(es) become clinically detectable. Thus the growth fraction is highest when the tumor first develops at a microscopic level. Once most tumors become macroscopic, greater than 1 cm^3, the growth fraction is relatively low. In practice, the smaller the tumor, the better chance of a favorable response to chemotherapy.

Some drugs are most active against cells in a specific phase of the cell cycle (cell cycle-dependent, phase-specific). These drugs only kill a limited number of cells with any single drug administration because at the time of administration only a limited number of tumor cells will be in the phase of the cell cycle in which the drug acts. The number of cancer cells killed depends on the amount of time the tumor cells are exposed to the drug, which is related to the area under the curve for the drug being administered. The area under the curve may be increased by prolonging exposure of the cells to the drug by administering the drug multiple times or as a constant rate infusion. Normal cell toxicity also increases when cell cycle-dependent, phase-specific drugs are administered more frequently or via a constant rate infusion because a greater number of normal cells also enter the phase of the cell cycle in which the drug acts. Drugs that work in this fashion are also termed 'schedule-dependent' because changing the schedule of administration profoundly alters the drug's effect. This group of drugs is most active in tumors where many cells are actively dividing. Classic examples of cell cycle-dependent, phase-specific drugs are the antimetabolites.

'Cell cycle-phase nonspecific' drugs do not require tumor cells to be actively dividing in order to cause lethal cell damage (so theoretically are active against resting cells). However, ultimately, the damaged cell must undergo division for the lethal effect to be expressed (so the drugs do not actually kill cells in the resting phase unless they start multiplying again). Because the degree of cell kill is dependent on the number of cells damaged, which in turn is dependent on the maximum drug concentration achieved (C_{max}), these drugs are also called 'dose-dependent'. Drugs in this category include the alkylating agents, antitumor antibiotics and platinum analogs.

A third classification of drugs based on the cell cycle is sometimes separated from the cell cycle-phase nonspecific group. Named the nonselective, phase-nonspecific group, it is small, consisting of nitrogen mustard and the nitrosoureas which are known to damage both normal and tumor stem cells.

IMPORTANT PRINCIPLES OF TREATMENT IN CANCER CHEMOTHERAPY

Dosing principles

The objective of anticancer chemotherapy is to use a dose regimen that combines maximum antitumor effect with minimal normal tissue toxicity. Unfortunately, because their actions on dividing cells are not specific to malignant cells, cytotoxic agents often have a small therapeutic index with acute toxicity affecting principally the gastrointestinal tract and bone marrow (see below). The recommended dose rate for many drugs is the maximally tolerated dose (MTD). The MTD may be defined differently in different studies but is generally described as the dose that has been shown to result in mild-to-moderate but sublethal toxicity in a significant percentage of patients, or serious toxicity to approximately 5% of normal animals of that species.

In a theoretical system, cell kill by cytotoxic agents follows first-order pharmacokinetics, i.e. the same proportion of cells in a tumor is killed with each dose (Fig. 15.2). The underlying assumptions of this system are that all the malignant cells grow at a constant rate, are equally chemosensitive and receive equal drug distribution. In practice, this does not occur and a log kill in the order of 2–4 is achieved by a single effective drug treatment. Cytotoxic agents often have a steep dose–response curve and should be used at the highest dose possible to achieve the highest log cell kill possible. However, a single dose of drug is highly unlikely to eradicate all the cells in a malignant cell population. Where treatments are repeated, agents should be given at the shortest time intervals possible, to avoid significant tumor cell repopulation. In practice, dose frequency is limited by toxicity to normal tissues and time for their recovery.

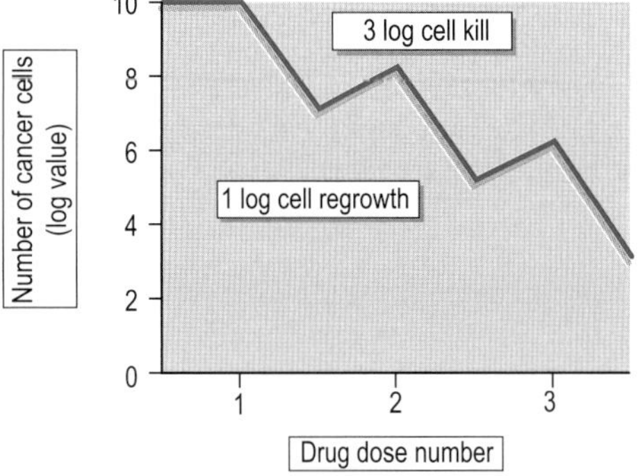

Fig. 15.2 **Chemotherapeutic agents act according to first-order kinetics, i.e. they kill a constant proportion of tumor cells with each dose. When regrowth between doses is less than cell killing, therapy is successful.**

Dose rates for cytotoxic drugs are usually calculated according to body surface area (BSA) in square meters (m^2), as this permits better matching of dose to the animal's capacity to metabolize drug than dosing per unit of bodyweight. However, it may be more appropriate to calculate dose rates according to bodyweight in kilograms where processes independent of metabolic rate are important for elimination of drugs such as melphalan. In comparison to bodyweight, BSA tends to overdose small animals and underdose large ones and for small animals, <10 kg, it may be safer to dose some drugs according to bodyweight.

Most cytotoxic drugs are administered systemically either as tablets PO or solutions by intravenous injection or infusion. In some circumstances drugs may be administered locally or regionally by:

- regional perfusion, e.g. of a limb or organ
- intracavitary injection of liquid formulations
- intratumoral injection of liquid formulations
- superficial application of creams
- implantation of slow-release solid formulations.

The rationale of local drug administration is to achieve high drug concentration over time in the tumor with low systemic exposure and minimum systemic toxicity. Extended low-dose systemic exposure from slow-release formulations may also be active against metastatic disease.

Agent selection

Treatment regimens which combine several different drugs are often more effective than single agents and may delay or avert the onset of clinical drug resistance. When using multiple drugs sequentially or in combination, the agents used should have activity against the specific malignancy and, if possible, have different or nonoverlapping dose-limiting toxicities, different mechanisms of action and not be subject to predictable cross-resistance.

Drug resistance

Resistance of tumor cells to cytotoxic drugs is the major barrier to successful treatment of cancer with chemotherapy. Drug resistance may be intrinsic or acquired during treatment and can be categorized in three ways:

- kinetic resistance
- biochemical resistance
- pharmacological resistance.

Kinetic resistance

Kinetic resistance occurs as a result of a small growth fraction. In large primary tumors a large proportion of cells are in the G_0 phase which is especially a problem for cell cycle phase-specific agents. In some circumstances this may be overcome by reducing tumor bulk (e.g. by surgery, radiotherapy) or theoretically by including drugs active against cells in G_0 phase, although in practice this has had limited success. Another approach is to schedule drugs to synchronize cell populations and increase cell kill. Practical applications of this theory are lacking.

Biochemical resistance

Biochemical resistance is due to numerous cellular biochemical mechanisms, including:

- decreased drug accumulation (decreased uptake or increased efflux from cells)
- altered drug metabolism
- altered drug targets
- enhanced nucleic acid repair capacity.

One well-known mechanism of resistance is increased drug efflux mediated by a membrane transport protein, P-glycoprotein (P-gp). Increased cellular levels of P-gp confer multidrug resistance (MDR), in which cells are resistant to multiple drugs of differing chemical classes, such as anthracycline antibiotics, vinca alkaloids and taxanes. In dogs with lymphoma, the presence of P-gp in primary tumor tissue has been shown to indicate a poor prognosis for survival. In some dogs treated with chemotherapy for lymphoma, the level of P-gp in the tumor cells at relapse is higher than at diagnosis. These observations suggest that P-gp may be an important mediator of drug resistance in canine lymphoma. MDR may also be mediated by other transport proteins, such as the multidrug resistance-associated protein (MRP), and by other unrelated mechanisms. P-gp mediated MDR has been overcome in vitro by agents blocking P-gp function. However, their use in veterinary medicine, and indeed the role of P-gp in veterinary clinical multidrug resistance, has yet to be clearly defined.

Pharmacological resistance

Pharmacological resistance is caused by poor or erratic drug absorption, metabolism or excretion, or drug interactions. Some forms of pharmacological and biochemical resistance may be overcome by increasing the drug dose, providing that toxicity to the recipient is minimal or nonexistent at the current dose.

Chemotherapy toxicity

In chemotherapy, toxicity is the major factor limiting maximum drug dose rates. Overall prevalence of chemotherapy-induced toxicity has been estimated to be between 5% and 40% for veterinary patients (75–100% for people).

Cytotoxic agents are most harmful to rapidly dividing cells. Clinically significant acute toxicity most commonly affects the bone marrow and the gastrointestinal system. Some drugs have other drug-specific or species-specific toxicities, with or without myelotoxicity or enteric toxicity.

Acute, low-grade gastrointestinal toxicity lasting 1–3 days, e.g. inappetence or mild vomiting, does not usually warrant dose modification. In previously susceptible animals or with certain drugs (e.g. cisplatin) more severe anorexia or vomiting may be prevented through use of antiemetics (e.g. metoclopramide or ondansetron). Management of diarrhea is usually symptomatic. Severe gastrointestinal toxicity may warrant 25–50% reduction of subsequent doses or discontinuation of the drug.

Hematological toxicity, especially neutropenia and occasionally thrombocytopenia, is common following administration of many cytotoxic drugs. In the majority of cases this is subclinical, manifest as cytopenia on routine blood cell counts, and may not require dose adjustment, depending on the count. Recovery of normal granulocyte numbers from acute neutropenia is usually, but not always, rapid (within a week). Subsequent myelosuppressive treatments should be delayed until the neutrophil count is in excess of 2–3 10^9/L. Clinically significant hematological toxicity is usually due to severe neutropenia which can result in a life-threatening sepsis. Febrile neutropenic patients require careful assessment and active therapy, guidelines for which may be found in current oncology texts. In animals which have suffered severe neutropenia, reduction of subsequent drug doses by 25–50% is warranted.

A grading scheme for adverse events following chemotherapy has been published by the Veterinary Co-operative Oncology Group. Whilst this is not entirely relevant to day-to-day veterinary practice, it does set out standard criteria for reporting adverse events in clinical trials and studies.

Dysfunction of organs involved in drug metabolism and excretion, principally liver and kidney, may warrant drug dose adjustment. There are no established guidelines for dose reduction but in general, doses should be reduced in proportion to the degree of organ dysfunction. This is probably most important in renal failure where serum creatinine may be used as a guide to degree of renal dysfunction. Discontinuation of a specific drug should be considered upon the occurrence of a non-dose-related toxicity such as anaphylaxis. Similarly, discontinuation should be considered if evidence of chronic/cumulative toxicity is found, e.g. doxorubicin-induced cardiotoxicity or cisplatin-induced nephrotoxicity.

Many drugs cause vesicant (blistering) or irritant tissue damage if extravasated. These include:

- actinomycin D
- BCNU
- dacarbazine
- doxorubicin
- etoposide
- mechlorethamine
- vinblastine
- vincristine.

There is no agreed best remedy for extravasation of most drugs and readers are encouraged to consult current oncology texts for further advice. Management of extravasation of specific drugs is also discussed in the relevant section later in this chapter. Extravasation is best prevented by:

- adequate patient restraint during drug infusion
- careful attention to correct IV catheter placement. Vesicant/irritant drugs should be administered through the side arm of a drip set connected to an IV catheter with rapidly flowing fluid of appropriate type
- vigilant monitoring of the animal/injection site during drug infusion
- prompt discontinuation of infusion if extravasation is suspected.

Acute tumor lysis syndrome, uncommon in dogs and very rare in cats, should be distinguished from drug toxicity. The syndrome is most commonly reported in patients treated for lymphoma or leukemia and is best characterized as a metabolic disturbance associated with hyperuricemia and electrolyte disturbances. Specific management of this syndrome is detailed in current oncology texts.

Cytotoxic agents may impair fertility and breeding of animals undergoing chemotherapy is probably unwise. Where possible, avoid cytotoxic drug administration during the proliferative phase of wound healing.

Cytotoxic drugs rarely cause alopecia in cats and dogs but some coat and hair changes may occur. In cats, loss of whiskers is a common sequela to chemotherapy. Certain breeds of dog, particularly poodles and old English sheepdogs, may lose significant amounts of coat and some breeds, e.g. golden retrievers may lose the long hairs from their coat. Hyperpigmentation of the skin may also occur.

Be aware that, in view of the seriousness of the indications for use of cytotoxic agents, there are few, if any, absolute contraindications to their use. Contraindications noted below for each drug should be viewed as warnings and the treatment risks and benefits carefully considered for each patient.

DRUG HANDLING

There are remarkably few data linking health worker disease with occupational exposure to cytotoxic agents. However, given that many cytotoxic agents are carcinogenic with no known risk-free dose, or may cause local toxicity or allergic problems, consideration of safe work practices is warranted. For oncology nurses, a strong link exists between safe work practices and reduced drug exposure, as indicated by urinary excretion of cytotoxic agents.

Exposure may be through skin or mucous membrane absorption, inhalation, ingestion or needle-stick injury. Exposure may occur during preparation, administration, spillage or disposal of agents.

Acceptable safe work practices will differ between different centers depending on local and regional legislative requirements, the oncology case load of the clinic and other factors such as availability of cytotoxic reconstitution services and cytotoxic waste disposal facilities.

A complete review of safe drug handling is beyond the scope of this chapter and the reader is encouraged to consult the references for more detailed advice. Practices using cytotoxic drugs regularly should establish a set of local rules and guidelines on the handling, administration and disposal of these agents.

Common sense dictates the following general guidelines.

- An area of the practice should be designated as a cytotoxic drug preparation area. Ideally this should be a low-traffic, draft-free space. If use of chemotherapy is significant (daily/weekly) then a laminar flow biological safety cabinet should be used or the agents purchased in reconstituted, ready-to-administer form.
- Do not consume or prepare food or smoke cigarettes in drug preparation areas.
- Avoid aerosol formation in all phases of drug preparation; Luer-Lok syringes are recommended to prevent separation of the syringe from its attachment. Venting needles may be used to withdraw solutions from vials.
- Minimum protective clothing requirement for avoiding direct drug contact during preparation or delivery is to wear no-powder latex gloves of suitable thickness for protection against inadvertent contact with chemotherapy agents. Specialized cytotoxic protective clothing, including gloves, armsleeves and full-length gowns, is available and its use is advisable.
- Tablets formulated with an outer coating covering the active ingredient are not hazardous to handle but gloves are recommended for administration of tablets. The tablets should not be broken.
- Use a designated chemotherapy waste disposal container for contaminated waste, preferably one suitable for sharps.
- Ensure that a procedure is in place for managing spills and biological wastes of hospitalized patients.
- It may be prudent to consider absolving pregnant women from work with cytotoxic agents.

STABILITY OF INJECTABLE CYTOTOXIC DRUGS

The duration of stability of an injectable agent after partial use of the manufacturer's container is important for veterinary clinicians. Many data sheets or product inserts indicate that drugs should be refrigerated and used within a short period (often 24 h) of opening or reconstitution. This recommendation may not relate to the drug's chemical stability but be directed towards ensuring that bacteria entering the solution during opening or reconstitution do not multiply and reach dangerous numbers before administration of solution to the patient.

In this chapter, guidance regarding injectable drug storage is derived from a variety of sources, as well as manufacturers' data sheets. The reader is encouraged to familiarize themselves with data sheets for each product. Where manufacturers' recommendations are exceeded, it is assumed that opening or reconstitution procedures have been performed aseptically.

COMPOUNDING DRUGS

Compounding is increasingly important in daily veterinary practice in response to pet owner demands for state-of-the-art veterinary care and unmet needs for veterinary drugs. Since no chemotherapy drugs are manufactured for use in veterinary patients, orally administered chemotherapy agents are often formulated by manufacturers in tablets or capsules too large for veterinary patients. While compounding drugs into smaller capsules, more dilute solutions or into different formulations (liquid, suspension or transdermal gel) facilitates appropriate dosing and client administration, it may compromise stability, potency and absorption and also raises health and safety issues (see above). Not every drug can be reformulated due to issues with solubility, stability and palatability. Ideally, compounded drugs should be scientifically tested for stability, potency and absorption prior to administration. Since this scenario is unlikely, veterinarians should be cautious when prescribing compounded drugs and monitor carefully for response to therapy and development of adverse events.

The compounded drug may not have the anticipated therapeutic effect. Compounding drugs from unapproved (bulk) substances may also compromise patient safety since there are no regulatory controls in place to ensure safety and purity of the final formulations compounded from bulk substances. The Food and Drug Administration (FDA) considers compounding from bulk substances illegal.

The purpose of government approval of drugs is to ensure adequate quality control during drug manufacturing to protect consumers against ineffective drugs or, worse, harmful drugs. Every jurisdiction has its own specific requirements on compounding. Generally, the approach taken by the FDA is broadly reflected elsewhere so this will be outlined here.

In the United States, compounding is legal when the following criteria are met. The drug being compounded must be:

- prescribed by a licensed veterinarian
- approved for use in the United States and compounded from a 'finished dosage form' but not from bulk substances
- unavailable as an approved drug for animal use in the required dosage form and concentration
- compounded by a licensed pharmacist or veterinarian for a specific patient
- compounded within the context of a veterinarian–client–patient relationship.

Compounding of drugs not approved for use in the United States is considered illegal by the FDA unless the drugs have been obtained from a foreign country through government channels. Veterinarians prescribing compounded medications are not protected by the laws governing 'extra-label' drug usage since these laws safeguard veterinarians only for the usage of drugs approved in other species.

CYTOTOXIC DRUG CLASSES

TUBULIN-BINDING AGENTS

All chemotherapy drugs in the class known as the tubulin-binding agents or plant alkaloids are derived from plants and bind to tubulin, an intracellular microfilament. Vincristine, vinblastine, vinorelbine and paclitaxel exert their antineoplastic effect via disruption of normal tubulin assembly. Although etoposide binds tubulin, its antineoplastic effect is mediated through inhibition of topoisomerase II, a DNA replication enzyme.

Mechanism of action

Vincristine, vinblastine and vinorelbine are similar with regard to their mechanism of action since the source of both vincristine and vinblastine is the periwinkle plant and vinorelbine is a semisynthetic derivative of vinblastine. These drugs are viewed as cell cycle phase-specific drugs with activity in the M phase of the cell cycle. The mitotic spindle formation is blocked which causes an accumulation of cells in mitosis. The drugs bind to α/β-tubulin dimers, preventing their polymerization and thereby blocking formation of microtubules. Cytolytic effects are also exerted at other phases of the cell cycle as a result of disruption of normal microtubule function.

Because platelets and megakaryocytes are rich in tubulin, vincristine and vinorelbine bind them avidly.

Table 15.1 Available formulations of commonly used chemotherapy drugs

Generic name	Trade name	Manufacturer	Formulations
Actinomycin D	Cosmegen	Merck	0.5 mg vials
BCNU Carmustine	BiCNU	Bristol Myers Squibb	100 mg vials
Bleomycin	Blenoxane	Bristol Myers Squibb	15, 30 U per vial
Carboplatin	Paraplatin	Bristol Myers Squibb	50, 150, 450 mg vials
CCNU Lomustine	CeeNU	Bristol Myers Squibb	10, 40, 100 mg vials
Chlorambucil	Leukeran	Glaxo Wellcome	2 mg tablets
Cisplatin	Platinol	Bristol Myers Squibb	10, 50 mg vials
Cyclophosphamide	Cytoxan	Bristol Myers Squibb	100, 200, 500 mg, 1, 2 g vials, 25 and 50 mg tablets
Cytoside arabinoside	Cytosar-U	Pharmacia & Upjohn	100, 500 mg, 1, 2 g vials
Dacarbazine	DTIC-Dome	Bayer	100, 200 mg vials
Doxorubicin	Adriamycin	Pharmacia & Upjohn	10, 50, 100 mg vials
	Rubex	Bristol Myers Squibb	
Epirubicin	Not available in USA		
Etoposide	VePsid	Bristol Myers Squibb	100, 150, 500 mg vials, 1 g vials
	Etopophos	Bristol Myers Squibb	50 mg capsules
Hydroxyurea	Hydrea	Bristol Myers Squibb	10, 50, 100 mg vials
	Droxia	Bristol Myers Squibb	
Idarubicin	Idamycin	Pharmacia & Upjohn	
Ifosfamide	Ifex	Bristol Myers Squibb	1, 3 g vials
5-Fluorouracil	Adrucil	Roche	500 mg vial
L-asparaginase	Elspar	Merck	10,000 IU/vial
Colapase	Levnase	Aventis	
Melphalan	Alkeran	Glaxo Wellcome	2 mg tablets
Methotrexate	Methotrexate	Immunex	50, 100, 150, 200 mg vials 2.5 mg tablets
Mitoxantrone			
Mitozantrone	Novantrone	Immunex	20, 25, 30 mg vials
Paclitaxel	Taxol	Bristol Myers Squibb	30, 100, 300 mg vials
Plicamycin			
Mithramycin	Mithracin	Bayer	2.5 mg vials
Vinblastine	Velban	Lilly	10 mg vials
	Velbe (in Europe)		
Vincristine	Oncovin	Lilly	1, 2, 5 mg vials

Vincristine is believed to be responsible for an increase in platelet release from bone marrow after administration. Vincristine binds platelets more avidly than vinblastine and consequently has theoretical advantage over vinblastine in the management of thrombocytopenia.

Mechanisms of drug resistance

Two types of biochemical resistance have been described in tumor cells insensitive to vincristine. First, mutations in α- or β-subunits of tubulin lead to decreased binding of vincristine to tubulin, resulting in resistance to inhibition of microtubule formation. Tumor cells also become resistant to the vinca alkaloids through development of multiple drug resistance mediated by P-gp.

Vincristine

Other names

NCS-67574, LCR, VCR, Oncovin®

Clinical applications

Vincristine is widely used in veterinary oncology. Almost all combination chemotherapy protocols for canine, feline and ferret lymphoma incorporate vincristine into the drug cycle. Remission can be induced with vincristine-containing protocols in cases of chronic lymphocytic leukemia and acute lymphoblastic leukemia. Single-agent vincristine is the treatment of choice for transmissible venereal tumor and results in a durable complete remission in over 90% of cases. Vincristine is a component of the VAC protocol (vincristine, doxorubicin (Adriamycin®), cyclophosphamide), which has shown some efficacy against soft tissue sarcomas, including hemangiosarcoma.

Vincristine and prednisone have also been shown to increase the platelet count in patients with immune-mediated thrombocytopenia compared to treatment with prednisone alone. Following administration of vincristine, a mild transient decrease occurs in platelet count followed by a peak platelet count 8 days after drug administration to normal dogs. Platelets formed following administration of vincristine showed normal aggregation in vitro. Similarly, clot retraction and buccal mucosal bleeding time were normal in vincristine-treated dogs. Vincristine is not believed to have major effects on wound healing.

Formulations and dose rates

Vincristine must be stored at 2–8°C to maintain potency and will degrade if exposed to light.

DOGS
- 0.5–0.75 mg/m² IV bolus, once weekly or according to protocol being used
- Doses as low as 0.02 mg/kg have been used to stimulate platelet production

CATS
- 0.025 mg/kg or 0.5 mg/m² IV bolus, once weekly or according to protocol being used

FERRETS
- 0.75 mg/m² IV bolus

Vincristine should never be administered intrathecally.

Pharmacokinetics

In normal dogs, the disappearance of tritiated vincristine from the plasma is biphasic, with an initial $t_{1/2}$ of 13 min and a second-phase $t_{1/2}$ of 75 min. Highest tissue levels achieved are in spleen (2.28 ng/g tissue). Levels in brain and cerebrospinal fluid are undetectable. Hepatic metabolism and rapid biliary excretion are followed by 70% of administered drug being excreted in feces. Only 15% of the drug is excreted in urine. Oral absorption is poor.

Adverse effects

- Vincristine should never be administered intrathecally.
- Myelosuppression is rarely reported when vincristine is used as a single agent in dogs. However, neutropenia is sporadically severe in cats 4–9 days following drug administration.
- Like any chemotherapy drug, vincristine can cause gastrointestinal signs. Anorexia seems to be most common in the cat and vomiting in the dog.
- Neutropenia can occur in susceptible dogs, e.g. certain collies, due to a mutation in the canine MDR1 gene causing a P-glycoprotein defect which also confers susceptibility to toxic effects of ivermectin.
- Vincristine is not believed to have major effects on wound healing.
- Constipation is reported to occur in both dogs and cats following administration of vincristine, but appears more common in cats.
- In humans, the dose-limiting toxicity of vincristine is a peripheral neuropathy. The effects are believed to be limited to peripheral nerves because vincristine does not penetrate the blood–brain barrier. Vincristine interrupts microtubular function, resulting in an inability to maintain axonal membrane integrity. Dogs appear to be relatively resistant to the neuropathic effect of vincristine, but a single case has been reported following 16 weekly doses of 0.5 mg/m².
- Extravasation of vincristine during infusion results in local tissue necrosis and sloughing. If extravasation is suspected, the infusion should be immediately discontinued but the infusion catheter left in place and an attempt made to aspirate fluid from the site to decrease the remaining drug. Warm compresses should be applied to the area for 15 min q.6 h for 3 d. The author also applies a solution (Synotic®) containing dimethyl sulfoxide, fluocinolone acetonide and flunixin meglamine (1 mL per Synotic® vial) applied topically q.12 h for 3–5 days following drug extravasation. Owners should wear gloves when applying the solution.
- Hyaluronidase has been reported to decrease the tissue damage following vincristine extravasation. 300 U of hyaluronidase are injected into the catheter, if still present, or into the indurated area in six aliquots using a 25-gauge needle. The injection may be repeated weekly.
- Administration of vincristine changes the morphology of bone marrow cells within 24 h of administration. The predominant changes are seen in erythroid cells. Abnormalities included increased numbers of cells in metaphase, fragmented nuclei and atypical nuclear configurations. An increased M : E ratio was seen 24 h post-vincristine.

Known drug interactions

The manufacturer's recommendations indicate that vincristine should not be given in combination with L-asparaginase because of severe myelosuppression; consequently some veterinary oncologists recommend spacing drug administration by 12–48 h. Neutropenia is seen in up to 50% of dogs at some centers treated with L-asparaginase and vincristine, although it rarely results in clinical signs. In one study which evaluated 147 dogs, neutropenia occurred in 40% of those receiving the combination of drugs, irrespective of the interval between administration of the two drugs. Hospitalization was necessary in 16% of dogs.

Vinblastine

Other names

NSC-49842, vincaleukoblastine, VLB Velban, Velbe (Europe)

Clinical applications

In cases of vincristine intolerance, vinblastine is typically substituted in combination chemotherapy protocols. Careful monitoring must be undertaken when making this substitution because life-threatening myelosuppression may occur. Use of vinblastine has been described in dogs with lymphoma and tonsillar squamous cell carcinoma. Vinblastine is currently being investigated as a treatment for canine mast cell tumors along with prednisone and appears to have efficacy in this disease. Optimum treatment protocols have yet to be defined.

Formulations and dose rates

Vinblastine must be stored at 2–8°C to maintain potency and will degrade if exposed to light.

DOGS

- The standard dosage of vinblastine is 2 mg/m^2 IV bolus every 10–14 days. Intrathecal administration of vinblastine to dogs resulted in severe neurological impairment and death in one-third of dogs

Pharmacokinetics

Using tritiated vinblastine, a biphasic clearance of vinblastine from plasma of normal dogs was identified. Initial rapid clearance occurred in 24–30 min and slower elimination over 4–7 h. Up to 80% of drug was protein bound. The majority of vinblastine was excreted in bile and metabolized in the intestinal tract. A smaller amount of unmetabolized vinblastine is excreted in urine. Vinblastine is poorly absorbed orally.

Adverse effects

- Although the dose-limiting effect of vinblastine is myelosuppression, with the nadir of leukopenia in dogs occurring 4–7 days following drug administration (mean occurrence of neutropenia, day 5), toxicity is typically mild. In a study of dogs with mast cell tumors, the most common toxicity was mild thrombocytopenia. Neutrophil reconstitution takes place 7–14 days after administration. Overall hematological toxicity was 10% of all complete blood counts.
- Gastrointestinal signs, such as vomiting and constipation, may also be seen.
- Like vincristine, vinblastine causes local tissue necrosis if the drug is extravasated. Management of a suspected extravasation is identical to that of vincristine.
- Vinblastine is not believed to have major effects on wound healing.

Known drug interactions

There are no known major drug interactions.

Vinorelbine

Other names

Navelbine, KW-2307, CAS71486-22-1

Clinical applications

Vinorelbine is currently under investigation in veterinary oncology. In a phase I clinical trial, modest efficacy was found in dogs with macroscopic bronchoalveolar carcinoma.

Formulations and dose rates

DOGS

- 15–18 mg/m^2 appears to be the range of maximum tolerated dose in dogs. A starting dosage of 15 mg/m^2 as an intravenous infusion over 5 min has been recommended

CATS

- Use of vinorelbine has not been reported in cats

Pharmacokinetics

Vinorelbine is widely distributed into tissues except the central nervous system and is highly (90%) protein bound. Unchanged drug has a terminal half-life of 34.5 h in dogs. Clearance is 1.2 L/h/kg and has a volume of distribution of 49.6 L/kg. Especially high concentrations are achieved in lung tissue and the concentration in mammary tissue exceeds those in plasma. The chief mechanism for excretion of vinorelbine is via the feces. Urinary excretion represents less than 30% of drug elimination.

Adverse effects

- Myelosuppression occurred in 32% of dogs treated with vinorelbine in a phase I clinical trial.
- Gastrointestinal toxicity (vomiting, diarrhea, anorexia) occurred in 16% of dogs in a phase I clinical trial.
- Skin necrosis if the drug is extravasated has been reported in humans.

Known drug interactions

There are no known major drug interactions.

Etoposide

Other names

NCS-141540, VP-16-213, epipodophyllotoxin, EPE-ethylidene Lignan P

Clinical applications

Etoposide has demonstrated minimal anticancer activity in dogs with relapsed lymphoma. In humans, it is effective in germ cell and lung tumors. Use of etoposide has not been reported in cats.

Mechanism of action

Etoposide is a semisynthetic derivative of podophyllotoxin, an alkaloid from the May apple or mandrake plant. The drug acts by interfering with the breakage–reunion reaction of mammalian DNA topoisomerase II.

Mechanisms of drug resistance

Two biochemical mechanisms of resistance have been described for etoposide:

- increased drug efflux associated with increased levels of P-gp or MRP
- modifications in topoisomerase II and enhanced capacity to repair DNA strand breaks.

Formulations and dose rates

Unopened vials should be stored at 2–8°C. When diluted for administration, the solution is stable at 2–8°C for 48 h.

DOGS

- Maximum tolerated dose and optimal dose scheduling have yet to be determined for use of etoposide in the dog
- One published dose is 100 mg/m^2 given once or divided over 4 consecutive days
- Data from humans suggest that multiple doses given over several days are advantageous
- The drug has been diluted in 0.9% sodium chloride to a concentration of 1–2 mg/mL and infused over 15–30 min

Pharmacokinetics

Etoposide enters the cells by passive diffusion. In normal dogs administered 2 mg/kg of etoposide, the initial $t_{1/2}$ is 0.3 min. The terminal $t_{1/2}$ is 1.7 h. Approximately half of the drug is excreted in urine unchanged. Major metabolites are found in plasma, urine and bile. When administered orally, only 50% bioavailability has been demonstrated, with wide individual variability.

Adverse effects

The clinical usefulness of this drug in dogs is limited by the adverse reaction attributed to the vehicle, polysorbate 80. Dose-limiting toxicity in the dog is a moderate-to-severe cutaneous reaction characterized by moderate-to-severe pruritus, urticaria and swelling of the head and extremities and hypotension. Toxicity is not ameliorated by concurrent administration of steroids, antihistamines or a slow infusion rate.

Myelosuppression occurs in dogs when etoposide is administered chronically.

Known drug interactions

No clinically significant interactions have been identified.

Paclitaxel

Other names

NSC-125973, Taxol

Clinical applications

Clinical applications for paclitaxel are currently under investigation in veterinary patients and may be limited by the adverse reaction to the vehicle, Cremophor EL and alcohol. Paclitaxel, in combination with a platinum analog, is the first-line treatment in humans for advanced ovarian and breast carcinoma. It is an emerging therapy for human prostate cancer.

Mechanism of action

Paclitaxel is a cell cycle-specific drug resulting in an accumulation of cells in M phase. It enhances polymerization of tubulin, resulting in inhibition of DNA synthesis.

Mechanism of drug resistance

Two general mechanisms of resistance have been described: one mediated by the MDR gene and the other by structural alterations in the tubulin subunits.

Formulations and dose rates

Paclitaxel should be stored at room temperature. Refrigeration or freezing does not affect drug stability. Once diluted for administration, it is stable for up to 27 h under ambient temperature and light. The solution should be discarded if cloudy

DOGS

- In an effort to alleviate the vehicle-induced adverse reaction, paclitaxel has been diluted in 0.9% saline and infused over 3–6 h
- The maximum tolerated dose in the dog appears to be 170 mg/m^2
- Pretreatment with cimetidine, diphenhydramine and glucocorticoids is recommended to abrogate the vehicle-induced side effects

Pharmacokinetics

Pharmacokinetic information is lacking in the dog. In humans, pharmacokinetics are linear when the drug is given in 6–24 h infusions and nonlinear if shorter infusion times are employed. The area under the curve (AUC) correlates well with dose of drug administered. The volume of distribution is much larger than total body water, indicating protein binding. Disposition in plasma is characterized by a biexponential elimination model. Paclitaxel is not believed to cross the blood–brain barrier. The major route of excretion is biliary, with a small component of renal excretion.

Adverse effects

- Myelosuppression occurs 3–7 days following administration but the dose-limiting toxicity in the dog appears to be a reaction to the drug's vehicle.
- Cremophor EL and alcohol induce mast cell degranulation, causing hypotension, cutaneous erythema and pruritus.
- Alopecia is significant in dogs administered paclitaxel.

Known drug interactions

None have been reported.

ALKYLATING AGENTS

Mechanism of action

Alkylating agents react chemically with nucleic acids (DNA) and proteins but, in general, their cytotoxicity has been correlated most closely with their capacity to react with DNA. In DNA, alkylating agents react with guanine or cytosine bases, substituting alkyl radicals for hydrogen atoms. This may cause DNA strand breaks and, in the case of bifunctional alkylating agents (which have two alkyl groups, each of which can bind a DNA molecule), lead to DNA intra- or interstrand crosslinks or DNA–protein crosslinks. This prevents normal function of DNA (DNA replication and consequent RNA transcription and translation) at all phases of the cell cycle.

The agents are therefore cell cycle phase-nonspecific and the nitrogen mustard and the nitrosoureas are sometimes classified as nonselective, phase nonspecific. They are lethal to resting cells, although cell division is required for the lethal event to be expressed. Thus, this group of drugs may be effective against slowly growing as well as rapidly growing tumors.

Mechanisms of resistance

Numerous mechanisms of tumor cell resistance to alkylating agents have been described in vitro. Specific mechanisms include:

- decreased drug uptake
- increased repair of drug-induced damage
- increased drug inactivation
- increased inactivation of cytotoxic metabolites.

Drug-specific examples are listed below but knowledge of these mechanisms has not yet proven clinically useful to improve chemotherapy response.

Decreased drug uptake or accumulation by cancer cells has been linked to resistance to melphalan and mechlorethamine.

Increased repair of drug-induced damage is a mechanism of resistance to nitrosoureas mediated by increased cellular levels of O6-alkylguanine DNA alkyltransferase, which repairs O6-alkylguanine DNA intermediates. Depletion of O6-alkylguanine DNA alkyltransferase reverses drug resistance in vitro, but attempts to do so in vivo have so far proved too toxic for clinical use.

Increased drug inactivation resulting from alterations in metabolism involving thiol compounds such as glutathione has been documented for a variety of alkylating agents such as nitrosoureas, chlorambucil and melphalan. The clinical significance of glutathione-mediated drug inactivation is uncertain. Recent reports suggest that glutathione conjugation may also contribute to efflux of chlorambucil and melphalan from the cell by MRP. Human clinical trials designed to pharmacologically modify glutathione synthesis or inhibit glutathione *S*-transferase (which catalyzes conjugation of glutathione to drug substrates) have not yet yielded clear results.

Increased inactivation of cytotoxic cyclophosphamide metabolites by high levels of aldehyde dehydrogenase in tumor cells has been linked to resistance to cyclophosphamide. Although inhibitors of aldehyde dehydrogenase have been identified, their value in reversing clinical drug resistance is unknown.

BCNU

Other names

Carmustine

Clinical applications

BCNU is primarily indicated in humans for palliation of malignant glioma, multiple myeloma and lymphoma. Objective tumor shrinkage was observed in a dog with an astrocytoma. BCNU has also been combined with vincristine and prednisone for the treatment of canine lymphoma. Remission rate and duration of remission (86% and 183 days) were comparable to other multiagent protocols and neutropenia was the dose-limiting toxicity.

Formulations and dose rates

- 50 mg/m^2 administered IV over 20 min and repeated every 6 weeks
- There is no information available for cats

Pharmacokinetics
BCNU is a nitrosourea alkylating agent. It is relatively nonionized and lipid soluble and crosses the blood–brain barrier quite effectively. Intravenously administered BCNU is rapidly degraded to reactive intermediates with a half-life of approximately 15 min in humans. In studies on dogs, using radiolabeled BCNU, approximately 28–30% of the total radioactivity administered was excreted in the urine in 6 h.

Adverse effects
- Myelosuppression is dose limiting, with neutrophil nadir at 7–9 d and recovery delayed for 15 d, and was pronounced when BCNU was used in a multiagent protocol (vincristine, BCNU and prednisone) for lymphoma. Thrombocytopenia is also likely. In humans, bone marrow toxicity is cumulative and dose adjustments are considered on the basis of nadir counts from the prior dose.
- Pulmonary fibrosis was reported in one dog given eight doses of BCNU and is a common adverse effect related to cumulative dose in humans.
- Nausea and vomiting are common, dose-related effects in humans; hepatic and other toxicities are uncommon.
- Rapid administration may cause intense pain and burning sensation at the injection site.

Contraindications and precautions
BCNU should be used with caution in myelosuppressed patients.

Known drug interactions
As with other cytotoxic agents, the myelosuppressive effects of BCNU may be enhanced by other myelosuppressive drugs.

Busulfan

Clinical applications
Busulfan is an alkyl alkane sulfonate alkylating agent. It is selectively cytotoxic to myeloid cells, leaving lymphoid cells relatively undamaged. Busulfan is principally indicated for the treatment of canine chronic granulocytic leukemia. Its use against this disease in cats is said to be less successful. It may also be useful to treat polycythemia vera.

Formulations and dose rates

DOGS AND CATS
- 2–6 mg/m^2 PO q.24 h until the WBC count approaches the upper limit of the normal range, then either discontinue the medication or reduce the daily dose to maintain the count at or just below this level. In humans, the recommended maximum daily dose is 4 mg
- The blood count should be monitored weekly during induction of remission; if response is inadequate after 3 weeks, consider increasing the dose rate
- In humans, if maintenance therapy is required, a dose between 0.5 and 2 mg daily is usual, although much lower doses are adequate for some individuals

Pharmacokinetics
Busulfan is readily absorbed after oral administration. In rats, it is extensively metabolized, principally in the liver, and metabolites are excreted in urine.

Adverse effects
- Myelosuppression (particularly neutropenia and thrombocytopenia) is the most important toxicity. In humans, WBC counts may not start to fall until 2 weeks after beginning therapy and may continue to fall for 2 weeks after the last drug dose. Marrow recovery may not occur for 3–6 weeks after discontinuing therapy.
- Nausea and vomiting are unusual in humans.
- Suppression of gonad function occurs in males and females.
- Other uncommon adverse effects usually reported after prolonged therapy in humans include skin pigmentation, pulmonary fibrosis, adrenal insufficiency, ovarian suppression and secondary neoplasia.

Contraindications and precautions
Busulfan is contraindicated in patients with thrombocytopenia, neutropenia or pulmonary fibrosis.

Known drug interactions
Busulfan may exacerbate the pulmonary toxicity of other cytotoxic agents or radiation therapy.

CCNU

Other names

Lomustine

Clinical applications
CCNU is used in the treatment of human brain tumors, melanoma and as secondary therapy for lymphoma. The use of CCNU has recently been reported as a single agent for treating canine mast cell tumors, canine and feline lymphoma and possibly canine brain tumors. CCNU may also have efficacy against some sarcomas. Its exact role in these diseases has yet to be completely clarified but it will probably find utility as one component of a multidrug treatment regimen.

In the case of mast cell tumors, it should only be considered for the treatment of dogs with tumors unsuitable for surgery and radiation therapy. Anecdotal evidence suggests that it may be combined with vinblastine to treat these patients effectively, but it is not known whether this combination is more effective than CCNU alone.

Formulations and dose rates

DOGS
- 60–90 mg/m^2 PO every 3–8 weeks

CATS
- 50–60 mg/m^2 PO every 3–6 weeks

Pharmacokinetics
CCNU is a nitrosourea alkylating agent. After oral or intravenous administration, CCNU is rapidly broken down to various intermediates by hepatic microsomal metabolic transformation. Following oral administration, little or no parent drug is detectable in plasma. High lipid solubility and relative lack of ionization at physiological pH enable CCNU or its metabolites to readily cross the blood–brain barrier. In dogs given 450 mg/m^2 radioactively labeled CCNU intravenously, radioactivity rapidly entered cerebrospinal fluid. The primary excretion route in dogs is renal, with approximately 85% of administered radioactivity excreted within 24 h.

Adverse effects
- Neutropenia is the dose-limiting toxicity. Dogs treated with 5 mg/kg (approx. 150 mg/m^2) became neutropenic, with the nadir at 7 d (1×10^9 cells/L) and recovery by 20 d. More recently, in 17 dogs treated for mast cell tumor with CCNU 50 mg/m^2, the median neutrophil count after 7 d was 1.4×10^9 cells/L (mean, 1.7×10^9 cells/L). Five dogs developed fever, of whom four were neutropenic; all recovered with supportive care. In another study, in dogs with lymphoma treated with the same dose rate of CCNU, delayed and cumulative neutropenia and thrombocytopenia were observed.
- Unexplained fever has been reported as an uncommon idiosyncratic toxicity in dogs.
- Hepatotoxicity was reported in dogs treated in preclinical studies with more than 125 mg/m^2. CCNU hepatotoxicity is delayed, cumulative and dose related, but is uncommon in clinical cases. In approximately half of the dogs developing CCNU hepatotoxicity, it was fatal. Elevation of serum ALT activity may be an early marker of CCNU hepatotoxicity. Serum biochemical profiles should be monitored in dogs receiving CCNU.
- Gastrointestinal toxicity is mild and self-limiting.
- Evidence of renal toxicity, manifest as elevated plasma urea concentration, has been observed in preclinical studies with dogs.
- CCNU should be used with caution in myelosuppressed patients.
- CCNU toxicity may be exacerbated in patients with renal pathology that interferes with excretion.

Known drug interactions
As with other cytotoxic agents, the myelosuppressive effects of CCNU may be enhanced by other myelosuppressive drugs.

Chlorambucil

Other Names

Leukeran

Clinical applications
The combination of chlorambucil and prednisone is an effective treatment for chronic lymphocytic leukemia. It is easy to administer and there is a low probability of myelotoxicity.

Chlorambucil is also used as a component of maintenance therapy for lymphoma and may be substituted for cyclophosphamide in animals with cyclophosphamide-induced cystitis although this may not be necessary (see cyclophosphamide below).

Other neoplastic diseases for which chlorambucil may be useful include multiple myeloma (particularly in cats), polycythemia rubra vera, macroglobulinemia, ovarian adenocarcinoma and nonresectable mast cell tumors in dogs.

Chlorambucil is also commonly used in the management of immune-mediated disorders in cats.

Formulations and dose rates

Recommended dose rates vary widely, permitting considerable scope for dosage adjustment according to the needs of an individual patient.

DOGS AND CATS
- 2 mg/m^2 (up to 6 mg/m^2) or 0.2 mg/kg PO q.24 h or q.48 h
- 20 mg/m^2 or 1.4 mg/kg PO q.1–4 weeks

Pharmacokinetics
Chlorambucil belongs to the nitrogen mustard group of alkylating agents. It is well absorbed from the gastrointestinal tract of rats and humans and is mainly distributed to liver, kidney and plasma in the rat. In addition to a degree of spontaneous hydrolysis, the drug is extensively metabolized in the liver to phenylacetic acid mustard and its derivatives.

In humans, peak plasma levels occur 2–4 h after dosing with 0.6 mg/m^2 PO and the terminal half-lives of the parent drug and the chief metabolite, phenylacetic acid mustard, are 92 and 145 min respectively. Approximately 50% of the chlorambucil metabolic products are excreted in human urine in 24 h. There do not appear to be data available on chlorambucil metabolism in companion animals.

Adverse effects

- Myelosuppression occurs to a lesser extent with this drug than with other alkylating agents. Granulocytopenia may be slow in onset but is usually mild and quick to resolve. However, it may persist up to 10 d after the last dose of the drug. Prolonged pancytopenia has been reported in humans but not so far in animals.
- Alopecia and gastrointestinal effects are uncommon and generally mild.
- Canine cerebellar toxicity was noted in doses exceeding 8 mg/m^2 daily.
- Toxicities reported in humans but not yet in animals include bronchopulmonary dysplasia with pulmonary fibrosis, uric acid nephropathy and hepatopathy.
- Chlorambucil may raise serum uric acid levels.
- Chlorambucil is contraindicated in patients with bone marrow suppression or infection.
- Chlorambucil is potentially teratogenic and has been reported to cause permanent infertility when given to nonadult human males.

Known drug interactions

Chlorambucil may augment the myelosuppressive effects of other antineoplastic agents and other drugs that suppress bone marrow function, e.g. chloramphenicol, flucytosine, amphotericin B.

Cyclophosphamide

Other names

Endoxana, Cytexan

Clinical applications

Alone (rarely) or in combination with other drugs, cyclophosphamide is an important agent for treating lymphoproliferative disorders (lymphoma, leukemia, multiple myeloma), soft tissue sarcoma (hemangiosarcoma, synovial cell sarcoma), carcinoma (feline mammary malignancy, thyroid carcinoma) and transmissible venereal tumor. Cyclophosphamide has long been recommended as an adjunct to prednisone therapy for immune-mediated hemolytic anemia. However, mounting evidence suggests that it provides no additional benefit over prednisone for short-term management of this disease.

Formulations and dose rates

Available in tablet and injectable formulation. Tablets should be stored below 25°C but short exposures of up to 30°C are acceptable. Cyclophosphamide powder for injection may be reconstituted in an elixir for oral administration and is stable for 14 d at 4°C. It is reconstituted in sterile water for intravenous administration and is stable for 24 h at room temperature and 6 days at 4°C. Care should be taken in the handling and administration of such solutions for health and safety reasons

DOGS AND CATS

- 150–200 mg/m^2 IV per week
- 10 mg/kg IV per week, cats
- 50 mg/m^2 PO q.24 h or q.48 h to total dose of 200–300 mg/m^2 per week
- 250 mg/m^2 PO every 3 weeks

FERRETS

- 200 mg/m^2 IV once weekly
- 168–336 mg/m^2 IV or PO divided over 2–4 d

Pharmacokinetics

Cyclophosphamide is a prodrug and is metabolized to active alkylating agents, principally by microsomal enzymes in the liver. Phosphoramide mustard and acrolein, endpoints of the metabolic pathway, are believed to be primarily responsible for the antitumor activity and bladder toxicity respectively. Acrolein has been implicated in denaturation of microsomal cytochrome P450 enzymes.

Pharmacokinetic data from humans show that cyclophosphamide is well absorbed orally and from parenteral sites, with peak plasma concentration occurring at about 60 min after oral administration. The drug is widely distributed to tissues and has been found to cross the human blood–brain barrier in low concentrations. The serum $t_{1/2}$ of cyclophosphamide is variable, with values reported from 4 to 65 h. Parent drug and metabolites are detectable in plasma for up to 72 h and both are excreted in the urine, mainly within the first 24 h of treatment.

Adverse effects

- Myelosuppression is the most important toxicity. The neutrophil nadir occurs at 7–14 d following a single dose and recovery generally follows within 10 d but may be delayed for several weeks.
- Anorexia, salivation (presumably indicating nausea), diarrhea and emesis may be noted, especially after intravenous administration.
- Sterile hemorrhagic cystitis may occur after a variable number of doses (in approximately 10% of dogs treated for lymphoma with a protocol containing cyclophosphamide. It has also been observed acutely

after a single intravenous administration. The cystitis may be severe and intractable and there is no specific remedy but mild cases will resolve spontaneously over a few days to a few weeks. Cyclophosphamide should be discontinued if drug-induced cystitis occurs. Furosemide (2.2 mg/kg IV) administered intravenously concurrently with cyclophosphamide has been shown to decrease the frequency of sterile hemorrhagic cystitis.

- Bladder fibrosis and transitional cell carcinoma may also occur secondary to cyclophosphamide therapy. These and bacterial cystitis are the most important conditions to distinguish from cyclophosphamide-induced cystitis.
- Other reported adverse effects include alopecia, diarrhea and secondary malignancy (lymphoproliferative, bladder). Pulmonary infiltrates and fibrosis and hyponatremia are yet to be reported in veterinary patients.
- Cyclophosphamide should be used with caution in patients who have undergone previous radiotherapy, or with impaired renal or hepatic function.
- The safe use of cyclophosphamide in pregnancy is uncertain; it is potentially teratogenic and embryotoxic.
- Cyclophosphamide may be associated with male sterility.

Known drug interactions

- Chronic use of barbiturates induces microsomal enzymes and thus may increase cyclophosphamide metabolism and hence its toxicity.
- Allopurinol and thiazide diuretics may exacerbate cyclophosphamide-induced myelotoxicity.
- Doxorubicin cardiotoxicity may be exacerbated by cyclophosphamide.
- Succinylcholine metabolism may be impeded and its effects prolonged as a result of cyclophosphamide-induced depletion of serum pseudocholinesterases. Digoxin absorption after oral administration may be impeded for several days after cyclophosphamide administration.

Ifosfamide

Other names

Ifex

Clinical applications

In humans, ifosfamide is active against soft tissue sarcomas and osteosarcoma. It also has activity against transitional cell carcinoma, pulmonary, ovarian and breast carcinoma and lymphoma. Only preliminary data are available on the use of ifosfamide in dogs. The antitumor activity appears not to be as high in dogs as in people. In one study, very little activity was seen against lymphoma and only moderate activity against soft tissue sarcomas.

Formulations and dose rates

- 350–375 mg/m^2 IV q.3 weeks with diuresis and mesna (sodium 2-mercapto-ethane sulfonate, Mesnex®) in dogs (see Pharmacokinetics section below). The recommended protocol for 0.9% NaCl fluid diuresis is 30 min at a rate of 18.3 mL/kg/h followed by ifosfamide diluted in 0.9% NaCl to a volume of 9.15 mL/kg infused over 30 min at a rate of 18.3 mL/kg. Additional diuresis is then administered for 5 h at 18.3 mL/kg. Mesna is administered 3 times at 20% of the ifosfamide dose. The first treatment is given before ifosfamide and the remaining two treatments 2 and 5 h after ifosfamide
- No dosing information is available for cats

Pharmacokinetics

Ifosfamide belongs to the nitrogen mustard group of alkylating agents. Like cyclophosphamide, ifosfamide is a prodrug and requires hepatic metabolism to active intermediates, but ifosfamide has a longer plasma half-life than cyclophosphamide. One of the metabolites is acrolein, the metabolite associated with the occurrence of hemorrhagic cystitis. Hemorrhagic cystitis occurs in all patients administered ifosfamide unless mesna is administered concurrently. In the urinary tract, mesna scavenges the toxic metabolites of ifosfamide, thus preventing hemorrhagic cystitits.

Adverse effects

- When used with appropriate mesna therapy, the dose-limiting toxicity is neutropenia. The nadir occurs 7 d following administration.
- Gastrointestinal toxicity has not been described in dogs receiving ifosfamide.
- Renal toxicity has been described in humans receiving ifosfamide, but does not appear to be a significant issue in dogs.

Contraindications and precautions

Ifosfamide should be used with caution in myelosuppressed patients.

Known drug interactions

As with other cytotoxic agents, the myelosuppressive effects of ifosfamide may be enhanced by other myelosuppressive drugs.

Mechlorethamine

Other names

Mechlorethamine hydrochloride, chloromethine hydrochloride, mustargen hydrochloride, chlorethazine hydrochloride, chlormethine (mustine) hydrochloride, nitrogen mustard, HN_2

Clinical applications

The major use of mechlorethamine is in the treatment of relapsed drug-resistant canine and feline lymphoma as part of the MOPP protocol (mechlorethamine, vincristine, procarbazine, prednisolone (or prednisone)). Mechlorethamine has been used topically in humans to treat mycosis fungoides and related cutaneous diseases. Due to the difficulties associated with drug handling, we cannot recommend topical therapy for veterinary patients with mycosis fungoides.

Formulations and dose rates

Preparation: 1 mg/mL in 0.9% w/v sodium chloride or 5% w/v glucose. Solutions decompose quickly and should be discarded if not used within 4 h (room temperature) or 6 h (4°C). Solutions should not be mixed with other drugs

DOGS AND CATS

- 3–6 mg/m^2 IV. The higher end of the dose range may be severely myelotoxic in both cats and dogs. 3 mg/m^2 IV on days 0 and 7 is recommended for use in the MOPP protocol
- Administer into injection port of rapidly running infusion of 0.9% sodium chloride at a rate of 60 drops per min

Pharmacokinetics

Mechlorethamine is the prototype drug in the nitrogen mustard group of alkylating agents. Nitrogen mustard undergoes rapid spontaneous hydrolysis after intravenous injection, disappearing from blood within approximately 10 min. In addition, it undergoes considerable enzymatic degradation. Less than 0.01% is excreted unchanged in urine.

Adverse effects

- Mechlorethamine is markedly vesicant and causes severe local reaction if extravasated.
- Nausea and emesis are common, usually lasting less than 12 h in humans. Consider pretreatment with antiemetic agents.
- Myelosuppression, with nadir at approximately 7 d.
- Other – diarrhea, oral ulcers, pulmonary infiltrates and fibrosis, leukemia, alopecia.
- Contraindications to use of mechlorethamine are severe neutropenia, thrombocytopenia, anemia and coexisting infection.

Known drug interactions

- Mechlorethamine is incompatible with methohexital sodium.
- As with other cytotoxics, the myelosuppressive effects of mechlorethamine may be enhanced by other myelosuppressive drugs.

Melphalan

Other names

L-PAM, L-phenylalanine mustard, L-sarcolysin, Alkeran

Clinical applications

Melphalan, in combination with prednisone, is the standard first-line treatment for canine multiple myeloma and has also been used in cats with multiple myeloma. In combination with actinomycin D, cytosine arabinoside and dexamethasone (D-MAC protocol), it has shown efficacy for canine lymphoma rescue therapy.

Melphalan has been used to treat canine ovarian, mammary, pulmonary and apocrine gland carcinomas and adenocarcinomas and osteosarcoma and is reported to be effective against feline chronic lymphocytic leukemia.

Formulations and dose rates

A number of different dosing regimens have been described for use in different protocols.

DOGS

- 0.63 mg/kg IV every 2–4 weeks
- 0.1 mg/kg PO daily for 10 d then 0.05 mg/kg/d
- 1.5–2 mg/m^2 PO daily for 7–10 d, repeat every 2–3 weeks if needed
- 20 mg/m^2 PO once weekly

CATS

- 10 mg/m^2 PO once weekly

For human patients, some authorities recommend adjusting the oral dose rate or duration until myelosuppression is detected in order to ensure that an effective dose has been administered. It is not known whether this recommendation might apply to companion animals. Anecdotal evidence suggests that cats may be more susceptible to melphalan-induced myelosuppression than dogs.

Pharmacokinetics

Melphalan is a member of the nitrogen mustard group of alkylating agents. Variable and incomplete oral absorption of melphalan has been reported in humans and is likely to occur in companion animals. Melphalan is thought to be degraded in vivo to two hydrolysis products and possibly three metabolites.

Pharmacokinetic studies were performed in beagle dogs dosed either orally or intravenously with 0.45 mg/kg (9 mg/m^2) melphalan. In dogs dosed orally 18 h after food was withheld, drug absorption was rapid, with maximum serum concentration occurring at 30 min. After intravenous administration, the parent compound was eliminated in two phases with α and β half-lives of 14 and 66 min respectively.

Elimination of metabolites from serum after either oral or intravenous administration was triphasic with half-lives ($t_{1/2}$) of 7–8 min, 2.8 h and 180 h. Urinary excretion was also triphasic, with 22% of the administered dose excreted by 4 h and 44% excreted by 11 d. By 5 d after administration, 22% of the administered dose was excreted in the feces, but only an additional 3% was excreted over the next 6 d.

Tissue distribution studies showed that half an hour after intravenous administration, the drug was principally found in liver, gallbladder, bile, kidney and urinary bladder, spleen, stomach contents and duodenal contents. At this time, approximately 11% of the administered parent compound was found in the bile. Melphalan and its metabolites or hydrolysis products were not sequestered in fat, nor did they cross the blood–brain barrier to any significant extent.

After intravenous administration of 0.63 mg/kg to dogs, the nadir of myelosuppression occurred at between 7 and 14 d. Up to 50% of animals had neutrophil counts of less than 1.5×10^9/L and platelet counts of less than 80×10^3/L.

Adverse effects

- Myelosuppression is a dose-limiting adverse effect. Cats may be more susceptible to this effect than dogs and care should be exercised when using melphalan to treat cats.
- Gastrointestinal effects may also occur (anorexia, vomiting, diarrhea).
- Pulmonary infiltrates and fibrosis have been reported in human patients but not yet in veterinary clinical practice.
- May raise serum uric acid levels.
- Melphalan should be used with caution in patients with pre-existing myelosuppression or infection, or renal dysfunction.
- Safe use during pregnancy has not been established. Gonadal function may be suppressed by melphalan.

Known drug interactions

- Melphalan is likely to augment the myelosuppressive effects of other antineoplastic agents and possibly other drugs that suppress bone marrow function, e.g. chloramphenicol, flucytosine, amphotericin B.
- As with other potent immunosuppressive drugs, live virus vaccines should be used with caution or not at all during therapy with melphalan.
- Enhanced nephrotoxicity has been reported in children treated with melphalan and cyclosporin but has not been reported in veterinary patients.

Procarbazine

Other names

Ibenzemethyzin, Natulane, Matulane, NSC 77213

Clinical applications

The primary indication for procarbazine is for treatment of lymphoma, in combination with mechlorethamine, vincristine, procarbazine and prednisolone (MOPP) (see Appendix). MOPP has been reported to be an effective rescue therapy for dogs and cats with relapsed lymphoma.

Formulations and dose rates

DOGS

- *In MOPP combination chemotherapy lymphoma rescue protocol*: 50 mg/m^2 PO q.24 h for 7–14 d every 4 weeks

CATS

- *In MOPP combination chemotherapy lymphoma rescue protocol*: 10 mg PO q.24 h for 14 d

Pharmacokinetics

Procarbazine is a nonclassic alkylating agent. It is extensively metabolized to active alkylating species in a multistep oxidative process chiefly involving the cytochrome P450 enzyme complex but also monoamine oxidase and other cytosolic enzymes. In the dog, the plasma $t_{1/2}$ is 12 min. The drug and its metabolites accumulate primarily in cerebrospinal fluid, liver, kidney, skin and intestines of animals. Metabolites are excreted chiefly in the urine. After administration of radioactively labeled procarbazine to dogs, approximately 75% of the administered radioactivity is excreted within 1 d and 90% within 4 d, the remainder being retained within the tissues. The mechanism of procarbazine cytoxicity is unknown.

Adverse effects

- Myelosuppression is dose limiting in dogs. One group observed that severe, sometimes fatal myelosuppression occurred in dogs given procarbazine 100 mg/m^2 daily and mechlorethamine 6 mg/m^2 on days 0 and 7. Dose reduction to 50 mg/m^2 and 3 mg/m^2 respectively markedly lessened the incidence of toxicity without affecting the median remission duration.
- In humans, nausea and vomiting are common for the first few doses until tolerance develops.
- CNS dysfunction (e.g. neuropathies, dizziness, somnolence, nervousness, ataxia, convulsions) is reported with varying incidences in humans.
- Various miscellaneous effects such as hypersensitivity reactions are uncommon in humans.
- Procarbazine is mutagenic, carcinogenic and teratogenic and is likely to cause irreversible inhibition of spermatogenesis, testicular atrophy and sterility.

Contraindications and precautions

Procarbazine should be used cautiously in patients with myelosuppression.

Known drug interactions

Various food and drug interactions may occur in humans (e.g. with alcohol, tricyclic antidepressants, sympathomimetics, tyramine-rich foods such as cheese or bananas, and CNS depressants). The clinical significance of these, especially in veterinary patients, is probably low.

Streptozocin

Other names

Streptozotocin, Zanosar

Clinical applications

Streptozocin may play a role in managing insulinoma in dogs with bulky, nonresectable tumors, metastatic disease, tumor-induced hypoglycemia or paraneoplastic peripheral neuropathy. In addition to insulinoma, streptozocin has been used to treat carcinoid and some lymphoproliferative diseases in humans.

Formulations and dose rates

Intravenous 0.9% NaCl is administered at a rate of 18.3 mL/kg per h for 3 h prior to administration of streptozocin. The streptozocin dose is 500 mg/m^2 administered in 0.9% NaCl at a rate of 18.3 mL/kg per h over 2 h. This is followed by 2 additional h of 18.3 mL/kg of 0.9% NaCl.

Pharmacokinetics

Streptozocin is a methylnitrosourea alkylating agent. Following IV administration, unchanged streptozotocin is rapidly cleared from the plasma. Metabolites persist in the plasma for up to 40 h and cross the blood–brain barrier. Streptozocin is directly toxic to pancreatic β-cells.

Adverse effects

- Proximal renal tubular necrosis resulting in renal failure occurs if adequate fluid support is not administered concurrently. (See Formulations and dose rates above.)
- Nausea and vomiting may be severe, but are uncommon. An ideal antiemetic protocol has not been described. Butorphanol (0.4 mg/kg IM, immediately following streptozocin administration) has been used with limited success.
- Increases in hepatic enzyme activities have been described.
- Hematological toxicity is rare and mild.

Contraindications and precautions

General contraindications include existing bone marrow, hepatic or renal dysfunction.

Known drug interactions

Streptozotocin destroys pancreatic β-cells and decreases insulin production. Glucose concentrations should be closely monitored in dogs receiving other diabetogenic agents.

Thiotepa

Other names

Thiophosphoramide, TESPA, TSPA

Clinical applications

Thiotepa is indicated for the treatment of superficial carcinoma of the bladder through intravesical administration and for control of malignant body cavity effusions through intracavitary administration. Its use in these situations has been reported in veterinary texts for some years, but reports in peer-reviewed journals are still lacking.

A high-dose regimen of thiotepa in combination with other drugs is indicated in the treatment of a variety of carcinomas and sarcomas in humans, in conjunction with bone marrow transplantation.

Formulations and dose rates

Solutions reconstituted in water are reported to be stable for 28 days at 2–8°C. Appearance of a precipitate in the solution indicates that thiotepa has polymerized; such solutions should be discarded.

- The dose rate for thiotepa in animals is uncertain. The human dose for intravesical administration is 30–60 mg in 40–50 mL water instilled into the bladder for 1 h, repeated weekly for 3–6 weeks
- A suitable canine dose is said to be 30 mg/m^2 in 30 mL water or 0.9% sodium chloride using the same time schedule as above
- Intracavitary dose rates of 25–30 mg/m^2 in 50–100 mL water, repeated as tolerated by blood leukocyte counts, are used in humans; this use is not well documented in dogs or cats

Pharmacokinetics

Thiotepa belongs to the aziridine group of alkylating agents. It is rapidly absorbed from administration sites, distributed systemically and metabolized by the hepatic cytochrome P450 enzyme complex to the polyfunctional alkylating agent, TEPA. Metabolites and unaltered drug are excreted in urine. Less than 1% of a systemically administered or intracavitary dose is recovered as unaltered drug in urine. Thiotepa's hydrophobicity and low molecular weight contribute to its rapid absorption across bladder epithelium and its consequent ability to cause systemic effects from this administration route.

Adverse effects

- Dose-limiting toxicity is myelosuppression, which may occur after intravesical administration. Nadir counts occur 1–2 weeks after administration to humans, with recovery usual by 4 weeks.
- A wide variety of other effects has been noted in humans. All are uncommon, except for amenorrhea and azoospermia.
- Thiotepa is teratogenic and carcinogenic in rats and mice and has been implicated in the development of secondary cancers in humans.
- General contraindications include existing bone marrow, hepatic or renal dysfunction.

Known drug interactions

- Thiotepa is unstable in acid urine, with $T_{90\%}$ of 3.3 min in urine pH 4 at 37°C.
- In general, thiotepa should not be given in conjunction with other alkylating agents, myelosuppressive agents or radiation therapy, as this may intensify the toxicities rather than enhance therapeutic response.
- Thiotepa is incompatible in solutions with mitoxantrone (mitozantrone).

ANTHRACYCLINE ANTIBIOTICS

The two most commonly used anthracyclines in veterinary patients are doxorubicin and mitoxantrone (mitozantrone). They are anticancer agents with a broad spectrum of activity, although mitoxantrone has a narrower spectrum of activity than doxorubicin. Doxorubicin and actinomycin D are derived from *Streptomyces* spp. Mitoxantrone, idarubicin and epirubicin are synthetic anthracycline analogs.

The vibrant color of these drugs results from their similar chemical structure. Idarubicin and epirubicin are drugs with a similar mechanism of action that have been used in veterinary clinical trials but are not commonly used in daily oncology practice.

Doxorubicin

Other names

Hydroxyl daunorubicin, NSC-123127, Adriamycin

Clinical applications

Doxorubicin is effective in controlling a wide variety of canine and feline tumors (Table 15.2). Lymphoma is especially sensitive to doxorubicin and the prognosis improves if the multiagent protocol includes doxorubicin.

Mechanism of action

Doxorubicin is a cell cycle-nonspecific drug but is most active in the S phase. The physical structure of doxorubicin allows it to intercalate into the DNA double helix, but the anticancer activity of the drug is believed to result from induction of free radical formation and from topoisomerase II-dependent DNA cleavage.

Mechanism of drug resistance

Because doxorubicin is a natural anticancer agent, resistance occurs via increased drug efflux mediated by P-gp or MRP. Tumor cells may also become resistant to doxorubicin by decreasing the activity of the target enzyme topoisomerase II. Increased glutathione activity in tumor cells will reduce organic peroxides to less toxic alcohols and decrease the effect of doxorubicin.

Formulations and dose rates

Doxorubicin must be given intravenously through a catheter to prevent extravasation. Storage of the readily dissolvable formulation is possible for 1 month at 4°C with retention of 98.5% potency. Doxorubicin solution can also be frozen – a 2 mg/mL solution stored at –20°C lost no potency after 30 d.

Table 15.2 Common tumors treated with doxorubicin

Tumor type	Protocol	Species	Median survival	Reference
Lymphoma	Single agent	Dog	230 days	Carter RF, Harris CK, Withrow SJ et al 1987 Chemotherapy of canine lymphoma with histopathological correlation: doxorubicin alone compared to COP as first treatment regimen. J Am Anim Hosp Assoc 23: 587-596
Lymphoma	Multiagent	Cat	6–9 months	Vail DM, Moore AS, Ogilvie GK et al 1998 Feline lymphoma (145 cases): proliferation indices, cluster of differentiation 3 immunoreactivity and their association with prognosis in 90 cats. J Vet Intern Med 2: 349-354
Lymphoma	Multiagent	Dog	9–12 months	Garrett LD, Thamm DH, Chun R et al 2002 Evaluation of a 6 month chemotherapy protocol with no maintenance therapy for dogs with lymphoma. J Vet Intern Med 16: 704-709
Osteosarcoma	Single agent following amputation	Dog	10–12 months	Berg J, Weinstein MJ, Springfield DS et al 1995 Results of surgery and doxorubicin chemotherapy in dogs with osteosarcoma. JAVMA 206: 1555-1560
Osteosarcoma	With platinum compound following amputation	Dog	10–12 months	Mauldin GN, Matus RE, Withrow SJ et al 1988 Canine osteosarcoma. Treatment by amputation versus amputation and adjuvant chemotherapy using doxorubicin and cisplatin. J Vet Intern Med 2: 177-180
Hemangiosarcoma	VAC protocol Vincristine, doxorubicin, cyclophosphamide	Dog	172 days	Hammer AS, Cuoto GC, Filppi J et al 1991 Efficacy and toxicity of VAC chemotherapy (vincristine, doxorubicin and cyclophosphamide) in dogs with hemangiosarcoma. J Vet Intern Med 5: 160-166
Hemangiosarcoma	With cyclophosph-amide following tumor excision	Dog	202 days	Sorenmo KU, Jeglum KA, Helfand SC 1993 Chemotherapy of canine hemangiosarcoma with doxorubicin and cyclophosphamide. J Vet Intern Med 7: 370-373
Hemangiosarcoma	Single agent following tumor excision	Dog	172 days	Ogilvie GK, Powers BE, Mallinckrodt CH et al 1996 Surgery and doxorubicin in dogs with hemangiosarcoma. J Vet Intern Med 10: 379-384
Vaccine-associated sarcoma	Single agent	Cat	Preliminary results indicate response	Poirier VJ, Thamm DH, Kurzman ID et al 2002 Liposome encapsulated doxorubicin (Doxil) and doxorubicin in the treatment of vaccine-associated sarcoma in cats. J Vet Intern Med 16: 726-731

In the USA, doxorubicin is available in a pegylated (stealth) liposome, Doxil® (Sequus Pharmaceuticals, Menlo Park, CA). Although this formulation of the drug is expensive, it has been shown to decrease cardiotoxicity, prolong drug circulation times and subsequent antitumor activity. The current recommended dosage of this product is 1.0 mg/kg intravenously every 3 weeks.

DOGS

- 30 mg/m^2, to a total cumulative dosage not greater than 240 mg/m^2
- The cumulative dosage is limited by development of dilated cardiomyopathy
- The meter-squared calculation has been shown to overdose small dogs (<10 kg), causing greater peak plasma concentrations, greater doxorubicin plasma area under the curve and longer $t_{1/2}$ than in dogs over 10 kg. In dogs less than 10 kg the recommended dosage is 1 mg/kg

CATS

- The optimal dose has not been determined
- Doses ranging from 20–30 mg/m^2 and 1 mg/kg have been recommended
- Because cats are relatively resistant to developing doxorubicin-induced cardiomyopathy, no cumulative dose recommendation has been made

FERRETS

- 20 mg/m^2 IV q.21 days
- 2.8 mg/kg IV q.21 days

Pharmacokinetics

Rate of administration of doxorubicin is important as the drug's toxic effects are related to its peak concentration. Rapid intravenous bolus will result in higher peak concentrations; consequently, it is typically recommended to dilute the drug in 0.9% sodium chloride and infuse over 30–60 min or to inject the solution into the side port of a fast-running IV saline drip over 30–60 min to minimize toxic side effects. Slower infusion rates also result in a greater area under the curve and a longer distribution phase than a faster infusion rate. Drug clearance is positively correlated with infusion rate. Doxorubicin is metabolized in the liver and excreted in the bile. In the dog, only 3% of the drug is excreted in the urine.

Adverse effects

- The most common signs of doxorubicin toxicosis in both the dog and cat are gastrointestinal – vomiting, diarrhea, colitis, anorexia and weight loss. These usually occur 3–5 d following treatment.
- Administration of doxorubicin has been shown to cause a dose-related increase of peripheral tissue histamine release and a secondary increase in catecholamine release. Clinical signs attributed to histamine release are pruritus, head shaking, urticaria, erythema and vomiting. Some oncologists recommend premedication with diphenhydramine in dogs or short-acting glucocorticoids in cats. These effects have been reported to be more frequent when a generic formulation of the drug is used.
- Clinically significant myelosuppression is uncommon in dogs given a standard dose of doxorubicin as a single agent. Dogs receiving doxorubicin in a multidrug protocol may experience severe myelosuppression. The nadir of neutropenia occurs 7–10 d post-treatment. In cats the nadir of neutropenia occurs between days 8 and 11 after treatment. RBC poikilocytosis occurs in cats following administration of doxorubicin but is clinically insignificant and not associated with anemia.
- Alopecia and hyperpigmentation of the skin occur in some dog breeds, especially poodles, old English sheepdogs and terriers. Dogs with long hair on the tail or legs (e.g. golden retrievers) lose the long hairs but not the entire coat. Cats receiving doxorubicin lose whiskers but loss of the entire hair coat is rare. These consequences of doxorubicin administration are insignificant to the patient but can be significant to the owners and should be discussed prior to drug administration.
- Doxorubicin-induced cardiomyopathy limits the total cumulative dose that can be administered in the dog (<240 mg/m^2). It typically occurs within 6–9 months following drug administration and in 3–18% of dogs receiving the drug. Clinical signs include: decreased amplitude of the R-wave, prolongation of the QRS complex, arrhythmias, conduction disturbances and overt congestive heart failure. The severity of the arrhythmia does not correlate with histopathological abnormalities. Decreased fractional shortening can be seen in dogs developing doxorubicin cardiomyopathy, but similar to ECG changes, the echocardiogram changes are not specific for doxorubicin cardiomyopathy. Histopathological evaluation of the myocardium demonstrates myocardial fiber degeneration, fibrosis and vacuolations. Elevations in cardiac troponins are currently being evaluated as potential markers of myocardial damage in dogs undergoing doxorubicin therapy.
- Dexrazoxane (ICRF-187, Zinecard®) has been shown to reduce or minimize doxorubicin-induced cardiotoxicity in dogs. It is administered at 10 times the doxorubicin dose by slow intravenous push, 30 min prior to commencing the doxorubicin infusion.
- Cats appear to be more resistant to the cardiotoxic effects of doxorubicin. However, echocardiographic changes consistent with doxorubicin cardiotoxicity have been demonstrated in normal cats chronically administered doxorubicin (cumulative dose 170–240 mg/m^2). Left ventricular internal dimension at end diastole and end systole increased significantly over time. Histopathological changes seen on examination of myocardium were similar to those in dogs. No clinical signs of congestive heart failure were seen.
- Mild renal insufficiency has been demonstrated in normal cats receiving doxorubicin. Increasing blood urea concentrations and decreasing urine specific gravity parallel a decrease in creatinine clearance. Histopathological changes consist of moderately thickened mesangial matrix, tubule lining cell necrosis and tubular regeneration in the inner cortex. Cause and effect have not been conclusively demonstrated.
- Perivascular administration of doxorubicin is a serious problem. Extravasation causes a severe perivascular slough that can lead to amputation of the affected limb. Initially no reaction will be evident but 5–7 d after administration, lameness may occur. The limb becomes progressively more swollen and eventually ulcerates. The ulcers enlarge insidiously, requiring debridement, multiple bandage changes and skin grafting. If extravasation is suspected, the infusion should be immediately discontinued but the infusion catheter left in place and an attempt made to aspirate fluid from the site to decrease the remaining drug. The area should be treated with topical ice for 15 min q.6 h to try and confine the extravasated drug locally. The use of dexrazoxane at a dosage of 400–600 mg/m^2 administered intravenously as soon as possible after extravasation has anecdotally been reported to decrease the sloughing associated with

doxorubicin. Dexrazoxane can be repeated 24 and 48 h following extravasation. It has been combined with topical ice and topical DMSO. Doxorubicin has been shown to have a detrimental effect on wound healing and this may contribute to the severity of the soft tissue reaction.
- Adverse reactions may occur with the pegylated liposome form of doxorubicin. In the dog, it causes a palmar-plantar erythrodysesthesia syndrome, which is diminished by the concurrent administration of pyridoxine. Clinically, dogs have erythema, scaling, crusting, alopecia and ulceration in addition to edema of the limb. Severe cases exhibit pruritus and pain. Cats have a milder form of the syndrome, with chin alopecia and occasional hair loss on the plantar surface of their paws but no ulcerations or pruritus.
- 'Radiation recall' is a phenomenon in which there is reactivation of latent radiation effects in a previously irradiated field induced by doxorubicin administration. It can occur with doxorubicin administered up to two decades following radiation therapy. This phenomenon has not been reported in veterinary patients, although it is believed to occur.

Known drug interactions

Heparin binds to and increases the clearance of doxorubicin; therefore, intravenous lines to be used with doxorubicin should be flushed only with saline to avoid this interaction.

Mitoxantrone (mitozantrone)

Other names

Dihydroxyanthracenedione, 1,4-dihydroxy-5,8-bis((2-((2-hydroxyethyl)-amino)-ethyl) amino) 9,10-anthracededione dihydrochloride, mitoxantrone hydrochloride

Clinical applications

In a phase I/II dose escalation study of mitoxantrone (mitozantrone) in dogs, an overall response rate of 18% was noted, with a response rate of 27% and 12% respectively in dogs and cats with lymphoma. In dogs with relapsed lymphoma, treated at a dosage of 6 mg/m^2, a 47% complete response rate has been reported. Some responses have been seen when mitoxantrone is used to treat sarcomas and carcinomas. Mitoxantrone may be combined with radiation therapy for the palliative management of oral squamous cell carcinoma in the cat (median survival 170 d).

Mechanism of action

Mitoxantrone binds to and inhibits nucleic acid synthesis. Cellular damage results from topoisomerase II-dependent DNA cleavage and is not cell cycle specific. The reduced capacity for mitoxantrone generation of free radicals is believed to result in decrease in cardiotoxicity compared to doxorubicin.

Mechanism of resistance

Decreased intracellular drug accumulation is possibly mediated by P-gp.

Formulations and dose rates

Mitoxantrone's usefulness is limited by its high cost and short storage time. The manufacturer recommends that unused drug should be discarded within 7 d of opening the vial and the package insert does not recommend freezing of the drug to prolong its shelf-life. However, in vitro cytotoxicity assays indicate no loss of cytotoxicity after four freeze–thaw cycles over 90 d, suggesting that unused drug may be frozen without loss of potency.

DOGS AND CATS
- 5–6 mg/m^2 at a 21-d interval when used as a single agent

CATS
- 5–6.5 mg/m^2 at a 21-d interval when used as a single agent

Pharmacokinetics

Mitoxantrone is poorly absorbed orally but rapidly absorbed if administered intraperitoneally. The drug is rapidly distributed, achieving high levels in erythrocytes, leukocytes and platelets and in tissues with high blood flow (liver, spleen and heart). However, it is slowly eliminated from these tissues. Mitoxantrone does not cross the blood–brain barrier. It is 78% protein bound, but other drugs do not influence binding. It is metabolized to the mono- and dicarboxylic acid derivatives and glucuronide conjugates of these acids. Dogs eliminate mitoxantrone and its metabolites slowly by both renal and biliary excretion, with the bilary route predominating.

Adverse effects

- Dogs experiencing toxicity after the first treatment with mitoxantrone may be more likely to show toxicosis with subsequent treatments than dogs without toxicity after the first treatment.
- Gastrointestinal toxicity is the most common adverse effect in dogs, with 15–30% of dogs experiencing mild, self-limiting vomiting, diarrhea, colitis or anorexia.
- Sepsis secondary to myelosuppression occurs in 6% of dogs treated.
- The nadir of leukopenia occurs 10 d following administration in dogs.

- Cardiotoxicity has not been reported in dogs treated with mitoxantrone and it does not seem to worsen mild doxorubicin-induced cardiotoxicity.
- Cats treated with mitoxantrone may experience gastrointestinal toxicity. Fewer than 20% of cats demonstrated vomiting, diarrhea or anorexia.
- Myelosuppression leading to sepsis occurs in approximately 10% of cats. The nadir of neutropenia in cats is not known.

Known drug interactions

Heparin binds to anthracyclines; therefore, intravenous lines to be used with mitoxantrone should be flushed with saline only to avoid this interaction.

Idarubicin and epirubicin

Mechanism of action

Idarubicin and epirubicin are doxorubicin analogs that induce DNA strand breakage via topoisomerase II- or free radical-mediated damage.

Mechanism of drug resistance

Drug resistance is mediated by P-gp and mutations in topoisomerase II.

Formulations and dose rates

Epirubicin is currently not available in the USA, although it is available elsewhere. Idarubicin is available in the injectable form only. See Table 15.3 for dose rates.

Pharmacokinetics

Unlike other anthracyclines, idarubicin has high oral bioavailability and can achieve therapeutic levels with oral administration. The LD_{50} of epirubicin in dogs is 2 mg/kg or 38 mg/m^2. In dogs, 90–95% of epirubicin is excreted in urine 4 h after administration. This differs from elimination in humans in whom epirubicin and its major metabolites are eliminated through biliary excretion and, to a lesser extent, by urinary excretion. Dogs may lack an enzyme required for glucuronidation of epirubicin, accounting for this difference in metabolism.

Adverse effects

- The most common adverse effect of idarubicin is anorexia, which occurs in 20% of cats.
- Leukopenia and vomiting are less common, but do occur.
- Epirubicin causes myelosuppression in dogs and the nadir of leukopenia occurs 6–10 d following administration.
- Cardiotoxicity of epirubicin in dogs may be less than that of doxorubicin.

Known drug interactions

No drug interactions have been identified for either epirubicin or idarubicin in dogs and cats but in people, cimetidine has been shown to decrease clearance of epirubicin.

Contraindications and precautions

Co-administration of cimetidine (400 mg twice daily for 7 d starting 5 d before chemotherapy) increased the mean AUC of epirubicin (100 mg/m^2) by 50% and decreased its plasma clearance by 30% in humans.

OTHER ANTITUMOUR ANTIBIOTICS

Plicamycin, actinomycin D and bleomycin are antitumor antibiotics isolated from *Streptomyces* spp. They are used infrequently in veterinary patients but may be useful in certain specific situations.

Plicamycin

Other names

Mithramycin, NSC-24559, aureolic acid

Clinical applications

Historically, plicamycin was used as an antihypercalcemic agent in cases of malignancy or rodenticide-induced hypercalcemia where hypercalcemia is refractory to

Table 15.3 Epirubicin and idarubicin

	Idarubicin	**Epirubicin**
Species	Cat	Dog
Dosage	2 mg/d for 3 d every 3 weeks	30 mg/m^2 every 21 d
Route of administration	Oral	Intravenous
Clinical application	Maintenance of remission in feline lymphoma Substitute for doxorubicin in lymphoma protocol	Single agent therapy of lymphoma Substitute for doxorubicin in lymphoma protocol

management with saline diuresis, furosemide, salmon calcitonin, prednisolone (prednisone) and appropriate chemotherapy. This use is now superceded by the bisphosphonate group of drugs. Plicamycin is not an effective antitumor drug.

Mechanism of action

Plicamycin binds to guanine-cytosine-rich regions of DNA. Inhibition of DNA-directed RNA synthesis appears to be the principal antitumor biochemical effect of plicamycin. The antihypercalcemic effect results from a decrease in osteoclast formation and inhibition of bone resorption. There is also an increase in the fractional excretion of calcium in the urine following plicamycin administration.

Mechanism of resistance

Although poorly studied, development of the multidrug resistance phenotype appears to confer drug resistance.

Formulations and dose rates

Prior to reconsititution, plicamycin should be stored at 2–8°C. The unused portion should be discarded immediately.

DOGS

- Typically prehydrated with 0.9% saline as part of the management of hypercalcemia
- The dose of plicamycin recommended is 25 µg/kg IV diluted in 250 mL of 0.9% saline and given over 1–4 h
- Serum calcium typically normalizes in 24–48 h, but it does not improve in all dogs. The decrease in serum calcium lasts 24–72 h
- Repeat dosing has been described in normal dogs but not in hypercalcemic dogs
- Multiple doses are used in humans at 4–7 d intervals to control hypercalcemia

CATS

- The effect of plicamycin in cats is unknown

Pharmacokinetics

Information on pharmacokinetic parameters of plicamycin in both humans and animals is unavailable. In humans, 40% of the drug is excreted in the urine 15 h following administration.

Adverse effects

- Dogs receiving plicamycin exhibit shivering, shaking and pain at the infusion site during infusion. Pyrexia can also occur.
- The recommended dose of plicamycin (25 µg/kg) causes mild gastrointestinal side effects in 33% of dogs and reduction of platelet count in a similar number of dogs.
- High-dose plicamycin (100 µg/kg) has been shown to cause fatal hepatocellular necrosis within 24 h of administration in dogs with malignancy but not normal dogs.
- In human cancer patients, repeat doses of plicamycin cause hypocalcemia, hypokalemia, thrombocytopenia, platelet dysfunction, proteinuria, azotemia and increased serum hepatic transaminase activity.

Known drug interactions

There are no known drug interactions.

Actinomycin D

Other names

NSC-3053, dactinomycin, actinomycin C_1, ACT-D, DACT

Clinical applications

Use of actinomycin D as a single agent or in combination protocols has been described in dogs with lymphoma. Results are highly variable, with response rates ranging from 0% to 83%. In a combination chemotherapy protocol, actinomycin D was less effective and resulted in a shorter median survival time than the same protocol with doxorubicin (median survival 309 d with doxorubicin versus 152 d for actinomycin). Actinomycin is a component of the DMAC protocol used for rescue therapy for dogs with relapsed lymphoma. (See Appendix.)

Mechanism of action

The most important biochemical effects of actinomycin D are binding to single- and double-stranded DNA and subsequent inhibition of RNA and protein synthesis. This effect is primarily cell cycle nonspecific, although maximum cell kill occurs in G_1.

Mechanisms of resistance

Decreased drug uptake through the plasma membrane and development of the multidrug resistance phenotype are proposed mechanisms of actinomycin D resistance.

Formulations and dose rates

Following reconstitution, actinomycin is stable for 2–5 months at room temperature but should be discarded after 24 h to prevent bacterial contamination.

DOGS

- 0.5–0.75 mg/m^2 q.21 days or as indicated in a multidrug protocol
- Actinomycin D is given as a slow intravenous bolus

Pharmacokinetics
The half-life of actinomycin D is 47 h in the dog. The drug distribution phase is estimated to be 3 h. There is rapid tissue uptake and excretion is via the biliary and urinary tracts. Although actinomycin D has high lipid solubility, no appreciable concentration of drug is detectable in the central nervous system because of its high molecular weight.

Adverse effects
- The most common toxicity with actinomycin D is gastrointestinal. Vomiting immediately following administration or vomiting 3–5 d following administration occurs in one-third of dogs.
- Myelosuppression is uncommon and the nadir of leukopenia occurs 5–7 d after drug administration.
- Drug extravasation results in soft tissue necrosis.
- Radiation recall is theoretically possible but has not been described in veterinary patients.

Known drug interactions
There are no known drug interactions.

Bleomycin

Other names

NSC-125066, BLM[2]

Clinical applications
Use of bleomycin has been described in squamous cell carcinoma, lymphoma and other carcinomas. Its high cost and short duration of effect limit its usefulness in veterinary patients.

Mechanism of action
Damage to DNA is the major mechanism of bleomycin cytotoxicity. Bleomycin also causes lipid peroxidation and oxidative metabolism of RNA. Bleomycin has a greater effect in the M and G_2 phases of the cell cycle.

Mechanism of drug resistance
Increased bleomycin inactivation, decreased intracellular drug accumulation and increased cellular DNA repair of damage have been identified as mechanisms of bleomycin resistance.

Formulations and dose rates

After reconstitution, the drug is stable for 4 weeks at 4°C. 1 unit of bleomycin is equivalent to 1 mg.

DOGS, CATS AND FERRETS
- 10–20 U/m^2 SC or IV once a week, not to exceed 200 mg/m^2

Pharmacokinetics
In normal beagles, bleomycin exhibits biphasic plasma elimination characteristics. The elimination half-life following IV injection is 1.0 h and after IM injection 1.1 h. The volume of distribution in the central compartment after IV administration is 0.125 L/kg. Bleomycin concentrates in the skin and lung, accounting for some of the clinical toxicity and efficacy.

Adverse effects
- Chronic administration in dogs results in interstitial pneumonitis, which is a potentially fatal dose-limiting toxicity.
- Cutaneous toxicity has also been described as footpad ulceration, nail deformities, pressure point sores and alopecia. Prior chemotherapy or radiation therapy may potentiate adverse effects.
- Myelosuppression is rare and mild, as are the gastrointestinal toxicities.

Known drug interactions
No clinically significant drug interactions have been reported.

PLATINUM ANALOGS

The platinum analogs are inorganic compounds that have an antitumor activity that is cell cycle phase nonspecific. Cisplatin was the first inorganic compound used as a chemotherapeutic agent in veterinary medicine but another platinum analog, carboplatin, is rapidly replacing cisplatin in clinical use because administration is more convenient.

Cisplatin

Other names

NSC-119875, *cis*-diamminedichloroplatinum (II), DDP, CACP

Clinical applications
Cisplatin is indicated primarily for treatment of canine osteosarcoma. Its efficacy as a single drug therapy for osteosarcoma has been well documented. Despite reports suggesting improved efficacy when cisplatin is used in combination with other drugs such as doxorubicin, the optimum adjuvant chemotherapy regimen for dogs with osteosarcoma has not been determined.

Other indications, more anecdotally, include squamous cell carcinoma, ovarian carcinoma, thyroid and nasal adenocarcinoma and mesothelioma. Intracavitary cisplatin infusions have been used to manage abdominal and thoracic effusions. Initial reports suggested useful activity against canine bladder tumors but more recent reports did not strongly support this use.

Intralesional cisplatin has been reported to be an effective treatment for sarcoids and squamous cell carcinomas in horses. Cisplatin is contraindicated in cats because at clinically useful doses it causes acute death as a result of severe respiratory toxicity.

Although cisplatin is efficacious in canine osteosarcoma and some carcinomas, it is largely being abandoned in favor of carboplatin. Carboplatin has fewer side effects and is simpler to use because cumbersome diuresis protocols are not required, resulting in the added potential benefit of less exposure of humans to toxic drugs.

Mechanism of action

Cisplatin is a cell cycle phase-nonspecific drug. However, its effects are greatest in the S phase. In plasma, the high concentration of saline maintains cisplatin in the uncharged and unreactive dichloro form. When cisplatin moves intracellularly, the low chloride concentration of the intracellular fluid favors the formation of the reactive charged aquated form. The reactive cisplatin molecule covalently binds to guanine-containing base pairs of the DNA molecule and consequently disrupts DNA function by forming both intra- and interstrand cross-links.

Mechanisms of drug resistance

Three main categories of drug resistance have been described for platinum complexes. First, decreased transport across the cell membrane results in resistance due to decreased intracellular drug accumulation. Second, platinum activity can be quenched by conjugation with thiourea or other sulfhydryl-containing proteins such as glutathione. Augmented repair of platinum-induced DNA adducts may also contribute to tumor resistance.

Formulations and dose rates

Cisplatin (1 mg/mL in 0.9% sodium chloride) was reported to be stable in plastic infusion bags for up to 14 d at 25°C and 37°C. Once reconstituted, the drug should not be stored in the refrigerator as it may precipitate at 4°C. Solutions in the concentration range of 0.1–0.2 mg/mL do not precipitate and are reportedly stable for 4 days at 4°C. If bacteriostatic water is used for reconstitution, a 1 mg/mL solution is stable for 72 h at room temperature or 3 weeks when frozen. Powder for injection and the injection formulation of the drug should be stored away from light. Cisplatin is sensitive to daylight but not adversely affected by artificial room lighting.

Intravenous

- Cisplatin is administered at a dose of 60–70 mg/m^2 IV to dogs
- Intravenous administration of cisplatin requires vigorous hydration with 0.9% saline to prevent nephrotoxicosis. One protocol used successfully administers cisplatin IV over 20 min after 0.9% saline is infused IV for 3–4 h at a rate of 18.3 mL/kg bodyweight per h. After the cisplatin infusion, saline infusion was continued at the same rate for an additional 1–2 h. Additional diuretic agents such as mannitol and furosemide may be used to supplement the diuretic effect of saline
- Experimentally, intraperitoneally administered methimazole has been used to protect against nephrotoxicity in dogs not receiving saline diuresis in conjunction with cisplatin therapy

Regional delivery

- Regional delivery of cisplatin has been investigated by some and may have a therapeutic advantage in specific cases
- This has been accomplished by direct injection of the drug in a matrix or suspended in medical-grade sesame oil to obtain sustained drug release in tumors in dogs, cats and horses. Sesame oil-cisplatin emulsion is prepared by sterilizing sesame oil and emulsifying 3.3 mg of cisplatin per mL of oil. The emulsion is administered at a dose of 1 mg/cm^3 of tumor. Saline diuresis is not required with this route of administration

Biodegradable sponges

- Cisplatin in biodegradable sponges has been implanted into the surgical wound following resection of osteosarcoma or soft tissue sarcomas in dogs, with an improvement in local control in cases of osteosarcoma

Intracavity

- Intracavity administration of cisplatin for treatment of mesothelioma and carcinomatosis has been successful in some dogs. The dose was 50 mg/m^2 into the pleural or peritoneal space and hydration with saline was used to prevent nephrotoxicosis
- For intrapleural administration, cisplatin was diluted in 250 mL/m^2 0.9% sodium chloride
- For intraperitoneal delivery 1 L/m^2 was infused over 15 min through a 16G catheter

Regional perfusion

- Intra-arterial administration of cisplatin has been used in dogs with long-bone osteosarcoma prior to limb-sparing surgery

Pharmacokinetics

In dogs, cisplatin exhibits a biphasic elimination profile. The initial plasma half-life is short (20 min), but the terminal phase is very long (120 h). Some 80% of a dose can be recovered as free platinum in the urine within 48 h of dosing in dogs. The long terminal phase results from concentration of the drug in liver, intestines and kidney. Cisplatin is also highly bound to serum proteins. After intravenous administration to dogs, plasma platinum elimination is biphasic, with α- and β-phase half-lives of less than 1 h and days respectively. Over 90% of plasma platinum is protein bound and consequently inactive. Free platinum elimination is also biphasic, with both phases less than 1 h. Platinum from cisplatin is rapidly distributed to most tissues, with highest levels in the kidney, liver, ovary, uterus, skin and bone. Tissue levels decline slowly and platinum may be detected in tissues 6 months after completion of a course of therapy.

Adverse effects

- The most important dose-limiting toxicity of cisplatin in dogs is cumulative nephrotoxicity, thought to be largely irreversible. The exact mechanism of cisplatin-induced nephrotoxicity is unknown but is probably related to its tubular secretion and interactions with other renal components such as the proximal nephron segment.
- Adequate pre- and post-treatment hydration decreases the urine concentration of platinum and does not change the pharmacokinetics of the compound. Nephrotoxicity may be exacerbated by concurrent administration of nephrotoxic drugs such as gentamicin, or by pre-existing diseases affecting the kidney (Table 15.4). For patients with cardiovascular impairment, less vigorous hydration regimens could be considered, or consideration given to substituting carboplatin for cisplatin.
- Cisplatin is a potent emetic. Acute vomiting, starting within 6 h of drug administration and lasting 1–6 h, is well documented and is a frequent adverse effect of cisplatin. Delayed nausea or vomiting may persist for days after drug administration.
- Anticipatory vomiting, a well-recognized phenomenon in human patients, has been noted anecdotally for some canine patients. Although nausea and vomiting are generally self-limiting, they may exacerbate nephrotoxicity if dehydration occurs.
- Pretreatment with butorphanol and dexamethasone greatly reduces the severity of this adverse effect (see Table 15.4); there is some evidence that treatment with the newer serotonin (5-HT_3) antagonists, such as ondansetron, is more effective, although expensive. Maropitant (Cerenia®) has been shown to be an effective anti-emetic in dogs treated with cisplatin (see Chapter 19).
- Myelotoxicity is generally mild to moderate. The neutrophil nadir in dogs is bimodal (days 6 and 15).
- Ototoxicity; high-frequency hearing loss is common in human patients but of negligible clinical significance in dogs.
- Other adverse effects occasionally reported in humans, such as anaphylaxis, severe electrolyte disturbances or peripheral neuropathies, are rarely recognized in veterinary medicine.

Contraindications and precautions

- Cisplatin is contraindicated in cats because of its severe pulmonary toxicity.
- Avoid using aluminum needles for reconstitution and administration as aluminum may react with cisplatin to form a black precipitate: any solution containing precipitates should be discarded.

Known drug interactions

- Cisplatin may form complexes with mannitol if stored as a mixture for several days; mannitol should therefore only be added immediately before administration.

Table 15.4 Prevention of cisplatin toxicity

Toxicity	Mechanism	Frequency of occurrence	Intervention
Renal	Damage to loop of Henle, distal tubules and collecting ducts. Decrease in renal DNA synthesis. Persistence of DNA-cisplatin adducts in renal tissue	Most common side effect. Seen in almost all dogs	Requires saline diuresis and diuretic agents for renoprotection Avoid use of other nephrotoxic agents Do not use in animals with pre-existing renal or urinary tract disease
Vomiting	Central vomiting via stimulation of the chemoreceptor trigger zone. Also induces release of serotonin in the gastrointestinal tract causing vomiting	Common	Antiemetic agents should be given pre-emptively to all dogs receiving cisplatin Butorphanol, metoclopromide, dexamethasone and ondansetron are useful
Hypomagnesemia	Cisplatin-induced renal damage allows excessive magnesium excretion	Rare in the dog	Monitor magnesium as required
Myelosuppression	Stem cell cytotoxicity. Nadir of leukopenia 6 and 15 d following administration	Common	Supportive care as required Monitor white blood cell count at anticipated nadir and prior to subsequent chemotherapy treatments

- Cisplatin is compatible with sodium chloride 0.9%. It may be incompatible with dextrose/saline combinations, 5% dextrose in water and metoclopramide, depending on pH, concentration, temperature and diluents.
- As with other cytotoxics, the myelosuppressive effects of cisplatin may be enhanced by other myelosuppressive drugs
- Serum levels of phenytoin may be reduced following cisplatin infusion.
- Caution should be used when combining cisplatin with other nephrotoxic drugs such as aminoglycosides or amphotericin B, as they may potentiate nephrotoxicity. The combination of cisplatin and piroxicam has been reported to be tolerated in dogs treated for oral malignant melanoma and squamous cell carcinoma although renal function must be monitored carefully.

Special considerations

There is a potential occupational risk to veterinary hospital staff involved in the care of dogs hospitalized for the administration of cisplatin. Cisplatin is excreted in urine and, in dogs receiving saline diuresis and diuretics, urine production is copious. Dogs receiving cisplatin should be allowed to urinate outdoors. When the inevitable urination occurs in the hospital, personnel wearing full personal protective equipment (gloves, gowns, face protection and foot covers) should clean up with absorbent disposable towels rather than flushing the urine down a drain, which may aerosolize the drug.

Carboplatin

Other names

CBDA, JM-8

Clinical applications

Carboplatin is a less potent, less emetogenic and much less nephrotoxic analog of cisplatin. Carboplatin has a similar spectrum of activity to cisplatin. Clinical trials demonstrate that carboplatin's efficacy is close to that of cisplatin for canine osteosarcoma. However, it should be used with caution as an alternative to cisplatin for dogs with renal disease, as it may exacerbate preexisting nephropathy. Carboplatin also has demonstrated some efficacy against canine melanomas and some carcinomas. However, transitional cell carcinoma of the bladder does not appear responsive to carboplatin.

In cats, carboplatin has been used to manage head and neck carcinomas and adenocarcinomas, mammary carcinomas and vaccine-associated sarcomas. Intralesional carboplatin has been reported as an effective agent for carcinomas and sarcomas in dogs and cats.

Mechanism of action

Carboplatin is similar to cisplatin in that it disrupts DNA function by covalent binding to the DNA base pairs. It is also a cell cycle-nonspecific drug.

Mechanisms of drug resistance

Like cisplatin, decreased transport of carboplatin across the cell membrane, augmented DNA repair and quenching of platinum reactivity by sulfhydryl compounds confer drug resistance.

Formulations and dose rates

Because aquation of carboplatin occurs more quickly in a high-chloride environment than in a low-chloride environment, it was originally thought that mixing carboplatin with any solution containing chloride should be avoided. This is now an outdated recommendation, since more recent reports show that carboplatin 1 mg/mL is stable in 0.9% sodium chloride for 24 h at 25°C and 4°C and 10 mg/mL is stable for at least 5 d at 4°C. For extended storage, however, water is a satisfactory diluent and indeed, one form supplied by the manufacturer is a 10 mg/mL solution in water.

DOGS

- 300 mg/m^2 IV over 15–60 min every 3–4 weeks

CATS

- 200 mg/m^2 IV over 15–60 min every 4 weeks

Pharmacokinetics

Pharmacokinetic parameters have been determined for 300 mg/m^2 of carboplatin administered over 30 min in tumor-bearing dogs. The volume of distribution at steady state was 39.3 L/m^2. Total body clearance was 119.8 mL/min/m^2. The area under the time–concentration curves was 1.85% dose-min/mL. Half-life was 233.1 min and 47% of the administered drug was eliminated in the urine in the first 4 h following administration. Half-life, area under the curve and total body clearance were not dose dependent.

Compared with cisplatin, the rate of aquation to the active form is slower, causing differences in the pharmacokinetic disposition and toxicity profile of the two drugs. One of the major degradation products is cisplatin. After intravenous administration of carboplatin to dogs, the plasma platinum elimination is biphasic, with α and β half-lives slightly longer than cisplatin.

Carboplatin does not bind to plasma proteins as extensively as cisplatin and remains in the plasma as free drug longer than cisplatin. Tissue distribution is similar to cisplatin. The major route of excretion is by glomerular filtration alone, with approximately 70% of an administered dose excreted in the urine within 4 d. Tissue levels decline slowly, similarly to cisplatin.

Adverse effects

- The dose-limiting toxicity of carboplatin is myelosuppression, occurring at different times in cats and dogs. In dogs, at a dose rate of 300 mg/m^2, neutropenia and thrombocytopenia occur with a nadir of 14 d. At this dose rate, the probability of a neutrophil count below 2×10^9 cells/L or a platelet count of less than 800×10^9 cells/L is approximately 10% or 20% for the first and second doses respectively. In normal cats, the neutrophil nadir occurs at approximately 17 d after doses between 150 and 210 mg/m^2 with neutropenia lasting from day 14 to day 25 post carboplatin administration. The platelet nadir may occur sooner at day 14. In tumor-bearing cats, the amount of carboplatin administered based on body surface area does not correlate with the severity of hematopoietic suppression. Area under the curve does correlate with severity of neutropenia and depends in part on glomerular filtration rate.
- Anorexia and emesis may occur for several days after treatment in dogs and cats, but are generally mild.
- Nephrotoxicity is generally not of veterinary clinical significance but has been reported in humans. Carboplatin may exacerbate pre-existing nephropathy and patients with renal dysfunction should be treated cautiously. No formula for dose reduction in the dog or cat has been developed but in humans the dose is decreased proportionately to the creatinine clearance.
- Hepatotoxicity is reported in about 15% of humans treated with carboplatin; neuropathies and ototoxicity are reported far less commonly than with cisplatin.
- Vascular access to previous carboplatin administration sites, especially where the drug was given as slow bolus IV injection, can be difficult, possibly because of thrombophlebitis caused by the previous drug dose. This may be avoided by diluting the drug prior to administration.
- Carboplatin is a mild irritant if extravasated.

Known drug interactions

- As with other cytotoxics, the myelosuppressive effects of carboplatin may be enhanced by other myelosuppressive drugs.
- The risk of developing ototoxicity or neurotoxicity is increased in humans previously treated with cisplatin.
- The immune response to vaccination may be modified if vaccines are administered to patients undergoing carboplatin therapy.

Contraindications and precautions

Aluminum can form a black precipitate with the platinum from carboplatin; hence the solution should not be administered through equipment made of aluminum. Solutions containing black precipitate should be discarded.

ANTIMETABOLITES

Antimetabolites are successful anticancer drugs because they interfere with DNA synthesis by competing with normal nucleotide for incorporation into the DNA molecule or inhibit enzymes responsible for synthesis of nucleotides. By definition, all antimetabolites exhibit their antineoplastic effect in the S phase of the cell cycle and are cell cycle phase-specific drugs. Duration of exposure of cancer cells to antimetabolites determines their toxicity.

Cytosine arabinoside

Other names

ARA-C, cytarabine, NSC-63878

Clinical applications

Cytosine arabinoside is used in veterinary practice as a component of multi-agent protocols for treatment of leukemia, either lymphoid or nonlymphoid, and lymphoma. Because it crosses the blood–brain barrier, cytosine arabinoside is useful for treatment and prevention of central nervous system lymphoma. It has been incorporated into some renal lymphoma protocols.

Mechanism of action

Cytosine arabinoside is a pyrimidine nucleoside antimetabolite. Intracellularly it is converted into cytarabine triphosphate, which competes with deoxycytidine triphosphate and inhibits DNA polymerase with resulting inhibition of DNA synthesis. It is a cell cycle-specific agent acting in the S phase.

Mechanism of drug resistance

The most frequent cellular abnormality leading to resistance is decreased activity of deoxycytidine kinase, the activation enzyme of cytosine arabinoside. Increased cytidine deaminase, the cytosine arabinoside degradation enzyme, decreased nucleoside transport sites and decreased intracellular deoxycytidine triphosphate pools have also been identified in resistant tumor cells. Normal dogs have low tissue levels of cytidine deaminase.

Pharmacokinetics

In the dog, cytosine arabinoside can be administered intravenously, intramuscularly or subcutaneously with no differences in pharmacological disposition. The plasma decay curve is biphasic, with calculated half-lives of 40 min and 2–2.5 h. By 5 h following administration, no more than 3% of the drug has been excreted and after 12 h only 10% is excreted. After 24 h, 40% of the drug was found in the urine and 35% in the feces. The drug is poorly absorbed orally and consequently is not administered orally.

Formulations and dose rates

As mentioned previously, duration of exposure of cancer cells to antimetabolites determines their toxicity. The longer the exposure of cancer cells to cytosine arabinoside, the greater number of cells likely to enter the S phase of the cell cycle, where the drug exerts its cytotoxic effect. Consequently, tumor kill will be greater if an equivalent dose is given as an infusion or multiple treatments rather than as a single dose. The toxicity will also be greater with multiple doses or infusion.

DOGS AND CATS

- Cytosine arabinoside can be administered either intravenously as a bolus or as a continuous rate infusion or subcutaneously
- Doses vary depending on the protocol, but up to 600 mg/m^2 can be given as a single dose or divided over 2–4 days

CATS

- *Feline acute lymphoid leukemia*: 10 mg/m^2 SC daily

Adverse effects

- Myelosuppression is the major adverse effect of cytosine arabinoside. It is both dose and schedule dependent. The nadir of leukopenia occurs 5–7 d following administration, with recovery at 7–14 days.
- Gastrointestinal toxicity, anorexia, nausea, vomiting and diarrhea have been reported to occur but are mild to moderate in severity and rarely require hospitalization.
- Rarely reported are hepatotoxicity, conjunctivitis, oral ulceration and fever.

Known drug interactions

Cytosine arabinoside may antagonize the anti-infective effect of gentamicin and flucytosine.

5-Fluorouracil

Other names

5-FU, fluorouracil, NSC-19893

Clinical applications

5-Fluorouracil is rarely used in the dog and is not recommended for use in cats due to neurotoxicity in this species. In humans, 5-fluorouracil with leucovorin rescue is a mainstay in the treatment of colon cancer. Basal cell carcinoma is treated with topical 5-fluorouracil. Treatment regimens for human pancreatic, breast and gastric carcinoma may include 5-fluorouracil. Two case reports of dogs with gastrointestinal adenocarcinoma showed clinical benefit from a treatment protocol containing 5-fluorouracil and cisplatin.

Mechanism of action

5-Fluorouracil is a fluorinated pyrimidine. This drug has two primary mechanisms of action capable of inducing cytotoxicity. First, 5-fluorouracil is phosphorylated to fluorouridine triphosphate, a fraudulent nucleotide, which is incorporated into RNA by RNA polymerase, inhibiting RNA synthesis and function. Fluorodeoxyuridine monophosphate inhibits thymidylate synthetase, depleting intracellular levels of thymidine monophosphate and thymidine triphosphate, which are essential for DNA synthesis.

Mechanism of drug resistance

Because 5-fluorouracil metabolism is intricate, mechanisms of drug resistance are complex. Changes in enzyme activity involved in 5-fluorouracil activation or degradation, the presence of salvage pathways that circumvent normal pyrimidine metabolism and inadequate intracellular pools of reduced folates all contribute to 5-fluorouracil resistance.

Formulations and dose rates

DOGS

- 5 mg/kg IV and 150–200 mg/m^2 IV weekly have been used safely
- Regional administration of 5-fluorouracil in a gel matrix has proved to be effective for the control of canine solar-induced squamous cell carcinoma

CATS

- Neurotoxicity prevents the use of intravenous or topical 5-fluorouracil in the cat

Pharmacokinetics

Some 21% of 5-fluorouracil is protein bound in normal dogs. The majority of 5-fluorouracil is metabolized to fluorodeoxyridine monophosphate in the liver or intestinal mucosa by dihydrouracil dehydrogenase. Unmetabolized drug attains high concentrations in the bone marrow. First half-life following a 10 mg/kg bolus of 5-fluorouracil was 3.4 min, terminal half-life was 23.5 min and volume of distribution 1.9 L/kg. In another normal dog study, pharmacokinetic analysis of a 30 mg/kg bolus injection of 5-fluorouracil resulted in a first-order elimination of drug from all compartments. The best-fit plasma level time area under the curve was 4024 g/mLxmin.

A proposed model of pharmacokinetics included flow-dependent clearance of 5-fluorouracil by the liver and linear elimination via the kidney. Total plasma clearance of 5-fluorouracil exceeds cardiac output and, consequently, extrahepatic pathways of disposition must be present to account for this phenomenon. Dose-dependent pulmonary extraction and clearance of 5-flourouracil has been demonstrated in the dog. As the dose of 5-fluorouracil increases, the percentage of drug cleared by the lung decreases. 5-Fluorouracil enters CSF and attains concentrations similar to plasma levels.

Adverse effects

- Some of the best information on 5-fluorouracil toxicity comes from cases of accidental ingestion in dogs. Accidental ingestion of 5-fluorouracil occurs in dogs exposed to their owner's topical 5-fluorouracil preparation. Exposure to more than 43 mg/kg resulted in death in all dogs exposed. Clinical signs of toxicosis occurred within 1 h of ingestion and included seizures, vomiting, tremors, respiratory distress, hypersalivation, diarrhea, depression, ataxia and cardiac arrhythmias.
- Temporary hair loss may occur in dogs receiving a nonlethal dose of 5-fluorouracil.
- Similar clinical signs as described above may occur when topical 5-fluorouracil is applied to dogs for the treatment of skin tumors.

Known drug interactions

Concurrent administration of cimetidine or α-interferon may decrease 5-fluorouracil clearance.

Gemcitabine

Other names

Gemzar, 2′- 2′-difluorodeoxycytidine, dFdC

Clinical applications

Only limited clinical response has been observed in dogs with lymphoma, oral melanoma, hepatocellular carcinoma and perianal squamous cell carcinoma.

Mechanism of action

Gemcitabine is a difluorinated pyrimidine analog of deoxycytidine. Once the drug enters the cell via facilitated nucleoside transport, it is metabolized to the active nucleoside form. During DNA synthesis the active metabolites are incorporated into the DNA molecule and ultimately block subsequent DNA replication.

Formulations and dose rates

DOGS

- 675 mg/m^2 IV q.2 weeks diluted in 10 mL/kg 0.9% NaCl and given over 30 min

CATS

- 250 mg/m^2 IV (preliminary information)

Pharmacokinetics

Dogs metabolize gemcitabine by a two-compartment model. The drug is deaminated and cleared through the kidneys. There is minimal protein binding. Half-life is 1.38 h. Approximately 76–86% of the dose is detected as metabolites in the urine 24 h after administration.

Adverse effects

- Rare and mild hematological toxicity.
- Mild gastrointestinal toxicity.

Known drug interactions

Use of low-dose (25–50 mg/m^2) gemcitabine twice weekly as a radiation sensitizer resulted in unacceptable hematological and local tissue toxicity.

Methotrexate

Other names

NSC-740, amethopterin, sodium methotrexate

Clinical applications

Methotrexate is a component of multidrug protocols for the treatment of canine and feline lymphoma and some soft tissue sarcomas. Its efficacy as a single agent in these neoplasms has not been demonstrated. It has also been used in the management of sclerosing cholangitis in cats.

Mechanism of action

Inhibition of dihydrofolate reductase by methotrexate leads to depletion of reduced folates, which are necessary for DNA synthesis. Polyglutamates of methotrexate and dihydrofolate inhibit both purine and thymidylate biosynthesis. Leucovorin is a reduced folate that has been used to rescue patients from methotrexate toxicity.

Mechanism of drug resistance

Multiple metabolic steps lead to methotrexate-induced cytotoxicity. Derangement in all phases of methotrexate transport and metabolism contribute to methotrexate resistance. Decreased transmembrane transport, decreased formation of polyglutamates, decreased binding to dihydrofolate reductase and upregulation of dihydrofolate reductase activity have been described in methotrexate-resistant tumors.

Formulations and dose rates

Methotrexate should be stored at room temperature and protected from light.

DOGS AND CATS
- 0.8 mg/kg or 2.5–5.0 mg/m^2
- Some veterinary oncologists recommend a maximum dose of 15 mg/dog
- Methotrexate is administered as an IV bolus and extravasation does not cause soft tissue necrosis
- A protocol for high-dose (3–6 g/m^2) methotrexate with leucovorin (a reduced folate) rescue has been used to treat dogs with osteosarcoma. The treatments were well tolerated but did not result in prolonged survival

Pharmacokinetics

Methotrexate is absorbed from the intestinal tract by a saturable transport mechanism. Small doses are well absorbed. Higher doses are incompletely absorbed. Methotrexate is loosely bound to albumin. Multiple drug half-lives occur in the plasma. In humans, the terminal half-life is 8–27 h. The primary route of methotrexate elimination is via renal excretion, which occurs in the first 12 h after administration. There is also enterohepatic circulation and metabolism of a small fraction of the drug within the gastrointestinal tract by intestinal flora. In the liver, methotrexate is converted to the polyglutamate form, which persists in the liver for months.

Adverse effects

- Gastrointestinal toxicity limits the clinical usefulness of methotrexate without leucovorin rescue in dogs.
- Neutropenia occurs 4–6 d after high-dose methotrexate treatment but is not common with low-dose therapy.
- Toxicoses reported in humans and not in veterinary patients include portal fibrosis, cirrhosis, pneumonitis and anaphylaxis.

Known drug interactions

- L-asparaginase has been reported to decrease methotrexate toxicity and antitumor activity in humans. Demonstration of a protective effect of L-asparaginase from methotrexate toxicity has been attempted but has not been successfully shown in dogs.
- High-dose toxicity to normal tissues can be blocked by leucovorin.
- Nonsteroidal anti-inflammatory drugs decrease renal clearance of methotrexate and increase its toxicity.
- In infusions, methotrexate is incompatible with bleomycin, 5-fluorouracil, prednisolone sodium phosphate, droperidol and ranitidine.

MISCELLANEOUS DRUGS

L-Asparaginase

Other names

Colaspase, l-ASP, crasnitin, asnase, amido hydrolase, NSC-109229 (*E. coli*), NSC-106997 (*Erwinia*), Crisantaspase/Erwinase

Clinical applications

The veterinary use of L-asparaginase has been in multidrug protocols for both canine and feline lymphoma. Its use in acute lymphoid leukemia and mast cell tumors has been proposed.

Mechanism of action

One approach to cancer therapy is to identify the differences between tumor cells and normal cells and to exploit those differences therapeutically. Although this is a rational approach, it has been difficult to identify consistent differences between the two types of cell and the only drug resulting from this approach has been L-asparaginase. L-Asparaginase is a cell cycle-specific drug, which exerts its activity in the G_1 phase of the cell cycle.

Normal cells can synthesize L-asparagine from glutamine and L-aspartic acid, but some tumor cells lack L-asparagine synthetase, the catalyst for L-asparagine production. The conversion of L-asparagine to aspartic acid and ammonia by L-asparaginase starves the tumor cells of L-asparagine. Depletion of L-asparagine inhibits protein synthesis and results in cytotoxicity. The most commonly used L-asparaginase formulation is purified from *Escherichia coli*. However, enzyme derived from *Erwinia carotovora* is also available.

Mechanism of drug resistance

Resistance to treatment with L-asparaginase arises from selection of a tumor cell population containing L-asparagine synthetase or a derepression of the synthetase as a result of a fall in intracellular L-asparagine levels. The patient's immune system also contributes to L-asparaginase resistance by producing antibodies with the capability to accelerate enzyme clearance and reduce therapeutic effectiveness.

Formulations and dose rates

Unreconstituted L-asparaginase should be stored at 4°C. Once reconstituted, the drug should be used within 8 h and discarded if the solution appears turbid. Some data exist to indicate that L-asparaginase may be stored for up to 14 d following reconstitution but this is not in accordance with the manufacturer's label.

DOGS, CATS AND FERRETS

- Both 400 IU/kg and 10,000 IU/m^2 have been recommended
- L-asparaginase is safe and effective when given IP, IM or SC. Intramuscular injections are associated with increased pain at the injection site when compared to SC injections but, in a group of dogs with lymphoma, dogs receiving IM L-asparaginase had longer remission and survival times than dogs receiving SC injections (191 versus 109 d and 286 versus 298 d respectively). Intravenous administration is associated with a high incidence of hypersensitivity reactions and therefore this route of administration is not recommended

Pharmacokinetics

Plasma L-asparaginase concentration has a primary half-life of 14–22 h in humans. L-asparaginase does not cross the blood–brain barrier but does deplete the CSF of L-asparagine and consequently has an antitumor effect in the central nervous system. The pharmacokinetics of L-asparaginase has not been extensively studied in dogs or cats. In a study of one dog with lymphoma treated with L-asparaginase, plasma levels of L-asparagine were undetectable and aspartic acid levels were markedly elevated 24 h after treatment. Urinary excretion of L-asparagine was also deceased. The half-life of the enzyme in this dog was 18–24 h, similar to the half-life in humans.

Adverse effects

- Toxicity of L-asparaginase is related to its immunogenicity and depression of protein synthesis leading to organ dysfunction (Table 15.5).
- Although L-asparaginase is a common component of feline lymphoma protocols, reports of toxicity in the cat are rare.

Known drug interactions

- The manufacturer's recommendations for vincristine indicate that vincristine should not be given in combination with L-asparaginase because of severe myelosuppression; consequently some veterinary oncologists recommend spacing drug administration by 12–48 h. Neutropenia is seen in up to 50% of dogs at some centers treated with L-asparaginase and vincristine, although it rarely results in clinical signs. In one study evaluating 147 dogs, neutropenia occurred in 40% of dogs receiving the combination of drugs, irrespective of the interval between administration of the two drugs. Hospitalization was necessary in 16% of dogs.
- Theoretically, depletion of L-asparagine induces tumor resistance to the effects of methotrexate but since they are not typically given together, this interaction is not clinically significant.

Table 15.5 L-asparaginase toxicity

Adverse effect	Frequency	Management	Comments
Myelosuppression	Rare	Supportive care	Not exacerbated by vincristine in dogs
Anaphylaxis	Rare?	Pretreatment with short-acting glucocorticoids and antihistamines	Usually occurs with repeated administrations, depends on route of administration, higher incidence if administered IV
Pancreatitis	Less than 5% of dogs treated	Supportive care	May occur without elevations in amylase and lipase because of decreased synthesis
Clinical coagulopathy due to decreased synthesis of clotting factors	Reported in normal dogs and dogs with lymphoma. Rarely occurs	Assess coagulation times if hemorrhage is seen	
Diarrhea, nausea, vomiting, anorexia, lethargy	Approximately 50% of dogs treated	None usually required Hospitalization rarely required	
Intramuscular injection site discomfort	Approximately 50% of dogs treated	None usually required	Consider intraperitoneal administration
Decreased hepatic protein synthesis	Rare	Supportive care. Monitor for coagulopathy and hepatic encephalopathy	Use with caution in dogs and cats with severe hepatic dysfunction

DTIC

Other names

Dacarbazine, imidazole carboxamide, DIC

Clinical applications

The primary indication for DTIC in humans is as a component of multiagent chemotherapy for malignancies, including Hodgkin's lymphoma, melanoma and soft tissue sarcoma. DTIC is not commonly used in veterinary medicine. Two reports described its use in combination with doxorubicin to treat dogs with lymphoma. Complete responses were observed in some individuals previously resistant to chemotherapy, suggesting a potential role in 'rescue' therapy. Its use as a single agent in canine lymphoma has not been evaluated, nor has its use in cats for any malignancy. Its value for treating melanoma and soft tissue sarcoma in animals is not known.

Mechanism of action

Dacarbazine was synthesized as a purine analog but its antitumor activity remains unknown. It is a cell cycle-nonspecific agent.

Mechanism of drug resistance

Because the mechanism of action is poorly defined, the mechanisms of resistance remain so also.

Formulations and dose rates

Dacarbazine should be stored at 2–8°C. Once reconstituted, it is stable for 8 h at room temperature or 72 h at 2–8°C. DTIC in aqueous solution (10 mg/mL) is stable for 72 h at 4°C in the dark. The solution readily undergoes photodecomposition if exposed to UV light and should be protected from daylight.

DOGS

- Intravenous infusion of 200 mg/m^2 q.24 h for 5 consecutive days is the standard dose regimen
- Reported dose rates vary from 133 to 200 mg/m^2 IV q.24 h for 5 d every 3–4 weeks
- One source recommends up to 250 mg/m^2 IV daily for 5 d every 3–4 weeks

CATS

- No dose rate has been reported for cats

Pharmacokinetics

DTIC is a prodrug and, as a result of the action of microsomal oxidases, is metabolically activated by N-demethylation to active alkylating metabolites and formaldehyde. In dogs, after IV administration of 20 mg/kg, clearance of DTIC from plasma is biphasic with α and β half-lives of 6 and 90 min. By 6 h after administration, the cumulative urinary excretion of DTIC is only 20% of the administered dose, suggesting rapid and extensive metabolism. Urinary excretion of DTIC and metabolites is thought to be by tubular secretion. DTIC enters the CNS only to a limited extent: after 10 min the CSF : plasma ratio is 1 : 7. The plasma half-life was increased in human patients with hepatic and renal dysfunction. In the dog, dacarbazine is 27% protein bound.

Adverse effects

- The adverse effects of dacarbazine as a single agent have not been investigated in the dog. When combined with doxorubicin, diarrhea, anorexia, fever, leukopenia and thrombocytopenia have been reported but cannot be directly attributed to dacarbazine.
- Pain occurs during IV infusion. This may be reduced by diluting the drug in 100–200 mL of 5% dextrose in water and infusing over 30 min rather than injecting rapidly. Extravasation may cause tissue damage.
- Severe myelosuppression is uncommon.
- Anorexia, nausea and vomiting, with onset 1–3 h after administration and duration up to 24 h; these may be reduced by pre-emptive treatment with anti-emetic medication. In humans, intensity of these effects decreases with each subsequent daily dose. Diarrhea is unusual.
- A mild flu-like adverse effect of DTIC observed in humans has not been reported for companion animals.

Contraindications and precautions

Dose reduction should be considered in animals with liver or kidney dysfunction.

Known drug interactions

DTIC precipitates with hydrocortisone sodium succinate but not hydrocortisone sodium phosphate.

Hydroxycarbamide (hydroxyurea)

Other names

NSC-23605, HU, HUR

Clinical applications

The principal use of hydroxycarbamide (hydroxyurea) has been the treatment of myeloproliferative syndromes in both the dog and the cat. Polycythemia vera, chronic granulocytic leukemia, essential thrombocythemia and basophilic leukemia in veterinary patients have been treated with hydroxycarbamide, with varying success.

Mechanism of action

Hydroxycarbamide (hydroxyurea) is a synthetic cell cycle-specific drug with its effect in the S phase. It inhibits ribonucleotide reductase activity, the rate-limiting catalytic enzyme in the de novo synthesis of deoxyribonucleotide triphosphates in DNA synthesis and repair.

Mechanism of drug resistance

Tumor cells achieve resistance to hydroxycarbamide (hydroxyurea) by increasing cellular ribonucleotide reductase activity.

Formulations and dose rates

Hydroxycarbamide is only available in capsules, which are too large for most veterinary patients. The capsules should be reformulated to ensure accurate dosing and prevent inadvertent overdosage.

DOGS AND CATS

- Because hydroxycarbamide (hydroxyurea) has an excellent oral absorption, it is typically given PO
- The dose should be adjusted to achieve the desired clinical effect, but a starting dose of 30 mg/kg for 7 d reduced to 15 mg/kg is the recommended starting point

Pharmacokinetics

Pharmacokinetic data are lacking in the dog and cat. In humans, the elimination half-life is 3.5–4.5 h. Pharmacokinetic studies are best described by a one-compartment model with parallel Michaelis–Menten metabolism and first-order renal excretion. A formula for dose adjustment with renal insufficiency has not been developed. Hydroxycarbamide (hydroxyurea) readily enters the CSF. Pathways for metabolism are undefined.

Adverse effects

- The dose-limiting toxicity is myelosuppression but it is uncommon with recommended doses.
- Macrocytic red blood cells have been reported in humans receiving chronic hydroxycarbamide (hydroxyurea) therapy and one of the authors has seen this in canine and feline patients.
- Paronychia is reported in cats receiving hydroxycarbamide but does not preclude its successful use in this species.
- Hydroxycarbamide is associated with an increased risk of developing leukemia in human patients but veterinary patients do not typically receive therapy for long enough to induce this problem.

Known drug interactions

No clinically significant drug interactions have been identified.

FURTHER READING

Allwood M, Stanley A, Wright P (eds) 2002 The cytotoxics handbook, 4th edn. Radcliffe Medical Press, Oxford

Bishop Y (ed.) 2005 Veterinary formulary, 6th edn. Pharmaceutical Press, London

Chabner B, Longo DL (eds) 1996 Cancer chemotherapy and biotherapy: principles and practice, 2nd edn. Lippincott-Raven, New York

Foye WO (ed.) 1995 Cancer chemotherapeutic agents. American Chemical Society, Washington, DC

Kitchell B, LaRue SM, Rooks RL 2000 Veterinary cancer therapy handbook: chemotherapy, radiation therapy and surgical oncology for the practicing veterinarian, 2nd edn. AAHA Press, Lakewood, CO

Lana SE 2003 Chemotherapy. In: Dobson J, Lascelles D (eds) BSAVA manual of canine and feline oncology, 2nd edn. BSAVA Publications, Quedgeley, Glos

Morris J, Dobson J 2001 Small animal oncology. Blackwell Science, Oxford

Morrison WB (ed.) 2002 Cancer in dogs and cats: medical and surgical management. Teton New Media, Jackson, WY

Ogilvie GK, Moore AS 1995 Managing the veterinary cancer patient. a practice manual. Veterinary Learning Systems, Trenton, NJ

Plumb DC 2005 Veterinary drug handbook, 5th edn. Blackwell, Oxford

Rosenthal RC, Michalski D 1991 Storage of expensive anticancer drugs. JAVMA 198: 144-146

Steel RT, Lachant NA 1995 Handbook of cancer chemotherapy, 4th edn. Little, Brown, London

Tennant B 2005 BSAVA small animal formulary, 5th edn. BSAVA Publications, Quedgeley, Glos

Vail DM 2004 Veterinary Co-Operative Oncology Group – common terminology criteria for adverse events (VCOG-CTCAE) following chemotherapy or biological antineoplastic therapy in dogs and cats v1.0. Vet Comp Oncol 2: 194-213

Withrow SJ, MacEwen G (eds) Clinical veterinary oncology, 3rd edn. WB Saunders, Philadelphia, PA

Safety/UK legislation

COSHH 2002 Control of Substances Hazardous to Health Regulations 2002. Approved Code of Practice and Guidance, 4th edn. HSE Books, London

HSE Information Sheet MISC615 2003 Safe handling of cytotoxic drugs. HSE, London

APPENDIX: COMMON CHEMOTHERAPY PROTOCOLS

Canine doses (feline doses). If a separate dose is not given for cats, the canine and feline doses are the same.

COP CHEMOTHERAPY

Weeks 1, 4, 7, 10, 13 and every 3 weeks if complete remission is sustained.
Cyclophosphamide 300 mg/m^2 PO

Weeks 1–4, 7,10, 13 and every 3 weeks if complete remission is sustained.
Vincristine 0.75 mg/m^2

Weeks 1–4
Prednisone 1 mg/kg PO daily. After 4 weeks, prednisone is administered at a rate of 1 mg/kg PO every other day for as long as complete remission is sustained.

MULTIAGENT PROTOCOL FOR LYMPHOMA UW- MADISON –25

Week 1
Vincristine 0.7 mg/m^2 (0.05–0.07 mg/m^2) IV
L-asparaginase 400 mg/m^2 IM

Week 2
Cyclophosphamide 250 mg/m^2 (200 mg/m^2) IV

Week 3
Vincristine 0.7 mg/m^2 (0.05–0.07 mg/m^2) IV

Week 4
Doxorubicin 30 mg/m^2 (25 mg/m^2) IV

Week 5
No chemotherapy

Weeks 6–9
Repeat weeks 1–4, deleting the L-asparaginase

Week 10
No chemotherapy

Week 11
Vincristine 0.7 mg/m^2 (0.05–0.07 mg/m^2) IV

Week 13
Cyclophosphamide 250 mg/m^2 IV (chlorambucil 1.4 mg/kg PO, once)

Week 15
Vincristine 0.7 mg/m^2 (0.05–0.07 mg/m^2) IV

Week 17
Doxorubicin 30 mg/m^2 IV
(methotrexate 0.5–0.8 mg/kg IV)

Week 19
Vincristine 0.7 mg/m^2 (0.05–0.07 mg/m^2) IV

Week 21
Cyclophosphamide 250 mg/m^2 IV
(chlorambucil 1.4 mg/kg PO, once)

Week 23
Vincristine 0.7 mg/m^2 (0.05–0.07 mg/m^2) IV

Week 25
Doxorubicin 30 mg/m^2 (25 mg/m^2) IV

Discontinue chemotherapy on week 25 if in complete remission. (For cats, if in complete remission at week 25, treatment should be continued at 3-week intervals following the same sequence of drugs in weeks 11–25. At the end of week 51, and if the cat continues in complete remission, treatment is continued at 4-week intervals substituting methotrexate for doxorubicin)

Prednisone start week 1
2 mg/kg PO q.24 h × 7 d
1.5 mg/kg PO q.24 h × 7 d
1.0 mg/kg PO q.24 h × 7 d
0.5 mg/kg PO q.24 × 7 d
Discontinue

(Cats – prednisone start week 1
2 mg/kg PO daily × 14 d
1 mg/kg PO daily × 7 d
1 mg/kg PO q.48 h for remainder of treatment)

LYMPHOMA RESCUE PROTOCOLS

MOPP chemotherapy

Day 1 and day 8
Methchlorethamine 3 mg/m^2 IV
Vincristine 0.7 mg/m^2 (0.25 mg/kg)

Days 1–14
Procarbazine 50 mg/m^2 PO (12.5–15 mg/cat daily)
Prednisone 30 mg/m^2 PO (5 mg/cat BID PO until protocol discontinuation)

Days 14–28
No chemotherapy
Repeat cycle beginning day 29

D-MAC

14-day cycle

Day 1
Dexamethasone, 0.23 mg/kg PO or SC
Actinomycin D 0.75 mg/m^2 as IV push
Cytarabine 200–300 mg/m^2 as IV drip over 4 h or SC

Day 8
Dexamethasone, 0.23 mg/kg PO or SC
Melphalan 20 mg/m^2 PO

16

Anticonvulsant drugs

Karen M Vernau and Richard A LeCouteur

Relevant physiology and pathophysiology

Seizure disorders are common in dogs and cats. Estimates of lifetime seizure frequency vary from 0.5% to 5.7% in dogs and 0.5% to 1.0% in cats. In humans, accurate seizure classification aids in the selection of the most effective anticonvulsant drug. For example, drugs used to manage petit mal (or absence) seizures may not be as effective in the management of grand mal (or generalized) seizures. Although many different types of seizures occur in dogs and cats, a universally accepted classification system has not been established. The most frequently recognized seizure type in dogs and cats is the generalized seizure; anticonvulsant drugs are evaluated primarily on their efficacy in the control of such seizures.

A seizure is the clinical manifestation of a paroxysmal cerebral disorder, caused by a synchronous and excessive electrical neuronal discharge, originating from the cerebral cortex. Cluster seizures are more than one seizure within a 24-h period. Status epilepticus is a continuous seizure, or two or more discrete seizures between which there is incomplete recovery of consciousness, lasting at least 5 min. Epilepsy is recurrent seizures from an intracranial cause. True epilepsy originates from a nonprogressive intracranial disorder. Symptomatic epilepsy is caused by progressive intracranial disease.

The normal brain is capable of initiating seizure activity in response to a variety of stimuli from within the nervous system and to many external influences. Disorders that induce seizures may arise either outside the nervous system (extracranial) or within the nervous system (intracranial). Extracranial causes may be subdivided into those that originate outside the body (e.g. toxic agents, including lead and organophosphates) and those that originate within the body but outside the nervous system (e.g. hypoglycemia, liver disease).

Intracranial causes of seizures are divided into progressive and nonprogressive diseases. Progressive diseases include inflammation (e.g. granulomatous meningoencephalitis), neoplasia, nutritional problems (e.g. thiamine deficiency), infection (e.g. feline infectious peritonitis, cryptococcosis, distemper), anomalous disorders (e.g. hydrocephalus, intra-arachnoid cyst), trauma and vascular diseases. Nonprogressive diseases include true epilepsy, such as inherited, acquired or idiopathic epilepsy. Inherited epilepsy is caused by a genetically determined intracranial disorder. Acquired epilepsy is caused by a previously active intracranial disorder, which is no longer active. Idiopathic epilepsy is where the cause and mechanism for the seizures are unknown.

Extracranial and intracranial diseases that cause seizures must be differentiated. Therapy for symptomatic epilepsy requires not only control of seizures but also specific therapy for the underlying disease. Further investigation of intracranial diseases by electroencephalography (EEG), magnetic resonance (MR) imaging, cerebrospinal fluid (CSF) analysis, biopsy (for cytology and/or histopathology) and serology may be indicated.

It is essential to approach symptomatic epilepsy as a manifestation of an underlying disease. Therapy is most effective when the underlying disease is diagnosed and treated. Therefore, a diagnosis should be established in a timely manner, before chronic anticonvulsant therapy is initiated. In some animals, the underlying cause of seizures may not be identified, as with true epilepsy. Regardless of the underlying cause, seizure management is based on control of seizures by selection and appropriate administration of anticonvulsant drugs. Adverse effects may limit the usefulness of an anticonvulsant drug; therefore, it is essential to study the mechanisms of action and drug interactions in the species in which the drug is to be used.

Clinical applications

While the ultimate goal of anticonvulsant therapy is to eradicate all seizure activity, this is rarely achieved. A realistic goal is to reduce the severity, frequency and duration of seizures to a level that is acceptable to the owner, without intolerable or life-threatening adverse effects on the animal.

Immediate, short-term (acute) anticonvulsant therapy is required to treat status epilepticus, cluster seizures and seizures resulting from some toxicities. Chronic anticonvulsant therapy is used in the management of epilepsy, where seizures are longer than 3 minutes' duration, are cluster seizures or occur more frequently than once every 4–6 weeks. Chronic anticonvulsant therapy may also be used as adjunctive therapy in animals with intracranial disease. Anticonvulsant drugs are most effective when started early in the course of a seizure disorder, since each seizure may increase the probability of additional seizures, because of effects such as kindling and mirror foci development in the brain.

Anticonvulsant drugs usually are contraindicated in animals with extracranial causes of seizures, except for animals with portosystemic shunts and occasionally in animals with toxicities. Animals with seizures from a progressive intracranial disease may require additional therapy to treat the underlying disease (e.g. neoplasia or inflammation). Therapy in these animals should be directed towards the underlying disease.

Successful anticonvulsant therapy depends on the maintenance of plasma concentrations of appropriate anticonvulsant drugs within a therapeutic range. Therefore, anticonvulsant drugs that are eliminated slowly are most efficacious. The elimination half-life of anticonvulsant drugs varies considerably between species. Few of the anticonvulsant drugs used for the treatment of epilepsy in people are suitable for use in dogs and cats. This is largely due to differences in the pharmacokinetics of drugs in animals when compared to humans. Some drugs are metabolized so rapidly in animals that consistently high serum concentrations are not maintained, even at very high doses. Pharmacokinetic data for, and/or clinical experience with, many anticonvulsant drugs are lacking in cats.

Phenobarbital and bromide are considered the anticonvulsant drugs most appropriate for management of chronic seizure disorders of dogs and cats.

Table 16.1 Recommended drug dosages

Drug	Recommended dosages
Phenobarbital	Dogs: 2–5 mg/kg q.12 h Cats: 1.5–2.5 mg/kg q.12 h
Potassium bromide	Dogs and cats: 35–45 mg/kg PO q.24 h or divided q.12 h Dogs: loading dose 400–600 mg/kg divided into four doses, given over 24 h
Sodium bromide	Dogs: 35–45 mg/kg PO q.12 h, reduce by 15% Dogs: loading dose 1200–1500 mg/kg over 24 h as a continuous-rate infusion of 3% NaBr in 5% dextrose in water
Felbamate	Dogs: 15 mg/kg PO q.8 h to a maximum of 300 mg/kg/d
Gabapentin	Dogs: 300 mg PO q.8 h, up to 1200 mg PO q.8 h over 4 weeks or 25–60 mg/kg divided q.8 h or q.6 h
Zonisamide	Dogs: 10 mg/kg PO q.12 h Cats: 5 mg/kg PO q.12 h
Levitiracetam	Dogs: 20 mg/kg PO q.8 h

ANTICONVULSANT DRUGS

Phenobarbital (phenobarbitone)

Clinical applications

Phenobarbital is a safe, effective and inexpensive drug suitable for chronic therapy of seizures in dogs and cats. It is a broad-spectrum anticonvulsant as it is effective for the treatment of multiple seizure types in cats and dogs. Phenobarbital is effective in controlling seizures in 60–80% of epileptic dogs, provided that serum concentrations of the drug are maintained within the therapeutic range (15–45 μg/mL or 66–200 μmol/L). Unlike other barbiturates (e.g. pentobarbital), phenobarbital suppresses seizure activity at subhypnotic doses.

Mechanism of action

The exact anticonvulsant mechanism of action of phenobarbital is not completely understood, although it is known to increase the seizure threshold required for seizure discharge and to decrease the spread of discharge to surrounding neurones.

Four potential mechanisms of action are:

- enhanced neuronal inhibition by increasing the activity of the inhibitory neurotransmitter γ-aminobutyric acid (GABA) in the central nervous system (CNS) at the postsynaptic membrane. By an allosteric effect, barbiturates increase the affinity of GABA for its own receptor and as a result the chloride ion channel

Table 16.2 Anticonvulsant therapy for status epilepticus

Drug	Recommended doses
Diazepam	Dogs and cats: 0.5–1.0 mg/kg IV bolus. Bolus may be repeated 2–3 times over several minutes to control seizures. Dogs: 0.5–1 mg/kg PR (2 mg/kg if receiving concurrent phenobarbital)
Phenobarbital	Dogs and cats: 2–4 mg/kg IV q.20–30 min. This dosage may be repeated q.20–30 min until a cumulative dosage of 20 mg/kg has been given. Once seizures are controlled a maintenance dosage of phenobarbital is used (2–4 mg/kg IV q.6 h for 24–48 h). Oral anticonvulsant therapy should be resumed or initiated q.12 h as soon as the animal is able to swallow
Pentobarbital	Dogs and cats: used when seizure activity continues beyond 10-15 min despite the above therapy. Dosages of 3–15 mg/kg IV are recommended. Must be given slowly, since diazepam and phenobarbital will potentiate its effects and respiratory depression may result. Once seizures are controlled, cardiorespiratory function should be assessed. It may be necessary to assist ventilation or to provide oxygen by mask or endotracheal tube

is open for a longer time, resulting in greater chloride flux and enhanced neuronal inhibition
- interaction with glutamate receptors to reduce neuronal excitotoxicity
- inhibition of voltage-gated calcium channels
- competitive binding of the picrotoxin site of the chloride channel.

Formulations and dose rates

Phenobarbital is a controlled substance, available as oral (tablets or elixir) or injectable preparation. The injectable form is intended for intravenous use but may be given intramuscularly. Trade names for phenobarbital in different markets include Epiphen®, Luminal®, Phenomav® and Bellatal®. A generic form of phenobarbital sodium also is available.

- For the chronic treatment of seizures in dogs dosing should begin at 2–5 mg/kg/day PO q.12 h. In dogs with frequent, severe or prolonged seizures, therapy may be initiated at a higher initial dosage. In some dogs or cats, the starting dosage may result in adverse effects. Should these adverse effects not resolve after 2 weeks of therapy, a reduction in dose may be indicated.

Cats: 1.5–2.5 mg/kg PO q.12 h

- Steady-state serum phenobarbital concentrations should be determined after 3 weeks of therapy. If a patient's seizures are adequately controlled, then serum concentrations may be determined again after 3–6 months, or more frequently should seizure activity resume at an unacceptable frequency. If a patient's seizures are not adequately controlled after 3 weeks of therapy, the dose of phenobarbital may be increased by 25% and serum concentrations should be determined again after 3 weeks of therapy at this higher dose. This process should be continued until the patient's seizures are controlled or until a patient fails phenobarbital therapy (i.e. becomes refractory). Dogs are refractory to phenobarbital therapy when seizure activity or unacceptable effects persist when plasma concentrations reach 35 μg/mL
- Dosages of phenobarbital as high as 18–20 mg/kg/day PO divided q.8 h or q.12 h are occasionally necessary to achieve seizure control in some patients, due to individual variations in drug metabolism. Adverse effects are often observed at dosages above 20 mg/kg/d
- Reductions in dosage should be made gradually as physical dependence may develop and withdrawal seizures may occur as serum levels decline. Therapy should not be discontinued abruptly, except in animals that develop fulminant liver dysfunction. Phenobarbital should be avoided in animals with hepatic dysfunction
- Phenobarbital may be administered IV for the treatment of toxic seizures or status epilepticus; however, a lag time of 20–30 min may be observed prior to maximal effect. Phenobarbital may be given at a loading dosage of 12–24 mg/kg IV to achieve therapeutic plasma concentrations more rapidly. A phenobarbital bolus may be given (2–4 mg/kg IV every 30 min), until a cumulative dosage of 20 mg/kg is achieved. The dosage should be decreased proportionately if the patient is receiving oral phenobarbital

Pharmacokinetics

Phenobarbital is rapidly absorbed after oral administration, although variation exists between animals. Bioavailability is high (86–96%) and peak plasma levels are achieved at 4–6 h after administration. Although it is widely distributed into tissues, lower lipid solubility means that it does not penetrate the CNS as rapidly as other barbiturates. After IV injection, therapeutic CNS concentrations are reached in 15–20 min. Administration with food reduces absorption by about 10%. Phenobarbital is metabolized primarily in the liver; 25% is excreted unchanged by the kidneys. Alkalinization of the urine will enhance elimination of phenobarbital and its metabolites. Plasma protein binding is approximately 45%.

The elimination half-life of phenobarbital ranges from 30 h to 90 h in dogs and from 3 h to 83 h in cats. The wide ranges are a result of several variables, including variation in drug dosages between studies and, more importantly, different dosing regimens between studies (single dose, a short course of several doses, or administered chronically). In addition, drugs capable of stimulating drug-metabolizing enzyme systems in the liver were included in some studies. In studies in cats, the use of different populations of cats appeared to be a factor contributing to the reported variability in elimination half-life.

In dogs, phenobarbital elimination half-life significantly decreases when administered chronically (47.3 ± 10.7 h when administered for 90 days versus 88.7 ± 19.6 h in a single-dose study). It increases its own rate of metabolism (autoinduction). Therefore the drug concentration of phenobarbital is expected to decrease in animals receiving chronic therapy and a dosage increase should be anticipated in patients after 3–6 months of therapy. In contrast, in cats, repeated phenobarbital administration does not alter serum steady-state concentration. However, large differences in phenobarbital elimination rates may exist between different populations of cats.

In dogs, the elimination half-life of phenobarbital is similar after oral or IV administration. Steady-state concentrations are achieved within 18 d of initiation of therapy. Therefore dosage adjustments should not be made until 3 weeks after treatment has commenced or been altered. The metabolism of phenobarbital is quite variable in dogs. Beagles metabolize phenobarbital more rapidly (32 h elimination half-life) than mixed-breed dogs. Clinical observations suggest that phenobarbital elimination half-life may be shorter in puppies.

Since there may be marked variations between the oral dosage of phenobarbital and the serum concentration, serum drug levels should be considered a guide to drug therapy alterations. Therapeutic serum phenobarbital concentrations for dogs and cats are estimated to be 15–45 μg/mL and 10–30 μg/mL respectively. Serum drug level monitoring should not be used as a substitute for clinical judgment. Expected therapeutic serum drug levels are average values and individual animals may have an optimal value.

Although pharmacokinetic studies in both cats and dogs suggest that once-daily dosing should be adequate to maintain appropriate serum concentrations, twice or even three times-daily dosing is usually recommended to decrease the fluctuations in serum drug levels and minimize adverse effects. When measuring serum drug levels it is recommended that blood be collected at a similar time in the daily administration cycle of phenobarbital. A blood sample should be collected within an hour before the next scheduled drug administration time (so-called trough levels). In a recent study, epileptic dogs receiving chronic phenobarbital therapy were shown to have minimal variations in serum phenobarbital concentrations throughout the day. Should other studies support these results, it may be acceptable to measure phenobarbital blood levels at any time during the day in chronically treated dogs. Serum separation tubes have been shown to falsely reduce drug concentrations and should be avoided for therapeutic drug monitoring.

In dogs that have an unacceptable level of seizure control, serum phenobarbital concentrations should be maintained between 30 and 40 μg/mL for 1–2 months before the maximal effects of the drug may be fully assessed. After this time, should frequency and/or severity of the seizures remain unacceptable, additional or alternative anticonvulsant medications may be considered.

Adverse effects

- Adverse effects that may be observed initially with phenobarbital therapy include sedation, ataxia, polydipsia, polyuria, polyphagia and weight gain.
  - Polyuria is caused by an inhibitory effect on the release of antidiuretic hormone.
  - Polyphagia may be caused by suppression of the satiety center in the hypothalamus.
  - Most dogs develop a tolerance to these effects after 2–4 weeks of therapy.
  - Unless sedation is extreme or persistent beyond 4 weeks, it should not be considered evidence of toxicity and does not warrant an adjustment in the dose.
  - Sedation at the initiation of therapy has been reported to be more severe in cats.
- Occasionally, dogs may appear hyperactive during the initial phase of therapy. This effect may be overcome by increasing the dose.
- The frequency of hepatoxicity is low in dogs. It is associated with chronic phenobarbital administration. Hepatotoxicity has not been reported in cats. Liver toxicity may be reduced in both species by avoiding combination therapy (i.e. concurrent use of more than one drug metabolized by the liver), by using therapeutic monitoring to achieve adequate serum concentrations at the lowest possible dosage and by evaluating serum biochemistry every 6 months.
- Induction of liver enzymes is common in dogs. Elevations of ALT, ALP and GGT frequently are noted in association with phenobarbital therapy. Enzyme elevations usually do not imply hepatic damage or dysfunction, although if ALT is disproportionately elevated in comparison to ALP, phenobarbital toxicity is possible. If there is doubt about whether hepatic dysfunction is present in an animal receiving anticonvulsant therapy, quantification of serum bile acids is recommended, which are not increased by phenobaribital therapy.
- Phenobarbital does not induce elevations in ALP or other liver enzymes in cats.
- In one study, serum albumin concentration decreased when phenobarbital therapy was initiated, but returned to pretreatment levels in most dogs when phenobarbital was discontinued. The significance of hypoalbuminemia without other indications of hepatic dysfunction is unknown.
- Blood dyscrasias such as neutropenia, thrombocytopenia, anemia and, in some cases, pancytopenia have been reported in dogs receiving phenobarbital. These adverse effects appear to be idiosyncratic or allergic and resolve once the drug is discontinued.
- Dyskinesia was associated with phenobarbital administration in one dog.
- Phenobarbital may increase the metabolism of thyroid hormones in liver and peripheral tissues and also may adversely impact thyroid-stimulating hormone concentrations.
- Regular monitoring is important to reduce the potential adverse effects. Animals should be examined by a veterinarian at least once every 6 months. A complete blood count, serum chemistry panel, urinalysis and serum phenobarbital concentration should be completed at least annually and if indicated, more frequently. Serum phenobarbital level should be maintained at 35 μg/mL or below to reduce hepatotoxicity.

Known drug interactions

- Hepatic microsomal P450 enzyme activity is accelerated by phenobarbital. This dose-related effect may enhance the biotransformation of other drugs, such as digoxin, glucocorticoids, phenylbutazone and some anesthetic drugs. As a result, the therapeutic efficacy of these drugs may be reduced in patients concurrently receiving phenobarbital.

- In contrast, drugs that inhibit hepatic microsomal enzymes (e.g. cimetidine) may inhibit phenobarbital metabolism and cause toxicity. Several cases of chloramphenicol-induced phenobarbital toxicity in dogs have been documented.
- Phenobarbital impairs the absorption of griseofulvin and therefore reduces the blood level and efficacy of this antifungal agent.
- Chronic phenobarbital treatment may influence the results of ACTH response tests, suggesting that this test should not be used to screen for hyperadrenocorticism in dogs receiving phenobarbital. Although plasma ACTH levels may be unchanged, not all studies have confirmed this observation. Similarly, dexamethasone suppression tests may be influenced in some, but not all, dogs chronically treated with phenobarbital.
- Total and free serum levothyroxine (thyroxine) concentrations may be reduced in dogs receiving phenobarbital.

Primidone

Clinical applications

Primidone is a deoxybarbiturate that is a structural analog of phenobarbital. Unlike phenobarbital, it is not a controlled substance; however, this is not sufficient justification to use primidone in preference to phenobarbital in dogs.

Fifty-two to 87% of epileptic dogs may be effectively controlled with primidone. In most dogs, primidone therapy has no advantage over phenobarbital for the treatment of seizures. In addition, adverse behavioral effects occur more frequently. There is a greater potential for hepatotoxicity with chronic primidone than with phenobarbital. There is anecdotal evidence that some dogs refractory to phenobarbital can be satisfactorily controlled with primidone. However, the efficacy of primidone in this situation remains unproven.

It was initially believed that primidone was toxic to cats; however, recent studies suggest that this is not the case. Although not widely used, primidone has been recommended by some authors for cats refractory to phenobarbital or diazepam therapy.

Phenobarbital blood levels are measured as a guide to primidone therapy. Target therapeutic ranges are the same as those for phenobarbital.

Formulations and dose rates

Primidone is not recommended in dogs and cats (except by some authors – see above). Trade names for primidone include Mylepsin® and Mysoline®.

DOGS

- Dosages vary from 29 mg/kg/d to 55 mg/kg/d divided q.8 h
- To change a dog from primidone to phenobarbital therapy, the conversion factor is 3.8 : 1, i.e. 250 mg of primidone to 65 mg of phenobarbital for an equivalent effect. Baseline phenobarbital concentrations should be determined prior to conversion and conversion should be progressive (e.g. 25% alteration each month) in patients whose seizure history includes prolonged or cluster seizures

CATS

- 40 mg/kg divided q.8 h

Pharmacokinetics

Primidone is rapidly absorbed after oral administration, achieving peak serum concentrations after 2 h. It undergoes hepatic oxidation and is excreted in the urine as unchanged primidone, phenylethylmalonamide (PEMA) and phenobarbital. All three compounds have anticonvulsant activity, although primidone contributes only 11% to the overall anticonvulsant effect and PEMA contributes 2%. Eighty to 85% of primidone's anticonvulsant activity is due to phenobarbital.

The half-life of primidone is 5 h in beagles and 10 h in mixed-breed dogs. Steady-state concentrations are achieved after 6–8 days of treatment. However, the half-life of primidone and PEMA decreases after 14–18 days of treatment. Plasma protein binding is 29%. Primidone reaches the CSF relatively slowly, with a mean penetration half-life of 43 min.

Cats metabolize primidone differently from dogs and plasma concentrations of primidone and PEMA may exceed the plasma concentration of phenobarbital. The safety of primidone at effective concentrations has not been established adequately for cats.

Adverse effects

Adverse effects are the same as those for phenobarbital.

- Hepatotoxicity and behavioral disturbances are more frequent with primidone than phenobarbital.
- ALT and ALP serum levels are abnormal more frequently in dogs receiving chronic primidone therapy than with any other commonly used anticonvulsants. In addition, hepatic cirrhosis secondary to chronic use of primidone has been documented.
- Idiosyncratic primidone hepatotoxicity also may occur.
- Sedative effects of primidone are more profound in cats than in dogs.

Known drug interactions

- The drug interactions described for phenobarbital also apply to primidone.
- Severe CNS depression and inappetance has been reported in dogs concurrently receiving primidone and chloramphenicol.

Bromide

Clinical applications

Bromide is a halide, discovered in 1826 by Balard. It was initially used as an anticonvulsant in humans by Sir Charles Locock in 1857. Bromide was the only effective anticonvulsant available until 1912, when phenobarbital was introduced. Bromide was used in dogs in 1907, but it was not until 1986 that interest in its use as an anticonvulsasnt was reported. Initially, bromide was used as an adjunct to phenobarbital in refractory epileptics. Recently, it has been used as a sole anticonvulsant therapy, particularly in dogs with hepatic dysfunction or in patients with mild seizures. Bromide is best suited for noncompliant owners because of its long half-life. Bromide is approved for use in several markets such as the UK (Epilease®) and Australia but is not approved in the USA.

Mechanism of action

The exact mechanism of anticonvulsant action of bromide is incompletely understood. The action appears to involve chloride ion channels which are an important part of the inhibitory neuronal network of the CNS. Their function is modulated by GABA. Increased chloride ion flow, as a result of activation of GABA receptors by barbiturates or benzodiazepines, results in increased neuronal inhibition and increases the threshold for seizures. Bromide appears to cross neuronal chloride channels more readily than chloride because it has a smaller hydrated diameter. By competing with chloride ions, bromide hyperpolarizes postsynaptic neuronal membranes and facilitates the action of inhibitory neurotransmitters. Barbiturates may act synergistically with bromide to raise the seizure threshold by enhancing chloride conductance via GABA-ergic activity.

Formulations and dose rates

Bromide is available as a potassium or sodium salt. Potassium bromide is available in tablet form in some countries such as the UK and Australia. Trade names include Epilease®, Bromapex® and Epibrom®. Where a veterinary formulation is not available (such as in the US), it may be formulated as a 200 mg/mL or 250 mg/mL solution of reagent-grade potassium bromide in syrup or distilled water. Alternatively, the powder may be placed in gelatin capsules.

Bromide is stable for more than 1 year at room or refrigerator temperature, in glass, plastic, clear or brown containers, when in solution with distilled water. The stability of bromide in syrup solution is unknown. Current recommendations include keeping the bromide syrup solution refrigerated and discarding it after 3 months.

Sodium bromide salt may be given to dogs that dislike the taste of the potassium salt or cannot tolerate it (e.g. because of hypoadrenocorticism). The dose of sodium bromide should be reduced by 15% compared to the potassium salt to account for the higher bromide content per gram (KBr = 67% bromide, NaBr = 78% bromide).

- Because reaching a steady state may require 2–3 months, a loading dose is recommended to achieve therapeutic concentrations more rapidly. The maintenance dose is designed to maintain concentrations achieved after loading. Alternatively, the maintenance dose may be given without a loading dose to allow more gradual accommodation to effective serum concentrations
- The appropriate dose of bromide depends on concurrent anticonvulsants, diet and renal function. The maintenance dosage of potassium bromide as a first-line anticonvulsant is 35–45 mg/kg/d PO q.24 h or in divided doses in dogs. Steady-state concentrations in dogs following 30 mg/kg q.24 h are 0.8–1.2 mg/mL. Bromide is not recommended in cats
- When used in conjunction with other anticonvulsants, the recommended dosage is 22–30 mg/kg PO q.24 h or divided (q.12 h)
- The authors' protocol loading dosage of potassium bromide is 400–600 mg/kg divided q.6 h, given over 24 h; stop when sedation occurs
- Serum bromide concentrations may be determined 1 month after a maintenance dosage is instituted, regardless of whether a loading dose was given. This approach will enable modification prior to steady state and prior to therapeutic failure or signs of adverse reactions. Recommended target ranges are controversial and depend on whether phenobarbital is given concurrently. Most laboratories use 1–3 mg/mL regardless of whether bromide is the sole agent or in combination with phenobarbital

Pharmacokinetics

The pharmacokinetics of bromide are not well established. Bromide is absorbed from the small intestine and peak absorption achieved 1.5 h after oral administration. It is not protein bound or metabolized and does not undergo hepatic metabolism. Therefore, bromide does not affect hepatic enzymes and is a useful anticonvulsant for dogs with hepatic disease.

The half life of bromide is longer in dogs than in humans (24.9 d versus 12 d). About 2–3 weeks of therapy are required before serum bromide levels enter the therapeutic range; steady-state levels are achieved in approximately 3–4 months. Higher serum concentrations may be required for seizure control if dogs are treated with bromide alone. The therapeutic range for potassium bromide when administered with phenobarbital is 0.8–2.4 mg/mL, or 0.8–3.0 mg/mL when used alone.

Distribution of bromide is to the extracellular space. Bromide is eliminated slowly from the body, perhaps because of marked reabsorption by the kidneys. Its rate of elimination can change with salt administration. Increased dietary salt will increase the rate of elimination of bromide and decreased dietary salt will result in the opposite effect.

The elimination of bromide in cats is faster than in dogs. The mean half-life is 1.56 weeks ± 0.38 weeks, or about 12 days, in cats. Following administration of 30 mg/kg orally for 8 weeks, the mean bromide concentration was 1.2 mg/mL (steady state).

Although bromide replaces chloride throughout the body, the sum of these two halides remains constant. Lower concentrations of bromide are found in the brain than are expected from measuring the serum chloride concentration as it appears that there is a barrier to the free passage of bromide across the blood–brain barrier. However, the concentration of bromide in the brains of dogs is higher than in humans. In humans the CSF to serum ratio is 31% whereas in dogs it is 87%. As a result, seizure control in dogs may be achieved at a lower serum bromide concentration than in humans. The potential for systemic toxicity may be lower in dogs than humans.

Adverse effects

- Clinical signs of bromide toxicity appear to be dose dependent and include polyphagia, vomiting, anorexia, constipation, pruritus, muscle pain, sedation and pelvic limb weakness.
- Asthma (may be fatal) is associated with bromide administration in cats.
- Ataxia and sedation are the major dose-limiting adverse effects in dogs.
- Other infrequently reported adverse effects in dogs include pancreatitis, increased attention seeking, aggression, coprophagia and hyperactivity.
- High-dose bromide therapy has been associated with thyroid dysfunction in humans and rats.
- Bromide toxicity was reported in a dog with renal insufficiency, resulting in decreased clearance of bromide and therefore a higher serum bromide concentration.
- Reduced seizure control was reported in a dog fed a high-chloride diet. Toxic concentrations of bromide may be reached rapidly when chloride intake is decreased.
- Bromide readily crosses the placenta in humans and may cause neonatal bromism. Because of the lack of information in dogs, bromide should be avoided in breeding animals.
- Sodium bromide should not be used in dogs with congestive heart failure, hypertension or liver failure.
- Potassium bromide should be used cautiously in dogs with hypoadrenocorticism.

Known drug interactions

- Bromide is not protein bound and is not metabolized, therefore it does not interact with many drugs. However, chloride-containing foods, food supplements, fluids, drugs and loop diuretics may enhance bromide elimination and lower serum bromide concentrations.
- Bromide is a product of halothane metabolism in dogs and therefore small increases in serum bromide may be noted after halothane anesthesia.
- Pseudohyperchloridemia occurs with bromide administration. Bromide ions interfere with colorimetric and automated ion-specific electrolyte analyzers used to measure chloride concentration.

Benzodiazepines

Clinical applications

A large number of benzodiazepine derivatives are used in human medicine. In veterinary medicine, diazepam is the most widely used. In dogs, the use of diazepam as an anticonvulsant is limited to treatment of status epilepticus, because of the significant first-pass hepatic clearance, rapid development of functional tolerance and short half-life of the drug. However, in cats, diazepam is effective as an acute and chronic anticonvulsant. Diazepam is the first-line treatment of choice for status epilepticus in both dogs and cats.

Clonazepam is more potent and longer lasting than diazepam and is used as both an acute and a chronic anticonvulsant in humans. In dogs, hepatic enzyme induction occurs within days to weeks, rendering clonazepam unsatisfactory as a chronic anticonvulsant. It may be useful in dogs as a chronic anticonvulsant if used as an adjunct to phenobarbital therapy, especially in cases of intractable epilepsy. There are no clinical evaluations of its use as an anticonvulsant in dogs. Because of the development of tolerance to the anticonvulsant effects of clonazepam in dogs, its clinical usefulness is limited.

Lorazepam is used as an acute anticonvulsant in humans. It is not as lipid soluble as diazepam. Pilot studies have shown that therapeutic concentrations are reached with IV but not per rectum therapy in dogs.

Midazolam is a water-soluble benzodiazepine. Since it is water soluble, it is much less irritating with IV or IM administration. It is most useful as an acute anticonvulsant in the treatment of status epilepticus.

Clorazepate is hydrolyzed in the stomach to nordiazepam, the active anticonvulsant. Nordiazepam is a major metabolite of diazepam. The short half-life of clorazepate in dogs and its confounding interactions with phenobarbital have rendered it of extremely limited usefulness as a maintenance anticonvulsant in dogs, even when used in combination with phenobarbital.

Mechanism of action

Benzodiazepines function as anticonvulsants by potentiating GABA-mediated neuroinhibition in the brain. In a mechanism of action similar to that of barbiturates, benzodiazepines increase the affinity of GABA for its own receptors and as a result, chloride flux is increased because of increased frequency of opening of the chloride ion channels. Tolerance to anticonvulsant activity of diazepam develops rapidly in dogs.

Formulations and dose rates

DIAZEPAM

Diazepam is available as both an IV and oral preparation. There are no veterinary-approved formulations of diazepam in the US and UK. In Australia the veterinary-approved formulation is Pamlin Injection®. One trade name for human-approved diazepam is Valium®. For administration per rectum, a gel formulation of diazepam (Diastat®) is available in some countries in a prefilled single dose syringe (5 mg/mL).

Status epilepticus

- An intravenous bolus of diazepam should initially be given at a dosage of 0.5–1 mg/kg. Onset of anticonvulsant activity occurs about 2–3 min after administration. This dosage may be repeated 2–3 times, or a constant rate IV infusion (1.0–2.0 mg/kg/h in dogs and 0.5–1.0 mg/kg/h in cats) may be given following the bolus
- When immediate venous access is not possible, diazepam may be given per rectum at a dosage of 2.0 mg/kg in dogs receiving phenobarbital and 0.5–1.0 mg/kg in dogs not receiving phenobarbital. Chronic use of phenobarbital reduces benzodiazepine blood levels and thus higher doses of diazepam are required in dogs receiving chronic phenobarbital. Diazepam may be administered up to three times per rectum in a 24-h period. Diazepam may cause agitation, sedation and ataxia in dogs. Therefore, owners should stay with their dog for about an hour after administration in case the dog has seizures requiring additional therapy and to ensure the dog's safety. In dogs, the per rectum method of administration is effective in managing cluster seizures at home
- Nasally administered diazepam attains therapeutic blood concentrations in dogs, but clinical use of this method of administration has not been reported
- Diazepam may be used as an alternative maintenance anticonvulsant in cats. Idiosyncratic fatal hepatic necrosis has been reported in cats. Liver enzymes should be evaluated prior to and 3–5 days after initiating therapy. Diazepam should be discontinued if liver enzyme elevations above baseline are detected
- Cats: 0.25–0.5 mg/kg PO q.8–12 h

CLONAZEPAM

- Dogs: 0.1–0.5 mg/kg PO q.8 h
- Cats: 0.05–0.2 mg/kg IV is recommended for treating status epilepticus (not available in the USA). IV clonazepam may have longer lasting effects than IV diazepam

LORAZEPAM

- Dogs: 0.2 mg/kg IV

MIDAZOLAM

- Dogs and cats: 0.25 mg/kg IV

CLORAZEPATE

- 1 mg/kg q.12 h PO for dogs receiving concurrent phenobarbital

Pharmacokinetics

After oral administration, diazepam is rapidly absorbed and metabolized to nordiazepam and oxazepam. These metabolites have one-third the anticonvulsant activity of diazepam. As a result of extensive first-pass metabolism, the bioavailability of unchanged diazepam is only 1–3%. However, the bioavailability of its active metabolites is 86%.

Diazepam rapidly penetrates the CSF and the onset of anticonvulsant activity after IV administration is 2–3 min, although brain concentrations decline rapidly after injection. After IV administration the half-life of diazepam, nordiazepam and oxazepam is 3.2 h, 3.6 h and 5.7 h respectively. The half-life of each drug is similar after oral administration.

Benzodiazepines are safer anticonvulsant drugs than barbiturates. The relationship between drug dosage and degree of CNS depression is curvilinear for benzodiazepines (proportionately greater dose increments are required to achieve profound CNS depression), whereas for barbiturates it is linear.

Although functional tolerance to diazepam is reported in dogs, in cats effective plasma concentrations of unchanged diazepam and its active metabolites may be maintained without development of tolerance.

Although clonazepam is rapidly absorbed after oral administration, bioavailability appears to be variable. In dogs, elimination half-life is dose dependent and ranges from 1 h (0.1 mg/kg) to 5.4 h (2.3 mg/kg). During continuous treatment with 0.5 mg/kg q.12 h for several weeks, the elimination half-life increased to between 6 h and 19 h in most dogs. With this dose, serum concentrations of 0.5 mg/L can be achieved, which are considered to be therapeutic in humans. Penetration into CSF is rapid. Because of saturation kinetics, the half-life increases considerably after several weeks of oral administration. However, functional tolerance develops in dogs within 2–5 weeks, although it is less rapid and less pronounced than with diazepam.

Midazolam is rapidly absorbed following IM administration, with peak plasma concentration in dogs occur within 15 min. Bioavailability of more than 90% is reported, with a mean elimination half-life of 56 min. Midazolam is biotransformed by hepatic microsomal oxidation followed by glucuronide conjugation. All metabolites are excreted in urine and bile. The half-life of the metabolites in dogs is 11 min. Midazolam has a wide margin of safety and a broad therapeutic index. The mean plasma elimination half-life in dogs is 53–77 min when given intravenously. These properties support the use of midazolam for the treatment of status epilepticus.

Adverse effects

- Idiosyncratic, fatal fulminant hepatic failure was reported in 11 cats treated with low-dose diazepam for behavioral disorders. Only one cat survived. Risk factors were not identified.
- Sedation is the most commonly reported adverse effect of all benzodiazepines.
- Diazepam acts as a skeletal muscle relaxant; therefore ataxia and weakness unrelated to sedation may occur.
- An interesting effect of diazepam, but not other benzodiazepines, is appetite stimulation in cats. This effect has been used therapeutically to encourage anorexic cats to eat (see Chapter 19).
- Occasionally, cats have an idiosyncratic behavioral reaction whereby they become hyperactive. This may be due to release of overt anxiety and hence release of the behavioral inhibition that maintained a tractable state in cats.
- Overtly friendly cats, particularly oriental breeds, may become excessively affectionate when treated with diazepam.
- Dogs may become aggressive when receiving clonazepam.
- Physical dependence to diazepam is reported in dogs. Clinical signs of diazepam withdrawal included tremor, weight loss, elevated body temperature and seizures.

Known drug interactions

- Benzodiazepines potentiate the action of other CNS depressants.
- Diazepam binds extensively to plasma proteins and should be used cautiously with other drugs that also have high plasma protein-binding activity.
- Benzodiazepines should be used cautiously with cimetidine. Cimetidine impairs hepatic microsomal oxidation of diazepam and prolongs its half-life and thus elimination from the body.

Phenytoin

Clinical applications

Although phenytoin is a very effective anticonvulsant in humans, it is not useful in dogs or cats because of marked pharmacokinetic differences between species. In dogs, the drug has a relatively short elimination half-life and, with repeated administration, enzyme induction leads to faster elimination. In one clinical study, seizure activity was adequately controlled in only one of 77 epileptic dogs treated with phenytoin.

Studies examining the clinical use of phenytoin in cats are lacking. The elimination half-life reported in cats is very long and even at low dosages, there is a high risk for the development of toxic drug levels.

A slow-release formulation of phenytoin (slow-release diphenylhydantoin, SR-DPH) has been used experimentally as an anticonvulsant in the Netherlands. Seizures were controlled similarly in dogs receiving SR-DPH and phenobarbital. However, dogs with refractory seizures already receiving phenobarbital had better control of their seizures when changed to SR-DPH.

Mephenytoin is a hydantoin derivative similar to phenytoin. Its anticonvulsant activity results from metabolism to nirvonal. Bone marrow dyscrasias preclude its common use in humans. Although isolated reports suggest that it may prove efficacious in dogs with epilepsy, hepatotoxicity, particularly when used in combination with phenobarbital, necessitates cautious use.

Mechanism of action

The major mechanism of action of phenytoin is suppression of repetitive action potentials by blocking sodium channels and decreasing inward flow of sodium. At high concentrations the release of serotonin and noradrenaline (norepinephrine) is inhibited. Phenytoin interacts with membrane lipids and may promote stabilization of membranes. It also may have other effects on neurotransmitters and the overall mechanism of action probably involves a combination of actions at several levels. Its effect on sodium channels is the basis for its use as an antiarrhythmic drug (see Chapter 17).

Formulations and dose rates

Phenytoin is not recommended as an anticonvulsant in dogs and cats.

Oral preparations of phenytoin are available in suspension, capsule and tablet forms. Trade names include Dilantin® and Epanutin®. The trade name of the slow-release formulation is Epitard 700® – this is not available in all markets.

- Dogs: 100–200 mg/kg/d divided q.8 h
- Epitard 700®: start at 50 mg/kg/d and increase the dosage over 4 weeks

Pharmacokinetics

Gastrointestinal absorption of certain formulations of phenytoin is poor in dogs, although the microcrystalline oral suspension is well absorbed. In dogs, phenytoin is rapidly metabolized and excreted, with a half-life of 3–7 h (compared to 7–42 h in humans). In cats the half-life is longer (24–108 h) due to their decreased ability to conjugate compounds with glucuronic acid.

The degree of protein binding of phenytoin is substantially lower in dogs than humans, a contributing factor to its rapid elimination in dogs. In addition, phenytoin is a potent microsomal enzyme inducer and chronic administration stimulates its own metabolism. In one study in dogs, the elimination half-life of phenytoin rapidly declined by 47–65% after initiation of treatment. After 1 week, serum concentrations were minimally detectable.

Because oral administration of phenytoin in dogs produces subtherapeutic and erratic serum concentrations, it is not possible to sustain adequate serum concentrations and therefore brain concentrations. As a result, phenytoin is not recommended as an anticonvulsant in dogs and further work is required before its use in cats is recommended.

Adverse effects

- In humans, phenytoin treatment is associated with a variety of side effects including ataxia, nystagmus, tremors, gingival hyperplasia, hepatitis, hirsutism, coarsening of facial features, mild peripheral neuropathy (long-term chronic use), abnormalities of vitamin D metabolism and birth defects (cleft palate).
- In dogs, adverse effects are uncommon. Gingival hyperplasia and hepatitis are reported.
- Phenytoin may cause hepatotoxicity in dogs, particularly if administered concurrently with phenobarbital or primidone.
  - Intrahepatic cholestasis has been observed in dogs treated with phenytoin in combination with phenobarbital.
  - Concurrent administration of phenobarbital may increase formation of epoxide intermediates of phenytoin, ultimately resulting in cholestatic injury.

Known drug interactions

In humans many drugs interact with phenytoin.

- Phenytoin blood levels are increased by phenylbutazone, halothane, diazepam, chlorpromazine, estrogens and chloramphenicol.
- Phenytoin may enhance the metabolism of dexamethasone.
- Phenytoin may increase blood levels of digitoxin.
- Phenytoin may decrease blood levels of phenobarbital.
  - The interaction between phenytoin and phenobarbital results in increased metabolism of both drugs in a seesaw fashion and the combined use of these drugs is discouraged. The combination also increases the risk of hepatotoxicity.

Carbamazepine

Clinical applications

Carbamazepine is a tricyclic compound used initially in the treatment of depression and trigeminal neuralgia in humans. It was subsequently found to be a useful anticonvulsant in people.

Although there are isolated reports of the use of carbamazepine as an anticonvulsant in dogs, appropriate studies of its clinical efficacy in canine or feline seizure control are lacking. The rapid metabolism in dogs makes it unsuitable as an anticonvulsant. However, successful long-term control of psychomotor seizures is reported in one dog, despite low to undetectable serum carbamazepine concentrations.

Mechanism of action

The chemical features and mechanism of action of carbamazine are similar to those of phenytoin.

Formulations and dose rates

The trade names of carbamazepine include Tegretol® and Epitol®.

DOGS

- 40–50 mg/kg q.8 h

CATS

- 25 mg/cat q.8 h

Pharmacokinetics

The pharmacokinetics of carbamazepine vary considerably between species and, like phenytoin, diazepam and valproic acid, it is eliminated more quickly in dogs than in humans. Oral absorption of carbamazepine solution is rapid in dogs. Absorption of tablets is slower and more erratic. The elimination half-life in dogs is 1.5 h. Daily treatment results in a pronounced and progressive decline in plasma levels from the second day of treatment. The elimination half-life of carbamazepine in dogs given 30 mg/kg q.8 h decreased to less than 1 h within 1 week of therapy initiation. Pharmacokinetic data are not available for the cat.

Adverse effects

- In humans the incidence and severity of adverse effects are relatively low but include diplopia, ataxia, vertigo, mild gastrointestinal toxicity, idiosyncratic blood dyscrasias (aplastic anemia, leukopenia) and skin rash.

- Carbamazepine induces secretion of antidiuretic hormone.

Known drug interactions

Because of induction of hepatic metabolism, the pharmacokinetics of other drugs undergoing hepatic metabolism are likely to be affected.

Valproic acid

Clinical applications

Valproic acid is an effective anticonvulsant in humans, particularly for petit mal or absence seizures, but it has not been extensively evaluated in dogs. Therapeutic blood levels in humans are 50–100 μg/mL. Since it is not possible to attain therapeutic blood levels even with high-dose therapy or sustained-release formulations, valproic acid is of limited usefulness in dogs. A clinical trial in the early 1980s suggested that valproic acid might have a role as an adjunctive anticonvulsant in dogs with refractory epilepsy but there has been no further work on its clinical efficacy. Reports of the clinical use of valproic acid in cats are lacking. Additional studies are necessary to evaluate the efficacy of this drug.

Mechanism of action

The anticonvulsant activity of valproic acid is similar to that of phenytoin, in that it prolongs recovery of voltage-activated sodium channels from inactivation.

Formulations and dose rates

The trade names of the drug include Valproate® and Depakene®.

DOGS

- 180 mg/kg divided PO q.8 h

Pharmacokinetics

Valproic acid is rapidly absorbed from the gastrointestinal tract. Bioavailability is 80% following oral administration. The half-life of valproic acid is much shorter in dogs than in humans (1.2–3.7 h versus 9–22 h). This species difference is in part due to the lower plasma protein binding of valproic acid in dogs (78–80% in dogs versus 80–95% in humans), permitting a more rapid elimination. Because of the lower plasma protein binding of valproic acid, higher concentrations of the drug are available to enter the CSF (20% versus 10% in humans) and lower plasma concentrations may therefore be sufficient for anticonvulsive effects. Valproic acid is extensively metabolized in the liver, predominantly by β-oxidation, and 3–7% is excreted unchanged in the urine. Some metabolites of valproic acid have anticonvulsant activity; however, they are much less potent than the parent compound. It is hypothesized that the concentrations of active valproic acid metabolites reached in the dog brain may be sufficient to have anticonvulsive properties.

Adverse effects

- In humans, valproic acid usually is well tolerated and relatively free of adverse effects. Adverse effects include thinning and curling of hair, nausea, vomiting, abdominal pain, tremor and weight gain.
- Idiosyncratic hepatotoxicity may occur.
- There is an increased incidence in spina bifida in children whose mothers ingested valproic acid during pregnancy.

Known drug interactions

Valproic acid may increase serum levels of phenobarbital.

Felbamate

Clinical applications

Felbamate is a dicarbamate anticonvulsant released for use in humans in 1993 for the control of partial seizures. Pharmacokinetic and toxicity studies in 40 beagles confirmed that felbamate has a wide margin of safety, with few adverse effects. Felbamate does not cause sedation and may be added to phenobarbital and/or bromide without potentiation of the sedative effect of these drugs. It is an effective anticonvulsant when added to phenobarbital and bromide; however, controlled clinical trials have not been completed. In dogs, a hemogram should be performed and liver enzymes measured regularly to monitor for bone marrow suppression and hepatotoxicity. This is especially important in animals receiving concurrent phenobarbital. It has not been evaluated in cats.

Mechanism of action

The mechanism of anticonvulsant action is unknown. Felbamate appears to inhibit excitatory neurotransmitters and to potentiate inhibitory neurotransmitters.

Formulations and dose rates

The trade name is Felbatol®.

DOGS

- 15 mg/kg PO q.8 h, with a maximum of 300 mg/kg/d

Pharmacokinetics

Felbamate is well absorbed after oral administration. Approximately 70% of orally administered felbamate is excreted unchanged in the urine. Hepatic metabolism does occur, resulting in liver enzyme induction and causing plasma levels of felbamate to decline with longer duration of drug administration. Peak plasma concentrations occur 3–5 h after oral dosing, with an elimination half-life of 5–6 h.

Adverse effects

- The toxicity is low; adverse effects in dogs are not evident with dosages below 300 mg/kg/d.
- Adverse effects at higher doses in dogs include ataxia, limb rigidity, tremors, salivation, emesis, reduction in bodyweight, elevation of ALT, liver disease and seizures.
- In humans, there is an increased incidence of aplastic anemia and liver toxicity.

Known drug interactions

None known.

Gabapentin

Clinical applications

In 1994 gabapentin was approved for use as an anticonvulsant for the control of partial seizures with or without secondary generalization in humans in the United States. Gabapentin is an analog of GABA and is generally used in addition to other anticonvulsant drugs in humans with intractable epilepsy, including generalized tonic-clonic and partial seizures. It is well tolerated in humans and has the advantage of not undergoing hepatic metabolism.

Although there are anecdotal reports of gabapentin as an anticonvulsant in dogs, studies of its clinical efficacy in dogs and cats are lacking.

Mechanism of action

Although the exact mechanism of its anticonvulsant action is not understood, gabapentin is known to bind to receptors in the brain and as a result inhibit voltage-dependent sodium currents. It also may enhance the release of GABA.

Formulations and dose rates

The trade name is Neurontin®.

DOGS

- 25–60 mg/kg PO divided q.6 h or q.8 h

Pharmacokinetics

Gabapentin is well absorbed after oral administration and is not plasma protein bound. In dogs, unlike humans, gabapentin is metabolized to *N*-methylgabapentin but it is not known whether this has anticonvulsant activity. In urine, *N*-methylgabapentin accounts for about 32% of a single 50 mg/kg oral dosage. Elimination is primarily by the kidney. In dogs the elimination half-life is 3–4 h compared to 5–6 h in humans.

Adverse effects

- In humans, reported adverse effects include excessive sedation, gastrointestinal irritation, ataxia and dizziness.
- In dogs sedation and gastrointestinal irritation are reported.
- The dosage is reduced in people with impaired renal function.

Known drug interactions

Pharmacokinetic drug interactions have not been reported in animals.

Zonisamide

Clinical applications

Zonisamide is a sulfonamide-based anticonvulsant approved for use in humans but not in animals. It is used most frequently as an add-on therapy for dogs already receiving anticonvulsants. Zonisamide should be used with caution in dogs with renal or hepatic impairment. There are few reports on the use of zonisamide in dogs and none in cats. Serum concentrations of zonisamide may be measured.

Mechanism of action

The mechanism of action is not known. Proposed mechanisms include: blockage of T-type calcium channels; alteration of dopaminergic metabolism in the CNS; scavenging free radical species; enhancement of the action of GABA in the brain; and inhibition of carbonic anhydrase activity.

Formulations and dose rates

The trade name is Zonegran®. Zonisamide is available as 25, 50 and 100 mg capsules. Due to its low solubility, a parenteral form has not been developed.

- **DOGS:** 10 mg/kg PO q.12 h
- **CATS** (anecdotal): 5 mg/kg PO q.12

Pharmacokinetics

Zonisamide is absorbed rapidly after oral administration. It has low plasma protein binding. Zonisamide is mostly excreted unchanged in the urine although about

20% is metabolized primarily by hepatic microsomal enzymes. It does not induce liver enzymes and the half-life in the dog is about 15 h.

Adverse effects

- Adverse effects in people include transient sedation, ataxia and loss of appetite.
- Zonisamide is contraindicated in animals with a known hypersensitivity to sulfonamides. The clinician should monitor the patient for the development of adverse effects associated with sulfonamides (keratoconjuctivitis sicca (KCS), bone marrow suppression, hypersensitivity reactions (particularly skin), polyarthritis, fever).

Known drug interactions

In people, the half-life of zonisamide is dramatically reduced when concurrent medications that stimulate hepatic microsomal enzymes are given.

Levetiracetam

Clinical applications

Levetiracetam is a relatively new anticonvulsant drug. It is approved for use in humans but not in animals. Levetiracetam is a pyrrolidone derivative drug, used primarily in dogs as an add-on anticonvulsant. There are no reports on its use clinically in dogs although there is a clinical trial underway at North Carolina State University.

Mechanism of action

The mechanism of action is not known.

Formulations and dose rates

The trade name is Keppra®. It is available in tablets (different color for each size) and a clear, grape-flavored liquid.

- Dogs and cats: 20 mg/kg PO q.8 h

Pharmacokinetics

Levetiracetam is rapidly absorbed after oral administration and about 90% is excreted in the urine. It is minimally protein bound (<10%). Some of the drug is metabolized by hydrolysis to the acid derivative. The half-life ranges from 2.3 to 3.6 h in dogs. The median half-life in cats is 5.3 h.

Adverse effects

- Sedation is the most common adverse effect noted in people and dogs.
- Restlessness, vomiting and ataxia are reported in dogs.

Known drug interactions

No drug interactions are known.

FURTHER READING

Boothe DM 1998 Anticonvulsant therapy in small animals. Vet Clin North Am Small Anim Pract 28(2): 411-448

Dewey CW, Kortz GD 2004 Alternative anticonvulsant drugs for dogs with seizure disorders. Vet Med September: 786-793

LeCouteur RA 1995 Seizures and epilepsy. In: Wheeler SJ (ed.) Manual of small animal neurology, 2nd edn. BSAVA Publications, Cheltenham, pp 95-111

Podell M 1998 Antiepileptic drug therapy. Clin Tech Small Anim Pract 13(3): 185-192

17

Drugs used in the management of heart disease and cardiac arrhythmias

Sonya G Gordon and Mark D Kittleson

BACKGROUND

Heart disease is an acquired or congenital abnormality of the cardiovascular system that can be structural, infective, degenerative, inflammatory and often genetic. Many heart diseases have a prolonged preclinical stage characterized by the presence of underlying cardiac disease and the absence of any clinical signs attributable to heart disease. During this stage the cardiovascular system adapts and compensates for the underlying abnormality in an effort to maintain a state that is free from clinical signs of cardiovascular disease. However, more often than not these adaptive mechanisms contribute to the eventual development of clinical signs and can thus be considered maladaptive. When heart disease is severe it overwhelms the ability of the heart and body to compensate and clinical signs of heart failure appear. Although not all heart diseases progress to a degree of severity that result in clinical signs, many do. The development of clinical signs attributable to heart disease identifies the development of heart failure and the onset of the clinical stage of heart disease.

Independent of underlying etiology (see Table 17.1) and species, heart failure is generally defined as the inability of the heart to deliver adequate quantities of blood to meet metabolic tissue demands with normal ventricular diastolic or atrial ('filling') pressures. Heart failure can be clinically classified as backward heart failure and forward heart failure. Backward heart failure almost always predominates and refers to elevated diastolic intraventricular and atrial pressures resulting in increased venous and capillary pressures causing the transudation of fluid into interstitial spaces (edema) or body cavities (ascites). Patients with backward heart failure often have increased systemic and pulmonary blood volumes and so are hypervolemic. They may be euphemistically called 'WET'. Backward heart failure can be subdivided into right, left and biventricular backward heart failure. The clinical presentations suggestive of left-sided congestive heart failure (CHF) are those commensurate with cardiogenic pulmonary edema in dogs and cats and pleural effusion in cats. Clinical signs consistent with right-sided CHF are those commensurate with ascites and pleural effusion. Forward heart failure refers to a lower than normal cardiac output resulting in poor peripheral perfusion. Patients with forward heart failure may be euphemistically called 'COLD'. Clinical presentations suggestive of forward heart failure are those commensurate with poor peripheral perfusion such as exercise intolerance, cold extremities and collapse.

Some medical therapies for heart failure are used independent of the underlying etiology (nonspecific) and some target specific abnormalities associated with the underlying etiology. For example, any patient with cardiogenic pulmonary edema will benefit from rest, oxygen and furosemide but only patients with diastolic dysfunction, such as feline hypertrophic cardiomyopathy, would be expected to benefit from a drug that improves relaxation, such as diltiazem. In addition, many drugs have more than one mechanism of action and so may be used for a variety of indications in different patients. For example, diltiazem is also used in the treatment of atrial fibrillation because as a Class IV antiarrhythmic it can slow down AV node conduction and slow ventricular response rate (heart rate). Finally, consideration must be given to potential side effects and drug interactions as well as client (cost and ease of administration) and patient (suspension, tablet) preferences.

THERAPEUTIC APPROACH TO HEART FAILURE

Clinically we predominantly manage patients with signs of backward heart failure. Isolated forward heart failure is rare. However, patients with signs of backward heart failure are at risk for forward heart failure and thus management of backward heart failure should include therapies targeting preservation of perfusion. In general,

Table 17.1 Causes of heart failure – pathophysiological classification

Heart failure can occur as a result of:

- **Primary reduction of myocardial contractility**
  - Dilated cardiomyopathy
  - Taurine deficiency
  - Chronic myocarditis (rare)
- **Systolic mechanical overload**

Pressure overloading
  - Aortic stenosis and pulmonic stenosis (rare)
  - Pulmonary hypertension

Volume overloading
  - Chronic degenerative valve disease
  - Mitral (rare) and tricuspid dysplasia (relatively rare)
  - Aortic or pulmonic insufficiency (rare)
  - Congenital left-to-right shunts, e.g. patent ductus arteriosus, ventricular septal defect (rare)
- **Diastolic mechanical inhibition**

Pericardial disorders, e.g. pericarditis, cardiac neoplasms
Ventricular myocardial disorders, e.g. feline hypertrophic and restrictive cardiomyopathies (rare)
- **Altered electrical function**

Dysrhythmias

the goal of heart failure therapies is to relieve/reduce clinical signs of backward heart failure, improve/preserve clinical signs of forward heart failure and prolong survival. Some medications work in more than one category, enhancing their potential clinical utility. For example, pimobendan reduces preload and afterload through mixed arterial and venous dilation, augments ventricular systolic function, may help palliate clinical signs attributed to pulmonary artery hypertension and have salutary effects on the maladaptive cytokine profile in heart failure.

Table 17.2 contains an overview of cardiovascular pharmacology. Agents are classified into categories based on mechanism of action. Table 17.3 contains a summary of cardiovascular medications used in the management of common small animal heart disease and is broken down by stage of disease, e.g. clinical versus preclinical. Tables 17.4a and 17.4b provide an overview of the common drugs and their indications in the management of cardiac disease in dogs (17.4a) and cats (17.4b).

Many drugs have more than one mechanism. For example, spironolactone is an aldosterone antagonist that acts as a potassium-sparing diuretic and a neuroendocrine modulator. Enalapril is an angiotensin converting enzyme (ACE) inhibitor with vasodilatory and neuroendocrine modulation properties. For the purpose of this chapter, an agent that has more than one effect will be mentioned in every appropriate section but the majority of the discussion and dosing recommendations will be covered in the section that represents its primary use. In addition, formulations and dose rates are not included for agents that currently have little to no clinical use in small animal veterinary medicine.

Therapeutic approach to backward heart failure (WET)

Relieve clinical signs of congestion

1. Abdominocentesis (dog) and pleurocentesis (cat, rarely dog) as required
2. Preload reduction
   a. Plasma volume reduction
      i. Diuretics such as furosemide, hydrochlorothiazide, spironolactone (especially right heart failure)
   b. Venodilation
      i. Nitroglycerine (topical), pimobendan
   c. Dietary sodium restriction
3. Inhibition of the renin-angiotensin-aldosterone system (RAAS)
   a. ACE inhibitors such as enalapril or benazepril
   b. Aldosterone antagonist such as spironolactone
4. Improve diastolic dysfunction if present
   a. Feline hypertrophic cardiomyopathy
      i. Calcium channel blocker such as diltiazem

Therapeutic approach to forward heart failure (COLD)

Improve forward cardiac output

1. Afterload reduction
   a. Contraindicated in feline obstructive cardiomyopathy and canine subaortic stenosis
      i. ACE inhibitors, hydralazine, amlodipine, pimobendan, Na nitroprusside (IV)
2. Augment systolic myocardial function in diseases characterized by systolic myocardial dysfunction
   a. Canine and feline dilated cardiomyopathy (DCM)
   b. Canine chronic valve disease (CVD)
      i. Pimobendan, dobutamine (IV), digoxin (weak inotrope)
3. Treat clinically important (hemodynamically significant) arrhythmias
   a. Tachyarrhythmias
      i. Ventricular
         Lidocaine (IV), procainamide, sotalol, amiodarone
      ii. Supraventricular (excluding sinus tachycardia)
         Digoxin, β-blocker, calcium channel blocker, amiodarone, sotalol
   b. Bradyarrhythmias
      i. Pacemaker

Table 17.2 Cardiovascular pharmacology overview

Category	Common drugs	Common indications
Afterload reducers	1. Hydralazine [O;****;2] 2. ACE inhibitor [O;*;2]: e.g. enalapril, benazepril 3. Calcium channel blocker: amlodipine [O;****;4] 4. Pimobendan [O;***;2] 5. Nitroprusside [I;*****;1]	1. Systemic hypertension 2. Systolic dysfunction: – Dilated cardiomyopathy (DCM) – Chronic valvular disease (CVD)
Preload reducers	A. Diuretics: 1. Furosemide [O,I,S,M;*****;5] 2. Spironolactone [O;*;1] 3. Thiazides [O;**;2] B. Venodilators 1. Nitroglycerin [I;T;*;1] 2. Pimobendan [O,**,2]	1. Left-sided and right-sided congestive heart failure (CHF) Note: spironolactone may be more useful in right heart failure
Positive inotropes (↑ strength of contraction)	1. Digoxin [O;1/4*;1] 2. Pimobendan [O; ****;5] 3. Adrenergic agonists: e.g. dobutamine [I;*****;4], epinephrine [1;***,2]	1. Systolic dysfunction: – DCM – CVD
Positive lusiotropes (improve relaxation)	1. Ca channel blocker: diltiazem [O;***;2] 2. β-blocker: atenolol [O;**;3], carvedilol [O;**;1]	1. Diastolic dysfunction: – Hypertrophic cardiomyopathy (HCM)
Positive chronotropes (↑ heart rate)	1. Adrenergic agonists: dobutamine [I;***;2], isoproterenol [I,****;2] 2. Anticholinergics [I,S,M;****;4]: atropine, glycopyrrolate	1. Hemodynamically important bradyarrhythmias, e.g. sinus bradycardia, AV block
Negative chronotropes	1. β-blocker [O;***;2]: atenolol, carvedilol 2. Ca channel blocker: diltiazem [O;***;3] 3. Digoxin [O;**;2] 4. Amiodarone [O;***;4]	1. Tachycardia: atrial fibrillation and other hemodynamically significant supraventricular arrhythmias Note: often require combination therapy, e.g. digoxin and diltiazem
Vasopressors (peripheral vasoconstriction)	1. Adrenergic agonists: dopamine, [I,***,2], epinephrine [I;***;2] 2. Vasopressin [I;***;3]	1. Hypotension that is <u>unrelated</u> to low cardiac output, e.g. shock, endothelial dysfunction
Neurohumoral modulators	1. β-blockers: carvedilol [O;***;4] 2. ACE inhibitors [O;****;5]: enalapril 3. Aldosterone antagonist: spironolactone [O;**;4] 4. Digoxin [O;**;2]	1. This category of medication is used in an attempt to delay the progression of both preclinical and clinical heart disease and combination therapy may be superior to monotherapy, e.g. ACE inhibitor + β-blocker Dog: DCM and CVD Cat: cardiomyopathies
<u>Antiarrhythmics</u>: Class I (#1–4) Class II (#5) Class III (#6&7) Class IV (#8) Other (#9)	1. Lidocaine [I;*****;5] 2. A Procainamide [I,M;***;4] B Procainamide [O;**;2] 3. Quinidine [O,I;***;2, only horses) 4. Mixelitine [O;***;2] 5. β-blockers [O;**;2] 6. Amiodarone [O,I;****;4] 7. Sotalol [O;****;4] 8. Ca channel blocker: diltiazem [O,I;***;4] 9. Digoxin [O;**;2]	1. Acute ventricular arrhythmias (VA) 2. A Acute supraventricular arrhythmias (SVA) B Chronic VA 3. Atrial fibrillation 4. Chronic VA (better in combination with 5) 5. Chronic SVA and VA (usually in combination) 6. Chronic and acute SVA and VA 7. Chronic VA (especially boxers) 8. Acute and chronic SVA 9. Chronic SVA (best in combination with 5 or 8)

[Route of delivery; Relative potency in category as monotherapy; Author preference/frequency of use within category], where route of administration (O, oral; I, IV; S, SQ; M, intramuscular; T, topical). Relative drug potency by effect within a category when used as monotherapy (****high, *low). Authors' preference by category (5 high, 1 low). If [O,**,4] is for the whole class it follows the class, e.g. ACE inhibitors, but if it is for a specific drug within a class it follows each drug, e.g. diuretics. Note potencies are for category that drug is listed in and authors' preference is for category effect and some drugs appear in more than one category because they have polypharmacy effects. For example, pimobendan is a strong positive inotrope and is our first preference in this category as an oral drug and although it is an afterload reducer and this is a desirable property, if we need to select an afterload reducer we would pick amlodipine empirically as it is more potent but we would still use pimobendan for its combination of effects in canine CHF.

Note: Most common SVA = atrial fibrillation.

Table 17.3 Summary of cardiovascular medications used in the management of common heart disease

Species		Disease	Preclinical Stage	Clinical Stage
Dog	Chronic valve disease	Sinus rhythm	NT [3], ACEI [2], β-blocker [2]	Diuretic (furosemide) [5]*, Pimobendan [5]*, ACEI [5], spironolactone [3], β-blocker [1]
		Atrial fibrillation or other supraventricular arrhythmias	NT [2], β-blocker [2]	As per sinus rhythm and add: amiodarone [3], digoxin [3], β-blocker [3], CCB [3] *Note: combination therapy may be necessary*
		Ventricular arrhythmias	NT [2], β-blocker [3]	As per sinus rhythm and add: sotalol [3], β-blocker & mexilitine [1]
		Left atrial enlargement causing left main stem bronchus compression	NT [2], ACEI [2], β-blocker [1–2]	As per sinus rhythm and add: theophylline SR [4], hydrocodone [3]
		Pulmonary artery hypertension		As per sinus rhythm: increase pimbendan dosing frequency to 3 times daily [4] and/or add sildenafil [3]
	Dilated cardiomyopathy	Sinus rhythm	NT [1], ACEI [4]*, β-blocker [2]	Diuretic (furosemide) [5]*, Pimobendan [5]*, ACEI [5]*, spironolactone [3], β-blocker [1]
		Atrial fibrillation or other supraventricular arrhythmias	NT [1], β-blocker [3], CCB [2]	As per sinus rhythm and add: amiodarone [3], digoxin [3], β-blocker [2], CCB [2] *Note: combination therapy may be necessary*
		Ventricular arrhythmias	ACEI [4], β-blocker [3]	As per sinus rhythm and add: amiodarone [3], sotalol [3], β-blocker & mexilitine [2], mexilitine [1]
Cat	Hypertrophic cardiomyopathy		ACEI [3], CCB [2], β-blocker [3]	Diuretic (furosemide) [5]*, ACEI [4]*, CCB [1], β-blocker [1–2]
	Intermediate or restrictive cardiomyopathy		ACEI [3], CCB [1], β-blocker [1]	Diuretic (furosemide) [5]*, ACEI [5]*, CCB [1], β-blocker [1]
	Dilated cardiomyopathy		ACEI [4], β-blocker [1] +/– taurine	Diuretic (furosemide) [5]*, ACEI [5]*, β-blocker [1]
	Arrhythmogenic right ventricular cardiomyopathy		ACEI [3–4], β-blocker [1]	Diuretic (furosemide) [4], ACEI [5], sotalol [3]

Note: *Clinical disease* is defined as the stage of disease when a patient ***has or had*** clinical signs attributable to their cardiovascular disease (e.g. cough due to cardiogenic pulmonary edema and or left atrial enlargement causing left main stem bronchial compression either at the time of the current exam or previously). Thus dogs with clinical disease may not have current clinical signs of disease if they are stable on medication. ***Preclinical disease*** is defined as the stage of disease when a patient has evidence of cardiovascular disease but currently or previously has no clinical signs that can be attributed to their underlying cardiovascular disease e.g. clinically normal dogs with heart murmurs characteristic of chronic valve disease or evidence of radiographic or echocardiographic left atrial enlargement who historically and currently have no clinical signs of cardiovascular disease. There is no definitive proof that any medication used during the preclinical stage of any listed disease can prolong the preclinical stage thus the numbers in [ ] represent the authors' views of current recommendations and no therapy is always an option.

Drugs are listed by class (e.g. angiotensin converting enzyme inhibitor) and if there is a preferred drug within a class it follows in brackets. Each class or specific drug listed is scored between 1 and 5 where [1] means rarely used and [5] means always used unless there is a clinical contraindication. Diuretic (furosemide) is always used if congestion is or was present. * denotes which medication should be used if number or medications to be used is limited. This summary is based on professional opinion/experience and currently available peer reviewed data and can be expected to evolve over time.

Angiotensin converting enzyme inhibitor (ACEI); beta-blocker (β-blocker); calcium channel blocker (CCB); no therapy (NT).

Table 17.4a Drugs commonly used for the therapy of canine heart failure

Drug	Preparation	Dosage	Indications (I) and potential toxicity (T)
AMIODARONE	Cordarone or generic (cheaper): 200, 400 mg tablets	DOG: 10-20 mg/kg q.24 h for 7-10 days then reduce to 3-15 mg/kg q.24-48 h chronically	I: hemodynamically significant ventricular or supraventricular arrhythmias (SVT, atrial fib) T: anorexia and elevated liver enzymes, neutropenia, etc. and potential proarrhythmic
AMLODIPINE Note: gradual uptitration required	Norvasc: 2.5, 5 mg tablets	DOG: 0.01-1 mg/kg PO q.12-24 h	I: hypertension T: hypotension
ATENOLOL Note: gradual uptitration required	Tenormin: 25, 50, 100 mg tablets	DOG: 6.25-12.5 mg q.12 h	I: diastolic dysfunction and hemodynamically significant ventricular or supraventricular arrhythmias (SVT, atrial fib) T: negative inotrope and chronotrope, beware decompensation
BENAZEPRIL	Lotensin: 5, 10, 20, 40 mg tablets	DOG: 0.3-0.5 mg/kg q.12-24 h	I: CHF (CVD, DCM), systemic hypertension T: beware azotemia and potential for interaction with NSAIDS
CARVEDILOL Note: gradual uptitration required	Coreg: 3.125, 6.25, 12.5, 25 mg tablets Note: can split in two but hard to split in 4. Can be formulated into suspension	DOG: 0.1-1 mg/kg PO q.12 h Note: 1 mg/kg is target dose and you will need to uptitrate to achieve this dose safely	I: occult systolic dysfunction (CVD, DCM) T: negative inotrope and chronotrope, beware decompensation
DIGOXIN	Lanoxin, Cardoxin, Digoxin USP: 0.125, 0.25, 0.5 mg tablets; 0.05 mg/mL and 0.15 mg/mL elixirs	DOG: 0.0055-0.011 mg/kg q.12 h or 0.22 mg/meter sq.body surface area q.12 h Note: err on low dose side to limit toxicity	I: heart failure, supraventricular tachyarrhythmias (SVT, atrial fib) T: GI (anorexia and vomiting), arrhythmias Note: toxicity potentiated by renal insufficiency
DILTIAZEM Note: gradual uptitration required	A. Nonsustained release: Cardizem: 30, 60, 90, 120 mg tablets B. Sustained release: Dilacor XR	DOG: 0.5-1.3 mg/kg orally q.8 h DOG: 2-4 mg/kg orally q.12 h	I: hemodynamically significant supraventricular arrhythmias (SVT, atrial fib) T: negative inotrope and chronotrope, beware decompensation
DOBUTAMINE	Dobutrex: 250 mg (20 mL) vial for injection	DOG: 2.5-20 μg/kg/min, constant rate IV infusion	I: severe systolic dysfunction (CVD, DCM) T: tachyarrhythmias
ENALAPRIL	Enacard: 1, 2.5, 5, 10 mg tablets	DOG: 0.25-0.5 mg/kg orally once or twice daily	I: CHF (CVD, DCM), systemic hypertension T: beware azotemia and potential for interaction with NSAIDS
FUROSEMIDE	Lasix: 12.5 [Vet] mg, 20, 40, 50 [Vet], 80 mg tablets; 1% syrup (10 mg/mL)	DOG: 2-6 mg/kg repeated q.2-12 h as needed (IV, IM, SQ, oral)	I: CHF T: hypotension, dehydration, hypokalemia, metabolic alkalosis
HYDRALAZINE Note: gradual uptitration required	Apresoline: 10, 25, 50 mg tablets	DOG: 0.5-3 mg/kg orally q.12 h (initial dose 0.5 mg/kg, titrate to effect or to at least 1 mg/kg q.12 h)	I: CHF, hypertension T: hypotension, GI
HYDROCHLOROTHIAZIDE (HCT) and SPIRONOLACTONE	Hydrodiuril, USP: 25, 50 mg tablets; Aldactazide: 25 mg HCT combined with 25 mg spironolactone	DOG: 2-4 mg/kg twice daily of either HCT or combined product Note: these are monotherapy doses	I: CHF T: hypotension, dehydration, hypokalemia, azotemia Note: reduce furosemide dose by 50% when starting HCT
LISINOPRIL	Zestril, Prinavil	DOG: 0.5 mg/kg PO q.24 h	I: CHF (CVD, DCM), systemic hypertension T: beware azotemia and potential for interaction with NSAIDS

Table 17.4a Drugs commonly used for the therapy of canine heart failure (*continued*)

Drug	Preparation	Dosage	Indications (I) and potential toxicity (T)
MEXILETINE	Mexitil: 150, 200, 250 mg capsules	DOG: 4-8 mg/kg PO q.8 h	I: hemodynamically significant ventricular arrhythmias T: anorexia and liver toxicity and potential proarrhythmic Note: may work best when combined with atenolol
PIMOBENDAN	Vetmedin: 1.25, 2.5, 5 mg capsules Note: not available in USA yet	DOG: 0.25-0.3 mg/kg PO q.12 h	I: CHF (CVD, DCM), pulmonary artery hypertension T: potential proarrhythmic?, hypotension
CLOPIDOGREL	Plavix 75 mg tablet	DOG: 1-2 mg/kg PO q.24 h Chronic (after 3 weeks) 1 mg/kg q.24 h Loading for acute effects (with in 90 min) 10 mg/kg PO	I: antiplatelet T: potential bleeding Note: If von Willebrand's deficiency is possible a VMB level should be determined before starting Plavix. Bleeding times are not sufficient
PROCAINAMIDE (sustained release)	Pronestyl SR or generic procainamide SR 250, 500, 750, 1000 mg oral 100 mg/mL, 10 mL vial or 500 mg/mL, 2 mL vial	DOG: 10-20 mg/kg PO q.8 h 5-25 mg/kg slow IV (10 min) 25-50 μg/kg/min as CRI to effect	I: hemodynamically significant ventricular and supraventricular (IV only) arrhythmias T: oral– anorexia, coat color change; IV –hypotension and potential proarrhythmic
NITROGLYCERIN	Nitrol, Nitro-bid, Nitrostat: one inch = 15 mg NTG; Minitran transderm patches 2.5, 5, 10, 15 mg/24 h	DOG: 4-12 mg (up to 15 mg) topically q.12 h	I: CHF T: hypotension
SILDENAFIL Note: gradual uptitration required	Viagra: 25, 50, 100 mg tablets	DOG: 0.25-3 mg/kg PO q.12 h	I: end-stage pulmonary artery hypertension T: hypotension Note: slow uptitration preferred but may be rapid in acute situation
SOTALOL	Betapace: 80, 160, 240 mg tablets	DOG: 0.5-2 mg/kg PO q.12 h	I: hemodynamically significant ventricular arrhythmias T: negative inotrope and chronotrope, beware decompensation, and potential proarrhythmic
SPIRONOLACTONE	Aldactone: 25, 50, 100 mg tablets	DOG: 0.25-1 mg/kg PO q.12 h antifibrotic effects DOG: 1-2 mg/kg PO q.12 h for diuretic effect	I: reverse remodeling, K-sparing diuresis, RAAS inhibition T: hyperkalemia especially when combined with an ACEI in the absence of furosemide

Echo sedation: (1) Preclinical young dog: combination of buprenorphine (0.007 mg/kg, IV or IM) and acepromazine (0.02–0.03 mg/kg, never >1 mg total, IV or IM). (2) Older or clinical dog: buprenorphine (0.007 mg/kg, IV or IM). (3) Dyspneic or very old clinical dog: butorphanol 0.2 mg/kg, IV or IM.
Taurine supplementation: Medium dog: 500 mg q.12 h; large dog: 1000 mg q.12 h.
L-carnitine supplementation: 1–3 g q.12 h.
Note: Therapeutic recommendations reflect the authors' opinion and are based on review of available data.

ii. Anticholinergics
Propantheline bromide
Atropine sulfate (IV)
iii. Sympathomimetics
Terbutaline
iv. Other
Theopylline

4. Treat pulmonary artery hypertension if present and contributing to clinical signs

a. Phosphodiesterase V inhibition
i. Sildenifil, pimobendan

Therapeutic approach for all heart failure (WET or COLD)

Agents in this category have the potential to prolong survival in all patients with clinical heart disease or heart failure. Medications that improve perfusion and/

Table 17.4b Feline cardiovascular medication chart

Drug	Class	Dose (per cat)	Dose (mg/kg)
Enalapril* or benazepril*	ACEI	PO: 1-2.5 mg q.12-24 h	PO: 0.2-0.7 mg/kg q.12-24 h
1. Diltiazem 2. Cardizem CD 3. Dilacor XR	Calcium channel blocker	1. PO: 7.5 mg q.8 h 3. PO: 30-60 mg q.12-24 h	2. PO: 10 mg/kg q.24 h
Atenolol*	β-blocker	PO: 3.125-12.5 mg q.12-24 h	PO: 1.1-2.5 mg/kg q.12-24 h
Atenolol, low dose*	β-blocker	PO: 1-3.125 mg q.24 h Uptitrate if well tolerated	
Furosemide*	Diuretic	PO: 3.125-12.5 mg q.12-48 h	PO: 1-2 mg/kg q.12-48 h IV/IM/SQ: 0.5-2 mg/kg PRN
Hydrochlorothiazide*	Diuretic	PO: 6.25-12.5 mg q.12 h	PO: 2-4 mg/kg q.12 h
Spironolactone*	Aldosterone antagonist	PO: 6.25 mg q.12 h	PO: 1-2 mg/kg q.12 h
Digoxin	Cardiac glycoside	PO: 0.031 mg q.24-48 h 1/4 of 0.125 mg tablet	
Aspirin	NSAID	PO: 81 mg q.3 d	PO: 25 mg/kg q.3 d
Sotalol*	Antiarrhythmic β-blocker	PO: 10 mg q.12 h	
Nitroglycerin paste	Vasodilator	Topical: 1/8-1/4 inch q.6-8 h	
Low molecular weight heparin	Antithrombotic		SQ: 100 IU/kg q.12-24 h
Butorphanol	Anxiolytic		IV/IM/SQ: 0.2 mg/kg PRN
Taurine	Amino acid	PO: 250-500 mg q.12 h	
Clopidogrel (Plavix)	Thienopyridine	18.75-75 mg PO q.24 h	

Can be formulated as a suspension by a formulation pharmacy.
Echo sedation medetomadine 20 μg/kg IM.
Note: Therapeutic recommendations reflect the authors' opinion and are based on review of available data.

or reduce congestion can be expected to reduce euthanasia-associated mortality.

Prolong survival

1. Inhibition of the RAAS
   a. ACE inhibitors
      i. Enalapril, benazepril
   b. Aldosterone antagonism
      i. Spironolactone
2. Inhibition of the sympathetic nervous system
   a. β-Blockers
      i. Atenolol and metroprolol (selective), propranolol (nonselective; unproven in dogs and cats)
   b. Adrenergic blockers (α- and β-blockade)
      i. Carvedilol
3. Improve diastolic function
   a. Feline hypertrophic cardiomyopathy (HCM)
      i. Calcium channel blocker such as diltiazem
      ii. β-Blocker such as atenolol (prolongs diastolic filling period)
4. Other
   a. Modulation of cytokine maladaption
      i. Pimobendan
   b. Prevention of thrombosis in heart diseases associated with increased risk
      i. Feline hypertrophic cardiomyopathy
         Antiplatelet agents such as clopidogrel
         Anticoagulants such as coumadin, heparin (IV, SQ) and low molecular weight heparin (IV, SQ)
   c. Antioxidants
      i. Carvedilol
      ii. Omega 3 fatty acid supplementation
   d. Complementary therapy
      i. Taurine
      ii. L-carnitine

Therapeutic approach for preclinical heart disease

Agents in this class target primarily mechanisms involved in the progression of heart disease. However, to date, no therapeutic agent has been demonstrated to delay the progression of any canine or feline preclinical heart disease and thus agents listed in this section are candidate therapies.

Prolong preclinical stage of disease

1. Inhibition of the RAAS
   a. ACE inhibitors
      i. Enalapril, benazepril
   b. Aldosterone antagonism
      i. Spironolactone

2. Inhibition of the sympathetic nervous system
   a. β-Blockers
      i. Atenolol and metroprolol (selective), propranolol (nonselective)
   b. Adrenergic blockers (α- and β-blockade)
      i. Carvedilol
3. Improve diastolic function
   a. Feline hypertrophic cardiomyopathy
      i. Calcium channel blocker such as diltiazem
      ii. β-Blocker such as atenolol
4. Other
   a. Prevention of thrombosis in heart diseases associated with increased risk
      i. Feline hypertrophic cardiomyopathy
         Antiplatelet agents such as clopidogrel
         Anticoagulants such as coumadin, heparin (IV, SQ) and low molecular weight heparin (IV, SQ)
   b. Antioxidants
      i. Carvedilol
      ii. Omega 3 fatty acid supplementation
   c. Complementary therapy
      i. Taurine
      ii. L-carnitine

WHICH THERAPY FOR WHICH CONDITION?

To date, there are few adequately powered prospective veterinary clinical studies to support definitive therapeutic recommendations regarding the treatment of clinical and preclinical heart disease secondary to any etiology. Evidence-based therapeutic recommendations for most cardiac diseases await adequately powered prospective clinical trials. Until that time, therapeutic decisions in patients with clinical signs of heart disease should be based on specific clinical signs, characterization of the underlying heart disease and individual response to therapy. In patients with preclinical heart disease therapeutic recommendations should be made based on the presence, severity and prognosis for the underlying cardiac disease. Finally, all therapeutic recommendations should be made in light of any important comorbidities and should be guided by follow-up evaluations as well as client and patient preferences.

The following classification system was modified from that of the American College of Cardiology and the American Heart Association.

Grade A evidence: Recommendations derived from multiple randomized clinical trials

Grade B evidence: Recommendations derived from small randomized trials and careful analysis of descriptive retrospective and case–control studies

Grade C evidence: Recommendations based on expert opinion and extrapolation from human and experimental literature

However, it is of interest to note that diuretics are inarguably useful to ameliorate clinical signs of congestion despite the absence of Grade A and Grade B data and remain a cornerstone of conventional CHF therapy independent of underlying etiology.

Canine dilated cardiomyopathy (DCM)

Preclinical

ACE inhibitors have been demonstrated to prolong the preclinical stage of DCM in some Doberman pinschers and may be more beneficial in males than females (Grade B evidence). There is overwhelming support for their use in human preclinical DCM and they are commonly used in preclinical canine DCM (Grade C evidence). As there is strong support in the human literature for the use of gradual β-blockade in human DCM, scientific rationale supports their potential utility in preclinical canine DCM (Grade C evidence). One small clinical trial, however, did not show any benefit.

Clinical

In addition to diuretics for the amelioration of clinical signs of congestion, there is strong evidence to support the use of ACE inhibitors and pimobendan in clinical canine DCM (Grade A and C evidence). Other agents may be useful in certain cases such as carnitine and taurine supplementation in cocker spaniels with clinical DCM (Grade B evidence). Gradual β-blockade improves mortality in people with DCM but has not been prospectively evaluated in the dog and carries a relative risk of decompensation in all patients with heart failure (Grade C evidence). Spironolactone has been demonstrated to reduce mortality in human patients with DCM and thus may be useful in clinical canine DCM but remains unevaluated in the veterinary literature at this time (Grade C evidence).

Canine chronic degenerative AV valve disease (CVD)

Preclinical

ACE inhibitors have been demonstrated *not* to prolong the preclinical stage of CVD (Grade B evidence). There is some scientific rationale and short-term canine clinical trials that suggest that gradual β-blockade may prolong the preclinical stage of CVD (Grade C evidence). Thus currently no medication has been proven to prolong the preclinical stage of canine CVD.

Clinical

In addition to diuretics for the amelioration of clinical signs of congestion, there is strong evidence to support the use of ACE inhibitors and pimobendan in clinical canine CVD (Grade A and C evidence). Gradual β-blockade may be useful, but has not been prospectively evaluated, in the dog and carries a relative risk of decompensation in all patients with heart failure (Grade C evidence). Digoxin and spironolactone have been demonstrated to reduce mortality and/or morbidity in human patients with clinical DCM. They therefore may be useful in clinical canine CVD but remain unevaluated in the veterinary literature (Grade C evidence).

Feline cardiomyopathies

Given the absence of clinical trial data on specific cardiomyopathies, comments will be made in general and any exceptions will be mentioned.

Preclinical

There are no definitive recommendations for any cardiomyopathy. In general, recommendations reflect the underlying severity of the cardiomyopathy in combination with an agent's safety, tolerability (dosing form and frequency) and potential to prolong the preclinical stage based on scientific rationale (Grade C evidence).

- There is no evidence that hypertrophic cardiomyopathy (HCM) benefits from diltiazem or an ACE inhibitor.
- Patients with hypertrophic obstructive cardiomyopathy (HOCM) may benefit from a β-blocker.
- There is no evidence that any drug alters the natural history of arrhythmogenic right ventricular cardiomyopathy (ARVC).
- If dilated cardiomyopathy (DCM) is due to taurine deficiency, taurine supplementation is generally curative (Grade B evidence). There is no evidence that any other intervention is beneficial.

Clinical

In addition to diuretics for the amelioration of clinical signs of congestion, there is evidence to support the use of ACE inhibitors in all feline cardiomyopathies (Grade B and C evidence). In addition, all cats with significant left atrial enlargement have an increased risk of thromboembolic complications and may benefit from thrombotic prophylaxis such as clopidogrel (Grade C evidence). Additional therapies may be indicated on an individual basis.

DRUGS USED TO TREAT HEART FAILURE

DIURETICS

EXAMPLES

Loop diuretics: furosemide, bumetanide, ethacrynic acid
Thiazide diuretics: hydrochlorothiazide, chlorothiazide
Potassium-sparing diuretics: spironolactone, triamterene, amiloride

Clinical applications

In most patients with heart failure, edema is primarily the direct consequence of an increase in blood volume. Blood volume may be increased by as much as 30% in dogs with severe heart failure. Diuretics decrease edema formation by decreasing this excess blood volume. The decrease in blood volume results in decreases in diastolic intraventricular, venous and capillary pressures.

Diuretics, especially the loop diuretics, are the most important and most efficacious class of drugs used for treating heart failure. Most heart failure patients, if left untreated, would die of severe edema or effusions. Consequently, the primary goal in these patients is to control the formation of edema and effusion. Although other agents, such as ACE inhibitors, nitrates and pimobendan, and sodium-restricted diets may be used for this purpose, their ability to control edema formation is at least one order of magnitude less than the loop diuretics such as furosemide.

Mechanism of action

Diuretics increase urine flow by increasing renal plasma flow or by altering nephron function. Diuretics that increase renal plasma flow by expanding plasma volume (e.g. mannitol, hetastarch) are contraindicated in patients with heart failure because they increase venous and capillary pressures and thus increase edema formation. Agents that alter nephron function increase urine production by interfering with ion transport or the action of aldosterone or antidiuretic hormone (ADH) within the nephron.

Agents that interfere with ion transport do so by altering (1) intracellular ionic entry, (2) energy generation and use for ion transport, or (3) ion transfer from the cell to the peritubular capillaries through the antiluminal membrane. Agents that interfere with ion transport also differ as to their site of action within the nephron. In general, agents that act on the loop of Henle are the most potent.

Three classes of diuretics are used clinically in dogs to treat heart failure: loop diuretics, thiazide diuretics and potassium-sparing diuretics. They differ in their ability to promote sodium and thus water excretion and in mechanism of action. The loop diuretics are the most potent and can be used in small doses in patients with mild to moderate heart failure and in higher doses in patients with severe heart failure. They can be administered orally for chronic administration or can be administered parenterally to patients with acute, severe heart failure. Thiazide diuretics are mildly to moderately potent agents. They are most commonly used in conjunction with a loop diuretic in patients with severe CHF that have become refractory to loop diuretics over time. Historically, the use of potassium-sparing diuretics has been reserved for those patients that become hypokalemic secondary to the use of other diuretics and for patients refractory to other agents because of an elevated plasma aldosterone concentration. In the latter situation, potassium-sparing diuretics are administered in conjunction with another diuretic, usually a loop diuretic. More recently, the potassium-sparing diuretic and aldosterone antagonist spironolactone has been used as an inhibitor of the renin-angiotensin-aldosterone system alone or in combination with an ACE inhibitor. If it is used in combination with an ACE inhibitor there is a risk of clinically significant hyperkalemia. This is minimized if furosemide is administered concurrently.

Adverse effects

Diuretic therapy has the potential to cause undesirable effects, primarily electrolyte disturbances, dehydration and prerenal and renal azotemia. The relative risks of azotemia are heightened when they are used concurrently with ACE inhibitors and/or nonsteroidal anti-inflammatories (NSAIDs) and other potential renal toxins. Diuretics may also increase the risk of digoxin toxicity.

Electrolyte abnormalities

- Electrolyte disturbances are less common in dogs and cats than they are in humans. However, they can occur, especially in those canine and feline patients that are not eating and/or drinking normally, or in patients administered acute, high-dose therapy.
- Cats appear to be more susceptible than dogs to becoming electrolyte depleted and dehydrated with diuretic therapy. This may be because of a species difference in drug effect but is more probably caused by the fact that cats tend to stop eating and drinking more readily when they are unwell.
- Hypokalemia is one of the more common undesirable effects. However, two studies have documented that the incidence of hypokalemia is low in dogs administered furosemide chronically and who are eating and drinking normally. Hypokalemia is always a significant risk, even in dogs that eat, when sequential nephron blockade is initiated with a rescue diuretic such as hydrochlorothiazide. Dogs that are hypokalemic and hypomagnesemic may not respond to potassium supplementation alone.
- Hyponatremia may occur in patients on high dose diuretic therapy. Patients with severe heart failure may also become hyponatremic through inappropriate antidiuretic hormone secretion and resultant water retention. It may be impossible to distinguish between these two causes in some heart failure patients. No primary corrective therapy is recommended.
- Hypomagnesemia may occur but the incidence in dogs with heart failure receiving diuretics is very low. In one study, there was no significant difference in serum magnesium concentration between control dogs and dogs with heart failure treated with diuretics ± digoxin. In another study of 113 dogs with heart failure, only four had a low serum magnesium concentration. Hypomagnesemia may accompany hypokalemia. Dogs that are hypokalemic and hypomagnesemic may not respond to potassium supplementation alone.

Note: electrolyte abnormalities can be profound when sequential nephron blockade is employed. Potassium supplementation may help with normalization of potassium concentrations. Hypochloremia and hyponatremia should not be corrected via supplementation of parenteral fluids.

Dehydration and prerenal azotemia

Subclinical hypovolemia (dehydration) is probably common in patients with severe heart failure that require maximum doses of diuretics to treat their heart failure. At times patients can become clinically dehydrated and, in some, prerenal azotemia will be present. If the patient is clinically affected (e.g. not eating), the diuretic dose must be reduced or discontinued temporarily and in some cases judicious intravenous fluid therapy must be employed. However, in patients that are not clinically affected by their dehydration and azotemia, the prerenal azotemia can be safely ignored as long as it is not severe or obviously progressive on serial analysis (e.g. urea <30 mmol/L).

Diuretic resistance

There are numerous factors that determine the response to diuretic therapy. These include the potency of the drug, the dosage administered, the duration of action of the drug, the route of administration, renal blood flow, glomerular filtration rate and nephron function. For example, furosemide must be delivered to its site of action in the loop of Henle to produce its effect. The number of molecules of furosemide that reach the site of action depends on the concentration of the drug in plasma and renal blood flow. The plasma concentration depends on the route of administration (intravenous administration will produce a higher concentration than oral administration) and the dose. The duration of effect will also determine the total diuretic effect produced in a certain time period.

Patients with CHF may become refractory to furosemide because of decreased delivery of the drug to the nephron as a result of reduced renal blood flow or hormonal stimulus for sodium and water retention. Drug delivery may be increased by administering a drug that may increase renal blood flow, such as an arterial dilator (e.g. hydralazine). However, afterload reduction with an arterial dilator must be done cautiously in patients with heart failure because of the risk of hypotension. Alternatively, a potent inotrope such as dobutamine (short term) or pimobendan (chronic) may improve cardiac output and thus renal blood flow. Delivery can also be increased by increasing plasma concentration. This is most readily accomplished by administering the drug parenterally (e.g. intravenous, intramuscular, subcutaneous). Administering the drug as a constant rate infusion (CRI) may be superior in the acute situation because it provides continual nephron delivery over the duration of the CRI, optimizing diuresis. However, a thoughtful bolus administration protocol works very well and does not require the special equipment that is needed for a CRI.

Heart failure and diuretic administration stimulate the RAAS, resulting in a marked increase in plasma aldosterone concentration. Aldosterone counteracts the effects of a diuretic and may contribute to diuretic resistance. Consequently, the administration of an ACE inhibitor will be beneficial if tolerated. Furosemide administration produces hypertrophy of the distal convoluted tubular cells and increases ion transport capacity in this region in rats. This shifts the dose–response curve to the right and downward in humans. If this also occurs in cats and dogs, it may also contribute to diuretic resistance.

It is possible that oral bioavailability of furosemide is decreased in patients with right heart failure. Gastroin testinal edema is the reputed offender in this scenario. However, it was documented in humans that massive fluid accumulation due to heart failure does not alter the pharmacokinetics of furosemide.

Loop diuretics

EXAMPLES

Furosemide (authors' preference), bumetanide, torsemide (torasemide), ethacrynic acid (not in dogs and cats)

Furosemide

Furosemide is a loop diuretic and the most commonly used diuretic for treating heart failure in the dog and cat. Other loop diuretics include ethacrynic acid, torsemide and bumetanide. Ethacrynic acid is not used. Bumetanide is a newer agent that is 25–50 times as potent as furosemide. Torsemide is also more potent than furosemide and has at least twice the duration of effect. There is little clinical experience with the latter two drugs in veterinary medicine. Furosemide remains the diuretic of choice in dogs and cats with heart failure.

Clinical applications

Furosemide is used as first-line therapy for treating all stages of acute and chronic heart failure secondary to all cardiac diseases except pericardial disease causing cardiac tamponade. However, pericardial effusion secondary to biventricular heart failure is managed in part with furosemide as required to control other clinical signs of congestion such as pulmonary edema. It is also used in noncardiac disease including treatment of hypercalcemia, management of ascites and edema associated with hepatic disease or nephrotic syndrome and in acute oliguric renal failure.

Mechanism of action

All loop diuretics inhibit sodium, potassium and chloride reabsorption in the thick portion of the ascending loop of Henle. In so doing, they inhibit sodium and obligatory water reabsorption in the nephron. The loop diuretics are capable of increasing the maximal fractional excretion of sodium from a normal of approximately 1% of filtered load to 15–25% of the filtered load, making them the most powerful natriuretic agents available.

Furosemide is a sulfonamide-type loop diuretic which, in addition to inhibiting sodium, potassium and chloride reabsorption in the loop of Henle, also decreases reabsorption of sodium and chloride in the distal renal tubule. Furosemide diuresis results in enhanced excretion of sodium, chloride, potassium, hydrogen, calcium, magnesium and possibly phosphate. Chloride excretion is equal to or exceeds sodium excretion. At a dose of 1.0 mg/kg to normal anesthetized dogs, furosemide increases sodium excretion approximately 17-fold. Potassium excretion is much less affected in dogs, at most twofold following furosemide administration. Magnesium excretion increases by a factor of 4 while calcium excretion increases 50-fold. Enhanced hydrogen ion excretion without a concomitant increase in bicarbonate excretion can result in metabolic alkalosis in dogs. This effect is rarely clinically significant, although it could be beneficial in dogs with pre-existing metabolic acidosis due to poor perfusion. Despite the increase in net acid excretion, urinary pH falls slightly after furosemide administration, while urine specific gravity is generally reduced to around 1.006–1.020.

In addition to its diuretic effects, furosemide acts as a mild systemic venodilator, decreasing systemic venous pressure before diuresis takes place (especially after intravenous administration). Furosemide decreases renal vascular resistance. Thus, it acutely increases renal blood flow (in the order of 50%) without changing glomerular filtration rate.

Furosemide increases thoracic duct lymph flow in dogs following high doses (8–10 mg/kg IV). This effect is independent of renal function as it occurs in nephrectomized animals. The basis for this effect is unexplained.

Furosemide acts as a bronchodilator in humans, horses and guinea-pigs. It can be administered as an inhalant in humans with asthma. Its bronchodilatory effects in dogs and cats are unknown. If it does have bronchodilatory effects in cats and dogs, it could have beneficial effects in cats with asthma and in dogs with chronic bronchitis but its use should not replace conventional therapy for these diseases. It does, however, offer an explanation for why some dogs with chronic valve disease that are not truly in heart failure and are coughing due to chronic bronchitis (small airway disease) may experience a reduction in their cough when treated with furosemide. Thus resolution or improvement of a cough following trial therapy with furosemide does not prove the patient was in heart failure. One needs to document radiographic resolution of a characteristic infiltrate in the therapeutic trial of this nature. It is important that dogs with heart disease (preclinical) that will not benefit from furosemide are not administered the drug chronically.

Formulations and dose rates

Furosemide is available in oral (tablets, suspensions) and parenteral formulations.

CANINE

Chronic heart failure

1 mg/kg PO q.12 h for mild heart failure to 5 mg/kg q.8 h (doses should be separated by at least 3 h but do not have to be exactly 8 h) for severe heart failure. When this dose fails to keep the patient free of clinical signs of congestion a second diuretic may be added (see hydrochlorothiazide). The need for the addition of a rescue diuretic is clinically relatively rare. In general, the goal with furosemide is to use the minimum dose necessary to keep the patient free of clinical signs of congestion. Dogs with mitral regurgitation secondary to CVD that are refractory to furosemide administration may also benefit from the administration of a systemic arteriolar dilator, such as amlodipine or hydralazine.

Acute heart failure

Severe pulmonary edema requires immediate intensive intravenous or intramuscular administration in dogs. Intravenous is preferred if feasible.

FUROSEMIDE DOSE SCHEDULE FOR SEVERE LIFE-THREATENING CARDIOGENIC PULMONARY EDEMA IN THE DOG

- Dependent on severity of respiratory clinical signs
- Guided by resting respiration rate with oxygen supplementation and thoracic radiographs when available
- For *severe life-threatening cardiogenic pulmonary edema* in the dog:

Initial dose: 4–6 mg/kg IV (IM if IV not feasible)
Then: 2–4 mg/kg IV q.1 h (or 1 mg/kg min CRI) until resting respiration rate (RR) ↓ by 20%
Then: 2–4 mg/kg IV q.2 h (or 0.5 mg/kg min CRI) until resting RR ↓ by 50%
Then: 2–4 mg/kg IV q.6–8 h (discontinue CRI at this time)
Then: switch to oral 2–4 mg/kg q.8–12 h

Note: For less severe edema use the lower end of the dose range and in older patients who are concurrently azotemic reduce the lower range doses in the schedule by 50%.

If dogs with respiratory distress fail to demonstrate a trend for improvement (reduced respiration rate) following 4–6 doses or 4–6 h of a furosemide CRI alternative differentials for respiratory distress should be considered and/or additional heart failure therapy should be initiated.

FELINE

Chronic heart failure

1 mg/kg PO every 1–3 d (mild heart failure) to 2 mg/kg twice to three times daily (severe heart failure) in most cases (doses should be separated by at least 3 h but do not have to be exactly 8 h). In general the goal with furosemide is to use the minimal dose necessary to keep the patient free of clinical signs of congestion. Some cats that are not amenable to oral administration may benefit from chronic client-administered subcutaneous injections. A higher oral dose may be considered in some cats that are not responding to a conventional dose. The need for the addition of rescue diuretics in the cat is exceedingly rare.

Acute heart failure

Severe pulmonary edema requires immediate intensive intravenous or intramuscular administration in cats. Intravenous is preferred if feasible.

FUROSEMIDE DOSE SCHEDULE FOR SEVERE LIFE-THREATENING CARDIOGENIC PULMONARY EDEMA IN THE CAT

- Dependent on severity of respiratory clinical signs
- Guided by resting respiration rate with oxygen supplementation and thoracic radiographs when available
- For *severe life-threatening cardiogenic pulmonary edema* in the cat:

Initial dose: 2–4 mg/kg IV (IM if IV not feasible)
Then: 1–2 mg/kg IV in 1–2 h
Then: 1–2 mg/kg IV in 2–4 h if resting respiration rate is not ↓ by 50%
Then: switch to oral at 1–2 mg/kg q.8–12 h once RR reduced by 50%

Formulations and dose rates—cont'd

Note: In general the doses at the lower end of the range are sufficient to resolve most cases of pulmonary edema in the cat. If cats do not stabilize or demonstrate a trend in respiratory rate reduction and effort following 2–3 doses of furosemide then alternative differentials for respiratory distress should be considered. For example, if asthma is possible start corticosteroids and/or bronchodilators and if pleural effusion is possible perform diagnostic/therapeutic pleurocentesis.

In general most cats with respiratory distress due to cardiogenic pulmonary edema can be stabilized with furosemide and good supportive care and will not require additional cardiovascular therapy until a safe echocardiogram can be performed. An echocardiogram can usually be safely performed, if available, 12–24 h after the respiratory rate has decreased by 30–50%.

Finally, a cat's initial response to the above therapeutic plan can be considered prognostic. That is, cats with cardiogenic pulmonary edema that fail to stabilize as outlined above often have a poorer long-term prognosis.

Pharmacokinetics

Furosemide is highly protein bound (86–91%). The ratio of kidney to plasma concentration is 5:1. A small amount of furosemide (1–14%) is metabolized to a glucuronide derivative in dogs but this metabolism does not take place in the liver. In dogs about 45% of furosemide is excreted in the bile and 55% in the urine. After intravenous administration, furosemide has an elimination half-life of approximately 1 h. Intravenously, furosemide's onset of action is within 5 min, peak effects occur within 30 min and duration of effect is 2–3 h. Also after intravenous administration, about 50% of the drug is cleared from the body within the first 30 min, 90% is eliminated within the first 2 h and almost all is eliminated within 3 h.

Furosemide is rapidly but incompletely absorbed after oral administration with a bioavailability of 40–50%. The terminal half-life after oral administration is biexponential. The initial phase has a half-life of approximately 30 min, the second a half-life of approximately 7 h. The initial disposition phase has the most effect on plasma concentration, with concentration decreasing from therapeutic to subtherapeutic within 4–6 h of oral administration. After oral administration, onset of action occurs within 60 min, peak effects occur within 1–2 h and duration of effect is approximately 6 h. In normal dogs, a dose of 2.5 mg/kg furosemide intramuscularly results in maximum natriuresis (beyond that dose there is no further increase in sodium excretion). This occurs at a plasma concentration of approximately 0.8 μg/mL. Because the diuretic effect of furosemide is dependent on its hematogenous delivery to the kidney, patients with decreased renal blood flow (e.g. those with heart failure) need a higher plasma concentration (higher dose) to produce the same effect observed in normal dogs. This is achieved by administering higher oral doses or administering the drug intravenously.

Experimentally induced moderate renal failure approximately doubles the serum half-life of furosemide in dogs and decreases renal clearance to 15% of control. Experimentally induced renal failure also markedly attenuates the diuretic effect of the drug to approximately one-third of control. A higher concentration of furosemide is required to produce the same diuretic effect in dogs with renal failure. However, the relationship between the rate of urinary furosemide excretion and diuresis remains constant. Consequently, the decrease in diuresis in dogs with renal failure appears to be due to a decrease in delivery of furosemide to the nephron. In canine patients with renal failure, two discordant effects interact on the diuretic effects of furosemide. First, the prolongation in half-life increases the serum concentration for any given chronically administered dose. This increases diuresis. Second, the diuretic effect for any given serum concentration is reduced. This complex interaction makes it much more difficult to determine an effective dose for furosemide in a patient with renal failure.

Cats are more sensitive to furosemide than dogs. The increase in urine volume is comparable between normal cats and normal dogs in doses from 0.625 mg/kg to 10 mg/kg IM. However, in cats sodium excretion is between 1.3 and 2.2 times (average 1.7 times) that seen in dogs at each dosage. The slope of the regression equation between furosemide dose and sodium excretion (mmol/kg) for cats is about twice that for dogs. Clinically, cats commonly require no more than 1–2 mg/kg q.12–24 h PO chronically for the treatment of pulmonary edema. However, higher doses may be needed in feline patients with severe heart failure because of reduced renal blood flow.

Adverse effects

Adverse effects shared with other diuretics are presented above.

- Furosemide has the potential for ototoxicity. However, when administered as the sole agent, doses in excess of 20 mg/kg IV are required to produce any loss in hearing ability in dogs. Doses in the 50–100 mg/kg range produce profound loss of hearing.
- Furosemide can potentiate the ototoxic and nephrotoxic effects of other drugs such as the aminoglycosides. Furosemide does not have direct nephrotoxic effects when administered by itself.
- Owners must be warned that high-dose furosemide therapy can produce profound dehydration in patients that stop drinking and so to markedly decrease the dose or stop the administration until they can talk to a veterinarian.

- Intensive intravenous dosing commonly results in mild to moderate hypokalemia (serum K^+ concentration 3.0–3.5 mmol/L), mild to moderate hyponatremia (serum Na^+ concentration 135–145 mmol/L) and mild to moderate dehydration. These may need to be addressed after the life-threatening pulmonary edema has been controlled. However, in dogs, electrolyte disturbances and dehydration are usually corrected when the dog feels well enough to eat and drink once the pulmonary edema has resolved. In addition, the electrolyte abnormalities and dehydration are usually not clinically significant unless severe overdosing has occurred. Consequently, aggressive fluid therapy for these abnormalities is not required and is often contraindicated because such fluid therapy can result in recrudescence of the heart failure. In cats, judicious administration of fluids may be required to rehydrate the patient after intensive diuresis because cats often do not restart eating and drinking as readily as dogs. Clinically significant electrolyte disturbances and dehydration are rare in dogs receiving long-term furosemide therapy unless maximal doses are employed and/or anorexia is present. These abnormalities may be more common in cats.

Known drug interactions

The natriuretic effect of furosemide is attenuated by aspirin administration in dogs. This drug interaction is possible with any NSAID by way of prostaglandin inhibition leading to reduced renal papillary blood flow. Indomethacin and aspirin completely inhibit the increase in renal blood flow observed after furosemide administration in dogs.

Special considerations

Furosemide injection contains the sodium salt of furosemide that is formed by the addition of sodium hydroxide during manufacturing. It should be stored at a temperature of 15–30°C and protected from light. Injections having a yellow color have degraded and should not be used. Exposure of furosemide tablets to light may cause discoloration. Discolored tablets should not be used. Furosemide injection can be mixed with weakly alkaline and neutral solutions having a pH of 7–10, such as 0.9% saline or Ringer's solution. A precipitate may form if the injection is mixed with strongly acidic solutions such as those containing ascorbic acid, tetracycline, adrenaline (epinephrine) or noradrenaline (norepinephrine). Furosemide injection should also not be mixed with most salts of organic bases, including lidocaine, alkaloids, antihistamines and morphine.

Thiazide diuretics

EXAMPLES

Hydrochlorothiazide, chlorothiazide

Clinical applications

The relative potency of thiazide diuretics when compared to furosemide is low in the dog and cat when they are used as monotherapy and thus they are rarely used as first-line diuretics in the dog and cat. Thiazides are primarily used in canine patients that have developed furosemide resistance. Dogs in heart failure are considered resistant to furosemide therapy when chronic oral furosemide at 4–5 mg/kg q.8 h fails to relieve clinical signs of congestion. In these cases the addition of a thiazide diuretic results in a synergistic drug–drug interaction as a result of sequential nephron blockade. This commonly results in restoration of diuresis and resolution of clinical signs. Sequential nephron blockade results from potentiation of thiazide diuretic effects due to upregulation of the specific exchange mechanism that is inhibited by thiazides in the distal convoluted tubule. This potentiation is the result of adaptations arising secondary to chronic furosemide therapy. Thus thiazides are commonly referred to as rescue diuretics.

Mechanism of action

The thiazides act primarily by reducing membrane permeability to sodium and chloride in the distal convoluted tubule. They promote potassium loss at this site and produce large increases in the urine sodium concentration but only mild to moderate increases in urine volume. Consequently, moderate renal sodium loss is produced. Thiazide diuretics increase renal sodium excretion from a normal value of about 1% to 5–8% of the filtered load. Thiazide diuretics also inhibit carbonic anhydrase in the proximal tubules but this effect varies considerably among the various agents. The thiazides are ineffective when renal blood flow is low, which may explain their lack of efficacy as a sole agent in patients with severe heart failure.

Thiazide diuretics decrease glomerular filtration rate, which may explain their lack of efficacy in patients with renal failure. It is unknown whether this is due to a direct effect on renal vasculature or is secondary to the decrease in intravascular fluid volume.

Thiazides are sometimes used to decrease the polyuria associated with diabetes insipidus; this effect is mediated through plasma volume reduction resulting in decreased glomerular filtration rate and enhanced proximal reabsorption of NaCl. Dietary sodium restriction can potentiate their beneficial effects in this setting.

Formulations and dose rates

Chlorothiazide is available in tablet and suspension formulations, hydrochlorothiazide in tablet form.

DOGS

Hydrochlorothiazide (preferred)

- 2–4 mg/kg PO q.12 h (monotherapy dose)

Note the authors' rescue diuretic of choice (see Diuretic resistance and furosemide formulation and dose rates) is hydrochlorothiazide, regardless of whether or not concurrent spironolactone therapy is employed. This is rarely required in the clinical setting (<15% of cases in the authors' experience)

Chlorothiazide (monotherapy dose)

- 20–40 mg/kg PO q.12 h

CATS

Hydrochlorothiazide (preferred)

- 1–2 mg/kg PO q.12 h

RULE OF THUMB: when a maximum chronic dose of furosemide (5 mg/kg PO q.8 h) alone or in combination with spironolactone fails to keep the patient free of cardiogenic edema or effusion, then hydrochlorothiazide can be initiated at 2 mg/kg q.12 h. However, when hydrochlorothiazide is initiated it is recommended by the author (Gordon) to reduce the daily dose of furosemide by approximately 50% (3 mg/kg q.12 h) and add a potassium supplement. The dose of spironolactone can be added at 0.5–1 mg/kg q.12 h to minimize potassium wasting.

Pharmacokinetics

In dogs, thiazides are well absorbed after oral administration. The action of chlorothiazide begins within 1 h, peaks at 4 h and lasts 6–12 h. Hydrochlorothiazide has an onset of action within 2 h, peaks at 4 h and lasts 12 h. The newer, more lipid-soluble thiazides (trichlormethiazide, cyclothiazide) have not been studied in the dog or cat.

Adverse effects

In addition to their effects on sodium and chloride, the thiazides also increase potassium excretion because of the increased sodium that reaches the distal tubular site of sodium-potassium exchange. Long-term thiazide administration can result in mild metabolic alkalosis associated with hypokalemia and hypochloremia in human patients. The effects in dogs and cats are less clear. These effects are potentiated when they are used concurrently with other loop diuretics such as furosemide. Although little can or should be done to normalize Na and Cl serum concentrations in this setting, K supplementation is often required to maintain the serum potassium concentration within the normal range. In addition, magnesium supplementation may be beneficial due to its positive correlation with potassium concentration.

Because thiazides are most commonly used as rescue diuretics in dogs with furosemide resistance, their relative potencies are profoundly augmented and they can cause marked diuresis resulting in prerenal azotemia. Therefore caution should be used when initiating rescue diuretic therapy, particularly in dogs with pre-existing azotemia. To minimize this risk when initiating thiazides as rescue therapy the author (Gordon) reduces the total daily dose of furosemide by approximately 50% (see Rule of Thumb). Follow-up re-evaluation should occur in 7–14 days or sooner if the patient is not doing well clinically and should include the revaluation of renal parameters and serum potassium concentration.

Potassium-sparing diuretics

EXAMPLES

Spironolactone (preferred), triamterene, amiloride

Clinical applications

This class of diuretics acts by inhibiting the action of aldosterone on distal tubular cells or blocking sodium reabsorption in the latter regions of the distal tubule and collecting tubules. In normal dogs, they can only increase the maximal fractional excretion of sodium to 2% of the filtered load. In dogs with heart failure, particularly those with ascites secondary to right heart failure, an increased plasma aldosterone concentration may be present and the effect of these diuretics may be enhanced. However, potassium-sparing diuretics are weak diuretics when used alone as diuretics and thus should never be used as sole agents in patients with heart failure. One should never rely on a potassium-sparing diuretic, such as spironolactone, to produce additional diuresis in a patient that is refractory to other diuretics. When potassium-sparing diuretics are administered with other diuretics, potassium loss is decreased, representing an additional benefit. Consequently, they can be administered to patients that become hypokalemic because of the administration of other diuretic agents.

Spironolactone

Spironolactone can be used in combination with other diuretics, primarily furosemide, to produce additional diuresis (generally a mild increase) or to decrease potassium excretion. In addition, as an aldosterone antagonist, spironolactone is considered a neuroendocrine modulator (aldosterone receptor blocker). One human study reported that low-dose spironolactone (subdiuretic doses) reduced heart failure mortality by approximately 18–40% and this effect was attributable to its neuroendocrine modulatory effects. Spironolactone is also used in the management of fluid retention associated with noncardiac disease such as hepatic disease and nephrotic syndrome. Spironolactone might be particularly useful as a diuretic in the setting of right heart failure causing ascites.

Triamterene

Triamterene is rarely used in dogs and cats and almost never as a sole diuretic agent. It is generally administered in combination with other diuretics, usually furosemide, to decrease potassium excretion in a patient that develops hypokalemia while on furosemide.

Mechanism of action

Spironolactone

Spironolactone is structurally similar to aldosterone and binds competitively to aldosterone's binding sites in the distal tubule. Due to its aldosterone antagonism spironolactone is also considered an inhibitor of the RAAS and thus a neuroendocrine modulator.

Triamterene

Triamterene is a potassium-sparing diuretic that is structurally related to folic acid. It acts directly on the distal tubule to depress reabsorption of sodium and decrease the excretion of potassium and hydrogen. It does not competitively inhibit aldosterone.

Formulations and dose rates

Spironolactone

Spironolactone is supplied as tablets. It is also supplied in a fixed combination with hydrochlorothiazide. The diuretic spironolactone dose for dogs is 2–4 mg/kg/d. Lower doses (0.5–1 mg/kg q.12 h) may be considered for inhibition of the RAAS.

Triamterene

Triamterene is supplied as capsules. It is also supplied in a fixed combination with hydrochlorothiazide. The oral canine dose is 2–4 mg/kg/q.24 h.

Pharmacokinetics

Spironolactone has a long half-life and so its onset of action is slow. In dogs its peak effect does not occur until 2–3 d after administration commences. The drug is extensively and rapidly metabolized to conrenone and other metabolites in plasma. These metabolites are pharmacologically active but much less so than the parent compound. The duration of effect for spironolactone is 2–3 d after cessation of drug administration.

Triamterene's action begins within 2 h, peaks at 6–8 h and lasts 12–16 h.

Adverse effects

The diuretic effects of potassium-sparing diuretics are generally too mild to produce any untoward effects. However, when combined with an ACE inhibitor whose mechanism of action also includes anti-aldosterone effects, the relative risk of hyperkalemia is increased. However, it is only clinically significant in patients who are not receiving furosemide concurrently.

Known drug interactions

The potassium-sparing property of spironolactone does not result in clinical hyperkalemia even when used in combination with an ACE inhibitor as long as furosemide is also given. However, in the authors' experience the combination of spironolactone and an ACE inhibitor (without concurrent furosemide administration) can result in clinically significant hyperkalemia and should thus be avoided.

POSITIVE INOTROPIC DRUGS

EXAMPLES

Oral: pimobendan (preferred), digoxin
IV: dobutamine (preferred), dopamine, epinephrine (adrenaline), milrinone, amrinone

As a class, with the exception of calcium-sensitizing aspect of agents such as pimobendan, the final common pathway for positive inotropy is dependent on increased concentrations of cytosolic calcium in cardiomyocytes. All drugs with this property have the potential to cause arrhythmias and increase myocardial oxygen consumption, negative properties which may be exaggerated in long-term therapy for the management of chronic heart failure. Thus any potential benefit must be weighed in relationship to these potential negative side effects.

Positive inotropy that is mediated through calcium sensitization (e.g. pimobendan) might thus be considered the safest form of positive inotropy. Positive inotropes include digitalis glycosides, sympathomimetics such as epinephrine (adrenaline), dobutamine and dopamine. Pure phosphodiesterase inhibitors such as milrinone and pimobendan, a calcium sensitizer/phosphodiesterase inhibitor, will be discussed in the section on inodilators.

Digitalis glycosides

Clinical applications

Historically, the digitalis glycosides were indicated for the treatment of heart failure characterized by systolic dysfunction (i.e. decreased myocardial contractility) and for the treatment of supraventricular tachyarrhythmias.

In dogs with heart failure, digitalis does not result in a clinically significant increase in myocardial contractility and currently there are more potent oral positive inotropes available (e.g. pimobendan). The current primary clinical indication for digoxin is for the management of clinically significant supraventricular arrhythmias such as atrial fibrillation where it is often used in combination with other antiarrhythmics such as β-blockers or diltiazem. Thus further discussion of digoxin will be covered in the antiarrhythmic section of this chapter.

Sympathomimetics

EXAMPLES

Dobutamine (preferred for acute inotropic support), adrenaline (epinephrine), dopamine

Clinical applications

Sympathomimetics are used to provide inotropic support for patients in acute cardiac failure. Most sympathomimetics have the ability to increase contractility about 100% above baseline, but many are unsuitable for treating heart failure because of other drug properties. Sympathomimetics such as dopamine, and particularly dobutamine, are less arrhythmogenic, produce a smaller heart rate increase and are more suitable for heart failure therapy than the classic sympathomimetics such as adrenaline (epinephrine) and noradrenaline (norepinephrine). The arrhythmogenic potential for all catecholamines is increased when dogs are anesthetized with drugs such as thiamylal and halothane. In this setting, the arrhythmogenic potential of adrenaline (epinephrine), dopamine and dobutamine is similar.

One of the major limitations of using sympathomimetics to treat patients with heart failure is the major alterations that occur in β-receptor density and sensitivity during subacute to chronic stimulation by endogenous or exogenous catecholamines such as occurs in the setting of chronic heart failure or prolonged use of the agent in question. Typically, the inotropic response to sympathomimetics decreases to 50% of baseline after a day or two of constant stimulation because of the decrease in β-receptor number and sensitivity. Consequently, one should generally not consider using a sympathomimetic for longer than 2 or 3 days for inotropic support and their effects may be reduced in chronic heart failure requiring higher doses.

Mechanism of action

In the heart, sympathomimetic amines increase contractility, conduction velocity and heart rate primarily by binding to cardiac β-adrenergic receptors. The increase in contractility is brought about by activation of adenyl cyclase within the cell. Adenyl cyclase cleaves adenosine triphosphate (ATP) to cyclic adenosine monophosphate (cAMP), which stimulates a cellular protein kinase system. Protein kinases phosphorylate intracellular proteins, such as phospholamban on the sarcoplasmic reticulum (SR), allowing the SR to bind more calcium during diastole and thereby release more calcium during systole. Cyclic AMP also affects L-type calcium channels to increase calcium entry into the cell during systole.

Dobutamine

Clinical applications

Dobutamine is preferred for acute or short-term inotropic support in heart failure characterized by systolic dysfunction.

In clinical situations, dobutamine can be used to treat acute or decompensated heart failure characterized by systolic dysfunction, such as DCM and most CVD, until inotropic support is no longer needed or until other longer-acting drugs have taken effect. It is also often used in anesthetized patients requiring inotropic support.

Mechanism of action

Dobutamine is a synthetic catecholamine. It stimulates β_1-adrenergic receptors, increasing myocardial contractility. It also weakly stimulates peripheral β_2- and α_1-adrenergic receptors. As this response is balanced, systemic arterial blood pressure is usually unchanged. Dobutamine is less arrhythmogenic than most of the other sympathomimetics in conscious animals. In vagotomized experimental dogs under anesthesia, dobutamine is as arrhythmogenic as adrenaline (epinephrine).

Formulations and dose rates

Dobutamine is supplied as 12.5 mg/mL in a 20 mL single use vial (250 mg/vial) and should be diluted appropriately for administration.

DOGS AND CATS (RARE)

- CRI = 2-40 μg/kg/min IV. Typically the CRI is initiated at the lower dose and increased every 2–10 min until desired effect (increase in systemic blood pressure) or toxicity is detected (worsening arrhythmias or clinically significant tachycardia)
- Doses of 5–20 μg/kg/min are generally adequate for conscious dogs in heart failure. Infusion rates of greater than 20 μg/kg/min often produce tachycardia and vomiting
- Lower doses 1–5 μg/kg/min IV are usually used in anesthetized patients who are not in heart failure
- Dobutamine can be used in combination with pimobendan in acute emergency situations
- Cats may be administered 5–15 μg/kg/min. It is however, rarely indicated because systolic dysfunction is rare in the majority of feline heart diseases
- The positive inotropic effect is dose dependent

Pharmacokinetics

Dobutamine must be administered as a CRI. A plateau plasma concentration is achieved within approximately 8 min of starting the infusion. Upon cessation of the infusion, dobutamine rapidly clears from the plasma with a terminal half-life of 1–2 min. The rapid clearance is due primarily to degradation of the drug by catechol-O-methyltransferase.

In experimental dogs, dobutamine produces dose-related increases in myocardial contractility, cardiac output, stroke volume and coronary blood flow, with no change in systemic arterial blood pressure. When administered to a patient with acute or chronic myocardial failure, it should increase contractility and cardiac output and decrease ventricular diastolic pressures, leading to a decrease in edema formation and normalization of systemic blood pressure if it is low. This has been poorly documented in dogs and cats with chronic myocardial failure but has been well documented in human patients. Failing myocardium responds much less avidly to positive inotropic agents than normal myocardium. Consequently, it is not unusual for echocardiographic measures of left ventricular function to change minimally following dobutamine administration in dogs with severe systolic dysfunction (e.g. DCM). This statement is true of all positive inotropes.

Dobutamine's effects on heart rate are generally less than those of other catecholamines. When studied in normal dogs and in dogs with experimental myocardial infarction, the heart rate did not increase at infusion rates less than 20 μg/kg/min. Dobutamine, however, does increase heart rate in a dose-dependent manner in dogs that are anesthetized.

Adverse effects

Dobutamine can exacerbate existing arrhythmias, especially ventricular arrhythmias. It can also produce new arrhythmias and increase heart rate.

Special considerations

The 12.5 mg/mL solution must be further diluted into at least 50 mL for administration. Once in an intravenous solution, the compound is stable at room temperature for 24 h.

Dobutamine should not be mixed with bicarbonate, heparin, hydrocortisone sodium succinate, cefalothin, penicillin or insulin.

Dopamine

Clinical applications

In cardiovascular medicine, dopamine is recommended for short-term use in animals with systolic dysfunction and in the management of acute oliguric renal failure, particularly in the dog. In addition, dopamine is often used as a pressor agent to manage inappropriate hypotension in both conscious and anesthetized patients.

Mechanism of action

Dopamine is the precursor of noradrenaline (norepinephrine). It stimulates cardiac α- and β-adrenergic receptors as well as peripherally located dopaminergic receptors. The reported effects of dopamine are dose dependent: where dopaminergic effects on renal blood flow occur at low doses 1–1.5 μg/kg/min, positive inotropic responses predominate at doses 5–10 μg/kg/min and pressor effects dominate at infusion rates greater than 10 μg/kg/min. The pressor effects are undesirable in the setting of decompensated heart failure and thus dobutamine is preferred in this setting. Dopaminergic receptors appear to be located most prevalently in the renal and mesenteric vascular beds, where they produce vasodilation and improve blood flow. As with dobutamine, all effects are attenuated over time and are reduced in dogs with heart failure relative to normal dogs.

Formulations and dose rates

Dopamine is supplied as 40 mg/mL in a 10 mL single use vial (400 mg/vial) and should be diluted appropriately for administration.

DOGS

- 1–10 μg/kg/min IV
- Low doses (1.0–1.5 μg/kg/min) cause renal vasodilation via specific dopaminergic receptors; therefore, dopamine is often used in the management of acute oliguric renal failure
- Medium doses (3–10 μg/kg/min) cause increased cardiac output with little effect on peripheral resistance or heart rate
- Doses higher than 10 μg/kg/min can be used but result in noradrenaline (norepinephrine) release and increased peripheral vascular resistance and heart rate (pressor effect)
- An initial dose of 2 μg/kg/min may be started and titrated upward to obtain the desired clinical effect (improved hemodynamics)

Pharmacokinetics

All sympathomimetics have a very short half-life (1–2 min). When administered orally, they experience rapid and extensive first-pass hepatic metabolism before they reach the circulation. Consequently, they must be administered intravenously as a CRI.

Special considerations

Dopamine is inactivated when mixed with sodium bicarbonate or other alkaline intravenous solutions. The solution becomes pink or violet. The product should not be used if it is discolored.

INODILATORS

EXAMPLES

Oral: pimobendan
IV: milrinone, amrinone

This class of agents has both positive inotropic and vasodilatory properties and they have been labeled inodilators as a reflection of the term 'inodilation' (coined by Lionel H Opie in 1989). Historically, short-term management of acute or decompensated heart failure characterized by systolic dysfunction benefited from a combination of dobutamine (inotrope) and sodium nitroprusside (vasodilator). Agents in this class combine these properties but are not as potent as a combination of dobutamin and nitroprusside. However, pimobendan is available in an oral formulation, making chronic therapy possible.

Pimobendan

Clinical applications

Pimobendan is a novel agent with properties that are desirable in the clinical management of canine heart failure secondary to both DCM and chronic CVD in dogs.

The efficacy of pimobendan in the treatment of heart failure arising from DCM and CVD has been evaluated thoroughly in dogs. Available prospective data support its ability to significantly reduce morbidity in dogs with heart failure secondary to these conditions. A prospective blinded placebo-controlled study by O'Grady et al demonstrated a doubling of overall survival in Doberman pinschers with heart failure secondary to DCM, from a mean of 63 ± 14 days (mean ± standard deviation) with furosemide, an ACE inhibitor and placebo, to 128 ± 29 days with furosemide, an ACE inhibitor and pimobendan at 0.25 mg/kg by mouth twice daily ($P = 0.04$). Additional studies suggest a survival benefit with the combination of pimobendan and furosemide when compared to an ACE inhibitor and furosemide (with or without digoxin) in dogs with heart failure secondary to DCM or CVD.

Other studies offer conflicting evidence with respect to the superiority of pimobendan over an ACE inhibitor for the treatment of heart failure secondary to CVD. Preliminary analysis of an ongoing study by O'Grady et al showed no survival advantage using pimobendan and furosemide compared to an ACE inhibitor and furosemide in dogs with heart failure due to CVD. Conversely, Smith et al and Lombard et al (VetScope study) demonstrated superiority of a combination of pimobendan and furosemide over an ACE inhibitor (ramipril or benazepril respectively) and furosemide for the treatment of heart failure due to CVD. Smith's study reported a significant reduction of overall adverse outcomes, including death from the CHF (euthanized or died) and treatment failure when furosemide and ramipril (48%) were compared to furosemide and pimobendan (18%) over 6 months of treatment. Lombard's study reported that the median survival (i.e. death or treatment failure) for dogs receiving pimobendan and furosemide was 415 days versus 128 days for those receiving benazepril and furosemide ($P = 0.0022$). In all three studies no significant adverse consequences occurred, which suggests that the combination of pimobendan and furosemide is superior to furosemide and an ACE inhibitor for the treatment of heart failure due to CVD.

To date, pimobendan appears to be safe and well tolerated in dogs with heart failure associated with CVD. Pimobendan in combination with an ACE inhibitor and furosemide has not been prospectively evaluated in comparison to an ACE inhibitor and furosemide in heart failure due to CVD. However, when used with concurrent therapy such as furosemide, an ACE inhibitor, digoxin, spironolactone, etc., it appears to be beneficial.

One of the authors (Gordon) has been using pimobendan (0.25–0.3 mg/kg PO) in addition to background heart failure therapy for > 6 years in over 300 dogs for the treatment of CHF from both DCM and CVD. In one unpublished study from these 300 dogs, survival and hemodynamic effects were reviewed in a subset of dogs with advanced heart failure due to CVD. In addition to pimobendan these dogs received furosemide (100%, at least 3 mg/kg PO q.12 h) and an ACE inhibitor (100%), spironolactone (>75%), a β-blocker (20%), digoxin (11%) and hydrochlorothiazide (3%). Hemodynamic effects were evaluated prior to initiation of pimobendan and approximately 45 days later. No significant changes in indirect systemic blood pressures, bodyweight, hematocrit, total solids, serum creatinine or electrolytes ($P = 0.05$) were detected. Blood urea nitrogen concentration increased significantly in some dogs (pre-pimobendan 29 mg/dL vs post-pimobendan 33 mg/dL, $P < 0.05$). Heart rate and respiratory rate were reduced and no changes occurred in the combined frequency of arrhythmias (i.e. ventricular premature beats, ventricular tachycardia, supraventricular premature beats, supraventricular tachycardia and atrial fibrillation) on electrocardiograms. A trend ($P = 0.059$) was noted in reduction of the dosage of furosemide administered to the dogs.

Certain echocardiographic parameters suggested improvement in systolic function, namely a reduction in left ventricular (LV) internal dimension in systole, reduction of LV end-systolic area and an increase in the percentage of LV area shortening. Reduction in the regurgitant fraction was suggested by a decrease in the radiographic vertebral heart score, a reduction in systolic left atrial diameter on echocardiography and a decrease in the M-mode derived ratio of left atrial to aortic size.

Taken together, these findings suggested that the addition of pimobendan to background heart failure therapy had no negative side effects and it enhanced systolic function, as well as reducing filling pressures. Although these beneficial effects were observed (on average) 45 days after initiating pimobendan, more recent experience and abstract data suggest that these effects may be apparent as soon as 24 h after starting the drug, which suggests a potential application in the treatment of acute, decompensated heart failure. The median survival of the dogs in the authors' 6-year study was 17 months (range 2–50 months). The median was estimated from a Kaplan Meier curve where mortality was the outcome variable and dogs were censored if still alive at the time of analysis (30% were censored).

The authors' clinical experience is in agreement with currently available prospective data supporting the efficacy of adjunctive pimobendan therapy in improving the quality and length of life in dogs with heart failure arising from both CVD and DCM. Pimobendan is easy to use clinically, requiring no additional monitoring, and enjoys excellent client compliance. Pimobendan works very rapidly and can be used during the initial, acute phase of heart failure treatment. Peak hemodynamic effects following oral administration on an empty stomach are achieved in 1 h and last 8–12 h. The rapid onset of action, low rate of side effects and decreased time of hospitalization with use of the drug have had a positive impact on the willingness of clients to pursue the treatment of heart failure in the clinic, as well as overall client satisfaction with chronic heart failure therapy. Ongoing studies will further define the survival benefits associated with the use of pimobendan in dogs with heart failure due to CVD.

Pimobendan has been licensed for use in dogs with CHF since 2000 in many countries around the world, including countries in Europe, Great Britain, Australia, Canada and Mexico and most recently the USA (2007). Pimobendan is produced and marketed under the trade name Vetmedin.

In summary, pimobendan is a novel agent with properties that are desirable in the clinical management of CHF secondary to both DCM and CVD in dogs. Review of available data supports that pimobendan is safe, well tolerated and leads to enhanced quality of life in dogs when used in combination with furosemide and other conventional heart failure therapies. Pimobendan prolongs survival in dogs with CHF from DCM and CVD and an ongoing study will offer additional insight into its effects on mortality in dogs with CHF due to CVD.

Mechanism of action

Inotropy

Pimobendan is a benzimidazole pyridazinone derivative and is classified as an inodilator (i.e. positive inotrope and balanced systemic arterial and venous dilator). In failing hearts it exerts its positive inotropic effects primarily through sensitization of the cardiac contractile apparatus to intracellular calcium. As a phosphodiesterase (PDE) III inhibitor it can potentially increase intracellular calcium concentration and increase myocardial oxygen consumption. However, the cardiac PDE effects of pimobendan are reportedly minimal at pharmacological doses in dogs with heart disease, which is a major advantage relative to other inotropic PDE inhibitors such as milrinone. Pimobendan's calcium sensitization of the contractile apparatus is achieved by enhancement of the interaction between calcium and the troponin C complex, resulting in a positive inotropic effect that does not increase myocardial oxygen consumption.

Overall, pimobendan enhances systolic function by improving the efficiency of contraction, limiting the potential arrhythmogenic side effects of other positive inotropes whose sole mechanism of action is to increase myocardial intracellular calcium. Calcium sensitizers such as pimobendan may thus represent the only class of inotropic agents that 'safely' augment contractility.

Vasodilation

Phosphodiesterase III and V are found in vascular smooth muscle. Inhibitors of PDE III such as pimobendan result in balanced vasodilation (combination of venous and arterial dilation) leading to a reduction of both cardiac preload and afterload, a cornerstone of therapy in heart failure. In addition, pimobendan may have some PDE V inhibition effects. PDE V concentrations are relatively high in the vascular smooth muscle of pulmonary arteries, so PDE V inhibition might help ameliorate elevations in pulmonary artery pressure (pulmonary hypertension) that tend to parallel long-standing elevations in left atrial pressure, a clinically important complication of CVD.

Cytokine modulation

The significance of alterations in proinflammatory cytokine concentrations such as tumor necrosis factor-β, interleukins 1β and 6 on the progression of heart failure has been documented in many forms of heart disease. Maladaptive alterations in these cytokine concentrations are associated with increased morbidity and mortality and pimobendan has demonstrated beneficial modulation of several such cytokines in various models of heart failure.

Antiplatelet effects

Pimobendan reportedly may have some platelet inhibitory effect in the dog. The clinical significance of this property is not yet clear.

Positive lusitropic effect

Positive lusitropic effects occur via PDE III inhibition in cardiomyocytes. Pimobendan increases intracellular cAMP, which facilitates phosphorylation of receptors on the sarcoplasmic recticulum and enhances the diastolic re-uptake of calcium and the speed of relaxation – a positive lusitropic property.

Formulations and dose rates

Pimobendan is supplied as hard gelatin capsules (most countries) containing 1.25, 2.5 mg or 5 mg pimobendan. In 2007 a new chewable formulation was released in the USA and Australia in the same sizes. Pimobendan is not stable in suspension and should not be reformulated in this manner. The labeled dose recommendation is 0.25–0.3 mg/kg q.12 h. Initial efficacy may be enhanced by administration on an empty stomach but once steady state is reached (a few days) it can be administered with food.

Pharmacokinetics

Bioavailability is reduced by food until steady state is reached in a few days. Consequently, the drug should be administered on an empty stomach at least 1 h before feeding for maximal effects when starting therapy. Peak hemodynamic effects following oral administration on an empty stomach are achieved in 1 h and last 8–12 h. Therefore it can provide rapid short-term support to dogs with acute or decompensated heart failure even though it is an oral preparation.

Adverse effects

Pimobendan is well tolerated clinically in dogs with heart failure.

- In the treatment of more than 300 dogs one of the authors (Gordon) has recognized systemic hypotension and sinus tachycardia once, which was resolved by dose reduction.
- Gastrointestinal signs including anorexia and vomiting are not statistically different in frequency from those reported with ACE inhibitor treatment in the same patient population.
- One case report documented chordal rupture in two dogs while using pimobendan for an off-label indication.
- One additional case report documented ventricular hypertrophy but the dogs in this study did not have heart failure and thus do not represent the patient population pimobendan is licensed to treat.
- No prospective randomized controlled blinded study in either human or veterinary medicine has reported an increase in the frequency of arrhythmias. Recently one small unpublished study suggested that pimobendan increases the number and complexity of ventricular tachyarrhythmias in dogs with DCM and one small prospective placebo controlled study reported no increase in arrhythmias (Holter) in dogs with CVD receiving pimobendan versus enalapril.
- According to the Canadian package insert:
  - suspected adverse effects that have been reported following clinical use in dogs include: systemic hypotension and tachycardia (usually dose dependent and avoided by reducing the dose), gastrointestinal problems (inappetence, anorexia, vomiting), nervous system/behavioral problems (uneasiness, inco-ordination, convulsions) and polyuria and polydypsia.
  - Arrhythmias and chordal rupture represent two additional potential adverse effects.
  - In addition, as for all positive inotropic agents, pimobendan should not be administered to patients with hypertrophic cardiomyopathy or patients with any type of outflow tract obstruction (e.g. subaortic stenosis, pulmonic stenosis).
  - There are no data on the safety of pimobendan in pregnant or lactating dogs.

Milrinone and amrinone

Mechanism of action

Milrinone and amrinone are bipyridine compounds. Bipyridine compounds increase myocardial contractility and produce mild systemic arteriolar dilation. Milrinone is about 30–40 times as potent as amrinone.

Bipyridine compounds primarily act as inhibitors of phosphodiesterase fraction III. Phosphodiesterase III is an intracellular enzyme that specifically hydrolyzes cAMP in myocardial and vascular tissue. When phosphodiesterase III is inhibited, intracellular cAMP concentration increases. This increase results in the same type of inotropic effect in the myocardium as is produced by sympathomimetics. The major difference is that bipyridine compounds 'bypass' the β-receptors and so there is no decrement in inotropic effect over time. Bipyridine compounds also produce arteriolar dilation, probably also mediated by phosphodiesterase inhibition. Milrinone also increases left ventricular relaxation and distensibility in human heart failure patients.

Cardiovascular effects of the bipyridine compounds are species dependent. Myocardial contractility increases to a similar degree as is observed following the administration of a β-agonist in dogs and cats (i.e. approximately 100% above baseline). Myocardial contractility increases only about 50% above baseline in nonhuman primates and presumably in humans. When amrinone is administered to rats, contractility only increases about

25% above baseline. Because of this marked species difference, data obtained from human patients given amrinone or milrinone cannot be extrapolated to dogs or cats.

Milrinone

Clinical applications

Milrinone is the preferred bipyridine compound but is rarely used clinically; for acute cardiovascular support, dobutamine is preferred. It is a bipyridine compound with pharmacological effects and clinical indications that are almost identical to amrinone. Milrinone is currently marketed for intravenous administration only. No clinical studies of the effects of intravenous milrinone administration for acute myocardial failure in dogs or cats have been performed. Clinical studies of the effects of chronic oral administration have been performed but this form of the drug has not been approved for veterinary use and is not available for human use.

Formulations and dose rates

Milrinone lactate is supplied in 10 mL and 20 mL single-dose vials containing 1 mg/mL. It can be diluted in 0.45% and 0.9% sodium chloride and 5% dextrose in water.

DOGS

- In normal anesthetized dogs, milrinone 30–300 μg/kg IV increases contractility by 40–120% while decreasing diastolic blood pressure by 10–30%
- Constant-rate intravenous infusions (1–10 μg/kg/min) increase contractility by 50–140%, with peak effect in 10–30 min
- Dogs with systolic dysfunction (predominantly from DCM) displayed improved echocardiographic parameters with milrinone 0.5–1.0 mg/kg q.12 h PO during a 4-week treatment regimen

Pharmacokinetics

Peak effect occurs within 1–2 min of starting an intravenous infusion and is reduced to 50% of maximum within 10 min of stopping the infusion. The effects are essentially gone in 30 min.

Adverse effects

Ventricular arrhythmias worsen in a small percentage of dogs.

Known drug interactions

Milrinone is chemically incompatible with furosemide and thus should not be administered in the same intravenous line without flushing adequately in between.

Amrinone

Clinical applications

Amrinone is used for short-term inotropic support in small animal patients with myocardial failure. It may be useful to supplant a sympathomimetic once β-receptor downregulation has become a problem. It is not commonly used as a first-line agent because of its expense.

Formulations and dose rates

Amrinone is supplied in 20 mL ampoules in a concentration of 5 mg/mL for administration as supplied or for dilution in 0.9% or 0.45% saline.

DOGS AND CATS

- Amrinone is marketed only as a solution for intravenous administration and so is useful only for short-term administration
- In dogs, the initial dose should be 1–3 mg/kg, administered as a slow intravenous bolus, followed by a CRI of 10–100 μg/kg/min. One-half the initial bolus may be administered 20–30 min after the first bolus
- The same regimen may be effective in the cat

Pharmacokinetics

In normal anesthetized dogs, an intravenous bolus of amrinone (1.0–3.0 mg/kg) causes contractility to increase 60–100%, systemic arterial blood pressure to decrease 10–30% and heart rate to increase 5–10%. The maximal contractility increase occurs within 5 min after injection and decreases 50% by 10 min. Effects are dissipated within 20–30 min. This short duration of effect necessitates administering the drug by constant intravenous infusion following the initial bolus injection. Infusion rates of 10–100 μg/kg/min in anesthetized experimental dogs increase contractility by 30–90% above baseline and in unanesthetized dogs by 10–80%.

In anesthetized dogs, an infusion of 10 μg/kg/min does not decrease systemic blood pressure, whereas 30 μg/kg/min decreases it by 10% and 100 μg/kg/min decreases it by 30%. Heart rate does not increase at 10 μg/kg/min but elevates by 15% at 30 μg/kg/min and increases by 20% at 100 μg/kg/min. In anesthetized dogs with drug-induced myocardial failure, amrinone infusions increase contractility by 40–200% above baseline and increase cardiac output by 80%. Constant infusions in dogs take about 45 min to reach peak effect. In experimental cats, amrinone infused at 30 μg/kg/min causes contractility to increase by 40% above baseline. Peak effect occurs 90 min after starting an infusion.

Studies have not been performed to determine the hemodynamic changes brought about by amrinone administration in dogs or cats with naturally occurring heart failure. On the basis of the information from normal dogs, however, clinical recommendations can be made. The drug has a wide margin of safety and the risk of toxicity is low. With milrinone (which has similar toxic effects in dogs as amrinone), exacerbation of ventricular arrhythmias may occur in about 5% of dogs treated for heart failure.

Special considerations

- Amrinone is incompatible with dextrose.
- The drug is prepared with the aid of lactic acid as a sterile solution of the drug in water. The commercially available injection is a clear yellow solution that is stable for 2 years from the date of manufacture.
- When the drug is diluted, it is stable for up to 24 h at room temperature or at 2–8°C under usual lighting conditions.
- Amrinone is chemically incompatible with furosemide and thus should not be administered in the same intravenous line without flushing adequately in between.

VASODILATORS

EXAMPLES

Pure vasodilators
Oral: calcium channel blocker (amlodipine) (preferred), hydralazine (preferred), prazosin, isosorbide mononitrate and dinitrate (nitrate)
IV: nitroprusside (nitrate; preferred)
Topical: nitroglycerine (nitrate; most likely ineffective)
Vasodilators with additional properties
Oral: pimobendan, ACE inhibitors, sildenifil
IV: milrinone

Tolerable vasodilation (preload and afterload reduction) represents a cornerstone of heart failure therapy in human and veterinary medicine. Vasodilator therapy was first introduced in human medicine in the early 1970s after it was noted that the acute administration of nitroprusside resulted in marked improvement in hemodynamics. The first reports of vasodilator use in veterinary medicine were published in the late 1970s and early 1980s. In addition, vasodilators are useful in the management of systemic hypertension.

Mechanism of action

Vasodilators are drugs that act on arteriolar or venous smooth muscle to cause smooth muscle relaxation (i.e. vasodilation) through a variety of mechanisms. Their hemodynamic effects depend on the vascular beds they influence (arterial or venous or balanced/mixed), as well as relative drug potency. The effect of these drugs on the pulmonary vasculature is erratic or insignificant. This discussion is therefore focused on systemic vascular beds. Two agents will be discussed as they relate to pulmonary hypertension (pimobendan and sildenafil).

In patients with heart failure, systemic arterioles are constricted (enhanced total peripheral resistance) so that a normal blood pressure (perfusion pressure) can be maintained when cardiac output is reduced. In addition, systemic veins are constricted so that blood volume is shifted from the peripheral to the central compartment in order to increase ventricular preload, producing volume overload hypertrophy (eccentric hypertrophy or dilation) and, in so doing, improve stroke volume and cardiac output. In patients with heart failure, these adaptive compensatory mechanisms ultimately become detrimental and maladaptive, contributing to the development of clinical signs consistent with heart failure.

Although systemic vasoconstriction is able to maintain a normal systemic blood pressure the relative increase in resistance to blood flow contributes to increased afterload. The normal systemic blood pressure and increased afterload decreases the effective transfer of mechanical energy into blood propulsion into the aorta. The net result is a decrease in stroke volume and an increase in energy consumption by the heart to generate stroke volume. Systemic venoconstriction in heart failure patients contributes to the increase in central blood volume. In heart failure patients, the ventricular chambers are unable to grow larger in response to this increase in volume (eccentric hypertrophy or dilation). Consequently, the increase in central blood volume and venoconstriction contributes to the increase in ventricular diastolic pressures and hence to the increase in edema and ascites formation.

Vasodilators are generally classified as arteriolar dilators, venodilators or combination (i.e. balanced) arteriolar and venodilators. Arteriolar dilators relax the smooth muscle of systemic arterioles, decreasing peripheral vascular resistance and impedance. This usually results in decreased systemic arterial blood pressure, systolic intraventricular pressure and systolic myocardial wall stress (or afterload). Thus, the force that opposes myocardial fiber shortening is reduced. This allows the heart muscle to shorten further and increases stroke volume. That reduces the work the heart has to do and increases tissue perfusion.

Arteriolar dilators are especially useful in patients with left-sided valvular regurgitation and left-to-right shunts. For example, in CVD, the left ventricle pumps blood in two directions: forwards into the systemic circulation and backwards through a leaky mitral valve. The percentage of blood pumped into the systemic circulation versus the percentage pumped into the left atrium depends on the relative resistances to blood flow. If resistance to blood flowing into the left atrium (e.g. 1000 $dyn.s.cm^{-5}.m^2$) is one half of systemic vascular resistance (e.g. 2000 dyn.s.cm^{-5}.m^{2}), twice as much blood will be ejected into the left atrium in systole as is ejected into the aorta (i.e. 67% of the stroke volume will be ejected into the left atrium and 33% will be ejected into the aorta). In dogs with severe CVD more than 75% of the total left ventricular stroke volume may go backward into the left atrium.

Resistance to blood flow into the systemic circulation depends primarily on the cross-sectional area of the systemic arterioles. Resistance to blood flow through a defect like a leaky mitral valve depends on the size of the defect. Defect size is relatively fixed (unless a surgeon intervenes) in the short term but does progress over time as the disease progresses. Systemic vascular resistance, however, is labile and can be manipulated with drugs. If an arteriolar-dilating drug is administered to a patient with CVD, the decrease in systemic vascular resistance (e.g. to 1000 dyn.s.cm^{-5}.m^{2}) will result in an increase in forward flow into the aorta and systemic circulation. This will result in a decrease in backward flow into the left atrium and so a decrease in left atrial and pulmonary capillary pressures. In this example, the percentage of the stroke volume ejected into the left atrium will decrease from 67% to 50%, which would represent a large change, but even modest reductions in regurgitation fraction (5%) would be clinically significant.

Venodilators relax systemic venous smooth muscle, theoretically redistributing some of the blood volume into the systemic venous reservoir, decreasing cardiac blood volume and reducing pulmonary and hepatic congestion. The net result is reduced ventricular diastolic pressures, decreased pulmonary and systemic capillary pressures and diminished edema and ascites formation. Consequently, venodilators are used in the same situations as diuretics and sodium-restricted diets.

Vasodilators are also classified according to their mechanism of action (Table 17.5). ACE inhibitors not only produce vasodilation, they inhibit the RAAS and are thus neuroendocrine modulators resulting in less sodium and water retention.

Therapeutic endpoints

The therapeutic endpoint of vasodilator therapy is reduction in edema (reduced pulmonary capillary pressure and venous pressures) for venodilators and improved forward perfusion (elevation of cardiac output) for arteriolar dilators in patients with diseases such as DCM. When regurgitation or left-to-right shunting is present, arteriolar dilators reduce pulmonary edema formation and improve forward flow.

While it may not be feasible to measure these parameters directly, close monitoring of clinical signs and radiographic appearance of the lungs is realistic. Therapeutic response is seen as a decrease in cough, return of normal respiratory rate and effort, improved capillary refill time and color (sometimes hyperemic), improved distal extremity perfusion and temperature, improved attitude and possibly exercise tolerance, resolution of ascites and radiographic resolution of the pulmonary edema or pleural effusion. Mean or systolic systemic arterial blood pressure is usually reduced by 10–20 mmHg after the administration of a potent arteriolar dilator. Mean systemic arterial blood pressure should be maintained above 60 mmHg.

Adverse effects

While vasodilators enable one to achieve better therapeutic results, with their use comes the potential for adverse effects. These drugs are often used in critically ill canine or feline patients or patients with multiple problems that may be on several medications at the time of evaluation or during the course of treatment. These patients, in general, are at greater risk for experiencing adverse effects from a drug.

Table 17.5 Vasodilator drugs commonly used in veterinary medicine

Vasodilator	Type (mechanism)	Route	Dose	
			Dogs	*Cats*
Pimobendan*	Balanced (inodilator)	PO	0.25-0.3 mg/kg q.12 h	
Amlodipine**	Arterial (Ca channel blocker)	PO	0.01-3 mg/kg PO q.12-24 h (usually 12)	0.625 mg/cat q.24 h
Hydralazine	Arterial (↑ PGI_2)	PO	0.5–3 mg/kg q.12 h	2.5–10 mg/cat q.12 h
Prazosin	Balanced (α_1-blocker)	PO	0.5–2 mg/dog q.8–12 h	0.6 cm/cat q.6–8 h
Nitroglycerin	Venous (cGMP formation)	Cutaneous	0.6 cm per 5 kg q.6–8 h	
Nitroprusside	Balanced (cGMP formation)	IV	1–15 μg/kg/min	
Benazepril*	Balanced (ACE inhibitor)	PO	0.3–0.5 mg/kg q.24 h	0.2–0.7 mg/kg q.24 h
Enalapril*	Balanced (ACE inhibitor)	PO	0.5 mg/kg q.12–24 h (usually used q.12)	0.5 mg/kg q.12–24 h

* Authors' preferred agents for HF.
** Authors' preferred agent for systemic hypertension.

The primary major adverse effect of systemic arteriolar dilator therapy is clinically significant hypotension (i.e. mean systemic blood pressure <60 mmHg). This is uncommon and usually occurs as an isolated event following administration of the first doses of the drug or during titration of the dose. It may only warrant a decrease in the dose rather than discontinuation of the drug. The additive effects of a diuretic and a vasodilator may be a factor in producing hypotension. In the authors' clinical experience, this generally only occurs if the patient is clinically dehydrated and severely volume depleted. Hypotension is more common and often more severe when two arteriolar dilators are administered concurrently.

It is important to recognize systemic arterial hypotension. If it is misinterpreted as incomplete response to medication or progression of the disease, further doses could result in added complications. Acute-onset weakness and lethargy following drug administration are the most common clinical signs of hypotension.

Hypotension is poorly defined in the medical literature or only defined as any systemic arterial blood pressure less than normal. However, in clinical patients the term hypotension probably should not be used to denote a mild to moderate decrease in blood pressure. Rather, it should be reserved to denote a systemic arterial blood pressure low enough to result in clinical signs.

To produce clinical signs, systemic arterial blood pressure must decrease to a point where blood flow is markedly reduced through particular vascular beds. When mean systemic arterial blood pressure decreases to less than approximately 50–60 mmHg, flow to renal, myocardial and cerebral vascular beds becomes compromised. Normal mean arterial blood pressure is 100–110 mmHg. Therefore, there is a blood pressure reserve of about 50 mmHg. Arteriolar dilators take advantage of this reserve in patients with heart failure and cause mild to moderate decreases or tolerable reductions in blood pressure as a therapeutic effect. In patients with heart failure it is common to decrease mean systemic arterial blood pressure to 70–80 mmHg. This is an expected and therapeutic effect and causes no clinical signs of hypotension. On the contrary, clinical signs are generally improved because of the enhanced systemic blood flow (tissue perfusion) achieved through a tolerable reduction in afterload (blood pressure).

PURE VASODILATORS

Calcium channel blockers

Amlodipine

Amlodipine is a dihydropyridine calcium channel blocker that primarily affects the calcium channels in vascular smooth muscle, specifically in systemic arteriolar smooth muscle. Calcium channel blockers as a class are considered vasodilators but individual agents have different relative potencies and additional effects. Calcium channel blockers are also class IV antiarrhythmics and positive lusitropic agents. For further discussion of these properties please refer to the antiarrhythmic and positive lusitropic sections of this chapter respectively.

Amlodipine is the only calcium channel blocker used in veterinary practice that has potent vasodilatory properties. Amlodipine is similar to nifedipine. Both drugs have primarily arteriolar dilating properties with little effect on cardiac conduction and mechanical properties in the doses used clinically. Because of its ability to relax the smooth muscle of systemic arterioles, amlodipine imparts benefits similar to hydralazine to patients with mitral regurgitation (i.e. reduce the amount of regurgitation). These benefits may be realized without the reflex tachycardia seen with hydralazine and the drug appears to be better tolerated by the gastrointestinal tract.

Clinical applications

Amlodipine is an arteriolar dilator frequently used to treat systemic hypertension in cats and dogs. It can also be used to treat severe mitral regurgitation in dogs, in a similar manner to hydralazine. In heart failure the dose must be titrated to an effective endpoint using systemic arterial blood pressure as a guide. In general, systolic blood pressure should decrease by 10–15 mmHg when an effective dose is being administered. This systemic hypotension is a relative contraindication to initiation of amlodipine in the treatment of heart failure. If the dose is not titrated up to an effective endpoint, most often an effective dose will not be achieved, resulting in no clinical benefit. Benefits of amlodipine over hydralazine appear to be less reflex tachycardia, fewer gastrointestinal side effects and a lower incidence of clinically significant hypotension.

One short term study documented a reduction in regurgitant fraction (74% to 63%) after an average dose of 0.25 mg/kg (range 0.13–0.53 mg/kg) PO q.24 h in 16 dogs with left heart failure secondary to CVD short term. No adverse effects were noted. Systolic blood pressure decreased from 140 mmHg to 134 mmHg.

Mechanism of action

Amlodipine is a calcium channel blocker that affects primarily the calcium channels in vascular smooth muscle, specifically in systemic arteriolar smooth muscle. It is similar to nifedipine. Both drugs have primarily arteriolar dilating properties, although amlodipine has even fewer negative inotropic effects than its parent compound.

Formulations and dose rates

Amlodipine is supplied as tablets containing the besylate salt of amlodipine (2.5, 5 and 10 mg tablets). To treat refractory pulmonary edema secondary to severe mitral regurgitation, the dose needs to be titrated. The starting dose can be as low as 0.1 mg/kg q.24 h and can peak as high as 0.5 mg/kg q.12 h. The same protocol can be used to treat systemic hypertension in dogs but the peak dose may be as high as 3 mg/kg q.12 h.

Pharmacokinetics

The pharmacokinetics of amlodipine have been studied in dogs. Bioavailability is about 90%, compared to bioavailability in humans of about 65%. Time to peak plasma concentration is 6 h in dogs and 8 h in humans. Following intravenous or oral administration, about 45% of the drug is excreted in the feces and 45% in the urine as metabolites. Only 2% of the drug is excreted unchanged. Initial metabolism involves oxidation of the dihydropyridine ring to the pyridine analog. Further metabolism involves side-chain oxidation and hydrolysis of one or both side-chain ester groups. Plasma half-life is similar to that in humans at about 30 h following intravenous administration. Volume of distribution is also similar to that in humans at 25 L/kg. Approximately 95% of amlodipine is protein bound in all species studied.

Adverse effects

Theoretically, amlodipine overdose can cause clinically significant systemic hypotension. In practice, this appears to be very uncommon. However, further experience with the drug is required before any definitive statements can be made. Amlodipine produces no electrocardiographic effects in humans administered the drug. Amlodipine and a β-blocker can be administered together. The drug has been too expensive to use in large dogs. However, a generic formulation has recently become available.

Hydralazine

Clinical applications

The primary indication for hydralazine administration in veterinary medicine is severe mitral regurgitation that is refractory to conventional therapy. Hydralazine is also very effective for treating canine and feline patients with severe aortic regurgitation and patients with a large ventricular septal defect. Hydralazine can also be used to decrease systemic blood pressure in dogs with systemic hypertension. Administration of an α-adrenergic blocking drug is frequently required when the drug is used to treat systemic hypertension to block the reflex increase in cardiac output brought about by the sympathetically mediated increase in contractility and heart rate.

Mechanism of action

Hydralazine directly relaxes the smooth muscle in systemic arterioles, probably by increasing the prostacyclin concentration in systemic arterioles. It also increases aortic compliance. Hydralazine has no effect on systemic venous tone. It decreases vascular resistance in renal, coronary, cerebral and mesenteric vascular beds more than in skeletal muscle beds. Hydralazine also reflexly increases myocardial contractility. This is most probably secondary to hydralazine-induced histamine release resulting in noradrenaline (norepinephrine) release.

Hydralazine is a very potent arteriolar dilator. In dogs it is able to decrease systemic vascular resistance to less than 50% of baseline in comparison to captopril, which can only decrease systemic vascular resistance by about 25%. Hydralazine's potency can be both beneficial and detrimental to its use. Its potency is of benefit because it results in good to profound improvement in the majority of patients in which it is indicated. Its potency can be detrimental if it results in systemic hypotension.

In small dogs with severe mitral regurgitation refractory to the administration of furosemide, regurgitant flow may constitute 75–85% of cardiac output. Left ventricular contractile function is usually normal or only mildly depressed. Consequently, the major hemodynamic abnormalities are caused by marked regurgitant flow through an incompetent mitral valve. The ideal treatment would be mitral valve repair but currently this is not technically feasible. Consequently, the theoretical treatment of choice is arteriolar dilator administration.

ACE inhibitors are usually the first choice for achieving mild arteriolar dilation. Hydralazine is more potent and is reserved for patients that are refractory to ACE inhibitors. Hydralazine decreases regurgitant flow, increases forward aortic flow and venous oxygen tension and decreases radiographic evidence of pulmonary edema. A therapeutic dosage decreases mean arterial blood pressure from 100–110 mmHg to 60–80 mmHg. These effects improve the quality of life and appear to prolong survival time.

In dogs with dilated cardiomyopathy, hydralazine also improves cardiac output but does not usually appreciably reduce edema formation. Consequently, the drug does not seem to improve the quality of life for the patient nor does it usually result in appreciable prolongation of life.

Formulations and dose rates

Hydralazine is available as tablets. The author (Kittelson) has witnessed a lack of response to some generic hydralazine products and does not recommend their use.

The effective dose is 0.5–3.0 mg/kg q.12 h PO. This dose must be titrated, starting with a low dose and titrating upward to an effective endpoint.

Dose titration

In dogs that are not being administered an ACE inhibitor, the starting dose of hydralazine should be 1.0 mg/kg. This can then be titrated up to as high as 3.0 mg/kg if no response is observed at lower doses. Titration in these animals can be performed with or without blood pressure measurement. If blood pressure cannot be monitored, titration is performed more slowly and clinical and radiographic signs are monitored. Baseline assessments of mucous membrane color, capillary refill time, murmur intensity, cardiac size on radiographs and severity of pulmonary edema are made.

A dose of 1 mg/kg is administered q.12 h PO and repeat assessments are made in 12–48 h. If no response is identified, the dose is increased to 2 mg/kg q.12 h and then to 3 mg/kg q.12 h if no response is seen at the previous dose. Mucous membrane color and capillary refill time will become noticeably improved in about 50–60% of dogs. In most dogs with heart failure due to mitral regurgitation, the severity of the pulmonary edema will improve within 24 h. In many of these dogs the size of the left ventricle and left atrium will decrease. In some dogs, improvement will not be great enough to identify with certainty. In those dogs the titration may continue, with the realization that some dogs will be mildly overdosed and clinical signs of hypotension may become evident.

Owners should be warned to watch for signs of hypotension and notify the clinician if they are identified. If a dog becomes weak and lethargic following hydralazine administration, the dog should be rechecked by a veterinarian but in almost all situations the dog should only be observed until the drug effect wears off 11–13 h later. The drug dose should then be reduced. In the rare event that signs of shock become evident, fluids and vasopressors may be administered. In human medicine, there has never been a death recorded that was secondary to the administration of hydralazine alone. The dosage record is 10 g. The authors have observed dogs becoming very weak following an overdose of hydralazine but have never observed a serious complication when the drug was not administered in conjunction with another vasodilator such as an ACE inhibitor.

More rapid titration can be performed if blood pressure monitoring is available. In this situation, baseline blood pressure is measured and 1.0 mg/kg hydralazine administered. Blood pressure measurement should then be repeated 1–2 h later. If blood pressure (systolic, diastolic or mean) has decreased by at least 15 mmHg, the dose administered (1.0 mg/kg) is effective and should be administered q.12 h from then on. If no response is identified, another 1.0 mg/kg dose should be administered (cumulative dose of 2.0 mg/kg) and blood pressure measured again 1–2 h later. This can continue until a cumulative dose of 3.0 mg/kg has been administered within a 12 h period. The resultant cumulative dose then becomes the dose administered q.12 h.

In dogs that are already receiving an ACE inhibitor, hydralazine must be added to the treatment regimen cautiously. ACE inhibition depletes the body's ability to produce angiotensin II in response to hydralazine-induced vasodilation. Severe hypotension can occur if the hydralazine dose is not titrated carefully. In general, the dosage should start at 0.5 mg/kg and the dose should be titrated at 0.5 mg/kg increments until a response is identified. Blood pressure monitoring is strongly encouraged in this situation. Referral to a specialist cardiologist or internist is also encouraged if feasible.

In dogs with acute, fulminant heart failure due to severe mitral regurgitation that are not already receiving an ACE inhibitor, hydralazine titration can be more aggressive. An initial dose of 2.0 mg/kg may be administered along with intravenous furosemide. This dose should produce a beneficial response in more than 75% of dogs. It may produce hypotension but the hypotension is rarely fatal, whereas fulminant pulmonary edema is commonly fatal.

Pharmacokinetics

Hydralazine is well absorbed from the gastrointestinal tract but undergoes first-pass hepatic metabolism. Although the kidney does not excrete hydralazine, its biotransformation is affected by renal failure, which may increase serum concentration. The vasodilating effect of hydralazine occurs within 30–60 min after oral administration and peaks within 3 h. The effect is then stable for the next 8–10 h, after which it rapidly dissipates. The net duration of effect is about 12 h.

Adverse effects

The most common side effects include first-dose hypotension and anorexia, vomiting and diarrhea.

- **Gastrointestinal.** Anorexia and/or vomiting occur in approximately 20–30% of patients. They are often intractable as long as the drug is being administered. Consequently, discontinuation of the drug may be necessary. Reducing the dose to 0.25–0.5 mg/kg q.12 h for 1–2 weeks and then increasing the dose to its therapeutic range may be effective in some cases.

- **Hypotension.** The most serious adverse effect is hypotension, indicated by signs of weakness and depression. In most cases, this does not require treatment and the signs will abate within 10–12 h after the last dose of hydralazine. The dose should then be reduced.
- **Reflex tachycardia.** When hydralazine is used as the only agent in patients with hypertension and normal cardiac function, hydralazine induces a reflex increase in sympathetic nervous system tone. The increased sympathetic drive increases myocardial contractility and heart rate. Consequently cardiac output increases dramatically, offsetting the effect of the arteriolar dilation. The net result is no change in systemic arterial blood pressure. When an α-adrenergic receptor blocker is added to the therapeutic regimen, the reflex effect is blocked and systemic arterial blood pressure decreases.

  Although hydralazine is not commonly used to treat hypertension in veterinary medicine, this same response would be expected in a patient that is misdiagnosed and receives hydralazine when it is not in heart failure.

  Reflex sympathetic tachycardia is not as common in heart failure patients as in patients with systemic hypertension. However, in one study, heart rate in dogs with mild to moderate heart failure increased from an average of 136 beats/min to 153 beats/min following hydralazine administration. In patients with heart failure, the sympathetic nervous system is already activated but the heart's ability to respond to the sympathetic nervous system is blunted or abolished. In fact, the heart's ability to respond to any type of stimulus is overwhelmed.

  Therefore, when hydralazine is administered to a patient with heart failure, systemic arterial blood pressure does decrease and a less profound increase in systemic blood flow is produced than that observed when the drug is administered to patients with systemic hypertension.

  Reflex tachycardia may be controlled by the addition of α-adrenergic blocking drugs or digoxin.
- **Increased renin release.** Rebound increases in renin and aldosterone secretion and decreased sodium excretion occur following hydralazine administration. The beneficial effect on regurgitant fraction usually outweighs these effects, however.

  One should remember that drugs like furosemide also increase renin release and so increase plasma aldosterone concentration. In people, systemic lupus erythematosus, drug fever and peripheral neuropathy have been reported.

Known drug interactions

Hydralazine administration may have beneficial effects on the pharmacokinetics and pharmacodynamics of other drugs.

- Increased renal blood flow caused by hydralazine administration can increase the glomerular filtration rate (if initially depressed) and thereby enhance digoxin excretion.
- Increased renal blood flow also improves furosemide delivery to the nephron. This increases furosemide's renal effects (increases natriuresis and diuresis), especially in patients that are refractory to furosemide administration because of decreased renal flow due to decreased cardiac output.

Prazosin

Clinical applications

Prazosin is an arteriolar and venodilatory agent. The hemodynamic effects of prazosin have not been documented in the dog or cat. In humans with heart failure, its administration decreases right and left ventricular filling pressures, edema and congestion and increases stroke volume and cardiac output. Prazosin is effective in reducing mean arterial blood pressure in some dogs with renal hypertension.

Mechanism of action

Prazosin acts primarily by blocking α_1-adrenergic receptors but also peripherally inhibits phosphodiesterase. Since prazosin does not block α_2-adrenergic receptors, noradrenaline (norepinephrine) release is still controlled via negative feedback. Reflex tachycardia is generally not seen. The vasodilating effects of prazosin become attenuated after the first dose in humans and in rats. This problem has markedly limited its use in human medicine. In rats, it is thought that this effect is brought about by stimulation of the RAAS.

Formulations and dose rates

Prazosin is supplied as capsules.

DOGS

- The starting dose is 1 mg q.8 h PO for dogs <15 kg and 2 mg q.8 h PO for dogs >15 kg
- The dose then needs to be titrated upward if the initial dose is ineffective, or reduced if hypotension occurs

CATS

- The preparation is not amenable for use in cats

Pharmacokinetics

Elimination and metabolism are primarily hepatic. No adjustment is made for renal insufficiency.

Adverse effects

Prazosin may cause first-dose hypotension, anorexia, vomiting, diarrhea and syncope.

Nitrates

> **EXAMPLES**
>
> **IV:** nitroprusside
> **Topical:** nitroglycerin

The organic nitrates, such as nitroglycerin, are esters of nitric oxide. Nitroprusside is a nitric oxide-containing compound without an ester bond. There are important differences in the biotransformation of these compounds but it is generally accepted that they share a common final pathway of nitric oxide (endothelium-derived relaxing factor) production and a common therapeutic effect. Organic nitrates, such as nitroglycerin, are explosive. They are rendered nonexplosive by diluting the compound with an inert recipient, such as lactose.

Mechanism of action

Nitrates relax vascular smooth muscle. They do this through a complex series of events. Nitrates are denitrated in smooth muscle cells to form nitric oxide (NO), which binds with the heme moiety on the enzyme guanylate cyclase. This causes activation of guanylate cyclase, which enzymatically forms cGMP from GTP. Cyclic GMP activates a serine/threonine protein kinase, which phosphorylates myosin light chains, resulting in smooth muscle relaxation. Cyclic GMP also stimulates calcium efflux and uptake by intracellular proteins and may inhibit calcium influx.

Clinical applications

Nitrates have been advocated as agents to produce systemic venodilation in dogs and cats with heart failure. Few studies have been performed to document the pharmacodynamics or establish the therapeutic dosage of the nitrates in dogs or cats. Nitrates can be administered orally, intravenously or transcutaneously to patients with heart failure. When administered transcutaneously or orally to humans, a low plasma concentration is achieved. Nitrates act primarily as venodilators at low plasma concentrations. When administered intravenously, a higher concentration is achieved and arteriolar dilation also occurs. Intravenous nitroglycerin is a potent venodilator with moderate arteriolar dilating properties.

Nitrates are well absorbed from the gastrointestinal tract but are rapidly metabolized by hepatic organic nitrate reductase. Consequently, bioavailability of orally administered nitrates is very low, typically less than 10%. In humans, the duration of effect after transcutaneous administration is 3–8 h.

Nitrate tolerance

The phenomenon of nitrate tolerance dates back to the 1940s. Munitions workers exposed to nitroglycerin commonly developed a headache on Monday that abated over the week as they developed tolerance. Over the weekend, their tolerance abated and on Monday, re-exposure again resulted in headache.

Tolerance to the organic nitrates is a common problem in human patients, occurring in up to 70% of individuals exposed to intravenous infusions of nitroglycerin. The exact mechanism is poorly understood, although two possible explanations have been proposed. The most popular theory is that sulfhydryl groups (thiols) are depleted with repeated exposure. Sulfhydryl groups are required for the metabolic conversion of nitroglycerin to nitric oxide. The second theory involves neurohormonal activation resulting in vasoconstriction and increased renal sodium retention.

Intermittent administration of nitrates prevents tolerance in human patients. However, this approach is limited by the fact that the hemodynamic benefit is interrupted. Concurrent administration of hydralazine with a nitrate appears to prevent nitrate tolerance in human heart failure patients. Hydralazine also prevents tolerance in a rat model of heart failure and in vitro in rat aortas rendered tolerant to nitrate in vivo. The results of the in vitro experiment suggested that the effect was due to inhibition of a pyridoxyl-dependent reaction, such as the catabolism of cysteine and methionine, which could enhance the availability of sulfhydryl groups.

Nitroglycerin

Clinical applications

In human patients with heart failure, transdermal administration of nitroglycerin primarily results in systemic venodilation. This effect results in a redistribution of blood volume from the central to the peripheral vascular compartments resulting in a decrease in diastolic intraventricular pressures and a reduction in the formation of edema fluid. Systemic vascular resistance is lowered to a lesser degree. The dosage required to produce a beneficial effect is highly variable from patient to patient and some patients are refractory to the drug. Tolerance develops quickly, within 18–24 h. A rebound increase in systemic vascular resistance is observed when nitroglycerin is withdrawn, which results in a decrease in cardiac output. There is no rebound effect on ventricular diastolic and atrial pressures.

Transdermal administration of nitroglycerin has been advocated for use in dogs and cats with heart failure. All references in the veterinary literature to the use of nitroglycerin, including dosing, are anecdotal. Nitroglycerin is most commonly administered in conjunction with furosemide, usually to patients with severe heart failure. Beneficial effects in this situation cannot be directly ascribed to nitroglycerin because it is well known that furosemide by itself can produce dramatically beneficial effects in these patients.

In our clinic, transdermal nitroglycerin is only rarely used in patients with heart failure. However, we have on occasion observed beneficial effects in dogs that were not responding or had become unresponsive to other cardiovascular drugs. Consequently, there may be a limited role for this drug in veterinary patients. Nitroglycerin is not a very effective drug and should never be administered as the sole agent to a patient with moderate to severe heart failure.

Formulations and dose rates

Nitroglycerin ointment is available in a 2% formulation to be spread on the skin for absorption into the systemic circulation. Numerous manufacturers also supply it in a transcutaneous patch preparation. Nitroglycerin is diluted with lactose, dextrose, alcohol, propylene glycol or another suitable inert excipient so that the medical-grade material usually contains about 10% nitroglycerin. It appears as a white powder when diluted with lactose or as a clear, colorless or pale yellow liquid when diluted with alcohol or propylene glycol. Nitroglycerin is also supplied as a liquid for intravenous administration. Extended-release preparations are supplied as capsules or scored tablets.

In dogs and cats, 2% nitroglycerin cream has been used (12 mm per 2.5 kg bodyweight q.12 h for dogs, 3–6 mm q.4–6 h for cats) but efficacy has not been documented. If transcutaneous nitroglycerin cream is used, it should be applied on a hairless area (usually inside the ear flap), using gloves, since transcutaneous absorption will occur in the clinician or owner as well as in the patient. Cutaneous absorption in a human can cause a profound headache and a very unhappy client. Transdermal patches have been used successfully in large dogs with dilated cardiomyopathy.

When nitroglycerin is administered intravenously it acts as a potent arteriolar dilator and venodilator. The onset of action after intravenous administration is similar to nitroprusside. Duration of effect is minutes so the drug must be administered by CRI. The recommended administration rate to start with in humans is 5 μg/min. This dose is increased in increments of 10–20 μg/min until an effect is identified. There is no fixed optimum dose. Effective doses in small animals have not been identified. To use this drug, a low starting dose would have to be identified and titrated upward as blood pressure was monitored.

In cats and dogs, extended-release nitroglycerin can be used to treat refractory heart failure alone or in conjunction with other vasodilators. Most experience has been garnered in dogs and cats with refractory ascites or pleural effusion. Anecdotal evidence would suggest that the time between fluid removal can be increased by several weeks if extended-release nitrogylcerin is used and in some cases use of the drug may eliminate the need for fluid removal altogether. The dose should be titrated, starting at 2.5 mg q.12 h orally in cats up to a maximum of 6.5 mg q.8 h PO. Small dogs can be treated the same as cats. In medium to large dogs, the dose is started at 6.5 mg q.12 h PO. The maximum dose is 9.0 mg q.8 h PO.

Mechanism of action

Nitroglycerin is an organic nitrovasodilator that possesses a nitrate ester bond. The biotransformation of nitroglycerin to nitric oxide is complex and not completely understood. Thiols (compounds containing sulfhydryl groups) appear to be important as intermediary structures.

Pharmacokinetics

Nitrates are metabolized in the liver by nitrate reductase to two active major metabolites: 1,2- and 1,3-dinitroglycerols. Although less active than their parent compounds, they may be responsible for some of the pharmacological effect.

Nitroglycerin has a very short half-life of 1–4 min. It is metabolized to 1,3-glyceryl dinitrate, 1,2-glyceryl dinitrate and glyceryl mononitrate. The parent compound is approximately 10–14 times as potent as the dinitrate metabolites but the metabolites have longer half-lives and are present in substantial plasma concentrations. The mononitrate metabolite is inactive. The onset of action with the transdermal route of administration is delayed and the duration of effect is prolonged. Transdermal systems are designed to provide continuous, controlled release of nitroglycerin to the skin, from which the drug undergoes absorption. The rates of delivery and absorption of the drug to the skin vary with the specific preparation. Individual manufacturers' information for a drug should be consulted for this information. However, one must remember that this information pertains to human skin and probably does not translate into the actual rate of delivery for a dog or a cat.

Special considerations

Nitroglycerin ointment should be stored in airtight containers at 15–30°C. Owners should be instructed to close the container tightly immediately after each use. Intravenous nitroglycerin solutions should be stored only in glass bottles because nitroglycerin migrates readily into many plastics. About 40–80% of the total amount of nitroglycerin in a diluted solution for IV administration is absorbed by the polyvinyl chloride (PVC) tubing of IV administration sets. Special non-PVC-containing administration sets are available.

Isosorbide mononitrate and dinitrate

Clinical applications

Isosorbide mononitrate and dinitrate are organic nitrates that can be administered orally, primarily to patients with severe, refractory heart failure. One study has documented that isosorbide mononitrate did not produce the expected shift in blood volume from the central thoracic space to the splanchnic space. As with other nitrates, one should never rely on the isosorbides to produce a clinically meaningful change in hemodynamics or produce clinically significant improvement.

Mechanism of action

This is the same as for other organic nitrates.

Formulations and dose rates

- Isosorbide dinitrate is supplied as 5, 10, 20, 30 and 40 mg tablets. Isosorbide mononitrate is supplied as 10 and 20 mg tablets
- The dose for both nitrates is in the 1–2 mg/kg q.12 h range

Pharmacokinetics

Isosorbide mononitrate has been studied in experimental dogs. In one study, a dose of approximately 1–2 mg/kg PO to dogs subjected to transmyocardial direct current shock produced acute hemodynamic effects that lasted only 2 h. This dose when administered over days, however, resulted in a chronic decrease in pulmonary capillary wedge pressure and a decrease in left ventricular volume and mass when compared to control dogs.

Nitroprusside

Clinical applications

Nitroprusside is a potent venodilator and arteriolar dilator. It may also increase left ventricular compliance. It is administered intravenously and is used only for short-term treatment of dogs with severe or fulminant heart failure. In one study in normal dogs, nitroprusside decreased systemic arterial blood pressure by 23% and increased cardiac output by 39%. This effect became attenuated over time. Because tolerance does not occur with nitroprusside, this attenuation of effect is probably due to reflex changes. As expected, left ventricular end-diastolic and end-systolic diameters decreased in one study, as did left ventricular end-diastolic pressure.

Nitroprusside is beneficial in dogs with experimentally induced acute mitral regurgitation (comparable to a patient with a ruptured chorda tendinea). In one study, a dose of 5 µg/kg/min reduced left ventricular systolic pressure 16% and decreased left ventricular end-diastolic pressure from 23 mmHg to a normal value of 10 mmHg. Left atrial pressure, left atrial diameter and left ventricular diameter also decreased. The left atrial ‘v’ wave decreased from 41 mmHg to 16 mmHg.

In humans with severe heart failure, nitroprusside can produce beneficial effects that are as good as or better than administration of intravenous furosemide. In one study, nitroprusside reduced pulmonary capillary pressure from 31 mmHg to 16 mmHg while increasing the cardiac index from 2.33 L/min/m^2 to 3.62 L/min/m^2. Furosemide (200 mg IV) in these same patients decreased pulmonary capillary pressure to 27 mmHg while the cardiac index did not change.

Nitroprusside, in combination with dobutamine, has been shown to be effective in dogs with severe heart failure due to DCM. Otherwise, all information is anecdotal. Available information suggests that nitroprusside can be very effective at improving the clinical signs of heart failure. Of course, nitroprusside only produces a temporary improvement that is readily reversible. When administration is discontinued, vasodilation rapidly disappears and a rebound increase in vasoconstriction, above that observed prior to drug administration, may occur. In human patients, when nitroprusside is discontinued after 24–72 h, pulmonary capillary and systemic arterial pressures return to pre-treatment values within 5 min. This occurs despite increases in urine volume and sodium excretion while on the drug. Consequently, other, longer-acting drugs must be administered while patients are weaned off the nitroprusside in order to maintain the improvement in hemodynamics.

Mechanism of action

Nitroprusside (sodium nitroferricyanide) produces nitric oxide in vascular smooth muscle. Unlike the organic nitrates, nitroprusside releases nitric oxide when it is nonenzymatically metabolized directly via 1-electron reduction. This may occur on exposure to numerous reducing agents and tissues such as vascular smooth muscle. The major difference between nitroprusside and the organic nitrates is that tolerance to nitroprusside does not develop.

Formulations and dose rates

Sodium nitroprusside is supplied as vials containing 50 mg of lyophilized dry powder for dilution in 5% dextrose in water.

The dose of nitroprusside is highly variable from patient to patient. In addition, the hemodynamic response can be varied depending on the amount of change in filling pressures and cardiac output desired. Consequently, the dosage range is large. Doses from 2–25 µg/kg/min reduce systemic arterial blood pressure in a dose-dependent manner in experimental dogs. However, the decrease in blood pressure with 25 µg/kg/min is only about 5 mmHg more than that observed with 10 µg/kg/min. Consequently, it does not appear that doses greater than 10 µg/kg/min provide much more benefit than those less than 10 µg/kg/min. In humans, the dosage rarely exceeds 10 µg/kg/min.

Pharmacokinetics

Nitroprusside is rapidly metabolized after intravenous administration, with a half-life of a few minutes. Consequently, no loading dose is required and any untoward effects of the drug can be rapidly reversed by discontinuing drug administration. When nitroprusside is metabolized, cyanogen (cyanide radical) is produced. This is converted to thiocyanate in the liver by the enzyme thiosulfate sulfurtransferase (rhodanase).

Adverse effects

- Adverse effects of nitroprusside are hypotension and cyanide toxicity.
- Nitroprusside-induced hypotension can be rapidly (1–10 min) reversed by discontinuing drug administration.
- Sodium nitroprusside infusions in excess of 2 μg/kg/min generate cyanogen in amounts greater than can be effectively buffered by the normal quantity of methemoglobin in the body. Deaths due to cyanogen toxicity can result when this buffering system is exhausted. In humans, this has only been reported in patients receiving infusion rates of 30–120 μg/kg/min. However, increased circulating cyanogen concentration, metabolic acidosis and clinical deterioration have been observed at infusion rates within the therapeutic range.
- In humans, it has been recommended that an infusion rate of 10 μg/kg/min should not last for longer than 10 min. Cyanogen toxicity can be manifest as venous hyperoxemia (bright red blood as a result of the inability of oxygen to dissociate from hemoglobin), lactic acidosis and dyspnea. Administration of thiosulfate and of hydroxycobalamin have been reported to prevent cyanide toxicity. In the presence of thiosulfate, cyanogen is converted to thiocyanate, which is excreted in the kidneys.
- Thiocyanate toxicity can occur, especially in patients that have a decrease in GFR, are on prolonged infusions or are receiving thiosulfate. Neurological signs occur in humans at a serum concentration of 60 μg/mL and death can occur at concentrations above 200 μg/mL. As for other hypotensive agents, nitroprusside increases plasma renin activity.

Special considerations

Sodium nitroprusside is sensitive to light, heat and moisture. Exposure to light causes deterioration that may be observed as a change in color from brown to blue caused by reduction of the ferric ion to a ferrous ion. If not protected from light, approximately 20% of the drug in solution in glass bottles will deteriorate every 4 h when exposed to fluorescent light.

The drug deteriorates even faster in plastic containers. Consequently, sodium nitroprusside should be protected from light by wrapping the bottle with aluminum foil. When adequately protected from light, the solution is stable for 24 h. Nitroprusside reacts with minute quantities of a variety of agents including alcohol, forming blue, dark red or green products. The solution should be discarded if this occurs.

VASODILATORS WITH ADDITIONAL PROPERTIES

Inodilators

EXAMPLES

Oral: pimobendan
IV: milrinone, amrinone

This class of agents has both positive inotropic and vasodilatory properties and has been labeled inodilators as a reflection of the term 'inodilation' coined by Lionel H Opie in 1989. All properties of this class are discussed in detail in the inodilator section of this chapter (p. 398).

Angiotensin-converting enzyme (ACE) inhibitors

EXAMPLES

Enalapril (preferred), benazepril (preferred), ramipril (preferred), lisinopril, captopril

In general, all ACE inhibitors have similar effects on hemodynamics. ACE inhibitors are modest balanced venodilators with important neuroendocrine modulatory effects. Thus further discussion of ACE inhibitors will be covered in the neuroendocrine modulation section of this chapter.

Sildenafil

Sildenafil (Viagra®) is an orally active phosphodiesterase V inhibitor (PDE Vi). Phosphodiesterase V is found in a relatively high concentration in lung and erectile penile tissue and is elevated in humans with pulmonary hypertension. Pulmonary hypertension (PH) is a clinically important disease in the dog with high morbidity and mortality rates. Canine PH is most often a sequel of other disease processes and thus requires a balanced therapeutic approach which targets the underlying etiology as well as palliation of clinical signs. An important goal of therapy is to reduce pulmonary artery pressure. Conventional systemic arteriolar dilators have no preferential effect on pulmonary vasculature and thus have no benefit and may worsen clinical signs. PDE Vi prevents degradation of cGMP resulting in relaxation of pulmonary vascular smooth muscle and, to a lesser degree, systemic vasodilation (preferential pulmonary vasodilation). Sildenafil is currently the most extensively researched of the PDE V inhibitors and has been shown to improve both exercise tolerance and quality of life in humans with pulmonary hypertension resulting in its FDA approval for treatment of this disorder in humans.

Viagra® was recently re-released as Revatio® (which is more expensive). Sildenafil is now available as a generic preparation in some countries further reducing its cost although documentation of efficacy of the generic formulations has not been reported. Clinical improvement in humans has been documented at multiple doses ranging from 20 mg to 80 mg three times a day. Because higher doses do not increase the efficacy, the currently recommended dose in humans is 20 mg every 8 h.

Formulations and dose rates

CANINE

- 0.25–3.0 mg/kg PO

Empirically, the authors start at a dose of approximately 5 mg/dog and titrate. In oxygen-dependent dogs, initiation of the target dose of approximately 3 mg/kg may be indicated and well tolerated based on the authors experience. Uptitration can occur over days to weeks if patients are not oxygen dependent. Due to cost the authors have not used doses greater then 25 mg/dog. Oral sildenafil liquid dosage forms have been reported to be stable and have been used in people. Therefore suspension formulations can be used in dogs and greatly facilitate cost effective accurate dosing.

Adverse effects

None have been documented in the dogs managed by the author (>25 dogs). One retrospective canine study also reported no adverse side effects and clinical improvements in 10 dogs with PH receiving a median dose of approximately 2 mg/kg every 8–24 h.

Known drug interactions

Due to the nature of canine PH, sildenafil has been used in combination with many other medications including conventional heart failure medications (diuretics, ACE inhibitors, pimobendan) with no recognized adverse effects.

NEUROENDOCRINE MODULATION

Agents in this group address the maladaptive changes associated with the progression of heart disease in the RAAS and sympathetic nervous system.

EXAMPLES

Oral: ACE inhibitors (preferred), aldosterone antagonist (e.g. spironolactone) (preferred), β-blockers (preferred), digoxin, neutral endopeptidase inhibitors, angiotensin receptor blockers

Angiotensin-converting enzyme (ACE) inhibitors

EXAMPLES

Enalapril (preferred), benazepril (preferred), ramipril (preferred), lisinopril, captopril

There are five ACE inhibitors that have been used in dogs and cats: captopril, enalapril, lisinopril, benazepril and ramipril. Generally these drugs have similar effects. The primary difference is in duration of effect and potential side effects. Captopril, the original ACE inhibitor, is short-acting, lasting less than 3–4 h, and has more side effects than the other ACE inhibitors. It is therefore now rarely used. The effects of enalapril and ramipril last 12–14 h. Lisinopril and benazepril are thought to be the longest-acting ACE inhibitors; once-daily use is advocated in humans and animals. Benazepril is excreted primarily via hepatic metabolism versus renal filtration (others) and thus may be better tolerated in patients with pre-existing renal disease particularly when a low dose is required.

Clinical applications

The primary clinical indication for ACE inhibitors is for the treatment of heart failure in dogs, cats and people. ACE inhibitors are also frequently used for the management of systemic hypertension in people. However, their efficacy in systemic hypertension in dogs and cats when used as monotherapy has been disappointing.

A more recent indication for ACE inhibitors in dogs, cats and people is in the treatment of a variety of renal diseases with emphasis on protein-losing glomerulopathy. Given the subject matter of this chapter, these indications will not be discussed in detail but the reader is directed to additional reading on the subject including the *ACVIM consensus statement on management of proteinuria in dogs and cats*. In brief, there is evidence that use of ACE inhibitors (benazapril) will attenuate the progression of renal failure in cats with significant proteinuria. However, the evidence that they are beneficial in cats with little proteinuria (the majority of cats) has not yet been established by appropriate large-scale clinical trials. There is probably no disadvantage to using ACE inhibitors in cats with renal failure as there may be some benefit provided the cat can be pilled easily and the owner can afford the treatment. However, dietary change (reduction in phosphate) carries significantly greater potential benefits in slowing the progression of renal failure and ACE inhibitor therapy should not be regarded as a substitute for it. Treating cats and dogs that are severely azotemic or that have prerenal azotemia with ACE inhibitors may actually speed their demise.

Mechanism of action

The RAAS plays an important role in regulating cardiovascular homeostasis in normal individuals and patients with heart failure. Renin is released from the juxtaglomerular apparatus in response to sympathetic stimulation and to decreased sodium flux by the macula densa. In the plasma, renin is a protease that acts on the glycoprotein angiotensinogen to form the polypeptide angiotensin I. Angiotensin converting enzyme (ACE) cleaves two amino acids from the decapeptide angiotensin I to form the octapeptide angiotensin II. This conversion primarily occurs in the vascular endothelium of the lung although other vascular beds are involved.

ACE inhibitors bind to the same site on ACE as angiotensin I, effectively arresting its action. This site contains a zinc ion and ACE inhibitors contain a sulfhydryl, carboxyl or phosphoryl group that interacts with this site. The relative potency of these compounds depends on the affinity of the compound for the active site. ACE inhibitors that are more tightly bound to the active site tend to be more potent. They also tend to have a longer duration of effect.

The effects of ACE inhibitors occur as a result of the decreased concentration of circulating angiotensin II. Angiotensin II has several important effects in patients with heart failure.

- It is a potent vasopressor.
- It stimulates the release of aldosterone from the adrenal gland.
- It stimulates vasopressin (ADH) release from the posterior pituitary gland.
- It facilitates the central and peripheral effects of the sympathetic nervous system.
- It preserves glomerular filtration when renal blood flow is decreased via glomerular efferent arteriolar constriction.
- It stimulates hypertrophy and thus contributes to maladaptive remodeling in heart failure.

ACE inhibitors have several effects in patients with heart failure. Balanced vasodilation (arteriolar and venodilation) occur as a direct result of the decreased concentration of angiotensin II. Consequently, ACE inhibitors are generally classified as vasodilators. ACE inhibitors also decrease activation of the RAAS and this is their most important role.

The effects of ACE inhibitors become evident at different times following the onset of administration. Arteriolar dilation is observed after the first dose is administered, while the lessening of sodium and water retention takes days to become clinically significant. Since most dogs presenting for severe heart failure are dying from pulmonary edema, the ACE inhibitors are poor emergency heart failure drugs and their potential to cause adverse renal effects is enhanced when aggressive parenteral furosemide is used. Thus this author does not initiate or continue ACE inhibitor therapy when intravenous furosemide is being used.

The ability of ACE inhibitors to decrease plasma aldosterone secretion may become attenuated or lost with time. In one study of cavalier King Charles spaniels with severe mitral regurgitation, enalapril significantly decreased plasma aldosterone concentration after 3 weeks of administration. However, 6 months later the plasma aldosterone concentration had increased to an even higher level than at baseline. These dogs were also on furosemide at 6 months, which may have contributed to the increase. However, it is known that other enzymes, such as chymase, are capable of converting angiotensin I to angiotensin II and so may contribute to the lack of prolonged effect.

In most canine patients the arteriolar dilating effect of ACE inhibitors is relatively mild when compared to the more potent arteriolar dilators like amlodipine and hydralazine. In general, ACE inhibitors can decrease systemic vascular resistance by 25–30% while hydralazine can decrease it by 50%.

Benefits

Clinical cardiovascular disease

The clinical benefits of ACE inhibitors in heart failure are well documented in human and canine studies and are considered a class effect. Thus if enalpril has been shown to be beneficial one could use benazepril and expect the same effect. In human medicine there are currently head to head ACE inhibitor trials under way that may address potential differences in efficacy between ACE inhibitors. In general, ACE inhibitors improve clinical signs and improve quality of life in dogs and cats with heart failure due to diverse causes. The improvement in clinical signs is primarily due to reduction in capillary pressures and edema formation and to increased perfusion of vascular beds. ACE inhibitors are one of the few drug types used to treat heart failure that have been proved to both improve symptoms and prolong life in humans and to prolong the time until treatment failure in dogs.

A number of studies have evaluated enalapril's efficacy in dogs with dilated cardiomyopathy and with primary mitral regurgitation and heart failure. In the first study (IMPROVE: invasive multicenter prospective veterinary evaluation of enalapril study) it was shown that measurements of acute hemodynamic variables in dogs in heart failure generally did not change but chronic measures of clinical status did. A second study (COVE: co-operative veterinary enalapril study group) examined 211 dogs at 19 centers. In this blinded and placebo-controlled clinical trial, dogs on enalapril again improved clinically when compared to those on placebo over a 28-day period. There were 141 dogs with primary mitral regurgitation and 70 with dilated cardiomyopathy as the primary diagnosis.

A third study (LIVE: long-term investigation of veterinary enalapril study) continued to examine 148 dogs from the COVE and IMPROVE studies for up to 15.5 months. Dogs remained in the study until they developed intractable heart failure (n = 48), died of heart failure (n = 17), died suddenly (n = 10), died of a noncardiac cause (n = 4), dropped out of the study for other reasons (n = 48) or the study ended (n = 21). Dogs administered enalapril remained in the study significantly longer (169 days) than dogs administered the placebo (90 days). Most of this benefit occurred in the first 60 days. After that, dogs in both groups either developed intractable heart failure or died at a similar rate. When divided into dogs with mitral regurgitation and those with dilated cardiomyopathy, the dogs with dilated cardiomyopathy receiving enalapril remained in the study significantly longer than those receiving placebo while the dogs with mitral regurgitation did not. Enalapril has been shown to be beneficial in dogs with mitral regurgitation but of less benefit for the group as a whole than might have been expected. In general, some dogs with mitral regurgitation have dramatic responses to an ACE inhibitor, many improve clinically but a significant number have little response.

A more recent clinical trial compared the effects of benazepril to placebo in 162 canine patients (37 with dilated cardiomyopathy and 125 with primary mitral regurgitation) with mild to moderate heart failure. Most dogs were already being treated for heart failure with diuretics and vasodilators, including other ACE inhibitors. Benazepril (0.25–0.5 mg/kg/day) increased time to treatment failure or death (428 days) when compared to placebo (158 days). The percentage of dogs surviving without being withdrawn from the study because of worsening heart failure 1 year after the onset of the study was 49% in the benazepril group and 20% in the placebo group. From these data it appears that benazepril produces benefits similar to other ACE inhibitors in dogs with heart failure.

The results of these studies are quite clear. ACE inhibitors, despite the fact that they produce minimal hemodynamic change, result in clinical improvement in dogs with heart failure due to mitral regurgitation or dilated cardiomyopathy. ACE inhibitors appear to perform better in dogs with DCM but are clearly efficacious in many dogs with mitral regurgitation. However, in general and in both diseases, the clinical response is not profound. Rather, in most cases ACE inhibition results in mild and gradual improvement, which helps to stabilize the clinical course of the patient and improve the quality of life.

More recently, pimobendan has been demonstrated to be superior to a variety of ACE inhibitors for the treatment of canine heart failure (see p. 398). Based on all currently available data it is one of the author's (Gordon) opinion that optimum canine heart failure therapy from 2007 involves a combination of an ACE inhibitor and pimobendan as well as furosemide at a dose that controls signs of congestion.

Preclinical cardiovascular disease

Studies have been performed in humans to determine if starting ACE inhibitor therapy with enalapril in patients with left ventricular dysfunction but without evidence of heart failure is beneficial. Benefit has been defined as reduction in mortality, reduction in the incidence of heart failure and reduction in the hospitalization rate. In a study of human patients with chronic cardiac disease, 4228 patients with ejection fractions less than 35% (comparable to a shortening fraction below 15%) were randomized to receive either placebo or enalapril. They were followed clinically for an average of 37 months. During this time there was no reduction in mortality associated with enalapril administration. There was a reduction in the incidence of heart failure and in hospitalizations for heart failure (the drug delayed the onset of heart failure). These latter findings should be expected for any drug meant to effectively treat heart failure.

A recent study examined the effects of administering either enalapril or placebo to 237 cavalier King Charles spaniels with myxomatous mitral valve disease and mitral regurgitation over 2 years. Dogs at entry had to have a heart murmur due to mitral regurgitation, with or without radiographic evidence of cardiomegaly. Enalapril, when compared to placebo, had no effect on how soon these dogs went into heart failure. Consequently, there is no current indication for administering an ACE inhibitor to dogs with mitral regurgitation prior to the development of heart failure. These results were more recently confirmed in an all breed study.

Adverse effects

The potential risks of interfering with angiotensin II formation lie in its role of preserving systemic blood pressure and glomerular filtration rate (GFR) as renal flow decreases. Blocking angiotensin II action on peripheral arterioles can result in hypotension that leads to cerebral hypoperfusion. Dizziness is seen in 15%

of humans taking ACE inhibitors. The incidence of clinically significant hypotension in dogs appears to be much less, probably because dogs do not walk upright.

The second risk is seen in patients that are very dependent on angiotensin II to maintain GFR. Glomerular efferent arteriolar constriction maintains normal GFR in mild to moderately severe heart failure when renal blood flow is reduced. The primary stimulus for this vasoconstriction is increased plasma angiotensin II concentration, which is elaborated in response to the decrease in renal blood flow. Glomerular capillary pressure provides the force for filtration and glomerular capillary pressure is determined by renal plasma flow and efferent arteriolar resistance.

When renal plasma flow is low (as in heart failure) and potentiated by concurrent diuretic use, angiotensin II causes efferent arterioles to constrict, bringing glomerular capillary pressure back to normal. GFR is then preserved despite the decrease in renal blood flow and normal serum urea and creatinine concentrations are maintained. The filtration fraction (ratio of GFR to renal plasma flow) is increased. When an ACE inhibitor is administered, efferent arteriolar dilation must occur. In some patients this dilation appears to be excessive, resulting in a moderate to marked reduction in GFR and subsequent azotemia.

Those human patients that are at greatest risk for developing azotemia include patients with high plasma renin activity, low renal perfusion pressure, hyponatremia and excessive volume depletion. When angiotensin II concentration is decreased in at-risk patients, GFR becomes decreased and azotemia results. The azotemia is generally mild but occasionally can be severe in both human and canine patients.

Functional azotemia can occur secondary to the administration of any ACE inhibitor. The longer-acting agents (e.g. enalapril) may more frequently produce azotemia in human patients than the shorter-acting agents (e.g. captopril). However, in one study in rats, captopril produced a marked reduction in GFR while perindopril did not. Treatment consists of reducing the diuretic dose or stopping the administration of the ACE inhibitor. Although this functional azotemia may develop with greater frequency in at-risk patients, it should be stressed that azotemia sometimes develops in a canine patient that appears to have no risk factors other than heart failure.

Decreased GFR and an increase in serum urea and creatinine concentration are seen in 35% of human patients receiving ACE inhibitors. In most cases the increase in urea is mild and requires no intervention. In dogs, the incidence of clinically significant azotemia (plasma urea >35 mmol/L) is low. However, it occurs frequently enough that any veterinarian using these drugs should be aware of the potential occurrence of azotemia. Mild to moderate increases in plasma urea concentration (between 12 and 21 mmol/L) also occur at a low rate. In these patients, urea concentrations may increase without a concomitant increase in serum creatinine, or the increase in creatinine may be milder. As long as these patients continue to eat and act normally, these changes can generally be ignored.

Recommended guidelines for ACE inhibitor therapy with regards to azotemia based on human studies include the following.

- Identify high-risk patients (patients with moderate to severe dehydration, hyponatremia) before therapy.
- Ensure that the patient is not clinically dehydrated and ensure adequate oral fluid intake throughout therapy.
- Evaluate renal function at least once within 1 week after commencing therapy.
- Decrease the dose of furosemide if moderate azotemia develops or discontinue the ACE inhibitor if the azotemia is severe or if a reduction in furosemide dose does not improve renal function.
- Do not initiate or continue ACE inhibitor therapy when parenteral furosemide is required for severe or decompensated heart failure.
- Be cautious when combining an ACE inhibitor with agents that have potential renal toxicity or drugs that have the potential to also reduce GFR in susceptible patients such as all NSAIDs (see Chapter 13 for mechanism).

The prescribing information for one ACE inhibitor states that if azotemia develops the dose of diuretic should be reduced and if azotemia persists the dose should be reduced further or discontinued. This implies that diuretic administration should be discontinued permanently. Recommendations to permanently discontinue furosemide therapy in a patient with a clear history of moderate to severe heart failure are not tenable. In human medicine, the recommendation is to discontinue diuretic therapy for 24–48 h if needed, not permanently.

It is important to warn owners of the clinical signs of severe azotemia (usually anorexia and other gastrointestinal signs) and to measure serum creatinine and/or urea concentrations within the first week of ACE inhibitor therapy.

If a patient develops severe azotemia, it is usually wise to discontinue ACE inhibitor therapy and ensure that the patient is not significantly dehydrated.

If dehydration is moderate to severe, it is advisable to reduce the furosemide dose or discontinue its administration for 1–2 days and administer intravenous fluids cautiously.

Once the dog is stable, reassess the need for an ACE inhibitor. If the ACE inhibitor was being administered because of its potential (rather than actual) benefits and the patient does not require its administration it is advised not to attempt to readminister the ACE inhibitor.

If the patient is refractory to furosemide administration there are several options

- Initiate pimobendan if the patient is not already receiving it.
- Readminister the ACE inhibitor but at a lower dose and then try to gradually titrate the dose into the therapeutic range.
- Use a short-acting ACE inhibitor, such as captopril, if a longer-acting agent, such as enalapril, lisinopril, or benazepril, was administered initially.
- Add a thiazide diuretic.
- Add hydralazine or amlodipine.

One study of human patients with heart failure has documented that captopril acutely decreases the natriuretic and diuretic effects of furosemide. In this study, furosemide increased sodium excretion 623% above baseline while captopril plus furosemide only increased it 242% above baseline. Urine volume increased 225% above baseline with furosemide but only 128% above baseline in patients receiving both furosemide and captopril. This was an acute study. The chronic effects of administering captopril to patients stabilized on furosemide are unknown. This finding suggests that an ACE inhibitor should not be administered to a patient with severe, acute heart failure that needs the diuretic effect of furosemide to maintain life.

Known drug interactions

The arteriolar dilating effect of enalapril, and probably other ACE inhibitors, is attenuated by the concomitant administration of aspirin in humans. ACE inhibitors also decrease the breakdown of bradykinin, which stimulates prostaglandin synthesis. The predominant effect of prostaglandins in the systemic circulation is vasodilation. In one study in humans, the normal decrease in systemic vascular resistance induced by an ACE inhibitor was blocked by the concomitant administration of aspirin. However, a study has been performed in experimental dogs with heart failure in which low-dose aspirin produced no decrease in hemodynamic response to enalaprilat. In addition, the potential renal adverse effects associated with ACE inhibition may be potentiated by concurrent use of any NSAID particularly in dogs with heart failure receiving furosemide.

The combination of an ACE inhibitor and spironolactone has the potential to cause clinically significant hyperkalemia. There is only one retrospective report of the relative safety of this combination in dogs with heart failure who are also receiving concurrent furosemide. However, the author (Gordon) has observed clinically significant hyperkalemia when an ACE inhibitor and spironolactone were administered to a dog not receiving concurrent furosemide.

Enalapril

Enalapril is structurally and pharmacologically similar to captopril but contains a disubstituted nitrogen rather than the sulfhydryl group. The lack of the sulfhydryl group may result in decreased risk of certain side effects in humans, such as taste disturbances and proteinuria. These adverse effects have not been documented in dogs or cats administered ACE inhibitors.

Formulations and dose rates

The veterinary formulation of enalapril maleate is supplied as tablets. The human formulation is also supplied as tablets. There is also a formulation of enalapril maleate and hydrochlorothiazide that contains 10 mg enalapril maleate and 25 mg hydrochlorothiazide in one tablet. Enalaprilat is available for intravenous injection as enalaprilat in 0.9% alcohol at a concentration of 1.25 mg/mL of anhydrous enalaprilat.

DOGS

- Dose range studies have been performed with enalapril in dogs with surgically induced mitral regurgitation and heart failure. In these dogs, a dose of 0.5 mg/kg enalapril PO produced a greater decrease in pulmonary capillary pressure than a dose of 0.25 mg/kg. A dose of 0.75 mg/kg produced no better response. After 21 days of administration, the 0.5 mg/kg q.24 h dose produced a significant decrease in heart rate while the 0.25 mg q.24 h dose did not. Consequently, the enalapril dose is 0.5 mg/kg
- Whether this dose should be administered q.12 h or q.24 h is debatable. The package insert recommends starting with dosing q.24 h, increasing to q.12 h if the clinical response is inadequate
- Based on the pharmacodynamics presented below, we generally start the drug by administering it twice a day to dogs in heart failure, at approximately 12 h intervals

CATS

- PO: 1–2.5 mg/cat q.12–24 h
- PO: 0.2–0.7 mg/kg q.12–24 h

Pharmacokinetics

Enalapril is the ethyl ester of enalaprilat. It has little pharmacological activity until it is hydrolyzed in the liver to enalaprilat. Enalapril is available commercially as the maleate salt. Enalapril maleate is absorbed better from the gastrointestinal tract in dogs than enalaprilat. The affinity for enalaprilat for the angiotensin I binding sites on ACE is approximately 200,000 times that of ACE.

In dogs, enalapril maleate achieves peak concentration within 2 h of administration. Bioavailability is approximately 60%. Enalapril is metabolized to enalaprilat. Peak serum concentration of this active form occurs 3–4 h after an oral dose. The half-life of accumulation is approximately 11 h and duration of effect is 12–14 h. Steady-state serum concentration is achieved by the fourth day of administration. Excretion of enalapril and enalaprilat is primarily renal (40%) although 36% is excreted in the feces. Approximately 85% of an oral dose is excreted as enalaprilat.

The pharmacodynamics of enalapril have been examined in experimental dogs. A dose of 0.3 mg/kg administered per os results in approximately 75% inhibition of the pressor response to angiotensin I. This effect lasts for at least 6 h and is completely dissipated by 24 h after administration. A dose of 1.0 mg/kg produces only slightly better inhibition (approximately 80%) for at least 7 h. About 15% inhibition is still present 24 h after oral administration.

Adverse effects

The adverse effects of enalapril are the same as for all ACE inhibitors, as outlined above. Chronic high-dose enalapril toxicity appears to be confined to the kidneys. In healthy dogs administered doses up to 15 mg/kg/d over 1 year, drug-induced renal lesions are not seen. High-dose (30–60 mg/kg/d) enalapril administration to dogs results in dose-related renal toxicity. At 30 mg/kg/d, increasing degrees of renal damage are observed that are shown to be a direct nephrotoxic response of enalapril itself on proximal tubular epithelium. This damage is permanent only when potentiated by marked hypotension. The damage is confined to the proximal tubules, primarily to the juxtamedullary regions of the cortex where necrosis of the tubular cells, but not the basement membrane, is present. Dogs that survive the initial insult to the proximal tubules undergo regeneration. A dose of 90–200 mg/kg/d is rapidly lethal through renal failure. The renal toxicity appears to be due to a direct nephrotoxic effect of the drug and to an exaggerated decrease in systemic blood pressure. Saline administration ameliorates the toxicity.

Benazepril

Benazepril can be used in dogs or cats with heart failure as any other ACE inhibitor. Benazeprilat has been studied in dogs with experimentally induced acute left heart failure. Benazeprilat decreased left ventricular end-diastolic pressure by approximately 15%, peripheral resistance by approximately 30% and aortic pressure by 30%. Cardiac output did not increase in these anesthetized dogs.

Formulations and dose rates

Benazepril

Benazepril is supplied as tablets and can be made into suspension by a formulation pharmacy.

DOGS

- PO: 0.3 mg/kg and 0.5 mg/kg q.24 h (some clinicians use it in advanced heart failure)

CATS

- PO: 1–2.5 mg/cat q.12–24 h
- PO: 0.2-0.7 mg/kg q.12–24 h

Benazeprilat

- Dog: 30 μg/kg IV

Pharmacokinetics

Benazepril is a nonsulfhydryl ACE inhibitor. Like enalapril, it is a prodrug that is converted to benazeprilat by esterases, mainly in the liver. Benazeprilat is approximately 200 times more potent as an ACE inhibitor than is benazepril. The conversion of benazepril to benazeprilat is incomplete and other metabolites are formed in the dog.

Benazeprilat is poorly absorbed from the gastrointestinal tract whereas benazepril hydrochloride is well absorbed in the dog. Bioavailability increases by about 35% with repeated dosing. Following the administration of oral benazepril, plasma benazeprilat concentration reaches peak concentration in plasma within 1–3 h. Benazeprilat is rapidly distributed to all organs except the brain and placenta. Benazeprilat is excreted approximately equally in the bile and the urine in dogs. The terminal half-life is approximately 3.5 h. There may be an additional slow terminal elimination phase in dogs that may have a half-life between 55 and 60 h. This combined excretion may allow better dosing control in patients with pre-existing renal insufficiency however benazepril is no more renal protective than any other ACE inhibitors at equipotent doses.

The pharmacodynamics of benazepril have been studied in dogs by measuring plasma ACE activity before and after various doses of the drug. A dose of 0.125 mg/kg benazepril q.24 h appears to be too low. It only inhibits plasma ACE activity to approximately 80% of baseline. A dose of 0.25 mg/kg decreases plasma ACE activity to less than 10% of baseline within 3 h of administration. This effect lasts for at least 12 h. By 16 h plasma ACE activity is back to 20% of baseline and by 24 h it is approximately 30% of baseline. Doses of 0.5 and 1.0 mg/kg cause the >90% suppression to last at least 16 h. When benazepril is administered chronically, doses from 0.25 mg/kg to 1.0 mg/kg produce indistinguishable effects at the time of peak effect (2 h after oral administration) and at trough effect (24 h after oral administration).

Adverse effects

Anticipated adverse effects would be the same as for other long-acting ACE inhibitors.

Lisinopril

Lisinopril is a lysine derivative of enalaprilat. It does not require hydrolysis to become active. It has a higher affinity for ACE than either captopril or enalapril.

Formulations and dose rates

Lisinopril is supplied as tablets.

DOGS AND CATS

- A clinically effective dose of lisinopril has not been identified
- The generally used dose in dogs is 0.5 mg/kg q.24 h PO. From pharmacodynamic data, a dose of 0.25–0.5 mg/kg q.12 h or 1.0 mg/kg q.24 h may be more effective
- The primary benefit of lisinopril may be in dogs with impaired liver function
- The major factor that retards its use is the fact that the studies to document its pharmacodynamics and efficacy in the dog and cat have not been performed

Pharmacokinetics

Lisinopril's bioavailability is 25–50% and is unaffected by feeding. Peak plasma concentration occurs 4 h after oral administration in dogs. Peak inhibition of the pressor response to angiotensin I occurs 3–4 h after oral administration. Peak ACE inhibition occurs 6–8 h after administration. Elimination half-life of lisinopril in dogs is about 3 h.

Lisinopril's effects last for 24 h but are substantially attenuated 24 h after oral administration in dogs. A dose of 0.3 mg/kg orally to dogs results in approximately 75% inhibition of the pressor response to angiotensin I 3 h after administration. This response decreases to about 60% inhibition by 6 h and to approximately 10% at 24 h. When a dose of 1.0 mg/kg is administered PO, more than 90% inhibition of the pressor response to angiotensin I is achieved 4 h after drug administration. This response is effectively unchanged 6 h after administration and is still approximately 40% inhibited 24 h after administration.

Adverse effects

The adverse effects of lisinopril are the same as those of the other long-acting ACE inhibitors.

Captopril

Formulations and dose rates

Captopril is supplied as tablets but is no longer a recommended ACE inhibitor in dogs or cats as more suitable products are now available on the veterinary market.

DOGS

- 0.5–1.0 mg/kg q.8 h PO
- Doses of 3.0 mg/kg q.8 h have been associated with glomerular lesions and renal failure in experimental dogs and in clinical canine patients
- In one study, the onset of activity of captopril was within 1 h following the first dose. Drug effect lasted less than 4 h. A dose of 1 mg/kg produced slightly greater effects than a dose of 0.5 mg/kg. A dose of 2 mg/kg produced no additional benefit

CATS

- 0.5–1.5 mg/kg q.8–12 h, determined from clinical experience

Pharmacokinetics

Captopril's affinity for ACE is approximately 30,000 times greater than that of angiotensin I. Captopril has a half-life in dogs of about 3 h. It is about 75% bioavailable in fasted dogs and 30–40% in fed dogs. Approximately 40% of circulating captopril is protein bound. Captopril is metabolized in the liver but almost all of the captopril and its metabolites are eliminated by the kidneys, principally via tubular secretion. In patients with decreased renal function, a decrease in dose interval or dose is recommended. The average total body clearance and the renal clearance of captopril are 600 mL/kg in the dog. The volume of distribution of captopril in the dog is 2.6 L/kg; the volume of the central compartment is about 0.5 L/kg.

Adverse effects

- Captopril is generally well tolerated in most patients. However, side effects can occur and include anorexia, vomiting, diarrhea, azotemia and hypotension.
- Gastrointestinal side effects appear to be more common in dogs administered captopril than in dogs administered other ACE inhibitors.
- In human patients, captopril produces fewer instances of azotemia and hypotension than do the longer-acting ACE inhibitors. Doses in excess of 2.0 mg/kg q.8 h can produce renal failure, hence should be avoided.

ALDOSTERONE ANTAGONISTS

EXAMPLE

Spironolactone

Spironolactone is an aldosterone antagonist and potassium sparing diuretic. It has potential beneficial effects on the progression of heart disease. For a full discussion of spironolactone see the diuretic section of this chapter.

β-BLOCKERS

EXAMPLES

Selective
Oral: atenolol, metoprolol
IV: esmolol
Nonselective
Oral: carvedilol, propranolol

Clinical applications and mechanism of action

Traditionally, β-blockers were considered indirect positive lusiotropes and class II antiarrhythmics. Discussion of these properties can be found in the positive lusiotropes and antiarrhythmics sections of this chapter respectively. However, there are also data that shows that the administration of β-blockers to human patients with heart failure due to systolic myocardial dysfunction results in improved myocardial function, exercise capabilities and prolonged survival. This effect is counter-intuitive, because β-blockers are negative inotropic agents; historically negative inotropic agents have been relatively contraindicated in heart failure characterized by systolic dysfunction.

The mechanism for the reported improvement in human patients with DCM may involve limiting the effects of chronic excessive adrenergic stimulation on cardiomyocytes. Elevated levels of circulating catecholamines (norepinephrine) are characteristic of chronic heart failure in humans and have been documented in canine patients with symptomatic spontaneous CVD in a chronic canine model of experimental mitral regurgitation and in spontaneous DCM. Catecholamines have been shown to reduce viability and protein synthesis in isolated adult human cardiomyocytes offering insight into one potential mechanism for impaired systolic function with CVD and DCM.

The reported beneficial effects of gradual β-blockade represent a biological effect that is not immediate upon initiation of therapy. In fact, the negative inotropic and chronotropic properties of these agents make decompensation a relative risk, in the short term, and mandate gradual initiation of therapy in the form of an uptitration protocol. However, improved systolic function and LV remodeling have been demonstrated in every human study greater than 3 months in duration.

When β-blockers are used in human patients with heart failure due to DCM, a low initial dose is administered orally to determine if the patient can tolerate any short term negative inotropic effects of the drug. If the patient does not deteriorate on the low dose, the dose is gradually increased (uptitrated) over 1–3 months, with the dose being increased by approximately 50–100% weekly. Eventually, doses 4–15 times the starting dose are administered. β-Blockers that have been used in humans include metoprolol, labetolol, carvedilol, bisoprolol and bucindolol. The starting dose for adult humans range from 1.25 mg PO for bisoprolol to 3.125 for carvedilol and 6.25 mg PO for metoprolol. The target dose in humans ranges from 5–10 mg PO per day for bisoprolol to 25 mg PO for carvedilol and 50–100 mg PO per day for labetolol and bucindolol.

Early evaluations of β-blockade for the treatment of heart failure focused on second-generation β_1-selective agents (metoprolol, atenolol) to avoid increases in afterload characteristic of nonselective β-blockade. However, β_1 and β_2 receptors are present in the myocardium and both are important in mediating adrenergic effects in cardiomyocytes. Additionally, in human heart failure, cardiac β_1 receptors are down-regulated while β_2 receptor numbers remain unchanged. Therefore, due to the relative increase in β_2 receptors, more comprehensive cardiac adrenergic blockade can be achieved with the use of nonselective β-blockers.

Carvedilol (Coreg®) is a third-generation nonselective β-blocker with α_1-blocking properties and ancillary antioxidant effects and thus combining the potential benefit of a nonselective β-blocker with the vasodilatory effects of an α_1-blocker. Additionally, the antioxidant properties may decrease the oxidant stress associated with progressive heart failure. Carvedilol is currently the only β-blocker approved by the American FDA for the treatment of human heart failure but the benefits of β-blockade are considered a relative class effect and number of different β-blockers are currently used for the treatment of human heart failure.

β-Blockers in canine DCM

Selective and nonselective β-blockers including carvedilol have been shown to significantly increase systolic function and survival in human patients with heart failure secondary to DCM. More recently, carvedilol has been shown to be superior to metoprolol with respect to survival in human DCM. One small prospective veterinary study evaluated the effect of carvedilol on survival in heart failure due to DCM in a small number of Doberman pinschers. No benefit was observed. However, the study had low statistical power due to small numbers of patients and used a low dose of carvedilol relative to more recently published canine pharmacokinetic and pharmacodynamic data. There are currently no data available to allow comment on the potential utility of β-blockade in the preclinical stage of canine DCM but their potential utility is rational based on the human model.

β-Blockers in canine CVD

High-dose atenolol (2–5 mg/kg PO q.24 h), a second-generation selective β-blocker, improved LV function in an experimental canine model of chronic mitral regurgitation (MR). The improvement was associated with enhanced innate contractile function of isolated cardiomyocytes due to an increase in the absolute number of contractile elements.

The reported beneficial effects of gradual β-blockade represent a biologic effect that is not immediate upon initiation of therapy. In fact, the negative inotropic and chronotopic properties of these agents make decompensation a relative risk in the short-term and mandate gradual initiation of therapy in the form of an up-titration protocol. Improved systolic function and LV remodeling have been demonstrated in every human study greater than 3 months in duration.

The left ventricular (LV) work associated with mitral regurgitation (MR) represents a model of pure volume overload because the excess volume is ejected into the relatively low pressure of the left atrium. In contrast, LV work associated with other forms of volume overload such as aortic insufficiency represents a combination of pressure and volume overload because the LV ejects the excess volume against relatively high aortic diastolic pressures. Although patients with chronic MR develop compensatory LV remodeling in the form of eccentric hypertrophy (dilation), the hypertrophic response is reportedly inadequate contributing to increased LV wall stress with commensurate increases in myocardial oxygen consumption. Researchers have suggested that inadequate hypertrophy is the result of the relatively low LV afterload in this condition. This premise argues against the primary utility of afterload reduction in patients with MR, and perhaps offers insight to the failure of afterload reduction to delay its progression. Additionally, reduced LV systolic function has been demonstrated in an experimental canine model of chronic MR and in chronic spontaneous human MR.

Incomplete understanding of the incessant progression of heart failure underlines the need for prompt intervention in mildly symptomatic patients in an attempt to decrease morbidity and mortality. This premise has been validated repeatedly in human heart failure studies with a number of agents including carvedilol. It is difficult to routinely diagnose canine patients with early (Class I & II) clinical signs of heart failure such as mild exercise intolerance. However, it is not uncommon to evaluate 'relatively' asymptomatic dogs with CVD that on further evaluation are found to have cardiac remodeling including, left atrial enlargement +/– left ventricular eccentric hypertrophy (dilation). A subset of these patients also demonstrate systolic dysfunction crudely based on an increased LV end-systolic diameter. The combination of non-selective β-blockade and afterload reduction in concert with the antioxidant properties offered by carvedilol is rational in dogs with chronic MR that are not yet in heart failure and might delay the development of overt clinical signs of heart failure in this population of dogs. Given the relative risk of decompensation associated with β-blockade in patients with CHF, gradual β-blockade is likely to have less risk in asymptomatic dogs with MR due to CVD.

Pharmacokinetics and pharmacodynamics

There are currently limited data on the pharmacokinetics and pharmacodynamics of carvedilol in dogs. The pharmacodynamics of chronic oral carvedilol administration in normal conscious dogs has been reported in two studies. The combined data evaluated dose ranges between 0.05–1.5 mg/kg and demonstrated the ability of carvedilol to offer significant β-blockade based on an isoproterenol challenge with little effect on systemic blood pressure and heart rate even at the highest dose reported. Additionally, one study reported a statistically significant correlation between plasma carvedilol concentration and the percent attenuation of an isoproterenol-induced tachycardic response. The study suggested that a plasma carvedilol concentration between 60 and 100 ng/mL may be necessary for near maximum β-blockade in healthy, conscious hound dogs. The pharmacokinetic profile of oral and intravenous carvedilol in healthy, conscious hound dogs was also reported, suggesting a 6-h dosing interval and a low and variable oral bioavailability (approximately 1/10th of that reported in humans). Conversely, the available pharmacodynamic data suggest a 12–24 h dosing interval is adequate to ensure β-blockade.

Another study reported the cardiovascular and renal effects of oral carvedilol (0.2–0.8 mg/kg q.24 h) in dogs with experimental MR and control dogs. The authors demonstrated β-blockade with oral carvedilol and suggested that a dose of 0.4 mg/kg PO q.24 h may be a reasonable target dose based on their pharmacokinetic data, cautioning against overzealous β-blockade in dogs with heart failure. However, the majority of investigators who have worked with an experimental model of MR in large dogs and demonstrated beneficial effects associated with β-blockade, alone or on a background of ACE inhibitor, have used atenolol at an initial dose of 12.5 mg/d (0.5–0.8 mg/kg PO q.24 h) gradually increasing to a target dose of 50–100 mg/d (2–5 mg/kg PO q.24 h) over a few weeks. The target dose was designed and proven to offer essentially complete, and likely nonselective (due to the size of the dose), β-blockade.

These data combined with the reported rise in norepinephrine in dogs with spontaneous CVD and the systolic dysfunction that is now recognized to occur in spontaneous primary human MR beg the question of whether or not β-blockade alone or on a background of neurohormonal modulation such as that offered by an ACE inhibitor, spironolactone, and/or digoxin can delay the progression of CVD in dogs. Although carvedilol is currently used by some clinicians for the treatment of CVD and other cardiac diseases, dosing until recently was empirical. The availability of pharmacokinetic and pharmacodynamic data in normal dogs and those with experimental MR greatly aids in the determination of an evidence based dose and dosing interval for carvedilol. However, based on evaluation of plasma carvedilol concentrations in normal conscious dogs, a reported target plasma carvedilol concentration of 50–100 ng/mL is recommended.

Clinically significant β-blockade is reported to occur at a plasma concentration >10 ng/mL. In this small number of dogs, those dosed above 0.5 mg/kg twice per day achieved a plasma concentration that should result in clinically significant β-blockade (>10 ng/mL) while those dosed at 0.3 mg/kg or below failed to achieve this level. However, to achieve close to maximum β-blockade doses >0.7–0.9 mg/kg or higher may be required.

One small prospective nonplacebo-controlled study in cavalier King Charles spaniels (n = 5) with preclinical compensated CVD reported that chronic oral carvedilol at approximately 1 mg/kg PO is safe and well tolerated when gradually uptitrated. There was no evidence of disease progression over the duration of this study (approximately 5 months). Some echocardiographic and gated radionuclide ventriculography parameters suggested a reduction in left atrial size, improvement in LV function and reduced filling pressures. However, there was no control group for comparison. In this study the plasma carvedilol concentration was >10 ng/mL. The true utility of carvedilol in dogs with CVD awaits prospective placebo-controlled studies.

There are no data to evaluate regarding the use of β-blockade in heart failure due to CVD (the clinical stage). The same precautions as those outlined for heart failure in general would be expected to apply. That is, β-blockers should not be initiated in dogs with decompensated heart failure due to CVD and initial dose and target doses may need to be lower in heart failure versus preclinical disease. In addition uptitration may need to be more gradual.

Formulations and dose rates

GENERAL COMMENTS

- β-Blocker therapy in patients with overt heart failure should not be attempted by anyone other than an individual who has experience with this form of therapy.
- Pre-existing bradycardia is a contraindication.
- The initial dose should be low and gradually increased over biweekly intervals.
- Adverse effects usually occur following a dose increase and may include development of signs of progressive heart disease.
- Acutely, all β-blockers are dose dependent negative inotropes and can therefore result in the occurrence of adverse signs suggestive of progressive heart disease following initiation or during uptitration. The dose should be reduced to the last tolerated dose (not abruptly discontinued) and therapy for heart failure should be initiated as required based on clinical signs.
- Any beneficial effect of β-blockade is not immediate but rather takes approximately 3 months. Maximum desirable effects may be achieved with the highest tolerated dose.
- β-Blockers should never be discontinued abruptly but rather weaned off should discontinuation be necessary.
- The authors' preferred β-blocker in patients with acquired heart disease is carvedilol.
- Plasma samples can be submitted to Auburn University Clinical Pharmacology Lab for determination of a plasma carvedilol concentration. Take the sample about 2 h after dosing. Target concentration is 50–100 ng/mL.
- In patients with preclinical CVD or DCM who have been receiving chronic β-blockers and then go on to develop heart failure, the following recommendations may prove useful.
  - If the heart failure is mild (outpatient treatment is possible) then the β-blocker should be continued at the same dose and heart failure therapy should be initiated including an ACE inhibitor, pimobendan and furosemide as needed to control signs of congestion.
  - If the heart failure is severe (hospitalization and IV furosemide are indicated) then the β-blocker dose should be reduced by 50% (β-blockers should not be discontinued abruptly) and heart failure therapy should be initiated including pimobendan and parenteral furosemide as needed to control signs of congestion and stabilize the patient. Once stable an ACE inhibitor can be added and eventually the β-blocker dose can be uptitrated to the previous dose if tolerated.
- Do not combine with other β-blockers, calcium channel blockers or sotalol (a class III antiarrhythmic with β-blocking properties).

CARVEDILOL FORMULATION AND DOSE RATES

Carvedilol is available as 3.125, 6.25, 12.5 and 25 mg tablets. A stability study has been reported and the drug can be reformulated into a suspension with simple corn syrup. The suspension has an expiration time of 90 d. Formulation of the suspension using the 25 mg tablets facilitates accurate dosing and uptitration and is cost effective, particularly for small dogs.

CARVEDILOL IN PRECLINICAL DCM

- The starting dose is 0.1 mg/kg (lower than that in dogs with preclinical CVD)
- Start at 0.1 mg/kg and increase by 50–100% every 2–3 weeks to a target dose of approximately 1 mg/kg (if possible)

CARVEDILOL IN CLINICAL DCM (HEART FAILURE)

- β-Blockers should not be routinely initiated in clinical DCM unless there is a specific indication such as a supraventricular arrhythmia (atrial fibrillation)

CARVEDILOL IN PRECLINICAL CVD

- The starting dose is 0.25 mg/kg
- Start at 0.25 mg/kg and increase by 50–100% every 2–3 weeks to a target dose of approximately 1 mg/kg (if possible)

Formulations and dose rates—cont'd

CARVEDILOL IN CLINICAL CVD (HEART FAILURE)

- β-Blockers should not be routinely initiated in clinical CVD unless there is a specific indication such as a supraventricular arrhythmia (atrial fibrillation)

Conclusions regarding β-blockade in heart disease/failure

There is an ongoing interest in β-blocker therapy for the treatment of canine heart disease (preclinical stage) and heart failure (clinical stage) due to both DCM and CVD. However, there is currently no evidence of efficacy in either disease. In general, β-blockers should not be initiated in dogs or cats with decompensated heart failure. That is, if the patient has severe clinical signs of backward (pulmonary edema) or forward (systemic hypotension) heart failure β-blockers should not be initiated. β-Blockers may be easier to initiate in the setting of stable canine heart failure if the patient is receiving pimobendan concurrently. There is one recent report of the advantage of this approach in the human literature. Any definitive recommendations regarding β-blockade for the treatment of canine clinical and preclinical disease await adequately powered prospective clinical trials.

Digoxin

The digitalis glycosides have effects on vascular baroreceptors. Baroreceptor function is abnormally reduced in human patients and experimental dogs with heart failure. This results in attenuated cardiac vagal tone and increased sympathetic activity. This maladaptive compensatory mechanism can be detrimental in patients with heart failure. The digitalis glycosides increase baroreceptor function in normal cats, dogs and humans. They decrease plasma catecholamine concentrations, directly recorded sympathetic nerve activity and plasma renin activity, which may all be related to increased baroreceptor activity and are thus considered neuroendocrine modulators.

However, clinical significance of this effect on morbidity and mortality in heart failure has not been demonstrated. This may be related to the relatively high rate of adverse or side effects associated with digoxin use and narrow therapeutic window. For additional information on other properties of digoxin see the antiarrhythmic section of this chapter.

Angiotensin receptor blockers

EXAMPLES

Irbesartan, losartan

Angiotensin II receptor blockers were developed for the treatment of systemic hypertension and heart failure in humans. They block only one type of angiotensin II receptor (AT_1) and do not potentiate bradykinin activity in contrast to the ACE inhibitors. Despite this, hemodynamic and clinical benefits in humans with heart failure appear to be similar to the ACE inhibitors. The drugs were primarily developed to avoid ACE inhibitor-induced coughing that occurs in humans; this is not a problem in dogs. Clinical use of these drugs will probably be limited to those patients that cannot tolerate ACE inhibitors. More recently these agents are being evaluated alone or in combination with an ACE inhibitor for the treatment renal disease.

Irbesartan is investigational in veterinary medicine. One reported canine dose is 30–60 mg/kg.

POSITIVE AGENTS (MEDICATIONS THAT IMPROVE VENTRICULAR RELAXATION)

This class of agents is used primarily in the treatment of diseases that are characterized by concentric ventricular hypertrophy such as feline hypertrophic cardiomyopathy, congenital canine subaortic stenosis and pulmonic stenosis.

EXAMPLES

Calcium channel blockers (diltiazem), β-blockers (atenolol)

Calcium channel blockers

EXAMPLE

Oral: diltiazem (preferred for this indication)

Diltiazem

Calcium channel blockers as a class are considered vasodilators but individual agents have different relative potencies and additional effects. Diltiazem is a calcium channel blocker that affects the calcium channels in cardiomyocytes and to a lesser extent vascular smooth muscle. Thus it is not used as a primary vasodilator. Calcium channel blockers including diltiazem are class IV antiarrhythmics and positive agents. For further discussion of the antiarrhythmic properties please refer to the antiarrhythmic section of this chapter (p. 424).

Clinical applications

Diltiazem is primarily used as an adjunctive agent to treat heart failure in cats with HCM. Its use for this purpose has decreased markedly over the past decade. It improves myocardial relaxation, reduces myocardial contractility and may reduce heart rate in these patients.

The improvement in myocardial relaxation may help decrease left ventricular diastolic pressure and so reduce pulmonary edema formation. Decreased myocardial contractility may reduce systolic anterior motion of the mitral valve. However, it usually does not do this as effectively as β-blocking drugs. Heart rate reduction may be beneficial in cats with sinus tachycardia or atrial fibrillation. Net beneficial effects include lessened edema formation. Rarely, left ventricular wall thickness decreases.

Diltiazem is also commonly used to decrease the ventricular rate in patients with atrial fibrillation, a common sequela of severe heart disease. A rapid heart rate induce myocardial failure in dogs. Consequently, rate reduction with diltiazem may be viewed as producing myocardial protection. Digoxin and β-blockers are used for this same purpose.

Mechanism of action

Diltiazem improves early diastolic left ventricular relaxation in hypertrophic cardiomyopathy. It may also decrease heart rate and reduce the degree of systolic anterior motion in cats with this disease. It does this by binding to L-type calcium channels in the heart and reducing systolic calcium entry into myocardial and automatic cells.

Formulations and dose rates

Diltiazem is a calcium channel blocker supplied as a tablet. There are also several extended-release formulations. Cardizem CD® is a dual release capsule that contains two types of bead of diltiazem hydrochloride. The beads differ in the thickness of the membranes that surround them. The manufacturer states that 40% of the beads are meant to dissolve within the first 12 h after oral administration and the other 60% (which are surrounded by a thicker membrane) are formulated to dissolve throughout the next 12 h. The net effect is a drug that lasts for 24 h in humans and in cats. Dilacor XR® is an extended-release capsule that consists of multiple 60 mg tablets contained in a swellable matrix core that slowly releases the drug over 24 h in humans and 12 h in cats. The total capsule contains either 120, 180 or 240 mg of diltiazem. The 60 mg tablets can be removed. The tablet can be cut in half or administered whole.

CATS

- The usual dose is 7.5 mg q.8 h. This may be increased to 15 mg q.8 h in refractory cases
- The extended-release formulation Dilacor XR® is dosed at 30–60 mg q.12 h
- The dose for Cardizem CD® is 45 mg (one-quarter of a 180 mg capsule) q.24 h

Pharmacokinetics

Diltiazem, when administered PO at a dose of 1 mg/kg to cats, has a bioavailability of 94%, a terminal half-life of 2 h and a volume of distribution of 1.9 L/kg. Peak serum concentration occurs 30 min after dosing and the serum concentration remains in the therapeutic range (50–300 μg/mL) for 8 h.

The bioavailability of Cardizem CD® is only 38%, necessitating a much higher dose for this product (10 mg/kg). The half-life is much longer, at 6.5 h, than that of the nonextended-release preparation and peak serum concentration does not occur until 6 h after drug administration. Serum concentration remains within therapeutic range for 24 h. Dilacor XR® (30 mg) produces significant decreases in heart rate and blood pressure in cats with HCM for 12–14 h.

Adverse effects

The primary adverse effects of diltiazem are seen with diltiazem overdose. Overdose results in decreased contractility, systemic vasodilation and bradycardia, which, if severe enough, results in cardiovascular collapse. Patients with myocardial failure and conduction system disease are more sensitive to the calcium channel-blocking properties of diltiazem and so are more prone to adverse effects than normal dogs or cats.

Known drug interactions

In general, diltiazem should not be administered in conjunction with a α-adrenergic blocking agent. However, this can be done safely in most cats with severe HCM. Still, if this is done, low doses of both agents should be administered initially and the doses titrated up to an effective endpoint.

β-Blockers

EXAMPLE

Atenolol

In addition to their neuroendocrine modulatory effects and antiarrhythmic effects (Class 2) all β-blockers have the potential to improve relaxation indirectly by slowing heart rate. However, unlike diltiazem they have no direct effects that improve relaxation and indirectly they slow the rate of relaxation. The heart rate-mediated beneficial effects on relaxation may, however, be clinically useful in stable heart failure characterized by systolic dysfunction. For further discussion on effects and dosing of β-blockers see the sections on neuroendocrine modulators (p. 412) and antiarrhythmics (p. 444) in this chapter.

NEW OR EXPERIMENTAL HEART FAILURE DRUGS

Because there is no cure for most cardiovascular diseases that result in heart failure, there are always new drugs being developed to treat cardiac disease and heart failure.

Some drugs eventually make it to the marketplace while others fall by the wayside during any phase of drug development. This section presents a few drugs that may become useful for treating heart failure in the future.

Aquaretics

Aquaretics are vasopressin receptor anatagonists, e.g. tolvaptan (OPC-41061). Tolvaptan is selective V_2 receptor antagonist, which is showing promise in the acute and chronic treatment of human CHF. In contrast to loop diuretics like furosemide, V_2 receptor antagonism has demonstrated free water excretion with little to no sodium loss. In addition, the water loss associated with V_2 antagonism has not been associated with activation of the RAAS in contrast to the loop diuretics. This novel class of agents may prove to be an addition to our pharmacological arsenal against CHF but recent evidence in human medicine suggests this agent is not useful above and beyond available diuretics.

Prostacyclin analogs

Prostacyclin analogs have been shown to improve symptoms and short-term survival in human patients with pulmonary hypertension. Epoprostenol (Flolan®) was the first available prostacyclin used to treat pulmonary hypertension in humans. It is administered via continuous rate intravenous infusion. Due to a very short half-life abrupt withdrawal is associated with increased morbidity and mortality. Adverse effects related to the drug are mild and dose related while sepsis and thrombosis are important adverse effects related to chronic central venous access.

Treprostinil (Remodulin®) has similar hemodynamic effects as epoprostenol but is administered as a constant rate subcutaneous infusion which lowers the risk of sepsis associated with direct venous access.

Intravenous iloprost has similar hemodynamic effects as epoprostenol with a longer half-life diminishing the adverse effects associated with abrupt withdrawal. Inhaled iloprost is also available and has a short half-life of 20–25 min requiring administration every 2–3 h.

Beraprost, the first orally stable prostacyclin analog, requires administration four times a day to maintain adequate blood levels.

Endothelin receptor antagonists

The pro-molecule big endothelin (ET)-1 is converted to functional ET by endothelin converting enzyme. ET is a potent vasoconstrictor and smooth muscle mitogen resulting in vascular hypertrophy. ET levels are elevated in humans with pulmonary hypertension and dogs with experimentally induced dirofilariasis.

Two types of ET receptors have been identified, ET_A and ET_B. ET_A receptors are located on vascular smooth muscle cells and mediate vasoconstriction and vascular smooth muscle proliferation while ET_B receptors are located on both endothelial and vascular smooth muscle cells and mediate vasodilation and vasoconstriction. ET_B receptors are upregulated in pulmonary hypertension.

The ET receptor antagonist bosentan (Tracleer®) competitively antagonizes the ET receptor types ET_A and ET_B, with slightly more affinity for ET_A receptors. Optimal dosage in humans is 125 mg every 12 h. In human studies, bosentan resulted in significant increases in exercise capacity. A potentially important adverse effect of bosentan therapy is elevations in hepatic enzyme activity that typically resolve with discontinuation of the drug but require monthly monitoring of serum biochemistries. Bosentan was developed initially for the treatment of heart failure but in clinical trials did not prove useful for this indication. The selective ET_A receptor antagonists, sitaxsentan and ambrisentan, are currently being evaluated in human clinical trials.

DRUGS USED FOR THE TREATMENT OF CARDIAC ARRHYTHMIAS

Relevant physiology and pathophysiology

Antiarrhythmic drugs are used to manage cardiac arrhythmias that arise as a result of an intrinsic cardiac defect (myocardial or electrical) or because of the effect of toxins such as drugs (e.g. digoxin toxicity) or endogenous factors (e.g. secondary to gastric dilation and volvulus). Different antiarrhythmic drugs have different mechanisms of action and will have varying efficacy depending on the type of arrhythmia present.

An understanding of the mechanisms by which action potentials are generated in the normal heart and in cardiac disease is essential to an understanding of the mechanism of action of antiarrhythmic drugs.

Cardiac muscle action potentials

Myocardium (Fig. 17.1A)

- Excitation of the myocardium results in:
  - influx of sodium through fast sodium channels
  - influx of calcium through slow calcium channels.
- This slow influx of calcium results in the long duration of cardiac action potentials relative to other excitable tissues. It also results in a long refractory period, as the fast sodium channels cannot be reactivated until the cell has been repolarized. Calcium influx also causes release of calcium from intracellular stores and activates the contractile mechanism.
- Repolarization is predominantly due to an outward potassium current.

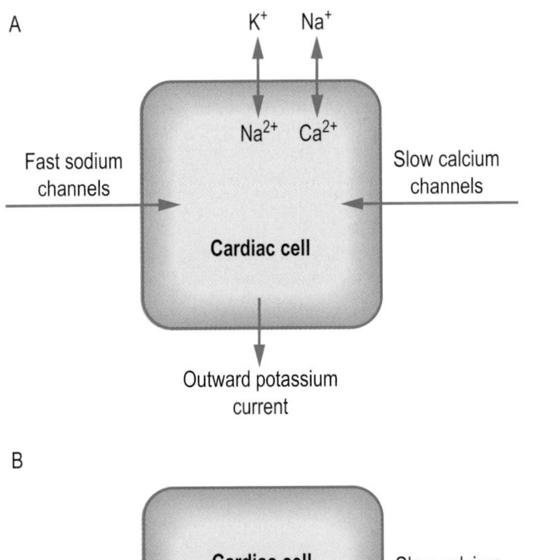

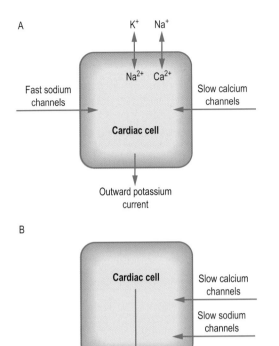

Fig. 17.1 Generation of action potentials in (A) normal myocardial cells and (B) normal pacemaker cells.

- During electrical diastole ionic balances are restored by membrane pumps that exchange sodium for potassium and calcium for sodium.

Pacemaker cells (SA and AV nodes), ischemic myocardial cells (Fig. 17.1B)

- The initial part of the action potential in these cells is due to a slow inward calcium current. This results in the initial part of the action potential being very slow, thus slowing conduction through the SA and AV nodes. This results in a delay between atrial and ventricular contraction, allowing time for adequate ventricular filling.
- Diastolic depolarization occurs because of a steadily declining outward potassium current and an increasing slow diastolic inward, predominantly sodium, current. The inward sodium current eventually reaches a threshold so that calcium ions start to flow in, hence initiating another action potential – automaticity.

Arrhythmias

Arrhythmias originate in either the atria (supraventricular arrhythmias) or the ventricles (ventricular arrhythmias). They can arise as a result of either the abnormal formation of impulses that arise from ectopic foci and have spontaneous activity or the abnormal propagation of impulses, where an extra anatomical or functional circuit exists so that the electrical impulse may take two possible pathways with different conduction velocities and refractory periods. The latter mechanism is termed re-entry.

Abnormal automaticity is a common form of abnormal impulse formation in small animals. In this abnormality, partly damaged cells become partially depolarized, attaining a resting membrane potential similar to automatic cells in the heart, such as the sinus node. When this occurs these cells attain the property of automaticity. When they depolarize at a rate faster than the normal pacemaker (i.e. automatic) cells, they take over control of the heart rate, sometimes for only one beat and at other times for long periods. All forms of abnormal impulse arrhythmia tend to be exacerbated by ischemia, high catecholamine concentrations and electrolyte imbalances, particularly decreased potassium and magnesium concentrations. Other forms of abnormal impulse formation are early and delayed or late afterdepolarizations and triggered activity.

DRUGS USED TO TREAT TACHYARRHYTHMIAS

The effective treatment of tachyarrhythmias is predicated on an accurate rhythm diagnosis and a working knowledge of the available antiarrhythmic drugs. The reader is referred elsewhere to learn rhythm diagnosis.

Classes of antiarrhythmic agents

The drugs used to treat supraventricular and ventricular tachyarrhythmias can be divided into separate classes based on their generalized mechanisms of action. Antiarrhythmic drugs exert their effects primarily by blocking sodium, potassium or calcium channels, or β-receptors. This classification scheme is somewhat helpful clinically when deciding to use particular drugs for specific arrhythmias. However, clinical experience with these drugs is the more important means of determining efficacy of various drugs to suppress different tachyarrhythmias. The common arrhythmias, the mechanisms responsible for their generation and the drugs most commonly effective clinically are listed in Table 17.6. The doses of the common antiarrhythmic agents are listed in Table 17.7.

Class I

Class I drugs are most frequently used to treat ventricular tachyarrhythmias, although they may also be used to treat supraventricular tachyarrhythmias. They are the

Table 17.6 Common arrhythmias and drugs used in their treatment

	Acute (intravenous)	Chronic (oral)
Ventricular arrhythmias: hemodynamically important VPCs or Vtach	1. Lidocaine (Class I) [5+] 2. Procainamide (Class I)[1+] 3. β-blockers (Class II) [1+]	1. Sotalol (Class III and II) [3+] 2. Amiodarone (Class III, II and IV) [2+] 3. Procainamide (Class I) [1+] 4. Mexiletine (Class I) [1+] 5. β-blockers (Class II) [1+] – not generally used as monotherapy but rather combined with a Class I
Supraventricular arrhythmias: hemodynamically importanty SVPBs or atrial fibrillation	1. Procainamide (Class I) [1+] 2. CCB: Diltiazem (Class IV) [2+] 3. β-blockers (Class II) [1+] 4. Quinidine (Class I, only horses) [1+]	1. Amiodarone (Class III, II and IV) [2+] 2. CCB: Diltiazem (Class IV) [2+] 3. β-blockers (Class II) [2+] 4. Digoxin (Class V) [2+] 5. Quinidine (Class I, only horses) [1+]
Both ventricular and supraventricular arrhythmias	1. Procainamide (Class I) [1+] 2. β-blockers (Class II) [1+]	1. Amiodarone (Class III, II and IV) [2+] 2. β-blockers (Class II) [1+]

Note: Class I antiarrhythmics work on Na^+ channels, Class II are beta-blockers, Class III work on K^+ channels (prolong action potential), Class IV are calcium channel blockers, Class V is digoxin and some agents have properties from more than one class. All agents are scored relative to how often they are used clinically to manage heart disease 1+ to 5+ where 5+ is the most common.

so-called 'membrane stabilizers'. Their common mechanism of action is the blockade of a certain percentage of the fast sodium channels in the myocardial cell membrane. Sodium channel blockade results in a decrease in the upstroke (phase 0) velocity of the action potential in atrial and/or ventricular myocardium and Purkinje cells. The upstroke velocity is a major determinant of conduction velocity. Consequently, class I drugs slow conduction velocity in normal cardiac tissue, abnormal cardiac tissue, or both.

Class I agents have variable effects on repolarization. Some of them prolong repolarization while others shorten it or have no effect. Primarily on the basis of differences in repolarization characteristics, class I agents are subdivided into classes Ia, Ib and Ic.

- Class Ia agents include quinidine, procainamide and disopyramide. These agents depress conduction in normal and abnormal cardiac tissue and prolong repolarization.
- Class Ib agents include lidocaine (lignocaine) and its derivatives, tocainide and mexiletine, along with phenytoin. Class Ib agents do not prolong conduction velocity in normal cardiac tissue nearly as much as class Ia drugs. They do, however, have profound effects on conduction velocity in abnormal cardiac tissue. They also shorten the action potential duration by accelerating repolarization. A greater degree of shortening occurs in fibers that have a longer action potential duration. Consequently, this effect is most profound in Purkinje fibers and does not significantly alter the effective refractory period of normal atrial and ventricular muscle. In contrast, class Ib agents may prolong the effective refractory period of damaged myocardium.
- Class Ic antiarrhythmic drugs include encainide and flecainide. These drugs slow conduction and have little effect on action potential duration.

Class II

Class II drugs are the β-adrenergic blocking drugs and are useful for treating both supraventricular and ventricular tachyarrhythmias. Although few tachyarrhythmias are the direct result of catecholamine stimulation, β-adrenergic receptor stimulation by catecholamines commonly exacerbates abnormal cellular electrophysiology. This can result in initiation or enhancement of a tachyarrhythmia. β-Blockers have additional properties including positive lusiotropy and neuroendocrine modulation in heart failure and further discussion of these uses can be found in the positive lusiotropy (p. 422) and neuroendocrine modulation (p. 412) sections of this chapter respectively.

Drugs that block β-adrenergic receptors do not have direct membrane effects at clinically relevant concentrations. Consequently, their action is indirect and related to blocking catecholamine enhancement of abnormal electrophysiology or related to other effects of the drug. An example of the latter is β-adrenergic receptor blockade resulting in a decrease in myocardial contractility and so in myocardial oxygen consumption. The resultant improvement in myocardial oxygenation might improve cellular electrophysiology and reduce arrhythmia formation.

Class II drugs are most commonly used to alter the electrophysiological properties of the AV junction in patients with supraventricular tachyarrhythmias. β-Receptor blockade at the AV junction results in an increase in conduction time through the AV junction

Table 17.7 Doses of common antiarrhythmic agents

Drug	Species	Route	Dose
β-blockers (Class II)			
Atenolol	Dog	PO	6.25 mg (0.25 mg/kg)–50 mg (1 mg/kg) q.12 h (total dose; start low; titrate)
	Cat	PO	6.25–12.5 mg q.12–24 h (total dose; start low; titrate)
Esmolol	Both	IV	0.25–0.5 mg/kg (single dose; maximum effect in 1–4 min); 10–200 µg/kg/min constant rate infusion
Propranolol	Dog	PO	0.1–2.0 mg/kg q.8 h (start low and titrate to effect in atrial fibrillation; higher doses used for other arrhythmias)
	Cat	PO	
	Both	IV	2.5–10 mg (total dose; start low; titrate)
			0.01–0.1 mg/kg (start low; titrate to effect for supraventricular arrhythmias)
Carvedilol*	Dog	PO	0.25–1.25 mg/kg q.12 h (total dose; start low and titrate, larger dogs and dogs with systolic dysfunction will not get to the highest dose)
Calcium channel blockers (Class IV)			
Diltiazem*	Dog	PO	0.5–1.5 mg/kg q.8 h (start low; titrate to effect for atrial fibrillation)
	Cat	IV	0.5–3 mg/kg (start low; titrate to effect for supraventricular tachycardia)
		PO	0.05–0.25 mg/kg (administer initial 0.05 mg/kg dose over 2–3 min; repeat every 5–10 min up to cumulative dose of 0.25 mg/kg)
			7.5–15 mg q.8 h (total dose)
Verapamil	Dog	IV	0.05–0.15 mg/kg (administer initial 0.05 mg/kg dose over 2–3 min; repeat every 5–10 min up to cumulative dose of 0.15 mg/kg)
Positive chronotropes			
Atropine*	Both	IV, SC	0.02–0.04 mg/kg
Glycopyrrolate*	Both	IV, SC	0.005–0.01 mg/kg
Isoproterenol	Both	IV	0.01–0.1 µg/kg/min (constant rate infusion; alternatively, dilute 1 mg in 500 mL of 5% dextrose or lactated Ringer's solution and infuse to effect)
Terbutaline	Dog	PO	2.5–10 mg (total dose; start low; titrate)
Other			
Digoxin	Dog	PO	0.22 mg/m^2 of body surface area q.12 h for dogs >20 kg
	Cat	PO	0.005–0.01 mg/kg q.12 h for dogs <20 kg
			0.03 mg/cat q.24 h for cats <3 kg
			0.03 mg/cat q.12-24 h for cats >3 kg
Ventricular antiarrhythmics			
Sotalol*	Dog	PO	1–3 mg/kg q.12 h
	Cat	PO	10 mg/cat q.12 h
Amiodarone* (supraventricular also)	Dog	PO	Loading dose: 10–20 mg/kg q.24 h × 7–10 days; maintenance dose: 5–15 mg/kg q.24 h
Lidocaine*	Dog	IV	Loading dose: 2–6 mg/kg (slow bolus); maintenance dose: 40–100 µg/kg/min
Mexiletine*	Dog	PO	5–10 mg/kg q.8 h
Phenytoin	Dog	PO	20–35 mg/kg q.8 h
Procainamide (supraventricular also)	Dog	PO	20–30 mg/kg q.6–8 h
		IV, IM	5–20 mg/kg (administer slowly; start low; titrate)
Quinidine (supraventricular also)	Dog	PO, IM	6–16 mg/kg q.6–8 h
Tocainide	Dog	PO	10–15 mg/kg q.8 h

* Agents commonly used by the authors for treatment of arrhythmias.

and an increase in the time that the AV junction is refractory to depolarization. Both changes effectively disrupt re-entrant circuits that use the AV node as part of the circuit. An increase in AV junctional refractoriness decreases the number of depolarizations reaching the ventricles from the atria in atrial fibrillation and flutter. Class II drugs are also used in combination with other agents to suppress ventricular arrhythmias.

Class III

Class III drugs act primarily by prolonging the action potential duration and refractory period. As such, they increase the fibrillation threshold and are used primarily to prevent sudden death due to ventricular tachyarrhythmias. They may, however, also have the ability to suppress ventricular arrhythmias. Examples of class III drugs are amiodarone, bretylium and sotalol. The use of these drugs is evolving in veterinary medicine.

Class IV

Class IV drugs are the calcium channel-blocking drugs. They are also known as calcium-entry blockers, calcium channel antagonists and slow-channel inhibitory blockers. They act by inhibiting the function of the slow

L-type calcium channels on cardiac cell membranes. Slow calcium channels are responsible for depolarization of sinus node and AV junctional tissues and for initiation of excitation–contraction coupling in myocardial cells. Calcium channel blockers have additional properties including positive lusiotropy and vasodilation and discussions of their utility in these settings can be found in the positive lusiotropy (p. 422) and vasodilator (p. 404) sections of this chapter respectively.

Calcium channel-blocking drugs slow the upstroke velocity of sinus node and AV junctional cell action potentials, resulting in slowing of sinoatrial and AV junctional conduction times. They may also slow the depolarization rate of the sinus node. Calcium channel-blocking drugs prolong the time for recovery from inactivation of the slow calcium channel and, as a result, markedly prolong the refractory period of the AV junctional tissue. Calcium channel-blocking drugs are also negative inotropic agents because of their effects on L-type slow calcium channels during phase 2 of the action potential in myocardial cells.

Because the primary effects of the calcium channel-blocking drugs are on the sinus node and the AV junction, these drugs are most effective for treating supraventricular tachyarrhythmias. Although they have been shown to suppress delayed afterdepolarizations (DADs) that occur secondary to digitalis intoxication and to depress automaticity in abnormally automatic cells, clinically they are generally considered not to be efficacious for treating ventricular tachyarrhythmias.

CLASS I ANTIARRHYTHMIC DRUGS

Lidocaine (lignocaine)

Clinical applications

Lidocaine (lignocaine) is used clinically to treat acute life-threatening ventricular arrhythmias in many different clinical settings. Its rapid onset of action, effectiveness, safety and short half-life make it ideal for acute interventions. Its short half-life also allows rapid changes in serum concentration so that lidocaine's effects can be titrated quickly. It is usually the most effective antiarrhythmic drug one can use to treat a ventricular arrhythmia. It does not affect supraventricular tachyarrhythmias.

Mechanism of action

Lidocaine is a class Ib antiarrhythmic agent that is also used for local anesthesia. It has little effect on atrial conduction or refractoriness and is not used for atrial tachyarrhythmias. Lidocaine can abolish both automatic and re-entrant ventricular arrhythmias. Lidocaine can abolish ventricular re-entrant arrhythmias either by increasing or decreasing conduction velocity within the circuit or by prolonging the refractory period.

The cellular actions of lidocaine are dependent on the extracellular potassium concentration. When the resting membrane potential is decreased, as when potassium concentration is high, lidocaine acts by suppressing the activity of fast sodium channels in a similar way to quinidine and procainamide. Lidocaine has more marked effects on automaticity, conduction velocity and refractoriness in damaged cells (where resting membrane potential is also often decreased) than in normal cells.

Lidocaine can also hyperpolarize partially depolarized cells and so can improve conduction in a region of damaged myocardium. Lidocaine's many potential effects on variables that cause re-entrant arrhythmias make it an especially effective drug for abolishing re-entrant arrhythmias. Lidocaine's ability to hyperpolarize partially depolarized cells gives it the ability to suppress arrhythmias due to abnormal automaticity in ventricular myocardium (e.g. accelerated idioventricular rhythm).

Although lidocaine has no direct effect on early afterdepolarizations (EADs), it may hyperpolarize or accelerate repolarization in cells with EADs, indirectly terminating the arrhythmia. However, in German shepherds with inherited ventricular arrhythmias due to EADs, lidocaine is not very effective. Lidocaine is effective at suppressing DADs due to digitalis intoxication. Because of this and because it is easy to use, lidocaine is the preferred drug for the acute termination of digitalis-induced ventricular tachyarrhythmias.

Formulations and dose rates

Lidocaine is supplied for intravenous administration in concentrations ranging from 10 mg/mL to 200 mg/mL. Concentrations above 20 mg/mL are used for infusion rather than bolus administration.

Lidocaine is administered parenterally because it has a short half-life and is extensively metabolized by the liver to toxic metabolites after oral administration. Although intramuscular lidocaine administration is feasible in the dog, clinical experience is limited at this time.

Lidocaine is generally administered as an initial intravenous loading dose followed by a constant intravenous infusion. If a loading dose is not administered, maximum infusion rates will take 1–2 h to achieve a therapeutic concentration. The initial loading dose in dogs is 2–4 mg/kg IV administered over 1–3 min, followed by an infusion of 25–100 μg/kg/min. The dose is titrated while observing the electrocardiogram. When the arrhythmia is suppressed, drug administration is discontinued. Half the initial loading dose may need to be repeated in 20–40 min if the arrhythmia recurs.

In cats the initial dose is 0.25–0.75 mg/kg IV, followed by an infusion administered at 10–40 μg/kg/min. Cats more commonly develop seizures with lidocaine. It must be used cautiously in this species.

Pharmacokinetics

Lidocaine's half-life in dogs is 90–100 min. Total body clearance is approximately 60 mL/min/kg. The liver primarily metabolizes lidocaine, with less than 5% of the clearance occurring through the kidneys. Clearance and half-life are prolonged by liver disease or poor hepatic perfusion (e.g. in heart failure, in shock and with propranolol administration). The volume of distribution is approximately 6 L/kg. Heart failure may also reduce the volume of distribution, resulting in a higher serum concentration. The therapeutic serum concentration is thought to be between 2 and 6 μg/mL.

Adverse effects

- Lidocaine exerts effects on the central nervous system when the serum concentration achieves a toxic concentration, producing signs of drowsiness, emesis, nystagmus, muscle twitching and seizures. Toxic effects can be particularly severe in the cat. Dogs administered infusion rates at the upper end of the dosage range are commonly sedated.
- Lidocaine can depress ventricular function in severe myocardial failure, produce atrioventricular block in conduction system disease and exacerbate sinus bradycardia and arrest in patients with sick sinus syndrome. It must be used with care in dogs with atrioventricular or ventricular conduction disorders, if at all.
- Lidocaine produces very few electrocardiographic changes except for a possible shortening of the Q-T interval. Unless the sinoatrial node is diseased, lidocaine does not affect its automaticity. It should be avoided in dogs with sick sinus syndrome. It does slow the rate of phase 4 depolarization in Purkinje fibers, resulting in a slowing of the rate of escape beats. For this reason, lidocaine (or for that matter any other antiarrhythmic drug) should never be administered to a patient dependent on an escape focus, such as a patient with a third-degree AV block. Lidocaine has fewer proarrhythmic effects than other antiarrhythmic agents.
- Treatment for toxicity is lidocaine withdrawal and, when necessary, intravenous diazepam administration (0.25–0.5 mg/kg IV) for seizure control.

Known drug interactions

Prolonged lidocaine infusions during concurrent propranolol administration prolong lidocaine's half-life.

Special considerations

Preparations containing adrenaline (epinephrine) used for local anesthesia should never be used intravenously. Lidocaine is absorbed by the PVC in the plastic bags used to store intravenous solutions.

Phenytoin

Clinical applications

Phenytoin may be effective in treating ventricular arrhythmias due to many causes but, because of dosing difficulties when administered intravenously, lidocaine is generally preferred for acute termination of ventricular arrhythmias. Phenytoin, however, may be useful for treating digitalis intoxication although generally lidocaine remains the preferred option. Because it can be administered orally, phenytoin can theoretically be administered prophylactically to patients that may be easily intoxicated with digitalis (e.g. severe myocardial failure patients).

Mechanism of action

Phenytoin, when used as an antiarrhythmic, shares many properties with lidocaine. It reduces normal automaticity in Purkinje fibers, abolishes abnormal automaticity due to digitalis intoxication and has effects identical to those of lidocaine on re-entrant arrhythmias. It can repolarize abnormal, depolarized cells, reduces sympathetic nerve effects and may modify parasympathetic nerve activity in digitalis toxicity.

Formulations and dose rates

Phenytoin is supplied as capsules. For parenteral administration, phenytoin sodium is supplied as injectable solutions of 50 mg/mL in 2 mL and 5 mL ampoules or vials.

The oral phenytoin dosage is 30–50 mg/kg q.8 h. Serious arrhythmias require intravenous treatment in intermittent doses of 2 mg/kg administered over 3–5 min to prevent hypotension and cardiac arrest from the propylene glycol vehicle. The total dose should not exceed 10 mg/kg. Because phenytoin in solution has a pH of 11.0, phlebitis will occur unless it is administered via a large vein and flushed immediately with normal saline.

Pharmacokinetics

Phenytoin absorption is erratic, slow and incomplete from both the gastrointestinal tract and intramuscular injection sites. The half-life is 3–4 h.

Adverse effects

Long-term phenytoin administration at 50 mg/kg q.8 h results in an increase in serum alkaline phosphatase concentration. Histological changes consist of increased hepatic cell size. This appears to be due to increased glycogen storage.

Known drug interactions

- The liver metabolizes phenytoin. Any drugs affecting microsomal enzymes will, therefore, also affect phenytoin metabolism.
- Chloramphenicol administration increases serum phenytoin concentration and in one study increased the half-life from 3 h to 15 h.

- Phenytoin may also decrease serum quinidine concentration.
- Phenytoin should not be added to intravenous fluids because of lack of solubility and resultant precipitation.

Quinidine

Quinidine is an optical isomer of quinine. It was originally prepared by Pasteur to treat malaria in 1853. It was not until 1918 that quinidine was recognized as an effective agent for treating atrial fibrillation in humans.

Clinical applications

Quinidine has been used most commonly for the long-term suppression of ventricular premature depolarizations and ventricular tachyarrhythmias. Chronic oral therapy of ventricular arrhythmias is most commonly aimed at preventing sudden death. Because quinidine does not appear to be very effective at preventing sudden death in dogs and, in humans, may increase the incidence of sudden death, use of this drug as a chronic agent has plummeted in the past 10 years.

Quinidine can also be used acutely to abolish ventricular arrhythmias and is occasionally effective in the control of atrial premature depolarizations and paroxysmal supraventricular tachycardia. However, other drugs (e.g. digitalis, β-blockers, calcium channel blockers) are generally more effective in the dog for supraventricular arrhythmias. Quinidine is ineffective in dogs with atrial fibrillation secondary to cardiac disease. However, it can be effective at converting atrial fibrillation to sinus rhythm in dogs without underlying cardiac disease (primary atrial fibrillation).

Mechanism of action

Quinidine is a class Ia antiarrhythmic agent that can be effective against automatic and re-entrant supraventricular and ventricular tachyarrhythmias in dogs. Its primary action is to decrease the movement of sodium through the fast sodium channel during phase 0. This results in a decrease in the upstroke velocity of the action potential and a consequent decrease in cardiac electrical impulse conduction velocity. This effect is enhanced by increasing extracellular potassium concentration because of the decreased resting membrane potential.

Quinidine prolongs the refractory period in atrial, ventricular and Purkinje cells, which can effectively interrupt re-entrant pathways. It also acts to decrease the slope of phase 4 and increase the threshold potential toward 0 in automatic cells. In so doing it suppresses normal automaticity in Purkinje fibers and suppresses cardiac excitability. Sinus node automaticity is unchanged or may even be increased owing to decreased vagal tone in normal patients (vagolytic effect).

There is a paucity of literature on the effects of quinidine on abnormal automaticity. Quinidine can suppress DADs in the Purkinje system but it can also increase the amplitude of DADs in atrial myocardium. Quinidine is used experimentally to produce EADs and so is unlikely to have beneficial effects with rhythms generated by this mechanism.

Formulations and dose rates

Quinidine is available as quinidine gluconate, quinidine sulfate and quinidine polygalacturonate. Quinidine sulfate and quinidine polygalacturonate are available as tablets. Quinidine gluconate comes as a solution for parenteral use.

DOGS

- Chronic oral dose for treating ventricular tachyarrhythmias: 6–16 mg/kg q.8 h. Quinidine sulfate is more rapidly absorbed than quinidine gluconate
- To convert atrial fibrillation to sinus rhythm in primary atrial fibrillation, doses ranging from 12.5 mg/kg q.6 h to 20 mg/kg q.2 h can be used. These doses are continued until conversion of the rhythm or until mild signs of toxicity are present
- Quinidine gluconate may be administered parenterally but rapid intravenous injections may cause dangerous hypotension. Lidocaine (lignocaine) and procainamide are preferred over quinidine for parenteral administration. The parenteral dose is 5–10 mg/kg IM or IV

Pharmacokinetics

Quinidine is about 85% protein bound and has a half-life of 5–6 h in the dog. A steady-state serum concentration is achieved approximately 24 h after initiating therapy but the serum concentration is commonly within the therapeutic range following the first dose. Pharmacokinetics have not been studied in cats.

Quinidine is metabolized in the liver to some cardioactive and some inactive metabolites and is also excreted by the kidneys. Renal disease and heart failure may increase the serum concentration. Microsomal enzyme-inducing drugs, such as anticonvulsants, may shorten the half-life of quinidine. Concomitant administration of the antacids aluminum hydroxide or magnesium oxide with quinidine decreases the maximum plasma quinidine concentration in dogs.

Adverse effects

- Gastrointestinal side effects have been reported to occur in approximately 25% of dogs administered quinidine. These appear to be direct effects of the drug on the gastrointestinal tract.
- Cardiovascular toxicity is frequently reported in human medicine and these findings have often been extrapolated to the veterinary literature. Quinidine toxicity is manifested as QRS and Q-T interval prolongation. However, clinically significant prolongation in the Q-T interval or QRS complex duration does not occur even in dogs that are seizuring due to toxicity.

- There is one report in the literature of a case of aplastic anemia in a dog treated with quinidine.
- The most important clinical problem is exacerbation of heart failure after quinidine administration. Presumably this is due to its negative inotropic effects. In general, quinidine use should be avoided in dogs with severe myocardial failure or in dogs that have, or have had, heart failure.
- Quinidine should not be used in cats.

Known drug interactions

Quinidine displaces digoxin from binding sites throughout the body and reduces digoxin renal clearance, resulting in a higher serum digoxin concentration. This is an important drug interaction and can lead to clinical signs of digitalis intoxication. Most of the digitalis toxicity in this situation is due to central nervous system stimulation (e.g. vomiting due to stimulation of the chemoreceptor trigger zone), since brain concentration of digoxin increases by 50% when quinidine is administered while digoxin concentration decreases in all other tissues, including myocardium.

Procainamide

Clinical applications

Procainamide is effective against ventricular tachyarrhythmias and may be effective against some supraventricular tachyarrhythmias in dogs. The authors have no experience using this drug in cats.

Although it is often effective at decreasing the frequency and rate of ventricular tachyarrhythmias, procainamide does not appear to be very effective at preventing sudden death in patients with severe underlying cardiac disease. It may have proarrhythmic effects in certain patients. Consequently, we do not recommend its use in Doberman pinschers and boxers with cardiomyopathy or dogs with subaortic stenosis that are prone to sudden death due to ventricular tachyarrhythmias.

Procainamide is more rationally used in dogs in the intensive care unit with malignant ventricular tachycardia that is unresponsive to lidocaine administration or in anesthetized dogs that have a serious ventricular tachyarrhythmia that is unresponsive to lidocaine.

Procainamide can also be used to treat a variety of supraventricular arrhythmias, including atrial fibrillation and supraventricular tachycardia due to pre-excitation syndrome. However, it is almost never the drug of choice for these arrhythmias.

Mechanism of action

Procainamide is a class Ia antiarrhythmic agent with properties very similar to those of quinidine. Procainamide decreases the upstroke velocity of phase 0 depolarization in normal action potentials and in action potentials produced by abnormal automaticity. This slows conduction in these tissues.

Re-entrant tachyarrhythmias may be terminated by procainamide either slowing conduction or producing a bidirectional block in the abnormal segment of the re-entrant pathway. This effect is enhanced as extracellular potassium concentration is increased. Therefore procainamide may be more effective in a patient with hypokalemia if the serum potassium concentration is normalized.

Procainamide shifts the threshold potential to more positive values. This reduces the excitability of cardiac tissue. It also increases the duration of repolarization and the effective refractory period. The increase in effective refractory period is greater than the increase in action potential duration. Theoretically, this function should increase fibrillation threshold and make procainamide an effective drug for preventing sudden death due to ventricular fibrillation. However, clinically this does not appear to be the case in human or veterinary medicine.

Procainamide can suppress digitalis-induced DADs. This should theoretically make it effective for treating digitalis intoxication-induced tachyarrhythmias. Although it does suppress these arrhythmias in dogs, a very high serum concentration is required. Procainamide was not effective against DADs produced by mechanisms other than digitalis intoxication in one in vitro study. The drug does not appear to suppress automatic atrial arrhythmias. Procainamide has vagolytic properties but these are less than those observed with quinidine and are rarely clinically significant.

Formulations and dose rates

Procainamide hydrochloride is available for oral administration in tablets or capsules and for parenteral administration. A sustained-release oral preparation is available.

Clinically, a dose of 20–30 mg/kg q.6 h PO for procainamide hydrochloride and q.8 h for the sustained-release preparation is generally used. We rarely observe any clinically significant toxicity at these doses and can usually document efficacy. There is a report of a young adult male Labrador retriever that required a dose of procainamide in the 30–40 mg/kg q.8 h PO range to control an arrhythmia associated with pre-excitation. No untoward effects were reported in this dog. Consequently, higher doses can be tried if the recommended dose is not effective.

When administered intravenously, intermittent boluses of 2–4 mg/kg should be injected slowly (over 2 min) up to a total dose of 12–20 mg/kg until the arrhythmia is controlled. This can be followed by a CRI of 10–40 μg/kg/min.

The sustained-release preparation has the same half-life as procainamide but has a longer time to peak concentration (longer absorption half-life). This enables 8-hourly administration. However, the peak serum concentration achieved with the sustained-release preparation is lower than the regular preparation when given at the same dose. Consequently, it has been recommended that the dose of the sustained-release preparation be higher.

Pharmacokinetics

Procainamide has a short half-life of approximately 3 h in the dog. The short half-life is problematic when administering procainamide orally to a dog. To maintain a serum concentration within the therapeutic range generally requires administering the drug at least q.6 h PO. The volume of distribution is approximately 2 L/kg. The vast majority of the drug is metabolized in the liver. Parenteral and oral routes of administration are used but intravenous injections must be administered slowly to prevent circulatory collapse from peripheral vasodilation and decreased cardiac contractility.

Humans commonly have beneficial effects from procainamide at lower doses and at a lower serum concentration than commonly seen in dogs. One reason for this may be because they metabolize procainamide to a metabolite, *N*-acetyl procainamide (NAPA), which has antiarrhythmic properties. Dogs cannot acetylate aromatic and hydrazine amino groups and so are incapable of producing NAPA.

Procainamide pharmacokinetics have not been studied in the cat.

Adverse effects

- Theoretically, procainamide can produce cardiotoxicity manifested as QRS and Q-T interval prolongation. However, this is almost never observed clinically.
- In humans, procainamide can have a proarrhythmic effect in some patients. This has never been documented in dogs, although it is suspected to occur.
- Toxic concentrations can depress myocardial contractility and produce hypotension. This only occurs with rapid intravenous administration.
- In humans, procainamide can cause systemic autoimmune reactions. Experimental dogs (beagles) given procainamide at 25–50 mg/kg q.6 h for 1–5 months developed antinuclear antibodies (ANA). This has not been reported in clinical patients, although the authors have observed two possible immune-mediated abnormalities in dogs receiving procainamide. One dog developed granulocytopenia that resolved when procainamide administration was discontinued. Another dog developed lymphadenopathy and a positive ANA test that resolved after procainamide administration was discontinued. Both dogs had been on procainamide for several years prior to these abnormalities occurring.

Special considerations

The intravenous preparation may become a light yellow color; it can still be used. If the solution becomes amber, however, the drug has deteriorated and the solution should not be used.

Disopyramide

Clinical applications

Because procainamide is as effective as disopyramide and is safer, disopyramide is almost never used in canine or feline patients.

Mechanism of action

Disopyramide is an oral antiarrhythmic agent with properties almost identical to those of quinidine and procainamide.

Formulations and dose rates

Disopyramide phosphate is supplied in capsules. When used as an antiarrhythmic in dogs, 7–30 mg/kg is administered q.4 h PO.

Pharmacokinetics

In the dog, disopyramide has a half-life of approximately 3 h, which makes effective dosing difficult. It is rapidly absorbed and its bioavailability is 70%.

Adverse effects

- In experimental dogs, all doses of disopyramide prolong the P-R interval. Doses of 15 and 30 mg/kg q.8 h prolong the Q-T interval while the 30 mg/kg q.8 h dose also prolongs the duration of the QRS complex.
- Doses of 15 and 30 mg/kg q.8 h significantly decrease the echocardiographic shortening fraction.
- Disopyramide is contraindicated in heart failure patients because it decreases myocardial contractility and increases peripheral vascular resistance, a potentially lethal combination.
- Disopyramide is such a potent negative inotropic agent that it is used in humans with HCM to reduce systolic anterior motion of the mitral valve.
- Disopyramide possesses significant anticholinergic properties that may produce toxic effects.
- It also decreases the serum glucose concentration in a dose-dependent manner (approximately 15% decrease at a dose of 30 mg/kg).

Mexiletine

Mexiletine is an analog of lidocaine that is not extensively metabolized on its first pass through the liver. It was first used as an antiarrhythmic agent in Europe in 1969.

Clinical applications

Mexiletine is indicated for chronic treatment of ventricular tachyarrhythmias in dogs but reports of clinical efficacy vary. One group of investigators reported limited success in suppressing ventricular arrhythmias with mexiletine in canine patients. In contrast, another group reported good efficacy. However, in the latter report, many dogs had what appeared to be benign and self-limiting ventricular tachyarrhythmias, so determining whether or not the drug was effective is difficult.

One investigator has reported that mexiletine appears to be effective at controlling ventricular tachyarrhythmias and preventing sudden death in Doberman pinschers with dilated cardiomyopathy. Although this has not been tested in any clinical trials, this report is encouraging and is consistent with the reported increase in the fibrillation threshold.

Mechanism of action

Mexiletine can interrupt re-entry circuits by slowing conduction and depressing membrane responsiveness, as for other class I drugs. Abnormal automaticity is suppressed by mexiletine. It can also suppress digitalis-induced DADs. Most important, mexiletine can increase the fibrillation threshold in the dog ventricle. In one study of experimental dogs with myocardial infarction, ventricular fibrillation or a rapid ventricular tachycardia could be induced in six of 10 dogs at baseline by stimulating the heart with two premature beats. These arrhythmias could not be induced after mexiletine administration.

Combination therapy is sometimes more effective than administration of one drug alone. A combination of mexiletine and quinidine was more effective at preventing induced ventricular arrhythmias in experimental dogs with myocardial infarction than was either drug alone in one study.

Formulations and dose rates

Mexiletine is supplied as capsules. The dose in dogs is 5–10 mg/kg q.8 h PO. An effective serum concentration may be achieved after three doses.

Pharmacokinetics

Mexiletine is well absorbed from the gastrointestinal tract in dogs, with a bioavailability of approximately 85%. Approximately 80% is excreted in the urine in dogs and 10% is metabolized by the liver and excreted in the feces. It has a plasma half-life of 3–4 h in the dog. Therapeutic serum concentration is thought to be between 0.5 and 2 fg/mL.

Adverse effects

Toxic effects can include vomiting and disorientation or ataxia but are uncommon at the suggested dosage range.

- A dose of 25 mg/kg PO to dogs can induce seizure activity.
- A dose of 40 mg/kg PO consistently produces ataxia, tremor and salivation within 10 min after administration. These signs last for up to 2.5 h. Tonic-clonic spasms often begin within 15–40 min after administration and last for up to 1 h.
- Vomiting and diarrhea can be seen at doses of 15–30 mg/kg.
- In humans, mexiletine has no effect on sinus rate, P-R interval and QRS duration in patients without pre-existing conduction system disease. In human patients with sinus node or conduction system disease, bradycardia and AV block can be produced. Mexiletine has been studied in normal dogs at doses ranging from 3 mg/kg to 15 mg/kg for 13 weeks. No effects on heart rate, P-R interval, QRS complex duration or Q-T interval were noted. No clinical signs of toxicity were seen.

Tocainide

Clinical applications

At present there are no indications for the use of tocainide in dogs or cats. Doses that are adequate to suppress arrhythmias result in unacceptable toxicity.

Mechanism of action

Tocainide is structurally similar to lidocaine. The major difference is that it is not metabolized extensively on first pass through the liver after absorption. Its actions on the normal action potential are almost identical to lidocaine. Although its effects on abnormal action potentials have not been well studied, they are likely to be similar to lidocaine's effects. Depression of the sodium current is more pronounced in abnormal than in normal myocardial tissue. Tocainide does increase the fibrillation threshold.

Formulations and dose rates

Tocainide is supplied as tablets. Clinical experience with the use of tocainide in small animal veterinary medicine is limited. Doses required to adequately suppress ventricular arrhythmias in Doberman pinschers range between 15 and 25 mg/kg q.8 h PO. These doses produce a serum tocainide concentration between 6.2 and 19.1 μg/mL 2 h after dosing and between 2.3 and 11.1 μg/mL 8 h after dosing. Apparently, smaller doses are not effective.

Pharmacokinetics

The half-life of the drug after oral administration is dose dependent. After oral doses of 50 and 100 mg/kg the half-life is 8.5 and 12 h respectively. These doses are much higher than those used clinically, so the half-life of the drug at clinical doses is unknown but probably shorter. Tocainide is metabolized by the liver and excreted in the urine. About 30% of an intravenous dose is excreted unchanged in the urine. Therapeutic plasma concentration is thought to be in the range 4–10 μg/mL.

Adverse effects

- At doses adequate to suppress arrhythmias:
  - about 25% of dogs acutely develop anorexia
  - about 10–15% develop central nervous signs of ataxia or head tremor.
- Chronically, these doses produce the intolerable side effects of:
  - corneal dystrophy in 10–15% of dogs
  - renal failure in about 25% of dogs within 4 months.
- Consequently, it does not appear that tocainide should be used in dogs for the suppression of ventricular arrhythmias and the prevention of sudden death.
- In humans, tocainide produces little effect on the electrocardiogram in patients without conduction system disease. It has been documented to produce asystole when administered concurrently with a β-adrenergic blocking agent in human patients with sinus node dysfunction. It produces no adverse effects in human patients with pre-existing conduction abnormalities.

CLASS II ANTIARRHYTHMIC DRUGS (β-ADRENERGIC BLOCKERS)

Class II antiarrhythmic drugs competitively bind with β-adrenergic receptors and so are termed β-blockers. All β-blockers exert their antiarrhythmic effects by inhibiting the effects of the adrenergic system on the heart. Cardiac adrenergic stimulation increases the heart rate, increases the conduction velocity through all regions of the conduction system and myocardium and decreases the refractoriness of cardiac tissues. In addition, it enhances normal automaticity of subsidiary pacemaker tissue.

Three types of β-receptor, termed β_1-, β_2- and β_3-receptors, are present in the body. The β_1- receptors are primarily located within the heart and adipose tissue. Stimulation of these receptors results in increases in heart rate, myocardial contractility, atrioventricular conduction velocity and automaticity of subsidiary pacemakers.

The β_2-receptors are primarily located in bronchial and vascular smooth muscle, where they produce relaxation. However, β_2-receptors also occur in the sinus and AV nodes, where they contribute to the increase in heart rate and increased conduction velocity. They are also present in myocardium, where stimulation results in increased contractility. In addition, they are present in kidney and pancreas, where they mediate renin and insulin release.

The β_3-receptors have only been recently discovered and appear to depress myocardial contractility. See Chapter 4 for further detail.

Classes

Numerous β-blockers are marketed for pharmacological use. They differ in their abilities to block β-receptor types. Some, in addition to their ability to block β-receptors, can also stimulate β-receptors mildly. Some are said to have membrane-stabilizing effects but these effects occur only at very high doses. Consequently, this is of no clinical significance. Some β-blockers also weakly inhibit α-receptors and so have mild vasodilating properties.

Many β-blockers have been developed to selectively block β_1-adrenergic receptors. This is primarily because bronchospasm develops in humans with asthma who receive a β_2-adrenergic blocking drug. Dogs do not develop asthma so there is no advantage in using a specific β_1-blocking drug in this species. However, it is a reason to use a specific β_1-blocking drug in cats with asthma. Drugs that block β_2-receptors also limit the ability of patients with diabetes mellitus to respond to hypoglycemia with glycogenolysis. Consequently, drugs that block β_2-receptors should be avoided in diabetic patients. Drugs that block β_2-receptors also have the potential of blocking the peripheral vasodilating response to β-agonists. As a result, peripheral vascular resistance may increase.

In veterinary medicine, very few individuals have any clinical experience with the vast majority of β-blockers. The three primary drugs in veterinary use today are propranolol, atenolol and carvedilol (see β blocker section of this chapter p. 419). The drugs are equipotent but their pharmacokinetics differ. Esmolol, a β-blocker with a very short half-life, is also used on occasion as an intravenous agent for short-term management of arrhythmias.

Clinical applications

In veterinary medicine, β-blockers are used to treat both supraventricular and ventricular tachyarrhythmias and prevent sudden death due to ventricular tachyarrhythmias. They are also used to treat HCM in cats. They are occasionally used to treat systemic arterial hypertension and more recently preclinical and clinical heart disease. They may be more effective in cats than dogs for controlling blood pressure. However, amlodipine is more effective than propranolol for this purpose in cats. β-Blockers are usually ineffective for treating systemic hypertension secondary to renal disease in dogs.

As antiarrhythmic drugs, β-blockers are most commonly used to slow the ventricular rate in patients with atrial fibrillation, to abolish supraventricular tachycardia and HCM, to slow the sinus rate in cats with hyperthyroidism, to prevent sudden death in dogs with severe subaortic stenosis and to chronically treat ventricular tachyarrhythmias. They are used either as sole agents or in combination with other antiarrhythmic drugs. They are also used to treat the cardiac effects of pheochromocytoma in combination with prazosin.

Mechanism of action

Drugs that block β-adrenergic receptors do not produce many of the specific cellular membrane changes observed with other antiarrhythmic drugs. At doses that induce β-adrenergic blockade, there is no change in resting membrane potential, amplitude of the action potential or velocity of depolarization. In the dog, however, atenolol does prolong the refractory period. This change, along with the inhibition of sympathetic input, reduces the ability of induced premature beats to produce ventricular tachycardia and fibrillation in experimental dogs 7–30 days following induced myocardial infarction, at a time when ventricular arrhythmias are caused by re-entry.

With all β-blockers, no simple correlation between dose or serum concentration and therapeutic effect exists. The serum concentration required to produce a beneficial effect depends on the prevailing sympathetic tone and on β-adrenergic receptor density and sensitivity. These variables vary widely from patient to patient.

In addition, the pharmacokinetics of β-blockers can differ substantially between patients. In humans, there can be a 20-fold difference in plasma concentration between patients receiving the same oral dose. In one study in normal dogs, a five-fold difference between dogs administered the same dose was reported. Because hepatic blood flow is a major determinant of propranolol clearance and half-life, this variability can be expected to be even greater in cardiac patients where hepatic blood flow is compromised. Consequently, the dose required to produce a therapeutic effect varies substantially. Because of this, the dosage must be titrated to an effective endpoint in each patient.

Adverse effects

In patients subjected to chronic increases in circulating catecholamine concentrations and increased sympathetic nervous system activity (e.g. patients with heart failure), β-adrenergic receptors decrease in number, internalize into the cell membrane and become less efficient at producing cAMP. These changes are commonly lumped together and termed receptor downregulation. In these patients, fewer receptors are available for drug binding. However, many of these patients are very dependent on stimulated β-receptors to maintain myocardial contractility. Acute administration of medium-to-high doses of a β-blocker to patients with compromised myocardial function (e.g. patients with dilated cardiomyopathy) dependent on β-receptor stimulation can result in lethal decreases in contractility and heart rate.

Propranolol

Clinical applications

Propranolol is indicated in canine and feline patients with ventricular and supraventricular tachyarrhythmias. It is commonly used with digoxin to slow the ventricular rate in patients with atrial fibrillation. It is effective for terminating and preventing the recurrence of supraventricular tachycardia.

Propranolol can be effective as the sole agent for terminating ventricular tachyarrhythmias but is generally more effective when used in combination with other antiarrhythmic agents. Propranolol is effective for decreasing the sinus rate in patients with hyperthyroidism, pheochromocytoma and heart failure. Few antiarrhythmic drugs can be used in cats. Propranolol has been used to treat both supraventricular and ventricular tachyarrhythmias in cats with moderate success.

Mechanism of action

Propranolol is the prototype β-receptor blocking agent. It reduces catecholamine-dependent automatic (normal and abnormal) rhythms and slows conduction in abnormal ventricular myocardium. Propranolol also increases the refractory period and slows conduction velocity in AV nodal tissues. This slows the ventricular response to atrial fibrillation and flutter and effectively abolishes supraventricular arrhythmias due to AV nodal re-entry.

By reducing contractility, propranolol reduces myocardial oxygen consumption, which may reduce myocardial hypoxia and arrhythmia formation in patients with subaortic stenosis. Propranolol also abolishes supraventricular and ventricular tachyarrhythmias due to pheochromocytoma and thyrotoxicosis.

Propranolol, like any β-blocker, produces dose-dependent decreases in myocardial contractility. This does not occur after an intravenous dose of 0.02 mg/kg in normal dogs (this would be comparable to an oral dose of 0.2 mg/kg). An intravenous dose of 0.08 mg/kg (comparable oral dose = 0.8 mg/kg) decreases dP/dt, an index of myocardial contractility, by approximately 30%.

Propranolol has a profound effect on peripheral vascular resistance in normal, conscious experimental dogs. At an intravenous dose of 0.02 mg/kg, peripheral vascular resistance increases to almost twice the baseline. There is no further increase with a dose of 0.08 mg/kg. These effects have not been studied in dogs with heart failure but it is apparent that larger doses of propranolol must be avoided in these patients. Propranolol appears to have a greater effect on the sinus rate in normal dogs than drugs that specifically block β_1-receptors. This is probably because β_2-receptors are also present in the sinus node and help modulate the sinus rate.

Formulations and dose rates

Propranolol hydrochloride is available as tablets for oral administration and ampoules for intravenous administration.

The dose of propranolol depends on the situation for which it is used. In dogs with atrial fibrillation due to severe underlying cardiac disease, the oral dose is 0.1–0.5 mg/kg q.8 h. At this dose range, the negative inotropic effects of propranolol appear to be negligible. We have never witnessed exacerbation of heart failure at this dose range in dogs with dilated cardiomyopathy or severe mitral regurgitation, even when the patient was not being administered a concomitant positive inotropic agent, like digoxin.

In canine patients with supraventricular or ventricular tachyarrhythmias and normal myocardial function, doses as high as 2 mg/kg q.8 h are well tolerated and often required. Doses in this range are contraindicated in patients with severe myocardial failure. Duration of drug effect is longer than the drug's half-life because of active propranolol metabolites and receptor binding of the drug. Consequently, administering the drug q.8 h appears to be effective. The feline oral dose is 2.5–10 mg q.8 h for control of tachyarrhythmias.

The intravenous dose in dogs is administered as intermittent boluses to effect. The initial IV dose is 0.02 mg/kg and the total dose should not exceed 0.1 mg/kg. Intravenous doses of propranolol must be administered cautiously to heart failure patients because a decrease in contractility may acutely worsen hemodynamics. The therapeutic endpoint is abolition or improvement of a tachyarrhythmia, slowing of the sinus rate or slowing of the ventricular response to atrial fibrillation.

Pharmacokinetics

Propranolol is lipid soluble and so is almost completely absorbed by the small intestine. It is largely metabolized by the liver. Oral propranolol undergoes a variable but extensive first-pass hepatic metabolism. As a result, its bioavailability for the first dose ranges from only 2% to 17% for oral administration in the dog. Serum half-life after the first dose is about 1.5 h in the dog. Chronic oral dosing increases half-life to about 2 h and results in serum concentrations 1.25–10 times greater than after initial doses due to an increase in bioavailability. This increase is probably due to saturation of first-pass metabolism.

Adverse effects

- Patients with myocardial failure or heart failure due to severe volume overload may have their heart failure exacerbated by propranolol, especially if it is administered intravenously. These patients usually receive propranolol for control of heart rate and only low oral doses are generally needed. If acute heart failure is precipitated it cannot be reversed by catecholamines, so calcium, glucagon or digitalis must be used.
- Propranolol should not be administered to patients with conduction disturbances or abnormal inherent pacemaker function. Propranolol will exacerbate sinus node dysfunction in patients with sick sinus syndrome. It will also exacerbate AV nodal dysfunction in patients with first- and second-degree AV block, potentially creating third-degree AV block. In patients with third-degree AV block, it will decrease the rate of the subsidiary pacemaker, a potentially lethal effect.
- Propranolol should not be used in patients with asthma or chronic lower airway disease, as increases in lower airway resistance may occur with β-blockade.
- Propranolol should also be used with caution in diabetic patients receiving insulin because propranolol reduces sympathetic compensation for hypoglycemia.
- Acute propranolol withdrawal may exacerbate the original problem for which the drug was being administered, so gradual withdrawal should be performed. As an example, the authors have witnessed sudden death in one boxer dog with ventricular arrhythmia following the acute cessation of propranolol administration.
- β-Blockers should not be administered to patients with hyperkalemia because the β-blockade reduces the potassium flux from intravascular to extravascular spaces.

Known drug interactions

Digitalis plus propranolol can cause varying degrees of AV block.

Special considerations

The intravenous preparation of the drug rapidly decomposes in alkaline solutions.

Atenolol

Clinical applications

Atenolol has clinical indications in both dogs and cats. In dogs, it is most commonly used in conjunction with digoxin to slow the heart rate in patients with atrial fibrillation. It is also used in dogs to treat supraventricular tachycardia and ventricular tachyarrhythmias and in an attempt to prevent sudden death in dogs with severe subaortic stenosis. Its most common indication in cats is to decrease systolic anterior motion of the mitral valve in feline HCM and to treat ventricular tachyarrhythmias.

Mechanism of action

Atenolol is a specific β_1-adrenergic blocking drug. It has the same potency as propranolol but different pharmacokinetics.

Formulations and dose rates

Atenolol is supplied as tablets. It is also supplied as a solution for IV injection. The IV dosage for dogs and cats is not known.

DOGS

- 6.25–50 mg/dog q.12 h PO. In humans, q.24 h dosing is adequate to maintain efficacy. Because of its shorter half-life in the dog, it is recommended that atenolol be administered q.12 h to dogs
- In large dogs with atrial fibrillation, the starting dose is 12.5 mg q.12 h PO. The dose is titrated upward until the heart rate is above 160 beats/min. In small dogs, the starting dose is 6.25 mg q.12 h PO
- If used to treat ventricular arrhythmias in dogs without underlying myocardial failure or in an attempt to prevent sudden death in dogs with subaortic stenosis, the dose should be at the higher end of the dosage range

CATS

- In hypertrophic cardiomyopathy, atenolol can be used to decrease the subaortic pressure gradient that occurs secondary to systolic anterior motion of the mitral valve. The starting dose is 6.25 mg q.12 h PO. It is then titrated upwards to as high as 25 mg q.12 h PO

Pharmacokinetics

Atenolol is more water soluble than propranolol. In the dog, bioavailability appears to be approximately 80%. Atenolol is eliminated unchanged in the urine. There is very little hepatic metabolism. The half-life of atenolol is longer than the half-life of propranolol, being 5–6 h in the dog. This is somewhat shorter than the half-life in humans, which is 6–9 h. In the cat, atenolol has a half-life of 3.5 h. Its bioavailability is high at 90% and the pharmacokinetic variability from cat to cat is small. When administered to cats at a dose of 3 mg/kg, atenolol attenuates the increase in heart rate produced by isoprenaline for 12 but not for 24 h.

Esmolol

Clinical applications

Esmolol has several clinical indications. It can be used for the acute termination of supraventricular tachycardia. It can also be used, at low doses, to decrease acutely the heart rate of dogs with severe tachycardia (heart rate >250 beats/min) due to atrial fibrillation. It has been administered to cats with HCM to determine if β-blockade will reduce the dynamic left ventricular outflow tract obstruction due to systolic anterior motion of the mitral valve.

Mechanism of action

Esmolol is an ultra-short-acting (half-life <10 min) β_1-adrenergic blocking drug used for intravenous administration.

Steady-state β-blockade is produced within 10–20 min after starting intravenous administration of esmolol in dogs. After discontinuation of drug administration, no detectable β-blockade is apparent at 20 min post-infusion, regardless of the dose administered. Esmolol decreases the sinus node rate. At an infusion rate of 25 μg/kg/min, approximately 30% of the effect of isoprenaline-induced tachycardia is inhibited. This value increases to approximately 60% with a 50 μg/kg/min dose and to approximately 70% with a 100 μg/kg/min infusion rate.

Myocardial contractility is depressed with esmolol. In normal conscious dogs, an infusion rate of 10 μg/kg/min does not change dP/dt. An infusion rate of 40 μg/kg/min decreases dP/dt by approximately 30% and an infusion rate of 160 μg/kg/min decreases it by 50%. Because esmolol only blocks β_1-adrenergic receptors, it produces no increase in peripheral vascular resistance.

Formulations and dose rates

Esmolol hydrochloride is supplied as a solution for injection and a concentrated solution for dilution in solution for intravenous infusion.

DOGS

- Esmolol can be administered in two different ways. An initial loading dose of 0.25–0.5 mg/kg (250–500 μg/kg) can be administered intravenously as a slow bolus over 1–2 min followed by a constant rate infusion of 50–200 μg/kg/min. Alternatively, a CRI of 10–200 μg/kg/min can be started without a loading dose. In this manner, maximal effect should be apparent within 10–20 min. With the loading dose, an effect should be apparent more quickly
- An initial loading dose and the high end of the dosage range should only be used in dogs with normal cardiac function. In dogs with severe dilated cardiomyopathy or severe mitral regurgitation and atrial fibrillation with a very fast ventricular rate, esmolol should be infused only (no loading dose). The infusion should start at 10–20 μg/kg/min and be titrated upward every 10 min to an effective endpoint

Pharmacokinetics

Esmolol has the basic structure of a β-adrenergic blocking drug but it contains an ester on the phenoxypropanolamine nucleus that is rapidly hydrolyzed by RBC esterases. The major metabolite of esmolol is ASL-8123 which has a half-life in dogs of 2.1 h. This metabolite has one-1500th the β-blocking activity of esmolol, which is clinically insignificant.

Carvedilol

See Neuroendocrine modulator section (p. 412).

CLASS III ANTIARRHYTHMIC DRUGS

There is increasing evidence in human medicine that class I antiarrhythmic agents are ineffective for preventing sudden death. In some instances they may actually increase the incidence of sudden death in patients with organic heart disease and ventricular arrhythmias. Because of this, the use of these drugs in human medicine has plummeted within the past 10 years. At the same time, the efficacy of other drugs has been examined more vigorously. Class II antiarrhythmics (β-blockers) are effective agents for preventing sudden death in human patients with myocardial infarction. As class III drugs act primarily by prolonging the refractory period, they theoretically reduce the propensity for micro re-entrant circuits to develop and so make it more difficult for ventricular fibrillation to develop.

Amiodarone

Clinical applications

It has been suggested that amiodarone may be useful in dogs with DCM that are at risk of sudden death. There have been no controlled studies but anecdotal evidence suggests it is effective. More recently, amiodarone has been reported to be beneficial in atrial fibrillation and may result in conversion to sinus rhythm in as many as 25% of dogs. Amiodarone is potentially useful and may become more popular in small animal medicine as veterinarians gain more experience with the drug.

Mechanism of action

Amiodarone is a benzofurane derivative. It is structurally related to levothyroxine (thyroxine) and has a high iodine content. It is metabolized to desethylamiodarone in the dog. Desethylamiodarone has important antiarrhythmic effects because of its ability to block fast sodium channels. It is more effective than amiodarone at suppressing ventricular arrhythmias 24 h after myocardial infarction in experimental dogs.

Amiodarone was first introduced into human medicine in 1961 as an antianginal agent. Its antiarrhythmic properties were recognized in 1970. Since then, it has been used for this purpose extensively in human medicine in European countries. It is currently being used more frequently in human medicine in the USA to treat patients at risk of sudden death due to ventricular arrhythmia. This increased use is primarily a result of reports of proarrhythmia and increased mortality in patients with ventricular tachyarrhythmias receiving class I antiarrhythmic agents and of the recognition that antifibrillatory actions may be more important than antiarrhythmic action in preventing sudden death.

Electrophysiologically, amiodarone's primary effect is to prolong the refractory period of atrial and ventricular myocardium and the AV junction without changing resting membrane potential when administered chronically. This may result in an increase in the P-R interval and the Q-T interval on the ECG. Because of its effect on refractory period in myocardium, amiodarone has a marked antifibrillatory effect. Consequently, its primary clinical use is to prevent sudden death. In automatic cells, amiodarone reduces the slope of phase 4 of the action potential. This results in a decrease in the sinus rate. Amiodarone can also suppress tachyarrhythmias. Prolongation of the refractory period can interrupt re-entrant circuits. In addition, amiodarone has sodium channel-blocking properties (class I effects), which can slow conduction and interrupt re-entrant circuits. Amiodarone also noncompetitively blocks α- and β-receptors and appears to have some ability to block slow calcium channels.

Formulations and dose rates

Amiodarone is supplied as tablets. The effective dose in the dog is unknown. Because of its bizarre and variable pharmacokinetics, predicting the ultimate serum concentration is difficult and predicting the myocardial concentration impossible. For years, amiodarone was administered to humans at higher doses than are currently used. More recently, lower doses have proved to be efficacious. This was discovered through clinical use.

Because amiodarone has not been used extensively in clinical veterinary medicine, it is unknown whether or not lower doses than those used in experimental studies are effective. It is known that an oral dose of approximately 10 mg/kg/d to experimental dogs increases the defibrillation threshold after 9 d.

No established relationship between plasma concentration and efficacy in humans exists. However, a plasma concentration below 1 mg/L is often not effective and a plasma concentration above 2.5 mg/L is usually not needed. A plasma concentration above 2.5 mg/L is associated with a higher incidence of side effects in humans.

It is known that the plasma concentration was 1.9 ± 1.1 mg/L within 3 weeks in experimental dogs administered 40 mg/kg/d PO for 10 d followed by 30 mg/kg/d PO for 4 d followed by 20 mg/kg PO d for 6 weeks. It is also known that this dose was effective in preventing inducible ventricular tachycardia/fibrillation in these dogs with experimentally induced myocardial infarction. From these data, it would appear that this dose regimen might be effective in clinical canine patients. However, lower doses were not tested in this study so it is unknown if a lower dose might have been equally effective.

The dose regimen outlined above resulted in a plasma concentration above 2.5 mg/L in some dogs. This may suggest that a lower dose might be safer. One veterinary clinician has reported that a dose regimen of 10–15 mg/kg q.12 h (20–30 mg/kg/d) PO for 7 d followed by 5–7.5 mg/kg q.12 h (10–15 mg/kg/d) PO improved ventricular arrhythmias in a few dogs.

Pharmacokinetics

Amiodarone has unusual pharmacokinetics. After repeated administration, the drug has a long half-life of

3.2 days in the dog. It is very lipophilic and accumulates to up to 300 times the plasma concentration in adipose tissue. Once drug administration is discontinued, amiodarone is cleared rapidly from all tissues except adipose tissue.

Myocardial concentration of the drug is approximately 15 times that of plasma. The long half-life of the drug means that it takes a long time to produce a significant effect once administration starts. It also takes a long time for the drug effect to dissipate once administration is discontinued. For example, the time to reach one-half of the peak value ultimately achieved for the increase in left ventricular refractory period in dogs is 2.5 days. The time to come down to one-half the peak value after drug administration is discontinued is 21 days in dogs. Because of the long time to onset, loading doses of amiodarone are commonly administered in human medicine. In humans it may take 1–3 weeks to observe onset of action, even with loading doses. Antiarrhythmic effects are present for weeks to months after discontinuing the drug in humans.

Adverse effects

- Numerous side effects of amiodarone have been reported in the human literature. In humans who receive more than 400 mg/d of amiodarone (400 mg is approximately 6 mg/kg/d), 75% experience adverse reactions and 7–18% discontinue the drug because of side effects. Most of the adverse sequelae occur after 6 months of drug use.
- Adverse reactions in humans consist of neurological problems (20–40%), gastrointestinal disturbances (25%), visual disturbances including corneal microdeposits (4–9%), dermatological reactions including photosensitivity and blue discoloration of the skin (5%), cardiovascular reactions including congestive heart failure and bradycardia (3%), abnormal liver function tests (4–9%), pulmonary inflammation and fibrosis (4–9%) and hypothyroidism and hyperthyroidism.
- Pulmonary fibrosis is the most common severe sequela of amiodarone administration in humans. Pulmonary fibrosis, heart failure and elevation of liver enzymes necessitate discontinuing the drug in humans. Pulmonary toxicity appears to be multifaceted but inhibition of phospholipase A with resultant phospholipidosis is one mechanism responsible for producing pulmonary lesions.
- Amiodarone's side effect profile in dogs is poorly documented.
  - In two studies elevated liver enzymes and neutropenia were reported in some dogs. The liver enzymes returned to normal following discontinuation of the medication in most dogs.
  - Gastrointestinal disturbances have also been reported.
  - The authors can find no studies of chronic toxicity of amiodarone in dogs.
  - Comparable lung changes to those seen in humans are induced in rats and mice.
  - Dyslipidic lesions can be produced in the gastrointestinal tract of dogs by amiodarone administration but only at very high doses (>50 mg/kg/d for 30 d).
  - It is also known that amiodarone increases the phospholipid content of feline myocardium. Consequently, it is suspected that chronic amiodarone toxicity could occur in dogs and cats.
- Amiodarone can result in either hypothyroidism or hyperthyroidism in humans. Amiodarone inhibits T4 and T3 secretion from canine thyroid glands. Consequently, thyroid function should be monitored when amiodarone is chronically administered in veterinary patients.

Known drug interactions

- Amiodarone alters the pharmacokinetics and increases the serum concentrations or the effects of several drugs in humans, including digoxin, quinidine, procainamide, phenytoin and warfarin.
- Amiodarone administration increases the bioavailability of diltiazem and decreases total body clearance and volume of distribution of the drug in the dog. This results in an increased serum diltiazem concentration and could produce a toxic concentration. This combination should be used cautiously and the dose of diltiazem reduced.

Bretylium

Clinical applications

Bretylium was first developed as an antihypertensive agent. In 1966, it was noted that it increased the fibrillation threshold. Since then, it has found limited usefulness as an antiarrhythmic and antifibrillatory agent in human medicine.

Bretylium is used for the emergency treatment of life-threatening ventricular tachycardia or ventricular fibrillation that recurs despite direct current shock and lidocaine. It is generally ineffective against supraventricular arrhythmias. Bretylium appears to have no use as an agent to produce chemical defibrillation in dogs.

Mechanism of action

Bretylium's primary effect is prolongation of the action potential and refractory periods in myocardium. It also decreases the disparity in action potential duration between normal and diseased myocardium. Bretylium is taken up by and concentrated in adrenergic nerve terminals. This initially results in noradrenaline (norepinephrine) release and a brief sympathomimetic effect. This is followed by an inhibition of noradrenaline release.

Bretylium's major effect on cardiac tissues is to prolong the action potential and refractory period of atrial and ventricular myocardium and Purkinje fibers. In so doing, it increases the fibrillation threshold. Bretylium produces a biphasic effect on impulse initiation and conduction and on hemodynamics. Sinus rate, myocardial contractility and blood pressure increase transiently for 10–15 min. These variables then tend to decrease as sympathetic tone decreases. These anti-adrenergic effects prolong atrioventricular conduction time in dogs.

Formulations and dose rates

Bretylium tosylate is supplied as a solution for intravenous administration. Because the oral route results in erratic absorption, bretylium is only administered intravenously.

DOGS

- 2–6 mg/kg IV. This dose increases the fibrillation threshold to 5–18 times the baseline
- In experimental dogs, this dose is effective at preventing ventricular fibrillation and tachycardia when administered every 12 h chronically. This, however, is not a practical means of treating canine patients
- When bretylium is administered to dogs during cardiopulmonary resuscitation, the antifibrillatory effects are not immediate. Lidocaine produces a more rapid but less pronounced antifibrillatory effect. A combination of lidocaine (2 mg/kg) and bretylium (5 mg/kg) may have a more beneficial effect than either drug alone

Pharmacokinetics

In the dog, bretylium has a biological half-life of approximately 16 h. However, plasma concentration declines rapidly after intravenous administration of 15 mg/kg from approximately 20 μg/mL at 6 min to less than 2 μg/mL after 1 h. The drug is cleared from the body through renal elimination. The antifibrillatory action correlates with myocardial concentration, which increases slowly after intravenous administration to reach a peak 1.5–6 h after dosing.

Adverse effects

- Toxicity is rare, although hypotension can occur. Blood pressure should be monitored and dopamine or noradrenaline (norepinephrine) administered if systolic blood pressure falls below 75 mmHg.
- Transient hypertension and arrhythmia exacerbation may occur after the initial dose because of noradrenaline (norepinephrine) release from nerve terminals.

Sotalol

Sotalol is a class III antiarrhythmic with important β-blocking properties but should not be substituted for a pure β-blocker. The information provided on this drug in this chapter is based on studies in experimental animals, on reports of its use in human medicine, on limited clinical experience and on anecdotal reports from individuals who have used the drug. Sotalol is potentially a very useful drug in small animal veterinary medicine but this potential has not yet been fully explored.

Clinical applications

In human medicine, sotalol is effective for treating various arrhythmias. It is not as successful as quinidine at converting primary atrial fibrillation to sinus rhythm. It is, however, as effective as quinidine at preventing recurrence of atrial fibrillation after electrical cardioversion. Sotalol is effective at terminating supraventricular tachycardia due to AV nodal re-entry or pre-excitation in humans. In human patients with ventricular tachycardia, sotalol may be one of the more effective agents for terminating or slowing the tachycardia. It also appears to be efficacious for preventing sudden death. These effects, however, are not profound and have required large clinical trials to reach statistical significance.

A major indication in veterinary medicine is boxer dogs with severe ventricular tachyarrhythmias and syncope. Sotalol is very effective at suppressing the arrhythmias and stopping the syncopal events in this breed. The authors have limited experience with sotalol for the treatment of supraventricular arrhythmias and ventricular arrhythmias in other breeds.

Mechanism of action

Sotalol is a potent and nonselective β-adrenergic blocking drug that also prolongs the action potential duration and increases the refractory period of both atrial and ventricular myocardium (class III effect). In human medicine it is useful for treating a variety of arrhythmias and for increasing the fibrillation threshold.

Sotalol is marketed as the racemic mixture of its stereo isomers, D- and L-sotalol. The D-isomer has less than one-50th the β-blocking activity of the L-isomer. The L-isomer's potency is similar to that of propranolol. The D- and L-isomers both prolong action potential duration and refractoriness. The increase in action potential duration is caused by blockade of potassium channels.

Sotalol, when administered intravenously or at high doses orally, increases the Q-T interval on the ECG in experimental dogs. As for any β-blocker, the heart rate is decreased with sotalol administration. It also prolongs the AV nodal refractory period and the P-R interval because of its β-blocking effect. Sotalol increases the atrial and the ventricular fibrillation threshold in experimental dogs. The effect on atrial refractoriness should make it a good drug for preventing atrial fibrillation in dogs, especially those with primary atrial fibrillation after cardioversion. The effect on the ventricular fibrillation threshold should make it an effective agent for preventing sudden death in dogs. Its effects on defibrillation are less well understood. In one study, sotalol decreased the success rate for defibrillation, while in another study, it decreased the energy required for defibrillation.

The hemodynamic effects of sotalol are mixed. Because it is a β-blocker, a decrease in myocardial contractility is expected and has been identified in anesthetized, experimental dogs with normal hearts and in experimental dogs after myocardial infarction. However, in isolated cardiac tissues, sotalol does not have any negative inotropic effect and may have a modest (20–40% increase) positive inotropic effect in catecholamine-depleted experimental cats. This effect may be caused by the prolongation of the action potential allowing more time for calcium influx in systole.

In experimental dogs, sotalol has less of a negative inotropic effect than propranolol. In humans with compromised myocardial function, sotalol can induce or exacerbate heart failure but the incidence is much lower than one might expect. In one study, heart failure was aggravated by sotalol in only 3% of human patients. The potential negative inotropic effects of sotalol could theoretically produce myocardial depression and produce or aggravate heart failure in small animal patients. As in human patients, if one uses this drug, the dose must be carefully titrated and canine or feline patients with moderate to severe cardiac disease must be monitored carefully.

Formulations and dose rates

Sotalol hydrochloride is supplied as tablets. Sotalol is marketed as D,L-sotalol. Both the D-and L-isomers prolong action potential duration, while the L-isomer is responsible for the β-blocking properties of the drug.

Doses used in experimental dogs

In one study in experimental dogs, sotalol successfully converted atrial flutter to sinus rhythm in 14 of 15 dogs at a dose of 2 mg/kg IV administered over 15 min. Quinidine only converted nine of the 15 dogs at a dose of 10 mg/kg IV over 15 min. In another study to examine sotalol's ability to terminate and to prevent atrial fibrillation, it was administered intravenously to dogs with induced atrial fibrillation. At a dose of 2 mg/kg IV, sotalol did not terminate or prevent atrial fibrillation. At a cumulative dose of 8 mg/kg, however, it terminated the arrhythmia in seven of eight dogs and prevented its reinduction in all eight dogs. This effect was due to a prolongation of atrial refractory period.

A high dose of D-sotalol is required to suppress the formation of ventricular arrhythmias in experimental dogs. This compound has no β-blocking activity and one would expect that a lower dose of the racemic mixture would be effective. In one study of conscious experimental dogs 3–5 d after myocardial infarction, four doses of 8 mg/kg D-sotalol administered intravenously successfully prevented the induction of ventricular tachycardia by programmed electrical stimulation in six of nine dogs and slowed the rate of the tachycardia in two of the three remaining dogs.

D-sotalol is also effective in increasing the ventricular fibrillation threshold in experimental dogs with myocardial infarction. Again, the dose required to produce this beneficial effect appears to be quite high, although the data are conflicting and lower doses were not used in most studies. In one study that examined conscious dogs, four doses of 8 mg/kg of D-sotalol PO were administered over 24 h. This dose prevented ventricular fibrillation secondary to ischemia produced distal to a previous myocardial infarction. The use of lower doses was not reported. In another study using conscious dogs subjected to distal myocardial ischemia and infarction, sotalol was administered at 2 mg/kg and at 8 mg/kg intravenously. Although the two groups were not reported separately, it appears that both doses prevented ventricular fibrillation and sudden death. In the group of dogs given sotalol, 13 of 20 dogs survived while only one of 15 dogs given a placebo lived.

Clinical experience with sotalol doses

Boxers with severe ventricular arrhythmias and syncope without severe myocardial failure often respond favorably to the administration of sotalol. Syncopal episodes cease and a marked reduction in ventricular arrhythmias occurs. The dose ranges from 40 mg to 120 mg q.12 h (approximately 1–4 mg/kg q.12 h) PO. This dose is comparable to the human pediatric dose of 50 mg/m^2 of body surface area q.12 h PO. The dose is generally titrated, starting at 40 mg q.12 h. If that dose is ineffective the dose is increased to 80 mg in the morning and 40 mg in the evening, followed by 80 mg q.12 h.

Sotalol may, in some circumstances, be used cautiously in dogs with moderate to severe myocardial failure. The authors recommend that **patients with moderate to severe myocardial failure be monitored very carefully during the initial stages of sotalol administration**. If this cannot be done, sotalol should not be used. In dogs with myocardial failure, the most common response to a relative overdose is weakness, presumably secondary to a low cardiac output. In patients in heart failure, exacerbation of edema can occur. In most cases, withdrawal of the drug should be the only action required if evidence of low cardiac output or exacerbation of the edema becomes apparent. If this does not suffice or if the clinical abnormalities are severe, the administration of a bipyridine compound, calcium or glucagon may be beneficial. Administration of a catecholamine, such as dobutamine or dopamine, will not produce the desired response, since β-receptors are blocked by sotalol.

Pharmacokinetics

In experimental dogs, sotalol is rapidly absorbed from the gastrointestinal tract and has a bioavailability in the 85–90% range. Less than 1% of the drug is metabolized. Elimination is via renal clearance and is linearly related to the glomerular filtration rate. Consequently, the drug dose must be reduced in patients with compromised renal function due to any cause. Sotalol is not protein bound in plasma of dogs. The elimination half-life is 4.8 ± 1.0 h. The apparent volume of distribution is in the 1.5–2.5 L/kg range.

Following oral administration of sotalol at 5 mg/kg q.12 h for 3 d (when steady state is reached in experimental dogs), the plasma concentration is in the 1.1–1.6 mg/L range. In humans given the same dose, the plasma concentration is in the 2–3 mg/L range. This discrepancy probably occurs because the elimination half-life in humans is longer (7–18 h). This suggests that the dose in dogs should be roughly double that used in humans. The human dosage recommendation is to administer 40–80 mg q.12 h as an initial dose. This dose then can be increased as necessary every 3–4 d. The maximum dose is 320 mg q.12 h. Assuming an average weight of 70 kg for humans means the dose starts at approximately 0.5–1.0 mg/kg q.12 h and can achieve a maximum dose of approximately 5 mg/kg q.12 h.

A plasma concentration of 0.8 mg/L is needed to produce half-maximal β-adrenergic blockade in experimental dogs. This suggests that a dose of 5 mg/kg q.12 h PO to a dog should result in near-maximal blockade. The plasma concentration required to prolong cardiac refractoriness is higher. In humans, a plasma concentration of 2.6 mg/L is necessary to increase the Q-T interval. Doses between 2 and 5 mg/kg q.12 h PO in humans prolong the Q-T interval by 40–100 ms. In experimental dogs, a dose of 5 mg/kg q.12 h PO also prolongs the Q-T interval.

Adverse effects

- Adverse effects of sotalol in humans are related to the negative inotropic effects of sotalol and to its ability to prolong the Q-T interval. As stated earlier, the negative inotropic effects appear to be minor and very few human patients experience exacerbation of heart failure.
- The most dangerous adverse effect of sotalol in humans is aggravation of existing arrhythmias or provocation of new arrhythmias.
- Excessive Q-T interval prolongation can provoke torsades de pointes in humans. Torsades de pointes has also been produced in experimental dogs but appears to be more difficult to invoke in dogs. For example, one canine model requires that the dog be bradycardic from experimentally induced third-degree AV block and hypokalemic (serum potassium concentration in the 2.5 mEq/L range) before sotalol can cause this serious arrhythmia. The arrhythmia in this model can be terminated with intravenous magnesium administration (1–2 mg/kg/min for 20–30 min).
- Sotalol apparently can also induce other forms of ventricular tachyarrhythmia because of the prolongation of the Q-T interval.
- As for any other β-blocker, withdrawal of sotalol should be performed gradually over 1–2 weeks because of 'upregulation' of β-receptors. Sudden cessation of use can produce fatal ventricular arrhythmias. The drug should not be used in patients with conduction system disease such as sick sinus syndrome, AV block or bundle branch block.

CLASS IV ANTIARRHYTHMIC DRUGS

Description and discovery

Class IV antiarrhythmic drugs are the calcium channel-blocking drugs. These are also known as calcium entry blockers, slow channel blockers and calcium antagonists. Verapamil, the prototype calcium channel blocker, was discovered in 1963. It was being developed as a coronary vasodilator and was discovered to have negative inotropic properties. The negative inotropism could be neutralized by the addition of calcium, β-adrenergic agonists and digitalis glycosides – measures that increase calcium flux into myocardial cells. It was subsequently discovered in 1969 that verapamil and other drugs with similar effects selectively suppressed transmembrane calcium flow. Today, at least 29 different calcium channel blockers are used in clinical human medicine worldwide. In veterinary medicine, only verapamil and diltiazem have been used with enough frequency to make recommendations regarding therapy of arrhythmias.

Classification and mechanism of action

Calcium channel blockers have a variety of chemical structures. They can be classified into three groups: the phenylalkylamines, the benzothiazepines and the dihydropyridines. The phenylalkylamines include verapamil. Diltiazem is a benzothiazepine. The dihydropyridines include nifedipine and amlodipine.

The primary sites of action for calcium channel blockers in cardiovascular medicine are the L-type calcium channels in cardiac cells and in vascular smooth muscle cells. In the heart, calcium channel blockers directly decrease myocardial contractility and slow sinoatrial depolarization and atrioventricular conduction. In vascular smooth muscle, calcium channel blockers produce relaxation of systemic arterioles, resulting in a decrease in peripheral vascular resistance.

The ability of calcium channel blockers to affect these sites varies tremendously. Verapamil binds equally well to cardiac and vascular smooth muscle sites, producing profound electrophysiological changes, depression in myocardial contractility and vasodilation. The dihydropyridines have very little effect on cardiac calcium channels but have profound effects on vascular smooth muscle. Diltiazem is somewhere between these two extremes, with profound electrophysiological changes, an intermediate effect on cardiac function and a mild effect on vascular smooth muscle. In conscious dogs, nifedipine and verapamil increase the heart rate. This is presumably due to reflex increase in sympathetic tone caused by vasodilation. Diltiazem has little effect.

Myocardial contractility is increased reflexly by nifedipine, decreased directly by verapamil and not changed by diltiazem in the normal cardiovascular system. When the autonomic nervous system is blocked with propranolol and atropine, all three drugs decrease contractility and heart rate. The variable effects are due to slight differences in L-type channel subunit structure between different sites that result in marked differences in channel pharmacology.

Calcium channel-blocking agents that affect myocardial channels block the slow inward calcium current during phase 2 of the cardiac cell action potential. This results in a decrease in myocardial contractility. This may be beneficial in certain circumstances, such as in feline patients with HCM and dynamic subaortic stenosis. In human patients with normal myocardial function, the negative inotropic effect is generally offset by reflex increase in sympathetic tone. However, in human patients with myocardial dysfunction the negative inotropic and negative chronotropic effects of a drug such as verapamil cannot be offset by a sympathetic nervous system that is already maximally stimulated. The resultant decrease in contractility and heart rate following calcium channel blockade can be clinically significant.

Slow calcium channel activity is responsible for depolarization in the sinus and AV nodes. Calcium channel blockers prolong AV conduction, slow the ventricular response to supraventricular tachyarrhythmias such as atrial fibrillation and abolish supraventricular arrhythmias when caused by re-entry through the AV node. The depolarizing currents of the sinus node and the atrioventricular junction are, at least in part, carried by calcium. Calcium channel blockers have the potential to decrease sinus rate in patients with tachycardia but reflex increases in sympathetic tone due to decreased vascular resistance commonly overcome this effect. This effect can be lethal in patients that are dependent on escape rhythms to maintain heart rate (e.g. canine patients with third-degree AV block).

Clinical applications

Calcium channel blockers are highly effective for treating paroxysmal supraventricular tachycardia. Diltiazem is particularly useful for slowing ventricular rate in patients with atrial fibrillation. Experimentally, calcium channel blockers are effective for suppressing accelerated idioventricular rhythms in dogs following shock-induced myocardial injury and myocardial infarction. They have also been effective at suppressing digitalis-induced ventricular arrhythmias in conscious experimental dogs. To our knowledge, however, no reports exist in the veterinary literature concerning the use of calcium channel blockers to suppress ventricular arrhythmias in canine patients.

The dihydropyridines are not useful for treating arrhythmias. Instead, they are used to treat heart failure secondary to mitral regurgitation as well as systemic hypertension in dogs and cats.

Verapamil

Clinical applications

Verapamil is indicated for the acute termination of supraventricular tachycardia in the dog. Although other indications may exist, the authors have not used this drug to treat any other arrhythmia and there are no reports of its use for other indications in the veterinary literature. The experimental literature suggests that verapamil may be effective for terminating accelerated idioventricular rhythm in intensive care patients and for treating digitalis-induced ventricular tachyarrhythmias.

Mechanism of action

The ability of verapamil to terminate supraventricular tachycardia is probably due to its effects on the AV junctional tissue. Most probably, most supraventricular tachycardias that respond to verapamil use the AV junction as part or all of a re-entrant loop. Verapamil has the ability to slow conduction through the AV junction and to prolong the refractory period of this tissue at clinically relevant doses and plasma concentrations. Prolongation of conduction and refractoriness are classic means of terminating re-entrant arrhythmias.

Formulations and dose rates

Verapamil hydrochloride is supplied for intravenous use in ampoules and tablets for oral administration.

For the acute termination of supraventricular tachycardia, the intravenous dose ranges from 0.05 to 0.15 mg/kg. The initial dose of 0.05 mg/kg should be administered over 1–2 min while the ECG is monitored. If this initial dose is not effective, the same dose should be repeated 5–10 min later. If the arrhythmia still is not terminated, a last dose of 0.05 mg/kg (total dose = 0.15 mg/kg) should be

Formulations and dose rates—cont'd

administered 5–10 min after the second dose. This dosage schedule is effective at terminating supraventricular tachycardia in approximately 85% of dogs. The effect following termination of administration is short-lived, often lasting less than 30 min. For longer control, the initial bolus injections can be followed by a constant infusion of verapamil at 2–10 μg/kg/min.

Pharmacokinetics

In dogs, verapamil is absorbed well (more than 90%) but undergoes extensive first-pass hepatic metabolism so that bioavailability is only 10–23%. Verapamil is metabolized to several active and inactive metabolites. Most of the metabolites are excreted in bile. The half-life of verapamil is 1.8–3.8 h in anesthetized experimental dogs and the volume of distribution 2.6 ± 1.0 L/kg. The effective plasma concentration is probably in the range 50–200 ng/mL. A plasma concentration of approximately 100 ng/mL increases the P-R interval in normal dogs and a plasma concentration of approximately 200 ng/mL will produce second-degree AV block. Myocardial concentration of the drug is linearly related to plasma concentration and is approximately nine times the plasma concentration. Left ventricular and AV nodal region concentrations are greater than the atrial concentration.

Adverse effects

- Verapamil can depress cardiac contractility and cause peripheral vasodilation. It should not be used in patients with severe myocardial failure or patients in heart failure unless hemodynamic monitoring can be done and calcium or catecholamines can be administered immediately.
- In mild to moderate myocardial failure patients, verapamil may increase cardiac output by dilating arterioles.
- Occasionally, severe hypotension and cardiovascular collapse can be induced in dogs with normal cardiac function, especially if the drug is administered too quickly.
- Verapamil should not be used in patients with sick sinus syndrome or AV block because of its ability to depress automaticity in these diseased tissues.
- Adverse effects can be reversed by calcium or catecholamine administration. Catecholamine administration is more effective than calcium for treating calcium channel blocker-induced AV blocks in experimental conscious dogs.

Known drug interactions

- Verapamil and β-blockers should not be used together for several reasons.
  - Coadministration of verapamil and β-blockers results in additive negative inotropic, chronotropic and dromotropic (conduction properties) effects on the heart. This produces profound myocardial depression, prolonged AV nodal conduction and depressed heart rate, resulting in severe cardiovascular depression.
  - Verapamil can increase the bioavailability of some β-blockers by decreasing first-pass hepatic metabolism.
  - Addition of β-blocker administration to dogs with a stable plasma concentration of verapamil results in an increase in the plasma verapamil concentration.
- Coadministration of verapamil and lidocaine to isoflurane-anesthetized experimental dogs produces profound cardiovascular depression and severe systemic hypotension.
- Cimetidine decreases total body clearance of verapamil. This increases the plasma concentration of intravenously and orally administered verapamil. This effect probably occurs because of cimetidine's ability to inhibit hepatic microsomal enzymes.
- Verapamil increases the serum digoxin concentration in humans and probably does the same in dogs. The increase is thought to be due to reduced renal and extrarenal clearances of digoxin.

Diltiazem

Clinical applications

The clinical pharmacology of diltiazem when used to treat heart failure in cats is described earlier in the chapter (p. 422).

Diltiazem is also popular for decreasing ventricular rate in dogs with atrial fibrillation. In most canine patients, digoxin is administered first and the heart-rate response determined once a therapeutic serum concentration is achieved. If an adequate response is not achieved, diltiazem can be added to treatment protocol. Diltiazem can also be used in dogs to treat supraventricular tachycardia.

Mechanism of action

Diltiazem slows AV conduction and prolongs the AV refractory period to a similar degree to verapamil. It has minimal effects on myocardial contractility at clinically relevant plasma concentrations in normal dogs. Diltiazem's effects on peripheral vascular smooth muscle are mild, although it is a potent coronary vasodilator.

In normal experimental dogs, one study found that diltiazem (0.8 mg/kg IV) did not alter left ventricular myocardial contractility but did decrease peripheral vascular resistance and increased the heart rate in response to a reflex increase in plasma catecholamine concentrations. These effects resulted in increased cardiac output. In the same study in experimental dogs with pacing-induced myocardial failure, however, the effects were very different. In these dogs, diltiazem decreased myocardial contractility and did not change the heart rate. The net result was a decrease in cardiac output. Another study identified similar findings in dogs with left ventricular volume overload induced by creating an aortocaval fistula. Consequently, diltiazem must be administered cautiously to dogs with moderate to severe myocardial failure or heart failure.

Formulations and dose rates

The formulations of diltiazem available are discussed earlier in the chapter (p.423) as well as appropriate doses for cats.

DOGS

- To decrease ventricular rate in dogs with atrial fibrillation, an initial dose of 0.5 mg/kg q.8 h PO should be administered. If the heart rate does not decrease adequately, the dose can be increased to 1.0 mg/kg q.8 h PO and finally to 1.5 mg/kg q.8 h PO. In general, the heart rate should be decreased to less than 160 beats/min. At these doses, diltiazem appears to have no or negligible negative inotropic effects, since exacerbation of heart failure at this dose is rare
- For acute termination of supraventricular tachycardia, a dose of 0.1–0.25 mg/kg can be administered intravenously over 2–5 min
- Diltiazem can also be used for the chronic control of supraventricular tachycardia. Doses higher than those used for heart rate control in atrial fibrillation are commonly needed to suppress supraventricular tachycardia. Doses as high as 4 mg/kg q.8 h PO may be required for this purpose in dogs without significant ventricular dysfunction. In general, the dose should be titrated, starting at a dose of 1 mg/kg q.8 h PO
- Diltiazem at doses ranging from 2–4 mg/kg q.8 h should probably not be administered to dogs that have moderate to severe myocardial failure or dogs with significant cardiac compromise

Pharmacokinetics

In normal experimental dogs, diltiazem is rapidly absorbed from the gastrointestinal tract, reaching a maximum plasma concentration approximately 30 min after oral administration. Bioavailability of the tablets is approximately 24% in dogs. The volume of distribution is 7.6 ± 1.1 L/kg. Approximately 70% of the drug is protein bound. The elimination half-life has been estimated to be 2.3 h and 4.2 h in two different studies. The effective plasma concentration for terminating supraventricular tachycardia is probably in the 50–200 ng/mL range. For controlling the ventricular rate in atrial fibrillation, a lower plasma concentration may be efficacious.

An oral dose of approximately 4 mg/kg results in a plasma concentration of 162–176 ng/mL 1 h after administration in dogs. Administration of a sustained-release diltiazem preparation at approximately 4 mg/kg q.8 h results in steady plasma concentrations between 60 and 100 ng/mL. Intravenous administration of a dose of 0.2 mg/kg results in an average plasma concentration of 138 ng/mL 1 min after administration. An infusion rate of 7 μg/kg/min produces a plasma concentration of 140 ± 23 ng/mL.

Adverse effects

The primary adverse effects of diltiazem are seen with diltiazem overdose. Overdose results in decreased contractility, systemic vasodilation and bradycardia, which, if severe enough, result in cardiovascular collapse. Patients with myocardial failure and conduction system disease are more sensitive to the calcium channel-blocking properties of diltiazem and so are more prone to adverse effects than normal dogs or cats.

Known drug interactions

In general, a β-blocker should not be administered in conjunction with diltiazem because of the possibility of increasing plasma concentrations of both drugs and because of the potential for negative inotropic effects, exacerbation of heart failure and death. However, this can be done safely in most cats with severe HCM although low doses of both agents should be administered initially and the doses titrated up to an effective endpoint.

DIGITALIS GLYCOSIDES

Cardiac glycosides, digitalis glycosides and digitalis are terms used to identify a spectrum of compounds that are steroid derivatives with the ability to mildly increase myocardial contractility and elicit characteristic electrophysiological responses. The most frequently used compounds are digoxin, an extract from the leaf of the *Digitalis lanata* plant and digitoxin, which is extracted from the *Digitalis purpurea* plant. Both plants are from the foxglove family.

A cardiac glycoside consists of a steroid nucleus combined with a lactone ring and a series of sugars linked to the carbon 3 of the nucleus. The steroid nucleus and the lactone ring are termed an aglycone. The number of sugar moieties is a major determinant of drug half-life, although other factors also change half-life. The lactone ring is crucial for inotropic activity.

Clinical applications

Historically, the digitalis glycosides were indicated for the treatment of myocardial failure (i.e. decreased myocardial contractility) and supraventricular tachyarrhythmias. In dogs with myocardial failure, digitalis does not routinely result in a clinically significant increase in myocardial contractility and there are now more potent oral positive inotropes available. Currently the primary clinical indication for digoxin is for the management of clinically significant supraventricular arrhythmias such as atrial fibrillation where it is often used in combination with other antiarrhythmics such as beta blockers or diltiazem.

The digitalis glycosides are moderately effective (usually in combination with other antiarrhythmics) for the treatment of supraventricular tachyarrhythmias, including control of ventricular response rates in atrial fibrillation. If the decrease in heart rate in patients with atrial fibrillation is inadequate (ventricular rate >160 beats/min) and or the initial documented heart rate is >200 bpm, an additional antiarrhythmic agent should be initiated such as a low dose of a β-adrenergic blocker or diltiazem, or amiodarone to produce the desired decrease in heart rate.

Digoxin is the only digitalis glycoside discussed in this chapter as it is virtually the only compound of this type used in veterinary medicine.

The ability of digoxin to improve quality and quantity of life is controversial in both human and veterinary medicine. A large clinical trial designed to answer the question of digoxin's efficacy in human patients was completed in 1997. The results lead to the following editorial comment: 'Digoxin's inability to substantially influence morbidity or mortality eliminates any ethical mandate for its use and effectively relegates it to be prescribed for the treatment of persistent symptoms after the administration of drugs that do reduce the risk of death and hospitalization'. This comment adequately reflects the current majority opinion on the use of digoxin for the treatment of heart failure in dogs and cats, particularly as other medications are demonstrated to have good efficacy in this setting (ACE inhibitors, pimobendan).

Mechanism of action

Antiarrhythmic effects

The current primary indication for digoxin in veterinary medicine is for the management (usually in combination with other antiarrhythmics) of supraventricular arrhythmias, including atrial fibrillation. Digitalis glycosides increase parasympathetic nerve activity to the sinus node, atria and AV node when the digitalis serum concentration is within the therapeutic range. By so doing, they decrease the sinus rate and are capable of abolishing supraventricular premature depolarizations and some supraventricular tachycardias. Cardiac glycosides also produce direct effects that help slow AV nodal conduction and prolong the AV nodal refractory period. The direct and indirect effects of the digitalis glycosides on the AV node are most commonly used to slow the ventricular response to atrial flutter and fibrillation.

Baroreceptor/neuroendocrine modulatory effects

The digitalis glycosides also have effects on vascular baroreceptors. Baroreceptor function is abnormally reduced in human patients and experimental dogs with heart failure. This results in attenuated cardiac vagal tone and increased sympathetic activity. This maladaptive compensatory mechanism can be detrimental in patients with heart failure. The digitalis glycosides increase baroreceptor function in normal cats, dogs and humans. They decrease plasma catecholamine concentrations, directly recorded sympathetic nerve activity and plasma renin activity, which may all be related to increased baroreceptor activity, and are thus considered neuroendocrine modulators. However, the clinical significance of this effect on morbitiy and mortality in heart failure has not been demonstrated. This may be related to the relatively high rate of adverse or side effects associated with digoxin use and narrow therapeutic window.

Positive inotropic effects

The digitalis glycosides are weak positive inotropic agents when compared to inodilators (e.g. pimobendan, milrinone) and β-agonists (e.g. dobutamine). The positive inotropic effect is caused by digitalis poisoning the Na^+,K^+-ATPase pumps on myocardial cell membranes. Digitalis competitively binds to the site on this pump to which potassium normally attaches and effectively stops pump activity. A therapeutic concentration of digoxin 'poisons' approximately 30% of the Na^+,K^+-ATPase pumps in the myocardium. Thus, the cell loses some of its ability to extrude sodium from the intracellular space during diastole, resulting in an increase in intracellular sodium concentration. The cell exchanges the excess intracellular sodium for extracellular calcium via the Na^+/Ca^{2+} cation exchanger or by reducing the exchange of intracellular calcium for extracellular sodium. The net result is an increase in the number of calcium ions within the cell. In a normal cell, these excess calcium ions are bound by the sarcoplasmic reticulum during diastole and are subsequently released on to the contractile proteins during systole, causing increased contractility. This effect is reduced by myocardial failure.

Diuretic effects

Investigators have examined the renal effects of a digitalis glycoside (ouabain) and found it to have diuretic properties. There are Na^+,K^+-ATPase pumps present on the basolateral aspect of renal tubular epithelial cells which promote renal tubular reabsorption of sodium.

In one study, digitalis increased sodium excretion 284% above baseline in experimental dogs with heart failure. This would translate into percentage of filtered sodium load increasing from 1% to approximately 4%, making digoxin a slightly better diuretic than spironolactone.

Formulations and dose rates

Digoxin is available as tablets (preferred), capsules, suspension, elixir and as an injectable formulation. Tablets are better tolerated than the alcohol-based elixir. In the authors' opinion use of the injectable formulation has no place in clinical veterinary medicine.

The therapeutic range for digoxin is based on evaluation of serum trough concentration (6–8 h after a dose) in patients at presumed steady state (i.e. 3–7 d after initiation or any change in dose). However, if a patient presents with signs of possible toxicity a serum level can be obtained immediately. The reported target therapeutic serum concentration is 1–2 ng/mL, where <0.5 ng/mL is subtherapeutic. However, some dogs will demonstrate signs of toxicity at serum levels of 2 ng/mL. Currently, most cardiologists aim for a serum concentration of 0.5–1.5 ng/mL. Serum concentrations above 2.5 ng/mL are considered toxic.

Starting dose

DOGS

- Because of the variability in pharmacokinetics from animal to animal and the narrow therapeutic range for serum concentration, digoxin administration to any animal should be viewed as a pharmacological experiment. An initial dose should be chosen and administered and serum concentration measured 3–5 d after starting treatment to determine if the chosen dose has resulted in a therapeutic serum concentration
- In dogs weighing less than 20 kg the initial starting dose of digoxin can be based on bodyweight at 5–10 μg/kg q.12 h PO (0.005–0.01 mg/kg q.12 h)
- In dogs weighing more than 20 kg, the dosage should be based on body surface area (so as not to overdose): 0.22 mg/m^2 of body surface area q.12 h PO

CATS (Rarely Used)

- The initial starting dose for normal cats is approximately 30 μg (0.03 mg) administered q.48 h for cats weighing less than 3 kg, 30 μg (0.03 mg) q.24 h for cats weighing 3–6 kg and 30 μg (0.03 mg) q.12–24 h for cats weighing more than 6 kg

Factors that alter dosage

Commonly, the initial starting dose of a digitalis glycoside needs to be modified because of factors that alter the pharmacokinetics of the drug. In one study in which digoxin dose (0.005–0.23 mg/kg/d) was plotted against serum concentration in dogs with heart failure, the correlation coefficient was only 0.39 (1.0 is a perfect correlation). This weak correlation was statistically significant, meaning that drug dosage is a factor determining serum concentration. However, the poor correlation indicates that the digoxin dose rate is only one factor among a number of other variables that determines serum concentration. These variables must be considered when administering digoxin.

- Renal failure reduces renal clearance, total body clearance and volume of distribution of digoxin, resulting in an increased serum concentration of the drug. There are no data to correlate degree of azotemia and serum digoxin concentration in dogs or cats. Consequently, whenever possible, digoxin should be avoided in dogs with any degree of renal failure. If digoxin must be administered, it is best to start at a very low dose and titrate upward, if necessary using the measured serum concentration as a guide.
- Because most of a digitalis glycoside is bound to skeletal muscle, dogs or cats that have lost significant muscle mass (decreased volume of distribution) have increased serum concentrations for any given dose. Consequently, for patients that are cachectic, the dose must be reduced. Older dogs commonly have decreased muscle mass and impaired renal function, so digoxin dosing in these patients must be performed cautiously.
- Digoxin is poorly lipid soluble. Consequently, dosing should be based on a lean bodyweight estimate. Lean bodyweight is an estimate of the weight that an obese patient *should* weigh.
- Digoxin does not distribute well into ascitic fluid. Consequently, the dose of digoxin must be reduced in patients with ascites if total bodyweight is used to calculate the dose. In general, patients with mild ascites should have their dose reduced by 10%, those with moderate ascites by 20% and patients with severe ascites by 30%.
- Hypokalemia predisposes to digitalis myocardial toxicity. Digitalis and potassium compete for the same binding site on the membrane Na^+,K^+-ATPase pumps. Hypokalemia leaves more binding sites available for digitalis. Hyperkalemia displaces digitalis from the myocardium.
- Hypercalcemia potentiates the positive inotropic and toxic effects of digitalis.
- Although hypothyroidism has been reported to reduce renal clearance of digoxin in humans, this does not appear to be the case in dogs. In one study, acute and chronic digoxin pharmacokinetics were measured in dogs before and after experimental induction of hypothyroidism. There was no difference between the groups. Consequently, it is not necessary to adjust the digoxin dose in hypothyroid dogs.
- Myocardial failure increases the sensitivity of the myocardium to the toxic effects of digitalis. Failing myocardial cells are usually thought to be overloaded with calcium. Digitalis may cause further calcium loading. Calcium-overloaded cells may

become electrically unstable, resulting in ectopic tachyarrhythmias.

- The administration of other drugs concurrently with digitalis may affect the serum concentration of digoxin.
  - Quinidine is the classic example. It displaces digoxin from skeletal muscle binding sites and reduces its renal clearance, resulting in an increased serum digoxin concentration. Quinidine probably also displaces digoxin from myocardial binding sites. This may lessen the direct cardiac toxicity of digoxin and decrease its positive inotropic effect. In general, the combination of digoxin and quinidine should be avoided. If both drugs must be used together, the rule of thumb in human medicine is to reduce the digoxin dosage by 50%. Since serum digoxin concentration approximately doubles following quinidine administration in dogs, this recommendation appears to be valid in veterinary patients.
  - In humans, there are reports of numerous other drugs that increase the serum concentration of digoxin, including oral aminoglycosides (neomycin), amiodarone, anticholinergics, captopril, diltiazem, esmolol, flecainide, ibuprofen, indomethacin, nifedipine, tetracycline and verapamil.
- Digoxin pharmacokinetics are not significantly altered in cats with compensated heart failure receiving furosemide and aspirin. This is despite increases in serum urea and creatinine concentrations.

Dosing strategy

In general, patients should be evaluated carefully before digoxin is administered. Factors that alter the dosage should be noted and an initial dose chosen. The patient should be monitored during the initial course of therapy for signs of toxicity or improvement. A decrease in heart rate or resolution of an arrhythmia are measurable benefits in patients with tachycardia or arrhythmia.

Clinical responsiveness due to improved hemodynamics in patients with heart failure is the desired endpoint of digitalis administration but can be difficult to identify, for several reasons. First, other drugs are generally administered with digoxin, so it may be impossible to identify the beneficial drug. Second, many dogs do not respond to digoxin, so clinical resolution may never occur. The dosage in the latter case should not be increased unless the serum concentration has been measured and documented to be subtherapeutic (i.e. less than 0.5 ng/mL).

Each case should have a serum digoxin concentration measured 3–7 d after initiating therapy and 6–8 h after the last dose (trough concentration) or immediately any time toxicity is suspected. The therapeutic range for serum digoxin concentration is somewhat controversial, although it is generally considered to be between 0.5 and 2.0 ng/mL. However, some dogs will demonstrate toxicity at serum concentrations of 2 ng/mL. A serum concentration above 2.5 ng/mL should be regarded as toxic. If such an elevation is identified in a patient, digoxin administration should be discontinued until the serum concentration is below 1.5 ng/mL. The dosage should be reduced accordingly several days later.

Pharmacokinetics

Approximately 60% of digoxin tablet formulations is absorbed, while about 75% of the elixir is absorbed. There is very little hepatic metabolism, so that almost all of the absorbed drug reaches the vascular system. In serum, an average of 27% of digoxin is bound to albumin. The volume of distribution is 12–15 L/kg. In normal young dogs, serum half-life of digoxin is 23–39 h although much interpatient variability exists. Theoretically, it takes about five half-lives to reach steady state, so it is commonly thought that five half-lives are required to achieve serum concentrations of between 1.0 and 2.0 ng/mL (which is generally considered to be the therapeutic range). However, this is not the case.

The canine maintenance dose of digoxin generally achieves a serum concentration of 1.5–2.0 ng/mL. The serum concentration after two half-lives (75% of steady state) should be 1.1–1.5 ng/mL and after three half-lives (87.5% of steady state) 1.3–1.75 ng/mL. Consequently, maintenance doses should theoretically achieve a therapeutic serum concentration within 2–4 d. In one study of dogs given 0.022 mg/kg digoxin every 24 h, the serum concentration was within therapeutic range by the second day. On the basis of these data, maintenance doses of digoxin in dogs should be used to achieve a therapeutic serum concentration in almost all situations. Loading doses designed to achieve a therapeutic concentration within a shorter period are not recommended in dogs and cats.

Digoxin is primarily excreted via glomerular filtration and renal secretion. About 15% is metabolized in the liver. Bile duct ligation increases the half-life of digoxin from an average of 26 h to 35 h in experimental dogs.

The half-life is extremely variable from cat to cat, ranging from 25 h to 50 h in one study and from 39 h to 79 h in another report. In a more recent study, the half-life in a group of six normal cats ranged from 30 h to 173 h with a mean half-life of 82 h. The half-life of digoxin increases dramatically with prolonged oral administration. The elixir form results in serum concentrations approximately 50% higher than those achieved with the tablet. However, cats generally dislike the taste of the alcohol-based elixir. When digoxin tablets are administered with food to cats, serum concentration is reduced by about 50% compared to the concentration without food.

Adverse effects

In normal beagle dogs, a serum concentration of digoxin that exceeds 2.5 ng/mL generally produces clinical signs of toxicity. However, dogs and cats may show clinical evidence of toxicity at a serum concentration less than 2.5 ng/mL and occasionally a dog will show no clinical signs of toxicity at a serum concentration greater than 2.5 ng/mL.

The incidence of digoxin toxicity in veterinary medicine is not well documented. In one canine study, 25% of dogs receiving digoxin had a serum concentration in the toxic range while 24% had a subtherapeutic concentration. In this author's experience, clinically significant digitalis toxicity such as anorexia is common but may be minimized if lower doses targeting lower serum concentrations are employed. Doberman pinschers may be particularly sensitive to the anorectic side effects of digoxin. Toxicity may occur even in patients that were previously documented to be in a therapeutic range due to progressive muscle wasting, progressive azotemia or accidental overdose. This highlights the importance of good client communication with respect to dosing instructions.

Clinical signs of toxicity

Problems from digitalis intoxication fall into three general classes: those referable to the central nervous system (common), those to the gastrointestinal system (most common) and those to the myocardium – arrhythmias (common). Most dogs intoxicated with digoxin appear depressed. Humans experience malaise and drowsiness and have headaches. Anorexia and vomiting are the common manifestations of digitalis intoxication and are probably due to the direct effect of the digitalis molecule on the chemoreceptor trigger zone (CTZ). In one study, normal dogs with a serum concentration of digoxin in the 2.5–6.0 ng/mL range decreased their food intake to about 50% of normal while maintaining a normal water intake while dogs with a serum concentration above 6.0 ng/mL stopped eating, decreased their water intake to less than one-third of normal and vomited. In clinical practice, a serum concentration of digoxin above 3.0–4.0 ng/mL usually produces anorexia and vomiting. Body temperature also decreases in digitalis intoxication. In one study of healthy beagle dogs, body temperature decreased by approximately 1°C in dogs with moderate toxicity and 1–3°C in dogs with severe toxicity.

In general digoxin toxicity is potentiated by agents that reduce GFR (e.g. enalapril), hypokalemia, azotemia and in cachetic patients.

Autonomic manifestations

Autonomic tone of the heart is increased with digitalis toxicity. Increased vagal tone can result in a decrease in sinus node rate and altered AV nodal conduction and refractoriness, although compensatory increased sympathetic tone can counter these effects. Consequently, sinus node rate is variable in dogs with digitalis intoxication. In one study of normal dogs administered toxic doses of digoxin for 2 weeks, the heart rate initially decreased from baseline values of 90–130 beats/min to 50–90 beats/min after intravenous administration of digoxin but returned to baseline by 24–48 h after dosing. Despite continued administration of toxic doses, the heart rate remained at baseline values or was mildly decreased. During the periods of most severe toxicity, the heart rate increased to 130–190 beats/min.

However, it should be remembered that increased vagal tone predominates at the AV nodal level. Consequently, regardless of baseline heart rate, first-degree AV block is a common finding in dogs with digoxin toxicity. Second-degree AV block may also occur, especially after prolonged intoxication, while third-degree AV block is rare.

Myocardial toxicity

Myocardial toxicity is the most serious complication of digitalis administration. A toxic serum concentration disrupts the normal electrical activity of the heart in several ways. Increased sympathetic nerve activity can result in increased normal automaticity and exacerbate other arrhythmic mechanisms. In dogs, blockade of the sympathetic nervous system increases the dose of digitalis required to produce arrhythmias. Digitalis also slows conduction and alters the refractory period, making it easier for re-entrant arrhythmias to develop.

Late (delayed) afterdepolarizations, where the diastolic membrane potential oscillates, eventually reaches threshold potential and depolarizes the cell, appear to be the most important reason for the development of arrhythmias in digitalis intoxication. The ECG counterpart of this depolarization would be a premature beat. Late afterdepolarizations are attributed to cellular calcium overload and are more easily induced in myocardium that has been stretched (analogous to a ventricle with an increased end-diastolic pressure) and in a hypokalemic environment. Myocyte calcium overload occurs when too many Na^+,K^+-ATPase pumps are poisoned. Digitalis cardiotoxicity occurs when 60–80% of Na^+,K^+-ATPase pumps are inhibited.

Clinically, myocardial toxicity can take the form of almost every known rhythm disturbance. In the dog, ventricular tachyarrhythmias and bradyarrhythmias are most common. The ventricular tachyarrhythmias consist of ventricular premature depolarizations, ventricular bigeminy and trigeminy and ventricular tachycardia. The common bradyarrhythmias are second-degree AV block, sinus bradycardia and sinus arrest, which occur because of increased vagal tone. Digitalis can also induce supraventricular and junctional tachyarrhythmias, as well as other arrhythmias.

Digitalis intoxication also appears to cause abnormal myocardial function and myocyte damage. In isolated hearts, digitalis intoxication results in an increase in diastolic tension (diastolic dysfunction) and a decrease in developed (systolic) tension (myocardial failure). In normal dogs, severe digoxin toxicity results in an increase in serum creatine kinase concentration and histological evidence of myocardial degeneration and necrosis.

Renal toxicity

Digoxin toxicity also causes renal damage. In one study, there was hydropic degeneration and epithelial necrosis in the proximal tubules and in the medullary collecting ducts. This resulted in increases in serum concentrations of urea nitrogen and creatinine. There was a direct correlation between the degree of elevation in serum concentration and the severity of the tubular damage.

Electrolyte abnormalities

A digitalis overdose can produce hyperkalemia and hyponatremia. In one study, moderate toxicity (serum digoxin concentration 2.5–6.0 ng/mL) resulted in a serum concentration of sodium between 130 and 145 mEq/L with a normal serum potassium concentration. Severe toxicity (serum digoxin concentration >6.0 ng/mL) produced a serum sodium concentration in the 110–130 mEq/L range and serum concentration of potassium anywhere from 3.2 to 7.7 mEq/L. These electrolyte abnormalities are probably caused by digitalis inhibition of the Na^+,K^+-ATPase pumps throughout the body.

Treatment of digitalis intoxication

The mainstay of treating digitalis intoxication is discontinuing drug administration. Because the half-life of digoxin in a normal dog is between 24 and 36 h, it should take between 1 and 1.5 days for the serum concentration to decrease to one-half the original concentration. Half-life is commonly prolonged in older animals and diseased animals. Consequently, the time to reach one-half the original concentration is prolonged.

Gastrointestinal signs related to a digitalis overdose are treated by drug withdrawal and correction of fluid and electrolyte abnormalities. Conduction disturbances and bradyarrhythmias usually require only digitalis withdrawal, although atropine administration is occasionally needed. Ventricular tachyarrhythmias are generally treated aggressively, especially when ventricular tachycardia is present. Lidocaine is the drug of choice for treating these ventricular tachyarrhythmias. It decreases sympathetic nerve traffic and can abolish reentrant arrhythmias and late afterdepolarizations.

Phenytoin can be used to treat digitalis toxicity in the dog. It has similar properties to lidocaine. When administered intravenously, the drug vehicle can produce hypotension and exert a depressant effect on the myocardium. The total intravenous dose is 10 mg/kg, given in 2 mg/kg increments over 3–5 min. Phenytoin can also be administered orally (35 mg/kg administered q.8 h) either to treat a digitalis-induced ventricular tachyarrhythmia or to prevent these tachyarrhythmias.

Serum potassium concentration should always be determined in patients intoxicated with digitalis. If serum potassium is less than 4.0 mEq/L, potassium supplements should be administered, preferably in intravenous fluids. Potassium competes with digitalis for binding sites on the Na^+,K^+-ATPase pumps and provides a more suitable environment for the antiarrhythmic agents to work.

Orally administered activated charcoal avidly binds digoxin and is useful after accidental ingestion or administration of a large oral dose. It decreases digoxin absorption up to 96%. Colestyramine, a steroid-binding resin, may also be useful early after digoxin ingestion but only decreases absorption 30–40%.

F_{ab} fragments of digoxin-specific antibodies (e.g. Digibind®) are used in humans to bind digoxin in the bloodstream and thus remove it from myocardial binding sites. This may be a useful means of treating life-threatening digitalis intoxication in veterinary medicine but it is very expensive. There have been two reports of its use in dogs. In one it cost US$1200 to treat a 23 kg Labrador retriever. The F_{ab} fragment binds with the antigenic epitope on the digoxin molecule. This complex cannot bind to Na^+,K^+-ATPase pumps and is cleared by glomerular filtration. This results in rapid resolution of clinical signs. The measured serum concentration of digoxin may increase or decrease after administration of Digibind®, depending on the type of assay used. Some assays measure total serum digoxin concentration and some measure primarily free serum concentration. Serum concentration of free digoxin decreases rapidly to very low concentrations after administration of Digibind® while total serum concentration of digoxin (free plus digoxin bound to F_{ab}) increases to 10–20 times the baseline after Digibind® administration. The dose of Digibind® can be calculated if either the dose of digoxin ingested or the serum digoxin concentration is known.

The body load of digoxin (mg) is calculated by one of the following methods:

Amount of ingested digoxin (mg) × bioavailability of digoxin = mg × 0.6 [Serum concentration (ng/mL) × volume of distribution (12 L/kg) × weight (kg)]/1000

The dose of Digibind® is then calculated as follows:

$$\frac{\text{mol. wt } F_{ab}\ (50000)}{\text{mol. wt digoxin } (781)} = 64 \times \text{body load (mg)}$$

$$= F_{ab} \text{ dose (mg)}$$

Each vial of Digibind® contains 40 mg of F_{ab} fragments, so the number of vials is calculated by dividing the F_{ab} dose by 40. For example, a 25 kg dog is presented with a serum digoxin concentration of 7.5 ng/mL and the owner thinks that it ingested 10 0.25 mg tablets. Using serum concentration, the body load is 2.25 mg. Using the owner's information, the body load is 2.5 mg. Using the serum concentration to calculate the body load gives a F_{ab} dose of 144 mg, or 3.6 vials. The four vials will cost approximately US$2000.

Combination antiarrhythmic therapy

At times, combinations of two antiarrhythmic drugs may be more effective than one drug alone. For example, the combination of digoxin and a β-blocker or digoxin and diltiazem is often more effective at controlling the ventricular rate in patients with atrial fibrillation than is digoxin alone. At times, using digoxin with quinidine may be more effective for converting primary atrial fibrillation to sinus rhythm than using quinidine alone. However, this is an example of a combination where toxicity can also be produced. Because quinidine decreases renal clearance of digoxin and displaces it from its non-CNS binding sites, serum digoxin concentration commonly doubles when quinidine is added. This can result in clinical signs of digoxin intoxication due to increased CTZ stimulation. Paradoxically, there may, however, be a concurrent reduction in digoxin's cardiac effects, as its capacity to bind to cardiac receptors will be reduced by the quinidine.

Another example of the combination of two drugs causing clinical problems is the combination of a β-blocker and a calcium channel blocker. Both drug types can produce negative inotropic effects. In combination, this effect is exacerbated and can result in a severe decrease in contractility, worsening of heart failure and even death.

Combination therapy may be more effective for treating some ventricular arrhythmias. Many veterinary cardiologists have for years had the clinical impression that the combination of a class I antiarrhythmic agent and a β-blocker is more effective at controlling ventricular arrhythmias than either agent alone. In one experimental study using dogs, the combination of quinidine and propranolol was more effective than either drug alone at preventing ventricular fibrillation. Most veterinary cardiologists prefer to use a combination of procainamide and propranolol or atenolol. In experimental studies, the combination of two class I agents may be more effective at controlling ventricular arrhythmias in dogs than either drug alone. An example is the combination of mexiletine and quinidine. In one study of experimental dogs with myocardial infarction, mexiletine controlled the ventricular arrhythmia in only one of 13 dogs and quinidine successfully suppressed the arrhythmia in only three of 13 dogs. The combination, however, was efficacious in eight of the 13 dogs.

Another example is the combination of mexiletine and sotalol. Mexiletine decreases the Q-T interval in experimental dogs that have a prolonged Q-T interval because of sotalol administration. One might think that this would counteract the antiarrhythmic efficacy of sotalol. However, in one study, the combination of these two drugs in experimental dogs was more effective at preventing ventricular tachycardia and more effective at slowing the rate of the ventricular tachycardia than was either drug alone. It is worth noting, however, that in this study sotalol was more effective than mexiletine at preventing ventricular fibrillation either alone or in combination with mexiletine.

DRUGS USED TO TREAT BRADYARRHYTHMIAS

Anticholinergic drugs

EXAMPLES

Anticholinergic agents, such as atropine and glycopyrolate, can be used diagnostically and therapeutically in veterinary patients with bradyarrhythmias

Clinical applications

Increased vagal tone can cause sinus bradycardia, periods of sinus arrest and second-degree AV block. Whenever a patient presents with one of these abnormalities, an assessment of the response to the administration of an anticholinergic agent is indicated, especially if clinical signs are caused by the bradyarrhythmia. Generally, atropine is administered either subcutaneously or intravenously to determine if a bradyarrhythmia is vagally induced.

Dogs with vagally mediated sinus node depression (either sinus bradycardia or arrest) respond to atropine administration by increasing their sinus rate to more than 160 beats/min. Dogs with intrinsic sinus node disease (sick sinus syndrome) may have no response to atropine administration or may have a partial response (e.g. the heart rate may increase to 110 beats/min). Second-degree AV block disappears following atropine administration to dogs with vagally mediated second-degree AV block. Although we commonly administer atropine to dogs with third-degree AV block to assess their response, we have never identified a dog that had a significant response.

Vagal tone can be increased by numerous factors. Anesthesia, central nervous system lesions, abnormal carotid sinus function (hypersensitive carotid sinus syndrome in humans), respiratory disease and abdominal disease are common. Often the cause is unknown (idiopathic). Parenteral anticholinergic therapy can be used to control bradyarrhythmias in situations where vagal tone is increased for only a short period (e.g. during anesthesia) or can sometimes be used for home therapy if the owner can administer an injection. This is no more involved than teaching a client to administer insulin to a pet with diabetes mellitus.

Oral administration of anticholinergic agents can also be tried in these patients. Some patients do very well on oral anticholinergic therapy. However, oral anticholinergic therapy is not always successful and parenteral administration, administration of a sympathomimetic or pacemaker implantation may be required. The oral anticholinergic drugs can be ranked in order of effect. Drugs with weak anticholinergic effects are commonly used as antidiarrheal drugs in veterinary medicine. They include isopropamide iodide and propantheline bromide. These drugs are only rarely effective for chronically treating vagally induced bradyarrhythmias. Atropine and glycopyrolate are more potent vagolytics and much more effective agents.

Formulations and dose rates

Atropine

When administered subcutaneously, 0.04 mg/kg should be administered and the dog should be placed in a cage for 30 min before reassessing the cardiac rhythm. For intravenous administration, 0.04 mg/kg is also administered but the rhythm can be reassessed in 5–10 min.

Atropine tablets used to be available and in the authors' experience were often effective. They are no longer manufactured but can occasionally be found. The parenteral atropine solution can also be administered PO but is extremely bitter. To administer it PO, it must be diluted in a sweet substance, such as corn syrup, to disguise the taste. The authors have found that a dose of 0.04 mg/kg q.8 h can be effective.

Glycopyrolate is available as 1 mg and 2 mg tablets. Although this product should be effective, the authors have little experience with its use.

Adverse effects

Vagolytic substances can produce side effects. These include:

- mydriasis
- constipation
- dry mouth
- keratoconjunctivitis sicca.

In the authors' experience, however, these side effects are often remarkably inapparent.

Sympathomimetic drugs

Isoprenaline (isoproterenol)

Clinical applications

Sympathomimetics can also be used to treat bradyarrhythmias. Isoprenaline (isoproterenol) is a pure β-agonist that stimulates both β_1- and β_2-adrenergic receptors (see Chapter 4). In so doing, it increases the sinus node rate, increases the rate of subsidiary pacemakers in the heart and increases conduction velocity in the AV node.

Isoprenaline can be used temporarily to increase the heart rate in dogs with sick sinus syndrome or third-degree AV block. This is done only in dogs that are severely bradycardic or are symptomatic. Isoprenaline is infrequently used in the author's clinic to increase the heart rate in dogs that are waiting to have a pacemaker implanted. It is more frequently used in dogs that become severely bradycardic under anesthesia prior to pacemaker implantation.

Formulations and dose rates

Isoprenaline is administered intravenously as a CRI at a dose of 0.05–0.2 μg/kg/min. The dose must be titrated and the lowest effective dose should be used. Oral administration of isoprenaline is not effective because it is almost completely metabolized by the liver before it reaches the systemic circulation.

Adverse effects

- Isoprenaline stimulates β-receptors in systemic arterioles, producing vasodilation. This can cause hypotension.
- Isoprenaline can also stimulate tachyarrhythmias.

β_2-Agonists

Clinical applications

Numerous drugs that stimulate β_2-receptors are available. These drugs are used as bronchodilators and are effective after oral administration. They are generally formulated not to produce many cardiac effects. However, this is impossible since β_2-receptors are present in the heart and play an important role in modulating the sinus rate. Consequently, these drugs can also be used to treat bradyarrhythmias. Most of the authors' experience is with the use of terbutaline in dogs with vagally mediated sinus bradycardia and sinus arrest. In these dogs, terbutaline can be effective at increasing the sinus rate and eradicating the sinus pauses.

Formulations and dose rates

Terbutaline is supplied as tablets. The dose must be titrated, usually starting with 2.5 mg q.8 h per dog PO and increasing as needed. Side effects include hyperactivity and gastrointestinal disturbances.

Adverse effects

Terbutaline should be used cautiously, if at all, in dogs with mitral regurgitation due to myxomatous mitral valve degeneration. The authors have not noted complications with this drug in this setting but have noted acute pulmonary edema, possibly secondary to ruptured chordae tendineae, in dogs treated with salbutamol (albuterol), another β_2-agonist.

ANTICOAGULANTS

EXAMPLES

Unfractionated heparin, low molecular weight heparin, warfarin

Unfractionated heparin

Unfractionated heparin (heparin), a water-soluble mucopolysaccharide, was first discovered in 1916. It was named heparin because of its abundance in liver. It was initially used to prevent the clotting of shed blood, which eventually led to its use in vivo to treat venous thrombosis.

Clinical applications

Heparin is used in the treatment of disseminated intravascular coagulation (DIC) and thromboembolic disease. Its prophylactic use has been recommended in severe immune-mediated hemolytic anemia (IMHA) to decrease the potentially harmful effects of thromboplastic substances released from hemolyzed red blood cells and to minimize the danger of developing pulmonary thromboembolism. However, controlled studies are lacking and the prophylactic use of heparin in IMHA is not universally accepted.

Heparin has been used in the management of cats with thromboembolic disease secondary to hypertrophic or restrictive cardiomyopathy. It has been given with acepromazine as an empirical, unproven treatment to promote collateral vasodilation and prevent growth of the thrombus.

In the management of DIC, heparin is used to activate antithrombin in blood products prior to administration to the patient. Antithrombin, an α_2-globulin acute-phase protein produced in the liver, is the natural inhibitor of serine proteases in the coagulation pathways (factors II, IX, X, XI, XII and kallikrein). It has little or no activity against factor VII. When a patient is in a hypercoagulable state and prothrombin is being actively converted to thrombin, the antithrombin concentration will be low (<80%). The affinity of antithrombin for serine proteases is enhanced 100-fold by administration of heparin.

Heparin has been reported to be ineffective in patients with DIC and to be the cause of hemorrhagic complications in these patients. However, it is believed that most of the poor responses to heparin are the result of its administration when there are inadequate circulating concentrations of antithrombin. In the absence of antithrombin, heparin has only weak antithrombotic effects. These are related to heparin–heparin cofactor II activity against thrombin. When administered alone (i.e. without additional antithrombin) heparin can actually diminish antithrombin concentrations.

Low-dose heparin has also been recommended as adjunctive therapy for severe pancreatitis in dogs but its efficacy is unknown and its use is not recommended in all cases.

Heparin can be administered to test for lipoprotein lipase activity. If serum lipids do not increase 15 min after intravenous administration of 100 U/kg heparin, this is suggestive of lipoprotein lipase deficiency.

Mechanism of action

Heparin inhibits coagulation by several mechanisms. It binds with and enhances the potency of plasma antithrombin III, which inhibits several coagulation factors (see above). Inhibition of thrombin and factor X probably accounts for most of heparin's anticoagulant effect. Antithrombin rapidly inhibits thrombin only in the presence of heparin. Heparin increases the rate of the thrombin-antithrombin reaction at least 1000-fold by serving as a catalytic template to which both the inhibitor and the protease bind. Binding of heparin also induces a conformational change in antithrombin that makes the reactive site more accessible to the protease.

Heparin also inhibits prothrombin activation and platelet aggregation. By inhibiting the activation of factor XIII (fibrin-stabilizing factor), heparin also prevents the formation of stable fibrin clots. While heparin will inhibit the reactions that lead to clotting, it does not change clotting factor concentration. Heparin will prevent the growth of existing clots but will not lyse clots.

Formulations and dose rates

Heparin is available in ampoules in a range of concentrations (1000–40,000 U/mL) as well as in prefilled syringes (various concentrations and amounts) and premixed with saline and half-normal saline in 250 mL, 500 mL or 1000 mL containers.

Thromboembolic disease

- 100–200 U/kg IV loading dose then 100–300 U/kg SC q.6–8 h

Low-dose prophylaxis

- 50–75 U/kg SC q.8–12 h

DIC

- 50–200 U/kg into plasma or whole blood to be transfused then 50–100 U/kg SC q.8 h once the antithrombin concentration is greater than 60%

Pharmacokinetics

Heparin is not absorbed from the gut if given orally; it therefore must be given parenterally to be effective. If sufficient antithrombin is present, anticoagulant activity begins immediately after intravenous injection and up to 1 h after subcutaneous injection.

Heparin is extensively protein bound, primarily to fibrinogen, low-density lipoproteins and globulins. It does not cross the placenta or into milk in any appreciable amounts. Heparin in humans appears to be cleared and degraded primarily by the reticuloendothelial system. A small amount of nondegraded heparin also appears in the urine. In humans the serum half-life averages 1–2 h and is dependent on the dose administered. The half-life in humans may be shorter in patients with pulmonary thromboembolism and prolonged in patients with renal failure and hepatic cirrhosis.

Adverse effects

- The most common adverse effects associated with heparin therapy are bleeding and thrombocytopenia. In human medicine, major bleeding occurs in 1–33% of patients receiving various forms of heparin therapy. Mild thrombocytopenia occurs in a small proportion of human patients 2–15 d after commencement of therapy; in these patients therapy can be continued if the platelet count does not fall below 100×10^6/L. In rare cases, severe immune-mediated thrombocytopenia can occur.
- Hypersensitivity reactions may occur if heparin is of bovine or porcine origin.
- Uncommon adverse effects reported in humans include:
  - osteoporosis and spontaneous vertebral fractures after long-term therapy
  - hyperkalemia as a result of heparin inhibiting the synthesis of aldosterone.
- In humans, mild increases in alanine aminotransferase enzyme concentrations are common.
- Intramuscular injection can result in hematoma formation. Hematomas, pain and irritation may also occur after deep SC injection.
- Because heparin does not cross the placenta and has not been associated with fetal abnormalities (in contrast to warfarin), it is used for anticoagulation in human pregnancies. However, its safety in pregnancy has not been established. Indeed, it has been reported that fetal mortality or prematurity occurs in one-third of pregnancies where heparin has been used.

Known drug interactions

- Heparin sodium is incompatible with the following solutions or drugs:
  - sodium lactate 1/6 mmol/L
  - aminoglycosides
  - chlorpromazine HCl
  - codeine phosphate
  - cytarabine
  - daunorubicin HCl
  - diazepam
  - doxorubicin HCl
  - droperidol HCl ± fentanyl citrate
  - erythromycin
  - hyaluronidase
  - levorphanol bitartrate
  - pethidine HCl (meperidine HCl)
  - methadone HCl
  - morphine sulfate
  - pentazocine lactate
  - phenytoin sodium
  - polymyxin B sulfate
  - vancomycin sulfate.
- There is conflicting information on compatibility, or compatibility is dependent on diluent or concentration, for:
  - dextrose-saline combinations
  - dextrose in water
  - lactated Ringer's solution
  - saline solutions
  - ampicillin sodium
  - cefalothin sodium
  - dobutamine HCl
  - hydrocortisone sodium succinate
  - methicillin sodium
  - oxytetracycline HCl
  - penicillin G sodium/potassium
  - tetracycline HCl.
- Heparin should be used with caution with other drugs that change coagulation status of platelet function, e.g.:

- NSAIDs
- warfarin.
- Heparin may antagonize the effects of:
  - corticosteroids
  - insulin
  - ACTH.
- Heparin may increase the plasma concentration of diazepam.
- Heparin's actions may be partially antagonized by
  - antihistamines
  - intravenous nitroglycerin
  - propylene glycol
  - digoxin
  - tetracyclines.
- Heparin decreases TSH and levothyroxine (thyroxine) concentrations, possibly as a result of interference with the binding of these hormones to proteins.

Low molecular weight heparins (LMWH)

EXAMPLES

Dalteparin (Fragmin®), enoxaparin (Lovenox®)

The LMWH or fractionated heparins represent an alternative to unfractionated heparin. These agents are similar in size to heparin but maintain a peptide sequence that prevents the activation of factor X. They inhibit thrombin IIa to a lesser degree and are frequently expressed as anti-Xa:anti-IIa activity ratios. Because they have less activity towards factor IIa, the PT will not be prolonged significantly and monitoring is not required. Instead, anti-Xa activity can be monitored. LMWH has a higher bioavailability and longer half-life than heparin in people, allowing q.12–24 h dosing. LMWH have minimal antiplatelet effects in humans compared to heparin. They do, however, exhibit fewer although similar proaggregating effects in humans with hypersensitive platelets. They are more expensive than heparin but can be administered subcutaneously. Both dalteparin and enoxaparin have been used in cats at 100 IU/kg SQ q.24–12 h and 1.0–1.5 mg/kg SQ q.24–12 h respectively. Efficacy can be monitored by determination of anti-Xa:anti-IIA ratios. The ratios for dalteparin and enoxaparin are 2:1 and 3:1 respectively. As with heparin, the most common side effect is bleeding.

One study reported the pharmacokinetics of dalteparin in normal cats. A dose of 100 IU/kg SQ q.24 h for 5 d achieved an anti-Xa activity in the human therapeutic range by 4 h after the dose was given and fell below the human therapeutic range by 4–8 h. Another study reported the effects of enoxaparin at 1 mg/kg SQ q.12 h and dalteparin at 100 IU/kg SQ q.12 h. Peak anti-Xa activity occurred by 4 h and returned to baseline by 8 h. However, peak anti-Xa activity was not within the human therapeutic range. Together, these studies suggest that a dosing interval of 8 h may be optimum. However, the correlation between thrombus prevention and therapeutic range of anti-Xa activity is not strong. Thus to better evaluate these agents in cats at risk for aorticothromboembolism (ATE), anti-Xa effects would need to be evaluated in this patient population and ultimately a prospective clinical trial would be required. One retrospective study failed to demonstrate a significant reduction in recurrence rate or improved survival in cats at risk for ATE receiving warfarin or dalteparin.

Warfarin

Clinical applications

Warfarin is used prophylactically to prevent thromboembolism in cats with hypertrophic and unclassified cardiomyopathy.

Mechanism of action

Warfarin interferes with the cyclic interconversion of vitamin K and vitamin K epoxide by inhibiting epoxide reductase (Fig. 17.2), thus inhibiting the production of vitamin K-dependent coagulation factors (II, VII, IX, X). These factors require activation from precursor coagulation proteins to activated coagulation proteins. Activation occurs via γ-carboxylation by carboxylase enzymes located in hepatocytes; vitamin K is an essential cofactor for this reaction.

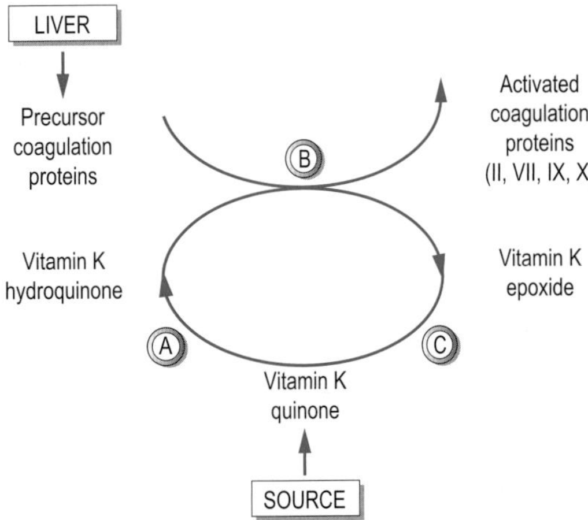

Fig. 17.2 Metabolic pathway for vitamin K. A, reductase reaction; B, linked γ-carboxylation and epoxidation reaction; C, epoxide reductase reaction.

Formulations and dose rates

There is a large interpatient variation in dose response to warfarin. A 20-fold variability in dose response has been reported in humans, and veterinarians using warfarin clinically have observed significant variability in cats. Thus careful patient monitoring is essential and initial hospitalization while the dose is being stabilized is recommended. One-stage prothrombin time is the most common coagulation test used to monitor warfarin therapy. Time of drug administration and blood sampling should be standardized to optimize interpretation of results. Veterinarians are advised to consult relevant references to ensure they are familiar with appropriate protocols for monitoring warfarin therapy.

Warfarin is available in tablet and injectable formulations. The initial dose in cats is 0.5 mg q.24 h PO. If used in dogs to prevent thromboembolism, an initial dose of 0.1–0.2 mg/kg PO has been recommended.

Pharmacokinetics

Pharmacokinetic data for warfarin in cats have not been determined. In humans it is rapidly and completely absorbed after oral administration. It is highly protein bound (approximately 99% in humans) but there are wide species variations in the degree of protein binding – for example, it is less protein bound in horses than in rats, sheep and swine. Comparative data are lacking for companion animal species.

Warfarin is predominantly metabolized in the liver to inactive metabolites that are excreted in urine and bile. Metabolites excreted in bile undergo enterohepatic recycling and are eventually eliminated in urine. The plasma half-life may be several hours to several days, depending on the patient and possibly on the species.

Adverse effects

Dose-related hemorrhage can be a serious complication.

Known drug interactions

Numerous drugs interact with warfarin and may affect the patient's response to the drug.

- In humans potentiated anticoagulant effects may occur with:
  - anabolic steroids
  - several antimicrobial drugs (chloramphenicol, erythromycin, metronidazole, tetracycline, trimethoprim/sulfamethoxazole)
  - several antifungal drugs (fluconazole, ketoconazole, miconazole)
  - antiulcer drugs (cimetidine and omeprazole)
  - thyroid medication (levothyroxine (thyroxine), propylthiouracil)
  - amiodarone
  - danazol
  - NSAIDs
  - quinidine.
- In humans decreased anticoagulant effects may occur with:
  - barbiturates
  - carbamazepine
  - corticosteroids
  - griseofulvin
  - estrogen-containing products
  - rifampicin (rifampin)
  - spironolactone
  - sucralfate
  - vitamin K
  - mercaptopurine.

ANTIPLATELET DRUGS

EXAMPLES

Aspirin, thienopyridines (clopidogrel (Plavix®), ticlopidine (Ticlid®))

ASPIRIN

See Chapter 13.

THIENOPYRIDINES

These agents induce specific irreversible platelet membrane ADP receptor antagonism. They are direct antiplatelet drugs and inhibit primary and secondary platelet aggregation in response to many agonists and thus prolong mucosal bleeding times. Antiplatelet effects are greater than those with aspirin. The ADP-induced conformational change of glycoprotein IIb/IIIa complex is also inhibited which reduces binding of fibrinogen and von Willebrand factor. Platelet release action is also impaired, decreasing the release of proaggregation and vasoconstrictive agents (e.g. serotonin, ADP, thromboxane).

Clopidogrel

Clopidogrel is a second-generation agent with increased potency relative to ticlopidine. A short-term pharmacodynamic study in normal cats reported that clopidogrel caused inhibition of platelet aggregation to ADP and serotonin by >90% and a 3.9-fold increase in mucosal bleeding time at 18.75, 37.5 and 75 mg/cat PO q.24 h. Maximum effects were present by 3 d and were lost 7 d following discontinuation of drug administration. No adverse effects were noted in the study or in 30 clinical feline patients receiving daily therapy for 18 months. There was no difference in antiplatelet efficacy between doses and thus the lowest dose (1/4 of a 75 mg tablet (18.75 mg/cat q.24 h) is recommended.

Canine starting doses are reported to be 2 mg/kg once daily. Doses as low as 1 mg/kg may be sufficient for chronic therapy (i.e. after at least 3 weeks of therapy). If rapid platelet inhibition is desired (i.e. within 90 min) then a loading dose of approximately 10 mg/kg could be used and was found to be safe and effective in six dogs.

However, if there is a possibility of von Willebrand's deficiency, then von Willebrand's levels should be checked (bleeding times are not sufficient) before starting any antiplatelet drug, including clopidogrel.

Ticlopidine

This was the first drug in this class to be used in people. A short-term pharmacodynamics study in normal cats demonstrated good antiplatelet effects but most cats had severe gastrointestinal side effects, limiting clinical utility.

FURTHER READING

ACVIM 2005 Consensus statement on management of proteinuria in dogs and cats. J Vet Int Med 19: 377-385

Arsenault WG, Boothe DM, Gordon SG, Miller MW 2005 Pharmacokinetics of carvedilol in healthy conscious dogs. Am J Vet Res 66(12): 2172-2176

Bach FJ, Rozanski EA, MacGregor J, Betkowski JM, Rush JE 2006 Retrospective evaluation of sildenafil citrate as a therapy for pulmonary hypertension in dogs. J Vet Intern Med 20: 1132-1135

Feldman BF, Kirby R, Caldin M 2000 Recognition and treatment of disseminated intravascular coagulation. In: Bonagura J (ed.) Current veterinary therapy XIII. WB Saunders, Philadelphia, pp 190-194

Goodwin JC, Hogan DF, Green HW 2007 The pharmacodynamics of clopidogrel in the dog. Abstract. ACVIM Forum

Gordon SG, Bahr A, Miller MW, Boothe DM, Glaze K 2005 Short-term hemodynamic effects of chronic oral carvedilol in cavalier King Charles spaniels with asymptomatic degenerative valve disease (abstract). J Vet Int Med 19(3): 417-418

Gordon SG, Arsenault WG, Longnecker M, Boothe DM, Miller MW, Chalkey J 2006 Pharmacodynamics of carvedilol in healthy conscious dogs. J Vet Int Med 20(2): 297-304

Harpster NK, Batey CJ 1995 Warfarin therapy of the cat at risk of thromboembolism. In: Bonagura J (ed.) Current veterinary therapy XII. WB Saunders, Philadelphia, pp 868-873

Hogan DF 2006 Prevention and management of thromboembolism. In: August JR (ed.) Consultations in feline internal medicine, volume 5. Elsevier Saunders, Philadelphia, pp 331-345

Kittleson MD 1998 Diagnosis and treatment of cardiac arrhythmias. In: Kittleson MD, Kienle RD (eds) Small animal cardiovascular medicine. Mosby, St Louis, MO

Lefebvre HP, Toutain PL 2004 Angiotensin converting enzyme therapy for the treatment of renal diseases. J Vet Pharmacol Therap 27: 265-281

Lombard CW, Jons O, Bussadori CM 2006 Clinical efficacy of pimobendan versus benazepril for the treatment of acquired atrioventricular valvular disease in dogs. J Am Anim Hosp Assoc 42: 249-261

Opie LH, Gersh BJ (eds) 2005 Drugs for the heart, 6th edn. Elsevier Saunders, Philadelphia. (This is a human reference text but good resource for cardiovascular drugs.)

Papich MG 1995 Incompatible critical care drug combinations. In: Bonagura J (ed.) Current veterinary therapy XII. WB Saunders, Philadelphia, pp 194-199

Plumb DC 2000 Veterinary drug handbook, 3rd edn. Iowa State University Press, Ames, IA

Roland R, Gordon SG, Bahr A, Miller MW 2006 Acute cardiovascular effects of oral pimobendan in dogs with heart failure due to chronic valve disease (abstract). J Vet Int Med 20(3): 731

Rush JE, Freeman LM, Brown DJ, Smith FWK 1998 The use of enalapril in the treatment of feline hypertrophic cardiomyopathy. J Am Anim Hosp Assoc 34: 38-41

Saunders AB, Miller MW, Gordon SG, Van De Wiele C 2006 Oral amiodarone therapy in dogs with atrial fibrillation. J Vet Int Med 20(4): 921-926

Smith PJ, French AT, Van Israel N et al 2005 Efficacy and safety of pimobendan in canine heart failure caused by myxomatous mitral valve disease. J Small Anim Pract 46: 121-130

18

Drugs used in the management of respiratory diseases

Philip Padrid and David B Church

INTRODUCTION

The term 'respiratory disease' includes any disorder of the pulmonary tree, including infectious and noninfectious disease(s) of the nasal cavity and sinuses, posterior oropharynx, larynx, trachea, bronchi, lung parenchyma and pleural cavity. This chapter will concentrate primarily on the drugs used to treat respiratory disease in dogs and cats in which the primary cause is not due to infectious or parasitic agents. The reader is referred to other chapters of this book for specific methods of treating viral, bacterial, fungal and parasitic infections of the respiratory tract. Additionally, respiratory dysfunction due to pulmonary congestion and edema as a result of primary or secondary heart failure will also be covered in other appropriate chapters.

CLINICAL SIGNS OF RESPIRATORY DISEASE

Regardless of the cause, inflammation and/or obstruction of the respiratory tract results in a relatively small number of clinical signs. These include sneezing, reverse sneezing, coughing, gagging, nasal discharge, noisy breathing, increased (rarely decreased) rate of breathing, increased or decreased depth of breathing, lethargy and exercise intolerance. Most respiratory disorders will cause some combination of these signs to occur simultaneously. In order to make rational choices for the treatment of both the signs and the underlying cause(s) of these signs, it is helpful to briefly review the relevant pathophysiology.

Pathophysiological regulation of airway size

The diameter of an airway has a profound effect on the amount of air that can travel through that airway as well as the speed with which that air travels.

There are two important clinical messages:

1. decreased airway diameter results in increased airflow velocity. This, in turn, causes a drop in airway pressure
2. small changes in airway diameter result in enormous changes in the amount of air that can pass through that airway.

Many respiratory diseases cause airway narrowing from edema, mucus formation or cellular infiltration. Normal volumes of air may not be able to flow easily on a breath-by-breath basis and the airways may be prone to collapse. This phenomenon is one of the causes of noisy breathing, tachypnea, sneeze, cough, lethargy and exercise intolerance. Therefore, drug therapy that results in an increase in airway diameter may minimize or even abolish these clinical signs.

Airway diameter is also determined by physiological bronchial tone mediated through nervous airway smooth muscle innervation. In dogs and cats the primary *efferent* system is parasympathetic and the major neurotransmitter is acetylcholine.

The mechanisms involved in cholinergic bronchoconstriction are complex and incompletely understood. Intracellular effects depend in part on modifications of intracellular levels of cyclic adenosine monophosphate (cAMP) and cyclic guanosine monophosphate (cGMP). The effects of these two second messengers are reciprocal; hence increased concentrations of one are associated with decreased concentrations of the other. Cyclic AMP is increased by β_2-receptor stimulation and decreased by activation of α-receptors. In contrast, activation of H_1-receptors, muscarinic effects of acetylcholine and a variety of different inflammatory mediators and increased intracellular Ca^{2+} concentrations all increase cGMP levels.

Acetylcholine's actions are mediated via a number of mechanisms, which are not all cAMP or cGMP dependent. These include increasing intracellular concentrations of inositol 1,4,5-triphosphate (ITP) and diacylglycerol (DAG) as well as promoting calcium influx through L-type calcium channels. The ITP effects are thought to be responsible for the initial phase of bronchial smooth muscle contraction, mediated via a transient increase in intracellular calcium concentration released from the sarcoplasmic reticulum. While this process appears to be cAMP dependent, it has been postulated that a cholinergically mediated decrease in cAMP is the cause of the increased intracellular ITP concentration. However, while this first phase may be cAMP independent, the maintenance of bronchoconstriction appears to involve both ITP- and DAG-modifying cAMP levels through unknown mechanisms.

Acetylcholine-mediated basal airway tone is minimal in dogs and results in only mild bronchoconstriction in resting feline airways. However, unlike the dog, there are at least five receptor types in feline airways that respond to parasympathetic input. One receptor type, the irritant receptor, is located beneath the respiratory epithelium and has been found in cat airways as far distally as the alveoli. The increased types and distribution of ACh-responsive receptors are likely to at least partly explain the severity of clinical signs associated with feline bronchitis compared with canine bronchitis.

Although resting airway tone in dogs is minimal, canine airways are more responsive than feline airways to acetylcholine. However, canine airways (in relation to their body surface area) are enormous compared with feline airways and changes in bronchomotor tone in dogs result in relatively trivial *clinical* changes compared with the cat.

The sympathetic system also mediates airway caliber and tone. These actions are mediated via β_1- and β_2-adrenergic bronchodilation and α_1-adrenergic bronchoconstriction, as well as possibly α_2-adrenergic reduction of parasympathetic bronchoconstriction. Variations in the density of β_1- and β_2-receptors within cat airways contribute to the increased responsiveness of cat airways to naturally occurring and drug-induced changes in bronchomotor tone compared with the dog.

A third nervous system, the nonadrenergic, noncholinergic (NANC) system, further mediates bronchomotor tone through various neurotransmitters, such as vasoactive intestinal peptide.

BRONCHODILATOR DRUGS

The use of bronchodilators in various disease states is based on the assumption that clinically significant bronchoconstriction exists. The degree of resting bronchomotor tone and the reactivity of airway smooth muscle in response to different disease states and airborne agents are species specific. For example, as previously mentioned, there is minimal bronchomotor tone in healthy dogs at rest. In contrast, cats have a greater degree of bronchomotor tone at rest that can be reversed with vagolytic agents.

In general, bronchoconstriction is not an important cause of clinical signs in dogs with bronchopulmonary disease. For example, less than 15% of dogs with chronic bronchitis have increased airway resistance (a measure of increased bronchomotor tone) that can be reversed with bronchodilator agents. In contrast, cats develop naturally occurring and clinically significant bronchoconstriction which in severe cases of allergic inflammation can be life-threatening.

Bronchodilator drugs can be classified as β-receptor agonists, methylxanthine derivatives and anticholinergics. As mentioned above, adrenergic stimulation can result in α_1-adrenoreceptor mediated bronchial constriction, α_2-adrenoreceptor mediated bronchodilation, probably through inhibition of cholinergic bronchoconstriction, or bronchodilation through activation of β_2-adrenoreceptors. The bronchodilatory effects of β_2-adrenoreceptors are mediated not only through increasing cAMP concentrations but also, perhaps more importantly, through a cAMP-independent pathway that involves activation of a large-conductance calcium-activated potassium channel. Activating this channel allows an extracellular potassium efflux, increase in transmembrane potential and hence a reduction in calcium influx through the voltage-dependent L-type calcium channels, thus resulting in bronchodilation.

ADRENERGIC AGONISTS

All adrenergic agonists have variable α- and β-receptor affinity. In view of the distribution of α- and β-receptors, nonselective β-receptor agonists such as isoprenaline (isoproterenol) or mixed α- and β-receptor agonists such as adrenaline (epinephrine) are more likely to produce cardiovascular side effects than similarly administered selective β-agonists. Consequently, drugs with preferential affinity for β_2-receptors are likely to provide more effective bronchodilation with fewer side effects.

Aerosol delivery

Even when selective β_2-agonists are used, the preferential activation of pulmonary β_2-receptors may be enhanced by inhalation of small doses of the drug in aerosol form. This approach typically leads to rapid and effective pulmonary β_2-receptor activation with low systemic drug concentrations.

Aerosol administration relies upon the delivery of drug to distal airways, which in turn depends on the size of the aerosol particles and various respiratory parameters such as tidal volume and inspiratory flow rate. Even in such co-operative patients as humans, only approximately 10% of the inhaled dose enters the lungs. Recent studies in cats have demonstrated that passive inhalation through a mask and spacer combination (Aerokat®) is an effective method of delivering sufficient medication to be clinically effective. Preliminary studies and anecdotal evidence suggest that dogs may be treated equally effectively using a similar system.

The two principal β_2-agonists currently marketed in preparations that can be readily and regularly used in small animals are terbutaline sulfate and salbutamol (albuterol) sulfate.

Terbutaline sulfate

Mechanism of action

Terbutaline is a selective β_2-receptor agonist that produces relaxation of smooth muscle found principally in bronchial, vascular and uterine tissues. The exact mechanism by which activation of β_2-receptors results in smooth muscle relaxation is poorly understood although it seems certain to involve changes brought about by increased intracellular cAMP. It has been postulated that the elevated cAMP levels inactivate the enzyme responsible for activating myosin. Since the inactive myosin is unable to interact with actin, smooth muscle contraction cannot occur.

Formulations and dose rates

Terbutaline is available as a tablet, an elixir and an injectable preparation suitable for subcutaneous or intramuscular use. The dose rate has been reported from as low as 0.01 mg/kg given subcutaneously or intramuscularly up to 0.1–0.2 mg/kg/8 h for the dog and cat given orally.

Pharmacokinetics

The pharmacokinetics of terbutaline in dogs and cats have not been described. In humans, around 45% of an oral dose is absorbed; peak bronchial effects occur within 2–3 h and last approximately 8 h. When administered subcutaneously, there is a more rapid onset of activity (15 min) with a peak effect after 30–60 min and duration of 4 h. Approximately 60% of administered terbutaline is excreted unchanged in the urine, while the remainder undergoes hepatic conjugation to inactive metabolites.

Adverse effects

- At usual doses, terbutaline has little effect on β_1-receptors so direct cardiostimulatory effects are unlikely. However, terbutaline should always be used with care in patients who may have increased sensitivity to adrenergic agents – in particular, patients with pre-existing cardiac disease, diabetes mellitus, hyperthyroidism, hypertension and seizure disorders.
- All β_2-agonists may lower plasma potassium; hence, in at-risk patients receiving long-term terbutaline therapy, it may be prudent to monitor plasma potassium levels. In clinical practice and experimentally, it is rare to find β_2-agonist associated hypokalemia in dogs and cats.

Known drug interactions

- Terbutaline used with other sympathomimetics increases the risk of adverse cardiovascular effects, as does its concurrent use with digoxin, tricyclic antidepressants and monoamine oxidase inhibitors. These potential effects are more likely in patients with pre-existing cardiac disease, especially hypertrophic cardiomyopathy.
- Use with various inhalation anesthetics may predispose the patient to ventricular arrhythmias.

Salbutamol (albuterol) sulfate

Mechanism of action

Salbutamol (albuterol) is a selective β_2-receptor agonist with pharmacological properties similar to terbutaline.

Formulations and dose rates

Salbutamol is available as a tablet, syrup, as well as various inhalants. The oral dose rate in the dog is 0.02 mg/kg/12 h. This dose should be maintained for 5 days and if there has been no improvement and no adverse effects, the dose may be increased to 0.5 mg/kg/8–12 h. In animals that respond at this higher dose, the dose should be reduced progressively until the lowest effective dose has been determined. However, because the inhaled form of salbutamol is now available for use in veterinary practice, there is little advantage to using the oral preparation.

The inhaled form of salbutamol comes as a single strength 17 g metered dose inhaler and delivers 90 µg per actuation of the device. Additionally, salbutamol can be included in discus or dry powder forms with other inhaled medications, including fluticasone hydrochloride (Advair®). Currently, however, there is no practical method to deliver the discus or powder form of the drug(s) to dogs and cats.

Pharmacokinetics

The pharmacokinetics of salbutamol in dogs and cats have not been studied. In humans, when administered by inhalation, salbutamol produces significant bronchodilation within 15 min that lasts for 3–4 h. It is also generally well absorbed orally and may have bronchodilatory effects for up to 8 h. Anecdotal experience with this drug in clinical practice suggests a similar pharmacokinetic profile in cats. Salbutamol undergoes extensive hepatic metabolism. After oral administration approximately 58–78% of the dose is excreted in the urine over 24 h, with 60% of the drug in an inactive form.

Adverse effects

- Occasional but not common adverse effects include skeletal muscle tremors and restlessness, which generally subside after 2–3 days.
- As with terbutaline, care should be exercised when administering salbutamol to patients with preexisting cardiac disease, diabetes mellitus, hyperthyroidism, hypertension and seizure disorders.

Known drug interactions

Salbutamol's potential interactions are similar to those of terbutaline.

METHYLXANTHINES

The methylxanthines share several pharmacological actions of therapeutic interest. They relax smooth muscle, particularly bronchial smooth muscle, stimulate the central nervous system and are weakly positive chronotropes and inotropes, as well as mild diuretics. However, in small animal practice the methylxanthines have been used primarily as bronchodilators.

Theophylline and aminophylline

Chemical structure

Caffeine, theophylline and theobromine are three naturally occurring methylxanthines. While all three alkaloids are relatively insoluble, the solubility can be enhanced by the formation of complexes with a wide variety of compounds. The best known of these complexes is aminophylline, which is the ethylenediamine complex of theophylline with differing quantities of water of hydration. Each 100 mg of hydrous and anhydrous aminophylline contains 79 mg and 86 mg of theophylline respectively. Conversely, 100 mg of theophylline is equivalent to 116 mg of anhydrous aminophylline and 127 mg of hydrous aminophylline. When dissolved in water, aminophylline readily dissociates to its parent compounds.

Mechanism of action

Although theophylline produces bronchial smooth muscle relaxation, importantly it is considered a less potent bronchodilator than the β-agonists. Theophylline has also been credited with producing centrally mediated increased respiratory effort at any given alveolar PCO_2, improved diaphragmatic contractility and reduced diaphragmatic fatigue, mild increases in myocardial contractility and heart rate, increased central nervous system (CNS) activity, increased gastric acid secretion and mild diuresis. These effects have not been demonstrated in dogs or cats and must be recognized as an extrapolation from other species.

A number of mechanisms have been proposed to explain these various effects. These have included inhibition of phosphodiesterases with a resultant increase in intracellular cAMP, direct and indirect effects on intracellular calcium concentration, uncoupling of intracellular calcium concentration and muscle contractile elements and competitive inhibition of adenosine receptors.

Interestingly, at therapeutic concentrations of theophylline, only adenosine receptor blockade has been reliably demonstrated. Consequently many investigators suggest that this is the most likely explanation for theophylline's varied effects. However, it should be noted that, at present, the exact mechanism by which theophylline causes bronchodilation is far from resolved.

Formulations and dose rates

Because of theophylline's relatively low therapeutic index and pharmacokinetic characteristics, dose rates should be based on lean body mass. The dose rate of theophylline varies depending on the preparation used. In standard preparations the recommended dose rate in dogs is 10 mg/kg/6–8 h PO and cats 4 mg/kg/8–12 h PO. When using sustained-release preparations, a dose of 20 mg/kg/12 h for dogs and 25 mg/kg/24 h for cats should be considered. Although there have been reports of varied bioavailability with different proprietary forms of sustained-release preparations, Theo-Dur® and Diffumal® have both reliably been shown to have bioavailability greater than 95% in dogs.

- The dose rate of aminophylline is 11 mg/kg/8 h in dogs PO and 5–6 mg/kg/12 h PO in cats

Pharmacokinetics

The pharmacokinetics of theophylline have been extensively studied in a number of species. Because theophylline is not water soluble it can only be given orally. After oral administration peak plasma rates occur within 1.5 h; rate of absorption is limited principally by dissolution of the dosage form in the gut. Bioavailability in both cats and dogs is generally >90% when nonsustained-release preparations are used. However, sustained-release preparations may have a more variable bioavailability. One study in dogs suggested that four different sustained-release preparations had bioavailability varying from 30% to 76%; however, other investigators found bioavailability to be greater than

95% in studies using two of these four products. In general, the anhydrous theophylline tablet is preferred.

Theophylline is only weakly protein bound (7–14%), with a relatively low volume of distribution (0.82 L/kg in dogs, 0.46 L/kg in cats). Because of this low volume of distribution and theophylline's poor lipid solubility, it is recommended that obese animals be dosed on a lean body mass basis. Additionally, a chronopharmacokinetic study in cats showed that evening administration is associated with better bioavailability and fewer fluctuations in plasma drug levels.

In humans, theophylline is mainly metabolized in the liver. Reported elimination half-lives are 5.7 h in the dog and 7.8 h in the cat. Renal clearance of parent compound contributes only about 10% of total plasma clearance. In humans there are marked variations in plasma half-life between individuals and it seems likely that similar variation exists in dogs and cats, although to date this has not been investigated.

Adverse effects

- Although theophylline can produce CNS stimulation and gastrointestinal disturbances, usually these effects are associated with excessive dosing and resolve with a dose adjustment.
- Seizures or cardiac arrhythmias may occur in severe toxicity.

Known drug interactions

- Theophylline's effects may be diminished by phenytoin or phenobarbital and enhanced by cimetidine, allopurinol, clindamycin and lincomycin.
- The effects of theophylline and β-adrenergic blockers may be antagonized if they are administered concurrently.
- Theophylline increases the likelihood of arrhythmias induced by adrenergic agonists and halothane.
- Theophylline increases the likelihood of seizures with ketamine.

ANTICHOLINERGICS

Mechanism of action

There are cholinergic nerve fibers within the brainstem at the level of the nucleus ambiguous, as well as within the vagus nerve via the dorsal motor nucleus. Nervous impulses traverse through parasympathetic ganglia within the airway wall; postganglionic nerve fibers innervate the submucosal glands and airway smooth muscle. When activated, the endings of these nerve fibers release acetylcholine and can result in mucus secretion and smooth muscle contraction (bronchoconstriction).

Additionally, there is cholinergic innervation of the lung and this is mediated through three muscarinic receptors (M1, M2, M3). Interestingly, the M2 receptor is antagonistic in that stimulation of M2 receptors causes inhibition of further acetylcholine release. Atropine is the classic anticholinergic compound and blocks muscarinic receptors nonselectively. Since concurrent blockage of M2 and M3 receptors is likely to have antagonistic effects on acetylcholine secretion, drugs that selectively block activation of M3 receptors (tiotroprium bromide) have been developed. Interestingly, while in humans drugs that block cholinergic pathways are effective in the treatment of COPD, this class of drug has not demonstrated similar efficacy in treating dogs or cats with bronchial disease.

In the authors' experience, the primary indication for anticholinergic drug therapy in veterinary respiratory medicine is to pretreat cats with existing bronchial disease prior to anesthesia to decrease excessive mucoid secretions that would otherwise result from tracheal intubation. It may also be helpful as an adjunctive bronchodilator for patients with pre-existing asthma for which bronchoscopy is planned.

TOPICAL ANTI-INFLAMMATORY THERAPY

Oral and parenteral corticosteroids are commonly used by veterinarians to treat a number of pulmonary disorders in dogs and cats, including allergic rhinitis, bronchitis, asthma and eosinophilic pneumonia (PIE syndrome). This class of drugs is effective for this purpose but the list of side effects is long and ranges from annoying (increased urination) to life-threatening (pancreatitis, diabetes mellitus). Inhaled steroid medications have the advantage of significant clinical efficacy without the systemic side effects of the oral or parenterally administered medications. The most commonly used inhaled corticosteroid is fluticasone proprionate.

Fluticasone proprionate

Fluticasone proprionate is a synthetic corticosteroid that has 18-fold greater affinity for the corticosteroid receptor compared with dexamethasone, the reference standard for corticosteroid potency. Similarly to oral and parenteral corticosteroids, fluticasone activates the glucocorticosteroid receptor present on virtually all cells within mammalian systems. Binding of the steroid to this receptor results in a new molecular complex that itself binds to promoter-enhancer regions of target genes, resulting in up- or downregulation of the gene and its product. Fluticasone, like other corticosteroids, acts to inhibit mast cells, eosinophils, lymphocytes, neutrophils and macrophages involved in the generation and exacerbation of allergic airway inflammation by transcriptional regulation of these target genes. Preformed and newly secreted mediators including histamine, eicosanoids, leukotrienes and multiple cytokines are inhibited as well.

Fluticasone is a large molecule and acts topically within the airway mucosa. Because there is poor absorption across gut epithelium there is minimal oral systemic bioavailability, thus plasma levels do not predict therapeutic effects. This explains the lack of systemic side effects but it also suggests that clinically effective absorption into the airway mucosa is delayed. Optimal clinical effects therefore may not occur for 1–2 weeks.

Fluticasone has been used to treat cats with bronchial asthma since at least 1993. The first systematic published report of the use of this drug for this purpose was in the year 2000. Since then, a number of manuscripts have demonstrated the clinical effectiveness of fluticasone to treat dogs and cats with allergic rhinitis, bronchitis and asthma (naturally occurring and experimentally induced). There have been no controlled published studies to determine the optimal dose or interval for use of fluticasone in dogs or cats. However, there are anecdotal reports (by one of the authors) that reference more than 500 small animal patients treated with fluticasone over a period covering 1995–2006. Dosage recommendations are therefore based on these anecdotal reports and are supported by more recent published studies.

Formulations and dose rates

Inhaled corticosteroids come in multiple forms. However, only the metered dose inhalers (MDI) combined with a spacer and mask appropriate for the size of the patient's muzzle are currently suitable for use in small animal patients. Fluticasone comes in three strengths: 44/110 and 220 μg per actuation. The authors have found that 44 μg dosing twice daily does not consistently result in acceptable clinical responses in either dogs or cats of any size. For cats and dogs less than 12 kg, 110 μg given twice daily frequently results in clinical responses equivalent to that achieved by administration of oral doses of prednisone 5 mg PO BID. Dogs larger than 12 kg may need twice this dose, or 220 μg inhaled BID.

The choice of spacer is clinically significant because the efficacy of a spacer as a delivery device affects the amount of drug available to the patient. Most mammalian species including dogs and cats have a tidal volume of 10–20 mL inspired air/kg of bodyweight. Currently, only the Aerokat® and Aerodawg® brand (Trudell Medical Inc, Ontario) spacers have been designed specifically based on the tidal volume characteristics of small animals. Using these spacer devices, dogs and cats will inhale the majority of drug propelled into the spacer by breathing 7–10 times through the spacer– mask combination after actuation of the MDI. As previously mentioned, it may take 1–2 weeks to reach maximal clinical efficacy due to the large size of the molecule and slow penetration into airway mucosa.

ANTITUSSIVES

Relevant pathophysiology

The cough reflex is complex, involving the central and peripheral nervous systems as well as the smooth muscle of the bronchial tree. Chemical or mechanical irritation of the epithelium within bronchial mucosa causes bronchoconstriction, which in turn stimulates cough receptors located within the tracheobronchial tree. Afferent conduction from these receptors occurs via the vagus nerve to centers within the medulla that are distinct from the actual respiratory center.

The drugs that can affect this complex mechanism are quite diverse. For example, coughing as a result of bronchoconstriction may be relieved by bronchodilators acting simply to dilate airways, while other antitussive agents act primarily on the peripheral or central nervous system components of the cough reflex. Generally, however, the most effective antitussives elevate the threshold for coughing by poorly understood centrally mediated mechanisms.

Clinical applications

Almost any respiratory tract disorder involving any level of the large and small airways can result in coughing. This should normally be viewed as a protective physiological process resulting in clearance of thick and tenacious secretions produced by chronic airway inflammation. Thus, cough suppression as a single therapeutic agent is relatively contraindicated when cough is associated with mucus production. In investigating any animal with suspected respiratory disease, it is important to establish if the animal gags, chokes or swallows after coughing. If the answer to any of these questions is yes, it is likely mucus is being produced and brought to the caudal pharynx. In these cases, cough suppression as a single treatment modality is likely to be contraindicated.

However, once mucus production is diminished or resolved, cough suppression may be desirable. Chronic coughing tends to increase airway inflammation, increasing the risk of a vicious cycle in which the cough causes mucosal irritation. This can result in further coughing. Consequently, cough suppression may be particularly helpful for selected patients, including dogs with tracheobronchial collapse or dogs recovering from the acute phase of the kennel-cough complex.

Additionally, there are cases when the cough is so frustrating for owners that euthanasia of the pet is being considered. Cough suppression may be life saving in this instance.

Typically, drugs used to suppress coughing are categorized as narcotic (opioid) or nonnarcotic (nonopioid). Unfortunately, although many nonopioid antitussives can be effective in experimental situations, these same drugs are not predictably effective in naturally occurring clinical situations. Consequently, in the authors' opinion, generally narcotic antitussives are needed to achieve effective cough suppression.

NONOPIOID ANTITUSSIVES

Dextromethorphan hydrobromide

Mechanism of action

Dextromethorphan hydrobromide is a semisynthetic derivative of opium that acts centrally to elevate the cough threshold. It does not have addictive, analgesic or sedative action and in usual doses does not produce respiratory depression or inhibit ciliary activity. Although dextromethorphan is the D isomer of the codeine analog, and thus levorphanol, it binds to central binding sites that appear to be distinct from standard opioid receptors. The nonopioid nature of these sites is reinforced by the inability of naloxone to reverse dextromethorphan's effects.

Formulations and dose rates

Dextromethorphan is generally marketed in over-the-counter formulations (usually syrups or lozenges) combined with various antihistamines, bronchodilators and mucolytics. A dose of approximately 2 mg/kg PO has been suggested, although, as with most of the antitussive agents, higher doses are often required. Antitussive effects may persist for up to 5 h. In the authors' experience, the effectiveness of dextromethorphan is significantly less than that of the various opioid antitussives. Its main advantage is its ease of availability and lack of accountability to federal agencies for its use, although generally this is more than offset by its lack of clinical efficacy!

Pharmacokinetics

There appears to be no information available on the pharmacokinetics of dextromethorphan in cats and dogs. In humans, onset of action is 30 min.

Adverse effects

Adverse effects of dextromethorphan are confined to CNS depression and this has only been reported at extremely high doses.

OPIOID ANTITUSSIVES

Codeine phosphate

Mechanism of action

Codeine has extremely low affinity for standard CNS μ, κ and δ opioid receptors. Its antitussive activity probably involves distinct codeine-specific receptors. Ligation of these receptors reduces the sensitivity of the cough center to afferent impulses.

Formulations and dose rates

Codeine phosphate is available as 30 mg and 60 mg tablets as well as being present in many mixed analgesic preparations. Codeine phosphate is a schedule II drug and is subject to the Controlled Substance Act of 1970 (USA). The starting antitussive dose has been as low as 0.1–0.3 mg/kg/8–12 h and as high as 1–2 mg/kg/6–12 h. Whatever the starting point, the dose may need to be increased to achieve a satisfactory effect.

Pharmacokinetics

Because of its reduced first-pass hepatic metabolism in comparison to other opioids, codeine has a high bioavailability. Oral administration of codeine provides around 60% of its parenteral efficacy. Once absorbed, codeine is metabolized by the liver, with the largely inactive metabolites excreted predominantly in the urine.

In humans, approximately 10% of administered codeine is demethylated to form morphine and both free and conjugated forms of morphine can be found in the urine of patients receiving therapeutic doses of codeine. In humans, codeine's plasma half-life is around 2–4 h.

Adverse effects

- Codeine is generally well tolerated, although adverse effects are possible especially at higher dose rates.
- Sedation is the most common side effect in the dog.
- CNS stimulation may be seen in cats.
- Constipation is common when codeine is given for more than a few weeks.

Hydrocodone tartrate

Mechanism of action

Hydrocodone has increased antitussive properties compared to codeine. In humans, it has been suggested that hydrocodone may have twice the antitussive potency of morphine. The mechanism of this effect seems to be direct suppression of the cough center within the medulla. Hydrocodone may also reduce respiratory mucosal secretions through undetermined mechanisms.

Formulations and dose rates

The starting dose rate in dogs is 0.22 mg/kg/6–12 h PO. For dogs with intractable cough (tracheal collapse, left mainstem bronchial collapse due to enlarged left atrium) the dose of hydrocodone often needs to be increased to 0.45–0.9 mg/kg/6–12 h. Hydrocodone is marketed in combination with homatropine as both an elixir and tablet formulations. The addition of homatropine may be intended to dissuade inappropriate use of the drug for pleasure and usually does not cause significant untoward side effects in dogs or cats. In the authors' experience this is the most effective and safe cough suppressant available for use in the canine species.

Pharmacokinetics

In humans, hydrocodone is well absorbed orally, with a serum half-life of 3.8 h. In dogs the antitussive effect generally lasts between 6 and 12 h. Owners may be instructed to note the duration of action in their pet. Dosing intervals are then based on these observations.

Adverse effects

Adverse effects include:

- sedation
- constipation
- other gastrointestinal side effects including borborygmus and diarrhea.

Dihydrocodeine tartrate

Mechanism of action

Dihydrocodeine also acts centrally to raise the cough threshold. Its other CNS activities seem to be markedly less than those of codeine.

Formulations and dose rates

Dihydrocodeine is marketed as an elixir, which is relatively palatable and well absorbed. A starting dose rate of 2 mg/kg/8–12 h PO is recommended, although higher doses may be required for satisfactory therapeutic effect.

Pharmacokinetics

In humans, dihydrocodeine is well absorbed after oral administration. It has a serum half-life of about 3.8 h and its antitussive effects last for 4–6 h. The antitussive action appears to persist for 6–12 h. Unfortunately there is no information available on the pharmacokinetics of dihydrocodeine in dogs.

Adverse effects

Although constipation has been reported in humans, it is an unusual occurrence and adverse effects are generally extremely uncommon.

Butorphanol

Mechanism of action

Butorphanol is a very effective antitussive as well as an analgesic. In dogs it is 100 times more potent as a cough suppressant than codeine and four times more potent than morphine. It has been shown to elevate the CNS respiratory center threshold to carbon dioxide but, unlike other opioid agonists, it does not suppress respiratory center sensitivity. In the authors' experience butorphanol is most helpful as an antitussive given parenterally to treat acute intractable cough.

Formulations and dose rates

The antitussive dose of butorphanol in dogs is 0.55–1.1 mg/kg/6–12 h orally or 0.055–0.11 mg/kg/6–12 h subcutaneously.

Pharmacokinetics

Butorphanol is well absorbed orally but a significant first-pass effect results in less than 20% appearing in the systemic circulation. Peak serum levels are attained at 1 h in dogs when the drug is given subcutaneously. The half-life is less than 2 h and duration of action is approximately 4 h in the canine species. It is well distributed and in humans approximately 80% protein bound. Butorphanol is extensively metabolized in the liver and predominantly excreted in the urine.

Adverse effects

Adverse effects include:

- sedation
- anorexia
- occasionally diarrhea.

MUCOLYTICS

Relevant pathophysiology

Mucus is a normal protective coating of the respiratory system from the nasal cavity through to the larger bronchioles. It acts as a barrier to infectious and irritating particles. It also provides airway humidification and participates in maintaining an ideal environment for ciliary movement. Mucus is produced by submucosal glands and goblet cells within the surface epithelium of airways. Although submucosal glands produce a far greater volume of mucus compared to the goblet cells, both of these mucus-secreting tissues respond to direct contact with a variety of substances such as smoke, sulfur dioxide and ammonia. Direct innervation is predominantly cholinergic.

The viscosity of pulmonary mucus secretions depends on the concentration of mucoproteins and DNA. Mucus chains are cross-linked by disulfide bonds and it is this chemical bond that is affected by some mucolytic agents (see *N*-acetylcysteine below). The feline species is somewhat unique in forming sialic acid residues within the mucus strands and this imparts a particularly viscous nature to feline mucus. While mucoprotein is the main determinant of viscosity in normal mucus, in purulent inflammation the mucus concentration of DNA increases (because of increased cellular debris) and so does its contribution to viscosity. Importantly, although water is incorporated into the mucus gel matrix during mucus formation, topically applied water is not absorbed into the already formed mucus plug.

Clinical applications

Dogs and cats with lower airway inflammatory diseases will produce large amounts of relatively viscous inflammatory exudate and mucus which is firmly attached to the lining of bronchioles and bronchi. By effectively increasing bronchial wall thickness, this thick adherent mucus can exacerbate the 'lumen-narrowing' effects of bronchial constriction, enhance the overall inflammatory process and potentiate persistent coughing. In this situation, mucolytic therapy has theoretical value in facilitating resolution of the inflammatory airway disease.

In general, mucolytic drugs act by altering mucus structure through changes in pH, direct proteolysis and/or disruption of disulfide bond linkages. The two most frequently prescribed mucolytic drugs in veterinary practice are described below. It is also worth remembering that normal saline, directly administered to the airways by nebulization, is an effective mucolytic and expectorant.

Bromhexine hydrochloride

Bromhexine hydrochloride is a synthetic derivative of the alkaloid vasicine.

Mechanism of action

Bromhexine decreases mucus viscosity by increasing lysosomal activity. This increased lysosomal activity enhances hydrolysis of acid mucopolysaccharide polymers, which significantly contribute to normal mucus viscosity. It should be remembered that, in purulent bronchial inflammation, bronchial mucus viscosity is more dependent upon the large amount of DNA present. As bromhexine does not affect the DNA content, its mucolytic action is limited in these situations.

It has also been suggested that bromhexine increases the permeability of the alveolar–capillary barrier, resulting in increased concentrations of certain antibiotics in luminal secretions. Furthermore, over time (2–3 d), bromhexine results in a significant increase in immunoglobulin concentrations and a decline in albumin and β-globulin concentrations in respiratory secretions. The increased immunoglobulins are IgA and IgG; IgM levels remain unchanged. It has been hypothesized that because of these effects concurrent administration of bromhexine and an antimicrobial agent will facilitate treatment of infectious tracheobronchitis.

Formulations and dose rates

The mucolytic dose of bromhexine hydrochloride in dogs and cats is 2 mg/kg/12 h PO for 7–10 d, then 1 mg/kg/12 h for a further 7–10 d.

Pharmacokinetics

Following oral administration, bromhexine is rapidly absorbed, with peak plasma levels being reached within 1 h. As it is lipophilic, it is rapidly redistributed, undergoes extensive hepatic metabolism and is excreted via the urine and bile.

Adverse effects

Adverse effects to bromhexine are extremely uncommon.

Acetylcysteine

Acetylcysteine is the *N*-acetyl derivative of the naturally occurring amino acid L-cysteine.

Mechanism of action

When administered directly into airways, acetylcysteine reduces viscosity of both purulent and nonpurulent secretions. This effect is thought to be a result of the free sulfhydryl group on acetylcysteine reducing the disulfide linkages in mucoproteins, which are thought to be at least partly responsible for the particularly viscoid nature of respiratory mucus. The mucolytic activity of acetylcysteine is unaltered by the presence of DNA and increases with increasing pH.

Formulations and dose rates

Mucolytic

For effective mucolytic activity, an acetylcysteine solution should be nebulized and administered directly to the respiratory mucosa as an aerosol. The dose rate in dogs and cats is 5–10 mg/kg for 30 min every 12 h. Additionally, there is at least one report of improved gas exchange in dogs with experimentally induced bronchoconstriction treated with oral acetylcysteine.

Acetylcysteine is available as 10% and 20% solutions of the sodium salt in various sized vials. This solution can be readily used in a nebulizer undiluted, although dilution with sterile saline will reduce the risk of reactive bronchospasm.

Pharmacokinetics

When given orally, acetylcysteine is well absorbed; when given by nebulization directly into the respiratory tract, most acetylcysteine is involved in the sulfhydryl-disulfide reaction and the remainder is absorbed. The absorbed drug is metabolized via deacetylation to cysteine in the liver.

Adverse effects

Unfortunately, acetylcysteine appears to irritate respiratory tract epithelium and many dogs and cats develop cough and/or bronchoconstriction when acetylcysteine is administered directly into the respiratory tract. Consequently, its use in animals with bronchoconstrictive airway disease must be carefully monitored.

Known drug interactions

Solutions of acetylcysteine are incompatible with:
- amphotericin B
- ampicillin sodium
- erythromycin lactobionate
- tetracycline and oxytetracycline
- hydrogen peroxide.

EXPECTORANTS

Expectorants are drugs used to produce an increased volume of respiratory secretions that can theoretically be coughed out more easily. Although drugs in this class are used in an enormous number of over-the-counter medications, a Food and Drug Administration advisory review panel found no well-controlled studies that documented the effectiveness of expectorants in managing chronic obstructive pulmonary disease (COPD) in man. Likewise, there are no current data available to suggest that expectorants are effective adjunctive treatments for dogs and cats with disorders of the respiratory tract. However, because this class of drug is used with such regularity, a brief discussion is appropriate.

Guaifenisin

The most commonly prescribed expectorant is guaifenisin. An older name for this drug is glycerol guaiacolate; it was isolated from guaiac resin in 1826. When given in large amounts, guaifenisin acts as an emetic; it is likely that it stimulates a gastropulmonary vagal reflex. It may also be absorbed into bronchial mucosal glands and exert a direct mucotropic effect.

The dose required to stimulate production of mucus and respiratory tract secretions is probably equivalent to the dose needed to produce emesis; this is far higher than the 400–1600 mg/d range of dosing most commonly prescribed. Thus, at doses recommended to treat humans with COPD the effect of guaifenisin is likely equivalent to placebo.

ANTILEUKOTRIENES

Clinical applications

Leukotrienes belong to a family of inflammatory mediators that are derived from arachidonic acid and are known collectively as eicosanoids. Arachidonic acid is metabolized to various prostaglandins and thromboxanes through the action of cyclo-oxygenase as well as various leukotrienes through the action of the lipoxygenase system.

The 5-lipoxygenase enzyme catalyzes the conversion of arachidonic acid to 5-hydroperoxy-eicosatetraenoic acid (5-HPETE) and then to leukotriene A4 (LTA_4). LTA_4 is then converted to LTB_4 or conjugated to LTC_4. LTC_4 is converted to LTD_4 and this is metabolized to LTE_4. The leukotrienes LTC_4, LTD_4 and LTE_4 are collectively known as the cysteinyl leukotrienes and play an important role in airway inflammation. They produce mucus hypersecretion, increased vascular permeability and mucosal edema, induce potent bronchoconstriction and act as chemoattractants to inflammatory cells, particularly eosinophils and neutrophils.

The cysteinyl leukotrienes act via two types of cell surface receptor: cys-LT_1 and cys-LT_2. While the cys-LT_2 receptor is mainly responsible for the effects of cysteinyl leukotrienes on pulmonary blood vessels, cys-LT_1 receptors mediate most of the effects of cysteinyl leukotrienes on airways.

Zafirlukast, montelukast, zileuton

Mechanism of action

All three products are competitive, highly selective and potent oral inhibitors of production or function of LTC_4, LTD_4 and LTE_4. Specifically, zileuton blocks leukotriene biosynthesis by inhibiting production of the 5-lipoxygenase enzyme while both montelukast and zafirlukast block adhesion of leukotrienes to their common leukotriene receptor (cys-LT_1).

In man, leukotrienes inhibit asthmatic responses to allergen, aspirin, exercise and cold dry air. Additionally. leukotriene blockade has been shown in many clinical trials to decrease the amount and frequency of administration of corticosteroids in steroid-dependent human asthmatics.

Few studies have investigated the role of leukotrienes in canine or feline airway disease. Because dogs do not develop naturally occurring asthma as do cats, the few studies that have been done have focused on feline airways. LTE_4 is found in increased concentrations in urine of asthmatic humans and is a commonly used marker for increased production of LTC_4 and LTD_4 in people with asthma. No such increase in urinary LTE_4 was found in 20 cats with signs of bronchial disease or cats with experimentally induced asthma. More recently, in another experimental model of feline asthma, no increase in cysteinyl leukotrienes was found in either urine or bronchoalveolar lavage fluid after challenge exposure to sensitizing antigen. Additionally, zafirlukast did not inhibit airway inflammation or airway hyperreactivity in this feline asthma model. There is no current evidence that drugs that affect leukotriene synthesis or receptor ligation will play a significant role in the treatment of feline or canine respiratory disease.

Formulations and dose rates

Drugs that block leukotrienes are available in pill form. There is at least one author who claims efficacy in treating feline asthma with zafirlukast (1–2 mg/kg BID) and montelukast (0.5–1.0 mg/kg SID).

Pharmacokinetics

The pharmacokinetics of these drugs in dogs and cats have not been reported. In humans, they are well absorbed orally, although the presence of food can reduce absorption by up to 60%. They are highly protein bound, extensively metabolized by the liver and undergo predominantly biliary excretion.

Adverse effects

- As only limited experience of these drugs in dogs and cats is available, the prevalence, type and severity of adverse reactions associated with their administration cannot be documented.
- In humans, leukotriene receptor antagonists have occasionally been associated with elevated hepatic enzyme levels, although active hepatic disease is uncommon. Human case reports have also suggested a rare association between the leukotriene receptor antagonists and Churg–Strauss syndrome. This is a rare condition involving vasculitis-associated asthma, eosinophilia and pulmonary infiltrates. The cause and effect association remains controversial, as most of the affected patients were receiving steroids prior to starting leukotriene receptor antagonist therapy. Consequently, it seems plausible that most of the cases were actually Churg–Strauss syndrome suppressed by the oral steroids, which became unmasked when the steroids were withdrawn.

FURTHER READING

Barnes PJ, Belvisi MG, Mak JC et al 1995 Tiotropium bromide, a novel long-acting muscarinic antagonist for the treatment of obstructive airways disease. Life Sci 56(11-12): 853-859

Bjermer J 2001 History and future perspectives of treating asthma as a systemic and small airways disease. Respir Med 95(9): 703-719

Boothe DM 2004 Drugs affecting the respiratory system. In: King LG (ed.) Respiratory disease in dogs and cats. WB Saunders, St Louis, MO, pp 229-252

Dye JA, McKiernan BC, Jones SD et al 1990 Chronopharmacokinetics of theophylline in the cat. J Vet Pharmacol Ther 13(3): 278-286

Kirschvink N, Leemans J, Delvaux F et al Bronchodilators in bronchoscopy-induced airflow limitation in allergen-sensitized cats. J Vet Intern Med 19(2): 161-167

Kirschvink N, Leemans J, Delvauz F et al 2006 Inhaled fluticasone reduces bronchial responsiveness and airway inflammation in cats with mild chronic bronchitis. J Feline Med Surg 8(1): 45-54

Norris CR, Decile KC, Berghaus LJ et al 2003 Concentrations of cysteinyl leukotrienes in urine and bronchoalveolar lavage fluid of cats with experimentally induced asthma. Am J Vet Res 64(11): 1449-1453

Padrid PA 2000 Feline asthma. Vet Clin North Am Small Anim Pract 30(6): 1279-1293

Padrid PA 2006 Use of inhaled medications to treat respiratory diseases in dogs and cats. J Am Anim Hosp Assoc 42(2): 165-169

Padrid PA, Hornof WJ, Kurpershoek CJ, Cross CE 1990 Canine chronic bronchitis. A pathophysiologic evaluation of 18 cases. J Vet Intern Med 4(3): 172-180

Petruska JM, Beattie JG, Stuart BO et al 1997 Cardiovascular effects after inhalation of large doses of albuterol dry powder in rats, monkeys and dogs: a species comparison. Fundam Appl Toxicol 40(1): 52-62

Reinero CR, Byerly JR, Berghaus RD et al 2005 Effects of drug treatment on inflammation and hyperreactivity of airways and on immune variables in cats with experimentally induced asthma. Am J Vet Res 66(7): 1121-1127

Ueno O, Lee LN, Wagner PD 1989 Effect of N-acetylcysteine on gas exchange after methacholine challenge and isoprenaline inhalation in the dog. Eur Respir J 2(3): 238-246

19

Gastrointestinal drugs

Alexander J. German, Jill E. Maddison and Grant Guilford

ANTIEMETIC DRUGS

Vomiting may occur as a sequel to primary or secondary (nonenteric) gastrointestinal disease. Antiemetic therapy should only be considered as symptomatic therapy. The clinician's attention should primarily be directed at determining and resolving the underlying disease process. A great variety of drugs have been found to be useful in treating vomiting due to different causes. However, no single drug is effective for all types of emesis.

Given that they are a symptomatic therapy, antiemetics are often used in combination with other drugs and clinicians should be aware of potential drug interactions that may arise. For example, metoclopramide may affect the absorption of other drugs and have an impact on efficacy (see below). Therefore, these drugs must be used with due care.

Clinical applications

Antiemetics are indicated to:

- control vomiting, especially when profuse and protracted vomiting may lead to fluid, electrolyte or acid–base disturbances or is causing distress to the patient or owner
- prevent vomiting predicted to occur with use of emetic drugs, e.g. cisplatin, amphotericin.

Use of antiemetics is not necessary if vomiting is intermittent, the patient is not distressed and correction of fluid and electrolyte imbalances can easily be achieved.

Inappropriate use of antiemetics

Use of antiemetics in the following situations is inappropriate:

- gastrointestinal obstruction – antiemetics may delay diagnosis
- gastrointestinal toxicity – antiemetics may prevent the patient from eliminating the toxin
- systemic hypotension – the phenothiazines and α_2-adrenergic antagonists, when used in high doses, can intensify hypotension.

Relevant pathophysiology

Antiemetic drugs may have central or peripheral actions (Fig. 19.1).

Initiation of vomiting

Vomiting is initiated by either humoral or neural pathways. The humoral pathway involves stimulation of the chemoreceptor trigger zone (CTZ) by blood-borne substances, while the neural pathway is through activation of the vomiting center.

Vomiting center

All animal species that vomit have a brainstem 'vomiting center' – a group of several nuclei that act in concert to co-ordinate the somatomotor events involved in expelling gastric contents. Nonvomiting species (such as rodents and rabbits) also have the brainstem nuclei and motor systems necessary for emesis but lack the complex synaptic interaction among nuclei and viscera required for a co-ordinated reflex.

The concept of a discrete vomiting center within the reticular formation of the medulla oblongata has been challenged. However, whether it is a discrete anatomical center or represents sequential activation of a series of effector nuclei, the important concept is that the medulla has a central co-ordinating role in emesis.

The vomiting center receives input from vagal and sympathetic neurones, the CTZ in the area postrema, the vestibular apparatus and the cerebral cortex. It may also be stimulated directly by blood-borne toxins that can cross the blood–brain barrier.

The receptors that have been identified as important in the vomiting center are 5-hydroxytryptamine (5-HT)$_{1A}$, α_2-adrenergic receptors and neurokinin-1 (NK$_1$) receptors which are receptors for substance P. Drugs such as buspirone act as antiemetics by acting as antagonists at 5-HT$_{1A}$ receptors. Antiemetics such as prochlorperazine block α-adrenergic receptors. Maropitant (Cerenia®) acts at NK$_1$ receptors.

Central stimulation

Central stimulation of the vomiting center occurs via higher centers in the central nervous system. Stimuli include nervousness, unpleasant odors, pain and psychogenic factors. Opioids and benzodiazepine receptors

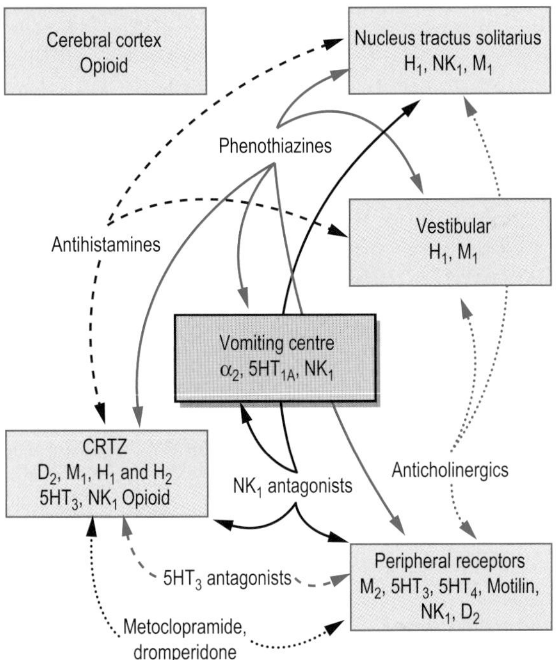

Fig. 19.1 **Diagrammatic representation of receptors involved in emesis and sites of action of antiemetics.**

have been implicated in centrally initiated vomiting but have not been well characterized pharmacologically.

The role of opioid receptors in emesis is confusing. Various studies have demonstrated that opioids have an emetic action in dogs and cats. However, opioids have been used in humans and animals to reduce nausea and vomiting associated with cancer chemotherapy. This apparent paradox is caused by a differential effect of opioids on the CTZ and the vomiting center. If an opioid penetrates the vomiting center it may strongly block the vomiting reflex. However, if an opioid penetrates the CTZ first it will initially cause vomiting before blocking the vomiting center. Morphine has been demonstrated to have this dual effect (although it may also cause vomiting because of histamine release).

Centrally induced vomiting may also occur as a result of direct stimulation of the vomiting center by increased cerebrospinal fluid pressure, encephalitis or CNS neoplasia.

Vestibular apparatus

Labyrinthine impulses associated with motion sickness and middle-ear infection also stimulate the vomiting center via neural pathways arising from the vestibular system. The CTZ is involved in this pathway in the dog but not in the cat.

The neuronal pathways for motion sickness have not been completely characterized. M_1-cholinergic, H_1-histaminergic and NK_1 receptors must be involved in the dog because antagonists at these receptors are very effective antiemetic agents. D_2-dopaminergic, α_2-adrenergic and 5-HT_3 receptors are not involved.

Chemoreceptor trigger zone (CTZ)

The CTZ is located in the area postrema in the floor of the fourth ventricle. It has no blood–brain barrier, thus allowing access to toxins and chemicals normally excluded from the CNS by the blood–brain barrier. The CTZ is stimulated by endogenous toxic substances produced in acute infectious diseases or metabolic disorders such as uremia and diabetic ketoacidosis and by drugs and other exogenous toxins.

A variety of neurotransmitters and their receptors are important in the CTZ, including dopamine, adrenaline (epinephrine), 5-HT, acetylcholine, histamine, encephalins and substance P. Species differ in the relative importance of some neurotransmitter–receptor systems. For example, apomorphine, a D_2-dopamine receptor agonist, is a potent emetic in dogs and humans but not in the cat, monkey, pig, horse or domestic fowl. This suggests that D_2-dopamine receptor antagonists such as metoclopramide might not be very useful as antiemetics in the cat.

In contrast, xylazine, an α_2-adrenergic agonist, is a more potent emetic in the cat than the dog. Cytotoxic drug-induced emesis has been shown to be mediated directly by 5-HT_3 receptors in the CTZ of the cat, in contrast to the dog, in which peripheral visceral and vagal afferent 5-HT_3 receptors are activated.

Histamine receptors have not been demonstrated in the CTZ of the cat. Studies based on eliminating the emetic response to parenterally administered compounds by lesioning the CTZ suggest that the CTZ may be less sensitive to emetic compounds in the cat than in the dog. Alternatively, other sites for the origin of emesis may be more important in the cat than the dog.

Peripheral receptors

Peripheral receptors are located mainly in the gastrointestinal tract, particularly the duodenum but also in the biliary tract, peritoneum and urinary organs. The receptors may be stimulated by distension, irritation, inflammation or changes in osmolarity.

Afferent receptors

Of the many afferent receptors found in the gut, 5-HT_3 receptors play an important role in initiation of vomiting by cytotoxic drugs. Cytotoxic drugs cause 5-HT release from enterochromaffin cells that activates 5-HT_3 receptors on vagal afferent fibers. 5-HT_3 receptor antagonists are very effective antiemetics for cytotoxic drug-induced vomiting. However, the role of 5-HT_3 receptors in other disorders of the gut has yet to be ascertained.

Efferent receptors

Vagal efferent receptors and myenteric neurones initiate the complex excitation and inhibition of visceral smooth muscle that culminates in emesis. Receptors involved include D_2-dopaminergic, 5-HT_4 serotonergic, M_2-cholinergic, NK_1 and motilin receptors.

CLASSES OF ANTIEMETICS

Phenothiazines

EXAMPLES

Prochlorperazine (e.g. Stemetil®, Compazine®, Darbazine®), chlorpromazine (e.g. Thorazine®)

Clinical applications

Phenothiazines are broad-spectrum antiemetics that have efficacy against vomiting initiated by central and peripheral stimuli.

Mechanism of action

Phenothiazines antagonize α_1- and α_2-adrenergic receptors, D_2-dopaminergic receptors, H_1- and H_2-histaminergic receptors and muscarinic cholinergic receptors (weakly). They therefore have antiemetic activity (see Fig. 19.1) at the CTZ (D_2-receptors, H_1- and H_2-receptors and muscarinic cholinergic receptors) and at high doses at the vomiting center (α_2-receptors).

Prochlorperazine is a piperazine phenothiazine with less sedative action than other phenothiazines such as acepromazine and chlorpromazine. In contrast to acepromazine, chlorpromazine has antiemetic efficacy at doses low enough to avoid sedation.

Formulations and dose rates

In most countries, prochlorperazine is only available in human-approved formulations (e.g. Stemetil®, Compazine®) such as prochlorperazine edisylate (injectable or oral syrup), prochlorperazine maleate (tablets) or prochlorperazine base (rectal suppositories). There are few, if any, countries where chlorpromazine is available as a veterinary-approved product.

DOGS AND CATS

Prochlorperazine

- 0.1–0.5 mg/kg IV, IM, SC q.6-8 h
- 0.5–1.0 mg/kg PO q.8-12 h

NB: Intramuscular injection may be painful but not to a degree that precludes administration by this route in most patients if necessary.

Chlorpromazine

- 0.1–0.5 mg/kg IM, SC q.8 h

Pharmacokinetics

Little information is available regarding the pharmacokinetics of prochlorperazine in animals, although it is believed to follow the general pattern of metabolism and elimination of other phenothiazine agents, i.e. metabolism in the liver with both conjugated and unconjugated metabolites eliminated in the urine. Although chlorpromazine is absorbed well from the gastrointestinal tract, it has a high first-pass metabolism. In the circulation, chlorpromazine is highly bound to plasma proteins – in humans the half-life is 36 h.

Adverse effects

- Phenothiazines may cause hypotension because of central effects and an α-adrenergic receptor-blocking action resulting in arteriolar vasodilation. Therefore, they should not be included at high doses in a therapeutic regime until dehydration is corrected by intravenous fluid therapy. They should not be given as an undiluted intravenous bolus.
- Sedation may occur at high doses.
- Similarly to other phenothiazines, it is believed that prochlorperazine may lower the seizure threshold. There is anecdotal evidence in the literature that this occasionally occurs.
- Extrapyramidal reactions such as rigidity, tremors, weakness and restlessness may occur at high doses.

Known drug interactions

- It has been stated that phenothiazines should not be given within 1 month of worming with an organophosphate agent as the effect of either drug may be potentiated. Whether this is a realistic clinical problem is debatable.
- Other CNS-active drugs such as barbiturates, narcotics and anesthetic agents may cause additive CNS depression.
- Quinidine given with phenothiazines may cause additive cardiac depression.
- Antidiarrheal mixtures containing kaolin and pectin and antacids may cause reduced absorption of orally administered phenothiazines.
- Increased blood concentrations of both drugs may occur if propranolol is administered with phenothiazines.
- As phenothiazines block α-adrenergic receptors, if adrenaline (epinephrine) is administered concurrently, unopposed β-adrenergic effects will occur, causing vasodilation and tachycardia.
- Phenytoin metabolism may be decreased if given concurrently with phenothiazines.
- The following drugs that might conceivably be used concurrently with prochlorperazine or chlorpromazine (other drugs may also be incompatible) are

reported to be incompatible in solution: amphotericin B, ampicillin sodium, chloramphenicol sodium succinate, dimenhydrinate, hydrocortisone sodium succinate, penicillin G sodium, phenobarbital sodium. Chlorothiazide sodium and methicillin are also incompatible with chlorpromazine. In addition, do not mix with other drugs or diluents containing parabens as preservatives.

Metoclopramide

Clinical applications

Metoclopramide is indicated for control of vomiting associated with:

- various emesis-inducing disorders involving either stimulation of the CTZ or depressed gastrointestinal motility
- cancer chemotherapy
- gastroesophageal reflux
- decreased gastric emptying associated with:
  - inflammatory gastrointestinal disorders
  - gastric ulcers
  - gastric neoplasia
  - autonomic neuropathy (diabetes mellitus)
  - postoperative gastric dilation and volvulus surgery/intervention
  - abnormal gastric motility.

Although metoclopramide is sometimes recommended for endoscopic procedures to facilitate passage of the endoscope through the pylorus, this effect was not confirmed in a well-controlled study of the effect of pharmacological agents on the ease of endoscopic intubation in dogs. In fact, increased antral motility caused by metoclopramide makes endoscopic intubation more difficult.

Mechanism of action

Centrally, metoclopramide antagonizes D_2-dopaminergic receptors and 5-HT_3 serotonergic receptors and has a peripheral cholinergic effect. The antiemetic properties of metoclopramide may be related to 5-HT_3 receptor antagonism rather than D_2-receptor antagonism, even though it has been classified for many years as an antidopaminergic drug. The evidence supporting reassessment of its mode of action includes the observation that analogs of metoclopramide have been developed that are effective antiemetics but show little or no dopamine antagonism. They are very specific 5-HT_3 antagonists and it is therefore believed that the serotonin-antagonist effects of metoclopramide account for a large part of its antiemetic effects. However, antidopaminergic mechanisms are still believed to play a role in the antiemetic action of metoclopramide.

Metoclopramide is commonly believed to cause increased gastric emptying, primarily through antagonism of peripheral D_2-receptors, although enhanced cholinergic activity may also be involved. However, there is evidence from some animal studies that the gastrointestinal effects of metoclopramide may be disassociated from its dopamine receptor-blocking action. Intact vagal innervation is not necessary for enhanced motility but anticholinergic drugs will negate its effects. Metoclopramide has also been demonstrated to have anticholinesterase effects and there are suggestions that this drug sensitizes gastrointestinal smooth muscle to the effects of acetylcholine.

Gastrointestinal effects include increased tone and amplitude of gastric contractions, relaxation of the pyloric sphincter and increased duodenal and jejunal peristalsis. Gastric emptying and intestinal transit times can be significantly reduced. There is little or no effect on colonic motility.

A beneficial effect of metoclopramide could not be demonstrated in dogs with gastric dilation and volvulus and delayed gastric emptying treated with metoclopramide postsurgically. However, as the study involved use of liquids rather than solids, it might have been difficult to demonstrate an effect even if gastric motility was enhanced.

Metoclopramide will also increase lower esophageal pressure and reduce gastroesophageal reflux. This effect is abolished by diphenhydramine. The increased lower esophageal pressure induced by metoclopramide is not sufficient to prevent gastric reflux in anesthetized dogs, although it does lower the risk.

Studies have indicated that metoclopramide has a biphasic effect on ureteral motility, increasing motility at low doses and inhibiting it at high doses. Semen volume is reported to be reduced in dogs treated with metoclopramide but sperm number was not significantly affected.

Formulations and dose rates

Metoclopramide is available as a veterinary preparation in tablet and injectable formulations in some countries (e.g. Australia) but only as a human preparation in others (e.g. USA, UK). Metoclopramide is photosensitive and should be stored in light-resistant containers at room temperature.

DOGS AND CATS

- 0.2–0.5 mg/kg IM, SC, PO q.6–8 h
- 1–2 mg/kg IV infusion over 24 h

The efficacy of metoclopramide is believed to be enhanced by administering 1–2 mg/kg/d by a constant-rate infusion instead of intermittent boluses.

When used to treat disorders of gastric motility and esophageal reflux, metoclopramide should be administered at a dose of 0.2–0.5 mg/kg PO 30 min before meals.

Pharmacokinetics

Metoclopramide is well absorbed from the gastrointestinal tract in humans and dogs. In humans, bioavailability can be reduced by up to 30% in some patients as a result of first-pass metabolism; this effect is quite variable among individuals. One study suggested that similarly, in dogs, the liver plays an active role in reducing the systemic availability of metoclopramide after oral administration. In a study of two greyhounds, bioavailability of metoclopramide after oral administration was about 48%. Bioavailability after intramuscular injection in humans is 74–96%.

The plasma half-life of metoclopramide in the dog is approximately 90 min. In contrast to humans, in whom glucuronidation and sulfate conjugation are the major metabolic pathways, *N*-demethylation is more important for metoclopramide metabolism in dogs.

Adverse effects

Side effects are uncommon but occur more often in cats than in dogs.

- Metoclopramide may cause (infrequently) mental changes ranging from hyperactivity to depression.
- Cats will infrequently show disorientated or frenzied behavior.
- Metoclopramide should not be used when gastrointestinal hemorrhage, obstruction or perforation is suspected.
- This drug is relatively contraindicated in patients with seizure disorders.
- Use with caution in patients with renal insufficiency because some reports suggest that metoclopramide reduces renal blood flow and may exacerbate pre-existing disease.

Known drug interactions

- Excellent synergy (as a result of their different modes of action) can be obtained in the management of persistent vomition using metoclopramide and phenothiazines concurrently. However, because of the potential for enhanced CNS effects, metoclopramide should be used with care with phenothiazines, butyrophenones and opioid analgesics.
- Anticholinergic drugs (e.g. atropine) and narcotic analgesics may negate the effects of metoclopramide on gastrointestinal tract motility.
- The gastrointestinal stimulatory effects of metoclopramide may affect absorption of many drugs. Drug products that disintegrate, dissolve or are absorbed in the stomach, such as digoxin, may be absorbed less, although the increased vigor of antral contractions can also hasten disintegration.
- Metoclopramide may enhance the absorption of drugs that are absorbed primarily in the small intestine, e.g. cimetidine, aspirin, tetracyclines, diazepam.
- Given that metoclopramide can accelerate the absorption of nutrients, insulin requirements may be influenced in diabetic animals.
- Metoclopramide antagonizes the antiprolactinemic effects of cabergoline.

Domperidone

Clinical applications

Domperidone is a dopamine antagonist at D_2-receptors which has similar actions to metoclopramide. It does not appear to cross as readily into the CNS as metoclopramide and therefore is believed not to have the same CNS effects as that drug. However, extrapyramidal adverse effects have been observed in some human patients.

Mechanism of action

Domperidone is a dopamine antagonist in the CTZ and GI tract. It also is an α_2- and β_2-adrenergic antagonist in the stomach.

Formulations and dose rates

Domperidone is not available as a veterinary preparation in any market but is available as a human preparation (Motilium®) and used quite extensively in some European countries. It is available as 10 mg tablets and a 1 mg/mL suspension and in some markets as suppositories and an oral suspension.

DOGS AND CATS

- 2–5 mg per animal q.8 h

Pharmacokinetics

Domperidone is absorbed from the GI tract but has an oral bioavailability of only 20% in the dog. This is presumably due to a high first-pass effect. The drug is highly protein bound (93%). Peak levels occur about 2 h after dosing. Metabolites are excreted in urine and feces.

Adverse effects

- There is little information on the use of domperidone in veterinary medicine.
- It may cause gastroparesis.
- Because domperidone is a potential substrate of P-glycoprotein, it should be used with caution in herding breeds such as collies which may have the gene mutation that causes a nonfunctional protein.
- The drug is teratogenic at high doses in mice, rats and rabbits.

- Because dopamine is involved in prolactin production, domperidone may increase prolactin levels resulting in galactorrhea or gynecomastia.
- There may be an impact on fertility as a result of domperidone's effect on prolactin levels.
- Injectable formulations have been associated with cardiac arrhythmias in human patients with cardiac disease or hypokalemia.
- Rarely, somnolence or dystonic reactions have occurred in people.

Known drug interactions

Domperidone should not be used with dopaminergic drugs such as dopamine or dobutamine.

NK_1 receptor antagonists

EXAMPLE

Maropitant (Cerenia®)

Clinical applications

Maropitant is the first drug of its class registered (in some markets) for veterinary use. It is indicated for the prevention and treatment of general emesis in the dog and the prevention of motion sickness in the dog.

In laboratory studies, the drug was highly effective in preventing and treating vomiting induced by apomorphine (centrally acting purely at the CTZ), cisplatin (central and peripheral emetic stimulus) and ipecac (peripheral emetic stimulus) at a dose of 1 mg/kg SC or 2 mg/kg PO.

Efficacy has also been demonstrated in field studies. Maropitant was significantly more effective in reducing emetic events in dogs treated for acute vomiting than metoclopramide; the proportion of dogs not vomiting within 24 h was 92% for maropitant and 50% for metoclopramide, a difference that was statistically significant. In relation to prevention of cisplatin-induced emesis, only two of 39 dogs treated with maropitant 1 h prior to cisplatin treatment vomited compared with 39 of 41 dogs who vomited when treated with saline alone prior to cisplatin treatment. Maropitant was also successful in treating cisplatin-induced vomiting, i.e. when the drug was given *after* cisplatin-induced vomiting commenced.

Maropitant also has efficacy in preventing motion sickness but a higher dose is required. In a small field study, motion sickness was prevented in the majority of (but not all) dogs with recurrent and persistent motion sickness only at a dose of 8 mg/kg PO. The higher dose of maropitant required to prevent emesis associated with motion sickness is likely to be related to the different input to the vomiting center (vestibular system), compared with the neural and humoral inputs associated with general emesis.

Mechanism of action

Maropitant is a selective antagonist of substance P at the NK_1 receptor. Some studies would suggest the antagonism is competitive. However, other studies suggest the inhibition is nonsurmountable. It inhibits the final common pathway involved in activating the vomiting reflex in the CNS and is effective against emesis induced by both peripheral and central stimuli.

Formulations and dose rates

DOGS

Prevention or treatment of emesis due to central or peripheral stimuli

- 2 mg/kg PO, once daily for up to 5 d
- 1 mg/kg SC, once daily for up to 5 d

Prevention of motion sickness

- 8 mg/kg PO, once daily for a maximum of two consecutive days

Pharmacokinetics

Oral bioavailability is 23.7% at a 2 mg/kg dose rate and 37% at 8 mg/kg. The difference suggests that first-pass metabolism is proportionally greater at the 8 mg/kg dose, possibly due to saturation of a high-affinity, low-capacity enzyme system (or efflux pump system) limiting access of the drug to the systemic circulation at the 2 mg/kg dose. Feeding does not affect oral bioavailability at the 2 mg/kg dose rate. Bioavailability when given subcutaneously is 90.7%.

Maropitant is metabolized by first-order kinetics in the liver by two enzyme systems: CYP2D15 (high affinity, responsible for >90% of clearance) and CYP3A12 (low affinity, high capacity). Hepatic clearance is the major route of excretion; there is no evidence of excretion of active drug or its major metabolite.

Adverse effects

Post-dosing emesis occurs in approximately 8% of dogs treated at the 8 mg/kg dose rate for the prevention of motion sickness. This is believed to be due to a local effect of the drug on the GI tract and can be reduced by dosing after consumption of a small amount of food.

Known drug interactions

- In laboratory and field studies significant drug interactions are unlikely to occur due to its margin of safety and well-characterized pharmacokinetics.
- Significant hepatic dysfunction could interfere with metabolism and elimination of maropitant but the

wide margin of safety for the drug suggests that this may not have clinically relevant adverse effects.

5-HT_3 antagonists

EXAMPLES

Ondansetron (Zofran®), granisetron (Kytril®), dolasetron (Carpuject®, Anzemet®, Anemet®, Zamanon®) and tropisetron

Clinical applications

The 5-HT_3 receptor antagonists are extremely potent (and expensive) antiemetics used in the management of cancer therapy-induced emesis in humans. Their clinical efficacy is orders of magnitude better than metoclopramide (e.g. 100 times better in the ferret) and they are often used in cases when 'first-line' antiemetics (e.g. metoclopramide or chlorpromazine) are ineffective. In this regard, these drugs can often control vomiting in puppies with parvoviral gastroenteritis. They have been used occasionally in dogs to control cisplatin-induced emesis but cost is prohibitive for most veterinary clinical situations.

Mechanism of action

5-HT_3 receptors are located in the CTZ and, peripherally, on vagal nerve terminals and on enteric neurones in the gastrointestinal tract. Although initially 5-HT_3 antagonists were thought to have a central action on the CTZ, recent work suggests that their main effect is through antagonism of peripheral 5-HT_3 receptors in the gut. This is supported by work demonstrating that chemotherapy-induced vomiting is caused by serotonin release from small intestinal enterochromaffin cells.

Formulations and dose rates

Most veterinary experience has been with ondansetron; most of the other drugs have not had extensive use at the current time. No veterinary formulations of any of these drugs are available.

ONDANSETRON

Ondansetron is available both as injectable and as tablet formulations.

DOGS

Prevention of cisplatin-induced vomiting

- 0.5 mg/kg IV as a loading dose and then 0.5 mg/kg/h as an infusion for 6 h
- 0.1 mg/kg PO q.12–24 h or at 30 min prior to and 90 min after cisplatin infusion

For intractable vomiting, when first-line drugs are ineffective

- 0.1–0.176 mg/kg q.6–12 h as a slow intravenous push
- 0.5–1.0 mg/kg PO once or twice daily

CATS

The use of ondansetron in cats is controversial and many pharmacologists do not recommend its use in this species.

OTHER 5-HT_3 ANTAGONISTS

Dolasetron is also available as both injectable (0.625 mL ampoules) and tablet (50 mg and 100 mg strength) formulations. The size of tablets is inconvenient for most cats and dogs, such that oral ondansetron preparations are preferred.

- 0.5–0.6 mg/kg IV, SC or PO q.24 h

Adverse effects

- Experimental studies suggest that 5-HT_3 antagonists are very safe in animals, showing minimal toxicity at doses up to 30 times greater than those needed to abolish vomiting.
- Given that ondansetron, and related products, are potent antiemetics, their use may mask signs of ileus or gastrointestinal distension. These drugs should be used with caution in cases where gastrointestinal obstruction cannot be excluded because appropriate therapy may be delayed.
- In humans, constipation, headaches, occasional alterations in liver enzymes and rarely hypersensitivity reactions have been reported.
- Dolasetron has also been associated with ECG interval prolongation (of the P-R, Q-T and J-T segments), whilst arrhythmias and hypotension have also been reported for ondansetron.
- Safety of this drug group during gestation has not been clearly established, so the drug should be used with caution in pregnant animals.
- Ondansetron is a potential substrate of P-glycoprotein. Given that some rough collies have a mutation causing a nonfunctional protein, these dogs and associated breeds may be more sensitive to the effects of 5-HT_3 antagonists.

Anticholinergics

EXAMPLES

Atropine, butylscopolamine (hyoscine), propantheline, isopropamide

Clinical applications

Anticholinergics are mainly used for their antispasmodic and antisecretory actions for some types of diarrhea. Given that their use is contradicted in many circumstances, they should be used with caution. These drugs have also been used frequently in the past as antiemetics but usually inappropriately. They are usually not effective unless vomiting is initiated by smooth muscle spasm (an extremely uncommon occurrence). They do not stop vomiting caused by stimulation of peripheral receptors by other means such as inflammation. Those anticholinergic drugs that can cross the blood–brain barrier (e.g. hyoscine) are effective for motion sickness through antagonism of M_1-receptors in the vestibular apparatus.

Anticholinergics have been used in the management of pancreatitis on the basis that they may reduce pancreatic secretion. However, no appreciable benefit has been demonstrated experimentally or clinically from this treatment. In fact, some clinicians consider that their use is contraindicated in pancreatitis because they cause thickening of pancreatic secretions.

Mechanism of action

Anticholinergics act as antagonists at central and peripheral muscarinic receptors (M_1 and M_2). Quaternary ammonium antimuscarinics, such as butylscopolamine and propantheline, do not cross the blood–brain barrier, so have a predominantly peripheral action, and CNS side effects are minimal.

Formulations and dose rates

Atropine sulfate is available as an injectable preparation. No veterinary-approved preparations of propantheline are available, but generic human tablet formulations can be used (7.5 mg, 15 mg). In some countries, butylscopalamine is available, as both injectable and oral preparations (Buscopan®) and also in an injectable formulation in combination with metamizole (dipyrone) (Buscopan Compositum®; 4 mg/mL butylscopalamine, 500 mg/mL metamizole); the latter is a pyrazoline drug with anti-inflammatory, analgesic and antipyretic properties.

Atropine
- The standard dose rate is 0.02–0.04 mg/kg, IM or SC

Propantheline
- The dose for both dogs and cats is 0.25 mg/kg PO q.8 h

Butylscopalamine
- In dogs, the primary indication is as a long-acting antispasmodic at a dose of 0.5 mg/kg IM or PO q.12 h (sole preparations) or 0.1 mg/kg IV or IM (in combination with metamizole)

Adverse effects

- The major problem with anticholinergics is that they also affect M_2-receptors, potentially causing delayed gastric emptying and ileus. This may potentiate vomiting and exacerbate gastric hypomotility, which occurs in many disorders causing vomiting. These drugs should also be avoided in cases suspected to have gastrointestinal obstruction.
- Overuse can result in gastric atony and intestinal ileus, which may predispose to absorption of endotoxins through damaged mucosa.
- Antimuscarinic agents should be used with caution in cases with known or suspected enteric infections, because the reduction in motility may prolong the retention of the causative agent.
- Antimuscarinic agents should also be used with caution in animals with hepatic or renal disease, hyperthyroidism, congestive heart failure, hypertension, concurrent myasthenia gravis, prostatic hypertrophy and in geriatric or pediatric patients.
- Side effects are those expected for antimuscarinics, e.g. xerostomia, dry eyes, hesitant urination, tachycardia and constipation. CNS side effects include stimulation, drowsiness, ataxia, seizures and respiratory depression; however, these effects are unlikely with the quaternary ammonium antimuscarinics. Ocular side effects of this group include mydriasis, cycloplegia and photophobia; again, these side effects are less likely with quaternary ammonium antimuscarinics.

Known drug interactions

- Antimuscarinics can enhance the actions of thiazide diuretics and sympathomimetics and antagonize the effects of metoclopramide.
- Antihistamines, procainamide, quinidine, meperidine, benzodiazepines and phenothiazines can all potentiate the effects of anticholinergics.
- Adverse effects can be exacerbated by corticosteroids, primidone, nitrates and disopyramide.

Antihistamines

EXAMPLES

Diphenhydramine (Benadryl®), dimenhydrinate (Dramamine®)

Clinical applications

Antihistamines are primarily indicated for treatment and prevention of motion sickness in the dog.

Mechanism of action

Antihistamines block histamine receptors in the CTZ and vestibular pathways. Histamine receptors in CTZ are involved in motion sickness in the dog but not in the cat.

In addition to its antihistaminergic effects, diphenhydramine has substantial sedative, anticholinergic, antitussive effects and local anesthetic effects. The anticholinergic action may in fact be the main mechanism by which it is effective in motion sickness, as there are muscarinic receptors in the vestibular system.

Formulations and dose rates

DOGS AND CATS

Diphenhydramine
- 2–4 mg/kg PO, IM q.8-12 h

Dimenhydrinate
- 4–8 mg/kg PO, IM q.8 h

Pharmacokinetics

The pharmacokinetics of these drugs have not been studied in domestic species. In humans diphenhydramine is well absorbed after oral administration but systemic bioavailability is only 40–60% because of first-pass metabolism. Diphenhydramine and dimenhydrinate are metabolized in the liver and largely excreted as metabolites in urine.

Adverse effects

- CNS depression (e.g. lethargy, somnolence, paradoxical excitement – cats). The sedative effects may diminish with time.
- Anticholinergic effects (e.g. dry mouth, urinary retention).
- Gastrointestinal side effects (e.g. vomiting and diarrhea) are uncommon, but have been reported.
- These drugs should be used with caution if pyloric or proximal intestinal obstruction is suspected.
- Use with caution in patients with hyperthyroidism, seizure disorders, cardiovascular disease, hypertension and closed-angle glaucoma; signs of ototoxicity may also be masked by these drugs.

Known drug interactions

Increased sedation can occur if antihistamines are combined with other CNS-depressant drugs. Antihistamines may counteract the anticoagulatory effects of heparin or warfarin. Diphenhydramine may exacerbate the effects of adrenaline (epinephrine).

ANTIULCER DRUGS

Clinical applications

Antiulcer drugs are useful in the specific management of gastrointestinal ulceration and reflux esophagitis. They are not usually needed for treatment of simple acute gastritis.

Relevant pathophysiology

The protective barrier that prevents gastric mucosa from being damaged by gastric acid includes the following factors.

- Mucus, with bicarbonate incorporated into the mucosal gel layer.
- High epithelial turnover (thus a high metabolic rate and oxygen requirement).
- Tight junctions and lipoprotein layer of epithelial cells.
- A rich vascular supply.
- Prostaglandins – PGE series and PGI_2 are protective:
  - inhibit gastric acid secretion
  - maintain mucosal blood flow
  - involved in secretion and composition of healthy mucus
  - may be intercellular messengers for stimulus of mucosal cell turnover and migration.

Gastrointestinal ulceration may be associated with a number of events.

- Drugs (aspirin, phenylbutazone, corticosteroids)
- Uremia (toxins, increased gastrin)
- Liver disease (cause not known)
- Stress
- Increased production of HCl (mast cell tumor at any site, gastrin-producing tumor of the pancreas (Zollinger–Ellison syndrome))
- Hypotension, e.g. during surgery, hypoadrenocorticism
- Spinal cord disease

Interruption of the gastric mucosal barrier allows back-diffusion of gastric acid into the submucosa, which causes mast cell degranulation, resulting in histamine release and subsequent further stimulation of acid production by gastric parietal cells, which enhances inflammation and edema in the submucosa. The aim of antiulcer therapy is to repair the mucosal barrier directly, reduce the amount of gastric acid produced or neutralize its effect and hence stop the vicious cycle of gut damage.

A number of classes of antiulcer drugs are available and numerous agents are available within each class. There are differences in mechanism of action amongst groups and in potency amongst individual agents. However, there is little information as to whether the reported differences in potency relate to real differences in clinical efficacy. An example is a recent study in healthy laboratory dogs, which examined changes in luminal pH after administration of four acid-blocking drugs: ranitidine, famotidine, omeprazole and pantoprazole. Famotidine, pantoprazole and omeprazole significantly suppressed gastric acid secretion, compared with saline solution, as determined by median 24-h pH, and percentages of time pH was ≥3 or ≥4. However, ranitidine did not. Of the four agents examined, twice-daily omeprazole was most effective in suppressing gastric acid secretion. Although this suggests that proton pump inhibitors are the agents of choice, the study involved healthy laboratory animals and it is not clear whether the criteria used in the study (luminal pH) were those which were most important in determining clinical efficacy.

CLASSES OF ANTIULCER DRUGS

Histamine-receptor antagonists

EXAMPLES

Cimetidine (Zitac®, Tagamet®), ranitidine (Zantac®), famotidine (Pepcid®), nizatidine (Axid®)

Clinical applications

The histamine-receptor antagonists have efficacy in treating gastric ulceration caused by a variety of disorders, including nonsteroidal anti-inflammatory drugs (NSAIDs) and uremia. However, they do not appear to be effective in preventing NSAID-induced ulcers. Ranitidine and nizatidine are also used as prokinetic agents (see below).

Mechanism of action

These drugs act as competitive inhibitors at the histamine (H_2) receptors on gastric parietal cells. H_2-receptors, when occupied by histamine and in the presence of acetylcholine and gastrin, stimulate maximal acid secretion. The H_2-receptor is the dominant receptor for stimulation of acid secretion. H_2-receptor antagonists cause a 70–90% decrease in gastric acid production. Ranitidine is reported to suppress gastric acid production to a greater extent than cimetidine (90% versus 75%); similarly, famotidine is more effective at suppressing acid secretion than is ranitidine. However, this does not appear to result in improved clinical efficacy in dogs. By decreasing the amount of gastric acid produced, H_2-antagonists also proportionally decrease pepsin secretion.

Cimetidine and famotidine have no effect on lower esophageal pressure or gastric emptying time and none of these agents affects pancreatic secretion or biliary secretion. However, ranitidine and nizatidine increase lower esophageal sphincter pressure and have anticholinesterase activity which significantly enhances gastrointestinal motility (by increasing the amount of acetylcholine supplied to muscarinic receptors). Nizatidine may also have direct agonist effects on M_3-muscarinic receptors. In fact, nizatidine is more commonly used primarily for its prokinetic activity than as an acid-blocking drug.

Cimetidine has an apparent immunomodulatory effect as it has been demonstrated to reverse suppressor T cell-mediated immune suppression by blocking H_2-receptors on suppressor T lymphocytes. It also increases lymphocyte response to mitogen stimulation. This effect has been used clinically in the treatment of malignant melanomas in people and gray horses. Cimetidine also possesses weak antiandrogenic activity.

Formulations and dose rates

DOGS AND CATS

Cimetidine
- 5–10 mg/kg PO, IV q.6–8 h

Ranitidine
- 1–2 mg/kg PO, SC, IV q.8-12 h

Famotidine
- 0.5–1.0 mg/kg PO, IV q.12–24 h

Nizatidine
- 2.5–5.0 mg/kg PO, IV q.12–24 h

Pharmacokinetics

Cimetidine

Oral bioavailability of cimetidine is reported to be 95% and serum half-life 1.3 h. Inhibition of gastric acid secretion peaks at 75% within 1.5 h and 50% inhibition lasts about 2 h after an oral dose. The effects of the drug are gone after 5 h. Concurrent administration with food delays drug absorption.

Cimetidine decreases hepatic blood flow and inhibits hepatic microsomal enzymes. This can affect the metabolism of other drugs, although the clinical significance of this is uncertain. In humans, cimetidine is both excreted unchanged by the kidneys and metabolized in the liver. More drug is excreted by the kidneys when administered parenterally than when given orally.

Ranitidine

In dogs, the oral bioavailability of ranitidine is approximately 80% and serum half-life is 2.2 h. Food does not affect absorption. Inhibition of gastric acid production peaks at 90% and 50% inhibition lasts about 4 h.

Ranitidine does not inhibit hepatic microsomal enzymes to the same extent as cimetidine. In humans, ranitidine is both excreted in the urine via glomerular filtration and tubular secretion and metabolized in the liver to inactive metabolites.

Famotidine

Famotidine is not completely absorbed after oral administration but hepatic first-pass metabolism is minimal. In humans, the oral bioavailability is approximately 40–50%.

Nizatidine

In dogs, oral absorption is rapid and almost complete and there is minimal hepatic first-pass metabolism. Although food improves oral bioavailability, the difference is not thought to be clinically relevant. Nizatidine is metabolized in the liver to a number of metabolites and at least one of these may have activity.

Adverse effects

- In animals, adverse effects appear rare at the doses commonly used.
- In humans, side effects of cimetidine such as gynecomastia and antiandrogenic activity and CNS signs (mental confusion, lethargy and seizures) have been reported.
- Occasionally, agranulocytosis may occur.
- Transient cardiac arrhythmias may occur if cimetidine, ranitidine or famotidine are given intravenously.
- Long-term used of H_2-antagonists could cause hypoacidity and bacterial overgrowth in the stomach but there is no clinical evidence that this is a serious concern. There is no evidence that rebound hypersecretion occurs after stopping therapy with cimetidine or ranitidine.
- Cimetidine has been reported to cause a cutaneous drug eruption in a cat.
- The dose of the H_2-antagonists should be reduced by 50% in patients with impaired renal function.

Known drug interactions

- Cimetidine can decrease hepatic microsomal enzyme systems and thus theoretically can decrease hepatic metabolism of various drugs, including benzodiazepines, barbiturates, propranolol, calcium channel blockers, metronidazole, phenytoin, quinidine, theophylline and warfarin. This has been demonstrated in the dog in a study of the pharmacokinetics of verapamil when cimetidine was administered concurrently. The clinical significance of this effect has not been established, although there are anecdotal reports of cimetidine therapy adversely affecting dogs receiving phenobarbital. Ranitidine inhibits microsomal enzyme systems to a much lesser (5–10-fold) degree.
- Cimetidine and ranitidine may decrease the renal excretion of procainamide.
- Famotidine may exacerbate leukopenias if given concurrently with other bone marrow-suppressing agents.
- Nizatidine may increase salicylate levels in patients taking high doses of aspirin.
- Anticholinergic agents (e.g. atropine and propantheline) may negate the prokinetic effects of ranitidine and nizatidine.
- The increased intragastric pH associated with H_2-antagonist administration may reduce the absorption of drugs that require an acid medium for dissolution and absorption, such as ketoconazole.
- It is recommended that at least 2 h elapses between dosing with cimetidine and giving antacids, metoclopramide, digoxin or ketoconazole.

Sucralfate

Clinical applications

Sucralfate is indicated for the symptomatic treatment of gastric ulceration from various causes. In humans, sucralfate is as effective as antacids or H_2-receptor antagonists in healing ulcers. It does not appear to be successful, however, in preventing corticosteroid-induced ulceration in dogs subjected to spinal surgery. Its efficacy in preventing NSAID-induced ulcers is unproven in the dog. Sucralfate has also been used to treat oral and esophageal ulcers and esophagitis.

Mechanism of action

Sucralfate is composed of sucrose octasulfate and aluminum hydroxide, which dissociate in the acid environment of the stomach. Minimal systemic absorption of either compound occurs. Sucralfate is structurally related to heparin but does not possess any appreciable anticoagulant activity. It is also structurally related to sucrose but is not used as a sugar by the body.

When given orally, sucrose octasulfate reacts with hydrochloric acid and is polymerized to a viscous sticky substance that binds to the proteinaceous exudate usually found at ulcer sites. Because of electrostatic charges, sucralfate preferentially adheres to ulcerated tissues. It protects the ulcer against hydrogen ion back-diffusion, pepsin and bile and therefore promotes ulcer healing. The aluminum hydroxide theoretically neutralizes gastric acid but this antacid activity is not believed to be clinically important.

It was believed that the formation of a physical protective barrier was the major mechanism by which sucralfate assisted ulcer healing. However, it is now believed that the major drug actions of sucralfate are related to stimulation of mucosal defense and reparative mechanisms, possibly related to stimulation of local PGE_2 and PGI_2 production. Sucralfate also inactivates pepsin, adsorbs bile acids and is believed to be cytoprotective by stimulating prostaglandin synthesis. It does not significantly affect gastric acid output but may slow gastric emptying appreciably.

Formulations and dose rates

LARGE DOGS
- 1 g PO q.8 h

SMALL DOGS
- 0.5 g PO q.8 h

CATS
- 0.25–0.5 g PO q.8–12 h

It is preferable to administer sucralfate at least 60 min prior to feeding.

Pharmacokinetics

Only 3–5% of an oral dose of sucralfate is absorbed and this is excreted unchanged in urine within 48 h. The remainder of the drug is excreted in feces within 48 h. Sucralfate binds to the ulcer site for up to 6 h after oral dosing.

Adverse effects

- Because very little drug is absorbed systemically, no systemic toxicities have been reported.
- The only reported side effect in humans is constipation.

Known drug interactions

- Recommendations vary concerning whether concurrent administration of H_2-antagonists decreases sucralfate dissolution. Although it was believed that sucralfate required an acid environment for dissolution, a study in rats indicated that sucralfate prevented mucosal injury in both acidic and neutral environments. However, as there are no definitive studies in dogs and cats, it is probably prudent where practical to administer sucralfate 30 min before an H_2-antagonist if both drugs are used.
- Sucralfate may have the ability to bind other drugs but no clinically important drug interactions have been reported. However, it is recommended that drugs such as tetracyclines, digoxin, fluoroquinolones and aminophylline should not be given within 2 h of administering sucralfate.
- Sucralfate can bind to and interfere with the absorption of fat-soluble vitamins (e.g. A, D, E and K). Therefore, avoid giving this medication concurrently with enteral feeding preparations.

Misoprostol

Clinical applications

Misoprostol (Cytotec®) is a synthetic prostaglandin (PGE_1). In human medicine, there are conflicting data about whether misoprostol is as effective as H_2-antagonists in healing ulcers. It is, however, most useful for prevention of NSAID-induced ulceration and its efficacy in this regard has been demonstrated in dogs. This contrasts with the lack of prophylactic efficacy of other antiulcer drugs. However, some studies suggest that it may not be effective in preventing gastric ulceration caused by high-dose glucocorticoid therapy (e.g. methylprednisolone).

Other less common uses include intravaginal administration in conjunction with PGF_2 for pregnancy termination in dogs (mid to late gestation). It has also been reported to be effective in reducing ciclosporin-induced toxicity and one study suggested some efficacy in treatment of atopic dermatitis in dogs.

Mechanism of action

Misoprostol has gastric antisecretory and mucosal protective effects as it acts as a synthetic replacement for PGE_1. PGE_1 inhibits hydrochloric acid through a direct action on gastric parietal cells, by suppressing the activation of histamine-sensitive adenylate cyclase. It also inhibits gastrin secretion and increases gastric mucus formation. It increases blood flow to the mucosa, which increases the oxygen and nutrient supply to the healing mucosa, ultimately enhancing epithelialization.

Formulations and dose rates

Misoprostol is not currently approved for veterinary use in any country. Although the most common recommendation is for q.8 h dosing, a recent study examining effects on aspirin-induced gastric ulceration suggested that q.12 h dosing was as effective.

DOGS
- 2–5 μg/kg PO q.8–12 h

Pharmacokinetics

Misoprostol pharmacokinetics are similar in dogs and humans. It is absorbed extensively after oral administration in dogs, although there is significant first-pass metabolism. It undergoes rapid esterification to its free acid, which is the active form. It is further metabolized in several tissues (biotransformed via oxidation to inactive metabolites) and is excreted mainly in urine. Both misoprostol and its acid are relatively highly protein bound. In humans the serum half-life of misoprostol is about 30 min and its duration of pharmacological effect 3–6 h.

Adverse effects

- Misoprostol can induce parturition or abortion as a result of luteolysis and myometrial contractions and is therefore contraindicated in pregnant animals unless intended as an abortifacient.
- Diarrhea, abdominal pain, flatulence and vomiting are relatively frequent side effects, although they are often transient and resolve over several days. They can be minimized by dosage adjustment and giving the dose with food.
- Life-threatening diarrhea has been reported in humans with inflammatory bowel disease, so it would be prudent to avoid or use the drug with caution in dogs with this disorder.
- Misoprostol should not be used in patients with known hypersensitivity to prostaglandins or prostaglandin analogs.
- Some prostaglandins and prostaglandin analogs (although not misoprostol to date) have precipitated seizures in epileptic humans.

Known drug interactions

- The presence of food decreases the rate but not extent of drug absorption.
- Bioavailability is reduced by concomitant use of antacids but this may not be clinically significant.
- Magnesium-containing antacids may exacerbate diarrhea induced by misoprostol.

Special considerations

Pregnant women should handle the drug with caution (check label warning).

Proton pump inhibitors

EXAMPLES

The main agent used in veterinary medicine is omeprazole (Prilosec®, Losec®). Other drugs in this group are now used in humans (e.g. lansoprazole, pantoprazole) but there is limited information about their use in companion animals.

Clinical applications

Omeprazole has slightly greater efficacy in promoting ulcer healing in humans than H_2-antagonists but is more expensive. Its use in veterinary medicine is usually restricted to refractory ulcers or ulcers associated with gastrinomas or mastocytosis. However, some veterinary gastroenterologists use omeprazole as their first-choice antiulcer drug. Such an approach is supported by the study previously referred to assessing efficacy and duration of gastric acid suppression, by measuring luminal pH, in healthy research dogs; omeprazole and pantoprazole were more effective than either famotidine or ranitidine. Nevertheless, given that the study was in healthy dogs, it is not clear whether the differences noted relate to clinical efficacy.

Excellent long-term clinical outcomes have been reported in humans and dogs with nonresectable gastrinomas treated with omeprazole. Omeprazole has been reported to be useful in dogs in management of severe erosive esophagitis, gastritis or gastric ulcer disease refractory to therapy with H_2-receptor antagonists and sucralfate. It has been used successfully to treat severe erosive esophagitis in one cat but had no effect in two similarly affected cats.

One recent study demonstrated that omeprazole has some efficacy in preventing exercise-induced gastritis in racing Alaskan sled dogs. In another study, omeprazole did not reduce mechanically induced gastric ulceration or prevent aspirin-induced gastritis in dogs, although there was a trend that suggested that omeprazole was more effective than cimetidine in this regard. However, a further study demonstrated limited efficacy, in both treating and preventing gastric mucosal lesions, in dogs with acute degenerative disc disease treated with corticosteroids.

Mechanism of action

Omeprazole, a substituted benzimidazole, is a proton pump inhibitor that binds to and irreversibly blocks H^+/K^+-ATPase, thereby blocking gastric acid secretion. Omeprazole inhibits gastric acid secretion stimulated by any secretagogue, in contrast to H_2-receptor antagonists, which only suppress gastric acid production stimulated by histamine. Because it is a weak base, omeprazole accumulates in the acid compartment of the parietal cell; therefore its effect persists after the drug is no longer detectable in blood. Omeprazole is inactive at physiological pH and so does not affect ATPase elsewhere in the body.

Omeprazole has a longer duration of action than the H_2-antagonists and most recommendations are for once-daily dosing. However, a recent study reported that twice-daily omeprazole maintained gastric lumen $pH > 3$ throughout a 24-h period, whereas q.24 h dosing did not. Whether it is necessary to maintain $pH > 3$ to achieve effective ulcer healing is not clear. Given the cost and convenience of once-daily dosing, this protocol is likely to remain the most common approach, with more frequent dosing used for refractory cases only.

The antisecretory effects increase with each dose until the drug attains a steady-state inhibition. In dogs, gastric acid output is reduced by about 30% in the first 24 h after an oral dose of 0.7 mg/kg and after five doses gastric acid production is almost completely inhibited.

Formulations and dose rates

Omeprazole is labeled for equine use in some countries but not, to the authors' knowledge, for small animal use. The drug is rapidly degraded by acid, so is formulated as 20 mg enteric-coated granules in a gelatin capsule. For dogs less than 20 kg, the enteric-coated granules must be repackaged in a gelatin capsule.

DOGS
- 0.5–1.0 mg/kg PO q.24 h (for ulcer management). Consider q.12 h dosing in refractory cases. A pragmatic dosing schedule has been recommended as follows:
  one 20 mg capsule daily for dogs weighing more than 20 kg
  0.5 × 20 mg capsule daily for dogs weighing less than 20 kg
  0.25 × 20 mg capsule daily for dogs weighing less than 5 kg
- 0.7–2.0 mg/kg PO q.12–24 h (for esophagitis)

CATS
- 0.7 mg/kg PO q.24 h (for ulcer management).

Pharmacokinetics
Omeprazole is rapidly absorbed from the gut and distributed widely but primarily in gastric parietal cells. It is metabolized extensively in the liver to at least six different metabolites, which are excreted principally in the urine and also via bile into feces. Significant hepatic dysfunction can reduce the first-pass effect of the drug, increasing the systemically available drug and prolonging its duration of action. Omeprazole inhibits hepatic microsomal enzymes to a similar degree to cimetidine.

Adverse effects
- There is limited information on veterinary use of omeprazole but anecdotal reports suggest that it is well tolerated in dogs and cats.
- The main potential side effects include gastrointestinal signs (anorexia, nausea, vomiting, flatulence, diarrhea), hematological abnormalities, urinary tract infections, proteinuria and CNS disturbances.
- Long-term therapy has been reported to cause reversible gastric hypertrophy in dogs because of the trophic effect of gastrin. Gastric hypertrophy has not been detected in dogs treated for 20 d.
- In rats, long-term therapy is reported to cause gastric hypertrophy and carcinoids. Similar changes have been found with long-term ranitidine therapy. There is a concern that similar changes may develop after long-term therapy in other species. However, given that similar changes have not been detected in humans, the relevance of this side effect is not clear. Nevertheless, as in humans, most clinicians do not recommend extending therapy beyond 8 weeks, unless the benefits outweigh potential risks.

Known drug interactions
- Inhibition of P450 hepatic enzymes may decrease hepatic clearance of some drugs such as diazepam, phenytoin and warfarin.
- Drugs that require a low pH for optimal absorption (e.g. ketoconazole, ampicillin) may have reduced absorption, as omeprazole increases gastric pH.
- In humans, omeprazole can occasionally cause bone marrow suppression, which may be exacerbated if used with other drugs that also suppress hematopoiesis.

Nonsystemic antacids

EXAMPLES

Nonsystemic antacids include a variety of oral preparations that contain aluminum hydroxide, calcium carbonate and magnesium compounds.

Clinical applications
Nonsystemic antacids are probably most frequently used in the management of uremia, as aluminum hydroxide binds phosphate, thus reducing hyperphosphatemia as well as having an antacid effect.

Mechanism of action
Nonsystemic antacids act to neutralize hydrochloric acid, bind bile acids, decrease pepsin activity and possibly stimulate local prostaglandin (PGE_1) production. Preparations are usually a combination of aluminum hydroxide and magnesium hydroxide to maximize the buffering capabilities of each compound. Magnesium causes increased bowel motility and aluminum causes decreased motility, which is another reason why the two are usually combined. Both magnesium hydroxide and calcium carbonate have a short, rapid effect; aluminum hydroxide has a slow, persistent effect.

Administration of antacid medications poses difficulties in veterinary patients because of the high volume and frequency of treatment required to prevent rebound acid secretion. Nevertheless, the clinical efficacy of antacid tablets was recently shown to be similar to higher doses of antacid liquids or cimetidine in humans.

Formulations and dose rates

Although inexpensive, nonsystemic antacids must be administered orally (which may be difficult in a vomiting patient) and frequently, which results in poor owner compliance.

- Dosages are empirical as no specific dosages have been defined for animals

Tablets (e.g. aluminum hydroxide 500 mg) can be administered at 10–30 mg/kg PO q.8 h

For liquid preparations (e.g. aluminum hydroxide gel 4% w/v), usual doses are generally in the order of 5–10 mL PO q.8 h

To be effective, antacids must be administered at least every 4 h

Adverse effects

- Calcium-containing antacids tend to promote constipation; magnesium promotes looser feces and aluminum reduces gastric motility and delays gastric emptying.
- If antacids are administered infrequently they may actually result in increased gastric acid production.
- Administration of excessive calcium-containing antacids may predispose to renal calculi.
- Hypophosphatemia and accumulation of aluminum are potential sequelae with long-term use of aluminum-containing antacids.

Known drug interactions

Antacids will interfere with gastric absorption of concurrently administered drugs such as digoxin, tetracyclines and fluoroquinolones.

THERAPY FOR ERADICATION OF *HELICOBACTER* SPP

Helicobacter pylori is the major cause of pyloric ulcer disease in humans. A number of *Helicobacter* species have been shown to colonize the gastric mucosa of cats and dogs, including *H. felis* and *H. heilmanii*, and gastric spiral organisms are often identified during histopathological inspection of gastric mucosal biopsy specimens procured from both symptomatic and asymptomatic companion animals. Therefore, it remains controversial as to whether or not *Helicobacter* species are a significant cause of disease in small animals. Certainly, disease is not the result of simple infection and disease pathogenesis is likely more complicated. Instead, it is thought that these organisms are normal commensal bacteria and that most dogs and cats can tolerate their presence. Current theories on the pathogenesis of *Helicobacter*-associated gastritis center on the hypothesis that disease manifests after a breakdown in mucosal tolerance to *Helicobacter* species. As a consequence, many clinicians choose to eradicate *Helicobacter* species in patients with chronic vomiting and biopsy-proven gastric inflammation.

Treatment usually involves administering a combination of antibacterial and acid-blocking drugs. Numerous combinations have been suggested, but those which have been critically evaluated include the following.

- Amoxicillin (20 mg/kg PO q.12 h for 14 d), metronidazole (20 mg/kg PO q.12 h for 14 d) and famotidine (0.5 mg/kg PO q.12 h for 14 d) in dogs.
- Clarithromycin (30 mg PO q.12 h for 4 d), metronidazole (30 mg PO q.12 h for 4 d), ranitidine (10 mg PO q.12 h for 4 d) and bismuth subsalicylate (40 mg PO q.24 h for 4 d) in *H. heilmanii*-infected cats.
- Azithromycin (30 mg PO q.24 h for 4 d), tinidazole (100 mg PO q.24 h for 4 d), ranitidine (20 mg PO q.24 h for 4 d) and bismuth subsalicylate (20 mg PO q.12 h for 4 d) in *H. heilmanii*-infected cats.
- Amoxicillin (20 mg/kg PO q.8 h for 21 d), metronidazole (20 mg/kg PO q.8 h for 21 d) and omeprazole (0.7 mg PO q.24 h for 21 d) in *H. pylori*-infected cats.
- Amoxicillin (20 mg/kg PO q.12 h for 14 d), clarithromycin (7.5 mg/kg PO q.12 h for 14 d) and metronidazole (10 mg/kg PO q.12 h for 14 d) in *H. pylori*-infected cats.

Thus if a decision is made to eradicate *Helicobacter* species, use of one of the above protocols is recommended.

DRUG COMBINATIONS

Hyoscine and dipyrone

Spasmogesic®, Buscopan® and other trade names describe drug combinations containing the anticholinergic hyoscine and the NSAID dipyrone. Although this combination is relatively commonly used in small animals, its value in the management of gastrointestinal disease is questionable.

The potential concerns with anticholinergic usage in the management of vomiting or diarrhea are discussed elsewhere in this chapter. The potential adverse effects from dipyrone are discussed in Chapter 13 on NSAIDs.

PROKINETIC DRUGS

Treatment of certain conditions such as delayed gastric emptying and suboptimal colonic motility is facilitated by the use of prokinetic drugs. These include metoclopramide (discussed previously), ranitidine (again described previously), erythromycin and cisapride.

Cisapride was previously the prokinetic of choice in small animals. However, this drug was recently implicated in causing adverse cardiac events in people. This is unfortunate given that, in most cases, the patients had pre-existing risk factors and/or were receiving other medications known to inhibit the hepatic CYP3A4 enzyme system and metabolism of cisapride. However, despite this, cisapride has recently been withdrawn from the market in many countries, including the USA and UK. Given that the drug is no longer widely available, its use can no longer be considered. Further, related novel compounds developed as alternatives to cisapride (e.g. prucalopride) have failed to gain approval for similar reasons.

Tegaserod (Zelmac®) is an aminoguanidine indole derivative of serotonin, which has recently become available in North America. It acts as a selective partial agonist highly selective for 5-HT_4 receptors; various studies have demonstrated prokinetic effects including stimulation of peristaltic activity in vitro, increased canine intestinal and colonic motility and transit, reduced visceral afferent firing or sensation in response to distension in animals, accelerated gastric, small bowel and colonic transit in healthy patients and increased small bowel transit in human patients with constipation-predominant irritable bowel syndrome. Thus, in time it may prove to be a suitable alternative to cisapride. However, the authors are not aware of any clinical trials of this drug in companion animals and more work is required before its use can be recommended in veterinary patients.

Erythromycin

Clinical applications

Erythromycin has antibacterial activities (not discussed further here) but at subantimicrobial doses can also be used as a prokinetic. It is used most commonly to improve the rate of gastric emptying, but may also be beneficial in the treatment of esophageal reflux.

Mechanism of action

Erythromycin is a macrolide antibiotic which, at doses below the level required for antimicrobial activity, has prokinetic activities. In many species (e.g. cats, rabbits and humans), the effect is due to the drug acting on motilin and 5-hydroxytryptophan (5-HT_3) receptors, thus stimulating migrating motility complexes and antegrade peristalsis. However, the mechanism of action in dogs is less well understood, but it is most likely via action on 5-HT_3 receptors. Gastric emptying is enhanced by stimulating antral contractions, whilst lower esophageal pressure is also increased. However, given that erythromycin has most effect in stimulating interdigestive activity, beneficial effects on gastric emptying during the digestive phase are less clear.

Formulations and dose rates

Erythromycin is available in numerous preparations as different esters, including erythromycin estolate, erythromycin ethylsuccinate, erythromycin lactobionate and erythromycin gluceptate. Erythromycin is also available as the base form. Oral preparations (tablets, capsule and suspension) are used most commonly for the prokinetic effects. Tablets and capsules usually contain erythromycin as base, stearate ester or ethylsuccinate ester; the suspension usually contains erythromycin ethylsuccinate. It is likely that pharmokinetics and toxicity vary depending upon the exact ester used.

DOGS AND CATS

- 0.5–1.0 mg/kg PO q.8 h

Pharmacokinetics

Erythromycin is absorbed after oral administration in the upper small intestine and a number of factors may influence bioavailability. These include the form of the drug, acidity of the gastrointestinal tract, presence of food and gastric emptying time. Given that the base is acid labile, it should be administered on an empty stomach. Erythromycin is partly metabolized in the liver to inactive metabolites, although most is excreted unchanged through the biliary route. Some active erythromycin is reabsorbed after biliary excretion, potentially prolonging the activity of each dose. The elimination half-life in cats and dogs is estimated to be 60–90 min.

Adverse effects

- The main side effect of erythromycin is vomiting, although this is less common when administered at the doses used for prokinetic effect, and enteric-coated products may further reduce the frequency of vomiting. Other gastrointestinal signs can also be seen, including anorexia and diarrhea.
- When used for its prokinetic effects, clinical signs may deteriorate rather than improve because the drug can stimulate the emptying of larger than normal food particles from the stomach.
- In humans, erythromycin estolate is occasionally associated with cholestatic hepatitis, although such an adverse effect has not been reported in a veterinary species. Nevertheless, as a precaution, this drug should not be given to patients with pre-existing hepatic dysfunction.
- Erythromycin should not be used in patients who are hypersensitive to it.

Known drug interactions

- Erythromycin may increase gastrointestinal absorption of digoxin, potentially leading to digoxin toxicity.

- Erythromycin may increase serum concentrations of theophylline and terfenadine. In humans, this effect is particularly important because this combination has been associated with the development of fatal arrhythmias.
- The metabolism of methylprednisolone may be inhibited and the clearance of theophylline may be increased by concurrent erythromycin administration. The significance of the former interaction is not clear, whilst the interaction with theophylline may lead to theophylline toxicity and close pharmacological monitoring is recommended.
- Erythromycin may prolong prothrombin times and lead to bleeding when given to a patient previously stabilized on warfarin.
- Other reported human drug interactions of erythromycin include ciclosporin, carbemazepine and triazolam. However, the significance of such interactions for veterinary species is less well established.
- Administration of erythromycin may falsely elevate serum concentrations of ALT and AST if colorimetric assays are used and urinary catecholamine measurements may be altered in a similar manner.

LAXATIVES, ENEMAS AND BOWEL CLEANSERS

These drugs are commonly used to evacuate the large bowel and the main pathological indications are constipation and obstipation.

LAXATIVE THERAPY

A number of groups of laxative drugs exist, including bulk-forming laxatives, emollient laxatives, lubricant laxatives, hyperosmotic laxatives and stimulant laxatives.

Bulk-forming laxatives

Most of the available agents in this group are dietary fiber supplements which contain poorly digestible polysaccharides and celluloses. These are mainly derived from cereal grains, wheat bran and psyllium. This group of agents can either be given in a purpose-formulated 'prescription' diet or as a preparation added to the existing diet. Examples include psyllium (Vetasyl®, Metamucil®, Genifiber®, etc.) and sterculia (Peridale®). Dietary fiber supplements are usually well tolerated, more effective and more physiological than the other groups of laxatives.

Psyllium

- **DOGS:** 5 mL (1 teaspoonful) to 30 mL (2 tablespoonfuls) PO q.12–24 h
- **CATS:** 5–20 mL (1–4 teaspoonfuls) PO with each meal

Sterculia

DOGS and CATS

- <5 kg: 1.5 g PO q.24 h
- 5–15 kg: 3 g PO q.12–24 h
- >15 kg: 4 g PO q.12–24 h

Emollient laxatives

Emollient laxatives are anionic detergents that reduce surface tension, thus increasing the miscibility of water and lipid digesta. This thereby increases lipid absorption and impairs the absorption of water. There is some evidence that docusate sodium (dioctyl sodium sulfosuccinate), the main agent used in this group, also increases colonic mucosal cell cAMP concentration and thus increases both ion secretion and fluid permeability. Most of the effect of this drug is local, although some drug is absorbed from the small intestine and then excreted into bile.

Docusate is present as the sole agent in enemas (e.g. Fletcher's enemette, Dioctynate®, Enema-DSS®, Docusoft®, Ther-evac®) and some oral preparations (tablets, capsules and syrups of various strengths) or in combination products with dantron, a fecal softener (e.g. 'co-danthrusate', Docusol®; 50 mg dantron and 60 mg docusate/5 mL). The enema preparations are all veterinary-licensed products, but the oral preparations are not.

Clinical efficacy has not been established definitively. Nevertheless, they are safe agents when used in healthy well-hydrated individuals. However, these preparations should be avoided in patients with pre-existing electrolyte or fluid deficits. These drugs have few reported side effects when used at recommended doses; cramping, diarrhea and intestinal mucosal damage have been reported, whilst liquid oral preparations can sometimes cause pharyngeal irritation. Concurrent administration of mineral oil is not recommended, because enhanced absorption of the oil may occur. If overdose occurs, it is advisable to monitor hydration and systemic electrolyte status. If concurrent administration is essential, it is advisable to stagger dosing by at least 2 h.

Docusate sodium (dioctyl sodium sulfosuccinate)

- **DOGS:** 50–300 mg PO q.12–24 h; 10–15 mL of a 5% solution mixed with 100 mL of water and instilled per rectum
- **CATS:** 50 mg PO q.12–24 h; 2 mL of a 5% solution mixed with 50 mL of water and instilled per rectum

Lubricant laxatives

As their name suggests, these agents have lubricating properties. They impede colonic water absorption and make it easier for feces to be passed. Some reports have suggested that up to 60% of these preparations may be absorbed, although most reports dispute these findings. Examples include paraffin (mineral oil) and white soft paraffin (white petrolatum). These agents have only moderate effects and are only likely to be of use in mild cases of constipation. Preparations of paraffin include generic preparations (e.g. liquid paraffin) and white soft paraffin (Katalax®).

In humans, use of these drugs is contraindicated in young or old patients, debilitated patients and pregnant patients. In addition, these agents should be avoided in patients with pre-existing dysphagia, regurgitation or vomiting. The main side effect is lipoid pneumonia secondary to inhalation (paraffin is tasteless and may not elicit normal swallowing when syringed). When significant quantities of mineral oil are absorbed, granulomatous reactions may develop in the liver, spleen and mesenteric lymph nodes. Long-term use is not recommended since it may predispose to malabsorption of fat-soluble vitamins (vitamins A, D, E and K), although the significance of this has not been determined clinically. Docusate sodium should not be administered concurrently with mineral oil, because it may enhance absorption.

DOGS
- Use liquid paraffin (mineral oil) 15–30 mL (1–2 tablespoonfuls) PO per meal, as required

CATS
- Adult cats: 1 inch of white soft paraffin paste PO q.12–24 h
- Kittens: 0.5 inch of white soft paraffin paste PO q.12–24 h

Hyperosmotic laxatives

Hyperosmotic laxatives consist of agents which are poorly absorbed in the gastrointestinal tract but osmotically active. Lactulose is a nondigestible carbohydrate used for both treatment of constipation and management of hepatic encephalopathy (see below). Polyethylene glycol 3350 (PEG) also acts as an osmotic agent and is commonly included in bowel-cleansing solutions used prior to lower bowel colonoscopy. Most preparations used for this purpose also contain sodium sulfate, which minimizes sodium absorption and other electrolytes (e.g. bicarbonate, potassium and chloride) to maintain isotonicity and prevent any net gain or loss in the secretion of water or electrolytes in the intestine.

A variety of preparations of PEG are available, e.g. Golytely®, Klean Prep®, Colyte® and Nulytely®. PEG should not be administered to animals with gastric retention, suspected gastrointestinal obstruction, bowel perforation, megacolon or in patients with reduced swallowing function (which may predispose to inhalation pneumonia). Occasional vomiting may be seen, especially if the maximal dose has been administered. Otherwise, this drug preparation is very well tolerated. Given that gastrointestinal motility is affected, the absorption of other drugs may be affected by administration of bowel cleansers.

DOGS
- Withhold food for 18–24 h prior to colonoscopy. Give 2–3 doses of 20–30 mL/kg, 4–6 h apart, by orogastric intubation. Prior to the procedure, a warm water enema should be administered

CATS
- Withhold food for 18–24 h prior to colonoscopy. Give 2 doses of 30 mL/kg, 4–6 h apart, by orogastric intubation. Prior to the procedure, a warm water enema should be administered

Stimulant laxatives

This group stimulates propulsive motility and the main agent used in companion animals is bisacodyl (Ducolax®). The exact mechanism of action is unclear; the two putative mechanisms are promoting peristalsis through direct stimulation of intramural neural plexuses and increasing fluid and ion accumulation in the large intestine and thus increasing catharsis. This drug can be given as sole therapy, or in combination with other laxative preparations such as fiber supplements. The drug is reported to be minimally absorbed after oral administration and onset of action is 6–10 h. Relatively few side effects have been reported but include cramping, nausea and diarrhea. Stimulant laxatives are contraindicated in cases of intestinal obstruction not caused by constipation, when rectal bleeding is present or if intestinal perforation is suspected. Bisacodyl should not be given concurrently with milk or antacids as both can cause premature disintegration of the enteric coating. Further, this drug should not be administered concurrently with other oral medications (e.g. not ≤2 h), because its effect on gastrointestinal motility may affect absorption. Daily administration is inadvisable because of potential injury to myenteric neurones when used chronically.

DOGS
- 5–20 mg PO q.24 h

CATS
- 2–5 mg PO q.24 h

ANTIDIARRHEAL DRUGS

For most cases of acute diarrhea, the mainstay of therapy is to replace fluid losses, modify the diet and treat the specific cause (infectious, immune-mediated, etc.) where possible. Treatment of diarrhea does not often require use of drugs but they may be considered when relief of discomfort will benefit the patient, provided that their use does not risk exacerbating the diarrhea or causing systemic effects.

MOTILITY-MODIFYING DRUGS

Intestinal transit time is predominantly determined by the balance between peristalsis, which moves ingesta in an aboral direction, and segmental contractions, which narrow the bowel lumen and increase the resistance to flow. Peristalsis is influenced by the cholinergic system and gut hormones such as motilin. Segmental contractions are cholinergic dependent.

Although it is theoretically possible to reduce diarrhea by either decreasing peristalsis or increasing segmental contractions, reducing peristalsis is of little clinical benefit and is generally contraindicated. This is because, in most cases of diarrhea, the gut is hypomotile, not hypermotile, and peristalsis and segmental contractions are already reduced.

Gastrointestinal motility may be modified by two groups of agents: opioids, which increase segmental contractions, and anticholinergic drugs, which decrease both segmental contractions and peristalsis.

Opioids

EXAMPLES

Diphenoxylate (Lomotil®), loperamide (Imodium®), paregoric

Clinical applications

These drugs may be effective for the symptomatic treatment of diarrhea as they increase segmental contractions, thus delaying gut transit time. They may relieve abdominal pain and tenesmus and reduce the frequency of defecation, although convincing clinical efficacy has not been observed in many veterinary patients.

They are rarely required, however, in management of diarrhea in small animals. Acute diarrhea is usually self-limiting with appropriate treatment and chronic diarrhea does not usually respond to such therapy and requires a definitive diagnosis to be established to allow specific treatment to be instituted.

The use of motility modifiers is not without risk as the diarrhea may be beneficial in removing toxins and slowing transit may be counterproductive. Reduced motility may allow enterotoxin-producing organisms to remain in the small intestine, resulting in increased fluid loss. In addition, in cases of diarrhea caused by invasive bacteria, diarrhea probably has a protective function in hastening elimination of organisms. Slowing transit time may prolong the time bacteria are resident in the bowel, resulting in a greater opportunity for proliferation, invasion of the mucosa and absorption of toxic products. However, loperamide appears to be antisecretory and therefore may have value in treating animals with secretory diarrhea due to *Escherichia coli*. Anecdotally, opioids appear to be useful in the management of fecal incontinence in some patients.

Mechanism of action

Opioids increase the amplitude of rhythmic contraction and decrease propulsive contractions. They directly affect intestinal smooth muscle, producing both tonic and phasic contractions of the circular muscle. They also act centrally and on synapses to augment segmentation. They either have no effect on longitudinal muscle or they relax it. The net effect of these actions is to inhibit flow of intestinal contents, delay gastric emptying and increase the tone of the ileocolic valve and anal sphincter.

Some opioids, such as loperamide and to a lesser extent diphenoxylate, also increase fluid and water absorption, possibly by a calcium-blocking effect or by inhibition of calmodulin, the intrinsic calcium-binding protein. Loperamide and diphenoxylate also inhibit the activity of secretagogues such as *E. coli* enterotoxin, vasoactive intestinal peptide, bile acids and PGE_2. Finally, opiates may also enhance mucosal absorption in the gastrointestinal tract.

Lomotil® contains atropine as well as diphenoxylate. This is to discourage abuse of the drug by people. At therapeutic doses of Lomotil® the atropine has no clinical effect.

Formulations and dose rates

There are no currently approved veterinary formulations of these drugs. Human formulations are available; paregoric is available as a liquid. Diphenoxylate and loperamide are available in tablet and liquid forms. Use of diphenoxylate in cats is not recommended.

DOGS AND CATS

Paregoric
- 0.05–0.06 mg/kg PO q.8 h

Loperamide
- 0.1–0.2 mg/kg PO q.8 h

DOGS ONLY

Diphenoxylate
- 0.1 mg/kg PO q.8 h

Pharmacokinetics

There are few data on the pharmacokinetics of the opioid agents in small animals. The morphine in paregoric is absorbed in a variable fashion from the gastrointestinal tract and rapidly metabolized in the liver, resulting in serum concentrations that are much lower than those produced by morphine administered parenterally.

In humans diphenoxylate is rapidly absorbed. Onset of action occurs about 45 min after dosing and lasts for 3–4 h. In dogs, it has been stated that loperamide has a faster onset and longer duration of action than diphenoxylate, although published clinical studies confirming this appear to be lacking.

Adverse effects

- In dogs, the most common side effects of opiates are constipation, sedation and bloating. Overdosage with these medications can lead to significantly reduced gastrointestinal motility (i.e. ileus) and delayed absorption.
- Signs of systemic opioid intoxication may occur with use of the opioid antidiarrheals, particularly in cats.
- Neurological disturbances such as ataxia, hyperexcitability, circling, head pressing, vocalization and prostration may occur with overdosage. In dogs there has been a suggestion that collies may be more sensitive to the toxic effects of loperamide.
- Treatment of side effects or overdosage involves use of the opioid antagonist naloxone and recovery is usually uneventful.
- Massive overdoses with the diphenoxylate/atropine preparations may also lead to atropine toxicity.

Known drug interactions

- Other CNS depressants such as anesthetic agents, antihistamines, phenothiazines, barbiturates and tranquilizers may cause increased CNS or respiratory depression when used with opiate antidiarrheal agents.
- Opiate antidiarrheal agents are contraindicated in patients receiving monoamine oxidase inhibitors, e.g. l-deprenyl (selegiline), within at least 14 d. However, the significance of this interaction in veterinary species is not clear given that this drug group is rarely used.
- Plasma amylase and lipase concentrations may be increased for up to 24 h after the administration of opiates.

Anticholinergic drugs

Anticholinergics have little use in the management of diarrhea in small animals, although they are frequently prescribed, usually in combination products. As discussed previously, most diarrheal disorders in small animals are associated with a hypomotile rather than a hypermotile gut and the risk with anticholinergics is that they will produce a dynamic ileus, especially if electrolyte imbalances such as hypokalemia are also present. Anticholinergics reduce but do not abolish peristalsis and substantially decrease segmental contractions. As long as some peristaltic activity is present, no matter how weak, it can propel liquid ingesta along the flaccid intestine and diarrhea will occur.

Although anticholinergics reduce gastric secretions, including protein exudation induced by histamine, they have little effect on intestinal secretions.

They may be justified in the short term for relief of pain and tenesmus associated with large bowel inflammatory disease. They also may be indicated in stress-induced colitis where cholinergic mechanisms might be involved.

Adsorbents and protectants

Kaolin and pectin

Kaolin and pectin are in many preparations that are widely used for the management of diarrhea in small and large animals. They are purported to soothe irritated gastrointestinal mucosa and bind toxins and pathogenic bacteria. However, their clinical efficacy is unproven. There is no evidence that kaolin and pectin reduce gastrointestinal fluid or electrolyte loss and kaolin may in fact increase fecal sodium loss.

Many preparations contain combinations of kaolin and pectin and/or antibacterials and/or anticholinergics. As discussed previously, the value of the latter two types of compound in the treatment of diarrhea is limited in small animals and may be detrimental.

Montmorillonite

Montmorillonite (Diarsanyl®) is an intestinal adsorbent/protectant, which is used in the symptomatic treatment of companion animals with diarrhea. It is a trilamellar smectite clay, with a similar mechanism of action to that of kaolin. However, it is reported to have superior adsorbent properties. Most preparations of montmorillonite also contain simple sugars and electrolytes. No adverse affects are known, but are likely to be similar to that of kaolin preparations. Overdosage would be expected to cause constipation. The main formulation (Diarsanyl®) is a paste in 10 mL, 24 mL and 60 mL multidose syringes. Each 10 mL of paste contains 4.5 g of montmorillonite and the recommended dose rate is as follows.

DOGS
- <7 kg: 1 mL PO q.12 h
- 7–17 kg: 2 mL PO q.12 h
- 18–30 kg: 4 mL PO q.12 h
- 31–60 kg: 10 mL PO q.12 h

CATS
- 1 mL PO q.12 h

Activated charcoal

Activated charcoal has been used for many years in the treatment of toxicosis. The drug is not absorbed from the gastrointestinal tract and is thought to have a local effect, by adsorbing toxic substances and binding bacterial toxins. However, it is not reported to be effective for mineral acids or alkalis and, in fact, there is limited work supporting its efficacy. Recommended dosages are in the range of 2–8 g/kg as an aqueous suspension per os. For example, administering 10 mL/kg of a 20% slurry provides a dose equivalent to 2 g/kg. Given the volumes involved, this drug is usually given by oro- or nasogastric intubation.

Very rapid administration may induce emesis and charcoal can cause effects on fecal characteristics (e.g. diarrhea, constipation, black feces). Aside from these, there are no reported systemic adverse effects. Finally, activated charcoal can permanently stain objects with which it comes into contact and the powder has a tendency to float over wide areas. Therefore, care is advised during preparation.

Bismuth subsalicylate

Bismuth subsalicylate is reported to be an effective agent for treatment and prevention of enterotoxigenic diarrhea. Nausea, abdominal pain and diarrhea are reduced in humans with infective diarrhea treated with bismuth-containing products. Bismuth subsalicylate has modest antibacterial effects against enteropathogens such as *E. coli*, *Salmonella* spp and *Campylobacter jejuni*. However, it is sometimes used in combination protocols for the eradication of *Helicobacter* species. The salicylate moiety is believed to decrease intestinal secretion by inhibiting prostaglandin production and inhibiting generation of cAMP by the enterotoxin.

Preparations which contain bismuth subsalicylate (Pepto-Bismol®, Peptosyl®) can be clinically useful in the management of acute diarrhea. However, such conditions usually resolve with appropriate nondrug therapy.

Reported side effects in humans include nausea and vomiting. Long-term use of bismuth-containing products is not recommended as the drug can be neurotoxic and is contraindicated in patients with renal impairment. Further, given that bismuth is radio-opaque, it may interfere with radiographic studies of the gastrointestinal tract. Overdosage can result in salicylate toxicity, especially in cats. A safe dose in dogs and cats is 0.25 mL/kg q.4–6 h. Dosages greater than 0.7 mL/kg could result in toxicity. Aside from this, changes in fecal characteristics can be seen, i.e. color change to black or green-black.

Sulfasalazine

Clinical applications

Sulfasalazine is indicated in the treatment of chronic colitides (e.g. inflammatory bowel disease) in dogs and (less commonly) cats. Although well-controlled studies have not been performed in small animals, uncontrolled studies and widespread clinical use indicate that the drug has convincing clinical benefit in patients with chronic colitis. It is not a panacea, however, and a number of animals do not respond or relapse during or after therapy.

Preparations containing only 5-aminosalicylic acid (5-ASA) (mesalazine, mesalamine) are now used in human and veterinary medicine in the treatment of ulcerative colitis. 5-ASA appears to retain the effectiveness of sulfasalazine but reduces (but does not eliminate altogether) the incidence of side effects by dispensing with the sulfonamide entity. The drug is administered as a suppository or as an enteric-coated tablet to ensure that the majority of drug reaches the colon. Other drugs used in human colitis include olsalazine, which is two molecules of 5-ASA linked by an azo bond. The clinical value of this drug in veterinary medicine has yet to be established.

Mechanism of action

Sulfasalazine is a combination of sulfapyridine and 5-ASA, which is cleaved by colonic bacteria, resulting in sulfapyridine being absorbed and ASA excreted in feces. Given that the colonic concentrations of both sulfapyridine and 5-ASA are higher than when given orally as individual agents, it is not entirely established which is responsible for the clinical effects. However, 5-ASA is probably the active ingredient, as a result of antiprostaglandin and antileukotriene activity. In addition, this agent is thought to have oxygen free radical-scavenging actions, to interfere with phagocytic chemotaxis and function and to inhibit cytokine and immunoglobulin production. NSAIDs such as aspirin that inhibit prostaglandin but not leukotriene synthesis are ineffective in treating colonic inflammation and may actually worsen inflammatory bowel disease.

Formulations and dose rates

Sulfasalazine is available as tablets or liquid. Various dosage regimens have been successfully used.

DOGS

- Some clinicians recommend a dose of 10–15 mg/kg PO q.8–12 h for 2 weeks, then tapered to the lowest effective dose
- Other reports suggest that higher doses are required, e.g. 20–50 mg/kg (up to a maximum of 1 g) PO q.8 h; from 2–4 weeks, attempts can be made to taper the dose gradually (e.g. by reducing 25–50% of the dose every 2–4 weeks) to the lowest effective dose
- Therefore, it is usually recommended to start at a low dose (e.g. 12.5 mg/kg PO q.8 h) and increase this after 4 weeks if it has been ineffective
- Olsalazine is used in dogs that cannot tolerate sulfasalazine. The recommended dose is 10–20 mg/kg PO q.8 h

CATS

- 10–20 mg/kg PO q.24 h. The reduced dosing interval is used in light of increased sensitivity to salicylates in this species

Pharmacokinetics

After oral administration approximately 20–30% of the drug is absorbed in the small intestine. Some of this absorbed drug is believed to be excreted unchanged into the bile. Unabsorbed and biliary excreted drug is cleaved in the colon by bacterial flora. Because the colonic microflora is required to cleave the drug, sulfasalazine is not effective against small bowel inflammation. The sulfapyridine component is rapidly absorbed but only a small percentage of the 5-ASA is absorbed; both are metabolized in the liver and excreted in the urine. Olsalazine is poorly absorbed and that which is absorbed is rapidly eliminated. Approximately 98% of an oral dose is thought to reach the colon.

Adverse effects

- The major adverse effect, although uncommon, is keratoconjunctivitis sicca. Should decreased tear production be recorded, this can be resolved by reducing the dose or discontinuing the drug altogether.
- Other occasional adverse effects include vomiting, allergic dermatitis, cholestatic jaundice, hemolytic anemia and leukopenia.
- Drug hypersensitivity manifested as lethargy, pyrexia, arthralgia and cutaneous drug eruption can occur with sulfonamide drugs and has been reported with the use of sulfasalazine.

Known drug interactions

- Sulfasalazine may displace other highly protein-bound drugs such as methotrexate, warfarin, phenylbutazone, thiazide diuretics, salicylates and phenytoin. The clinical significance of these interactions has not been established.
- Sulfasalazine may decrease the bioavailability of folic acid or digoxin. Antacids may decrease the oral bioavailability of sulfasalzine if administered concurrently.
- Antacids may decrease the oral bioavailability of sulfasalazine if administered concurrently.
- As with other sulfonamides, sulfasalazine may affect blood thyroid concentrations, e.g. decreased total and free T4, increased cTSH.
- Olsalazine may causes increases in plasma concentrations of ALT and AST.

APPETITE STIMULANTS

The main appetite stimulants used in companion animals are the H_1-receptor antagonists cyproheptadine and diazepam. In both drugs, the appetite stimulation is effectively a 'side effect' of the indication for which they were predominantly designed.

Cyproheptadine also has serotonin antagonist and calcium channel-blocking properties. It is indicated for short-term use as an appetite stimulant in cats; profound anorexia or chronic nutritional disorders are better managed with more intensive nutritional support, i.e. tube feeding. The drug is well absorbed, almost completely metabolized in the liver and metabolites are excreted in the urine. The main side effects are sedation and anticholinergic effects (dry mucous membranes, mydriasis); occasional reports of hemolytic anemia have been described.

Diazepam is used mainly for its anticonvulsant, anxiolytic and skeletal muscle relaxant properties. However, when used IV, it can be an effective appetite stimulant in cats. Again, only short-term (and preferably single) use is recommended. The IV preparation should be injected slowly, since rapid administration may cause marked excitation. Thrombophlebitis has also been reported. The drug should be used with caution in patients with pre-existing or suspected renal or hepatic insufficiency. The main side effects include muscle fasciculations, weakness, ataxia, behavior changes and excessive sedation. Fulminant hepatic necrosis has also been described in cats after oral administration (usually for >5 d). Given that the IV preparation is used for appetite stimulation, the significance of this finding is unclear. Nevertheless, cautious use is recommended.

CATS

Cyproheptadine

- 1–4 mg per cat PO q.12–24 h

Diazepam
- 0.05–0.4 mg/kg IV. Eating may begin shortly after administration so have a food supply ready

Oxazepam
- 2 mg per cat PO q.12 h

DRUGS USED FOR MANAGEMENT OF HEPATIC DISEASE

URSODEOXYCHOLIC ACID (URSODIOL)

Clinical applications

Ursodeoxycholic acid (ursodiol) is a naturally occurring bile acid found in the bile of the Chinese black bear. Black bear bile has been used for many years by practitioners of Eastern medicine and has been commercially synthesized and available for use as a hepatoprotective agent in Japan since the 1930s. Since the 1970s ursodeoxycholic acid has been used in Western human medicine for dissolution of gallstones. More recently, it has been used in the management of chronic hepatic diseases in humans such as primary biliary cirrhosis, biliary disease secondary to cystic fibrosis, nonalcoholic steatohepatitis, idiopathic chronic hepatitis, autoimmune hepatitis, primary sclerosing cholangitis and alcoholic hepatitis. However, its therapeutic efficacy in some of these disorders has not been firmly established.

In veterinary medicine, ursodeoxycholic acid has been used in the management of dogs with chronic hepatitis and cats with lymphocytic plasmacytic cholangitis. It is believed to be most beneficial in disorders where bile toxicity plays an important role in the ongoing pathology. The efficacy of ursodeoxycholic acid in veterinary patients has not been definitely established, although anecdotal reports suggest it may have some benefit in patients with chronic inflammatory hepatobiliary disease. It may be of some benefit in slowing disease progression, especially if used at an early stage of the disease. Some authors recommend ursodeoxycholic acid treatment for all cats with cholangiohepatitis where extrahepatic biliary obstruction has been eliminated.

Mechanism of action

Ursodeoxycholic acid decreases intestinal absorption and suppresses hepatic synthesis and storage of cholesterol. This is believed to reduce cholesterol saturation of bile, thereby allowing solubilization of cholesterol-containing gallstones. It has little effect on calcified gallstones or on radiolucent bile pigment stones and therapy is only successful in patients with a functioning gallbladder.

Ursodeoxycholic acid, a relatively hydrophilic bile acid, is also believed to protect the liver from the damaging effects of hydrophobic bile acids, which are retained in cholestatic disorders. Hydrophobic bile acids can be cytotoxic through detergent-like and nondetergent-like actions. The mechanisms responsible for this hepatoprotective effect in humans have not been fully elucidated and are controversial but they are believed to involve replacement of the more hydrophobic bile acids, increased bile flow (choleresis) and immunomodulation. Ursodeoxycholic acid may also inhibit ileal uptake of toxic secondary bile acids formed by bacterial modification of primary bile acids in the gut lumen. The hepatoprotective effect may, however, be less in cats and dogs than in humans as the major circulating bile acid in dogs and cats is taurocholate. This is more hydrophilic and less hepatotoxic than the major circulating bile acids in humans.

Choleresis results from protonation of unconjugated ursodeoxycholic acid when it is secreted into bile, resulting in the generation of a bicarbonate ion. Protonated ursodeoxycholic acid is passively absorbed by biliary epithelial cells, resulting in the net secretion of one bicarbonate ion, which then serves as an osmotic draw for biliary water secretion. Induced choleresis may protect the hepatocytes from potentially toxic substances normally secreted into bile such as copper, leukotrienes, cholesterol and bilirubin.

The immunomodulatory effects of ursodeoxycholic acid are believed to involve decreased immunoglobulin production by B lymphocytes, decreased interleukin-1 and -2 production by T lymphocytes, decreased expression of hepatocyte cell surface membrane HLA class I molecules and possibly stimulation of the hepatocyte glucocorticoid receptor.

Formulations and dose rates

Currently, no veterinary preparations are available but a variety of human products exist, including both tablet (250 mg; e.g. Destolit®, Urso®) and capsule formulations (300 mg; e.g. Ursofalk®, Actigall®). The exact choice of product depends upon the size of patient and ease of dosing with a particular type of preparation.

DOGS AND CATS
- 10–15 mg/kg q.24 h or divided and given q.12 h

It is recommended that ursodeoxycholic acid be administered for 3–4 months, after which the patient should be reassessed for improvement in biochemical markers of hepatocellular pathology. If there has been improvement treatment is continued but if there has been no improvement or progression, either treatment should be terminated or additional therapies such as glucocorticoids or colchicine added.

Pharmacokinetics

Ursodeoxycholic acid is well absorbed from the small intestine in humans, with over 90% of the administered dose being absorbed. It is extracted from the portal circulation and conjugated with either taurine or glycine and excreted into bile. Only very small amounts enter the systemic circulation and minimal amounts are detected in urine. It undergoes enterohepatic circulation; at each cycle some of the free and conjugated drug is degraded by gut bacteria, oxidized or reduced to less soluble compounds and eliminated in the feces.

Adverse effects

- Ursodeoxycholic acid appears to be well tolerated by dogs and cats; vomiting and diarrhea are reported rarely.
- There is some concern in human patients that taurine depletion may be potentiated by chronic treatment with ursodeoxycholic acid. This may be important in cats, who are obligate taurine conjugators. This potential for taurine depletion may be exacerbated in some cats with hepatobiliary disease, who have increased urinary excretion of taurine-conjugated bile acids. Dogs are less likely to become taurine depleted by this mechanism as they can shift to glycine conjugation.
- Ursodeoxycholic acid should not be used in patients with extrahepatic biliary obstruction, biliary fistulas, cholecystitis or pancreatitis.

Known drug interactions

Aluminum-containing antacids or colestyramine resin may bind to ursodeoxycholic acid, thus reducing its efficacy. Ursodeoxycholic acid dissolves more rapidly in bile and pancreatic juice; therefore, administration with food may improve absorption and is recommended.

Colchicine

Clinical applications

Colchicine is used in the management of gout in humans, providing acute relief of symptoms as well as prophylaxis. It has also been used for the treatment of fibrosing liver diseases such as primary biliary cirrhosis, alcoholic liver disease, cryptogenic liver fibrosis and liver cirrhosis. However, two recent meta-analyses have demonstrated limited efficacy of this drug, but more adverse events. Thus, this drug is likely to fall from favor in human hepatology. In veterinary medicine it has been used in the management of amyloidosis and chronic hepatic fibrosis. There is anecdotal evidence from a few case studies that colchicine may improve liver function and slow the progression of hepatic fibrosis. However, controlled clinical trials are lacking and, given recent findings in human studies, it should therefore be used cautiously or avoided altogether.

Mechanism of action

Collagen secretion from lipocytes requires microtubules, the assembly of which is inhibited by colchicine, thereby interfering with the transcellular movement of collagen. The drug increases collagenase activity and may therefore promote degradation of existing collagen, although collagen already cross-linked cannot usually be degraded. It has anti-inflammatory effects by inhibiting leukocyte migration, which may suppress fibrogenesis. It may also have a direct hepatoprotective effect by stabilizing hepatocyte membranes. Colchicine is also reported to block synthesis of serum amyloid A by hepatocytes, thus preventing amyloid formation. The mechanism of its apparent efficacy in gout is poorly understood.

Formulations and dose rates

Various colchicine preparations are available in tablet form, usually in either 0.5 mg or 0.6 mg sizes (dependent upon manufacturer). Injectable formulations may be available, but most experience in veterinary species is with oral dosing. Doses in dogs have been extrapolated from the human literature. Its use in the cat has not been reported. Colchicine is marketed in combination with probenecid in some countries – this combination should be avoided as probenecid can cause nausea, vomiting and lethargy.

DOGS

- 0.025–0.03 mg/kg/d

Pharmacokinetics

No information is available on the pharmacokinetics of colchicine in dogs and cats. Data derived from humans and laboratory animals indicate that the drug undergoes first-pass metabolism after absorption from the gut, the metabolites, as well as unchanged drug, being resecreted into the gut in bile and then reabsorbed. Colchicine is concentrated in leukocytes. Its plasma half-life is about 20 min; leukocyte half-life is 60 h.

Colchicine is deacetylated in the liver as well as being metabolized in other tissues. Most of the dose is excreted in the feces, with a small amount excreted in urine, particularly in patients with hepatic disease.

Adverse effects

- Because of the limited veterinary experience with colchicine, little is known about its potential toxicity in dogs and cats.
- In humans, the therapeutic window for colchicine is quite narrow, with toxic effects occurring after only small overdoses.
- Nausea, vomiting and diarrhea have been reported in dogs.
- Bone marrow suppression has occurred in humans after prolonged use.
- Myopathy and peripheral neuropathy have been reported rarely in humans.

- Severe local irritation occurs if the drug is inadvertently administered perivascularly. Thrombophlebitis has also been reported.
- Colchicine is contraindicated in patients with serious renal, gastrointestinal or cardiac disease and should be used with caution in patients with less severe disease of these organs.
- Colchicine is teratogenic in mice and hamsters; therefore it should not be used in pregnant patients unless the benefits outweigh the risks.
- Colchicine may decrease spermatogenesis.
- Safety for nursing neonates is unknown as it is not known whether it is excreted in milk.

Known drug interactions

- NSAIDs, especially phenylbutazone, increase the risk of thrombocytopenia, leukopenia or bone marrow suppression when used concurrently with colchicine.
- Many antineoplastic and other potentially marrow-suppressing drugs may cause additive myelosuppression when used concurrently with colchicine.
- Colchicine may enhance the activity of sympathomimetic drugs and CNS depressants, although the clinical significance of this interaction is not known
- Colchicine may cause false-positive results for erythrocytes on urine dipsticks and may elevate serum ALP concentrations.

Penicillamine

Penicillamine is a degradation product of penicillin but has no antimicrobial activity. It was first isolated in 1953 from the urine of a patient with liver disease who was receiving penicillin.

Clinical applications

Penicillamine is a monothiol chelating agent which is used in veterinary medicine in the treatment of copper storage hepatopathy (e.g. Bedlington terriers), lead toxicity and cystine urolithiasis. It has also been used in the management of rheumatoid arthritis in humans.

Mechanism of action

Penicillamine chelates several metals, including copper, lead, iron and mercury, forming stable water-soluble complexes that are excreted by the renal route. It also combines chemically with cystine to form a stable, soluble, readily excreted complex.

Although it usually takes months to years for hepatic copper levels to decrease, clinical improvement is often seen in Bedlington terriers after only a few weeks, suggesting that the drug has beneficial effects other than copper depletion. Penicillamine induces hepatic metallothionein, which may bind and sequester copper in a nontoxic form. It may also have antifibrotic effects as it inhibits lysyl oxidase, an enzyme necessary for collagen synthesis, and directly binds to collagen fibrils, preventing cross-linking into stable collagen fibers. However, its efficacy as an antifibrotic agent in humans is doubtful and it has not been evaluated in veterinary medicine.

Penicillamine may have immunomodulatory effects and has been demonstrated to reduce IgM rheumatoid factor in humans with rheumatoid arthritis. However, its mechanism of action in this disease remains uncertain.

Formulations and dose rates

Penicillamine is available as tablets and capsules.

DOGS AND CATS

Copper-associated hepatopathy

- 10–15 mg/kg PO q.12 h on an empty stomach. However, if gastrointestinal adverse effects are experienced, these may be reduced if it is given with food, although absorption may be reduced. Alternatively, reduce dose and gradually build up to full dose

Cystine urolithiasis

- 15 mg/kg PO q.12 h (same comments as above if toxicity experienced)

Lead toxicity

- 110 mg/kg/day divided q.6–8 h. Reduce dose to 33 mg/kg/d if gastrointestinal adverse effects occur

Adverse effects

- Gastrointestinal tract adverse effects are common, resulting in nausea and vomiting. Smaller doses on a more frequent basis may alleviate adverse effects. Alternatively, the drug can be given with food, although this will reduce absorption.
- Other adverse effects observed infrequently or rarely include:
  - fever
  - lymphadenopathy
  - skin hypersensitivity reactions
  - immune-complex glomerulonephropathy.
- Leukopenia, aplastic anemia and agranulocytosis have been reported in humans.

Known drug interactions

Administration of penicillamine with gold compounds, cytotoxic or immunosuppressant drugs or phenylbutazone may increase the risk of hematological and/or renal adverse effects. Zinc (or other cationic minerals) may decrease the efficacy of penicillamine when given concurrently.

Zinc

Zinc is a nutritional metal agent that is used to reduce copper toxicity in breeds with copper-associated hepatopathies, e.g. Bedlington terrier. It is also reported to have antifibrotic functions. The effect of copper toxicosis relates to the ability of zinc to inhibit the absorption of copper in the gastrointestinal tract. For liver disease, zinc supplementation is often provided as part of a purpose-formulated prescription diet. However, oral and injectable forms are also available and usually include either zinc acetate or zinc sulfate. Zinc acetate is the preparation most commonly used for hepatic disorders.

Large doses of zinc can cause gastrointestinal signs, including vomiting, whilst hemolysis can occur after administration of large doses or if serum concentrations exceed 1000 µg/dL. Penicillamine and ursodeoxycholic acid can decrease zinc absorption, whilst zinc salts can reduce the absorption of tetracycline and fluoroquinolones (e.g. enrofloxacin). It is recommended to stagger dosing by at least 2 h.

Formulations and dose rates

DOGS

Copper-associated hepatopathy

- 5–10 mg/kg (of elemental zinc) PO q.12 h. Start at the higher end of the dose range for the first 3 months, then reduce dose to 50 mg PO q.12 h for maintenance. Separate the dose from feeding by 1–2 h. Monitor plasma zinc concentrations every 2–3 months and aim for plasma zinc concentrations of 200–400 µg/dL

Hepatic fibrosis

- 10 mg/kg (of elemental zinc) q.24 h PO, aiming for plasma zinc concentrations between 200–300 µg/dL

S-adenosyl methionine (SAMe)

S-adenosyl methionine (SAMe) is an endogenous molecule which is synthesized, from methionine, by many cells in the body. However, the enzyme SAMe synthetase is found in the liver and is the rate-limiting step for SAMe synthesis in the face of hepatic compromise. SAMe is an essential factor in three major biochemical pathways (most important in the liver), namely transmethylation, transsulfuration and aminopropylation. SAMe functions as a donor of methyl groups and is thus essential for the activation or elimination of many substances. For transsulfuration, SAMe generates sulfur-containing compounds, which are important for conjugation reactions and for synthesis of glutathione (GSH). The latter is also essential for numerous metabolic processes and detoxification reactions; conversion of SAMe to GSH requires folate, cyanocobalamin and pyroxidine. Ample SAMe is usually synthesized but, with hepatic disease or if toxic substances are present, conversion to GSH may be reduced. Administration of exogenous SAMe increases hepatic and red blood cell GSH concentrations, whilst this compound also inhibits apoptosis secondary to the presence of alcohol or bile acids in hepatocytes. Other effects include antidepressant activity, possibly due to increased serotonin turnover, and increased dopamine or noradrenaline (norepinephrine) release.

Oral bioavailability is reported to be 1% and the amount absorbed can be reduced further in the presence of food. Once absorbed, SAMe enters the portal circulation and is metabolized in the liver.

Clinical applications

SAMe is most frequently used as adjunctive therapy for a variety of hepatic disorders (canine chronic hepatitis, hepatic lipidosis, cholangiohepatitis, etc.). It may also be beneficial in the treatment of certain hepatotoxic disorders, most notably paracetamol (acetaminophen).

Formulations and dose rates

No pharmaceutical preparations exist; SAMe is considered to be a nutritional supplement. Therefore, potency, purity, safety and efficacy may vary across the various preparations. Specific animal products exist, e.g. Denosyl®, Zentonil® and Hepatosyl®.

DOGS AND CATS

- Calculate daily dose based upon 17–20 mg/kg PO q.24 h (or divided twice daily), rounded to the closest tablet size. The product should be administered on an empty stomach, ≥1 h before feeding
- Or, dose according to the following regimen: 5.5 kg, 90 mg PO q.24 h; 5.5–11 kg, 180 mg PO q.24 h; 11–16 kg, 225 mg PO q.24 h; 16–29.5 kg, 450 mg PO q.24 h; 29.5–41 kg, 675 mg PO q.24 h; 41 kg+, 900 mg PO q.24 h

Adverse effects

SAMe appears relatively safe for use in small animals and adverse effects are minimal. In humans, oral dosing may cause anorexia, nausea, vomiting, diarrhea, flatulence, constipation, dry mouth, insomnia, headache, sweating and dizziness.

Known drug interactions

Concurrent use of pethidine (meperidine), monoamine oxidase inhibitors (e.g. selegiline), serotonin reuptake inhibitors (e.g. fluoxetine) and other antidepressants (e.g. amitryptiline, clomipramine) could cause additive serotonergic effects.

Silymarin

Milk thistle, *Silybum marianum*, is a flower used for thousands of years for medical purposes. Three biochemicals of interest have been isolated from the milk thistle: silychristine, silydianin and silybin. The mixture of these three substances is called 'silymarin'. Silymarin has been traditionally used in the treatment of liver disease but while it has recently been advocated for use in pets, all scientific information available concerns human use. The biological mechanism of action is yet unknown but several theories exist. Silymarin may:

- control hepatic cell membrane permeability and thus prevent toxin penetration
- inhibit the cytotoxic, inflammatory and apoptotic effects of tumor necrosis factor
- inhibit lipid peroxidase and β-glucoronidase and act as a free radical scavenger and antioxidant
- reduce hepatic collagen formation
- increase hepatic glutathione content.

Clinical applications

Controlled studies demonstrating the efficacy of silymarin are lacking and formulations are not standardized. However, it is used commonly in the treatment of human and companion animal hepatic disorders. It is most commonly utilized in the treatment of chronic hepatopathies, although it may also be suitable for acute hepatic disease and as a hepatoprotective agent against a variety of hepatotoxic substances (such as *Amanita phalloides*).

Formulations and dose rates

No pharmaceutical preparations exist and, as with SAMe, silymarin is considered to be a nutritional supplement. Therefore, potency, purity, safety and efficacy may vary across the various preparations. A variety of preparations exist, including tablets and capsules in various strengths, e.g. from 150 mg to 1000 mg.

DOGS AND CATS

- 20–50 mg/kg PO q.24 h

Adverse effects

- There are no reported absolute contraindications for silymarin and this drug is well tolerated by the oral route.
- Overdoses rarely cause significant morbidity. The main signs seen in these situations are gastrointestinal.

Known drug interactions

- Silymarin may inhibit the cytochrome P450 enzyme 2C9, such that drugs with narrow therapeutic ranges should be used with caution, e.g. warfarin, amitriptyline and verapamil.
- Silymarin may also inhibit cytochrome P3A4, but this interaction has not yet been found to be significant.
- Finally, silymarin may increase the clearance of drugs which undergo hepatic glucuronidation, e.g. paracetamol (acetaminophen), diazepam and morphine.

Lactulose

Lactulose is a synthetic derivative of lactose, consisting of one molecule of galactose and one molecule of fructose. This disaccharide cannot be digested by enzymes of the mammalian digestive tract, allowing the colonic microflora to convert it to low molecular weight acids (lactic, formic and acetic acid). These acids both increase osmotic pressure (thus drawing water into the intestine and having a laxative effect) and cause an acidifying effect. By acidifying the colonic contents, ammonia (NH_3) is trapped as ammonium (NH_4^+) and, in this form, cannot be absorbed across the intestinal wall. Less than 3% of this drug is absorbed, the drug is not metabolized and is excreted unchanged in the urine within 24 h.

Clinical applications

The main use of lactulose is to reduce blood ammonia concentrations in the treatment of hepatic encephalopathy. It can also be used as an osmotic laxative for the treatment of constipation.

Formulations and dose rates

The commercially available preparations are viscous sweet liquids and have an adjusted pH of 3–7.

DOGS

- 5–30 mL PO q.6–8 h initially, then adjust the dose to achieve 2–3 soft stools per day
- For encephalopathic coma, first empty and clean the lower bowel with repeated warm water enemas, then use 18–20 mL/kg of a solution containing 3 parts lactulose and 7 parts warm water, as a retention enema. Replace every 4–8 h

CATS

- For hepatic encephalopathy: 0.25–5mL PO q.8–12 h. Again, modify the dose to achieve soft stools
- For encephalopathic coma, first empty and clean the lower bowel with repeated warm water enemas, then use 18–20 mL/kg of a solution containing 3 parts lactulose and 7 parts warm water, as a retention enema. Replace every 4–8 h
- For constipation, 0.5 mL/kg q.8–12h PO

Adverse effects

- The main adverse effects are gastrointestinal, e.g. flatulence, gastric distension and cramping.
- The main side effect of overdose is diarrhea.
- Use cautiously in patients with pre-existing fluid and electrolyte imbalances.

- Cats do not like the taste of lactulose and it can be difficult to administer this drug to some patients.

Known drug interactions

- Do not use lactulose and other laxatives concurrently.
- In theory, the use of some antibacterials (e.g. neomycin) could eliminate the bacteria that convert lactulose to low molecular weight acids that exert an osmotic effect. However, this has not appeared to be a clinical concern since synergy has been reported when lactulose and antibiotics are used concurrently.
- Nonabsorbable oral antacids may reduce colonic acidification and might reduce the efficacy of lactulose.

EMETIC AGENTS

In some circumstances, most notably after recent ingestion of toxic compounds, drugs are required to induce vomiting. A number of household products have been used for the purpose, most notably strong salt (sodium chloride) solutions, hydrogen peroxide and washing soda crystals. In addition, the sedative drug xylazine may be effective for this purpose in cats. However, the most commonly used pharmaceutical agents are syrup of ipecacuanha (ipecac) and apomorphine.

Emetic agents rarely eliminate more than 80% of the ingested material and more commonly only 40–60%. Therefore, it is advisable to use other symptomatic therapies in conjunction with emetic agents.

Ipecac syrup

Clinical applications

Ipecac syrup is derived from the roots and rhizomes of certain plants; it contains two active alkaloid agents: emetine and cephaeline. The main indication of this agent is to induce vomiting, after the ingestion of toxic compounds or after a drugs overdose.

Mechanism of action

The major alkaloids of ipecac (emetine and cephaeline) are thought to be the pharmacologically active agents and have both local and central activity. Locally, they produce an irritant effect on the gastric mucosa, whilst centrally they stimulate the chemoreceptor trigger zone. The medullary regions must be responsive for vomiting to be elicited. When vomiting occurs, contents from both the stomach and small intestine are evacuated. Vomiting usually occurs with 10–30 min of administration in both dogs and cats.

Formulations and dose rates

There are no veterinary-approved formulations, but a variety of human preparations are available (e.g. Ipeca®, Ipecacuanha tincture®, Ipecavom®, Ipetitrin®, etc.) containing various concentrations, e.g. 1.5%, 1.75% and 2%.

DOGS

- 1.0–2.5 mL/kg PO (to a maximum of 15 mL) as a single dose. Repeat after 20 min if no response. If the stomach is empty, give 5 mL/kg of water immediately afterwards. If vomiting does not occur after the second dose, subsequently perform gastric lavage to retrieve the ipecac

CATS

- 1.0–3.3 mL/kg PO as an initial dose. It may be prudent to dilute the dose 50:50 with water, to minimize the adverse effect of the taste. Repeat with a second dose 20 min after the first if vomiting does not occur; subsequently perform gastric lavage to retrieve the ipecac

Pharmacokinetics

There are few data available on the pharmacokinetics of ipecac syrup. Apparently, there is great interindividual variability in the proportion absorbed amongst patients.

Adverse effects

- Emetics are contraindicated in patients that are hypoxic, dyspneic, unable to swallow, hypovolemic or comatose.
- Emetics should not be given to animals which have ingested strong acids or alkalis because the contents of the vomitus may cause further damage to esophageal, pharyngeal or oral tissues.
- Given the risk of aspiration, emetics should not be given after ingestion of petrolatum or related compounds because the risk of subsequent aspiration outweighs the potential toxicity.
- The syrup is clear, with a mild odor. It has an unpleasant taste and, as a consequence, may be difficult to administer successfully to cats.
- Although side effects are uncommon, occasional side effects include salivation, lacrimation, protracted vomiting, diarrhea and lethargy.
- Overdosage of ipecac has been known to lead to cardiotoxicity (e.g. arrhythmias, hypotension and fatal myocarditis).

Known drug interactions

- Use of emetics in the face of strychnine intoxication, or with other CNS stimulants, may precipitate seizures.
- Activated charcoal may adsorb ipecac syrup and, as a result, these drugs should not be administered con-

currently. Instead, ipecac syrup should be given first and activated charcoal only administered once vomiting has occurred.
- The efficacy of ipecac may be decreased by dairy products and carbonated beverages.

Apomorphine

Clinical applications

Apomorphine is used as an emetic agent in dogs, where it is considered to be the drug of choice for this purpose. Its use is controversial in cats.

Mechanism of action

Apomorphine stimulates dopamine receptors in the chemoreceptor trigger zone and thereby induces vomiting. Although it may have both stimulatory and inhibitory effects within the CNS, stimulatory effects predominate. However, depression of medullary centers may lead to respiratory depression.

Formulations and dose rates

No veterinary licensed products are available, but there are a number of human preparations.

DOGS

- 0.03–4 mg/kg IV or 0.04–0.08 mg/kg IM or SC, as a single dose

CATS

- 0.04 mg/kg IV, or 0.08 mg/kg IM or SC as a single dose. However, use in this species is controversial and many do not recommend it
- If vomiting does not occur after administration, it is inadvisable to administer repeated doses as they are unlikely to be effective and signs of toxicity may occur

Pharmacokinetics

Apomorphine is slowly absorbed after oral administration and efficacy is unpredictable by this route. As a result, parenteral (or subconjunctival) administration is preferred. Emesis usually occurs rapidly after intravenous administration, whilst therefore may be a delay of 5 min after intramuscular injection. Although conjunctival administration is effective, response is less predictable and injected routes are preferred.

Adverse effects

- Emetics are contraindicated in patients that are hypoxic, dyspneic, unable to swallow, hypovolemic or comatose.
- Emetics should not be given to animals which have ingested strong acids or alkalis because the contents of the vomitus may cause further damage to esophageal, pharyngeal or oral tissues.
- Given the risk of aspiration, emetics should not be given after ingestion of petrolatum or related compounds because the risk of subsequent aspiration outweighs the potential toxicity.
- The principal adverse effect is protracted vomiting. Excitement, restlessness, CNS excitement/depression and cardiorespiratory depression may occur if an overdose is administered. The CNS adverse effects can be reversed by naloxone, although this drug cannot usually block the vomiting.
- Apomorphine should not be used in cases of oral opiate or other CNS depressant (e.g. barbiturate) toxicity.
- Apomorphine is contraindicated in patients hypersensitive to morphine.
- The use of this drug is controversial in cats and many clinicians believe that xylazine and ipecac syrup are both more effective.

Known drug interactions

- Drugs with antidopaminergic effects may antagonize the effect of apomorphine, e.g. phenothiazines.
- Additive CNS, cardiac and respiratory adverse effects may develop if apomorphine is administered concurrently with opiates.

FURTHER READING

Hall JA, Washabau RJ 2000 Gastric prokinetic agents. In: Bonagura J (ed.) Current veterinary therapy XIII. WB Saunders, Philadelphia, PA, pp 614-617

Leveille-Webster C 2000 Ursodeoxycholic acid therapy. In: Bonagura J (ed.) Current veterinary therapy XIII. WB Saunders, Philadelphia, PA, pp 691-693

Plumb DA 2005 Plumb's veterinary drug handbook, 5th edn. Blackwell Publishing, Ames, IA

Washabau RJ, Elie MS 1995 Antemetic therapy. In: Bonagura J (ed.) Current veterinary therapy XIII. WB Saunders, Philadelphia, PA, pp 679-684

20

Drugs used in the management of thyroid and parathyroid disease

Boyd Jones and Carmel T Mooney

THYROID DISEASE

Drugs used to treat thyroid disease include those used to replace thyroid hormone in hypothyroid states and those administered to block thyroid hormone production or secretion in hyperthyroidism. Hyperthyroidism is one of the most common endocrinopathies in the cat and hypothyroidism is a relatively common acquired disease in the adult dog. Less commonly in both species, hypothyroidism occurs as a congenital disease due to a defect in thyroid-stimulating hormone (TSH) or thyroid hormone production. In order to understand the indications for and action of the drugs used in the management of thyroid disease, an understanding of normal thyroid physiology is important.

Relevant physiology/pathophysiology

Thyroid hormone synthesis

The synthesis of thyroid hormones is dependent upon a readily available supply of iodine in the diet. Dietary iodine is absorbed in the small intestine, converted to iodide, bound to plasma proteins and transported to the thyroid gland. The concentration of inorganic iodide in canine plasma is 10–20 times that found in humans and the dietary iodine requirements are greater in the dog than in man.

After iodide has passed across the follicular cell membrane, against a gradient – an energy-requiring process – it undergoes enzymatic oxidation by thyroid peroxidase and is bound to tyrosine residues on thyroglobulin, a glycoprotein synthesized by the thyroid follicular cells and stored in the colloid. Iodination of tyrosine residues within thyroglobulin results in mono-iodotyrosine (MIT) and di-iodotyrosine (DIT).

Iodothyronines are formed by the coupling of two DIT molecules to form thyroxine (T_4) or the coupling of one DIT and one MIT molecule to form tri-iodothyronine (T_3). In response to a stimulus for secretion of thyroid hormone, iodinated thyroglobulin in the colloid is engulfed by pinocytosis to form a colloid droplet within a follicular epithelial cell. This droplet then fuses with a lysosome to form a phagolysosome, after which thyroglobulin undergoes proteolysis, the peptide linkages within the thyroglobulin being cleaved and resulting in the formation of T_3 and T_4. Metabolically active T_3 and T_4 are then released.

Thyroid hormone secretion and transport

Thyrotropin-releasing hormone (TRH) stimulates pituitary secretion of TSH, modulating the response of the TSH-secreting cells (thyrotropes) to the normally suppressive effects of circulating thyroid hormone. Thyroid hormones have a negative feedback on TRH by reducing hypothalamic production of TRH and increasing TRH degradation in the pituitary and hypothalamus.

TSH, a glycoprotein, is synthesized and secreted by thyrotropes in the adenohypophysis. TSH stimulates thyroid hormone synthesis and secretion and has various tropic effects on the thyroid gland. The direct negative feedback of thyroid hormones on thyrotropes is the primary control mechanism for TSH synthesis and secretion. Deiodination of T_4 to T_3 occurs in the pituitary and is thought to be important in the feedback control.

Serum thyroid hormones are highly protein bound, with only the unbound or 'free' hormone being metabolically active. In the dog, thyroxine-binding globulin (TBG) binds approximately 60% of T_4, compared to 72% in man. Other binding proteins and the relative amount of thyroxine bound to each in the dog include thyroxine-binding prealbumin (17%), albumin (12%) and an α_1-protein, possibly high-density lipoprotein-2 (11%). T_3 is bound to albumin and one globulin fraction. The binding affinity of these proteins for T_3 is much less than that for T_4. The protein bound fraction serves as a buffer against rapid changes in free thyroid hormone concentrations.

In both dogs and cats approximately 0.1% of T_4 is circulating in the free form. The free hormone enters cells and is responsible for the metabolic effects of thyroid hormone, as the actions of thyroid hormone are basically intracellular and bound hormone cannot cross cell membranes.

Although the thyroid gland secretes T_4 and T_3 in a ratio of approximately 4 : 1, peripheral 5′ deiodination of T_4 by the enzyme 5′ deiodinase accounts for 40–60%

of T_3 produced in the dog. Since T_3 is roughly 3–5 times more potent than T_4, the major actions of thyroid hormones are mediated by T_3 acting intracellularly.

Although T_3 is more biologically active, most T_3 is present in the intracellular compartment. Consequently, serum concentrations of T_4 are more representative of the total thyroid hormone status of the animal than serum T_3 measurements.

Thyroid hormone-binding protein concentration and affinity are lower in dogs compared to humans, which accounts for the lower total thyroid hormone concentration in the dog. It also accounts for the relatively short half-life of T_4 of 10–16 h in dogs compared to approximately 7 d in humans. The plasma half-life of T_3 in the dog is estimated to be 5–6 h compared to 24–36 h in humans.

The metabolism of the thyroid hormone that is not deiodinated includes conjugation to inactive sulfate or glucuronide and decarboxylated and deaminated metabolites. Fecal excretion via liver and bile is an important route of thyroid hormone excretion, accounting for 55% of T_4 and 30% of T_3 metabolized in the dog.

Hypothyroidism

Approximately 95% of cases of canine hypothyroidism arise because of a defect within the thyroid gland itself (primary hypothyroidism). The two most common causes are lymphocytic thyroiditis and idiopathic atrophy of the thyroid gland, each of which occurs with similar frequency. Rarely, hypothyroidism due to defective TSH secretion is reported in dogs and cats. Feline hypothyroidism is most common after surgical removal of the thyroid gland or after radio-iodine treatment for hyperthyroidism.

Hyperthyroidism

Hyperthyroidism occurs mostly in cats and is usually due to thyroid adenoma (adenomatous hyperplasia) or, more rarely, adenocarcinoma.

THYROID HORMONE REPLACEMENT THERAPY

Crude thyroid extract

Extract of thyroid tissue from animals (cows, sheep, pigs) was once used as thyroid hormone replacement therapy. However, the ratio of the T_4:T_3 content is nonphysiological, their concentrations variable and the shelf-life short. Additionally, as the material must be administered uncooked, the possibility of disease transmission is always a consideration. In view of these limitations and the ready availability of suitable alternatives, there are now no indications for its use.

Synthetic L-tri-iodothyronine (tri-iodothyronine, liothyronine)

Although T_3 is the active intracellular hormone, there are few specific indications for its use and no advantage in administering T_3 to the vast majority of patients with hypothyroidism. It is a potent form of replacement therapy and conversion from T_4 is not required. However, it circumvents normal physiological control and thus the risk of toxicity is greater. In addition, its shorter half-life means that adequate replacement therapy usually requires a minimum of thrice-daily dosing. Whilst its use is associated with normalization of circulating T_3, circulating T_4 concentrations remain subnormal. Additionally, some organs, specifically the cerebral cortex and pituitary gland, are dependent on an adequate supply of T_4 and may remain deficient if only T_3 is replaced.

T_3 has been recommended for use in dogs that may not convert T_4 to T_3 adequately, although this has never been convincingly demonstrated in dogs and cats. It is potentially of use in animals with severe small intestinal malabsorptive diseases as in these circumstances its improved absorptive characteristics (approximately 95% in humans) over T_4 may be beneficial.

Formulations and dose rates

- T_3 is available in 20 or 25 μg tablet form. The dose is 2–6 μg/kg, titrated to effect, administered every 8 h

Synthetic levothyroxine (L-thyroxine, thyroxine)

T_4 is the product of choice for the treatment of hypothyroidism in both dogs and cats for the following reasons.

- T_4 is the main hormone secreted by the thyroid.
- T_4 administration does not bypass the regulatory processes controlling the production of T_3 from T_4.
- Both circulating T_4 and T_3 are normalized.
- Synthetic T_4 is preferred as it has better bioavailability and results in more predictable thyroid hormone concentrations than crude thyroid products.

Formulations and dose rates

T_4 is available in tablet and liquid formulations in a range of sizes from 0.1 to 0.8 mg and a 1 mg/mL solution. The dose is 20–40 μg/kg once or twice daily or 0.2–0.5 mg/m^2 daily. The short half-life of T_4 would suggest that twice-daily administration is most appropriate and certainly results in less fluctuation of circulating T_4 concentrations

Formulations and dose rates—cont'd

compared to administration of the same total dose as a single daily bolus. However, the biological action of thyroid hormones far exceeds the plasma half-life and once-daily administration is successful in most hypothyroid dogs. The most common protocol is to administer T_4 at an initial dose of 20 µg/kg once daily with an initial maximum dose of 800 µg per dog.

The bioavailability of T_4 may be affected if it is given with food.

T_4 is also available as an injectable preparation for intravenous use. At a dose of approximately 4–5 µg/kg it has resulted in improvement in clinical signs within 30 h in a small number of dogs with myxedema coma thus far treated.

Pharmacokinetics

Thyroid hormones are absorbed from the gastrointestinal tract by passive diffusion. Most absorption occurs in the ileum and colon. Absorption is significantly modified by intraluminal factors (food, intestinal flora, etc.) and net absorption is low at approximately 10–50% with marked individual variation.

Increasing doses of T_4 are associated with a decrease in the biological half-life of the hormone, supportive of dose-dependent kinetics. There is some evidence to suggest that doubling the dose of T_4 results in an increase in peak circulating T_4 of approximately 50–60%.

Monitoring therapy

The success of T_4 replacement therapy is dependent on demonstrating a resolution of clinical signs and attainment of therapeutic thyroid hormone concentrations. Few studies have specifically examined both factors simultaneously. In one study of once-daily dosing, successful therapy was associated with a peak 4–6 h post-pill T_4 concentration of greater than 35 nmol/L. With divided daily dosing, peak values are invariably lower and pre-pill testing of circulating T_4 concentration is also recommended. Maintenance of elevated TSH concentrations may provide evidence of poor long-term compliance in medication administration.

It has previously been suggested that a minimum of 4–6 weeks is required before a steady-state condition is met and therapeutic thyroid hormone monitoring should not be attempted until then. However, there is limited change in circulating T_4 or TSH concentration after 2 weeks of therapy unless an actual dose adjustment is made, suggesting that therapeutic monitoring can be performed within 2 weeks of starting medication.

Although an improvement in the metabolic derangements associated with hypothyroidism is usually apparent within 2 weeks of adequate therapy, skin changes may take weeks to months to normalize. Similarly, although changes in circulating cholesterol concentration are rapidly corrected, the anemia associated with hypothyroidism can take weeks to resolve.

Adverse effects

T_4 replacement therapy is typically associated with circulating T_4 concentrations at the high end or above the reference range (50–100 nmol/L) yet clinical signs of thyrotoxicosis are rare. This apparent paradox is likely to be due to a number of factors, including the virtually unsaturable binding proteins, need for conversion of T_4 to T_3 for bioactivity and the rapid metabolism and excretion of thyroid hormones in dogs and cats. When clinical signs do occur, they include nervousness, hyperactivity, weight loss, polyphagia, polydipsia, polyuria, panting and fever. Diagnosis is confirmed by demonstrating an elevated serum T_4 concentration and by observing the amelioration of signs after discontinuation or decreasing the dose of the drug.

Gradual introduction of T_4 replacement therapy has been recommended in animals with a reduced ability to metabolize T_4 and an increased risk of thyrotoxicosis such as those with hypoadrenocorticism, diabetes mellitus, heart disease or in aged patients. A divided-dose protocol starting with 25% of the normal dose and increasing in 25% increments every fortnight is widely cited. However, such recommendations are usually made when the 'normal' dose used is at the higher end of the range and administered twice daily. Using the common protocol of 20 µg/kg once daily, there is minimal evidence of any untoward effects in hypothyroid animals with concurrent nonthyroidal disease.

Known drug interactions

- Concurrent therapy with drugs that induce hepatic microsomal enzymes (e.g. phenobarbital) may induce more rapid metabolism and necessitate a higher dose of replacement therapy.
- Hypothyroid dogs with diabetes mellitus tend to be insulin resistant and insulin requirements may decrease after thyroid hormone supplementation has commenced.
- A number of drugs can affect thyroid function in humans and lead to erroneous evaluation of thyroid function. These medications alter the synthesis, secretion, transport or metabolism of thyroid hormones or may directly inhibit the hypothalamic-pituitary axis. The effects of many drugs on thyroid function in dogs are becoming increasingly well understood. Such drugs include glucocorticoids, potentiated sulfonamides, phenobarbital and nonsteroidal anti-inflammatory drugs, although a range of other possibilities exist. The potential effect of these medications in altering the effect of administered T_4 concurrently is not yet known.

ANTITHYROID DRUGS

These drugs are indicated for the treatment of hyperthyroidism due to excessive autonomous secretion of thyroid hormone in adenomatous thyroid hyperplasia or, more rarely, functional thyroid adenocarcinomas. Cats are far more commonly afflicted with hyperthyroidism or thyrotoxicosis and, in some areas, adenomatous hyperplasia is the most common endocrinopathy encountered in cats.

In general, antithyroid medication is used in three ways.

- Long-term therapy for patients in which surgery or iodine-131 treatment is not possible.
- Short-term treatment before surgery to reduce the risk of cardiac and metabolic complications associated with anesthetizing hyperthyroid animals. Antithyroid medication is continued until the patient is euthyroid and then a thyroidectomy can be more safely performed.
- Short-term therapy to assess the effect of correcting thyrotoxicosis on renal function. The response to treatment can assist a final decision as to whether a more permanent treatment option such as iodine-131 or surgery is appropriate.

Thiourylene antithryoid drugs

The most important drugs available are the thiourylenes or thionamide drugs, which are derived from a sulfur-containing parent compound, thiouracil. Propylthiouracil, thiamazole (formerly methimazole) and carbimazole are used most commonly. Carbimazole, a carbethoxy derivative of thiamazole, is itself inactive, but is rapidly converted to thiamazole in vivo. Because of the severity and relatively high frequency of serious adverse reactions with propylthiouracil, this drug is no longer recommended as a means of controlling thyrotoxicosis in the cat.

Mechanism of action

The thiourylenes inhibit thyroid hormone synthesis by:

- acting as general inhibitors of thyroid peroxidase catalyzed reactions. This enzyme is involved in the oxidation of iodide and subsequent iodination of tyrosyl residues in thyroglobulin
- interfering with the coupling of MIT and DIT into T_4 and T_3 either through inhibition of thyroid peroxidase or through binding to thyroglobulin and altering its structure. This reaction is more sensitive to inhibition than the formation of iodotyrosines.
- inhibiting the peripheral conversion of T_4 to the more active T_3, although this effect is limited to propylthiouracil.

The thiourylenes do not affect the uptake of iodine or the release of preformed hormone from the thyroid gland.

Formulations and dose rates

Thiamazole

Thiamazole is available as 2.5 and 5 mg tablets. Induction doses of 2.5–5 mg/cat administered twice daily for 2–3 weeks are recommended. Induction doses of 5 mg administered once daily may also be effective in inducing euthyroidism, although a longer period of treatment (4 weeks) is required. The final maintenance dose is dependent on response but is usually 2.5 mg administered once or twice daily or 5 mg administered once daily.

Carbimazole

Carbimazole is available as 5 and 20 mg tablets. Induction doses of 10–15 mg divided twice or three times daily for 2–3 weeks are recommended. The maintenance dose is 5 mg administered either once or twice daily.

Pharmacokinetics

There is rapid and complete absorption of thiamazole and carbimazole after oral administration with oral bioavailability of approximately 80% in most hyperthyroid cats. Although possessing inherent antithyroid activity, carbimazole is almost totally converted to thiamazole soon after oral administration such that only thiamazole accumulates in the thyroid gland where it exerts its effect. This conversion results in a 10 mg dose of carbimazole being approximately equal to 6.1 mg of thiamazole. This may explain at least in part, the slight differences in dosage regimens recommended for the two drugs.

The pharmacokinetics of thiamazole are largely unaffected by hyperthyroidism or multiple dosing. The serum half-life of oral thiamazole in cats is approximately 4–6 h. Thiamazole is actively concentrated by the thyroid gland within minutes of absorption. Thus the effect of thiamazole is likely to be more prolonged than the half-life suggests. The intrathyroidal residence time may be approximately 20 h in cats, as it is in humans, and as such once-daily administration is frequently effective, particularly in the long-term management of the condition.

Monitoring therapy

Before treatment commences, circulating urea, creatinine and phosphate concentrations should be measured. If a hyperthyroid cat is azotemic before treatment, antithyroid drugs must be used with care as the reduction in glomerular filtration that can accompany the induction of euthyroidism may precipitate overt renal failure. The development of azotemia must also be considered a potential adverse reaction to antithyroid medication.

In general, the higher the pretreatment T_4, the longer it takes to achieve euthyroidism although in many cats 'biochemical euthyroidism' is achieved within days. Obvious regression of clinical signs lags behind the reduction in T_4 concentration but is generally apparent after 2–3 weeks. Consequently, monitoring should begin roughly 2 weeks after starting medication. If a circulating total T_4 concentration is below or within the low end of the reference range, the dose can be decreased by 2.5–5 mg to the final maintenance dose, or a surgical thyroidectomy performed. If thyroid hormone concentrations remain high, the duration of therapy is increased or the dosage is altered in 2.5–5 mg increments. The cat should be checked 2–3 weeks after each dose adjustment and thereafter, every 3–6 months.

Despite marked suppression of circulating total T_4 concentration, clinical signs of hypothyroidism do not develop. This is presumably because corresponding circulating T_3 concentrations, the more metabolically active hormone, remain within the reference range, possibly through increased extra- or intrathyroidal production of T_3. The latter may arise from intrathyroidal iodine deficiency or increased TSH production induced by antithyroid medication. In addition, circulating free T_4 concentration, the active portion of total T_4, appears to remain somewhat higher than the total hormone concentration during thiamazole therapy, suggesting a potential shift in the binding affinity of circulating proteins.

Medication should be stopped if serious adverse reactions occur and an alternative form of therapy should be sought.

Transdermal administration

Thiamazole can be incorporated into a pluronic lecithin organogel (PLO) for transdermal application. This route of administration may be of particular relevance for fractious or inappetant cats or those with concurrent gastrointestinal disease or drug-induced vomiting. The bioavailability of thiamazole administered by this route in healthy cats is variable but generally poor. However, administration of 2.5 mg twice daily in hyperthyroid cats has been shown to be effective although the time to achieve euthyroidism in the majority of cats is longer (approximately 4 weeks) than after oral administration. Interestingly, cats treated with oral thiamazole have a higher incidence of gastrointestinal adverse effects compared to cats treated with transdermal thiamazole.

Adverse effects

Thiamazole and carbimazole are safer and better tolerated than propylthioruracil although adverse reactions certainly can occur (Table 20.1).

Mild adverse effects occur in approximately 10–15% of cats and include anorexia, lethargy and vomiting.

Table 20.1 Adverse reactions associated with thiamazole therapy

Reaction	Approximate % of cases
Anorexia	10
Vomiting	10
Lethargy	10
Excoriations (facial)	2
Hepatopathy	1.5
Thrombocytopenia	2.5
Agranulocytosis	1.5
Leukopenia	4
Eosinophilia	10
Lymphocytosis	7
Positive ANA titer	50
Positive Coombs' test	1.5
Myasthenia gravis	<0.5
Hemolytic anemia	<0.5
Cold agglutinin-like disease	<0.5

These signs tend to occur within the first 4 weeks of therapy and are often transient, resolving despite continuation of medication. The gastrointestinal side effects are less common when thiamazole is administered transdermally. They also appear to be less common with carbimazole and this may be related to the fact that thiamazole has a more bitter taste whereas carbimazole is tasteless. In some cats, gastrointestinal signs persist, necessitating discontinuation of therapy.

Self-induced excoriations of the face and neck occur in a few cats within the first 3 months of therapy. Correction generally requires not only cessation of therapy but also glucocorticoid administration.

In the initial stages of therapy, development of mild eosinophilia, lymphocytosis and leukopenia with a normal differential count and without any clinical effect has been described in approximately 5–15% of cases. More serious hematological complications occur in <5% of cases, usually within the first 3 months of therapy. They include agranulocytosis and thrombocytopenia either alone or concurrently or, less commonly, immune-mediated hemolytic anemia. Hepatic toxicity (icterus and elevated liver enzymes) has been infrequently reported. For these serious reactions, withdrawal of the drug and supportive medication are required.

Approximately 50% of cats treated with thiamazole for more than 6 months develop serum antinuclear antibodies (ANA) although associated clinical signs of a lupus-like syndrome have not yet been observed. Serum ANA becomes negative in many of these cats if the dose of thiamazole is subsequently reduced.

Myasthenia gravis with characteristic transient muscle weakness and a cold agglutinin-like disease has been reported rarely after thiamazole treatment. A bleeding tendency has been anecdotally described but to date an explanation has been lacking.

Ipodate

Sodium or calcium ipodate, a cholecystographic contrast agent that reduces thyroid hormone production, has potential for the treatment of feline thyrotoxicosis, although experience with the drug is limited and complicated by lack of availability.

Mechanism of action

Although ipodate blocks the release of thyroid hormones as a consequence of the iodine released during its metabolism (ipodate is 63% iodine by weight), its major effect is to inhibit the outer-ring 5' deiodination of T_4 to T_3. Consequently, although circulating T_4 concentration may be unaffected by ipodate, there may be some clinical response as T_3 production is suppressed.

Formulations and dose rates

- 100 mg/cat divided twice daily is the recommended starting dose, administered orally

Adverse effects

No adverse side effects have been reported.

Stable iodine

Iodine is not indicated for the long-term medical management of cats with hyperthyroidism, but has been used (in combination with β-adrenergic blockers) for the presurgical treatment of cats unable to tolerate thiamazole or carbimazole. Its antithyroid effects are transient and inhibition only lasts for a short time (approximately 2–3 weeks). Iodine can be administered in conjunction with thiourylenes but this is rarely considered necessary because of their potency and efficacy when used alone.

Mechanism of action

Large doses of stable iodine acutely inhibit thyroid hormone synthesis (Wolff–Chaikoff effect) and thyroid hormone release. The former effect is mediated through inhibition of the enzyme thyroid peroxidase. These effects are not consistent and serum thyroid hormone concentrations, while often decreasing, rarely suppress markedly. Stable iodine purportedly reduces the size and vascularity of adenomatous thyroid tissue, although this is controversial.

Formulations and dose rates

- The current recommendation is to use potassium iodate at a dose of 21.25 mg three times daily for 10 days prior to surgery in cats with prior (10 d) and concurrent propranolol treatment

Adverse effects

Side effects include ptyalism and inappetence resulting from its unpleasant brassy taste. These can be minimized by placing the tablets in gelatin capsules before administration.

PARATHYROID DISEASE

Drugs used to treat parathyroid disease are rarely directed at the parathyroid gland itself but rather correct the derangements in calcium homeostasis resulting from both parathyroid and nonparathyroid disorders. Irrespective of cause, the principles of therapy for hypocalcemia and hypercalcemia remain the same. In order to understand the indications for and actions of the various drugs used, an understanding of normal calcium homeostasis and the diseases that potentially result in hypo- and hypercalcemia is important.

Relevant physiology/pathophysiology

Calcium homeostasis is controlled predominantly by parathyroid hormone (PTH (parathormone)), and the active form of vitamin D (1,25-dihydroxycholecalciferol ($1{,}25(OH)_2D_3$) or calcitriol) variously acting through the kidneys, gastrointestinal tract and bone. Phosphate homeostasis is similarly controlled although it is generally considered to be secondary to calcium. Calcitonin, produced by the parafollicular cells of the thyroid gland, may also affect calcium homeostasis, although its physiological role in dogs and cats is less clear.

Typically there are two parathyroid glands associated with each thyroid lobe (cranial or external and caudal or internal) although ectopic parathyroid tissue may also be found in both dogs and cats. The chief (or principal) cells form the major cell type of the parathyroid glands and their primary function is to secrete PTH. This hormone is an 84-amino acid, single-chain polypeptide secreted in response to low plasma ionized calcium concentration. Subsequently, calcium concentrations are increased through a concerted action on both bone and kidney, as follows.

- Stimulation of calcium and phosphate release from bone with the permissive presence of $1{,}25(OH)_2D$.
- Increased calcium reabsorption from the glomerular filtrate while phosphate reabsorption is inhibited.
- Stimulation of the enzyme 1 α-hydroxylase located in the proximal tubules of the kidney which in turn increases the synthesis of $1{,}25(OH)_2D$.
- As circulating calcium is increased, PTH release is inhibited.

Vitamin D is integral to normal calcium homeostasis. Vitamin D is a fat-soluble vitamin. The first step in its production involves conversion of cholesterol to 7-dehydrocholesterol in the skin, although it can also be obtained through the diet. Conversion then occurs in the liver in a nonrate-limiting step to 25-hydroxycholecalciferol. Subsequent conversion to its active form is regulated by PTH and occurs in the kidney. The major action of $1,25(OH)_2D_3$ is to stimulate intestinal calcium and phosphate absorption. It also acts to inhibit PTH secretion from the parathyroid glands and together with PTH promotes release of calcium and phosphate from bone.

Phosphate concentration also plays a role in regulating PTH secretion indirectly through its effect on calcium concentrations and directly by influencing PTH secretion and $1,25(OH)_2D_3$ production. Hypophosphatemia decreases PTH synthesis and stimulates renal production of $1,25(OH)_2D$ while hyperphosphatemia inhibits the activity of the renal 1-α-hydroxylase enzyme.

Derangements in calcium homeostasis

Primary parathyroid disorders are uncommon in dogs and cats but despite this, derangements in circulating calcium concentrations are relatively common. Spurious hypo- and hypercalcemia are possible and it is always recommended that any abnormality be confirmed as repeatable. In addition, most laboratory assessment of calcium is directed at measurement of total calcium, a measure of both the bound and unbound fraction. The unbound, free or ionized fraction constitutes approximately 50% of total calcium and is considered to be the biologically active portion. The remainder is divided into protein bound (approximately 40% of total calcium) and complex bound (approximately 10%). The majority of protein-bound calcium is bound to albumin whereas the complex fraction is associated with low molecular weight ligands such as bicarbonate, lactate, citrate and phosphate. Alterations in the complex but more particularly the protein-bound fraction can have significant effects on the total calcium concentration. As a consequence the existence of both hypo- and hypercalcemia should be confirmed by direct measurement of the active ionized portion. Calculation of the ionized fraction using formulae accounting for total protein and albumin concentrations is inaccurate by comparison and no longer recommended.

Hypercalcemia

Hypercalcemia can arise from a variety of causes (Table 20.2). In dogs hypercalcemia is most commonly associated with malignancy, hypoadrenocorticism, renal failure and primary hyperparathyroidism. In patients with impaired renal function, ionized calcium concentration is rarely elevated and the hypercalcemia associated with hypoadrenocorticism usually resolves rapidly with treatment of the adrenal insufficiency. However, in malignancy-associated hypercalcemia, primary hyperparathyroidism and vitamin D toxicosis, treatment directed towards lowering serum calcium concentration is generally required. This treatment is usually instituted whilst diagnostic evaluation for the underlying cause is ongoing and as such care must be taken to avoid any therapies that may interfere with such test results.

Table 20.2 Potential causes of hypercalcemia in dogs and cats. The disorders highlighted in bold are those that usually require specific therapy for hypercalcemia

Neoplasia
Lymphoma
Anal sac adenocarcinoma
Myeloproliferative disease
Other tumors
Primary hyperparathyroidism
Hypervitaminosis D
Granulomatous disease
Idiopathic (cats only)
Renal failure
Nutritional secondary hyperparathyroidism
Osteolytic/osteoporotic disease
Hypoadrenocorticism

In cats, hypercalcemia is most commonly associated with malignancy and renal failure although idiopathic hypercalcemia has become an increasingly recognized entity. Primary hyperparathyroidism and hypoadrenocorticism appear to be rare in cats.

Hypercalcemia is potentially toxic to many organs but its major effects are on the renal, neurological, cardiovascular and gastrointestinal systems. Most animals with a circulating total calcium greater than approximately 3.75 mmol/L will exhibit some clinical signs and require treatment and those with values greater than 4.50 mmol/L are usually severely affected. The rate at which calcium increases, the length of time it has been present and its underlying cause also play a role in the type and severity of the clinical signs. Although an increased risk of renal damage and a need for early therapeutic intervention have been suggested when the calcium phosphate product is high, recent studies suggest that this product is less useful in predicting renal damage than the absolute total calcium concentration alone.

Hypocalcemia

As with hypercalcemia, hypocalcemia can also arise from numerous causes (Table 20.3). However, clinical signs rarely become apparent until circulating total calcium concentration is less than 1.5 mmol/L. As a consequence, the majority of causes of hypocalcemia result in a clinically occult abnormality and specific treatment is not required providing the underlying cause is addressed. Puerperal tetany and hypoparathyroidism are the most common conditions associated with clini-

Table 20.3 Potential causes of hypocalcemia. The disorders highlighted in bold are those that require specific therapy for hypocalcemia. Those italicized may or may not require treatment depending on the severity of the hypocalcemia

Hypoparathyroidism
Eclampsia
Pancreatitis
Phosphate enema toxicosis
Ethylene glycol toxicity
Systemic inflammatory response syndrome
Tumor lysis syndrome
Malabsorption
Renal failure
Medullary carcinoma of thyroid

cal hypocalcemia. Given the large number of hyperthyroid cats in some countries that undergo bilateral thyroidectomy, iatrogenic hypoparathyroidism is relatively commonly encountered.

The clinical signs of hypocalcemia generally relate to the neuromuscular system. These signs include focal muscle spasms or fasciculations, tremors, twitching, tetany and generalized seizures. The number and severity of these signs relate to the magnitude of the hypocalcemia and the rate of change of ionized calcium. Once hypocalcemia induces neuromuscular signs, particularly tetany or seizures, prompt treatment is required.

TREATMENT OF HYPERCALCEMIA

Once persistent clinical hypercalcemia has been identified, treatment is warranted while the underlying cause is identified. Generally, short-term success is achieved using simple measures such as intravenous fluid therapy with or without diuretic administration. More prolonged control will require more specific intervention and currently bisphosphonates are the most appropriate and potent drugs available.

General supportive therapy

Intravenous fluid therapy

Many hypercalcemic animals are dehydrated when presented which exacerbates the hypercalcemia. Rehydration with mild volume expansion eliminates the effects of dehydration and promotes calciuresis.

Normal saline is the fluid of choice as it contains no additional calcium and it promotes calciuresis as sodium competes with calcium for tubular resorption. Potassium supplementation may be required.

Approximately 2–3 times maintenance (120–180 mL/kg/d) is required over the dehydration deficit (this can be replaced in the first 4–6 h).

Care should be taken to avoid volume overload.

Diuretic therapy

The loop diuretic furosemide enhances the effect of volume expansion by inhibiting calcium resorption in the thick ascending limb of the loop of Henle. By contrast, thiazide diuretics are unhelpful as they decrease calcium excretion, thereby promoting hypercalcemia. Furosemide may also protect against the risk of volume overload associated with saline diuresis.

Furosemide is initially administered intravenously as a 5 mg/kg bolus followed by a 5 mg/kg infusion or 2–4 mg/kg q.8–12 h.

The use of furosemide should only be considered once any dehydration deficits have been replaced and volume expansion instituted.

Glucocorticoids

Glucocorticoids decrease circulating calcium concentration potentially through a variety of mechanisms although few have been specifically evaluated in dogs or cats. Glucocorticoids counter the effect of $1,25(OH)_2D$ and enhance renal excretion of calcium. Glucocorticoids are also cytotoxic to neoplastic lymphocytes and can inhibit the growth of neoplastic tissue and consequently may decrease circulating calcium concentration in malignancy-associated hypercalcemia.

However, their use can interfere with diagnostic tests and may adversely affect the response to the treatment of some disorders producing hypercalcemia (e.g. various malignancies, granulomatous disorders due to infectious agents). As a result, the use of glucocorticoids in managing hypercalcemia is usually limited to the hypercalcemia associated with vitamin D intoxication (including granulomatous disease) or in cats with idiopathic hypercalcemia where glucocorticoids alone have reportedly been effective.

Prednisolone is the most common agent used at a dose of 1–2 mg/kg/12 h. Alternatively dexamethasone at a dose of 0.1–0.2 mg/kg/12 h can be used. These drugs are administered orally, subcutaneously or intravenously.

Adverse effects of glucocorticoids are described elsewhere (Chapter 11). However, it is worth noting here that glucocorticoids potentially increase the risk of calcium oxalate urolithiasis in hypercalcemia but this is usually countered by a decrease in the filtered load of calcium as the hypercalcemia itself is addressed. Additionally dexamethasone's long half-life markedly increases the likelihood of adverse effects when it is used for any significant period with dosing frequencies of less than 48 hourly.

Bisphosphonates

The bisphosphonates are pyrophosphate analogs that act as inhibitors of bone mineralization.

Bisphosphonates directly inhibit bone resorption by binding to hydroxyapatite crystals, thereby impeding calcium and phosphorus mineral dissolution. In addition, they inhibit osteoclastic activity and induce osteoclastic apoptosis. The aminobisphosphonates (bisphosphonates with a nitrogen atom on their side chain) such as pamidronate and alendronate are extremely potent inhibitors of bone resorption.

Clinical applications

In humans, bisphosphonates are used for the management of tumor-induced hypercalcemia, Paget's disease, osteolytic bone metastases of breast cancer and osteolytic lesions associated with malignant myeloma. In dogs, bisphosphonates are most commonly used for the treatment of malignancy-associated hypercalcemia and hyperparathyroidism. They do not interfere with diagnostic tests for malignancy and therefore they are most suitable for use in hypercalcemia when a definitive diagnosis has not been obtained. In cats, bisphosphonates have been recommended specifically for the treatment of odontoclastic resorptive lesions and idiopathic hypercalcemia.

Formulations and dose rates

Bisphosphonates are usually used intravenously although oral formulations are available. Pamidronate disodium is available as 15, 30 or 90 mg powder in vials with solvent in ampoules. Alendronate sodium is available as a 10 mg tablet.

Pamidronate is administered at a dose of 1.3 (1.0–2.0) mg/kg infused intravenously over 2 h in 150 mL 0.9% saline. Pamidronate has a relatively rapid onset of action within 48 h with a duration of effect spanning from 1 to up to 9 weeks. Repeated administration is possible but should be attempted cautiously as data are limited in small animals.

Oral alendronate has been recommended for the treatment of odontoclastic lesions and idiopathic hypercalcemia in cats, although experience is limited. Doses used range from 3 to 9 mg/kg once to twice weekly.

Pharmacokinetics

In humans, approximately 50–60% of pamidronate is absorbed by bone after intravenous administration. Pamidronate is slowly excreted unmetabolized in kidneys.

Adverse effects

- Use of pamidronate has been associated with the development of acute renal tubular necrosis and glomerulonephropathies in a small number of humans and purportedly also in dogs. It is recommended that its administration is preceded and followed by a minimum of 4 h of diuresis to avoid nephrotoxicity.
- Other potential adverse effects associated with the use of pamidronate include development of hypocalcemia, hypophosphatemia, hypomagnesemia and hypokalemia.

Calcitonin

Calcitonin acts mainly by inhibiting osteoclastic activity in bone although it may have some effect on reducing both calcium and phosphate resorption in the proximal renal tubules. In the treatment of hypercalcemia it is considered to have a rapid onset of action (hours) but only weak to moderate potency that is of short duration (days). Repeated use has been associated with reduced efficacy.

Formulations and dose rates

Synthetic or recombinant salmon calcitonin (salcatonin) is widely available as an injectable 50, 100 or 200 IU/mL solution. It has only been used in a small number of dogs and cats at dosages ranging from 4 to 8 U/kg every 8–24 h subcutaneously or intramuscularly.

Adverse effects

Data on adverse effects are limited due to the small number of cases treated. In humans its use has been associated with transient nausea, vomiting, abdominal pain, flushing and local skin reactions.

Miscellaneous drugs

Plicamycin (formerly mithramycin) is an antiresorptive drug that was the first-line agent for treating hypercalcemia in humans for many years.

In a small number of dogs where plicamycin has been used at a low dose of 25 μg /kg intravenously, calcium concentrations decreased within 12 h and remained suppressed for 1–3 d.

In humans, use of plicamycin is associated with a range of adverse effects including renal, hepatic and hematological reactions. Mild gastrointestinal side effects have been noted in dogs and acute hepatonecrosis has been reported with higher doses. As a consequence of limited data, this drug has not gained widespread use.

Intravenous administration of EDTA has been recommended for acute life-threatening hypercalcemia. However, given its potential nephrotoxicity and the availability of other calcium-lowering drugs, it can no longer be recommended in small animals.

Correcting acidosis or causing a mild alkalosis with intravenous bicarbonate reduces the clinical effects of hypercalcemia by shifting the ionized to the protein-bound fraction. However, the effect is mild and should not be relied on as sole therapy for hypercalcemia.

TREATMENT OF HYPOCALCEMIA

Once clinical signs of hypocalcemia develop, acute therapy with parenterally administered calcium is indicated to control the clinical signs. Depending on the underlying cause, continuing therapy may or may not be warranted.

Parenteral calcium preparations

Formulations and dose rates

Parenteral calcium preparations are most commonly supplied as the gluconate or chloride salt. When clinical signs are present, calcium is administered intravenously to effect. The recommended starting dose is based on the elemental calcium concentration (10–15 mg/kg) of the preparation. This dose is equivalent to 1.0–1.5 mL/kg of 10% calcium gluconate or 0.2–0.5 mL/kg of 10% calcium chloride. Calcium must be injected slowly to avoid cardiac toxicity. Once neurological signs have been controlled the injection is stopped. A single injection has a variable duration of action ranging from 1 to 12 h.

To avoid recurrence of clinical signs generally continued administration of calcium is required either until the cause has been identified and addressed or until oral calcium supplementation takes effect. This 'maintenance calcium infusion rate' is usually administered as a slow intravenous infusion at a dose of 60–90 mg/kg/d of elemental calcium. Normal saline is the diluting fluid of choice as precipitation of calcium salts occurs with fluids containing bicarbonate, lactate, acetate or phosphate. The elemental dose is achieved by using 25 mL of 10% calcium gluconate diluted in 250 mL of saline and infused at a rate of 2.5 mL/kg/h. As an alternative, subcutaneous injections of diluted calcium gluconate solutions have been recommended every 6–8 h. However, their repeated use should be avoided because of the risk of the development of iatrogenic calcinosis cutis.

Adverse effects

Adverse reactions are mainly related to the development of cardiotoxicity (manifest as bradycardia, ventricular premature contractions, sudden elevation of the ST segment or shortening of the Q-T interval). However, calcium chloride is extremely irritant if administered perivascularly and because of this, calcium gluconate is generally the preferred parenteral preparation.

Oral calcium preparations

If continued calcium supplementation is required, oral therapy is begun as soon as possible. High doses are used initially until vitamin D administration begins to take effect. High doses ensure that passive diffusion of calcium from the intestinal lumen to the circulation is maximized.

Formulations and dose rates

Numerous calcium salts are available although those with the highest calcium content are preferred. The initial starting dose of elemental calcium is 60–90 mg/kg/d. This is equivalent to 150–225 mg/kg/d of calcium carbonate or 450–700 mg/kg/d of calcium lactate. Tapering doses are instituted once vitamin D therapy has begun to take effect. Thereafter dietary supply of calcium is usually sufficient.

Adverse effects

Adverse reactions primarily relate to the potential development of hypercalcemia when calcium and vitamin D are supplemented concurrently. Calcium chloride is, however, specifically avoided because it tends to cause gastric irritation.

Oral vitamin D preparations

Maintenance therapy for hypoparathyroidism usually consists of a combination of oral vitamin D supplementation with initially concurrent calcium administration. Once the calcium and phosphorus levels are normalized maintenance therapy tends to be based around vitamin D supplementation alone. The most commonly recommended vitamin D preparations include ergocalciferol, dihydrotachysterol, calcitriol and alfacalcidol.

Ergocalciferol (vitamin D_2 or calciferol)

Formulations and dose rates

This is the cheapest and most readily available vitamin D preparation. However, extremely high pharmacological doses (4000–6000 IU/kg/24 h) must be employed in the absence of PTH to exert any biological effect. It is highly lipid soluble, requiring weeks to saturate body stores. Its effect usually becomes apparent after 5–14 days of therapy although on occasion it may take longer. The aim is to maintain circulating calcium concentrations within the low end of the reference range and this usually requires decreasing the dose to alternate-day administration. It has a long half-life, such that if hypercalcemia occurs and the drug is withdrawn, 1–4 weeks are required before its effects dissipate. As a consequence it is not recommended for use in dogs and cats.

Dihydrotachysterol

Formulations and dose rates

Dihydrotachysterol is a synthetic analog of vitamin D. It has a more rapid onset of action (1–7 d) and a shorter time for dissipation of effect in the event of toxicity (2-3 weeks) than ergocalciferol. It is available as a 0.25 mg/mL solution or 0.25 mg tablet. The initial dose is 0.03 mg/kg/24 h over 3 d, decreasing to 0.01 mg/kg/24–48 h depending on the circulating calcium concentration.

Adverse effects

As with all vitamin D preparations, development of hypercalcemia is the most serious adverse reaction.

Calcitriol

Calcitriol is the biologically active form of vitamin D and therefore has a more immediate onset of action (maximal effect in <4 d) and a much shorter time for dissipation of effect in the event of toxicity (1–7 d). It is therefore the drug of choice for the treatment of hypoparathyroidism. Calcitriol can also be used prior to surgical parathyroidectomy for treatment of hyperparathyroidism.

Formulations and dose rates

It is available as 250 or 500 ng capsules and is administered orally at an initial dose of 30–60 ng/kg/24 h. If administered at a dose of approximately 7.5 ng/kg/24 h in the 5–7 d preceding surgery for primary hyperparathyroidism, active calcium absorption will be expected in the immediate postsurgical period when the risk of hypoparathyroidism is high.

At lower dose (2.5–3.5 ng/kg/d) calcitriol inhibits PTH secretion and it is this dose that is recommended for renal secondary hyperparathyroidism although studies clearly evaluating its efficacy are lacking. The available capsule size limits the use of this drug at low doses or in small dogs or cats. Regular monitoring of circulating calcium concentration is required using the lowest possible dose to maintain calcium concentration in the lower end of the reference range.

Adverse effects

Hypercalcemia is the most common adverse reaction to the administration of calcitriol.

Alfacalcidol

Formulations and dose rates

Alfacalcidol requires 25-hydroxylation in the liver to produce active vitamin D. As this is not a PTH-dependent step, the drug is therefore considered similar to calcitriol and is used at the same dose. Although available as 250–1000 ng capsules, its availability as an oral solution (2 μg/mL) may provide some advantage when using low doses.

Table 20.4 Drugs available for the management of thyroid and parathyroid disease

Drug	Brand names	Manufacturer
Levothyroxine	Soloxine®	Daniels Pharmaceuticals
	Forthyron®	Eurovet Animal Health
	Leventa®	Intervet
	Thyroxyl®	Dechra Veterinary Products
Tri-iodothyronine	Tertroxin®	Glaxo Wellcome
Thiamazole (methimazole)	Tapazole®	Eli Lilly
	Felimazole®	Arnolds Veterinary Products
Carbimazole	Neomercazole®	Roche
Calcium ipodate	Orograffin®	Bristol-Myers Squibb
Pamidronate	Aredia®	Novartis
Alendronate	Fosamax®	MSD
Salcatonin	Miacalcic®	Novartis
	Forcaltonin®	Unigene UK
Dihydrotachysterol	AT10®	Bayer
Calcitriol	Rocaltrol®	Roche
Alfacalcidol	One-alpha®	Leo

Parathyroid hormone

Physiological replacement of PTH is the optimum treatment for hypoparathyroidism. Although synthetic PTH is available for use in humans, to date its use remains experimental, expensive and difficult to administer, as it requires repeated injections. Consequently, at present it is not effectively available for use in small animals.

FURTHER READING

Behrend EN 1999 Medical therapy of feline hyperthyroidism. Compend Cont Educ 21: 235-244

Daminet S, Ferguson DC 2003 Influence of drugs on thyroid function in dogs. J Vet Intern Med 17: 463-472

Hoffmann G, Marks SL, Taboda J, Hosgood GL, Wolfsheimer KJ 2003 Transdermal methimazole in cats with hyperthyroidism. J Fel Med Surg 5: 77-82

Hostutler RA, Chew DJ, Jaeger JQ, Klein S, Henderson D, DiBartola SP 2005 Uses and effectiveness of pamidronate disodium for treatment of dogs and acts with hypercalcemia. J Vet Intern Med 19: 29-33

Mooney CT 1997 Update on the medical management of hyperthyroidism. In: August JR (ed.) Consultations in feline internal medicine, 3rd edn. WB Saunders, Philadelphia, PA, pp 155-162

Peterson ME, Kintzer PP, Hurvitz AL 1988 Methimazole treatment of 262 cats with hyperthyroidism. J Vet Intern Med 2L 150-157

Sator LL, Trepanier A, Kroll MM, Rodan I, Challoner L 2004 Efficacy and safety of transdermal methimazole in the treatment of cats with hyperthyroidism. J Vet Intern Med 18: 651-655

Drugs used in the treatment of disorders of pancreatic function

David B Church

Pancreatic dysfunction in companion animals can be divided into three broad categories: a relative or absolute insulin deficiency due to reduced insulin secretion, insulin excess due to uncontrolled insulin secretion and insufficient synthesis and secretion of digestive enzymes from the exocrine pancreas.

RELATIVE/ABSOLUTE INSULIN DEFICIENCY (DIABETES MELLITUS)

A relative or absolute insulin deficiency will result in clinically significant carbohydrate, protein and lipid intolerance. These deficiencies may come about as a result of destruction of pancreatic islet tissue alone or in combination with any one of a number of so-called 'diabetogenic' factors which interfere with normal insulin activity and may predispose the islet tissue to further damage.

Insulin deficiency can be addressed through two main treatment strategies. One strategy consists of administration of various forms of exogenous insulin to provide systemic anabolic effects required for normal health as well as possibly reducing the demand placed upon any remaining functioning islets. The second strategy utilizes various agents which act to increase insulin secretions in response to standard insulinogenic stimuli. Of course, this latter strategy is predicated upon the presence of significant amounts of actual or potential insulin-secreting tissue.

INSULINS

Mechanism of action

The administration of suitable doses of insulin temporarily restores the ability to metabolize carbohydrates, fats and proteins, store hepatic glycogen, inhibit gluconeogenesis and ketosis, and promote intracellular movement of potassium. Consequently, when it is given in suitable doses at regular intervals to most patients with diabetes mellitus, blood glucose is maintained within a reasonable range, urine remains relatively free of glucose and ketones, and diabetic acidosis and coma are prevented.

Chemical structure

Insulin is a polypeptide hormone with a molecular weight of around 6000 consisting of a 21 amino acid (acidic) A-chain and a 30 amino acid (basic) B-chain linked by two sulfide bonds. Amino acid sequences vary between species although most commercial insulin preparations are composed of porcine, bovine, human or human analog forms that only vary by 1–3 amino acid residues.

Whatever the species of origin, commercial insulin preparations are available in various physicochemical formulations designed to modify the onset and duration of action of the insulin.

Insulin dissolved in water is known as soluble or neutral insulin and has the shortest duration of action, usually lasting no more than 6 h when injected subcutaneously.

Insulin can be precipitated with zinc and an excess of the basic peptide protamine to produce protamine zinc insulin or isophane insulin if there is no surplus of either protamine or zinc. In addition, when zinc alone is used to precipitate insulin this resultant insulin–zinc complex can also delay absorption from injection sites. When the insulin–zinc complexes are present in large crystals (ultralente), absorption is significantly delayed. When the insulin–zinc complexes are present in an amorphous form (semilente) the absorption is more rapid and when they are present in a mixture of 30% amorphous and 70% crystalline forms (lente), absorption is similar to isophane insulin preparations.

Pharmacokinetics

The absorption of unmodified insulin occurs relatively rapidly with the effects of subcutaneous insulin usually completed within 4–6 h. However, a number of different physicochemical modifications of the insulin complex structure can modify the rate of absorption, resulting in some insulins exerting their effects for up to 30 h after subcutaneous administration.

A fraction of the endogenous or exogenous insulin in plasma may be associated with certain proteins, chiefly α- and β-globulins. However, there is debate about whether these associations are of any importance for the transport of insulin, the bulk of which appears to circulate in an unbound form. Although there have been concerns regarding significant immune-mediated reactions to insulin and the subsequent development of circulating insulin antibodies, these rarely if ever seem to influence any aspect of insulin's biological activity or pharmacodynamic characteristics.

Insulin has a short half-life (less than 9 min in humans) and is principally metabolized by both the liver and kidney. Although peripheral tissues such as muscle and fat bind and inactivate insulin, this is of minor quantitative significance. Severe impairment of renal function appears to affect the rate of disappearance of circulating insulin, presumably as the kidney operates more closely to its maximum capacity to degrade insulin.

Adverse effects

Only soluble insulins should be administered intravenously. Intravenous administration of insulin suspensions can precipitate anaphylactic reactions and multiple organ failure.

In humans, hypersensitivity reactions to subcutaneously administered insulin have been reported and have included pruritus, rash, erythema and lipoatrophy. However, these have become very uncommon since the introduction of highly purified insulins and similar reactions are equally rare in companion animals.

Perhaps the most commonly encountered adverse effect of insulin is hypoglycemia. The fear of hypoglycemia dominates many veterinarians' approach to the management of diabetes, tending to result in lower doses of insulin being used and the common practice of tending to feed the patient before dosing with insulin. In reality, perhaps the most common reasons for hypoglycemia are failure to recognize a reducing insulin requirement as a result of returning endogenous insulin secretion and/or the practice of administering the total daily insulin dose every 24 h rather than dividing it and administering 12 hourly.

CLASSES OF INSULINS

Neutral or soluble insulin, insulin lispro

Clinical applications

Soluble insulin preparations can be used in conjunction with longer acting insulins to provide a more rapid onset of action. However, they are most commonly used to achieve some measure of glycemic control in diabetic patients with significant gastrointestinal dysfunction generally due to diabetic ketoacidosis or pancreatitis. These patients are likely to have severe metabolic perturbations and require intensive management of not only their insulin deficiency but also hydration status and concurrent electrolyte derangements.

Formulations and dose rates

The soluble insulins can be of bovine, porcine, human or human analog form and are all dissolved in an aqueous solution, making them the only form of insulin available for intravenous administration.

DOGS AND CATS

Intravenous infusion technique

As a slow intravenous infusion at a dose of 50 mU/kg/h until blood glucose is lowered to approximately 12–15 mmol/L, when the rate should be reduced to 25 mU/kg/h and a continuous glucose infusion started at a rate of approximately 150 mg/kg/h. At all times, the insulin and glucose dose may be modified on the basis of repeated estimation of the changes in blood glucose and plasma potassium concentrations. To facilitate accuracy, the insulin should be diluted to a concentration of **not less than** 50 mU/mL in any standard fluid bag. Concentrations lower than 50 mU/mL result in unacceptably high amounts of insulin adhering to the administration apparatus.

Intermittent intramuscular technique

An initial dose of 0.2 U/kg is given intramuscularly and followed by hourly intramuscular injections of 0.1 U/kg until the blood glucose returns to around 12–15 mmol/L, when the administration is changed to 8-hourly subcutaneous injections of 0.1–0.4 U/kg and a glucose infusion started at a rate of around 150 mg/kg/h. As with the intravenous infusion protocol, the insulin and glucose dose may be modified on the basis of repeated estimation of the changes in blood glucose and plasma potassium concentrations.

Isophane insulin

Clinical applications

The intermediate-acting isophane or NPH insulin is one of the traditional insulins of choice for the glycemic regulation of diabetes mellitus in dogs and cats. Peak activity time and duration of effect can be variable in both species although generally the best control is achieved with twice-daily dosing, matching the peak activity time of the insulin with the maximum hyperglycemic effects of the meal. An effective starting point is to administer insulin subcutaneously 12 hourly and feed the animal approximately 50% of the daily caloric intake approximately 1–2 h later.

Formulations and dose rates

As bovine and feline insulins vary by only one amino acid and human insulin differs by only one amino acid from both porcine and canine insulin, it is usually preferable to use isophane insulins of bovine origin in cats and porcine or human origin in dogs.

DOGS

- Approximately 0.5–2.0 IU/kg/24 h generally divided and given 12 hourly although the dose MUST be individualized on the basis of serial blood glucose estimations or regular estimates of circulating glycated proteins such as fructosamine or glycosylated hemoglobin

CATS

- Approximately 2–6 IU/cat/24 h divided and given 12 hourly although as with all insulin therapy in diabetic cats, the dose must be individualized and close monitoring is essential

Lente insulin

Clinical applications

The intermediate-acting lente insulin is one of the traditional insulins of choice for the glycemic regulation of diabetes mellitus in dogs and cats. Peak activity time and duration of effect can be variable in both species although generally the best control is achieved with twice-daily dosing, matching the peak activity time of the insulin with the maximum hyperglycemic effects of the meal. An effective starting point is to administer insulin subcutaneously 12 hourly and feed the animal approximately 50% of the daily caloric intake approximately 1–2 h later.

Formulations and dose rates

As bovine and feline insulins vary by only one amino acid and human insulin differs by only one amino acid from both porcine and canine insulin, it is usually preferable to use lente insulins of bovine origin in cats and porcine or human origin in dogs.

DOGS

- Approximately 0.5–2.0 IU/kg/24 h generally divided and given 12 hourly although the dose MUST be individualized on the basis of serial blood glucose estimations or regular estimates of circulating glycated proteins such as fructosamine or glycosylated hemoglobin

CATS

- Approximately 2–6 IU/cat/24 h divided and given 12 hourly although as with all insulin therapy in diabetic cats, the dose must be individualized and close monitoring is essential

Protamine zinc insulin

Clinical applications

Protamine zinc insulin generally lasts a little longer than either isophane or lente insulins. Consequently, it is generally used in those patients where the duration of activity of the so-called intermediate-acting insulins is insufficient to provide adequate glycemic control for 12-h periods. As insulins generally last for a shorter period of time in cats than dogs, protamine zinc insulin is more commonly used for treating diabetes mellitus in cats than dogs. Indeed, some endocrinologists prefer 12-h subcutaneous bovine protamine zinc insulin as the initial choice in treating diabetes mellitus in cats.

Formulations and dose rates

As bovine and feline insulins vary by only one amino acid and human insulin differs by only one amino acid from both porcine and canine insulin, it is usually preferable to use protamine zinc insulin of bovine origin in cats and when available, protamine zinc insulin of porcine or human origin in dogs.

DOGS

- Approximately 0.5–2.0 IU/kg/24 h generally divided and given 12 hourly although the dose MUST be individualized on the basis of serial blood glucose estimations or regular estimates of circulating glycated proteins such as fructosamine or glycosylated hemoglobin

CATS

- Approximately 2–6 IU/cat/24 h divided and given 12 hourly although as with all insulin therapy in diabetic cats, the dose must be individualized and close monitoring is essential

Ultralente insulin

Clinical applications

The longer duration of action of ultralente insulin makes it less suitable for achieving satisfactory glycemic control in most diabetics although it has been recommended in those patients where other insulin preparations have been shown to have an inadequate duration of action. Unfortunately, in dogs and cats ultralente insulins appear to be poorly absorbed and their use in managing all but the mildest forms of diabetes mellitus tends to be associated with high insulin doses and increased risk of hypoglycemia.

Formulations and dose rates

DOGS

- Approximately 0.5–2.0 IU/kg/24 h generally divided and given 12 hourly although the dose MUST be individualized on the basis of serial blood glucose estimations or regular estimates of circulating glycated proteins such as fructosamine or glycosylated hemoglobin

CATS

- Approximately 2–6 IU/cat/24 h. In some cats this may be as a once-daily dose although in many the dose is divided and given 12 hourly. As with all insulin therapy in diabetic cats, the dose must be individualized and close monitoring is essential

Special considerations

Due to the relatively slow onset of action of ultralente insulin, in most situations it may be advisable to use a diet relatively high in fiber and/or to encourage the patient to eat small amounts frequently rather than one or two large meals per day.

Insulin glargine

Clinical applications

Insulin glargine has been shown in humans to be a long-lasting, peakless insulin more closely resembling the profile of constitutive basal endogenous insulin secretion. In humans it has been shown to be beneficial in the management of both type 1 and type 2 (or insulin-dependent and insulin-independent respectively) diabetes mellitus with decreased incidence of hypoglycemic episodes and improved control when compared to at least one traditional intermediate-acting insulin (NPH).

In dogs and cats, insulin glargine generally lasts longer than either lente or protamine zinc insulins although this extended duration generally is not sufficient to justify once-daily administration. Consequently, it is generally used in those patients where the duration of activity of the so-called intermediate-acting insulins is insufficient to provide adequate glycemic control for 12-h periods. As insulins generally last for a shorter period of time in cats than dogs and a greater proportion of diabetic cats tend to have 'grazing feeding' patterns, making their insulin requirement more suited to an insulin with a relatively consistent effect over its duration of action, insulin glargine is more commonly used for treating diabetes mellitus in cats than dogs. Indeed, preliminary data suggest that when combined with appropriate dietary control, 12-hourly administration of subcutaneous insulin glargine to cats with diabetes mellitus is more likely to produce remission than similarly administered either lente or protamine zinc insulin.

Formulations and dose rates

Insulin glargine was developed by recombinant DNA technology and differs from human insulin by the substitution of glycine for asparagine at position 21 of the A-chain and the addition of two positively charged arginine molecules at the C-terminus of the B-chain. These changes result in glargine being relatively insoluble at neutral pH, leading to its microprecipitation in neutral pH, as is found in normal subcutaneous tissue. This microprecipitation delays absorption, resulting in insulin glargine being released from its subcutaneous site relatively consistently over an extended period. It is because of this tendency for a relatively stable activity profile over a reasonable period that glargine has been recommended for use in cats as either once- or twice-daily insulin. One recent preliminary study showed no difference in glycemic control between diabetic cats dosed with similar total daily doses of lente insulin given 12 hourly and glargine 24 hourly. Other investigators have reported improved remission rates in diabetic cats given 12-hourly glargine compared to those given either protamine zinc or lente 12 hourly. In both studies the numbers of animals enrolled were small and the results interpreted with caution. First, the small sample size may not have allowed for the contribution of confounding factors to the apparent differences and second, the studies may have been underpowered and thus unable to demonstrate real differences.

Nevertheless insulin glargine can effectively control diabetes mellitus in cats and offers a suitable alternative to the more traditional prolonged action insulins. Its apparent relatively peakless activity profile might make it particularly suitable for cats that tend to consume their daily caloric intake in regular amounts over a 24-h period. When administered once daily, it is at least as effective as twice-daily lente but the most recent results tend to suggest that optimum control is most likely to be achieved with twice-daily dosing.

DOGS

No published information is available on the use of glargine in dogs. Consequently currently its use should be considered as experimental and close monitoring would be strongly recommended.

- A standard dose of 0.5–2.0 IU/kg/24 h generally divided and given 12 hourly is recommended although the dose MUST be individualized on the basis of either serial blood glucose estimations or regular estimates of circulating glycated proteins such as fructosamine or glycosylated hemoglobin

CATS

- A starting dose of 1.0 IU/kg/24 h divided and given 12 hourly is recommended although as with all insulin therapy in diabetic cats, the dose must be individualized and close monitoring is essential

ORAL HYPOGLYCEMIC AGENTS

The so-called 'oral hypoglycemic agents' have been variably successful in treating canine and feline diabetes mellitus. Generally, they are unlikely to be effective in patients with an irreversible, absolute insulin deficiency. Consequently they have not been considered a worthwhile treatment option in dogs as, by the time canine diabetics present to a veterinarian, most have an irreversible absolute insulin deficiency. As this is not the case with feline diabetes mellitus, it is in this species that the use of oral hypoglycemics is most likely to be effective.

Sulfonylureas

Chemical structure

All drugs in this class are substituted arylsulfonylureas. They differ by substitution at the para position on the benzene ring and also at one nitrogen residue on the urea moiety. All the sulfonylureas currently used in small animals are from the so-called second-generation groups which contain a second benzene ring linked through the para position and a 6-carbon ring attached to the urea moiety.

Mechanism of action

The primary effect of sulfonylureas is the direct stimulation of insulin secretion from β-cells within pancreatic islets. This occurs through direct binding to cell membrane receptors, resulting in an increase in intracellular calcium and resultant increased release of presynthesized insulin granules. Extrapancreatic effects including increased peripheral insulin sensitivity and modification of hepatic gluconeogenesis and glycolysis have also been postulated, although these effects are unlikely to be clinically significant in the absence of any direct effect on insulin secretion. Consequently, the benefits of therapy with sulfonylureas are only likely in animals in which actual or potential insulin-secreting capacity is present.

Formulations and dose rates

CATS

- The recommended dose is 2.5–7.5 mg/cat/12 h of glipizide and glibenclamide and 0.625–2 mg/cat/24 h of glyburide. It is generally recommended to start at a lower dose and increase it to achieve a satisfactory effect. Doses need to be adjusted on the basis of changes in overall diabetic control which are generally best assessed using weekly fructosamine estimations

DOGS

- Although the sulfonylureas are far more commonly used in cats, one experimental study demonstrated that single doses of both glipizide at 180 μg/kg/12 h and glibenclamide at 90 μg/kg/12 h were effective in lowering blood glucose and increasing insulin concentrations in normal dogs

Pharmacokinetics

Limited information is available on the pharmacokinetics of sulfonylureas in cats although studies in normal cats suggested significantly increased insulin secretion within 7.5 min of glipizide administration with the hyperinsulinism persisting for up to 60 min.

In humans the half-lives of the second-generation sulfonylureas are short, generally 1.5–5 h, although their effects can last as long as 24 h. All the sulfonylureas are metabolized by the liver and the metabolites are excreted in the urine.

Adverse effects

Adverse effects of the sulfonylureas are relatively uncommon although reports of the prevalence of side effects have varied from none observed in 10 normal cats receiving various doses through to 16% of 50 diabetic cats showing adverse reactions. The signs included anorexia, vomiting, icterus and elevated liver enzymes, all of which were reversible with either reduction of dose or cessation of medication.

In humans nausea, vomiting, cholestatic jaundice, agranulocytosis, aplastic and hemolytic anemias and dermatological reactions have all been reported. Also, in around 5% of cases hyponatremia has been reported, possibly as a result of potentiation of antidiuretic hormone's effects on the renal collecting tubule.

Known drug interactions

A number of drugs may displace glipizide or be displaced by glipizide, thereby enhancing the pharmacological effects of both drugs. Relevent drugs include: chloramphenicol, nonsteroidal anti-inflammatory agents, sulfonamides and warfarin. Glipizide potentiates the effects of phenobarbital and glipizide's actions are enhanced by cimetidine.

Special considerations

Therapy with the sulfonylureas should only be continued whilst the diabetes is controlled. The sulfonylurea should be discontinued and insulin therapy initiated if the clinical signs deteriorate, ketoacidosis develops or marked hyperglycemia persists after 6–8 weeks of treatment.

Biguanides

Currently the most commonly used drug in this class is metformin (1,1-dimethylbiguanide) which has replaced the older, more toxic phenformin (phenethylbiguanide).

Mechanism of action

The mechanism of action of the biguanides remains incompletely understood although there is general agreement that it does not involve stimulation of insulin secretion. Depending on the experimental protocol used to explore its mechanism of action, it has been variably credited with inhibiting gluconeogenesis, stimulating peripheral glycolysis, utilizing the nonoxidative components of the glycolytic pathways, inhibiting intestinal carbohydrate absorption and producing an overall reduction in plasma fatty acids and bodyweight.

Formulations and dose rates

CATS

The dose of metformin remains controversial. An early study suggested that an oral dose of 2 mg/kg/12 h in cats would result in metformin plasma concentrations shown to be effective in improving glycemic control in noninsulin-dependent human diabetics. However, a later study suggested that healthy cats required oral doses of 5–10 mg/kg to achieve these presumed therapeutic plasma concentrations and provided no obvious explanation for the discrepancy. Interestingly, the latter study demonstrated limited efficacy at the higher dose rates in five diabetic cats (one cat died unexpectedly and the severity of the diabetes only improved temporarily in one of the four remaining cats). However, it is worth noting that none of the five received a low carbohydrate diet during the trial period. Additionally, six normal cats receiving 25 mg of metformin per cat once or twice daily consistently displayed lethargy and gastrointestinal side effects.

The level of adverse reactions and the apparent lack of activity when used at dose rates similar to those in humans suggest metformin should be administered with care in diabetic cats. If used at all, metformin should be given at a starting dose of 25 mg/cat/24 h and the dose increased gradually on the basis of changes in overall diabetic control that are generally best assessed using weekly fructosamine estimations and the prevalence of side effects.

Pharmacokinetics

In the only detailed study of the pharmacodynamics of metformin in cats, detailed analysis of both oral and intravenous metformin suggested a three-compartment model with a terminal phase half-life of around 11.5 h. The mean bioavailability of orally administered metformin was 48% and its excretion was predominantly renal.

Adverse effects

Because of its renal excretion, metformin should be used with care in patients with compromised renal function. In humans metformin can produce anorexia, vomiting and diarrhea in a proportion of patients and may result in lactic acidosis when given in high doses. Limited data in cats suggest they experience similar side effects although possibly at lower dose rates and with higher frequencies. Additionally, one diabetic cat receiving metformin died unexpectedly 11 d after starting the drug at a dose rate of 25 mg/cat once daily.

Special considerations

Therapy with the biguanides should only be continued whilst the diabetes is controlled. Metformin should be discontinued and insulin therapy initiated if the clinical signs deteriorate, ketoacidosis develops or marked hyperglycemia persists after 2–4 weeks of therapy.

Thiazolidinediones

The thiazolidinediones are a relatively new class of oral antidiabetic agents that include agents such as pioglitazone, rosiglitazone and darglitazone.

Mechanism of action

Although the precise mechanism of action of the thiazolidinediones is not known, at least part of their effect appears to be mediated through the activation of peroxisome proliferator-activating receptor gamma (PPAR-γ) and retinoic X receptor. These form a heterodimer that binds to the PPAR response element and activates transcription of genes involved in adipogenesis. Consequently the thiazolidinediones tend to increase fatty acid uptake in adipose tissue and reduce it in muscle. This may potentially increase overall insulin sensitivity as increased levels of fatty acids in muscle can interfere with insulin's action.

In addition to facilitating insulin-dependent peripheral glucose uptake, the thiazolidinediones also appear to inhibit hepatic glucose output by inhibiting both gluconeogenesis and glycogenolysis. There is also inconsistent evidence to suggest a possible role of the thiazolidinediones in enhancing peripheral glucose uptake through overexpression of GLUT1 and/or GLUT 4 receptors.

Pharmacokinetics

A study in five healthy cats revealed overall pharmacokinetics of troglitazone which were similar to those reported in a number of other species, including humans. Troglitazone has poor oral bioavailability (6.9%) which is also markedly variable between individuals. Its mean elimination half-life was 1.1 h with a steady-state volume of distribution of 0.23 ± 0.15 L/kg. Troglitazone undergoes extensive hepatic metabolism and is predominantly excreted in the bile.

Unfortunately there is little information on the pharmacodynamics of other thiazolidinediones although one report demonstrated significant improvement in carbohydrate and lipid metabolism in obese cats when darglitazone was administered orally at a dose of 2 mg/kg once daily.

Formulations and dose rates

CATS

- Based on experimental pharmacodynamic data in normal cats, troglitazone administered orally at 20–40 mg/kg/12–24 h should produce plasma concentrations which have been documented in humans as effective
- Another thiazolidinedione, darglitazone, has been shown to significantly improve carbohydrate and lipid metabolism in obese cats when given at a dose rate of 2 mg/kg/24 h. The report only documents the effects for a 42-d period and unfortunately currently no information is available on the efficacy or safety of either of these drugs or the described dose rates for long-term administration to normal or diabetic cats

Adverse effects

There is no information available on the adverse effects of troglitazone in cats. In humans, a proportion of patients develop variably severe hepatocellular damage. As this has been associated with an unacceptable number of fatalities, troglitazone has not been licensed for human use in either the UK or Australia and the prevalence of this problem resulted in its withdrawal from the US market. More recent thiazolidinediones such as pioglitazone and rosiglitazone appear to have similar potency to troglitazone and have not been associated with idiosyncratic hepatopathies in humans. However, their long-term administration has been linked to mild nonregenerative anemias and interestingly, in one report where darglitazone was administered to normal and obese cats, the investigators commented on a mild but significant reduction in the hematocrit of cats receiving darglitazone over a 42-d period.

Special considerations

Additional studies are needed to determine the efficacy and safety of the various commercially available thiazolidinediones in the treatment of feline diabetes mellitus.

α-GLUCOSIDASE INHIBITORS

Chemical structure

The α-glucosidase inhibitors acarbose and miglitol are complex oligosaccharides of microbial origin.

Mechanism of action

α-Glucosidase inhibitors bind competitively to the α-glucosidases glucoamylase, sucrase, maltase and isomaltase located within the brush borders of the small intestinal mucosa, inhibiting the conversion of complex carbohydrates and disaccharides to monosaccharides. These inhibitory effects delay and reduce postprandial glucose concentrations as well as decreasing insulin secretion.

Acarbose alone does not appear to be effective in treating diabetes mellitus but it can be used in conjunction with insulin and/or other oral hypoglycemic agents to achieve better diabetic control. However, a recent report suggests that while acarbose resulted in a demonstrable improvement in diabetic control in diabetic cats receiving a standard commercial diet, there was no significant effect of acarbose when the cats were fed a standard low-carbohydrate diet.

Formulations and dose rates

CATS

- The recommended dose is 12.5–25 mg/cat/12 h orally given with food. It is generally recommended to start at a lower dose and increase it to achieve a satisfactory effect. Doses need to be adjusted on the basis of changes in overall diabetic control and on the prevalence of side effects. As the effect of acarbose is entirely dependent upon its interaction with intestinal enzyme during the post prandial period, it is essential that it is only administered at the time of feeding

DOGS

- It is generally recommended to start with a low dose of 12.5–25 mg per animal per meal and increase this to 50–100 mg per meal over a 2-week period. Dose adjustment will be based on appropriate modification of diabetic control and the prevalence of side effects. As the effect of acarbose is entirely dependent upon its interaction with intestinal enzyme during the postprandial period, it is essential that it is only administered at the time of feeding

Adverse effects

Adverse effects of acarbose are common although, as it is not absorbed, they are predominantly confined to reversible gastrointestinal problems such as poorly formed stools, diarrhea, flatulence and weight loss. The prevalence and severity of the signs appear to be dose related. Although gastrointestinal signs were evident in approximately 35% of normal dogs receiving acarbose regardless of dose, these signs tended to resolve within 2–3 d of discontinuing the medication.

Special considerations

As mentioned above, the effect of acarbose requires it to be administered at the same time as the meal. While it may have a role to play in facilitating some level of improved control in diabetic dogs, recent reports suggest that the addition of acarbose is only likely to improve control of diabetes in cats if they are not being fed a low-carbohydrate diet.

EXOCRINE PANCREATIC INSUFFICIENCY

Relevant physiology/pathophysiology

The exocrine pancreas is an accessory digestive organ which, under complex neuroendocrine control, secretes fluid containing digestive enzymes and sodium bicarbonate into the intestinal lumen, resulting in digestion of food and neutralization of HCl of gastric origin. Three types of enzymes are secreted by the pancreas: amylases, lipases and proteases. The reserve capacity of the pancreas is enormous. Consequently, in the dog, protein digestion is not impaired until more than 90% of the gland is removed or destroyed.

In both dogs and cats, significant destruction of exocrine pancreatic tissue may occur, probably due to inappropriate activation of an immune-mediated inflammation. In a proportion of these patients the resultant destruction in digestive capacity will be clinically significant.

This clinically significant deficiency in exocrine pancreatic digestive secretions can be addressed utilizing a variety of commercially available exocrine pancreatic supplements.

It should be remembered that as there are often consequent derangements in the local intestinal environment as a result of the maldigestion, exocrine supplements are commonly used in conjunction with other treatment modalities aimed at addressing these abnormalities.

EXOCRINE PANCREATIC ENZYME REPLACEMENTS

Mechanism of action

The administration of suitable doses of an exocrine pancreatic enzyme supplement will result in the digestion of sufficient amounts of dietary fat (both triglycerides and long chain monoglycerides), proteins and carbohydrates to allow adequate intestinal absorption. As the exocrine pancreas is the sole source of the lipolytic activity of intestinal secretions, the actual lipolytic activity of the particular supplement chosen is a critical factor in determining therapeutic success. Consequently, when given on a regular basis to most patients with exocrine pancreatic insufficiency, digestive enzyme supplements with adequate concentrations of an active lipase should insure satisfactory caloric assimilation.

Formulations and dose rates

Most commercially available exocrine pancreatic enzyme supplements are composed of freeze-dried extracts of bovine or porcine exocrine pancreatic tissue and contain variable amounts of lipases, amylases and proteases. Numerous preparations are available and their composition, availability and formulation are quite variable. Although powders rather than enteric-coated product have been recommended, there are limited controlled studies in dogs to suggest that a particular formulation is necessarily better than another. What is critical in assessing the likely efficacy of these preparations is the enzyme activity present per unit weight of product and its method of presentation. Larger enteric-coated capsules or tablets may not be readily dissolved in the relatively acidic gastroduodenal environment of patients with exocrine pancreatic insufficiency, resulting in reduced delivery of active enzyme to the duodenum.

DOGS AND CATS

- Each milligram of most commercially available exocrine pancreatic supplements has not less than 20 USP units of lipase activity and not less than 100 USP units of protease and amylase activity
- An initial dose of around 280 mg/kg bodyweight of an exocrine pancreatic supplement per meal is generally recommended. In most cases once the clinical signs of malassimilation and steatorrhea have resolved, clinical remission can be maintained with approximately half this dose
- Some authors have recommended mixing the enzyme supplement with the food roughly 15–30 min prior to ingestion but no significant effect was shown when this practice was evaluated

Pharmacokinetics

In an attempt to minimize enzyme inactivation during passage through the stomach, a number of preparations are enteric coated. There is some controversy as to whether this is an advantage in dogs as (especially in the untreated exocrine pancreatic insufficiency patient) lack of alkaline-rich pancreatic secretions may result in generally lower pH levels in the duodenum, maintenance of the enteric coating and hence less enzyme availability. Although numerous publications recommend the use of nonenteric-coated preparations, there are few published controlled clinical data to support this hypothesis.

The enzymes are only active as intact molecules and consequently any absorption or distribution considerations are irrelevant to their therapeutic efficacy.

Adverse effects

In humans, reports of hypersensitivity reactions have included diarrhea, constipation, abdominal discomfort, and gum and perianal irritation.

FURTHER READING

Feldman EC, Nelson RW 2004 Feline diabetes mellitus. In: Canine and feline endocrinology and reproduction, 3rd edn. Saunders, Philadelphia, pp 539-579

Hoenig M, Ferguson DC 2003 Effects of darglitazone on glucose clearance and lipid metabolism in obese cats. Am J Vet Res 64: 1409-1413

Mazzaferro EM, Greco DS, Turner AS, Fettman MJ 2003 Treatment of feline diabetes mellitus using an α-glucosidase inhibitor and a low-carbohydrate diet. J Fel Med Surg 5: 183-189

Nelson R, Spann D, Elliott D, Brondos A, Vulliet R 2004 Evaluation of the oral antihyperglycemic drug metformin in normal and diabetic cats. J Vet Intern Med 18: 18-24

Weaver KE, Rozanski EA, Mahony OM, Chan DL, Freeman LM 2006 Use of glargine and lente insulins in cats with diabetes mellitus. J Vet Intern Med 20: 234-238

22

Drugs used in the treatment of adrenal dysfunction

David B Church

Diseases of the adrenal gland may result in inappropriately increased or decreased adrenocortical activity and/or similarly modified adrenal medullary activity. In small animals, dysfunction of the adrenal cortex is far more commonly encountered and this chapter will concentrate on drugs used to manage patients with abnormal adrenocortical activity due to either primary or secondary causes.

HYPERADRENOCORTICISM

Spontaneous hyperadrenocorticism in dogs and cats can be due to increased ACTH secretion from the anterior pituitary (PDH) or autonomous cortisol production from a functional adrenocortical neoplasm. Drugs used to control hyperadrenocorticism can be categorized into agents acting on the hypothalamic-pituitary axis to reduce ACTH secretion and drugs acting directly on the adrenal cortex to inhibit adrenal steroid synthesis.

DRUGS ACTING ON THE HYPOTHALAMIC-PITUITARY AXIS

Relevant pathophysiology

In the dog, corticotrophin-releasing hormone (CRH) stimulates release of ACTH from the pars distalis. Some investigators have indicated that CRH and/or ACTH release may be, at least partly, mediated by 5-hydroxytryptamine (5-HT).

ACTH is also secreted from the pars intermedia. This pars intermedia-derived ACTH is controlled by local dopamine levels which tonically inhibit ACTH secretion from the pars intermedia. It has been suggested that as dogs age, there is a decline in dopamine activity which may be, at least partly, a result of increased activity of enzymes involved in dopamine metabolism.

One of two major metabolic pathways for monoamines such as dopamine is oxidative deamination. This reaction is catalyzed by two isoenzymes of monoamine oxidase (MAO). While both isoenzymes (MAO-A and MAO-B) are present peripherally and inactivate monoamines of intestinal origin, the isoenzyme MAO-B is the predominant form in the striatum of the CNS. Consequently it is MAO-B which is responsible for most of the oxidative deamination of CNS-located dopamine.

As MAO activity reportedly increases with age, it has been suggested that, at least in some cases, PDH in the dog may be a result of dopamine depletion.

Additionally, it has been suggested dopamine depletion may increase CRH-stimulated ACTH secretion from the pars distalis, providing a further possible means by which agents which act as dopamine agonists or increase CNS dopamine levels may be helpful in managing PDH in dogs.

In summary, some investigators believe that in a proportion of canine PDH patients, excessive ACTH secretion is a result of uninhibited ACTH production from the pars intermedia. In these patients it is possible that dopamine agonists or inhibitors of dopamine metabolism within the CNS may reduce ACTH secretion and consequently improve the clinical signs of PDH in the dog.

Furthermore, in a small proportion of PDH patients, it has been hypothesized that increased 5-HT levels may be involved in elevated CRH or ACTH levels. If this is the case, drugs that block 5-HT activity may be helpful in managing these patients.

Cyproheptadine

Cyprohepatidine is also discussed in Chapters 7 (Behavior-modifying drugs) and 11 (Glucocorticosteroids and antihistamines).

Mechanism of action

Cyproheptadine's structure resembles the phenothiazine H_1-antagonists and has antiserotoninergic (anti-5-HT) activity. Like other H_1-antagonists, cyproheptadine acts by competing with histamine for H_1-receptor sites on effector cells. It also has potent 5-HT (serotonin) antagonist activity through its 5-HT_{2A} receptor-blocking action. In addition, it also has weak anticholinergic and central depressant properties.

As local levels of 5-HT could be involved in stimulating both secretion of CRH and/or ACTH, cyproheptadine may reduce ACTH production in some PDH patients.

Formulations and dose rates

The use of cyproheptadine for the control of PDH has not been extensively evaluated. However, in one of the few reports of its efficacy, doses of 0.3–3.0 mg/kg/24 h produced only variable clinical and biochemical responses in less than 10% of dogs with PDH.

Pharmacokinetics

The pharmacokinetics of cyproheptadine suggest it is well absorbed orally, undergoes extensive hepatic metabolism and that metabolites are predominantly renally excreted.

Adverse effects

At usual doses the most commonly reported adverse effects have been sedation, anticholinergic effects and polyphagia.

Known drug interactions

- Cyproheptadine may enhance CNS depression when used with sedatives.
- Monoamine oxidase inhibitors such as deprenyl may intensify cyproheptadine's anticholinergic effects.

Bromocriptine

Bromocriptine is also discussed in Chapter 7 (Behavior-modifying drugs).

Mechanism of action

Bromocriptine is an ergot-derived alkaloid with dopaminergic activity. It is a strong D_2-receptor agonist and a partial D_1-receptor agonist. These are the two major dopamine receptors found within the striatum of the CNS in humans and are presumed to be most important in the treatment of Parkinson's disease.

As a result of this dopamine receptor agonist activity, it has been postulated that bromocriptine may have some potential to lower ACTH secretion, particularly in PDH patients in which increased ACTH secretion may be a result of reduced dopaminergic activity at the pars intermedia.

It should be remembered that dopamine is an effective inhibitor of prolactin secretion from the anterior pituitary. This appears to be achieved either by a direct effect on the pituitary or by stimulation of postsynaptic dopamine receptors in the hypothalamus, resulting in release of prolactin-inhibitory factor.

Formulations and dose rates

Bromocriptine has been evaluated in the treatment of PDH in dogs with doses ranging from 0.01 to 0.1mg/kg/24 h either as a single dose or divided. Regardless of the dose, the efficacy has been low and the adverse effects frequent.

Pharmacokinetics

The pharmacokinetics of bromocriptine in dogs and cats have not been described. In humans approximately 30% of orally administered bromocriptine is absorbed and only 6% is available due to a significant first-pass effect. In humans the drug is highly protein bound, undergoes extensive hepatic metabolism with a half-life of 3–7 h.

Adverse effects

- Adverse effects are common with bromocriptine and generally are dose related.
- Most frequently encountered problems include anorexia, vomiting, diarrhea, generalized weakness and depression as well as hypotension.
- Rarely, profound hypotension may occur after the first dose. For this reason bromocriptine should be started at a low dose and with gradual increments after regular monitoring.
- Generally, the frequency with which adverse effects are encountered has limited the use of bromocriptine for the treatment of PDH.

Known drug interactions

The hypotensive effects of bromocriptine may be additive when used in conjunction with other hypotensive agents.

Selegiline (L-deprenyl)

Selegiline is also discussed in Chapter 7 (Behavior-modifying drugs).

Mechanism of action

Selegiline is 2-proponylphenethylamine, an irreversible inhibitor of MAO-B. It is a specific inhibitor of MAO-B, the enzyme that is predominantly responsible for catalyzing the metabolism of CNS dopamine.

In the dog, CRH stimulates release of ACTH from the pars distalis while local dopamine levels tonically inhibit ACTH secretion from the pars intermedia. As MAO activity reportedly increases with age, it has been suggested that at least in some cases, PDH in the dog may be a result of dopamine depletion.

By inactivating MAO-B, selegiline may increase CNS dopamine levels and decrease pars intermedia derived-ACTH.

Additionally, it has been suggested dopamine depletion may increase CRH-stimulated ACTH secretion from the pars distalis, providing a further possible means by which selegiline may reduce ACTH secretion in PDH patients.

Formulations and dose rate

The recommended treatment regimen for controlling PDH in the dog is a starting dose of 1 mg/kg/24 h. Over the ensuing 8 weeks the patient's response should be monitored and if after this time no improvement has been seen, the dose should be increased to 2 mg/kg/24 h. The manufacturers state that while increasing the dose from 1.0 to 2.0 mg/kg/24 h may not improve efficacy in a particular patient, 'favorable responses were seen in dogs treated at both 1.0 and 2.0 mg/kg in clinical trials'. However, subsequently two independent controlled clinical studies failed to show any consistent or significant response in 21 dogs with PDH receiving selegiline at the recommended dose rate for between 3 and 6 months. In these animals 'favorable' clinical responses were present in only three of the 21 patients and no animal showed a significant change in the results of their ACTH stimulation test or basal urinary corticoid:creatinine ratios.

Pharmacokinetics

In the dog, selegiline is absorbed rapidly with a bioavailability of around 10%, is extensively distributed and has a plasma half-life of approximately 1 h. In humans, selegiline undergoes hepatic metabolism to desmethylselegiline, methylamphetamine and L-amphetamine. Although desmethylselegiline is an active MAO-B inhibitor, neither methylamphetamine nor amphetamine is, although both are active CNS stimulants. All three metabolites are predominantly excreted in the urine.

Adverse effects

Adverse effects have been minimal and have included nonspecific gastrointestinal changes, disorientation, behavioral abnormalities and decreased hearing.

Known drug interactions

- In humans severe agitation, hallucinations and death have accompanied concurrent use of an MAO inhibitor and meperidine. The potential for this to also occur in dogs receiving selegiline and either meperidine or other opioids has not been clarified, although it would seem prudent to avoid this combination until the potential for adverse reactions has been clarified.
- In addition, in humans concurrent use of selegiline with serotonin reuptake inhibitors such as tricyclic or tetracyclic antidepressants should be avoided.

DRUGS ACTING ON THE ADRENAL CORTEX

Relevant physiology

ACTH stimulates the adrenal cortex to secrete glucocorticoids, mineralocorticoids and weak androgens such as androstenedione and dehydroepiandrosterone. Temporally, the response of adrenocortical cells to ACTH has two phases: an acute phase lasting minutes, which results in an increased supply of cholesterol substrate to the steroidogenic enzymes, and a chronic phase lasting hours or days that produces increased steroidogenic enzyme transcription. A summary of the pathways involved in adrenal steroid biosynthesis is shown in Figure 22.1.

Most of the enzymes required for biosynthesis of steroid hormones are members of the cytochrome P450 superfamily, a related group of mixed-function oxidases that are important in the biosynthesis of many compounds. The rate-limiting step in steroid biosynthesis is the mobilization of substrate cholesterol and its conversion to pregnenolone, a reaction catalyzed by the cholesterol side chain cleavage enzyme, designated $P450_{scc}$.

Although anatomically the adrenal cortex is divided into three zones – zona glomerulosa, fasciculata and reticularis – functionally it can be thought of as two compartments: the outer glomerulosa 'compartment' responsible for aldosterone production and the inner fasciculata/reticularis 'compartment' responsible for glucocorticoid and adrenal androgen production. Cells from the outer compartment have AgII receptors and aldosterone synthase ($P450_{aldo}$) while cells from the inner compartment lack AgII receptors and possess two enzymes which catalyze glucocorticoid synthesis: steroid 17α-hydroxylase and 11β-hydroxylase (see Fig. 22.1).

Interestingly, the blood supply to the adrenal cortex appears to be influenced by ambient ACTH levels. It has been known for some time that increased plasma concentrations of ACTH result in an elevation in adrenocortical blood flow. This stimulatory effect of ACTH on adrenal blood flow has been documented in a number of species, including both humans and the dog. Furthermore, there is experimental evidence to suggest that chronic elevations in plasma ACTH levels result in damage to the endothelial lining of the adrenocortical blood vessels, causing regional hemorrhage and potential necrosis of local adrenal tissue.

A number of drugs which either inhibit steroid synthesis or block steroid receptors have been suggested as possible treatments for hyperadrenocorticism in the dog and cat. Unfortunately, some of these suggested drugs, including etomidate, suramin, mifepristone and aminoglutethimide, have not been evaluated in hyperadrenocorticoid patients. Consequently, their value in the management of this condition remains a matter of speculation. There are, however, drugs that act on the adrenal cortex which have been used to treat hyperadrenocorticism in either dogs or cats. These drugs are discussed in the following section.

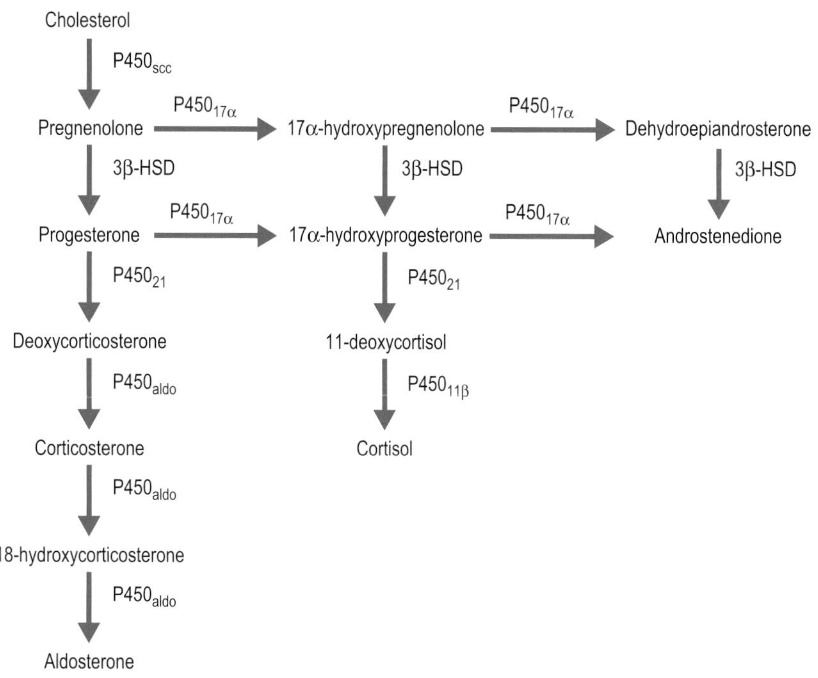

Fig. 22.1 **The steroidogenic pathways used in the biosynthesis of the corticosteroids, showing the structures of the intermediates and products. P450$_{scc}$, cholesterol side chain cleavage enzyme; 3β-HSD, 3β-hydroxysteroid dehydrogenase; P450$_{17\alpha}$, steroid 17α-hydroxylase; P450$_{21}$, steroid 21-hydroxylase; P450$_{aldo}$, aldosterone synthase; P450$_{11\beta}$, steroid 11β-hydroxylase.**

Trilostane

Mechanism of action

Trilostane, an androstane-carbonitrile compound, is a synthetic, orally active steroid analog. Trilostane has been traditionally thought of as a competitive, and therefore reversible, dose-dependent inhibitor of 3β-hydroxysteroid dehydrogenase, the enzyme that converts pregnenolone to progesterone. Inhibition of this enzyme results in reduced adrenocortical synthesis of both cortisol and aldosterone as well as increasing urinary excretion of 17-ketosteroids (see Fig. 22.1). The increased urinary excretion of 17-ketosteroids may be at least partly explained by increased corticoid synthesis in response to marked increases in ACTH secretion.

Interestingly, trilostane's mechanism of action in controlling canine hyperadrenocorticism may be more complex than originally proposed. Increasing evidence suggests its effects may be at least partly mediated through its capacity to modify other enzymes in the steroid synthetic pathway (including possible inhibition of 21-hydroxylase or 11β-hydroxylase) and/or upregulation of one of the isoforms of 11β-hydroxysteroid dehydrogenase, resulting in enhanced conversion of cortisol to its inactive metabolite cortisone. Additionally, some authors have speculated that the initial increased ACTH levels likely to be seen in a PDH patient receiving trilostane (due to the reduced cortisol levels) may result in adrenocortical damage through enhanced, ACTH-stimulated, adrenal blood flow with consequent hemorrhage and regional necrosis. This hypothesis is to some extent supported by the enhanced bilateral adrenomegaly and accompanying characteristic hypoechogenic adrenocortical margins that consistently accompany subacute trilostane treatment. It is also supported by the sporadic reports of adrenal hemorrhage and necrosis seen in the small proportion of dogs in which trilostane has created acute but long-term hypoadrenocorticism.

Using trilostane, the time to clinical remission and long-term survival rates are similar to those of mitotane. Clinical improvement is usually seen within 2 weeks of starting trilostane and in those dogs that respond to trilostane, adequate control is invariably achieved within 30 d of starting medication. In a recent report comparing survival times for PDH dogs, median survival time for those treated with trilostane was 662 days (range 8–1971) and for mitotane it was 708 days (range 33–1399). It is important to remember the required dose rate is variable and patients need to be monitored regularly with an ACTH stimulation test within 4–6 h of trilostane's administration if a consistent and satisfactory level of adrenal suppression is to be achieved.

Formulations and dose rates

Currently the suggested starting dose rate for dogs with PDH is 5–12 mg/kg once daily given with food. As trilostane is supplied in 30, 60 and 120 mg capsules, generally dogs weighing under 5 kg receive 30 mg per day, those between 5 and 20 kg receive 60 mg per day and those over 20 kg receive 120 mg per day. In some dogs twice-daily dosing has been explored in an attempt to achieve adequate adrenal suppression.

Because of individual variation it is imperative that each animal is re-evaluated regularly with both a clinical examination and ACTH stimulation test and the dose adjusted based on these findings. Generally control can be reliably achieved in approximately 80% of cases if dogs are re-examined and an ACTH stimulation test performed approximately 10–14 d, 30 d and 90 d after starting therapy. It is important that all ACTH stimulation tests are performed 4–6 h after trilostane administration and interpreted in conjunction with the clinical findings. If the post-ACTH cortisol concentration is below the sensitivity of the assay (generally 30 nmol/L) the trilostane dose may be reduced. If the post-ACTH cortisol concentration is more than 1.5 times the upper limit of the basal cortisol's normal range, then the dose of trilostane is increased. If the post-ACTH cortisol concentration is between these two values and the patient appears to be clinically well controlled then the dose should remain unaltered. If the post-ACTH cortisol suggests adequate adrenocortical suppression but clinical signs are not well controlled, sometimes improved control can be achieved by administering trilostane twice daily.

Estimating urinary corticoid:creatinine ratio has proved a poor method of monitoring trilostane therapy, at least partly because of increased urinary secretion of cross-reacting 17-ketosteroid metabolites. In the future estimation of endogenous ACTH values may be a valuable method of individualizing the trilostane dose.

Once the clinical condition of the animal and trilostane dose have been stabilized, dogs should be examined and an ACTH stimulation test performed every 3–6 months. Serum biochemistry (especially electrolytes) should be performed periodically to check for hyperkalemia.

Based on the results of these ACTH stimulation tests, regular dose adjustments can be made to achieve ongoing satisfactory adrenal suppression. In the author's opinion, 'satisfactory adrenal suppression' could be defined as basal and stimulated plasma cortisol levels within the relevant laboratory's normal range for basal plasma cortisol concentration.

Pharmacokinetics

In rats, monkeys and people, trilostane is rapidly absorbed after oral dosing, with peak blood concentrations occurring between 30–60 min after dosing in rats and 2–4 h in monkeys and humans. In healthy dogs peak trilostane concentrations are seen within 1.5 h and decrease to baseline values in approximately 18 h. Trilostane is variably absorbed after oral administration, at least partly due to its poor water solubility. Like other drugs with high lipid solubility, its oral bioavailability may be enhanced by administering the drug with food although at present this phenomenon has not been investigated.

Trilostane metabolism follows a triexponential algorithm with trilostane cleared from the blood after 7 h in rats and humans and 48 h in the monkey. Following the administration of trilostane to rats, the metabolite ketotrilostane is formed within a few minutes. Conversely, when ketotrilostane is given to rats, trilostane is rapidly formed, suggesting that these compounds exist in equilibrium in vivo. Both trilostane and ketotrilostane are biologically active with ketotrilostane having approximately 1.7 times the bio-activity of trilostane. Trilostane and ketotrilostane are metabolized into any one of four further metabolites. While excretion in rats is mainly via feces, in monkeys urinary excretion is more important. Unfortunately, no information is available on the excretion of trilostane and its metabolites in the dog.

Adverse effects

In general trilostane is well tolerated. Up to 10% of dogs receiving trilostane may develop mild side effects including lethargy, depression, inappetance, vomiting and diarrhea which are usually self-limiting or corrected by adjusting the total dose or dose frequency.

Clearly one of the difficulties is that these signs are relatively vague and while they may be attributable to a direct adverse drug reaction, they could also be caused by relative hypoadrenocorticism through either a direct effect of overdosage or possible adrenal necrosis. Given trilostane's relatively short duration of action, hypoadrenocorticism might not be considered an expected consequence. However, while it appears to be an uncommon event, it is particularly important for clinicians using trilostane to be aware of the potential for an animal receiving the drug to develop fulminant hypoadrenocorticism. It is because of this potential that patients should be monitored regularly to insure there is adequate adrenal reserve.

As trilostane may cause hyperkalemia caution should be exercised when using trilostane with a potassium-sparing diuretic such as spironolactone or ACE inhibitors. However a recent study suggested plasma aldosterone was not significantly different in trilostane-treated hyperadrenocorticoid dogs with hyperkalemia, subnormal post-ACTH or normal post-ACTH cortisol values and no correlation between potassium and aldosterone could be found. Additionally no unwanted drug interactions have been seen in dogs on trilostane receiving other medications such as various nonsteroidal anti-inflammatories, antibiotics, insulin and levothyroxine.

Ketoconazole

Mechanism of action

Ketoconazole is an imidazole compound primarily used as an antifungal agent (see Chapter 9: Systemic antifungal therapy). However, at doses higher than those recommended for antifungal activity, ketoconazole can inhibit steroid synthesis.

Ketoconazole is an effective inhibitor of adrenal and gonadol steroidogenesis primarily as a result of its inhibition of the 17-hydroxylation activity of $P450_{17\alpha}$. In other words, ketoconazole inhibits the conversion of progesterone and pregnenolone to 17α-hydroxyprogesterone and 17α-hydroxypregnenolone. At higher doses, ketoconazole also inhibits $P450_{scc}$, effectively blocking steroidogenesis in all primary steroidogenic tissues (see Fig. 22.1).

Formulations and dose rates

For the treatment of hyperadrenocorticism a dose of 15 mg/kg/12 h is generally recommended. Most authors suggest starting at a dose of 5 mg/kg/12 h for 7 d and if no adverse effects are noticed, increasing the dose to 10 mg/kg/12 h for 14 d and evaluating adrenal suppression with an ACTH stimulation test at the end of this period. Although a small number of cases will be 'adequately suppressed' (in the author's opinion, defined as a **post-ACTH** cortisol within the laboratory's normal range for **basal** cortisol) with this dose, most require 15 mg/kg/12 h.

Ketoconazole is more effectively absorbed in an acidic environment. Although the manufacturer recommends dosing with food to reduce the risk of GIT side effects, unfortunately, this is likely to reduce bioavailability.

The disadvantages of ketoconazole include its lack of efficacy in a high proportion of cases (reportedly ineffective in 25–50% of cases), the need for constant twice-daily dosing and in many countries its expense.

Pharmacokinetics

In the dog, oral bioavailability appears to be quite variable, with one report suggesting a range of 4–89% and peak serum concentrations in the range 1.1–45.6 μg/mL. Ketoconazole's absorption is enhanced in an acidic environment, however, and absorption may be facilitated by dosing after fasting. Ketoconazole is approximately 90% protein bound, undergoes extensive hepatic metabolism and these inactive metabolites are predominantly excreted in the feces via the bile.

Adverse effects

- Gastrointestinal effects including anorexia, vomiting and diarrhea are the most common adverse effects of ketoconazole administration. Although dividing the dose or dosing with food may reduce anorexia, the latter may reduce absorption.
- Hepatotoxicity has been reported in both dogs and cats and may be idiosyncratic or dose related.
- Thrombocytopenia is a rare adverse effect.
- There have been rare reports of changes in hair coat color in animals.

Known drug interactions

- Antacids, anticholinergics and H_2-blockers all increase gastric pH and may inhibit absorption of ketoconazole.
- Any agent that may produce adrenocorticolysis or inhibit steroidogenesis is likely to potentiate ketoconazole's inhibition of adrenal and gonadal steroidogenesis.
- In contrast, ketoconazole alters the disposition and extends the duration of activity of methylprednisolone and possibly other synthetic glucocorticoids.
- Ketoconazole may increase plasma concentrations of cisapride (with a resultant increased risk of ventricular arrhythmias).
- Ketoconazole may increase plasma concentrations of ciclosporin.
- Ketoconazole may decrease plasma concentrations of theophylline.
- Phenytoin and ketoconazole modify each other's metabolism.
- As ketoconazole is hepatotoxic it should not be administered with other hepatotoxic agents.

Mitotane

Mechanism of action

Mitotane is the *o,p'* isomer of DDD which is structurally related to chlorophenothane (DDT). By binding to and destroying mitochondria, mitotane's active metabolite exerts a direct cytotoxic effect on the adrenal cortex, resulting in relatively selective progressive necrosis of the zona reticularis and fasciculata. Mitotane also interferes with adrenal steroidogenesis by poorly understood mechanisms although inhibition of 11β-hydroxylase is likely to be involved.

Formulations and dose rates

Although there are numerous reports on how mitotane should be administered to dogs with PDH, many involve small variations around two basically different strategies. Both protocols involve creating profound adrenocorticolysis. However, in one the aim is to leave sufficient adrenocortical activity for normal day-to-day activities while the second attempts to achieve complete 'chemical adrenalectomy' and provide long-term glucocorticoid and mineralocorticoid supplementation as required.

Protocol 1

This protocol has two basic parts: a remission-inducing sequence and a remission-maintaining sequence.

Remission induction: The aim of this part of the treatment protocol is to create marked adrenocorticolysis resulting in an inability of the remaining adrenal tissue to mount any response to supraphysiological doses of ACTH. Additionally, most endocrinologists suggest an improved clinical response is achieved if both the basal and post-stimulation plasma cortisol concentrations remain within the bottom third of the normal range for basal plasma cortisol.

Specifically this goal is achieved by the oral administration of mitotane with a meal at a dose of 25 mg/kg/12 h for 5–7 d. At the end of this period an ACTH response test is performed not less than 36 h after the last mitotane dose. This timing recommendation is to insure the ACTH response test is evaluating the adrenocorticolytic effect of mitotane and not its inhibitory effects on steroidogenesis. If both basal and post-ACTH cortisol values are in the desired range, the treatment moves to the remission-maintaining stage; if not, the remission induction process is repeated.

Generally, satisfactory adrenocorticolysis is achieved with total mitotane doses of 250–700 mg. Furthermore, the total dose required for remission induction is usually an indication of the weekly dose required for remission maintenance.

As there is potential for either absolute or relative iatrogenic hypoadrenocorticism, it is prudent to provide owners with an oral glucocorticoid like prednisolone. This can then be used when there are suspected signs of hypoadrenocorticism or any acute non-adrenal illness. These are potentially critical situations in patients undergoing remission induction and administering prednisolone while awaiting veterinary attention substantially reduces the risk of a life-threatening problem developing.

Remission maintenance: Once satisfactory adrenocorticolysis has been achieved, remission is maintained by the weekly oral administration of mitotane at a dose of 30–100 mg/kg/week. Generally this is administered in two doses, each with a meal, on one day per week. Maintenance of remission is evaluated by regular ACTH stimulation tests or possibly urinary corticoid:creatinine ratios.

Protocol 2

Mitotane is administered at a dose of 50–75 mg/kg/24 h for 25 d. The dose is usually divided into three or four and given with food. Owners are instructed to stop mitotane administration if the dog becomes inappetent and to resume administration once it returns (generally in 2–3 d). When severe side effects are seen the mitotane dose should be reduced and/or the daily dose further subdivided.

On the **third** day, glucocorticoid and mineralocorticoid replacement is started. This consists of cortisone acetate at a dose of 1 mg/kg/12 h together with 9α-fludrocortisone at 7 μg/kg/12 h and sodium chloride supplementation at 50 μg/kg/12 h. All owners are given injectable glucocorticoid and mineralocorticoid supplements to be used if more than two successive oral replacement treatments are missed.

Effective complete chemical adrenalectomy is confirmed with an ACTH stimulation test 30 d after mitotane administration was begun and at this time the dose of cortisone is reduced to 0.5–1.0 mg/kg/24 h. Animals should be re-evaluated every 6 months or sooner if the owners suspect a relapse. Doses of 9α-fludrocortisone and NaCl are adjusted on the basis of plasma electrolytes while the cortisone acetate dose is reduced or stopped if there are any signs of hyperadrenocorticism.

With this protocol approximately 40% of dogs relapse and require further 25-d induction protocols.

Interestingly, in one large study of mitotane therapy in canine PDH, bigger dogs remained disease free for significantly longer than small dogs. This may indicate that small dogs require a higher dose of mitotane or a dose based on surface area. However, to date neither possibility has been evaluated.

Pharmacokinetics

The bioavailability of mitotane is poor, although this may be enhanced by administering the drug with food. Interestingly, mitotane's bioavailability appears to be higher in dogs with PDH. In dogs, peak plasma concentrations occur approximately 4 h after dosing with an elimination half-life after a single dose of 1–2 h. The rapidity of this calculated elimination time is somewhat misleading, however. Elimination from plasma will be prolonged after chronic dosing as the drug is slowly released from adipose tissue where it is present in high concentrations. This same phenomenon is present in humans, where plasma half-lives ranging from 18 to 159 d have been reported.

In humans, mitotane is predominantly metabolized by the liver and this is also likely to be the case in dogs. Consequently, any drug which enhances the hepatic microsomal system is likely to accelerate mitotane's metabolism. Additionally, mitotane may facilitate its own metabolism by activation of the hepatic microsomal enzyme system.

Adverse effects

- Adverse effects are relatively common in dogs receiving mitotane. Although many of these are due to acute glucocorticoid deficiency, mitotane itself can be associated with various gastrointestinal disturbances, behavioral changes, cranial nerve palsies and transient muscle weakness.
- In a small proportion of cases receiving mitotane, severe and irreversible glucocorticoid and mineralocorticoid deficiency will develop. This appears to be an idiosyncratic reaction and occurs independent of dose, age or severity of hyperadrenocorticism.

Known drug interactions

- As mitotane can induce hepatic microsomal enzymes, it may enhance the metabolism of a number of different drugs such as the barbiturates and warfarin.
- Mitotane also has its metabolism enhanced by the barbiturates; consequently animals on barbiturates will require higher doses of mitotane.
- Spironolactone has been shown to block the effects of mitotane.
- Diabetic patients may have their insulin requirement lowered by mitotane administration.

Metyrapone

Mechanism of action

Metyrapone or metopirone is 2-methyl-1,2-di-3-pyridl-1-propanone. It reversibly inhibits the synthesis of cortisol, cortisone and aldosterone by blocking enzymatic 11β-hydroxylation. The reduction in cortisol synthesis reduces corticosteroid feedback inhibition, leading to increased ACTH secretion which results in increased production of the 17-hydroxysteroids such as 11-deoxycortisol.

In humans, its long-term use for the treatment of PDH remains controversial as loss of adrenal blockade due to increased ACTH levels significantly limits its efficacy. How relevant this limitation may be in dogs and cats has not been evaluated.

Formulations and dose rates

Metyrapone has been used for the successful treatment of hyperadrenocorticism in the cat at an oral dose of 65 mg/kg/8–12 h. Only a small number of cases are cited and the follow-up periods were short, suggesting that this agent may have some potential in the short-term management of hyperadrenocorticoid cases.

Pharmacokinetics

No information is available on the pharmacokinetics of metyrapone in the dog or cat. In humans, it is well absorbed orally and is rapidly eliminated via the urine, mainly as an inactive glucuronide conjugate. In humans metyrapone has a short half-life of approximately 30 min. It has been suggested that an effective peak plasma concentration is 3.7 μg/L.

Adverse effects

- In humans occasional vomiting, nausea, abdominal pain, hypotension and hypoadrenalism have been noted.
- Although metyrapone blocks aldosterone synthesis, mineralocorticoid insufficiency is not common as there is increased production of 11-deoxycorticosterone which also has significant mineralocorticoid activity.

HYPOADRENOCORTICISM

Clinical applications

Hypoadrenocorticism is an uncommon condition in both the dog and cat which generally results in clinically significant loss of both mineralocorticoid and glucocorticoid activity through immune-mediated adrenocortical destruction. In most patients gastrointestinal signs dictate that in the early phases of treatment, medication is administered parenterally. Additionally, once the hypoadrencocorticoid patient is stabilized, glucocorticoid and mineralocorticoid replacement therapy almost always needs to be maintained for the remainder of the animal's life. Traditionally both a semiselective glucocorticoid and a semiselective mineralocorticoid are initially used together, with the former being discontinued in a proportion of patients after 1–2 months.

The glucocorticoid and mineralocorticoid potency of various natural and synthetic steroids is predominantly determined by their structure. An understanding of the biological effects of the various chemical substitutions can facilitate an understanding of which drug or drugs are likely to be most effective in the acute and long-term treatment of hypoadrenocorticism.

The structure of hydrocortisone and some of its major derivatives are shown in Figure 22.2. The 4,5 double bond and the 3-keto group on ring A are essential for both glucocorticoid and mineralocorticoid activity. An 11β-hydroxyl group is essential for glucocorticoid but not mineralocorticoid activity, while a 21-hydroxyl group appears to be necessary for mineralocorticoid but not glucocorticoid activity. Although a 17α-hydroxyl substitution is not essential for glucocorticoid activity, when it is present glucocorticoid potency is enhanced.

The placement of a double bond at the 1,2 position preferentially enhances glucocorticoid over mineralocorticoid action (examples include prednisolone, dexamethasone) and a 9-fluorination markedly enhances both glucocorticoid and mineralocorticoid activity (dexamethasone, 9α-fludrocortisone). Any substitutions at C16 on ring D virtually eliminate mineralocorticoid action (dexamethasone, betamethasone) while an 11-keto substitution (cortisone and prednisone) results in an inactive molecule which must be 11-hydroxylated to the biologically active compound (hydrocortisone and prednisolone respectively).

Hydrocortisone sodium succinate

Mechanism of action

Hydrocortisone sodium succinate (HSS) is the succinate ester of hydrocortisone or cortisol. Its chemical composition is pregn-4-ene3, 20-dione-2-(3-carboxy-1-oxopropoxy)-11β,17α-dihydroxy, monosodium salt.

Hydrocortisone or cortisol is the principal steroid produced by the adrenal cortex of dogs and cats. It has equipotent glucocorticoid and mineralocorticoid activity although it has only 25% of the glucocorticoid potency of prednisolone and less than 1% of the mineralocorticoid potency of 9α-fludrocortisone. However, at the recommended doses it provides sufficient glucocorticoid and mineralocorticoid activity to avoid the clinical consequences of hypoadrenocorticism and consequently can be effectively used in the short-term management of these patients.

Formulations and dose rates

HSS can be used for the acute treatment of spontaneous hypoadrenocorticism or as a supportive agent in the immediate postoperative management of a patient undergoing unilateral or bilateral adrenalectomy. It currently remains the only commercially available steroid

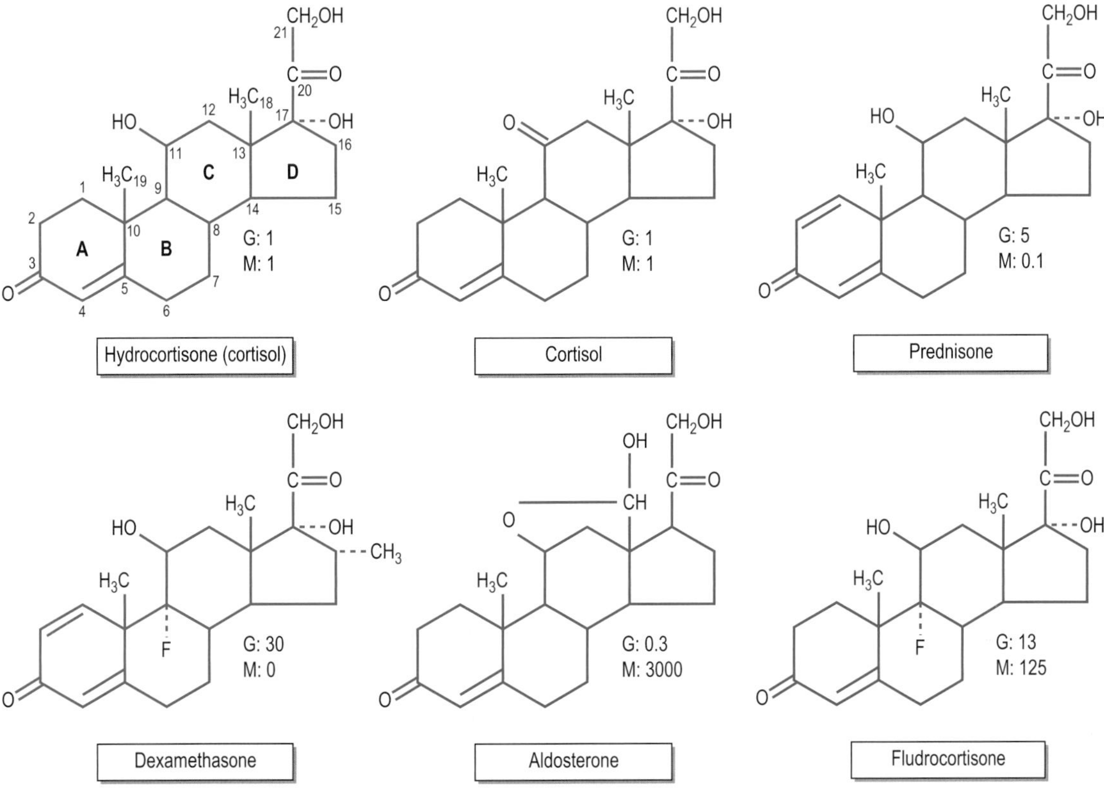

Fig. 22.2 Structure of natural and synthetic corticosteroids with their relative glucocorticoid (G) and mineralocorticoid (M) potency.

with equipotent glucocorticoid and mineralocorticoid activity which can be administered parenterally.

In adrenalectomy patients it can be given as a bolus before and after surgery (4–5 mg/kg) or, in the author's opinion, preferably as a continuous infusion of 0.5 mg/kg/h starting 1 h before induction and continuing for 12–24 h postoperatively. At this time it should be reduced to 0.25 mg/kg/h for a further 24 h or until the dog is eating and drinking and able to be changed to oral steroid supplementation.

In dogs with spontaneous hypoadrenocorticism which require supportive fluid therapy HSS should be given at a dose of 0.5 mg/kg/h until normal gastrointestinal function has returned, the dog is eating and drinking normally and can be changed to oral steroid supplementation.

As there is potential for HSS to adhere to plastic or glass at low concentrations, it is best to administer it in its own fluid bag made up to a concentration of 1 mg/mL. As HSS is incompatible with a variety of different solutions, including ampicillin sodium, it is best to dilute the HSS in normal saline.

Pharmacokinetics

As a water-soluble derivative of hydrocortisone, HSS can be administered intravenously. In humans HSS is relatively rapidly metabolized with excretion complete within 12 h of administration.

In normal dogs, stable plasma cortisol concentrations of approximately 750–900 nmol/L and 350–385 nmol/L were achieved within 3 h of starting a continuous intravenous infusion of HSS at 0.625 mg/kg/h and 0.313 mg/kg/h respectively. In dogs with hyperadrenocorticism the values were reduced by approximately 50% while in hypoadrenocorticoid patients, cortisol values were significantly higher. These variations in plasma cortisol concentrations in dogs with altered adrenal function suggest a positive correlation between previous cortisol exposure and the rate of metabolism of administered steroids.

Adverse effects

In humans there have been rare reports of anaphylactic reactions to the intravenous administration of HSS.

Cortisone acetate

Mechanism of action

Cortisone is a synthetic steroid with an 11-keto substitution. Once absorbed, it is rapidly activated to hydrocortisone by a distinct 11β-hydroxysteroid dehydrogenase operating in a reductive mode.

As cortisone is rapidly 11-hydroxylated to cortisol, it provides a complete replacement for any form of cortisol deficiency. As it has equipotent glucocorticoid and mineralocorticoid activity, it will also provide more mineralocorticoid activity than other synthetic glucocorticoids such as prednisolone. In addition, its shorter half-life and lower overall activity means it is less likely to create iatrogenic hyperadrenocorticism with long-term administration.

Formulations and dose rates

In patients with hypoadrenocorticism, orally administered cortisone acetate can be used as an effective long-term cortisol replacement. Depending on the country of origin, these can be supplied as 5 mg, 10 mg and 25 mg tablets. The dose in dogs is 0.5–1 mg/kg/12–24 h. The dose must be individualized according to the severity of the condition, the response obtained and what other glucocorticoid or mineralocorticoid is being concurrently administered.

Pharmacokinetics

There is little information available regarding the pharmacokinetics of cortisone in dogs. An early report suggested cortisone had a half-life of 1 h in normal dogs. A more recent study of eight dogs given approximately 1.25 mg/kg of cortisone acetate orally revealed rapid absorption, a peak plasma cortisol concentration of 300–500 nmol/L occurring approximately 1 h after dosing and plasma levels returning to baseline around 5 h after dosing. There was no effect of feeding on these parameters. However, the reports suggested that spontaneous hypoadrenocorticism delayed metabolism and/or excretion of adrenosteroids.

Adverse effects

Adverse effects are uncommon and are usually dose dependent.

9α-Fludrocortisone

Mechanism of action

9α-Fludrocortisone is synthetic adrenocortical steroid with a fluoride ion substituted at the 9α position and an 11β-hydroxyl group, giving it both glucocorticoid and mineralocorticoid potency. Because of the 9α fluoride substitution, 9α-fludrocortisone has potent mineralocorticoid activity while the 11-hydroxylation confers significant glucocorticoid activity. When compared to hydrocortisone, 9α-fludrocortisone has 10 times the glucocorticoid activity and 125 times the mineralocorticoid activity.

Formulations and dose rates

The dose of 9α-fludrocortisone is 10–30 μg/kg/24 h. Typically a lower dose is used to start with and it may be titrated up on the basis of clinical impression and plasma electrolyte concentrations. Dose adjustments are usually made after weekly electrolyte evaluations. Once they are stable and within the normal range, adjustments can be made every 3–4 months.

In patients receiving concurrent long-term 9α-fludrocortisone, it is not uncommon for the dose of 9α-fludrocortisone to increase over time, as there appears to be a reduction in its mineralocorticoid efficacy. In one study the daily maintenance dose increased from a median of 13 μg/kg to a final median dose of 23 μg/kg while the final dose of fludrocortisone administered to more than half the dogs ranged from 15 to 30 μg/kg/24 h. In another group of hypoadrenocorticoid dogs treated with 9α-fludrocortisone and considered well controlled clinically, 84% had hyponatremia, hyperkalemia and/or a subnormal sodium:potassium ratio. Unfortunately, titrating up the 9α-fludrocortisone dose in an attempt to normalize plasma electrolyte levels can result in excess glucocorticoid activity and dogs can develop signs of iatrogenic hyperadrenocorticism while still not having normal sodium and potassium levels. Reasons for this '9α-fludrocortisone creep' are not clear although poor compliance may play a role, as might tachyphylaxis.

A substantial proportion of patients receiving 9α-fludrocortisone do not require maintenance glucocorticoid supplementation after initial stabilization. In patients that do require glucocorticoids, cortisone acetate is the preferred choice in small dogs and cats to minimize the risk of overdosing. In these patients the 9α-fludrocortisone dose required to maintain normal electrolyte levels is generally at the lower end of the suggested dose range.

Pharmacokinetics

In humans 9α-fludrocortisone is well absorbed from the gastrointestinal tract with peak levels occurring approximately 1.7 h after dosing. Like most steroids (which, of course, act intracellularly) although the plasma half-life of 9α-fludrocortisone is 3–5 h, biological activity persists for 18–36 h.

Adverse effects

Adverse effects of 9α-fludrocortisone are generally associated with overdosing or sudden withdrawal.

Known drug interactions

Patients may develop hypokalemia if 9α-fludrocortisone is administered concurrently with amphotericin B or potassium-depleting diuretics such as thiazides and furosemide. In addition, it should be used cautiously in patients receiving digoxin.

Deoxycorticosterone pivalate

Mechanism of action

Deoxycorticosterone pivalate (DOCP) is a long-acting mineralocorticoid (see Fig. 22.1). As it has neither an 11β- nor a 17α-hydroxylation, theoretically it has little if any glucocorticoid activity. Mineralocorticoids act at the distal convoluted tubule to increase sodium resorption as well as increasing potassium and hydrogen excretion in exchange for sodium.

Formulations and dose rates

The recommended dose of DOCP is 2.2 mg/kg by intramuscular or subcutaneous injection every 25 d. Plasma electrolyte, urea and creatinine concentrations can be monitored every 2 weeks to determine the duration of action and to help individualize the dose. Once stabilized, it is prudent to check electrolytes every 3–6 months. While the manufacturer recommends 2.2 mg/kg/25 d and this is generally accepted as producing reliable mineralocorticoid control, in one study lower doses of between 1.4 and 1.9 mg/kg were found to be effective in controlling electrolyte concentrations. The same study also suggested that dose interval could range between 14 and 35 d in individual dogs. While it seems likely that there is room for some individualization of the dose, it is worth noting that the vast majority of dogs appear to have stable and adequate mineralocorticoid supplementation when receiving 2.2 mg/kg of DOCP every 3–4 weeks. Additionally DOCP appears to be an extremely effective mineralocorticoid and once the dose has been individualized, the dose rate and frequency remain unchanged over years.

As DOCP has predominantly mineralocorticoid activity, all dogs and cats treated with it should receive concurrent glucocorticoid supplementation. As this is a replacement for physiological requirements, the dose of glucocorticoid should be much lower than the traditional anti-inflammatory dose rates. As a general guide, the daily glucocorticoid requirement for dogs and cats is the equivalent of approximately 0.2 mg/kg/24 h of cortisol or 0.04 mg/kg/24 h of prednisolone. Consequently tablet size tends to dictate that in cats and at least small dogs, cortisone acetate is the preferred method of oral glucocorticoid supplementation.

Pharmacokinetics

The pharmacokinetics of DOCP have not been reported in dogs or cats. It is injected intramuscularly as a microcrystalline depot for slow dissolution into the circulation. In dogs, DOCP usually has a duration of action of 21–30 days.

Adverse effects

Adverse effects of DOCP are generally a result of overdosing although occasionally irritation at the site of injection may occur.

Known drug interactions

- Patients may develop hypokalemia if DOCP is administered concurrently with amphotericin B or potassium-depleting diuretics such as thiazides and furosemide.
- DOCP should be used cautiously in patients receiving digoxin.

Dexamethasone

Dexamethasone is a synthetic adrenal steroid with markedly potentiated glucocorticoid activity (approximately 30 times that of hydrocortisone) and little mineralocorticoid activity. The soluble esters of dexamethasone can be given intravenously and some clinicians advocate its parenteral use in the acute management of hypoadrenocorticoid patients. A detailed discussion of its pharmacology can be found in Chapter 11 (Glucocorticosteroids and antihistamines).

Prednisolone

Prednisolone is a synthetic adrenal steroid with moderately potentiated glucocorticoid activity (approximately five times that of hydrocortisone) and less than 10% of hydrocortisone's mineralocorticoid activity. Some clinicians advocate its use as a glucocorticoid supplement in the long-term management of hypoadrencorticism. A detailed discussion of its pharmacology can be found in Chapter 12 on immunomodulatory therapy.

23

Drugs and reproduction

Philip G A Thomas and Alain Fontbonne

INTRODUCTION

Normal function of the reproductive system is determined by complex interactions between higher centers, the hypothalamus, the pituitary gland, the gonads and the tubular reproductive tract. Drugs directed at a specific target inevitably cascade to affect other parts of the reproductive system. The clinician should select drugs with care, acknowledging that the potential benefit must exceed undesirable consequences.

Reproductive endocrinology in the dog and cat is largely extrapolated from other species. Given that carnivores have proved to be dramatically different in reproductive function from traditional experimental models, some of the physiology on which drug selection is based is tenuous. Drugs whose choice may be justified in farm animals or humans may be inappropriate for use in small animals.

Over the past 5–10 years, many new drugs have been applied to canine, and sometimes feline, reproduction. Some are not officially approved for use in companion carnivores; their use is only experimental at the moment and further clinical trials are necessary. The availability of these drugs varies in different countries. As a result the prevalence of their use and practitioners' knowledge about them vary greatly.

Most drugs used in reproduction are naturally occurring or synthetic analogs of endogenous hormones; therefore, a sound understanding of the structure and function of the native hormones is essential to sensible clinical selection of drugs.

Relevant physiology

General physiology

Gonadotropin-releasing hormone (GnRH) is secreted from hypothalamic nuclei into the portal hypophyseal circulation. GnRH acts on the pituitary gland to cause the release of stored gonadotropins, luteinizing hormone (LH) and follicle-stimulating hormone (FSH). Pulsatile release of LH and FSH induces steroid synthesis and gametogenesis by the gonad. Steroids mediate reproductive behavior and gametogenesis. Steroids and inhibin from the gonad have a negative feedback on the hypothalamus and pituitary gland. Estradiol has a brief positive feedback effect on gonadotropin secretion in preovulatory females, leading to the LH surge.

Male physiology

Testosterone is produced by Leydig (or interstitial) cells. Testosterone is necessary for male behavior, libido, function of the accessory sex glands and the production of spermatozoa and is involved, possibly with estradiol, in the negative feedback and regulation of pituitary LH secretion. Pulsatile secretion of LH acts on Leydig cells to regulate the conversion of cholesterol to pregnenolone which is a testosterone precursor. Prolactin may act synergistically with LH in testosterone production. FSH acts to induce aromatization of testosterone to estradiol.

Testosterone is converted to dihydrotestosterone by 5-α-reductase. The production of spermatozoa (spermatogenesis) requires FSH, testosterone and dihydrotestosterone. FSH acts on Sertoli cells to indirectly stimulate spermatogenesis. Sertoli cells produce inhibin which inhibits FSH secretion. Spermatogenesis occurs in waves as undifferentiated germ cells undergo terminal differentiation to become spermatozoa.

Female physiology

In the female, FSH acts on granulosa cells, which make up the wall of the ovarian follicle, to induce steroidogenesis, including estrogen synthesis. Estrogen is transported to luteal cells. A surge of LH is responsible for ovulation and luteinization of follicular cells to luteal cells, which produce progesterone. LH and prolactin are luteotrophs, which maintain the corpus luteum (CL).

In most domestic species, endogenous prostaglandin $F_{2\alpha}$ ($PGF_{2\alpha}$) is responsible for CL regression. In the bitch and queen, ovulation is always followed by prolonged diestrus, which is equivalent hormonally to pregnancy. In the queen, however, if no pregnancy follows ovulation, diestrus still exists but is shortened (pseudopregnancy). The role of endogenous $PGF_{2\alpha}$ has not been clearly determined in small animals.

The estrus cycle of the female dog occurs every 6–12 months in the following sequence.

- **Proestrus** (7–9 d): estradiol rises and falls, progesterone begins to rise, vaginal cornification begins and the bitch is attractive but not receptive to males.

- **Estrus** (7–9 d): progesterone continues to rise in response to the preovulatory LH surge that occurs about the beginning of estrus. The bitch is receptive to males. Ovulation occurs in response to the LH surge and occurs around 42–54 h post-LH surge. It has been shown, using ovarian ultrasonography, that there is no significant difference in the time of ovulation between the left and the right ovary. Ovulated eggs are primary oocytes that cannot be penetrated in vivo by the sperm until there is a complete resumption of meiosis. Maturation, including the second meiotic division, is complete after a further 54–75 h. Ovulated oocytes are fertilizable for approximately 2 d but there may be breed differences.
- **Diestrus** (57 d): progesterone is secreted throughout diestrus.
- **Pregnancy** (57–58 d from the first diestrus vaginal smear, 65 d on average from the LH surge): progesterone is secreted throughout pregnancy at levels indistinguishable from a nonpregnant diestrus.
- **Anestrus** (3–6 months): characterized by the absence of circulating steroid hormones and a quiescent endometrium.

The female cat (queen) is a seasonal breeder, requiring increasing day length to begin cycling. The queen is an induced ovulator, requiring mechanical stimulation of the vagina and cervix or copulation to ovulate. However, in specific cases (old queens, queens housed in catteries) spontaneous ovulation may occur in a minority of cases.

- **Copulation** is followed by an LH surge within minutes and cessation of estrus within 48 h. Ovulation occurs 30–50 h after copulation.
- **Nonovulatory estrus cycles** are normally followed during the breeding season by return to estrus within 7–21 d.
- **Ovulatory estrus cycles** are followed by pregnancy (63–68 d) or by nonpregnant diestrus (25–45 d), both of which are characterized by high circulating progesterone.

POLYPEPTIDE HORMONES

Endogenous polypeptides include GnRH, the gonadotropins, oxytocin and prolactin.

Relevant physiology

The peptide hormones are constructed from amino acids and are stored and secreted in response to specific triggers. Circulating polypeptide hormones bind to membrane receptors on target cells to activate adenyl cyclase and, via a second messenger, cytoplasmic protein kinase, to induce steroid synthesis and secretion.

Gonadotropin-releasing hormone (GnRH)

GnRH is a hypothalamic decapeptide. GnRH agonists have one or two amino acid changes in the GnRH chemical structure.

> **EXAMPLES**
>
> *GnRH* formulations include gonadorelin diacetate tetrahydrate (hypothalamic decapeptide) and gonadorelin HCl (hypothalamic decapeptide).
>
> *GnRH agonists* such as fertirelin acetate and buserelin often have increased GnRH receptor affinity. Several synthetic analogs such as lutrelin, deslorelin and nafarelin have recently been used experimentally for regulating the estrous cycle in bitches. More than 700 GnRH agonists have been synthesized.

Under normal conditions, GnRH or GnRH agonists are short acting drugs. When they are administered as subcutaneous implants they may be used as long-acting devices.

Mechanism of action

GnRH stimulates a surge release of endogenous FSH and LH from the anterior pituitary that acts to:

- cause follicular maturation, ovulation and progesterone secretion in the bitch and queen
- promote testosterone secretion in the male dog and cat.

GnRH agonists also stimulate, with different potencies, production and release of gonadotropins from the pituitary. Conversely, when used at sustained doses GnRH agonists reversibly inhibit (after a short period of stimulation) the gonadal axis by downregulating the anterior pituitary GnRH receptors.

Clinical applications

In bitches

- GnRH causes release of LH, which may induce ovulation in estrous bitches and will promote luteinization of follicular cysts in bitches with functional ovarian cysts.
- GnRH has been used experimentally to induce estrus in anestrus bitches.
- Postponement of puberty.

In queens

- GnRH-mediated release of FSH and LH will allow estrus induction in queens.
- GnRH will induce ovulation in queens.

In males

- Determination of the presence of testicles in cryptorchids (GnRH causes release of endogenous LH within 15 min, followed in males by release of testosterone).
- Promotion of descent of undescended testicles; however, there are no convincing data to support this claim.
- Libido stimulant in carnivores on the basis of scant evidence. More searching trials may not support this conclusion.
- Treatment of prostatic hyperplasia.
- Postponement of puberty.

Formulations and dose rates

IN BITCHES

Cystic ovarian disease

- 2.2 μg/kg IM daily for 3 d
- However, GnRH treatment enhances the production of progesterone by the ovaries. Therefore veterinarians must be aware that when there has been prolonged estrogen secretion by an ovarian cyst, GnRH treatment may lead to a cystic endometrial hyperplasia (CEH)-pyometra. It is highly recommended that the bitch be spayed or treated with an antiprogestin compound (see p. 532) just after GnRH treatment.

Estrus induction

- Pulsatile administration or continuous infusion (2.3–14 ng/kg/min for 7–9 d) resulted in estrus and ovulation in two out of four bitches in one study. Continuous administration for 7–14 d via osmotic mini-pumps has been reported to result in a high rate of fertile estrous induction. It is important to note that the administration of GnRH does not need to be pulsatile: constant infusion or release of GnRH analogs via mini-pumps or subcutaneous implants may lead to estrus induction and pregnancies, provided that the GnRH administration is stopped after ovulation to prevent premature luteal failure. However, estrus induction using short-acting GnRH or GnRH agonists intravenously is not clinically feasible due to the expense of pulsatile infusion pumps or the need for hospitalization during the intravenous infusion.
- A single subcutaneous injection of a sustained-release formulation of leuprolide actetate to anestrous bitches has been reported to result in an 83% ovulation rate and 78% pregnancy rate.
- Deslorelin, a GnRH analog, is manufactured in Australia as a biodegradable subdermal implant containing 2.1 mg of deslorelin. It induces a rapid and synchronous estrus. In preliminary studies, fertile estrus was also successfully induced after repeated intramuscular administration of 1.5 mg of deslorelin in three bitches. However, induction of estrus in bitches is not as reliable when deslorelin is administered by this route compared with subdermal implants. Individual differences in drug absorption and/or metabolism between bitches, or variable drug compounding, may explain these inconsistencies.
- Deslorelin has also been administered by submucosal implant. In order to be able to remove the implants easily to prevent secondary luteal failure, 2.1 mg deslorelin implants were inserted just beneath the vestibular mucosa on the inside of the vulva lips in eight anestrous bitches; 8/8 bitches came into heat within 6 d. The implants were removed 1 d after serum progesterone reached 2 ng/mL and 5/8 bitches became pregnant.

Suppression of reproductive function in bitches

- GnRH agonist implants induce prolonged and reversible estrus suppression in adult bitches and may be used for this application in the future. However, many treated bitches initially come into heat due to the primary activating effect of these drugs, a problem which has not yet been solved.

Postponement of puberty

- The administration of a GnRH agonist (GnRH ethylamide-A) in prepubertal male or female dogs daily for 23 months caused a reduction in testicular and prostatic volume, absence of secondary follicles in the ovary and hypotrophy of pituitary LH-secreting cells in both sexes. After cessation of treatment and a 14-month recovery period, fertility was completely restored. Pups from different breeds implanted with deslorelin around 4 months of age showed prolonged postponement of puberty without any estrus response at the time of implantation. A similar result was obtained after implantation of the azagly-nafarelin GnRH agonist in prepubertal bitches. Puberty was significantly delayed, without any alteration of growth or weight during treatment. In the following estrus after cessation of treatment, ovulation and luteal function were normal.

IN QUEENS

Estrus induction in the queen

- 1 μg/kg daily SC until signs of estrus are noted or for a maximum of 10 d

Ovulation induction in queens

- 5–25 μg/cat IM or 25–50 μg/cat IM at the peak of estrus

IN MALES

Promotion of libido

- 2.2 μg/kg IM once weekly for a month prior to breeding

Challenge testing

- 2.2 μg/kg IM
- Measure serum testosterone concentration immediately before and 1 h after GnRH administration

Cryptorchidism

- 50–750 μg IM 1–6 times at 48-h intervals. A recovery rate of 26.6% was observed only in animals less than 4 months old at the beginning of treatment. Note that this therapy is indicated only for testis retained at an inguinal or inguino-scrotal site and not for testis retained inside the abdominal cavity.

Suppression of reproductive function in male dogs

- Males implanted with deslorelin long-acting implants showed a decrease of serum testosterone to basal values (<1 ng/mL) within a mean of 17 d after implantation. After removal of the implant, spermatogenesis returned and fertility was restored. No adverse effects were observed in animals treated repeatedly. Similar suppressive and reversible effects on reproductive male function have been observed with implants containing the GnRH agonist azagly-nafarelin.

Control of prostatic disease
- Five adult dogs implanted with deslorelin at a dose of 0.5–1.0 mg/kg showed a significant 50% decrease in prostatic volume from week 6 to week 44.

Reduction of aggression
- Some studies suggest that prolonged use of deslorelin implants may reduce aggression in male dogs and cats.

Pharmacokinetics
Data are not available for the dog and cat. In the pig, distribution half-life to extracellular fluid after intravenous administration is 2 min and elimination half-life is 13 min.

Adverse effects
- None reported, although naturally occurring GnRH might induce a hypersensitivity reaction.
- However, when trying to prevent estrus in anestrous bitches, the use of GnRH agonists, especially deslorelin implants, may first induce heat as a result of the stimulatory effect of the drug on the pituitary. Some studies have shown that concomitant use of progestins may reduce this adverse reaction but not suppress it completely.

Contraindications and precautions
None reported.

Known drug interactions
None reported.

Gonadotropins

Gonadotropins include the pituitary gonadotropins, luteinizing hormone (LH) and follicle-stimulating hormone (FSH), and the nonpituitary gonadotropins, human chorionic gonadotropin (hCG) and equine chorionic gonadotropin (eCG), which is also called pregnant mare's serum gonadotropin (PMSG).

EXAMPLES

FSH has two subunits ($\alpha = 89$ amino acids and $\beta = 115$ amino acids). There are a variety of products available, which are biological products purified from the pituitary glands of farm animals and therefore contain some LH activity. 1 mg FSH-P contains 1 Armour unit, which may be 9.4–14.2 IU of FSH.

LH has two subunits ($\alpha = 89$ amino acids and $\beta = 115$ amino acids). LH is no longer available as a commercial product.

hCG is a high molecular weight glycoprotein secreted by the chorion of pregnant women and recovered from their urine. It has mostly LH-like but also has some FSH-like activity. 1 IU = 1 USP unit. 1 mg ≥1500 USP units. It is available as a purified biological.

eCG is a high molecular weight glycoprotein secreted by the endometrial cups of the pregnant mare with a long (>24 h) half-life. Several products have FSH-like as well as LH-like activities.

Mechanism of action
The gonadotropins are produced endogenously by the anterior pituitary and act with other hormones to promote folliculogenesis, spermatogenesis and steroidogenesis. They may not have all these effects when administered parenterally.

Clinical applications
In females
- Estrus induction in the bitch (FSH and hCG, eCG and hCG).
- Luteinization of follicular cysts (hCG).
- Estrus induction in anestrus queens (FSH and hCG).
- Ovulation induction in bitches and queens (hCG).
- Stimulation of progesterone release from luteal cells, including challenge testing to diagnose the presence of ovarian parenchyma (hCG).

In males
- Stimulation of testosterone release from Leydig cells, including challenge testing to diagnose the presence of testicular parenchyma (hCG).
- Cryptorchidism treatment (hCG).
- Enhancement of spermatogenesis (infertile male dogs): recent data suggest that this treatment is ineffective. This may be because repeated injections may lead to immuno-sensitization, thus decreasing the efficacy of gonadotropin administration.

Formulations and dose rates

IN FEMALES

Estrus induction in bitches
- The most widely studied gonadotropin for estrus induction in the dog is eCG. Protocols range from daily (20–40 IU/kg) to weekly (110 IU/kg) injections, often IM. However, premature luteal failure occurs frequently and, therefore, the pregnancy rates remain low. Ultrasonographic and histological studies have demonstrated that ovarian follicular dynamics differ widely from those at spontaneous estrous cycles. Furthermore, the likelihood of inducing cystic follicular degeneration is very high.

Formulations and dose rates—cont'd

For all these reasons, eCG is not recommended for use in bitches or queens.

Challenge testing for ovarian tissue

- This test may be used in cases where ovarian remnant syndrome in spayed females is suspected.
- hCG 100–1000 IU (bitch) or 50–100 IU (queen) IM when showing estrus signs and measure peripheral progesterone in 5–7 d. Progesterone above 1 ng/mL is consistent with functional ovarian tissue.

Luteinization of follicular cysts

- hCG 500 IU per dog IM and repeat in 48 h. However, as discussed previously, veterinarians must be aware that when there has been prolonged estrogen secretion by an ovarian cyst, GnRH treatment may lead to a CEH-pyometra. It is highly recommended that the bitch be spayed or treated with an antiprogestin compound (aglepristone) just after GnRH treatment.

Estrus induction in anestrus queens (many different protocols have been described)

- The preferred treatment is: eCG (100–150 IU IM) followed 5 d later by 1–3 daily injections of hCG (50–100 UI IM). This treatment leads to ovulation and pregnancy results similar to those observed with natural matings (over 80%)

Ovulation induction in queens

- 50–200 IU hCG at the peak of estrus. Ovulation generally occurs 24–36 h after injection

IN MALES

Challenge testing for testicular tissue

- hCG: 50 µg/kg (dog) or 250 µg (cat) IM. Measure serum testosterone concentration immediately before and 4 h after hCG.

Cryptorchidism treatment

- hCG: 500 IU per dog IM twice weekly for 4–6 weeks or 50 IU/kg IM every 2 d for 10 d followed by no treatment for 10 d, then 50 IU/kg IM every 2 d for 10 d. Animals should be aged less than 4 months at the beginning of treatment. The success rate is not defined, as most studies do not include any control group. In reality, there is no good evidence to support this treatment approach.

Stimulation of spermatogenesis

- FSH and eCG have been promoted as appropriate for use as stimulators of spermatogenesis, with or without concurrent hCG. There are no conclusive data to support this recommendation.

Pharmacokinetics

- **FSH, eCG:** no specific information is available.
- **hCG:** peak plasma levels at 6 h. Biphasic elimination from blood: the initial elimination half-life is 11 h and terminal elimination half-life is 23 h.

Adverse effects

- Repeated injections of exogenous gonadotropins may lead to the production of antibodies against FSH or LH, which may cross-react with the endogenous and exogenous hormones and lead to a subsequent decreased response to stimulation or subsequent infertility.
- **FSH** and **PMSG:** undesired superovulation, follicular cysts and cystic endometrial hyperplasia mediated by steroid production are possible and are more likely with higher doses and repeated administration.
- **hCG:**
  - Hypersensitivity
  - In humans, injection site pain, gynecomastia, headache, depression, irritability and edema have been reported.

Contraindications and precautions

- FSH and eCG
  - Do not use in bitches with cystic endometrial hyperplasia.
  - Adverse effects are likely to be exacerbated if gonadotropins are given concurrently with exogenous sex steroids or in the face of high levels of endogenous sex steroids.
- hCG: none reported.

Known drug interactions

None reported, but use of gonadotropins concurrently with sex steroids is likely to promote cystic endometrial hyperplasia in females.

Oxytocin

Oxytocin is a nonapeptide hormone synthesized in the hypothalamus and stored in the posterior pituitary gland. Oxytocin mediates contractility of the endometrium which has been prestimulated with estradiol. It stimulates contractility of the myoepithelial cells that surround mammary alveoli. It is measured in USP posterior pituitary units, where 1 unit = 2.0–2.2 mg of pure hormone.

Mechanism of action

Oxytocin causes contraction of uterine smooth muscle by increasing the sodium permeability of the uterine myofibrils. Presence of high peripheral estrogen levels reduces the threshold for oxytocin-induced smooth muscle contraction. A dose of 1 IU oxytocin IV (per bitch) will induce intrauterine pressure of over 100 mmHg in a pre-estrous bitch and 58 mmHg in an anestrous bitch, demonstrating that it is still active in the absence of estrogen.

Oxytocin facilitates some milk let-down without having galactopoietic ability. It is mildly antidiuretic.

Clinical applications

- To promote contraction of uterine smooth muscle to assist vaginal birth, to induce uterine evacuation in metritis and to assist uterine contraction following reduction of uterine prolapse.
- To promote milk let-down in bitches with adequate milk production.

Formulations and dose rates

Induction of uterine smooth muscle contraction (for dystocia, uterine evacuation or postpartum uterine contraction)

- Oxytocin is available as purified, pH adjusted or synthetic forms of the hormone for parenteral administration. A synthetic form is also available for intranasal administration.
- Doses recommended have ranged from 0.25–4 IU or 1–5 IU per bitch to 5–20 IU per bitch, repeated up to three times. In the queen, 2 IU maximum per queen and per injection IM or by IV infusion.
- It is important to use calcium gluconate 10% solution (1 mL/5.5 kg SC q.4–6 h) minimum 15 min before oxytocin even in eucalcemic bitches. If one treatment of oxytocin for dystocia is unsuccessful, repeated use must be questioned, given the likelihood of inducing tetanic uterine contraction and fetal death.
- There are no data supporting any specific regimen for use in dystocia. Indeed, since absolute oxytocin deficiency has not been demonstrated in the parturient bitch or queen, it is difficult to make a rational argument for its use.

For milk let-down

- In bitches with adequate milk production, milk let-down may be stimulated with intranasal oxytocin. There is little experimental evidence to support this protocol.

Pharmacokinetics

Oxytocin must be given parenterally because it is destroyed in the gastrointestinal tract. Onset of activity is 5 min after IM administration. Duration of activity is 13 min after IV bolus and 20 min after SC or IM administration.

Oxytocin is metabolized by the liver and kidneys and a circulating enzyme, oxytocinase, can destroy the hormone. A small amount is excreted unchanged in urine. The half-life is 3–5 min in humans and 20 min in goats.

Adverse effects

- Use in obstructive dystocia can cause uterine rupture.
- Overdose, either single large doses or multiple doses, will cause spastic, hypertonic or tetanic uterine muscle contraction with lack of orchestration of contractions. This may induce placental separation or damage without delivery, fetal distress or death and uterine rupture.
- Water intoxication is possible with large overdosage.

Contraindications and precautions

Oxytocin is widely overused and used in inappropriate situations.

- Obstructive dystocia.
- Any contraindication for vaginal delivery (e.g. relative or absolute oversize).
- Maternal toxemia.
- Underlying causes of dystocia (e.g. hypocalcemia) should be treated before use of oxytocin.

Known drug interactions

- Incompatible with fibrinolysin, noradrenaline (norepinephrine) bitartrate, prochlorperazine edisylate and warfarin sodium.
- If used with sympathomimetic agents, can result in postpartum hypertension.

Dopamine agonists and serotonin antagonists

Prolactin is a 198-amino acid glycoprotein synthesized by the lactotrophs of the adenohypophysis. Prolactin synthesis in pregnancy (from day 25–30 post-LH surge) and the postpartum period induces mammary development and lactation.

Prolactin is one of two luteotrophs in the dog (along with LH). Hypothalamic dopamine has inhibitory control over prolactin secretion at the pituitary level, so dopamine agonists inhibit prolactin secretion and dopamine antagonists such as the antiemetic domperidone (see Chapter 19) may increase prolactin secretion, resulting in gynecomastia. Serotonin inhibits dopamine secretion at the hypothalamus and therefore indirectly stimulates prolactin secretion.

EXAMPLES

Dopamine agonists act on D_2-dopamine receptors of the lactotrophic cells of the pituitary gland.

- Cabergoline (approved in Europe but not Australia, New Zealand or the United States)
- Bromocriptine

Antiserotoninergic compounds

- Metergoline. This compound also exerts a direct dopaminergic effect at high doses.

Mechanism of action

Cabergoline is a specific dopamine agonist. Bromocriptine mesylate is a synthetic ergot alkaloid derivative which, like cabergoline, directly inhibits prolactin by its action of D_2 pituitary receptors. Metergoline is a serotonin antagonist, which increases dopamine-inhibiting tone at the hypothalamus.

Clinical applications

- *Galactostasis:* dopamine agonists will prevent prolactin secretion and indirectly impede milk production.
- *Overt pseudocyesis or pseudopregnancy:* bitches exhibiting these signs have high peripheral prolactin concentrations, which can be treated with dopamine agonists.
- *Pregnancy termination:* dopamine agonists given systemically or orally during pregnancy, after day 30–40 post-LH surge, may induce abortion. Oral cabergoline or bromocriptine may be combined with cloprostenol (a synthetic prostaglandin analog) to reduce the dose of both drugs in the bitch and queen.
- *Estrus induction and reduced interestrus interval:* the action of dopamine agonists is not fully understood. They do not act only by reducing the level of serum prolactin. They may also directly stimulate the hypothalamic pituitary axis. Cabergoline and bromocriptine will reduce the interval between estrus by shortening both diestrus and anestrus, possibly by a dopaminergic action that is not related to the suppression of prolactin secretion. However:
  - the duration of treatment for estrus induction is much shorter in late versus early anestrus;
  - estrus induction in diestrus is unlikely to lead to a successful pregnancy, probably due to lack of uterine endometrial regeneration.
- *Treatment of pyometra.*
- *Pretreatment of mammary tumors.*

Formulations and dose rates

Galactostasis and pseudocyesis

- Cabergoline: 5 μg/kg/d PO for 5–10 d
- Bromocriptine: 50–100 μg/kg PO for 10–14 d. To reduce side effects, the dose can be given q.8–12 h. Dopamine receptors play an important role in the vomiting pathway (see Chapter 19). The emetic effect can be attenuated by gradually increasing the dose: 2.5 μg/kg q.12 h day 1, 5 μg/kg q.12 h day 2 and 10 μg/kg q.12 h day 3–5 or 3–10
- Metergoline: 0.1 mg/kg PO q.12 h for 8–10 d. Minimum 8 d required

Pregnancy termination in the bitch

- Cabergoline: 5 μg/kg/d PO for 5 d or 1.7μg/kg SC every 2 d for 6 d will induce abortion in 100% of bitches treated from 40 d post-LH surge, but only 25% of bitches from day 30
- Cabergoline (5 μg/kg/day PO for 10 d) plus cloprostenol (1 μg/kg/48 h SC for five injections) from day 28 post-LH surge will induce abortion in > 95% of bitches
- Bromocriptine at doses of 50–100 μg/kg PO twice a day for at least 5 and up to 10 d is not consistently effective in inducing abortion before day 40. This treatment should never be discontinued until termination of pregnancy has been confirmed. It is never effective before day 30

Pregnancy termination in the queen

- Use of dopaminergic drugs alone is not recommended for early pregnancy termination in queens, as variable efficacy is reported. However, after 40 d of pregnancy, cabergoline (5 μg/kg/d for 7 d) or bromocriptine (25–50 μg/kg q.8 h for 7d) will result in pregnancy termination, often associated with fetal expulsion. Combined treatment with $PGF_{2\alpha}$ begins earlier, on day 25 after first breeding. Abortion can be induced using three injections of cloprostenol (5 μg/kg) at 48-h intervals (d1, d3 and d5) associated with a daily oral administration of cabergoline (5 μg/kg for 7–10 d). This treatment does not lead to any side effect.

Estrus induction in bitches

- Dopamine agonists (bromocriptine, cabergoline) have been used successfully to induce estrus in bitches. Cabergoline-induced cycles have follicular development and ovulatory rates similar to those observed at natural cycles. However, if the level of estrus induction is high, regardless of the period of treatment within the estrous cycle, the stage of treatment appears to be important. Fertile estrus is more reliably obtained if the bitch is treated during late anestrus. Bromocriptine (250 μg/kg/d until proestrus occurred) induced a fertile estrus in 5/6 bitches. Cabergoline 5 μg/kg/d induces estrus within 30 d, with 75–85% whelping rate. In cases of prolonged anestrus (>8 months), daily treatment for 3 weeks with oral cabergoline (5 μg/kg) induced fertile estrus within one month in 70% of treated bitches.

Treatment of pyometra in bitches

- Combination treatment with oral cabergoline (5 μg/kg daily) and cloprostenol (5 μg/kg every third day) has been used to treat pyometra medically (in addition to appropriate antibacterial therapy) in bitches. Resolution was achieved in 21 of 22 treated bitches within 13 d. 11/21 bitches were mated at the next estrus and conceived. Cabergoline (5 μg/kg PO daily) and cloprostenol (1 μg/kg daily SC) for 7–14 d were also successful in 24/29 bitches

Treatment of pyometra in queens

- Cabergoline (5 μg/kg PO daily) and cloprostenol (1 μg/kg SC daily) until complete uterine emptying (in addition to appropriate antibacterial therapy) has been recommended

Pretreatment of mammary tumors

- Most mammary tumors are detected and surgically treated during diestrus when the mammary gland is enlarged and often partially filled with milk. Treatment with cabergoline 5–7 d before surgery will facilitate the surgical procedure because (a) mammary tumors can be more accurately palpated because the mammary gland is not enlarged, (b) there is reduced risk of a postsurgical reaction because milk does not contaminate the surgical site and (c) the bitch or queen recovers more quickly because the surgery is faster and the duration of anesthesia reduced. Furthermore, due to the decreased progesteronemia, it has been postulated that there may be a higher immunity in the operated bitch or queen

Pharmacokinetics

The duration of activity of bromocriptine in the dog is only about 8 h; in humans it has a biphasic half-life (4 h and 15 h). Bromocriptine pharmacology is not well described in the dog but in humans only 28% of an oral dose is absorbed and only 6% reaches systemic circulation. It is 90–96% bound to serum albumin and is metabolized by the liver.

Cabergoline binds to pituitary receptors for more than 48 h, making it long acting. Cabergoline has greater bio-activity and superior receptor (D_2) specificity than bromocriptine and a longer duration of action. Only a small percentage crosses the blood–brain barrier, resulting in a less emetic effect than bromocriptine.

Metergoline has a shorter half-life and is administred q.12 h.

Adverse effects

- Cabergoline may cause mild emesis and nausea. When used in prolonged treatments (>15 d), reversible coat color changes may occur due to tonic suppression of pituitary secretion of melanocyte-stimulating hormone (MSH).
- Bromocriptine causes nausea, vomiting, sedation, fatigue and hypotension. Because it is a potent emetic, its use is not recommended despite its low cost. If it is used, an increasing dose schedule can reduce the emetic effect (see above). It has often been stated that concurrent administration of bromocriptine with metoclopromide or metopimazine is inappropriate as both antiemetic drugs may increase release of prolactin. However, some authors recommend use of bromocriptine in association with metopimazine (0.25 mg/kg PO 15 min before bromocriptine administration) as, despite the concerns outlined above, in practice use of metopimazine does not appear to reduce the clinical success of bromocriptine.
- Metergoline, due to its antiserotoninergic action, should not be given to pseudopregnant bitches who exhibit strong behavioral manifestations, especially if they are nervous or restless. The drug may increase unpleasant behavior associated with pseudopregnancy even if it effectively stops lactation.
- Abortion induced prior to day 40 post-LH surge will be accompanied by serosanguinous vaginal discharge and after day 40 by fetal expulsion.

Contraindications and precautions

- If pregnancy is to be maintained, prolactin inhibitors are contraindicated during pregnancy.
- Bromocriptine is contraindicated in patients with liver disease and hypertension.

Known drug interactions

Phenothiazines, reserpine, amitriptyline and butyrophenones (e.g. haloperidol) will increase prolactin concentrations and doses of prolactin inhibitors may need to be increased.

Dopamine antagonists

Dopamine antagonists promote prolactin secretion. They include metoclopramide and phenothiazines. Metoclopromide may be successfully used in cases of hypogalactia to enhance milk production after a normal parturition or after surgical cesarean section in the bitch.

As metoclopramide blocks dopamine receptors, it may cause sedation and extrapyramidal effects although these effects are uncommon (see Chapter 19). Metoclopramide reduces renal blood flow which may exacerbate pre-existing renal disease.

Metoclopramide should not be used with antimuscarinic drugs (e.g. atropine) or narcotic analgesics. It may decrease cimetidine absorption. Phenothiazines may potentiate the extrapyramidal side effects of metoclopramide.

STEROIDS

Endogenous steroids include testosterone, estradiol, progesterone and cortisone. Steroid hormones are synthesized from cholesterol and immediately released. Circulating steroids bind to and penetrate cell membranes of target cells and then bind to intracytoplasmic receptors, inducing nuclear production of mRNA, which codes for new protein synthesis by the target cell.

Progesterone and the progestins

Progesterone is produced by the CL of the dog and cat and the placenta of the cat. Progestins are synthetic analogs. Both mimic the effects of the CL, producing signs of pseudopregnancy. Increasing knowledge regarding the adverse effects of progestins has led to most being contraindicated for use in small animal reproduction.

EXAMPLES

- Medroxyprogesterone acetate (MPA), proligestone and hydroxyprogesterone hexanoate are synthetic progestins that should not be used in small animal reproduction. Megestrol acetate (MA) is a synthetic progestin registered for use in bitches and queens.
- Delmadinone acetate is an antiandrogen and synthetic progestin registered for use in male dogs in Australia and New Zealand.
- Progesterone is the naturally occurring hormone and is available in an oil formulation.

Mechanism of action

All progestins have the following broad effects.

- Transformation of proliferative endometrium to secretory endometrium.
- Enhancement of myometrial hypertrophy.
- Inhibition of spontaneous uterine contraction.
- Negative feedback inhibition on the secretion of pituitary gonadotropins.
- Insulin antagonism.
- Antiestradiol and glucocorticoid activity with resultant adrenal suppression.

Different progestins may also exert an antiandrogenic effect, depending on their antigonadotrophic and androgenic receptor-binding ability. Medroxyprogesterone acetate, megestrol acetate, delmadinone acetate, clormadinone acetate and cyproterone acetate have been successfully tested for that purpose in the dog.

Clinical applications

In females

- Estrus suppression in bitches.
- Estrus postponement in the bitch and queen.
- Prevention of abortion in the bitch and queen.
- Treatment of infertility with shortened interestrus intervals.

In males

- Suppression of libido in male dogs.
- Treatment of prostatic hyperplasia in dogs.

Formulations and dose rates

IN FEMALES

Estrus suppression

- MA 2.2 mg/kg/d PO for 8 d, beginning in the first 3 d of pre-estrus, is 92% efficacious

Estrus postponement in the bitch

- MA 0.55 mg/kg/d PO for 32 d, beginning at least 7 d before the onset of the next anticipated pre-estrus

Estrus postponement in the queen

- 2.5 mg PO once weekly for up to 18 months
- MA should not be given to queens during estrus or diestrus, although its use has been recommended for estrus-cycle control during these times

Prevention of abortion

It has been proposed that a primary lack of progesterone, 'luteal insufficiency' or 'hypoluteoidism', is a cause of abortion and can be treated with progesterone. This use of progesterone is controversial. Authors disagree about its relative safety and efficacy and there are no accurate studies to support or refute its use. As such, the potential disadvantages of giving progesterone to pregnant animals may outweigh the perceived benefit.

Treatments that have been used include:

- progesterone in oil 2 mg/kg IM every 72 h, which will maintain serum progesterone at 10 ng/mL or higher (it can be measured by laboratory assays to assess adequacy of supplementation), but this may cause dystocia and masculinization of female fetuses
- in some countries, when available: oral micronized progesterone, 10–20 mg/kg every 8 h, until 58 d of pregnancy
- synthetic oral progestin altrenogest: 0.088 mg/kg daily (this drug cannot be measured by progesterone assays)

Treatment of infertility with shortened interestrus intervals in the bitch

- Megestrol acetate (2 mg/kg for 8 consecutive days) or clormadinone acetate (0.5 mg/kg for 8 consecutive days) have been used successfully to treat infertility associated with shortened interestrus intervals (<4 months) in 10 bitches. All treated bitches exhibited normal estrus within 3 months of treatment completion. 9/10 bitches became pregnant

IN MALES

Libido suppression in male dogs

- Delmadinone acetate 1–2 mg/kg IM or SC once and repeat if necessary in 3–4 weeks

Treatment of prostatic hyperplasia in dogs

- Delmadinone acetate 1–2 mg/kg IM or SC once and repeat if necessary in 3–4 weeks
- MA 0.11 mg/kg PO once daily

It is the author's opinion that finasteride (see below) or surgical castration might provide better options for this disease.

In recent experimental trials osaterone acetate (0.25 mg/kg daily for 7 d) was effective in treating prostatic hyperplasia without affecting libido or sperm quality

Pharmacokinetics

MPA has a duration of activity of at least 30 d in cats and has contraceptive effects for 3 months in humans. MA is well absorbed from the gastrointestinal tract, is metabolized in the liver and has a half-life of 8 d in the dog.

There is little information regarding the pharmacokinetics of delmadinone acetate.

In dogs, osaterone acetate has a long half-life (197 ± 109 h). The major route of excretion is in feces via bile.

Adverse effects

- In cats, MA may cause adrenocortical suppression and adrenal atrophy, as well as transient diabetes mellitus, weight gain, cystic endometrial hyperplasia, mammary hypertrophy and neoplasia and rarely hepatotoxicity.
- In bitches, MA may induce weight gain, lethargy, behavior change, cystic endometrial hyperplasia with mucometra, mammary enlargement and neoplasia,

acromegaly and adrenocortical suppression. High doses of progestins or repeated or prolonged exposure to moderate doses of progestins may: increase the incidence of uterine pathology, including the CEH-pyometra complex; increase secretion of growth hormone and thus the risk of acromegalic changes; increase the risk of local skin alterations when administered parenterally and promote weight gain. Their role in promoting mammary tumors after prolonged use remains unclear. For all these reasons, repeated progestin treatments are not recommended in females, especially in breeding bitches.

- Progestins at high doses given to male dogs (MPA 20 mg/kg SC; MA 4 mg/kg PO daily for 7 d) cause reduced sperm quality (which may be irreversible if sufficiently high doses are used for long periods) but do not affect libido.
- Delmadinone has a suppressive effect on both libido and spermatogenesis and return to normal function following use of delmadinone in male dogs is unpredictable.

Contraindications and precautions

- All progestins are contraindicated in pregnancy, diestrus, following estrogen administration and in animals with diabetes mellitus, mammary neoplasia or endometrial disease.
- Progestins should be used with care in any animal that will subsequently be used for breeding.

Known drug interactions

- Progestins in combination with corticosteroids may exacerbate adrenocortical suppression and diabetes mellitus.
- Estrogens will induce progesterone receptors on the endometrium so concurrent or prior use of estrogens with progestins is more likely to precipitate cystic endometrial hyperplasia.

Antiprogestins

EXAMPLES

The antiprogestin compounds that have been tested in small animal reproduction are mifepristone (RU 486) and aglepristone (RU 534).

Mechanism of action

Antiprogestins are synthetic steroids which have a high affinity for progesterone receptors, preventing progesterone from exerting its biological effects. They act as true receptor antagonists, preventing the uterine effects of progesterone without initially decreasing serum progesterone concentrations. The affinity of aglepristone for uterine receptors is three times greater than that of progesterone itself. Progesterone concentrations after treatment only decline to less than 3 nmol/L from 8 to 34 d. This may be due to premature luteolysis caused by increased endogeneous $PGF_{2\alpha}$.

Clinical applications

- Pregnancy termination in bitches and queens.
- Medical treatment of pyometra.
- Induction of parturition.
- Planning of an elective cesarean section.
- Treatment of feline mammary fibroadenomatosis.
- Treatment of hypersomatotropism (acromegaly). There are only preliminary experimental studies supporting this potential use.

Formulations and dose rates

Aglepristone is available as an injectable formulation in oil.

IN BITCHES

Pregnancy termination

- Aglepristone 10 mg/kg SC given twice, 24 h apart, is the recommended dose. Aglepristone can be used from the first to the 45th day of mating. However, it is preferable, to avoid failure due to a premature treatment, to wait until the end of estrus to use the protocol described above. Treatment before 25 d after mating results in nearly 100% in utero embryonic resorption. Treatment from 25 d after mating may lead to induced abortion within 7 d, with a prolonged vaginal discharge, mammary development and maternal behavior patterns. The effectiveness of aglepristone-induced abortion after 25 d is approximately 95%. To avoid in vivo intrauterine fetal mummification the manufacturer does not recommend induced abortion after 45 d of pregnancy. The interestrus intervals following induced abortion are usually significantly reduced by 1–3 months. Treatment does not seem to affect future reproduction in the aborted bitch.

Medical treatment of pyometra

In bitches with pyometra and serum progesterone levels above 1–2 ng/mL, aglepristone treatment causes the uterine cervix to open and uterine contractions, resulting in discharge of uterine contents and reduction of endometrial size. Broad-spectrum systemic antibacterials must be administered concurrently during the treatment period to prevent septicemia and any other related complications. When the pyometra has resolved, it is recommended to breed the bitch at the subsequent cycle to prevent recurrence. Aglepristone may be used in combination with prostaglandins or alone

- *Combination of aglepristone and $PGF_{2\alpha}$.* Most protocols recommend the use of aglepristone 10 mg/kg at day 1 (d1), d2, d8, d15 (with a final treatment on d29 if some vulvar discharge still persists). There are various dosing schedules for $PGF_{2\alpha}$ when used with aglepristone: cloprostenol (1 μg/kg SC daily from d3 to d7, or 1 μg/kg SC on d3 and d8), dinoprost (25 μg/kg SC three times daily, d3 to d7, or 25 μg/kg d3,d6 and d9). The addition of cloprostenol to the aglepristone therapy, compared with aglepristone alone, significantly improved the

Formulations and dose rates—cont'd

overall success rate in treating pyometra in bitches: 84.4% vs 60%

- *Combination of aglepristone and PGE_1*: the concomitant use of aglepristone 10 mg/kg at day 1 (d1), d2, d8, d15 (with a final treatment on d29 if some vulvar discharge still persists) and misoprostol (10 μg/kg PO q.12 h d3 to d12) leads to a significant clinical improvement in 75% of cases without the side effects of $PGF_{2\alpha}$
- *Use of aglepristone alone*: aglepristone 10 mg/kg has been used to treat open or closed pyometra at day 1 (d1), d2, d8 and d15 (with a final treatment on d29 if some vulvar discharge still persists). In cases of closed-cervix pyometra, a purulent vulvar discharge was observed from 36 to 48 h after the start of treatment, due to the induced opening of the uterine cervix. The pyometra resolved in most cases.

Induction of parturition

It may be desirable to induce parturition during daylight or working hours, thus facilitating its supervision by the bitch's owners. Although some success using aglepristone for this purpose has been reported, the studies have only been performed in beagle bitches. Therefore, it is too early to confirm the efficacy of the following experimental procedures.

- *Use of aglepristone plus oxytocin or $PGF_{2\alpha}$*: aglepristone (15 mg/kg SC) was administered at 58 d of pregnancy in 10 bitches; 24 h later, the bitches were treated SC with either oxytocin (0.15 UI/kg) or the synthetic prostaglandin alfaprostol (0.08 mg/kg) every 2 h until parturition. On average, parturition commenced 32 h (29.7–34.5 h) after aglepristone administration. In a further study using aglepristone and oxytocin with the same protocol, the onset of induced parturition in beagle bitches occurred between 29.7 and 32 h
- *Use of aglepristone alone*: aglepristone (15 mg/kg) was administered twice (q.9 h) at 58 d of pregnancy. Expulsion of the first pup occurred between 35 and 56 h after treatment (mean 41.0 ± 3.7 h)

Planning of an elective cesarean section

- Injection of 15 mg/kg aglepristone 18–24 h before a planned C-section may induce final fetal maturation, thus preventing the release of premature puppies. However, further studies are needed to confirm this hypothesis

Treatment of acromegaly (growth hormone excess)

- Acromegaly in dogs (but not cats) is almost always due to a progestin-induced hypersecretion of growth hormone (GH). In a recent study, preliminary data suggested that aglepristone may be effective in treating acromegaly in bitches

IN QUEENS

Induced abortion

- The dose is slightly higher than in dogs: two repeated SC injections 15 mg/kg at 24-h intervals between day 0 and day 45 after mating. The effectiveness of this protocol is greater before implantation (95%) than after implantation (85%). Termination of pregnancy is achieved in 50% of the queens within 3 d. In most cases, the following interestrus interval is significantly shortened and the queen rapidly comes into heat with high fertility.

Conservative treatment of pyometra

- The combination of aglepristone and $PGF_{2\alpha}$ described above may be successfully used in queens.

Treatment of mammary fibroadenomatosis

Different protocols have been published.

- 20 mg/kg (SC once a week) until complete mammary regression
- 10 mg/kg on two consecutive days, once weekly
- Usually a minimum of 4–6 weeks is needed for a complete mammary regression

Pharmacokinetics

There are no data on aglepristone pharmacokinetics in dogs and cats in the literature but they are probably similar to mifepristone. Enteric absorption of mifepristone after oral administration occurs very quickly. The transport of mifepristone in the blood occurs with a high binding affinity (98%) to plasma protein. Its plasma half-life is around 18 h. Its metabolism occurs mainly in the liver. Elimination occurs mainly in the feces, via the bile (90%), but also in urine (10%).

Adverse effects

Side effects that may be observed with aglepristone treatment include restlessness, anorexia, emesis, diarrhea, drop of rectal temperature, vulvar discharge. Metritis requiring specific therapy using $PGF_{2\alpha}$ developed in 5.7% (5/88) bitches treated for induced abortion.

Contraindications and precautions

None reported.

Known drugs interaction

None reported.

Testosterone and derivatives

Widely used in the past for a variety of conditions, testosterone is of no clinical use in small animal reproduction. The 19-nor-steroid mibolerone is the only related drug of use.

EXAMPLES

Testosterone cypionate, testosterone propionate and testosterone ethanate are synthetic esters of testosterone. Mibolerone or dimethyl-nortestosterone is a synthetic, androgenic, anabolic steroid.

Mechanism of action

Mibolerone blocks the release of LH from the anterior pituitary by negative feedback.

Clinical applications

Mibolerone is labeled in the USA for estrus prevention in bitches. Testosterone derivatives have been promoted as stimulants of libido, spermatogenesis and infertility, with no data supporting these claims.

Formulations and dose rates

For estrus postponement, beginning at least 30 d prior to pre-estrus in the bitch but not prior to the first estrus

- The dose of mibolerone is weight and breed dependent (0.5–12 kg, 30 μg/d; 12–23 kg, 60 μg/d; 23–45 kg, 120 μg/d; >45 kg, 180 μg/d; and German shepherd type-bitch, 180 μg/d PO)
- Treatment can continue for a maximum of 2 years. However, the drug is not recommended in bitches that will be mated.
- It has been proposed that mibolerone may be used for the same purpose in cats but this use is not recommended because of the narrow therapeutic index.

Pharmacokinetics

Mibolerone is well absorbed from the gastrointestinal tract, metabolized in the liver and excreted in the urine and feces.

Adverse effects

Mibolerone may induce:

- premature epiphyseal closure
- clitoral enlargement and vaginitis, especially in immature bitches
- abnormal behavior
- urinary incontinence
- riding behavior
- epiphora
- hepatic changes
- increased renal weight in adults.

Adverse effects usually resolve after discontinuation of therapy, with the exception of clitoral hypertrophy.

Contraindications and precautions

Mibolerone is contraindicated in:

- dogs with androgen-dependent conditions
- pregnancy (it causes masculinization of female fetuses)
- lactating bitches
- Bedlington terriers
- dogs with hepatic or renal disease.

Fatalities have been reported in cats treated with doses as low as 120 μg/d.

Known drug interactions

Mibolerone should not be used concurrently with progestins or estrogens.

Antiandrogenic drugs

EXAMPLES AND MECHANISMS OF ACTION

Flutamide is a nonsteroid pure antiandrogen drug that directly blocks androgenic receptors. It has no adverse effect on the hypothalamus-pituitary function. It has proved successful in reducing prostatic hyperplasia without alteration of semen or libido.

Finasteride is a 4-azasteroid synthetic drug that inhibits 5α-reductase, an enzyme responsible for the metabolism of testosterone to dihydrotestosterone in the prostate, liver and skin. Dihydrotestosterone is the primary intracellular hormone responsible for prostate development and function.

Clinical applications

These drugs are predominantly used for treatment of prostatic diseases in dogs, including canine benign prostatic hyperplasia.

Formulations and dose rates

Only finasteride will be discussed.

- 1 mg/kg daily PO for 21 weeks. Treated dogs had a marked decrease in prostate size 5–15 weeks after treatment began. The prostate size was significantly reduced (30% of the initial value) and fertility was fully restored after a 20–22 week recovery period
- Reduced doses of 0.1 mg/kg or 0.5 mg/kg daily PO for 16 weeks have proved to be effective (43% reduction of the prostatic volume). Finasteride treatment reduced the volume of the ejaculates without affecting sperm number, sperm defects, libido or fertility after artificial insemination

Pharmacokinetics

Finasteride is absorbed in humans from the gastrointestinal tract and absorption is unaffected by food. Of absorbed finasteride, 90% is bound to plasma proteins. It is metabolized by the liver and excreted in both urine and feces. The half-life is about 6 h. A single dose of finasteride in humans causes reduced dihydrotestosterone for about 24 h.

Adverse effects

- In humans, adverse effects reported are mild, including decreased libido, reduced volume of ejaculate and impotence.
- In dogs treated at 1 mg/kg/d PO for 21 weeks, no long-term effects of the drug were noted. After 5–15 weeks of treatment, sperm concentration increased and prostatic fluid volume decreased to the point that ejaculates were no longer collectable, in spite of

normal sexual behavior. However, 6–8 weeks after the cessation of treatment these effects were reversed, with treated dogs impregnating bitches.

Contraindications and precautions

- Do not use in females or in sexually immature animals.
- Use is contraindicated in dogs with severe hepatopathy.

Known drug interactions

None reported.

Estradiol and derivatives

EXAMPLES

Diethylstilbestrol (DES) is a synthetic nonsteroidal estrogen no longer available in the USA and available in Australia and New Zealand only as an oral preparation.

Estradiol benzoate, cypionate and valerate are estradiol esters. Estradiol cypionate is no longer available in Australia and New Zealand.

Estriol (Epiestriol) is labeled in European countries for use to treat urinary incontinence after spaying in the bitch.

Mechanism of action

Estrogens are necessary for the growth, development and function of the female reproductive tract and for secondary sexual characteristics. Estrogens cause proliferation and cornification of the vaginal epithelium, endometrial proliferation and increased uterine tone. They have a negative feedback effect on pituitary gonadotropin secretion. Estradiol mediates luteolysis via $PGF_{2\alpha}$ release in farm animals.

Estrogen effects outside the reproductive tract include calcium deposition, accelerated epiphyseal closure, anabolism, increased sodium and water retention. Excessive estrogen will affect oocyte transport in the oviduct as well as local oviductal conditions, including the function of local carbonic anhydrase.

Clinical applications

- *Estrus induction:* DES has been used for estrus induction in the bitch.
- *Mismating:* estradiol esters have been promoted as treatments for mismating. Doses are given below but this product is not recommended for this purpose. DES has been proposed as a treatment for mismating in the bitch but is not effective in its oral form.
- *Treatment of vaginitis in prepubertal or spayed bitches:* estrogens will increase the thickness of the vaginal mucosa and promote local resistance to infections.

Formulations and dose rates

Estrus induction in the bitch

- Anestrus bitches were given DES at 5 mg/d PO until 2 d after the first signs of pre-estrus. Duration of treatment was 6–9 d, with 5/5 bitches ovulating and conceiving following treatment

Estradiol esters for mismating in the bitch

- Estradiol cypionate (ECP) 0.44 mg/kg IM to a maximum of 1 mg once during estrus
- Estradiol benzoate 0.01 mg/kg SC on d3, 5 and 7 after mating

Estradiol esters for mismating in the queen

- 0.125–0.25 mg ECP within 40 h of mating

However, note that, due to a significantly increased risk of induced CEH-pyometra after estrogenic-induced abortion, the authors do not recommend the use of estrogens to treat mismating in the bitch and queen.

Treatment of vaginitis in bitches

- Low doses of oral DES (0.5–1 mg/animal) for 7 d, tapering the dose over 2 weeks, may be used in spayed bitches with vaginitis. Lifelong treatment may be required in some cases
- Estriol (0.5–1 mg PO daily) for 30 d may be a successful adjuvant therapy of prepubertal vaginitis in young bitches, or in the treatment of vaginitis in adult spayed bitches

Pharmacokinetics

DES is absorbed from the gastrointestinal tract, metabolized by the liver and excreted in the urine and feces. No specific information is available for estradiol esters; however, in humans, estradiol in oil is absorbed from intramuscular sites over several days and esterification slows absorption. Estrogens are stored in adipose tissue, metabolized by the liver and excreted in urine and also in bile, allowing reabsorption from the gastrointestinal tract.

Adverse effects

- Estrogens can cause bone marrow aplasia, which appears as an initial thrombocytosis and/or leukocytosis followed by aplastic anemia, thrombocytopenia and leukopenia. This effect can be idiosyncratic or dose responsive. Oral DES has not been shown to cause this side effect. The likelihood of toxicity of the estradiol esters depends on the type of ester and associated duration of action.
- Estrogens induce progesterone receptors on the endometrium and may therefore precipitate cystic endometrial hyperplasia. This effect is dose responsive and is pronounced if estrogens are administered before or coincident with exogenous or endogenous progesterone.
- Very high doses of DES administered to young bitches may induce malignant ovarian adenocarcinomas.
- Daily administration of DES in cats may induce pancreatic, hepatic and cardiac lesions.

Contraindications and precautions

- Estrogens should not be used: in diestrus, in pregnancy or prior to the use of exogenous progesterone in intact females.
- Administration of DES and estrogens during pregnancy causes fetal malformations of the urogenital system.
- Some estrogens are carcinogenic at low levels in laboratory animals.

Known drug interactions

- Rifampicin (rifampin) administered concurrently with estrogens may decrease estrogen activity by inducing microsomal enzyme activity and increasing estrogen metabolism.
- Oral anticoagulant activity may be decreased by concurrent administration of estrogens.
- Concurrent use of estrogens with glucocorticoids may increase glucocorticoid effects.

Antiestrogens

EXAMPLES

Clomifene actetate, tamoxifen acetate.

Mechanism of action

Most antiestrogenic drugs are receptor blockers, such as clomifene and tamoxifen citrate. However, they may also induce an estrogenic response, due to their partial agonist effect. The relative estrogenic-antiestrogenic effect depends on the species, organ and tissue considered. In bitches, tamoxifen seems to act predominantly as an estrogen agonist.

Clinical applications

The potential for tamoxifen to be effective in treatment of prostatic diseases in dogs is currently under investigation though its use remains experimental at present.

Formulations and dose rates

- Tamoxifen (2.5 mg/kg daily PO for 28 d) has been successfully used experimentally to reduce prostatic volume and testosterone concentration in dogs. A lower dose of 0.3 mg/kg daily PO for 30 d significantly reduced prostatic size. In the future, tamoxifen may have therapeutic applications in male dogs

Adverse effects

- Endometritis, pyometra and ovarian cysts developed in 9/20 bitches treated with tamoxifen (1 mg/kg PO q.12 h).
- Other side effects are vulvar swelling, vaginal discharge and urinary incontinence.

Dexamethasone

See Chapter 11 for further information on dexamethasone.

Clinical applications

Oral dexamethasone has been advocated as an abortifacient.

Just before parturition or before a cesarean section, late-term glucocorticoids may enhance the viability of pups by enhancing the maturation of fetal lungs, as has been shown to occur in humans. However there are no data yet to confirm this hypothesis.

Formulations and dose rates

Abortifacient

- Beginning on day 30 post-LH surge, dexamethasone 0.2 mg/kg/d PO q.12 h for 9.5 d decreasing from 0.16 to 0.022 mg/kg over the last five administrations is 100% efficacious in terminating pregnancy 7–15 d after the start of treatment

Adverse effects

With the dosing regimen described in the previous section, adverse effects were mild and included only transient and reversible polydipsia and polyuria.

EICOSANOID FATTY ACIDS

Endogenous eicosanoids relevant to reproduction include members of the prostaglandin (PG) family, which in turn belong to a family of acidic lipids whose basic structure is a 20-carbon unsaturated carboxylic acid. PGs are synthesized from available arachidonic acid derived from cell membrane phospholipids. Cyclo-oxygenase is necessary to transform arachidonic acid to PGs relevant to reproduction. Nonsteroidal anti-inflammatory drugs inhibit cyclo-oxygenase. Corticosteroids block PG synthesis by inhibiting release of arachidonic acid from cell phospholipids.

Prostaglandin F_{2a} and derivatives

$PGF_{2\alpha}$ is present in seminal plasma, is luteolytic and causes contraction of uterine smooth muscle. In farm animal species, $PGF_{2\alpha}$ is synthesized in the uterine endometrium and released in late diestrus and at parturition, causing luteolyis (CL regression). Luteolysis occurs in these species as a result of cell death and an anti-steroidogenesis effect mediated by protein kinase C. The role of $PGF_{2\alpha}$ in luteolysis in carnivores is poorly understood.

EXAMPLES

Dinoprost tromethamine is the tromethamine (THAM) salt of naturally occurring $PGF_{2\alpha}$. Cloprostenol is a synthetic analog of the F-class.

Mechanism of action

$PGF_{2\alpha}$ causes myometrial contraction, cervical relaxation and luteolysis in several species. Its specific mechanism of action in carnivores is poorly understood.

Clinical applications

- Abortion induction in the bitch and queen.
- Treatment of pyometra in the bitch and queen.
- Reduction of the duration of interestrus intervals.

Formulations and dose rates

Abortion in the bitch

- Natural or synthetic $PGF_{2\alpha}$ is rarely capable of inducing luteolysis in early pregnancy (before day 15–20).
- However, high doses (150–250 μg/kg q.12 h for 4–5 d) may be successfully used around day 15–25 of pregnancy. Lower doses (20 μg/kg q.8 h) around 20–21 d after ovulation induced abortion in 5/5 bitches
- Use of natural $PGF_{2\alpha}$: in mid-pregnancy (around day 30), abortion can be successfully induced using:
  - moderate doses: 30–50 μg/kg q.12 h for 5–9 d
  - increasing doses: starting 30–50 μg/kg then increasing to 100–200 μg/kg after several days
  - high doses: 200–250 μg/kg q.12 h for 4–7 d.
- However, side effects (emesis, salivation, defecation, respiratory distress) are often induced when using a high dose from the start of the treatment period. To avoid this a suggested protocol is repeated injections q.8–12 h, for 7 d or longer, initially using low doses (25 μg/kg) for 1 or 2 d, increasing to doses of 50 μg/kg and then increasing again to doses of 100 μg/kg after 4 d if higher doses are well tolerated by the bitch.
- Cloprostenol has been proved to be an efficient abortive agent: 2.5 μg/kg 3 injections at 48-h intervals after d25 of pregnancy.

Abortion in the queen

- Dinoprost 0.5–1.0 mg/kg SC once and repeated in 48 h will result in abortion (after d40) within 8–24 h. The protocol might work earlier in gestation, especially at higher and more frequent dosing, but is more reliable from d40 as the CL in the cat and dog is quite resistant to the effect of PGF prior to mid-gestation.
- Natural prostaglandins are better tolerated by queens than by dogs. Doses of up to 0.5 mg/kg q.8–12 h for 5 d may be used

Treatment of pyometra in the bitch

- Dinoprost (0.01–0.1 mg/kg q.8–12 h SC) until both uterine evacuation has occurred and serum progesterone is basal. The dose of dinoprost may be reduced by including cabergoline (5 μg/kg/d PO) in the regimen.

Treatment of pyometra in the queen

- Dinoprost 0.1 mg/kg SC on d1 then 0.25 mg/kg/d SC for 5 d, re-evaluate in 2 weeks and retreat if necessary. Lower doses of dinoprost (0.01–0.05 mg/kg SC q.4–6 h for 5–10 d) were well tolerated and proved efficient for treating pyometra in queens. In the majority of treated queens, uterine size decreased by 50% in 72–96 h.

Reduction of the duration of interestrus intervals in the bitch

- The use of long-acting $PGF_{2\alpha}$ fenprostalen (one injection SC 25 d after ovulation) significantly shortened the time to subsequent estrus by a mean of 80 d, with a normal conception rate.

Pharmacokinetics

In rats, dinoprost distributes very rapidly to tissues and has a serum half-life of minutes in cattle. No information is available on cloprostenol.

Adverse effects

- Dinoprost and cloprostenol may cause:
  - abdominal pain
  - emesis
  - defecation
  - urination
  - pupillary dilation followed by constriction
  - tachycardia
  - restlessness and anxiety
  - fever
  - hypersalivation
  - restlessness and panting.
- Adverse effects appear within 5–120 min and may last 20–30 min.
- Adverse effects are dose dependent, with the dinoprost LD_{50} being 5.13 mg/kg SC in the bitch.
- Prior atropine administration may attenuate adverse effects. Concurrent administration of atropine, metopimazine and prifinium bromide 15–20 minutes prior to prostaglandins administration has been proposed, by some authors, to reduce side effects. Butylscopolamine, when available, may also be an effective adjuvant therapy to reduce side effects of $PGF_{2\alpha}$.
- Fatalities have been reported. The authors do not recommend use of either natural or synthetic $PGF_{2\alpha}$ in English bulldogs, as this breed often reacts adversely to these drugs, with serious side effects and sometimes death.

Contraindications and precautions

- $PGF_{2\alpha}$ and synthetic analogs are contraindicated during pregnancy or in animals with hepatic, renal or systemic disease.
- Do not administer intravenously.
- Pregnant women or people with bronchial disease, including asthma, should not handle or administer these drugs.

Known drug interactions

- Concurrent use of progestins may reduce the efficacy of prostaglandins.
- Concurrent use of other ecbolic agents (e.g. oxytocin) may have additional myotonic effects.

MISCELLANEOUS DRUGS

Methylergometrine

Oral methylergometrine maleate (0.5 mL PO, q.8 h) has been proposed as an adjuvant therapy in cases of moderate uterine hemorrhage, for example after parturition.

In women, it displays a uterotonic effect, probably via a stimulation of myometrial α-adrenergic receptors. Its action remains effective for 4–6 h.

This drug should not be used with sympathomimetics, ergotamine or dopaminergic drugs. No adverse effect has been observed with the concomitant use of oxytocin. It should not be given during pregnancy.

Phenylpropanolamine

Phenylpropanolamine, an α-adrenergic compound commonly used to treat urinary incontinence in spayed bitches, has been proved to be effective in cases of retrograde ejaculation in infertile male dogs. The dose is 2 mg/kg q.24 h PO for 5 consecutive days or 3 mg/kg twice daily orally. The onset of action may take several days. Adverse effects may include restlessness, aggressiveness, irritability and hypertension.

Aromatase inhibitors

Aromatase inhibitors, such as formestane, exert an antiandrogenic effect by inhibiting the conversion of testosterone to estradiol 17β in peripheral tissues.

Recently, some of these compounds (4-androsten-4-ol-3,17-dione) have been successfully used experimentally to improve spermatogenic function in oligozoospermic and azoospermic dogs.

REFERENCES

Axner E 2006 Practical approach to physiology of reproduction in cats. In: Proceedings of the 5th EVSSAR Congress (European Veterinary Society for Small Animal Reproduction), April 7-9, Budapest, Hungary, pp 56-59

Baan M, Taverne MAM, Kooistra HS, de Gier J, Dieleman SJ, Okkens AC 2005 Induction of parturition in the bitch with the progesterone-receptor blocker aglepristone. Theriogenology 63: 1958-1972

Beaufays F, Onclin K, Lecouls G, Verstegen J 2004 Treatment of retrograde ejaculation in the male dog by phenylpropanolamine: a dose titration study. In: Proceedings of the 4th International Symposium on Canine and Feline Reproduction, August 4-6, São Paulo, Brazil, pp 170-172

Bhatti SFM, Duchateau L, Okkens AC, Van Ham LML, Mol JA, Kooistra HS 2006 Treatment of growth hormone excess in dogs with the progesterone receptor antagonist aglepristone. Theriogenology 66: 797-803

Bogaerts P 2006 Clinical approach to genital and mammary pathologies in cats. In: Proceedings of the 5th EVSSAR Congress (European Veterinary Society for Small Animal Reproduction), April 7-9, Budapest, Hungary, pp 68-76

Bouchard GF, Gross S, Ganjam VK et al 1993 Estrus induction in the bitch with the synthetic estrogen diethylstilboestrol. J Reprod Fertil 1(suppl 47): 515

Buff S 2004 Luteal insufficiency and abortion. In: Proceedings of the EVSSAR Congress (European Veterinary Society for Small Animal Reproduction), June 4-6, Barcelona, Spain, pp 79-81

Buff S, Fontbonne A, Saint-Dizier M, Guerin P 1998 Induction of estrus with oral administration of cabergoline. In: Proceedings of the 1st EVSSAR Congress (European Veterinary Society for Small Animal Reproduction), May 1-3, Barcelona, Spain, p 314

Corrada Y, Arias D, Rodriguez R, Spaini E, Fava F, Gobello C 2004 Effect of tamoxifen citrate on reproductive parameters of male dogs. Theriogenology 61: 1327-1341

Corrada Y, Hermo G, de la Sota PE, Garcia P, Trigg T, Gobello C 2006 A short term progestin treatment prevents estrous induction by a GnRH agonist implant in anestrous bitches. In: Proceedings of the 5th EVSSAR Congress (European Veterinary Society for Small Animal Reproduction), April 7-9, Budapest, Hungary, p 278

Davidson AP 2006 When and how caesarean section can be avoided (medical management of labor). In: Proceedings of the 5th EVSSAR Congress (European Veterinary Society for Small Animal Reproduction), April 7-9, Budapest, Hungary, pp 93-99

England GCW 1997 Effect of progestins and androgens upon spermatogenesis and steroidogenesis in dogs. J Reprod Fertil 51(suppl): 123-138

England GCW, Hewitt DA 1999 Mechanism and regulation of follicular growth. In: Proceedings of the EVSSAR (European Veterinary Society for Small Animal Reproduction) Annual Symposium, September 22nd , Lyon, France, p 51

England GCW, Russo M 2004 Treatment of spontaneous pyometra in the bitch with a combination of cabergoline and prostaglandin. In: Proceedings of the 4th EVSSAR Congress (European Veterinary Society for Small Animal Reproduction), June 4-6, Barcelona, Spain, pp 277-278

Feldman EC, Nelson RW 1989 Diagnosis and treatment alternatives for pyometra in dogs and cats. In: Kirk RW (ed.) Current veterinary therapy X. WB Saunders, Philadelphia, PA, pp 1305-1310

Fieni F 2006 Antiprogestins and obstetrics. In: Proceedings of the 5th EVSSAR Congress (European Veterinary Society for Small Animal Reproduction), April 7-9, Budapest, Hungary, pp 123-128

Fieni F, Fuhrer M, Tainturier D, Bruyas JF, Dridi S 1989 Use of cloprostenol for pregnancy termination in dogs. J Reprod Fertil 39(suppl): 332-333

Fieni F, Tainturier D, Bruyas JF et al 1996 Etude clinique d'une anti-hormone pour provoquer l'avortement chez la chienne. Recueil Med Vet 172(7/8): 359-367

Fieni F, Verstegen J, Heraud D, Onclin K 1999 Physiologie de la prolactine, pharmacologiedes antiprolactiniques et applications chez la chienne. Prat Med Chirurg Anim Comp 34: 187-199

Fieni F, Bruyas JF, Battut I, Tainturier D 2001 Clinical use of anti-progestins in the bitch. In: Concannon PW, England G, Verstegen J (eds) Recent advances in small animal reproduction. IVIS, NewYork

Fieni F, Marnet PG, Martal J et al 2001 Comparison of two protocols with a progesterone antagonist aglepristone (RU534) to induce parturition in bitches. J Reprod Fertil 57(suppl): 237-242
Galac S, Kooistra HS, Butinar J, Bevers MM, Dieleman SJ, Voorhout G, Okkens AC. Termination of mid-gestation pregnancy in bitches with aglepristone, a progesterone receptor antagonist. Theriogenology. 2000 Mar 1; 53(4): 941-50
Gobello C 2006 Dopamine agonists, anti-progestins, anti-androgens, long-term release GnRH agonist and anti-oestrogens in canine reproduction: a review. Theriogenology 66: 1560-1567
Gobello C, Castex G, Broglia G, Corrada Y 2003 Coat colour changes associated with cabergoline administration in bitches. J Small Anim Pract 44(8): 352-354
Gobello C, Castex G, Klima L Rodriguez R, Corrada Y 2003 A study of two protocols combining aglepristone and cloprostenol to treat open cervix pyometra in the bitch. Theriogenology 60: 901-908
Gorlinger S, Kooistra HS, van der Broek A, Okkens AC 2002 Treatment of fibroadenomatous hyperplasia in cats with aglepristone. J Vet Intern Med 16(6): 710-713
Hori T, Akikawa T, Kawakami E, Tutsui T 2002 Effects of administration of prostaglandin F2a - analogue fenprostalene on canine corpus luteum and subsequent recurrence of estrus and fecundity. J Vet Med Sci 64(9): 807-811
Iguer-Ouada M, Verstegen JP 1997 Effect of finasteride (Proscar, MSD) on seminal composition, prostate function and fertility in male dogs. J Reprod Fertil 51(suppl): 139-149
Inaba T, Tani H, Gonda M et al 1998 Induction of fertile estrus in bitches using a sustained-release formulation of a GnRH agonist (leuprolide acetate). Theriogenology 49: 975-982
Johnston SD, Root-Kustritz MV, Olson PN 2001 Canine and feline theriogenology. WB Saunders, Philadelphia, PA
Kawakami E, Hirano T, Hori T, Tsutsui T 2004 Improvement in spermatogenic function after subcutaneous implantation of a capsule containing an aromatase inhibitor in four oligozoospermic dogs and one azoospermic dog with high plasma estradiol-17β levels. Theriogenology 62: 165-178
Kützler MA 2005 Induction and synchronisation of estrus in dogs. Theriogenology 64: 766-775
Kützler MA, Wheeler R, Lamb SV, Volkmann DH 2002 Deslorelin implant administration beneath the vulvar mucosa for the induction of synchronous estrus in bitches. In Proceedings of the 3rd EVSSAR congress (European Veterinary Society for Small Animal Reproduction). 2002, Liège, Belgium, 96
Kützler M, Stang B, Waldvogel R, Holthofer P 2006 Administration of a single or multiple doses of injectable long-acting deslorelin (GnRH analogue) does not induce oestrus in bitches. In: Proceedings of the 5th EVSSAR Congress (European Veterinary Society for Small Animal Reproduction), April 7-9, Budapest, Hungary, p 280
Lange K, Günzel-Apel AR, Hoppen HO, Mischke R, Nolte I 1997 Effects of low doses of prostaglandin F2a during the early luteal phase before and after implantation in beagle bitches. J Reprod Fertil 51(suppl): 251-257
Lennoz-Roland M 2006 Practical uses of aglepristone: review of a recent expert meeting. In: Proceedings of the 5th EVSSAR Congress (European Veterinary Society for Small Animal Reproduction), April 7-9, Budapest, Hungary, pp 152-159
Ludwig C, Desmoulins PO, Flocxhay-Sigognault A, Driancourt MA, Hoffmann B 2006 Treatment with a subcutaneous GnRH agonist-containing implant down-regulates the hypothalamo-pituitary-gonadal axis of male dogs. In: Proceedings of the 5th EVSSAR Congress (European Veterinary Society for Small Animal Reproduction), April 7-9, Budapest, Hungary, p 317
Mimouni P, Noullet M, Albouy M, Sanquer A 2006 Treatment of benign prostatic hyperplasia with Osaterone acetate tablets: a study in breeding dogs. In: Proceedings of the 5th EVSSAR Congress (European Veterinary Society for Small Animal Reproduction), April 7-9, Budapest, Hungary, p 303
Morgan RV 1988 Handbook of small animal practice. Churchill Livingstone, New York
Okkens AC, Kooistra HS, Diele SJ, Bevers MM 1997 Dopamine agonist effects as opposed to prolactin concentrations in plasma as the influencing factor on the duration of anoestrus in bitches. J Reprod Fertil 51(suppl): 55-58
Olsen PN, Bowen RA, Husted PW, Nett TM 1986 Terminating canine and feline pregnancies. In: Kirk RW (ed.) Current veterinary therapy IX. WB Saunders, Philadelphia, PA, pp 1236-1240
Onclin K, Verstegen JP 1997 Termination of pregnancy in cats using a combination of cabergoline, a new dopamine agonist and a synthetic PGF_{2a} cloprostanol. J Reprod Fertil 51(suppl): 259-263
Plumb DC 2000 Veterinary drug handbook, 3rd edn. Iowa State University Press, Ames, IA, pp 194-195
Ponglowhapan S, Lohachit C, Swangchanuthai T, Trigg TE 2002 The effect of the GnRH agonist deslorelin on prostatic volume in dogs. In: Proceedings of the 3rd EVSSAR Congress (European Veterinary Society for Small Animal Reproduction), Liège, Belgium, p 150
Reynaud K, Fontbonne A, Marseloo N et al 2005 In vivo meiotic resumption, fertilization and early embryonic development in the bitch. Reproduction 130(2): 193-201
Romagnoli S 2004 Retrograde ejaculation. In: Proceedings of the 4th EVSSAR Congress (European Veterinary Society for Small Animal Reproduction), June 4-6, Barcelona, Spain, pp 233-239
Romagnoli S 2006 Deslorelin in small animal andrology. In: Proceedings of the 5th EVSSAR Congress (European Veterinary Society for Small Animal Reproduction), April 7-9, Budapest, Hungary, pp 204-207
Romagnoli S, Concannon PW 2003 Clinical use of progestins in bitches and queens: a review. In: Concannon PW, England G, Verstegen J (eds) Recent advances in small animal reproduction. IVIS, New York
Romagnoli S, Frumento P, Abramo F 2002 Induction of ovulation in the estrous queen with GnRH: a clinical study. In Proceedings of the 3rd EVSSAR congress (European Veterinary Society for Small Animal Reproduction). 2002, Liège, Belgium, 160-161
Romagnoli S, Fieni F, Prats A, Gardey L, Vannozzi I, Rota A 2006 Treatment of canine open-cervix and closed-cervix pyometra with combined administration of aglepristone and misoprostol. In: Proceedings of the 5th EVSSAR Congress (European Veterinary Society for Small Animal Reproduction), April 7-9, Budapest, Hungary, p 287
Root-Kustritz MV 2001 Use of supplemental progesterone in management of canine pregnancy. In: Concannon PW, England G, Verstegen J (eds) Recent advances in small animal reproduction. IVIS, New York
Rubion S, Desmoulins PO, Rivière-Godet E et al 2006 Treatment with a subcutaneous GnRH agonist containing controlled device reversibly prevents puberty in bitches. Theriogenology 66: 1651-1654
Salo F, Illas J, Arus J, Vinaixa F 2004 Use of tamoxiphen for treatment of two cases of benign prostate hyperplasia with prostatic cysts. In: Proceedings of the 4th EVSSAR Congress (European Veterinary Society for Small Animal Reproduction), June 4–6, Barcelona, Spain, p 301
Shille VM, Olsen PN 1989 Dynamic testing in reproductive endocrinology. In: Kirk RW (ed.) Current veterinary therapy X. WB Saunders, Philadelphia, PA, pp 1282-1288
Sirinarumitr K, Sirinarumitr T, Johnston SD, Sarkar DK, Kustritz MV 2002 Finasteride-induced prostatic involution by apoptosis in dogs with benign prostatic hypertrophy. Am J Vet Res 63(4): 495-498
Sutton DJ, Greary MR, Bergman JGHE 1997 The prevention of pregnancy in bitches following unwanted mating: a clinical trial using low dose oestradiol benzoate. J Reprod Fertil 51(suppl): 239-243
Trigg T 2004 Advances in use of the GnRH agonist deslorelin in control of reproduction. In: Proceedings of the 5th International Symposium on Canine and Feline Reproduction, August 4–6, São Paulo, Brazil, pp 49-51

Trigg TE, Wright PJ, Armour AF et al 2001 Use of a GnRH analogue implant to produce reversible long-term suppression of reproductive function in male and female domestic dogs. J Reprod Fertil 57(suppl): 255-261

Verstegen J 2000 Overview of mismating regimens for the bitch. In: Bonagura JD (ed.) Current veterinary therapy XII. WB Saunders, Philadelphia, PA, pp 947-954

Verstegen J 2003 Etiopathogeny, classification and prognosis of mammary tumors in the canine and feline species. In: Proceedings of the SFT Annual Conference, September 16–20. Columbus, USA, pp 230-242

Verstegen J 2003 The mucometra-pyometra complex in the queen. In: Proceedings of the SFT Annual Conference, September 16–20. Columbus, USA, pp 345-347

Verstegen J 2003 Estrous cycle regulation and estrus induction in the queen and pregnancy regulation and termination. In: Proceedings of the SFT Annual Conference, September 16–20. Columbus, USA, pp 334-339

Verstegen J, England G 2003 New hormones to control reproduction in dogs and cats. In: Proceedings of the 3rd EVSSAR Annual Symposium, September 6-7, Dublin, Ireland, pp 30-41

Veukenne P, Verstegen JP 1997 Termination of dioestrus and induction of oestrus in dioestrous nonpregnant bitches by the prolactin antagonist cabergoline. J Reprod Fertil 51(suppl): 59-66

Wanke M, Loza ME, Monachesi N, Concannon P 1997 Clinical use of dexamethasone for termination of unwanted pregnancy in dogs. J Reprod Fertil 51(suppl): 233-238

Wanke MM, Romagnoli S, Verstegen J, Concannon PW 2002 Pharmacological approaches to pregnancy termination in dogs and cats including the use of prostaglandins, dopamine agonists and dexamethasone. In: Concannon PW, England G, Verstegen J (eds) Recent advances in small animal reproduction. IVIS, New York

Wanke M, Loza ME, Rebuelto M 2004 Progestin treatment for infertility in short interestrous interval bitches. In: Proceedings of the 5th International Symposium on Canine and Feline Reproduction, August 4-6, São Paulo, Brazil, pp 71-72

Wehrend A, Hospes R, Gruber AD 2001 Treatment of feline mammary fibroadenomatous hyperplasia with a progesterone-antagonist. Vet Rec 148(11): 346-347

Wheaton LG 1989 Drugs that affect uterine motility. In: Kirk RW (ed.) Current veterinary therapy X. WB Saunders, Philadelphia, PA, pp 977-981

Winer N, Lopez P, Sagot P, Boog G 1993 Bases fondamentales et apllications obstétricales de la mifépristone ou RU486. Rev Fr Gynécol Obstétr 88(2): 73-77

Wright PJ, Verstegen JP, Onclin K 2001 Suppression of the oestrous responses of bitches to the GnRH analogue deslorelin by progestin. J Reprod Fertil 57(suppl): 263-268

24

Topical dermatological therapy

Ralf S Mueller

Skin diseases are common in small animal practice. Unlike most other organs, skin is readily visible and accessible so topical therapy can be a feasible treatment option for some disorders. This chapter serves as an introduction to topical therapy in small animal practice. After providing details on pathophysiology of the skin, practical tips on topical therapy will be followed by a discussion of the major ingredients in shampoos and conditioners. Relevant examples of creams and ointments and information on topical therapy of otitis externa complete the chapter. It is impossible to list the multitude of products available. Rather than discussing individual products, the focus of the chapter will be on ingredients commonly found in topical medications in most countries. The choice of individual products is up to the veterinarian and will depend on availability and personal experience.

Application of drugs to the skin surface is theoretically easy and limited more by owner and patient constraints than by inherent procedural problems. Owner concern over possible side effects of oral drugs has increased in recent years, resulting in an increased willingness to spend time and money on topical therapy. These products may improve the animal's skin condition, appearance and odor, and relieve pruritus.

However, the hair coat of small animals can limit the use of creams and ointments, especially with skin diseases affecting larger areas of the body. Many pets will try to remove topical agents by licking. This may remove most of the drug before penetration and render it useless. Systemic side effects may also occur due to ingestion of the drug or its vehicle.

Typically, creams or ointments are used in the treatment of otitis externa or localized skin lesions. When applying these agents, it is recommended the patient be distracted by feeding, playing or walking for the first 5–15 min after administration to avoid removal of the active drug prior to penetration into the skin and possible systemic adverse effects.

Relevant pathophysiology

The skin is the largest organ of the body. It is the anatomical and physiological barrier between the animal and the environment and as such has a multitude of functions, summarized in Table 24.1.

The skin consists of epidermis, dermis and subcutis or panniculus. The epidermis is the outermost part of the skin and is formed by several layers of keratinocytes situated on a basal membrane. The basal keratinocytes divide constantly and new keratinocytes gradually move outwards through the stratum spinosum, stratum granulosum and stratum corneum while differentiating into a dead horny cell or corneocyte, which is ultimately shed. Proliferation and differentiation are influenced by a multitude of factors such as hormones, vitamins, cytokines and physical or chemical insults.

The dermis is a part of the body's connective tissue system and provides the tensile strength and elasticity of skin. It contains hair follicles, arrector pili muscles, sebaceous and sweat glands, lymph and blood vessels and nerves.

The subcutis is usually the thickest layer of the skin. It functions as an energy reserve and has a role in thermogenesis, insulation and protective padding.

A disturbance of the cutaneous physiological balance often results in an influx of inflammatory cells and/or release of inflammatory mediators and cytokines in the epidermis and dermis. This leads to increased proliferation of keratinocytes and thus epidermal hyperplasia, which may lead to the clinical feature of scaling. Pathogenic microbial agents may proliferate on the surface of the stratum corneum or in the follicular lumen. They may eventually penetrate the epithelial barrier, causing ulceration or furunculosis. Pruritus, as well as visual changes in the skin and hair coat such as scaling, greasiness and odor, are often associated with chronic inflammation and/or infection and are major concerns for animal owners.

Practical tips for topical dermatological therapy

Shampoos, conditioners and moisturizers are suitable for decreasing or eliminating pruritus and odor temporarily and improving the appearance of skin and coat. If the inflammation and/or infection affects deeper layers of the skin, topicals may also be useful as concurrent therapy. However, they typically cannot penetrate to deeper layers and therefore are not effective as sole therapy in these cases.

Trade names of a selection of shampoos available in the USA, Europe and Australasia are given in Table 24.2

Table 24.1 Functions of the skin	
Sensory perception	Touch Pressure Itch Pain Heat Cold
Protection against	Physical insults Microbes Solar radiation Water loss
Secretion/excretion of	Sweat Sebum
Vitamin D production	
Immune regulation	
Temperature regulation	

and topical ear medications are listed in Table 24.3. Topical insecticides are frequently an essential part of flea or tick control in small animal practice. Repellants, adulticides and combinations of these agents with insect development inhibitors/growth regulators are available and are discussed in Chapter 10.

Topical therapy with shampoos and moisturizers is symptomatic. It is used as sole therapy to resolve clinical signs or as an adjunct to systemic drug therapy. Once clinical signs resolve, shampoos and moisturizers may be used to maintain clinical remission without need for systemic therapy.

The success of topical dermatological therapy will depend on several factors.

- The disease
- The patient

Table 24.2 Selected shampoos and conditioners available in Australia, Europe and the USA

Australia

Shampoos

* Dermocil (Illium; 0.5% hexetidine)
* Malaseb (Dermcare; 2% chlorhexidine, 2% miconazole)
* Pyoben (Virbac; 3% benzoyl peroxide)
* Pyohex (Dermcare; 3% chlorhexidine)
* Sebazole (Virbac; econazole nitrate, sulfur, sodium salicylate)
* Triocil (Parke-Davis; 0.5% hexetidine)
* Allergroom (Virbac; 5% urea, glycerin, lactic acid)
* Aloeveen (Dermcare; 2% colloidal oatmeal, aloe vera)
* Episoothe (Virbac; 2% colloidal oatmeal)

Conditioners

* Aloeveen (Dermcare; 2% colloidal oatmeal, aloe vera)
* Episoothe Conditioner (Virbac; colloidal oatmeal)
* Resisoothe (Virbac; fatty acids, vitamine E, oatmeal)

Europe

(Names and availability may differ in various European countries)

Shampoos

* Canoderm (Graeub, 3% benzoyl peroxide)
* Clorexyderm (Jacoby; 2% chlorhexidine)
* Etiderm (Virbac; 10% ethyl lactate, benzalconium chloride)
* Hexocil (Pharmacia & Upjohn; 0.5% hexetidine)
* Lactaderm (Chassot; 10% ethyl lactate)
* Malaseb (Dermcare; 2% chlorhexidine, 2% miconazole)
* Oxydex (3% benzoyl peroxide)
* Peroxyderm (Chassot, 2.5% benzoyl peroxide)
* Sebolytic (Virbac; omega-6 fatty acid, 2% salicylic acid, piroctonolamin, zinc gluconate, 0.25 tea tree oil)
* Sebomild P (Virbac; Piroctonolamin, omega-6 fatty acids, glycerin, lactic acid)
* Polytar (Stiefel, 4.5% tar)
* Allercalm, Episoothe (Virbac; 2% colloidal oatmeal)
* Allermyl (Virbac; omega-6 fatty acids, mono- and oligosaccharides, vitamin E, piroctonolamin)
* Sebocalm (Virbac; 10% sodium oleic sulfonate, 9% lauramide, 1% glycerin)

Conditioners/Sprays

* Allermyl Lotion (Virbac; omega-6 fatty acids, mono- and oligosaccharides, vitamin E)
* Dermacool Spray (Virbac; benzalconium chloride, hamamelis, menthol)
* Sebomild P Lotion (Virbac; vitamin E, piroctonolamin, glycerin, salicylic acid)

USA

Shampoos

* Benzoyl-Plus (EVSCO; 2.5% benzoyl peroxide and encapsulated Novasome moisturizer)
* ChlorhexiDerm (DVM; 2% chlorhexidine)
* Dermazole (Virbac; 2% miconazole)
* Hexadene (Virbac; 3% chlorhexidine, lactic acid, chitosanide)
* Imaverol (Janssen, 10% enilconazole)
* Malaseb (DVM; 2% chlorhexidine, 2% miconazole)
* Mycodex (SmithKline Beecham; 2.5% benzoyl peroxide)
* Miconazole shampoo (EVSCO; 2% miconazole and encapsulated Novasome moisturizer)
* OxyDex (DVM; 2.5% benzoyl peroxide)
* Pyoben (Virbac; 3% benzoyl peroxide)
* Allerseb T (Virbac; 4% coal tar, 2% sulfur, 2% salicylic acid)
* Dermapet (Dermapet; 2% sulfur, 2% salicylic acid)
* LyTar (DVM; 3% coal tar, 2% sulfur, 2% salicylic acid)
* NuSal-T (DVM; 3% salicylic acid, 2% coal tar, 1% menthol)
* Seba-Hex (EVCO; 2% chlorhexidine, sulfur, salicylic acid and encapsulated Novasome moisturizer)
* SebaLyt (DVM; 2% sulfur, 2% salicylic acid, 0.5% triclosan)
* Sebolux (Virbac; 2% sulfur, 2% salicylic acid)
* Seba Moist (EVSCO; 2% sulfur, 2% salicylic acid and encapsulated Novasome moisturizer)
* Sulf/OxyDex (DVM; 2.5% benzoyl peroxide, 2% sulfur)
* SeboRex (DVM; 3% salicylic acid, 2% sulfur, 1% chlorhexidine)
* Relief (DVM; 1% pramoxine, colloidal oatmeal)
* Allergroom (Virbac; 5% urea, glycerin, lactic acid)
* Dermal Soothe Shampoo (EVSCO; pramoxin, novasomes)
* Episoothe (Virbac; 2% colloidal oatmeal)
* Hydra Pearls Rehydrating Shampoo (EVSCO; Novasomes)
* HyLytefa (DVM; humectants, emollients and omega-6 fatty acids)

Conditioners/Sprays

* Dermal Soothe Spray (EVSCO; pramoxin, novasomes)
* Episoothe (Virbac; 2% colloidal oatmeal)
* Hydra Pearls Rehydrating Spray (EVSCO; Novasomes)
* HyLytefa (DVM; humectants, emollients and omega-6 fatty acids)
* Relief (DVM; pramoxine 1%, colloidal oatmeal)

Table 24.3 Selected topical ear medications (names and availability may differ in various countries)

* Aurimite (Schering Plough; pyrethrins, benzocaine)	* Otiprin (Vetoquinol; chloramphenicol, dexamethasone, lidocaine)
* Aurizon (Bayer; marbofloxacin, clotrimazole, dexamethasone)	* Otomax (Schering Plough; gentamicin, betamethasone, clotrimazole)
* Baytril Otic (Bayer; enrofloxacine, silver sulfadiazine)	* Otomite Plus (Virbac; pyrethrins)
* Bur-Otic (Virbac; hydrocortisone, Burrow's solution)	* Panolog (Fort Dodge; nystatin, neomycin, thiostreptone, triamcinolone)
* Cerumite (EVSCO; pyrethrins, squalene)	* Surolan (Jansen; miconazole, polymyxin B, prednisolone)
* Conofite Lotion (Schering Plough; miconazole)	* Synotic Otic (Fort Dodge; fluocinolone, dimethyl sulfoxide)
* Eradimite (Fort Dodge; pyrethrins)	* Tresaderm (Merial; thiabendazole, neomycin, dexamethasone)
* Fucidine (Graeub; fusidic acid, framycetin, nystatin, prednisolone)	* Tritop (Pfizer Animal Health; neomycin, isoflupredone)
* Gentocin Otic (Schering Plough; gentamicin, betamethasone)	
* Mita-Clear (Pfizer; pyrethrins)	

- The owner
- The environment

The disease

The pathomechanism of the skin disorder will determine whether an agent may be useful and if so, which one. **Seborrheic disorders** cause epidermal hyperplasia and hyperkeratosis, clinically evident as scaling. This may be primary or (much more commonly) secondary to a variety of underlying diseases such as infection, allergy, hormonal disorders and others. Secondary seborrhea will resolve after the underlying cause is appropriately treated. Seborrhea may benefit from keratoplastic and keratolytic agents such as sulfur, salicylic acid and tar.

Treating **bacterial infections** with appropriate antimicrobial agents will eliminate the organism and resolve secondary signs such as scaling or odor. Antibacterial agents such as ethyl lactate or benzoyl peroxide, and antifungal agents such as ketoconazole are available in shampoo formulations. Shampoos may also contain chlorhexidine, iodine and miconazole, which are antibacterial as well as antifungal. Additional antimicrobial agents in some topical products are benzalconium chloride, PCMX (para-chloro-meta-xylenol) and piroctonolamin.

Pruritic skin diseases such as hypersensitivity may be treated with nonspecific antipruritic agents such as oatmeal or emollient shampoos or conditioners in conjunction with regular moisturizing rinses or sprays. Fatty acids, vitamins, urea, lactic acid, glycerine and mono- and oligosaccharides may also be included in antipruritic shampoos and lotions.

Topical ear medications are indicated in almost every patient with otitis externa. If the ear canal is dry and scaly, ointments are more suitable than solutions or lotions. Otitis externa purulenta should be treated with solutions or lotions rather than ointments where possible. Almost all ear medications contain a glucocorticoid to suppress inflammation in addition to antimicrobial or antiparasitic drugs. Which particular product is most effective will depend on the underlying cause of the otitis as suggested by history, otoscopic examination, ear cytology, microbial culture and sensitivity and microscopic examination of debris for parasites.

The patient

Species, size, hair coat and temperament will determine the suitability of the patient for topical therapy. Cats tend to dislike immersion in water (with or without shampoo) or spraying and often express their displeasure aggressively. Dogs are more readily convinced to accept shampoos, sprays or moisturizers. In general, it is more difficult (and more expensive and time-consuming) to bath larger breeds than small or toy breeds. Long-haired and plush-coated breeds are more difficult to shampoo than short-coated breeds. Last but not least, some dogs enjoy their bath, others tolerate it and a small percentage dislike it enough to make the bath an unpleasant experience for all involved. It is essential to identify dogs in the last group early on as long-term shampoo therapy is an unrealistic goal for them and their owners.

The owner

Regular and long-term topical therapy requires time, dedication and money. Clear, simple, written instructions will avoid misunderstandings and good communication will ensure that owners unable to comply are identified early. Owners with a busy lifestyle may have more difficulty coping with long-term topical therapy than those with a more relaxed lifestyle. If the pet is considered a family member, the motivation to undertake treatment regimens will be higher. If, however, the patient has a low priority within the family, compliance may be problematical. If financial constraints are present, the author recommends using an inexpensive nonmedicated cleansing shampoo prior to the typically more expensive medicated product. This is more time-consuming but decreases the amount of medicated shampoo needed per bath and thus the long-term cost to the owner.

The environment

Climate and seasonal temperature will be relevant. Shampoo therapy for a Jack Russell terrier can be accomplished easily indoors but bathing a St Bernard regularly may be unrealistic during the cold seasons in temperate or colder climates, as most clients will shampoo big dogs outdoors.

Long-term maintenance

The author initially recommends shampooing once to twice weekly. Whether therapy will be continued beyond the first few weeks depends, of course, to a large degree on the efficacy of the treatment. Once the condition has responded to topical agents, it may be possible to taper therapy to weekly or fortnightly baths to maintain remission. Important to achieving long-term compliance is the ability to communicate well with the client and reassure them that they are contributing significantly to their pet's wellbeing.

Technical tips

It is important at the start of therapy that clients are shown in the clinic how to apply topical products. This applies particularly to creams, ear medication, sprays and spot-ons. If the owner does not feel comfortable spraying the animal, it may be more effective to schedule appointments for this to be done by a veterinarian or veterinary technician/nurse at regular intervals.

The method of administration of ear medications should be explained carefully and then demonstrated to the owner using one of the patient's ears. After the demonstration, the owner should treat the other ear under supervision of the veterinarian or veterinary nurse/technician to maximize compliance and minimize chances of procedural problems.

Specific tips for shampoo therapy

It is often not possible to demonstrate shampoo therapy in a clinical setting, so thorough oral and written instructions are crucial.

- Product warnings should be discussed prior to therapy.
- Grooming prior to shampooing reduces coat matting.
- Ocular ointments to protect the eyes are not only ineffective but may enhance the irritant potential of shampoo, perhaps by trapping irritant solution in the eye.
- It may be useful to remove debris and dirt with a nonmedicated shampoo before using a medicated shampoo. This decreases the amount of medicated shampoo required and thus treatment cost.
- Shampoo therapy is effective only if the right shampoo is used at the right frequency and for the right time. Most shampoos require a contact time of 10–15 min, a long time when trying to restrain a wriggly or bouncy animal. Contact times should be accurately timed using a watch or stopwatch.
- To facilitate patient compliance, the patient may be petted or massaged in the bath. In warmer climates it may be possible to play with the animal outside for 5–10 min once the shampoo has been applied and then return to the tub for the recommended 10 min of rinsing.
- Adverse reactions after shampoo use are rare. If there is concern that a patient may be at risk, shampoo reactions can be identified by 'patch testing'. The shampoo is applied to a small area of nonhaired skin on the ventrum, left on for 10 min and then rinsed off. The area is inspected regularly during the following 24 h for signs of inflammation. If inflammation is observed this indicates that this particular shampoo is not suitable for this patient. During shampoo therapy patients must be monitored as adverse effects may occur at any time. If the skin appears inflamed and/or the patient is irritated beyond the normal rubbing and shaking that occurs to assist drying in the first 5–20 min after a bath, topical therapy should be discontinued or different products used.
- The use of a whirlpool has been advocated for treatment of skin disease in dogs. In a double-blinded, randomized and placebo-controlled study, shampooing pruritic dogs in a whirlpool achieved better results than conventional shampoo therapy or water treatment alone. This effect was particularly pronounced in long-haired dogs.

Specific tips for application of topical preparations to the external ear canal

- Ear medications should be warmed to 'skin temperature' by placing them in a pocket for 5–10 min prior to administration.
- All attempts should be made to make the experience enjoyable. Patting, giving a treat or playing a game after every treatment may all be helpful.
- In pets with recurrent ear disease, it can be beneficial to handle the ears regularly twice weekly, even when the ears are healthy. Pretending to apply ear drops then rewarding with a game or treat can reduce the anxiety the pet associates with administration of ear drops.
- Animals should not be restrained by pulling or holding the affected and painful ear. If the pet struggles, altering the restraint method or seeking assistance may be necessary.
- Once the pet is appropriately restrained on the floor, table, chair or lap, the tip of the ear should be lifted to visualize the opening of the ear canal. Once the opening has been clearly identified, the top should be taken off the tube or bottle and the prescribed amount squeezed into the opening. Alternatively a syringe can be used to draw up the correct amount and then squirt the contents into the ear canal. Gently moving the ear will straighten the angle of the ear canal and assist the medication to reach the deeper

areas. If the pet shakes the head immediately when the drops are applied, swabs should be held over the opening to stop the drops being flicked out again.

- If the inner part of the pinna is affected, a very thin layer of medication should be applied to cover the affected area.
- After the drops are administered, the ear should be gently massaged for 1–2 min. The animal will then shake the solution from the ear. Excess medication may be removed with a tissue but only from the outside of the ear. Cotton swabs should never be pushed down into the ear canal as this will only force debris down further.

Special tips for application of topical drugs to smaller skin lesions

- Application of a thin layer of the cream or ointment to cover the affected area is sufficient; application of large amounts of the topical does not increase efficacy.
- Prevention of licking or rubbing is most important in the first 5–10 min after application and is best achieved by either feeding, walking or playing with the pet for the first 10 min after treatment.
- The frequency and duration of drug administration must be communicated clearly to the owner and should be adhered to. It is necessary to treat until clinical and microscopic remission (determined by impression smears or tape preparations) is achieved.

SHAMPOOS, MOISTURIZERS AND CONDITIONERS

Shampoos typically are soap or detergent based. Soaps are composed of sodium or potassium salts of high-molecular-weight aliphatic acids and emulsify skin oils and sebum with water to remove dirt. The associated alkaline reaction can be irritant. Thus, soaps are not commonly used in veterinary shampoo formulations.

Detergents are mild cleansing soap substitutes consisting of emollient oils, emulsifiers, surfactants and stabilizers and typically are tolerated well by sensitive or inflamed skin. Other added ingredients include antioxidants, conditioners, pH adjusters, preservatives, coloring agents and fragrances. Some shampoos also contain moisturizing agents such as glycerin, lactic acid, urea and essential fatty acids. 'Hypoallergenic' shampoos contain a smaller number of ingredients, presumably with a lower chance of an irritant or allergic reaction.

The pH of canine skin is less acidic than that of human skin and some companies attempt to formulate veterinary shampoos with a pH close to that of normal canine skin. However, in general the most important factor for pH determination is not the patient's skin pH but the qualities of the active ingredients and their solubility at various pH levels. Thus, the difference between human and veterinary shampoos with similar ingredients may not be sufficient to avoid use of human formulations in small animal patients.

Many ingredients, particularly tar, benzoyl peroxide and chlorhexidine, are difficult to formulate, package and keep in solution and therefore should be bought from reputable companies.

New technologies have led to formulation of shampoos where the active ingredients are trapped in microvesicles. Once the shampoo is applied to the skin, the lipid membrane of the microvesicles attaches to the skin and hair. A positive exterior charge contributes to binding to the negatively charged skin and hair. In the dry environment, the active ingredient is gradually released, leading to sustained activity. Microvesicles may contain water (e.g. Novasomes®, EVSCO) or active ingredients (e.g. Spherulites®, Virbac). The benefit of sustained action may be less pronounced with antibacterial shampoos, as one of the proposed mechanisms for antibacterial action is the pH change on the skin surface associated with shampooing. This pH change leads to a decrease in bacterial adherence and bacteria are easily removed from the skin surface.

Shampoos contain a variety of active ingredients singly or in combination.

Antiseborrheic agents

Sulfur

Clinical applications

Sulfur shampoos are indicated for the treatment of seborrheic dermatitis and primary seborrhea sicca and oleosa. If the seborrhea is secondary to another skin disease, treatment of the primary disorder will resolve the seborrhea. In pets with dry skin, the use of a moisturizer after the shampoo is recommended.

Mechanism of action

Sulfur is keratoplastic; it slows down the epidermal cell proliferation by a cytostatic effect on the basal cell layer. It is also keratolytic. Hydrogen sulfide and pentathionic acid are formed and cause damage to corneocytes and subsequent softening of the stratum corneum and shedding of cells. They are also responsible for the antibacterial and possible antifungal action of sulfur. Sulfur is not a good degreasing agent and is therefore not as drying as other antiseborrheic agents.

Adverse effects

- Occasionally, irritant reactions can occur. Dogs and cats may show pruritus and/or inflamed skin after shampooing.
- Sulfur can stain jewelry!

Known drug interactions

Sulfur has synergistic keratolytic activity with salicylic acid. Thus the two agents are frequently combined. The synergy is most pronounced when the concentrations are similar. Typically, shampoos contain 2% sulfur and 2% salicylic acid.

Salicylic acid

Clinical applications

Salicylic acid is usually combined with sulfur and is recommended for the treatment of seborrheic dermatitis and primary seborrhea sicca and oleosa. If the seborrhea is secondary to another skin disease, therapy of the primary disorder will resolve the seborrhea. In pets with dry skin, the use of a moisturizer after the shampoo is recommended.

Mechanism of action

Salicylic acid is keratolytic by lowering the pH of the skin, resulting in increased hydration of the keratin and swelling of the corneocytes. It also solubilizes the intercellular cement substance in the stratum corneum, facilitating desquamation. Salicylic acid does not change the mitotic rate of the basal keratinocytes. It is mildly antipruritic and anti-inflammatory.

Adverse effects

Occasionally, irritant reactions can occur. Dogs and cats may show pruritus and/or inflamed skin after shampooing.

Known drug interactions

Salicylic acid has synergistic activity with sulfur.

Tar

Tar shampoos are prepared typically from coal tar but may occasionally be derived from wood or bituminous tars (prepared from shale deposits). Distillates of coal contain some 10,000 different constituents and it is not clear which of these components are responsible for the clinical efficacy. It is possible that very potent and clinically efficacious components are not responsible for the smell of crude tar. The smell may influence owner compliance. Coal tar solution may be found in shampoo formulations and contains only 20% coal tar. Some products combine tar with sulfur and salicylic acid. Tar shampoos are now used less commonly than in the past as other effective products have been developed.

Clinical applications

A tar shampoo is recommended for the treatment of primary seborrhea oleosa. It is probably the most effective antiseborrheic shampoo available. Tar is not only keratoplastic and keratolytic but also degreasing. Dogs with normal or dry skin will often deteriorate without the concurrent use of a moisturizer to prevent excessive dryness. Greasy seborrhea, however, will respond better to tar shampoos than to sulfur or salicylic acid as the degreasing action removes the grease and debris caused by the disease.

Mechanism of action

Tar is keratolytic and keratoplastic, antipruritic, degreasing and vasoconstrictive. The exact mechanism of the keratolytic and antipruritic action is unknown. Tar suppresses epidermal growth and DNA synthesis. Crude coal tar and some of its photoreactive ingredients produce oxygen and superoxygen radicals and interstrand cross-links in DNA, causing the keratoplastic effect. In the human literature, the role of concurrent ultraviolet (UV) B radiation in enhancing this effect is controversial.

Adverse effects

- Irritant or allergic reactions are more common in shampoos with higher concentrations of tar (>2%) and 'patch testing' is recommended prior to the use of products containing tar.
- Folliculitis can be observed in some patients and should be considered if the patient seems to develop 'hive-like' reactions.
- Sun sensitivity may occur. Sparsely-haired dogs should not be allowed outside on the day of the bath.
- Tar products should not be used in patients with dry skin.
- Tar shampoos must not be used in cats.

Known drug interactions

- Tar induces microsomal drug-metabolizing enzymes. It has been suggested that even topically applied tar could influence the rate of biotransformation of concomitantly administered oral drugs in some patients.
- Coadministration of photosensitizing drugs such as sulfonamides and phenothiazines may aggravate the tendency of sun sensitivity in sunbathing, sparsely-haired dogs.

Selenium sulfide

Clinical applications

Selenium sulfide is an older antiseborrheic agent and is considered for severe cases of oily seborrhea nonresponsive to tar and/or sulfur/salicylic acid. It also has been used to treat cutaneous yeast infections.

Mechanism of action

Selenium sulfide interferes with hydrogen bond formation in the keratin and thus is keratolytic. It is keratoplastic by depressing epidermal cell turnover rate. Selenium sulfide is fungicidal at higher concentrations.

Adverse effects

Selenium sulfide is drying and may be irritant. It will also stain the coat and is thus not recommended as a first-line shampoo.

Antimicrobial agents

Benzoyl peroxide

Clinical applications

Benzoyl peroxide is indicated for superficial and deep pyodermas. Because of its presumed follicular flushing activity, it also is recommended in patients with demodicosis, acne, comedone syndromes and sebaceous adenitis. Benzoyl peroxide has prominent degreasing activity so it is the agent of choice for patients with greasy or oily skin. However, its use must be followed by a moisturizing rinse in any dog with normal or dry skin. It is generally used at concentrations of 2–3%.

Mechanism of action

Benzoyl peroxide is metabolized in the skin (predominantly in the upper layers of the epidermis) to benzoic acid and free oxygen radicals. The former lowers skin pH, the latter disrupts microbial cell membranes. Benzoyl peroxide has broad-spectrum antimicrobial activity that persists for 48 h even when conditions for bacterial growth are optimal. It has also been shown to be keratoplastic by inhibiting the epidermal metabolism and DNA synthesis.

Benzoyl peroxide has been shown to decrease metabolism of sebaceous gland cells in humans but whether sebum production is actually decreased is controversial. Free fatty acids decrease in sebum of human patients treated with benzoyl peroxide, presumably because of its antibacterial effect, as bacterial lipases are responsible for production of free fatty acids. Benzoyl peroxide is also believed to have a follicular flushing action.

Adverse effects

- Erythema, pain and pruritus can occur, especially in cats. This occurs more commonly when concentrations over 3% are used. Thus, most veterinary products have a benzoyl peroxide concentration of 2–3%.
- Ocular irritations have also been reported.
- Alone, benzoyl peroxide has no known carcinogenic effect. It is, however, a tumor promoter by enhancing chemical carcinogenesis with 7,12-dimethylbenzanthracene in hairless mice. Conversely, it appears to protect against ultraviolet carcinogenesis.
- Owners must be informed that benzoyl peroxide may bleach fabrics.

Chlorhexidine

Clinical applications

Chlorhexidine is indicated for dogs and cats with skin infections and dry to normal skin. It appears to have greater efficacy for bacterial infections, particularly *Staphylococcus* spp, than for yeast or dermatophyte infections. It is usually added in concentrations between 0.5% and 3%. Shampoos containing combinations of chlorhexidine and miconazole are available and have superior action against yeast and fungal infections compared to shampoos containing chlorhexidine only.

Mechanism of action

Chlorhexidine is a cationic surfactant synthetic biguanide with broad-spectrum antibacterial and less pronounced antifungal activity. It disrupts microbial cell membranes and coagulates cytoplasmic proteins. Chlorhexidine has a residual activity of several hours. It is nonirritant, nontoxic and works in organic debris.

Adverse effects

Irritant reactions may rarely be seen.

Ethyl lactate

Clinical applications

Ethyl lactate is used for mild superficial bacterial infections in normal to dry skin. Conflicting results are reported from various studies: some show it to be as effective as benzoyl peroxide, others that it is no more effective than water.

Mechanism of action

Ethyl lactate is metabolized to ethanol and lactic acid by bacterial lipases in hair follicles and sebaceous glands. Ethanol solubilizes lipids and lactic acid and lowers the skin pH, resulting in a bactericidal effect. Both agents are short-lived in vivo.

Adverse effects

Occasionally, patients show irritant reactions following treatment.

Iodine

Clinical applications

Iodine products are indicated for bacterial or fungal infections of the skin. However, they are considered to be cosmetically inferior to other equally effective products and thus are less commonly used.

Mechanism of action

Iodine is an excellent bactericidal, fungicidal, virucidal and sporicidal agent. Povidone-iodine is elemental iodine complexed with the carrier molecule pyrrolidone nitrogen, which augments sustained release, dispersibility and penetration. It must be diluted for proper dissociation of the complex. It has a mild degreasing activity.

Adverse effects

Iodine usage may cause irritations and cutaneous hypersensitivities, and stains light hair coats.

Triclosan

Clinical applications

Triclosan is an antibacterial ingredient in some shampoos used for seborrheic disorders and may be helpful in preventing infections of seborrheic skin.

Mechanism of action

Triclosan is a bisphenol disinfectant. It is bacteriostatic against predominantly Gram-positive bacteria and has been reported to be effective in treating meticillin-resistant staphylococcal infections at a concentration of 2%. At a concentration of 0.5% it was less effective than benzoyl peroxide or chlorhexidine in inhibiting the growth of *Staphylococcus intermedius*.

Miconazole

Mechanism of action

Miconazole inhibits the synthesis of ergosterol, a major component of fungal cell membranes. This interferes with the barrier function of the membrane and with membrane-bound enzymes.

Clinical applications

Miconazole is an azole derivative that, because of its poor oral absorption and rapid clearance, is used predominantly for topical treatment of localized superficial infections. A formulation containing chlorhexidine and miconazole has been shown in double-blinded studies to be effective in the treatment of canine *Malassezia* dermatitis. Miconazole in various ear medications is effective against yeasts complicating canine otitis externa. Miconazole also has activity against Gram-positive bacteria such as *Staphylococcus intermedius*, the predominant organism involved in bacterial skin infections in small animals.

Adverse effects

Irritation characterized by erythema, pruritus and occasionally exudation may rarely be seen.

Antipruritic and moisturizing agents

Emollients

Clinical applications

Emollients include fats such as lanolin, hydrocarbons such as paraffin, petrolatum and mineral oil, humectants such as carboxylic acid and lactic acid and oils such as olive, cottonseed, corn, almond, peanut and coconut oil. These agents are added to shampoos as vehicles and for their local effects in softening and protecting the skin.

Mechanism of action

Emollients soften the skin by forming an occlusive oil film on the stratum corneum, thus decreasing the transepidermal water loss.

Moisturizing agents

Clinical applications

Urea, glycerin and propylene glycol are classified as demulcent polyhydroxy compounds. They are added to many shampoos for protection and moisturizing of the skin. Essential fatty acids and colloidal oatmeal are also added to some products.

Mechanism of action

A demulcent is a high molecular weight compound in aqueous solution that coats the skin surface, thus protecting the underlying cells and alleviating irritation. Urea promotes hydration and is antibacterial. It accelerates the digestion of fibrin and is proteolytic; thus it helps in removal of excess keratin and crusting.

Glycerin is a popular vehicle as this trihydric alcohol is miscible with water and alcohol. It is a hygroscopic agent that is absorbed into the skin. Similarly, propylene glycol is a good vehicle, miscible with water and dissolving many essential oils. Linoleic acid is important for the barrier function of the stratum corneum, particularly in relation to transepidermal water loss.

Topical application of fatty acids has been shown to affect epidermal fatty acid concentrations and may hydrate the stratum corneum by reducing transepidermal water loss. Colloidal oatmeal hydrates the stratum corneum hygroscopically by attracting and binding water passing through the epidermis.

Adverse effects

Irritant and more commonly, allergic reactions are possible with oatmeal preparations.

Antipruritic agents

Hydrocortisone, antihistamines and aloe vera extracts have been incorporated in shampoos.

Clinical applications

Shampoos containing antipruritic agents are recommended for pruritic patients without secondary infection or seborrhea and dry to normal skin. Their long-term use depends on their efficacy in each patient; relief of pruritus may be negligible or the shampoo may be effective in controlling pruritus for up to 3 d.

Mechanism of action

Antihistamines and hydrocortisone presumably penetrate the epidermis and exert antihistaminic and anti-inflammatory effects in the upper dermis. Their mechanism of action is discussed in Chapter 11.

Systemic absorption of hydrocortisone from shampoo formulations used twice-weekly for 6 weeks has been shown to be clinically insignificant.

Aloe vera has been reported to have anti-inflammatory activity in rats as a result of inhibition of cyclo-oxygenase activity and neutrophil migration. Further studies are needed to evaluate the efficacy and side effects of these shampoos in small animal dermatology.

CREAMS, EMULSIONS AND OINTMENTS

Many creams and ointments are available and it is beyond the scope of this review to discuss them in detail. Most of these products are a combination of anti-inflammatory and antimicrobial agents, commonly glucocorticoids with antibacterials and/or antifungals in a base of solvents, emollients and moisturizing agents discussed above. They form a protective cover and, if occlusive, may prevent transepidermal water loss.

Because of the typically dense hair coat of small animals and their tendency to remove administered topicals by licking or rubbing, creams and ointments are useful for small, local lesions only. Pyotraumatic dermatitis or 'hot spots', skinfold pyoderma, otitis externa and feline acne are common examples of localized problems that may be successfully treated with creams, emulsions or ointments.

Numerous topical anti-inflammatory and antibacterial agents are available. The mechanism of action of most of these drugs is covered elsewhere in this textbook. However, some common ingredients of topical products are discussed below.

Mupirocin

Clinical applications

Mupirocin is an antibacterial agent recommended for localized bacterial infections in dogs and cats. It has been reported to be efficacious in the treatment of feline acne, even when *Malassezia* spp rather than bacteria were documented to be the etiological organism.

Mechanism of action

Mupirocin inhibits bacterial protein synthesis by binding to bacterial isoleucyl transfer RNA synthetase. It is mainly efficacious against Gram-positive aerobes such as staphylococci.

Adverse effects

Mupirocin is supplied as a 2% solution in a water-soluble ointment base of polyethylene glycol. The base can be toxic, especially in cats with impaired renal function, if large amounts are applied for extended treatment periods and the cat licks off some of the ointment.

Tacrolimus

Clinical applications

Tacrolimus is a macrolide immunomodulator synthesized by the fungus *Streptomyces tsukubaensis*. Tacrolimus is reported as an effective treatment for canine atopic dermatitis, perianal fistula and discoid lupus erythematosus. It is also used for other immune-mediated skin diseases such as pemphigus foliaceus in the dog. In veterinary medicine, tacrolimus is applied as a 0.1% ointment initially twice daily topically and then may be tapered down after disease remission to daily or once every alternate day.

Mechanism of action

Tacrolimus is a calcineurin inhibitor similar to ciclosporin and has numerous inhibitory effects on a number of immune cells such as lymphocytes, dendritic cells, mast cells and eosinophils. Its mechanism of action is discussed in more detail in Chapter 12.

Adverse effects

- Tacrolimus may cause a transient burning sensation in dogs and humans.
- When blood concentrations were measured in dogs, they were shown to remain below toxic levels and no hematological or biochemical abnormalities were reported.

TOPICAL THERAPY OF OTITIS EXTERNA

Ear preparations usually consist of a vehicle (such as oil, solution or ointment) and a variety of active ingredients, including anti-inflammatory, antimicrobial and/or antiparasitic agents. The detailed mechanism of action of the active ingredients is discussed in other relevant chapters. Owner education is crucial prior to topical therapy of otitis externa. Patients with otitis frequently resent administration of medication because of associated discomfort and pain. It may be necessary in severe cases to begin therapy with an ear flush under anesthesia to remove debris.

Clinical applications

Topical treatment of otitis externa is indicated when the external ear canal is inflamed and/or infected. However, otitis externa may be caused by a variety of conditions from allergies, hormonal disease and ectoparasites to foreign bodies and neoplasia. Symptomatic treatment may be successful in achieving temporary remission but without diagnosis and therapy of the primary disease, long-term success is highly unlikely. In addition, a careful assessment of potential middle ear involvement is indicated. Otitis externa without otitis media may usually be treated successfully with topical medications. If otitis media is present, long-term systemic therapy is often needed. Otoscopic examination may reveal a ruptured tympanum, indicating middle ear disease. However, otitis media has been reported in patients with intact ear drums. In these patients, the tympanum most likely has healed after initial trauma and infection of the middle ear. If clinical signs of otitis media such as Horner's syndrome or head tilt are not present, imaging methods such as radiography, computed tomography or magnetic resonance imaging may be needed to exclude otitis media in patients with recurrent otitis externa or ear disease unresponsive to appropriate topical therapy.

Glucocorticoids

Glucocorticoids are included in most products. Because of the anatomical structure of the external ear and the cartilaginous structures, inflammation and associated swelling of the aural epithelium lead to a smaller canal lumen, which decreases ventilation and contributes to the development and persistence of infection. The anti-inflammatory effects of glucocorticoids decrease exudation, swelling, scar tissue and proliferative changes, all of which help to promote drainage and ventilation.

Betamethasone valerate and fluocinolone acetonide are some of the more potent glucocorticoids found in ear medications. Moderately potent glucocorticoids include triamcinolone acetonide and dexamethasone. All of these are systemically absorbed and influence the pituitary-adrenal axis, thus long-term treatment with these drugs should be carefully considered. Once active inflammation is controlled, long-term and prophylactic therapy should utilize glucocorticoids of lower potency such as hydrocortisone.

Antibacterial agents

Antibacterial agents frequently included in topical ear medications include aminoglycosides such as neomycin or gentamicin, polymyxin, chloramphenicol, bacitracin, framycetin, enrofloxacin, marbofloxacin, miconazole, silver sulfadiazine, povidone-iodine, chlorhexidine and acetic acid. Before choosing an appropriate formulation, cytological evaluation of an ear swab is recommended and will identify inflammatory cells, cocci, rods and/or yeast organisms.

Cocci are typically *Staphylococcus* spp or *Streptococcus* spp. The former respond to most antibacterial agents. Miconazole and bacitracin are used most commonly in the author's practice for otitis externa complicated by coccal infection, as determined by cytology. When appropriate therapy based on cytology is not effective, bacterial culture and sensitivity are recommended to assist in the choice of antibacterial agents.

Rods are typically *Pseudomonas aeruginosa, Pasteurella multocida, Escherichia coli* or *Proteus* spp. Their response to antibacterial therapy is much more unpredictable and culture and sensitivity tests are recommended as a base for the selection of therapy even in patients not previously treated. If culture is not possible because of financial constraints, the most effective commercial ear preparations for rod infections in the author's practice contain gentamicin in combination with a potent glucocorticoid. *Pseudomonas* isolates are often susceptible to polymyxin B, but this antibiotic is inactivated by purulent discharge and thus should only be applied after thorough ear cleaning. Commercial products containing fluoroquinolones may also be effective.

However, if the tympanum is ruptured, most commercial preparations have ototoxic potential and alternatives need to be considered. Acetic acid at a concentration of 2% appears to be effective against *Pseudomonas aeruginosa*, but administration into ulcerated ear canals is not tolerated well. A solution of silver sulfadiazine at 1% (1 g of silver sulfadiazine in 100 mL of sterile water) administered twice daily has also been reported to be effective. In a more recent study, a solution containing 0.1% silver sulfadiazine also was effective but more liquid and thus easier to apply and disperse in the external canal.

Injectable ticarcillin or fluoroquinolones may be diluted with physiological saline solution and applied to the external ear canal. Ticarcillin is reconstituted to a concentration of 100 mg/mL. This solution is not stable at room temperature and should be frozen in aliquots (stable for 1 month) and thawed on the day of use. Enrofloxacin may be diluted to a 0.3–0.5% solution.

Antifungal agents

Yeast organisms, particularly *Malassezia pachydermatis*, are commonly involved in otitis externa. Dermatophytes and *Candida* spp are less frequently present. Clotrimazole and miconazole are most useful in the treatment of *Malassezia* otitis. Thiabendazole and nystatin have also been effective in some cases. Povidone-iodine or chlorhexidine may also be useful. In patients with chronic otitis externa and media due to yeast organisms, systemic antifungal medication with azoles may be used in combination with acetic acid flushes.

Antiparasitic agents

Antiparasitic agents such as pyrethrins, fipronil, selamectin, moxidectin, ivermectin or amitraz are indicated for mite infestations such as *Otodectes cynotis*. Recurrent clinical signs may be due to resistance of the mites. However, asymptomatic carrier animals are a potential source of reinfestation and all in-contact animals should be treated. *Otodectes cynotis* can be found on other body parts and whole-body treatments with effective miticidals may be needed to eliminate infection. Systemic therapy for ectoparasites is covered in Chapter 10.

Adverse effects

Ototoxicity is of concern with most commercial otic preparations if the tympanum is ruptured and penetration into the middle ear is possible. In patients with chronic otitis externa it may be difficult to evaluate the tympanum even under general anesthesia. However, as antimicrobial topical treatment is the most effective medical therapy for an infected otitis externa (oral antimicrobials do not achieve the same concentrations in the ear canal), the risk of ototoxicity has to be balanced against the benefit of eliminating the infection. Fortunately, ototoxicity does not occur frequently in small animal practice.

FURTHER READING

Ascher F, Maynard L, Laurent J et al 1990 Controlled trial of ethyl lactate and benzoyl peroxide shampoos in the management of canine surface pyoderma and superficial pyoderma. In: Von Tscharner C, Halliwell REW (eds) Advances in veterinary dermatology 1. Baillière Tindall, London, pp 375-382

Campbell KJ, Weisger R, Cross T et al 1995 Effects of four antibacterial soaps/shampoos on surface bacteria of the skin of dogs. In: Proceedings of the 11th Annual Meeting of the American Association for Veterinary Dermatology, Santa Fe, pp 43-44

Kwochka KW 1988 Rational shampoo therapy in veterinary dermatology. In: Proceedings of the 11th KalKan symposium, Columbus, Ohio, pp 87-95

Kwochka KW 1993 Keratinisation abnormalities: understanding the mechanism of scale formation. In: Ihrke PJ, Mason IS, White SD (eds) Advances in veterinary dermatology 2. Pergamon Press, Oxford, pp 91-111

Kwochka KW 1993 Topical therapeutics. In: Locke PH, Harvey RG, Mason IS (eds) Manual of small animal dermatology. British Small Animal Veterinary Association, Cheltenham, pp 220-232

Kwochka KW, Kowalski JJ 1991 Prophylactic efficacy of four antibacterial shampoos against Staphylococcus intermedius in dogs. Am J Vet Res 52: 115-118

Löflath A, von Voigts-Rhetz A, Jaeger K, Mueller RS 2006 The efficacy of a commercial shampoo and whirlpooling in the treatment of canine pruritus – a double-blinded, randomized, placebo-controlled, cross-over study. Vet Derm 17(3): 207-220

Scott DW, Miller WH, Griffin CE 1995 Small animal dermatology. WB Saunders, Philadelphia, PA, pp 188-209

25

Ocular clinical pharmacology

Robin G Stanley

SPECIAL CONSIDERATIONS IN OCULAR THERAPY

The eye can be treated by a number of different administration routes, including topically, subconjunctivally and systemically. When treating an eye condition, the clinician needs to consider the following factors: the location of the lesion, the tissue drug concentration required to be therapeutic, ease of application and the properties of the drug itself.

Lesion location and routes of administration

Topical ophthalmic therapy

Topical therapy in the form of drops, ointments, drug-impregnated inserts and contact lenses has the advantage of achieving high local drug concentrations and is indicated for medicating the eyelids, conjunctiva, deficiencies of the precorneal tear film, cornea, sclera and anterior uvea (Table 25.1). However, the constant turnover of the precorneal tear film means that drugs applied topically are soon washed out of the eye. In order to maintain high local drug concentrations, topical drugs need to be applied frequently.

Increased concentrations of drugs can be achieved by repeated applications of the drug. Repeated applications at 5 min intervals can usually be expected to maximize drug concentrations while minimizing drug irritation of the conjunctiva.

It is ideal to prolong the duration of the drug on the surface of the eye. This can be achieved by increasing applied drug concentration, increasing the viscosity of eye drops and using drug suspensions, emulsions and liposomes. Ointments tend to have much longer contact times on the eyeball and may be a better choice than drops if the owner is unable to medicate the eye frequently.

In some cases it may prove difficult to medicate small animal patients topically; therefore, therapy may have to be administered by subconjunctival injection or systemically.

Subconjunctival ocular injections

Subconjunctival injections can be given either under the eyeball conjunctiva (epibulbar) or underneath the conjunctiva lining the eyelid (subpalpebral). Subconjunctival injections are indicated for treatment of lesions in the cornea, sclera, anterior uvea and vitreous.

Injection underneath the conjunctiva allows drugs to bypass the epithelium, one of the main barriers that limit drug entry. Subconjunctival injection can be used in severe conditions that require high drug concentrations and also in animals that are difficult to treat. Significant systemic drug exposure occurs due to rapid absorption of subconjunctivally injected drugs into the ocular venous circulation.

Systemic therapy

Systemic administration is the optimal therapeutic route when treating the posterior segments of the eye (retina, choroid, optic nerve and vitreous). In a normal eye the blood–eye barriers limit the amount of drug penetration into the eye. However, if the eye is inflamed the normal impermeability of these barriers is greatly reduced, increasing drug concentration into the target tissues.

Systemic therapy can be used to treat conditions of the eyelids, sclera, uveal tract (both anterior and posterior), vitreous, retina, optic nerve and retrobulbar area. Apart from oral doxycycline, systemic therapy does not provide adequate therapy for diseases of the cornea and the conjunctiva. For specific therapeutic purposes, retrobulbar injections, retrograde infraorbital arterial injections and vitreous drug inserts may be used.

The indications for the different routes of administration are summarized in Table 25.2.

Combining routes of administration

In some cases combining different routes of administration will greatly improve therapeutic efficacy. Most commonly in ophthalmic practice, this is used in severe cases of uveitis, when corticosteroids are administered topically by epibulbar subconjunctival injection and orally.

Achieving adequate tissue concentrations

The eye is unique in its anatomy. The intraocular contents are among the best-protected structures in the body, protecting the eye from potentially dangerous substances in the environment or the blood.

The cornea and blood–eye barrier are the main factors that limit the amount of drug that can enter the eye.

Table 25.1 Topical ophthalmic preparations and common trade names

Drug	Trade name	Manufacturer
Corticosteroids		
1% prednisolone acetate	Prednefrin Forte	Allergan
0.1% phenylephrine		
0.1% dexamethasone alcohol	Maxidex	Alcon
1% hydrocortisone	Hycor Eye Ointment	Sigma
1% hydrocortisone	Hycor Eye Drops	Sigma
Corticosteroids and antibacterials		
0.25% prednisolone with neomycin, polymyxin B and sulfacetamide	Amacin	VR Laboratories
1% prednisolone and gentamicin	Optigentin-S	Jurox
Nonsteroidal anti-inflammatory drugs		
Flurbiprofen 0.03%	Ocufen	Allergan
Diclofenac 0.1%	Voltaren	Ciba-Vision
Ketorolac 0.5%	Acular	Alcon
Miscellaneous anti-inflammatory drugs		
Ciclosporin	Optimmune	Schering-Plough
Sodium cromoglycate 4%	Opticrom	Fisons
Anti-infective drugs		
Gentamicin	Soligental	Virbac
Tobramycin	Tobrex	Alcon
Ciprofloxacin 0.3%	Ciloxan	Alcon
Ofloxacin 0.3%	Ocuflox	Allergan
Fusidic acid	Conoptal	Boehringer Ingelheim
Cloxacillin	Orbenin	Pfizer
Polymyxin B, bacitracin	Neosporin Ointment	Wellcome
Natamycin 5%	Natacyn	Alcon
Aciclovir	Zovirax	Glaxo SmithKline
Mydriatics		
Atropine 0.5%, 1%,	Atropine	Sigma
Tropicamide 1%	Mydriacyl	Alcon
Miotics		
Pilocarpine 1–2% drops	PV Carpine	Sigma
Demecarium	Humorsol	MSD
Local anesthetics		
Proparacaine 0.5%	Opthaine	Allergan
Alcaine	Alcaine	Alcon
Glaucoma		
Dorzolamide	Trusopt	MSD
Brinzolamide	Azopt	Alcon
Dorzolamide/timolol	Cosopt	MSD
Latanoprost	Xalatan	Pharmacia & Upjohn
Travaprost	Travatan	Alcon
Bimatoprost	Lumigan	Allergan

Table 25.2 Suggested routes of administration for the eye

	Topical	Subconjunctival	Systemic
Eyelids	++	+	+
Conjunctiva	++	+	Doxycycline – cats
Cornea	+	++	+
Sclera	+	+	+
Iris, ciliary body	+	+	++
Vitreous		+	+
Retina			++
Optic nerve			++
Orbit/retrobulba			++

Other mechanisms that help to protect the eye include continuous turnover of the precorneal tear film, rapid turnover of intraocular fluids, active transport mechanisms within the eye that can eliminate substances, and marked anatomical and physiological compartmentalization within the eye. If a drug is unable to enter the eye for any of these reasons, its therapeutic efficacy will be greatly reduced.

Covered by the tear film, the cornea is the main barrier to topical drugs entering the eye. If the drug applied to the cornea is irritant, reflex tearing may wash it away before it has had a chance to penetrate.

The cornea is composed of lipid epithelium. This layer can be penetrated easily by fat-soluble compounds but is relatively impermeable to ionized compounds. In contrast, the stroma can be readily penetrated by ionized solutions but the passage of fat-soluble compounds is severely restricted. The innermost layer is Descemet's membrane and the corneal endothelium. This layer is also lipid and acts similarly to the corneal epithelium in relation to drug passage.

For drugs to be able to pass readily through the cornea they need to be able to convert between the ionized and nonionized forms. Drugs, such as chloramphenicol and atropine, which exist in equilibrium between the two forms can readily reach high intraocular concentrations. In some cases of corneal ulceration, where the epithelium has been removed, many water-soluble (ionized) drugs are able to penetrate readily into the eyeball.

Other factors that may affect the intraocular penetration of topically applied drugs include:

- the size of the drug molecule – the smaller, the better the penetration
- the drug concentration – the higher, the better the penetration. Clinically it is common to fortify antibacterials, such as gentamicin, that are used to treat serious corneal infections.

The blood–eye barrier acts to severely impede the transfer of blood-borne drugs into the eye. Fortunately, ocular inflammation reduces the blood–eye barrier, allowing penetration of drugs into the eye. As inflammation subsides, the impermeability of the blood–eye barrier is restored.

Drug characteristics

There are a number of drug factors that need to be considered when treating the eye, including drug pH, tonicity, viscosity and use of wetting agents.

Drug pH

Dogs have a tear pH of approximately 6.5. If a drug is to be nonirritant to the eye, the drug solution should be buffered to this pH. Some drugs, such as pilocarpine, can be very irritating and need to be buffered with the vehicle solution. Drug pH can affect drug penetrability and shelf-life.

Tonicity

Ophthalmic drugs should be isotonic with the precorneal tear film. Generally, small animals will tolerate a wide variation in tonicity. Some drugs need to be in relatively high concentrations to be effective but may be irritating. Ointments appear to be less irritating than drops for highly concentrated drugs.

Viscosity

Drugs that are contained in viscous vehicles have much longer contact times, resulting in greater intraocular penetration. This is seen most commonly in artificial tear preparations used to treat dry eye. Viscous preparations such as Visco Tears and Liquifilm Forte remain in contact with the cornea for substantially longer than normal artificial tears. As a result these drugs can be used less frequently, which in veterinary practice often means better owner compliance and improved clinical outcome.

Wetting agents

Drugs that act as wetting agents do so by reducing the surface tension. These compounds can be added to ophthalmic preparations to increase corneal penetration of ionized drugs.

ANTI-INFLAMMATORY OCULAR THERAPY

Inflammation occurs in many common ocular conditions and can be beneficial and protective. However, the eye is especially prone to excessive inflammation, which can destroy vision. Prompt and judicious use of anti-inflammatory drugs is essential in clinical ophthalmic practice.

Uncontrolled inflammation in the eye can result in a number of adverse sequelae, including vision loss from retinal and optic nerve damage, glaucoma from obstruction of aqueous outflow, cataract formation and phthisis bulbi (shrinkage of the eye). Such outcomes can be reduced by the correct use of anti-inflammatory drugs. In clinical ophthalmic practice anti-inflammatory drugs are generally underused.

Relevant pathophysiology

Ocular inflammation is generally considered to be primarily mediated by prostaglandins. Injury to cell membranes can cause release of arachidonic acid from the phospholipid layer of the cell membrane. This results in a cascade of reactions, ultimately leading to production of leukotrienes, prostaglandins and free radicals. The cascade can be blocked by use of corticosteroids and nonsteroidal anti-inflammatory drugs (NSAIDs). Corticosteroids act by inhibiting the release of arachidonic acid from the cell membrane (see Chapter 11). NSAIDs act by inhibiting the enzyme cyclo-oxygenase which converts arachidonic acid into prostaglandins and free radicals (see Chapter 13).

Specifically in the eye, anti-inflammatory drugs reduce vasodilation and vascular permeability of ocular blood vessels. They also reduce migration of inflammatory cells into the eye. Topical anti-inflammatory drugs can be used to reduce corneal vascularization and minimize scar tissue formation.

Clinical applications

Anti-inflammatory drug therapy is most commonly used for the treatment of uveitis (Table 25.3). It is also used to treat ocular inflammation caused by allergies and to reduce scarring following the healing phase of corneal ulceration.

CLASSES OF DRUGS USED TO TREAT OCULAR INFLAMMATION

Corticosteroids

Mode of action

The beneficial effects of corticosteroids in the eye include anti-inflammatory effects and reduction in the vascular and cellular response to injury.

Decreased vascular response

Decreasing the vascular response is an important effect in the eye. In inflammation, the blood–eye barrier is reduced. Clinically this manifests as aqueous flare (protein and inflammatory cells in the aqueous humor). In severe cases hyphema (blood in the anterior chamber)

Table 25.3 Clinical ophthalmic use of anti-inflammatory drugs

Drug	Dose	Comments
Acute uveitis		
Prednisolone acetate 1%	One drop to the affected eye 2–10 times daily depending on the severity of inflammation	
Atropine 0.5–1%	One drop q.8 h until the pupil is dilated, then q.24 h	
Betamethasone	3 mg by epibulbar subconjunctival injection	This modality is used when the uveitis is severe, or if the animal is difficult to treat
Prednisolone	1–2 mg/kg PO q.12 h for 3 d, then q.24 h for 5 d, then alternate days	
Chronic uveitis		
Prednisolone acetate	q.12–24 h	
Atropine	Alternate days as required to keep the pupil dilated	
Carprofen	2 mg/kg q.24 h PO for 1–2 months	Dogs only
Keratitis		
Prednisolone acetate	q.6–12 h	If the cornea is unhealthy of if corneal ulceration threatens consider a topical NSAID or ciclosporin
Prednisolone	1 mg/kg q.24 h for 5 d, then alternate days	

may develop. In animals with lighter-colored irises, blood vessel proliferation can be observed over the anterior iris surface – rubeosis iridis and preiridal fibrovascular membrane formation. These membranes can cause hyphema from bleeding inside the eye and if they grow across the iridocorneal drainage angle, glaucoma can result. Vision loss can also result from exudation of inflammatory fluid from the choroid causing retinal detachment.

Corticosteroids, when used topically, subconjunctivally and systemically, reduce the increased capillary permeability. This clinically can also reduce aqueous flare. Corticosteroids will also inhibit production of new blood vessels (preiridal fibrovascular membranes). Inflammatory retinal detachment can be minimized by systemic corticosteroid treatment, which reduces fluid and cellular exudation. When treating uveitis it is vital to use systemic anti-inflammatory therapy to protect the posterior segment, in particular the retina and optic nerve.

Anti-inflammatory effects

The major anti-inflammatory action of corticosteroids is inhibition of arachidonic acid release from damaged cell membranes and reduction in the production of prostaglandins, the main mediators of ocular inflammation. Other less important corticosteroid anti-inflammatory effects in the eye include reduced degranulation of inflammatory cells, such as mast cells and neutrophils, and thus reduction in the release of proteases, histamine and bradykinin.

Reduction of cellular response

Accumulation of inflammatory cells is observed in ocular inflammation. These can often be seen in dogs and cats as follicles in the conjunctiva and in cats as small nodules in the iris. Corticosteroids can help reduce ocular inflammation by reducing this cellular response.

Topical corticosteroids

Clinical applications

Topical corticosteroids are indicated for treatment of allergic conjunctivitis, inflammatory and immune-mediated corneal diseases (keratitis), episcleritis and anterior uveitis.

Topical preparations

The efficacy of a topical ophthalmic corticosteroid depends on its potency, concentration and penetrability.

Prednisolone acetate

1% prednisolone acetate has the best intraocular anti-inflammatory effect. It penetrates the cornea better than other preparations and persists longer in the cornea and aqueous than other preparations, resulting in the highest possible intraocular concentrations. This is the drug of choice to treat uveitis – inflammation inside the eye. It is usually administered 1–10 times daily into the affected eye, depending on the severity of the inflammatory disease.

Dexamethasone

Dexamethasone as a 0.1% suspension eye drop can be an effective topical anti-inflammatory. Dexamethasone does not penetrate the cornea as well as prednisolone acetate. For this reason it is not used as often in severe cases of intraocular inflammation (uveitis). Topical dexamethasone is used most commonly in cats and small dogs.

Hydrocortisone

Hydrocortisone has the least anti-inflammatory effect and does not penetrate the cornea well. It is most commonly used for the treatment of allergic conjunctivitis. In most cases hydrocortisone either as a drop or an ointment is not effective in treating uveitis.

Subconjunctival corticosteroids

In animals that are difficult to medicate topically, or when poor owner compliance is anticipated, depot corticosteroids can be given by subconjunctival injection, either under the conjunctiva of the eyeball (epibulbar) or under the eyelid conjunctiva (subpalpebral). Subconjunctival injections of corticosteroids are contraindicated in all cases where corneal ulceration threatens or is present and when infection is present in either the cornea or the conjunctiva.

After subconjunctival corticosteroid treatment, owners should be warned to watch closely for signs of infection such as increased levels of ocular discharge, blepharospasm, increased corneal opacification or increased ocular pain. Unlike topical corticosteroids, it is much more difficult to withdraw corticosteroids administered subconjunctivally should an infection or ulcer develop. If complications occur it is essential to recognize the problem quickly and if possible, attempt to surgically remove the residue of the subconjunctival injection.

The use of methylprednisolone by subconjunctival injection is not recommended as it can be associated with unsightly granuloma formation following administration.

Formulations and dose rates

DOGS

Betamethasone dipropionate 5 mg/mL and betamethasone phosphate 1 mg/mL

- 0.5–1.0 mL subconjunctivally

Dexamethasone phenylpropionate 2 mg/mL and dexamethasone sodium phosphate 1 mg/mL

- 0.5–1.0 mL subconjunctivally

Dexamethasone-21-isonicotinate 3 mg/mL

- 0.25–1.5 mL subconjunctivally

CATS

Betamethasone dipropionate 5 mg/mL and betamethasone phosphate 1 mg/mL

- 0.25 mL subconjunctivally

Dexamethasone phenylpropionate 2 mg/mL and dexamethasone sodium phosphate 1 mg/mL

- 0.25–0.5 mL subconjunctivally

Dexamethasone-21-isonicotinate 3 mg/mL

- 0.1–0.25 mL subconjunctivally

Systemic corticosteroids

Clinical applications

When treating uveitis it is important to treat the posterior segment of the eye. This requires systemic corticosteroids, as the other therapeutic routes are unlikely to reach the target tissue. For example, topical and subconjunctival therapies are unlikely to be effective for inflammatory conditions of the optic nerve so systemic therapy is indicated.

Formulations and dose rates

Prednisolone is the most common corticosteroid used systemically to treat ocular inflammation.

DOGS AND CATS

- 1.0–2.0 mg/kg q.12 h for 5 d, then q.24 h for 5 d, then q.48 h for 10–14 d

The dosage regimen may need to be varied depending on the clinical response. For longer-term control of inflammatory ocular conditions, NSAIDs may be preferred.

Contraindications and precautions

- Ophthalmic corticosteroids (either topical or subconjunctival) are contraindicated in all cases of corneal ulceration and any corneal wound or infection. Systemic corticosteroids at usual doses do not have much effect on the healing of noninfected corneal ulcers.
- Corticosteroids are contraindicated whenever there is any infection inside the eyeball, or in the eyelids.

Adverse effects

Potentiation of corneal ulceration

Topical corticosteroids should never be applied to an ulcerated cornea, or to a cornea that is likely to ulcerate. Topically applied corticosteroids can dramatically worsen corneal ulceration by retarding epithelial healing and can potentiate collagenases by up to 15 times. Collagenases, when released in controlled amounts, assist healing by allowing epithelial cells to slide across the ulcer bed. However, when mixed with corticosteroids, collagenase activity is greatly potentiated, resulting in rapid destruction of normal corneal structure. Clinically this is seen as a melting cornea. Systemic corticosteroids at normal doses seem to have no effect on corneal collagenase activity. However, it would be prudent to use a systemic NSAID drug rather than a corticosteroid when treating a melting cornea.

Before using a topical corticosteroid the clinician should always apply fluorescein stain to check for corneal ulceration.

Potentiation of infection

Like corticosteroids elsewhere in the body, topical corticosteroids greatly potentiate infection in the cornea. This is caused by decreased movement of leukocytes to the infected area and reduction in macrophage phagocytosis of bacteria.

Corneal stromal and epithelial degeneration

Prolonged topical corticosteroid treatment may potentiate degeneration of the corneal stroma and also in some cases the corneal epithelium as well. This usually results in corneal lipid degeneration. German shepherds treated with long-term topical corticosteroids for control of pannus frequently develop corneal lipidosis.

Delayed healing

Topical corticosteroids can greatly delay corneal healing. This is caused by reduced corneal epithelial migration and proliferation and reduction of corneal stromal collagen deposition.

Cataract formation

In humans, cataract formation is commonly seen following topical corticosteroid administration. This seems to be extremely rare in small animals. There are reports of cats developing cataracts following short- and long-term topical corticosteroid therapy. However, this is not recognized as a clinical problem in veterinary practice.

Systemic effects

Topical use of corticosteroids in dogs has been associated with suppression of the hypothalamic-adrenal axis and increased liver enzyme leakage. It has also been postulated that topical ophthalmic corticosteroids may occasionally cause iatrogenic hyperadrenocorticism.

The possibility of clinically important systemic effects should be considered when a potent topical corticosteroid such as prednisolone acetate 1% is used in a small dog or cat. Such potent topical corticosteroids contain 10 mg of prednisolone per milliliter. One drop to both eyes q.6 h results in administration of 5–6 mg of prednisolone per day, an amount sufficient to cause systemic effects in a small dog or cat.

Conditions where corticosteroids are of limited benefit

Ophthalmic corticosteroids are of limited benefit unless:

- an accurate diagnosis has been made
- infection can be ruled out as a cause of the inflammation
- any predisposing causes of inflammation such as dry eye or poor eyelid conformation have been corrected.

Corticosteroids and ophthalmology

Many eye diseases require frequent use of topical potent corticosteroids. The author observes on an almost daily basis cases where greater use of topical corticosteroids could and should have been used by referring veterinarians. The following are some myths that may be causing veterinarians not to use corticosteroids effectively.

1. **Corticosteroids can cause corneal ulcers.** NOT TRUE! Certainly topical corticosteroids can make an ulcer worse but they do not cause them. Something else needs to affect the cornea for an ulcer to develop. Always stain the cornea with fluorescein. If there is no dye uptake then it is safe to use a topical corticosteroid. Caution needs to be exercised when the cornea is inflamed, e.g. in keratitis, as these cases can easily ulcerate. In a case of keratitis the author might use topical ciclosporin or a NSAID. Caution is also needed in using a topical corticosteroid in cat eyes with a history of viral keratitis. Potent corticosteroids can reactivate latent viral infections.
2. **Antibacterial cover is required when ocular corticosteroids are used.** NOT TRUE! As long as the cornea is not ulcerated there is no need to use a topical antibacterial. In fact, use of topical antibacterial drugs will reduce the normally protective Gram-positive flora in the conjunctiva. This allows pathogenic Gram-negative bacteria to proliferate and also encourages development of bacterial resistance. In horses, use of combined antibacterial corticosteroid preparations increases the risk of fungal infection. Many veterinarians use a combined antibacterial corticosteroid ointment. However, in nearly all cases of uveitis the potency of the corticosteroid in these preparations is totally inadequate.
3. **Ointments are effective in treating inflammation.** NOT TRUE! All ophthalmic corticosteroid preparations contain hydrocortisone, using only 0.5–1.0% concentration. Remember that hydrocortisone is not nearly as potent as prednisolone acetate and does not penetrate as well. Treatment of keratitis, uveitis or episcleritis requires a topical corticosteroid in a drop form, such as prednisolone acetate 1% or 0.1% dexamethasone.

Nonsteroidal anti-inflammatory drugs

Prostaglandins are the most important mediators of ocular inflammation. Antiprostaglandin drugs such as NSAIDs can be used to suppress and hopefully control ocular inflammation. Most commonly, NSAIDs are used systemically for the longer-term control of uveitis or in combination with topical corticosteroids, when systemic corticosteroids are contraindicated or not desirable.

Clinical applications

NSAIDs are indicated in inflammatory conditions of the eye. As they usually have fewer adverse effects than corticosteroids, they are preferred for longer-term treatment and control of inflammatory conditions.

Used prior to intraocular surgery, NSAIDs limit intraocular inflammation and reduce corneal vascularization in cases where corticosteroid use is not desirable.

Topical NSAIDs

Topical NSAIDs have become more widely available in recent years. They are used prior to intraocular surgery to prevent intraoperative miosis and to minimize fibrin exudation. Topical NSAIDs have also been used to reduce corneal vascular reactions, especially when topical corticosteroids are contraindicated. Although topical NSAIDs are less likely to potentiate corneal ulceration than corticosteroids, in the author's opinion they should not be used when corneal ulceration is present.

NSAIDs used topically include flurbiprofen sodium, diclofenac and ketorolac (see Table 25.1). Frequency of administration varies with clinical application. For example, prior to intraocular surgery 1 drop is administered every 30 min for 2 h prior to surgery. In contrast, in the treatment of corneal vascular reaction and anterior uveitis, treatment frequency is q.6–24 h daily.

Systemic NSAIDs

Prolonged therapy is indicated for management of most cases of uveitis. Systemic NSAIDs are probably the most valuable therapeutic agents for the prolonged treatment of these cases. Dose rates, relevant pharmacokinetics and adverse effects are described in Chapter 13.

Carprofen

Carprofen has been shown both clinically and experimentally to be an effective anti-inflammatory drug in uveitis. Experimentally, carprofen was approximately 80% as effective as corticosteroids in inhibiting uveitis flare. Clinically, the author uses carprofen as the drug of choice for longer-term management of uveitis in dogs but not cats.

Flunixin meglumine

Flunixin is used to treat acute inflammatory eye conditions. It has also been used prior to surgery to reduce fibrin exudation and postoperative swelling. However, in the author's opinion, carprofen is a superior drug in all aspects for treatment of ocular conditions in small animals, with fewer side effects.

Aspirin

Aspirin is commonly used for the long-term treatment of chronic uveitis. In some cases, especially cats, therapy may be lifelong. Aspirin appears to be very effective in chronic uveitis but is not as effective as carprofen or flunixin meglumine in acute uveitis or flare-ups of chronic uveitis.

The author has found 10 mg/kg twice weekly to be very effective for chronic granulomatous uveitis in cats.

Other NSAIDs have not been evaluated for ophthalmic use.

Tissue plasminogen activator

Clinical applications

Tissue plasminogen activator (TPA) is used for dissolving intraocular fibrinous exudations. Fibrinous exudation occurs following trauma to the eye, following uveitis and during intraocular surgery (cataract and luxated lens removal).

Formulations and dose rates

DOGS AND CATS

- 10–25 μg dissolved in balanced salt solution injected into the anterior chamber

Adverse effects

- TPA may potentiate hyphema.
- TPA can dissolve fibrin holding corneal or scleral wounds together, causing wound breakdown. Therefore, any wounds sealed by fibrin should be sutured prior to use of TPA.

Immunosuppressive drugs – azathioprine

Clinical applications

Azathioprine is used in combination with corticosteroids for severe inflammatory conditions that are not controlled by corticosteroids alone. The most common ophthalmic indication for azathioprine is episcleritis and uveodermatological syndrome (Vogt–Koyanagi–Harada-like syndrome).

Mechanism of action

The mechanism of action of azathioprine is described in Chapter 12. As it is a slow-acting drug, a clinical response is not usually observed for 4–6 weeks. From an ophthalmic point of view, most eyes are damaged by the time azathioprine becomes clinically effective.

Formulations and dose rates

DOGS

- 1.0–2.0 mg/kg PO q.24 h

Often azathioprine is given on alternate days, with prednisolone given on the other day. Once good control is achieved, azathioprine may be required every 7–10 days to control the inflammatory disease.

Antihistamines

Histamines have a role in the mediation of ocular and adnexal inflammation. Clinically, antihistamines have been used topically for the treatment of allergic conjunctivitis and systemically prior to intraocular surgery. However, they are not commonly used in veterinary ophthalmology today.

Mast cell stabilizers

Sodium cromoglycate 4% (Opticrom®) is widely used in human ophthalmology to treat allergic keratoconjunctivitis. In the author's experience, it seems to have limited efficacy in dogs and cats.

ANTIBACTERIAL DRUGS

Clinical applications

Anti-infective agents are indicated in cases of proven or suspected ocular infections (Table 25.4). They may also be indicated for prophylactic use in cases where development of an infection could lead to loss of the eye, e.g. in deep corneal ulceration.

Generally, antibacterial drugs are grossly overused in clinical veterinary ophthalmic practice. The periocular and ocular structures are uniquely predisposed to infection, so veterinary practitioners are rightly concerned about the serious potential complications of ocular infection. However, many antibacterial drugs are used without justification. The decision to use an ocular antibacterial depends on a number of considerations.

It is important to do a thorough eye examination. In many cases ocular discharge may not be primarily due to an infection. Conditions such as dry eye or foreign bodies may be the primary cause of ocular irritation resulting in secondary infection. Before using antibacterials the clinician should:

- check underneath the eyelids and behind the third eyelid for foreign bodies
- examine the eyelids. Conditions such as entropion, ptosis, ectropion and extra eyelashes may predispose to ocular infection. Correcting an eyelid problem often resolves the secondary infection
- use diagnostic aids, such as Schirmer tear tests and fluorescein stain, to diagnose any underlying conditions such as dry eye
- flush the nasolacrimal duct if there is discharge coming from the nasolacrimal puncta. In cases of chronic ocular infection it is prudent to flush the nasolacrimal duct which can act as a reservoir of infection
- consider conjunctival cytology. Observation of many neutrophils and bacteria is indicative of infection.

Culture and sensitivity is usually not done in ophthalmic cases, unless there is an immediate danger to the eye such as a melting cornea, or in a chronic case where no underlying cause can be found and response to treatment has been poor.

Relevant pharmacokinetics

As previously discussed, the eye has several barriers that limit the penetration of drugs. These are the cornea, blood–aqueous and blood–retina barriers. Knowledge

Table 25.4 Suggested drugs for the treatment of ocular infections

Disorder	Recommended treatment
Eyelid blepharitis (usually a staphylococcal infection)	Fusidic acid ophthalmic ointment, q.12 h Enrofloxacin, 5 mg/kg PO q.24 h
Bacterial conjunctivitis – dog	Neosporin or Tricin ophthalmic ointment, q.8 h for 5 d
Bacterial conjunctivitis – cat	Doxycycline, 5 mg/kg PO q.12 h for 21 d
Corneal ulceration	Tricin or Neosporin ointment, q.8 h Atropine (use if the pupil is small), 1 drop q.8 h until the pupil is dilated Carprofen for secondary uveitis, 2–4 mg/kg PO q.24 h
Corneal ulceration – infected	Gentamicin – fortified, 1 drop q.2 h until the infection is controlled *or* Ofloxacin, 1 drop q.2–4 h until the infection is controlled, combined with Fusidic acid q.12 h, Atropine, 1 drop q.8 h until the pupil is dilated, Carprofen for secondary uveitis, 2–4 mg/kg PO q.24 h
Bacterial endophthalmitis	Ofloxacin, 1 drop q.2–4 h until the infection is controlled, combined with Fusidic acid q.12 h, Enrofloxacin, 5 mg/kg PO q.24 h
Dacryocystitis	Gentasone (gentamicin/dexamethasone), drops q.6 h Doxycycline, 2.5 mg/kg q.24 h
Orbital abscessation	Amoxicillin-clavulanate, 20 mg/kg PO q.12 h *or* Clindamycin, 5.5 mg/kg PO q.12 h for at least 3 weeks

of drug characteristics is required to select an appropriate antibacterial.

For topically applied drugs to penetrate the cornea, they must be able to pass through the lipid epithelium and endothelium as well as the hydrophilic corneal stroma. Antibacterials that have good penetration through the cornea include chloramphenicol, erythromycin, tetracyclines and fluoroquinolones.

The blood–aqueous and blood–retina barriers severely limit drugs given systemically that are not lipid soluble or are highly protein bound. However, if the eye is inflamed the blood–eye barriers break down. Drugs that have good intraocular penetration in normal eyes include chloramphenicol, lincomycin, sulfonamides and the fluoroquinolones. Drugs that are poorly liposoluble, such as ampicillin and amikacin, must be given by subconjunctival injection to achieve a therapeutic intraocular concentration.

ANTIBACTERIAL DRUG CLASSES

Aminoglycosides

Aminoglycosides, especially gentamicin, are commonly used in ophthalmology because of their efficacy against *Pseudomonas* spp. Because of widespread and often inappropriate use of gentamicin, bacterial resistance is increasing. For this reason it is judicious to restrict the use of aminoglycosides to severe, infected corneal ulcers. Culture and sensitivity is recommended because of gentamicin resistance and cross-resistance by *Pseudomonas* spp to other aminoglycosides.

Gentamicin

Although gentamicin is commonly used to treat corneal ulcers in veterinary practice, its use should be restricted to treatment of severe infected corneal ulceration. There is no benefit in using gentamicin as a prophylactic treatment for corneal ulceration.

Formulations and dose rates

DOGS AND CATS

For severe vision-threatening infections, such as a melting cornea, gentamicin should be used frequently, e.g. hourly, and as a fortified preparation. Commercially, gentamicin is available as a 3 mg/mL ophthalmic preparation.

When treating severe infected corneal ulcers, gentamicin can be fortified to a concentration of 10 mg/mL by adding injectable gentamicin to the ophthalmic preparation. Following systemic administration, relatively low concentrations of gentamicin are reached in the tears, cornea and anterior chamber.

Tobramycin

Tobramycin is very similar to gentamicin and can be fortified for use in serious infections.

Neomycin

Neomycin is usually combined with polymyxin and bacitracin in ophthalmic preparations (drops or ointments). It has been reported to cause local allergic reactions.

Bacitracin

Bacitracin is used in a number of eye preparations in combination with other antibacterials, usually neomycin and polymyxin. It has a bactericidal action, chiefly against Gram-positive organisms. There is limited penetration into the eye.

Chloramphenicol

Chloramphenicol is commonly used in ophthalmology as it can penetrate the intact cornea due to the high lipid solubility of the nonionized form. When administered systemically, it is able to penetrate the blood–aqueous and blood–retina barriers.

Chloramphenicol is bacteriostatic, with a broad spectrum of activity against both Gram-negative and Gram-positive organisms. It is not effective against *Pseudomonas* so is often used in combination with polymyxin B. Chloramphenicol is also effective against *Chlamydophila*.

Clindamycin

Clindamycin is usually used in ophthalmology for the treatment of *Toxoplasma* infections. Toxoplasmosis usually causes posterior chorioretinitis. Systemic clindamycin is selectively concentrated into the choroid and retina. Clindamycin can also be given as a subconjunctival injection. The usual dose is 35 mg per subconjunctival injection.

Clinical data have shown that oral clindamycin at a dose of 25 mg/kg/d for 14–42 d may reduce the ophthalmic signs of ocular toxoplasmosis in the cat.

Erythromycin

Erythromycin is available as a 0.5% ointment but is not commonly used. It is effective against Gram-positive organisms and *Chlamydophila*. Erythromycin has poor penetration of the blood–aqueous and blood–retina barriers.

Fluoroquinolones

Fluoroquinolones are effective against aerobic Gram-positive and Gram-negative bacteria. They are highly effective against all common ocular pathogens, including *Pseudomonas* spp. Fluoroquinolones penetrate the intact cornea and the blood–aqueous and blood–retina barriers well. Because of their wide spectrum of activity and their ability to penetrate into the eye, they are considered the treatment of choice for serious ocular infections, i.e. melting corneas (keratomalacia). Their use should be reserved for this purpose. One cause of melting corneas can be β-hemolytic *Streptococcus*. The fluoroquinolones do not have good efficacy against these organisms, so the author always uses topical fusidic acid in addition to a topical fluoroquinolone.

Ophthalmic formulations available include ciprofloxacin 0.3% and ofloxacin 0.3% administered every 1–2 h, with fusidic acid twice daily, until the infection is controlled.

Systemic fluoroquinolones are the drugs of choice for the treatment of suspected or confirmed intraocular infections. They penetrate well, are bactericidal and have a wide spectrum of activity. In rare cases systemic administration of enrofloxacin has caused blindness in cats. Affected cats may initially show pupillary dilation. If this is recognized, drug withdrawal and diuresis are recommended. Unfortunately, most affected cats develop irreversible blindness. This is specifically due to enrofloxacin toxicity in the photoreceptors in the retina. Older cats with reduced renal function and those cats treated with more than the recommended dose, especially those treated with 20 mg/kg, are more likely to develop blindness. For this reason, ophthalmologists do not use this drug in cats.

Fusidic acid

Fusidic acid has a predominantly Gram-positive spectrum of activity. It is usually indicated in staphylococcal infections of the conjunctival sac and eyelids (staphylococcal blepharitis). The drug is presented in a viscous base, giving a prolonged contact time. Therefore only twice-daily administration is required. When using topical fluoroquinolones to treat serious corneal infections, fusidic acid is also indicated to provide efficacy against *Streptococcal* spp.

Polymyxin B

Polymyxin B cannot be used systemically and is usually combined in ophthalmic preparations with bacitracin and neomycin. Polymyxin B does not penetrate the intact cornea or the blood–aqueous or blood–retina barriers. It is irritant if given by subconjunctival injection. Polymyxin B is effective against Gram-negative organisms, including *Pseudomonas* spp.

Tetracyclines

Tetracyclines are commonly used in ophthalmic practice. When given orally, they are partially excreted into the tear film and reach high therapeutic concentrations in the tear film and therefore the superficial cornea. This can be advantageous in dogs with ulcers that are difficult to treat with topical medications, as oral tetracyclines, particularly doxycycline, can provide excellent antibacterial coverage. The tetracyclines when given systemically are able to penetrate well into the eye due to their lipophilic nature. However, due to their large molecule size and lipophilic nature, tetracyclines when given topically do not penetrate the intact cornea well. Tetracyclines are bacteriostatic and effective against *Chlamydophila* and a number of Gram-positive and Gram-negative bacteria. They are considered to have little effect against *Pseudomonas* spp and resistance in *Staphylococcus* spp is increasing.

Doxycycline

Doxycycline is indicated for treatment of *Chlamydophila* infections. Topical therapy is not adequate as, even when conjunctivitis is the predominant clinical sign, *Chlamydophila* also can be found in the respiratory and urogenital tracts. To treat and eradicate *Chlamydophila* a 3-week course of doxycycline is indicated. Systemic doxycycline reaches therapeutic levels in the precorneal tear film and is then concentrated in the cornea and conjunctiva.

When used to treat chlamydial infections, doxycycline should be administered at 5 mg/kg q.12 h (twice the usual recommended dose at twice the recommended frequency) for 3 weeks. This regimen has been shown to eradicate *Chlamydophila*. It is also important to treat all cats in the affected cat's environment, as other cats can be carriers.

Doxycycline is also very useful clinically when treating corneal ulceration in dogs and cats. It can be used to supplement topical antibacterial therapy, but also can be used as the primary antibacterial when the animal is difficult to treat or when owner compliance is poor. It has been suggested in humans that doxycycline has a positive effect on corneal healing. It is the author's subjective impression that this is also the case in the treatment of corneal ulcers in small animals.

Sulfonamides

Sulfonamides are not commonly used in veterinary ophthalmic practice because they have been documented to cause keratoconjunctivitis sicca (dry eye) in dogs. Although this usually occurs after long-term systemic administration, dry eye has been seen to develop after use of trimethoprim/sulfadiazine for only 4 d. Dry eye has not been reported following topical use of sulfonamides.

ANTIFUNGAL AGENTS

Ocular fungal infections in small animals are rare. They occur more commonly in horses. Fungal infections are usually seen after injury to the cornea by vegetable matter or after prolonged use of a combined antibacterial-corticosteroid preparation. Fungal infections are characterized by slowly progressing corneal lesions that are usually white or yellow in color and unresponsive to intensive antibacterial therapy. Deep corneal scrapings or a corneal biopsy are usually required to obtain a positive culture.

There is very little information in the veterinary literature on the efficacy of drugs used to treat ocular fungal infections. Fungi can vary widely in their sensitivity to drugs so sensitivity testing is always indicated.

There are three main groups of antifungal agents: polyene antibacterials, pyrimidines and imidazoles. Other drugs used to treat fungal infections include iodine and silver sulfadiazine. Ophthalmic applications for these drugs will be discussed in this chapter. Information on mechanism of action and pharmacokinetics can be found in Chapter 9.

POLYENE ANTIBACTERIALS

Natamycin

Natamycin is available in a 5% suspension as an ophthalmic preparation. The preparation is generally well tolerated but the suspension may adhere to the ulcerated cornea. Natamycin has poor ability to penetrate the intact cornea. It must be administered up to six times daily.

Amphotericin B

Amphotericin B is effective against common systemic fungal infections such as cryptococcosis and blastomycosis. It is of limited use in intraocular fungal infections because it has very poor intraocular penetration through the cornea and the blood–eye barrier and because of its systemic toxicity.

Amphotericin can be used as a topical preparation but can be irritant and may cause toxicity to corneal and conjunctival epithelium. It is of limited use in the treatment of keratomycosis because it is not effective against *Aspergillus* spp, a common cause of keratomycosis.

PYRIMIDINE DERIVATIVES

Flucytosine

Flucytosine is of limited use in ophthalmic practice because of its limited efficacy against the filamentous fungi commonly isolated from keratomycosis.

IMIDAZOLE DERIVATIVES

Miconazole

Miconazole has been used to treat keratomycosis in animals. A commercially available intravenous preparation can be used subconjunctivally (5–10 mg q.24 h) as well as topically (1 drop six times daily). Miconazole is also available as a dermatological or vaginal cream. Both preparations appear to be well tolerated by the cornea.

Ketoconazole

Ketoconazole penetrates the eye well when administered either topically or systemically. Equine keratomycosis caused by *Aspergillus* spp appears to respond well to ketoconazole. A 1% solution is well tolerated by the eye after topical administration (one crushed ketoconazole tablet suspended in artificial tears). Ketoconazole has been reported to cause cataracts in dogs with long-term oral therapy.

Fluconazole

Fluconazole is available as an intravenous preparation and can be administered topically or as a subconjunctival injection. It has also been administered as an intracameral injection into the anterior chamber to treat deep-seated corneal fungal infections.

Itraconazole

Oral treatment with itraconazole is effective in treatment of experimental fungal keratitis in rabbits. Currently, there are no data to demonstrate that it is effective in treatment of keratomycosis in the dog or cat. In the horse 1% itraconazole with 30% DMSO in an ointment preparation results in high corneal concentrations of the drug and is well tolerated. Clinically this combination seems to have great efficacy in the treatment of fungal keratitis

OTHER ANTIFUNGALS

Povidone-iodine

Povidone-iodine diluted to a 1% concentration normal saline has been used in the treatment of equine keratomycosis. No data regarding its clinical efficacy are available.

Silver sulfadiazine

The author has found silver sulfadiazine to be extremely effective in the treatment of keratomycosis. It is available as a skin preparation usually used in the treatment of skin burns. It is usually well tolerated. Studies have shown that the silver is concentrated well in the cornea.

Directions for use involve applying a generous amount onto the affected cornea 4–6 times daily. Clinically the author has found this preparation to be useful in treating fungal keratitis.

ANTIVIRAL THERAPY

Ophthalmic viral infections are seen most commonly in cats and are usually due to feline herpes virus. Ophthalmic lesions caused by the virus include conjunctivitis, keratitis (usually ulceration) or a combination of corneal and conjunctival disease.

Antiviral therapy is of questionable value for the treatment of viral conjunctivitis. It is mainly indicated for active herpetic keratitis. Clinical signs of herpetic keratitis are dendritic (linear tree-branching ulceration) or geographic ulcers (a large superficial ulcer with loose epithelial edges). Clinical response to antiviral treatment regimens is variable.

All the antivirals used in veterinary practice are human preparations. Recently, many antivirals previously used to treat viral keratitis in humans have been withdrawn from the market and replaced by aciclovir. Unfortunately, aciclovir has much less efficacy against feline herpes virus infections than the drugs (idoxuridine and virabadine) it has replaced. In vitro testing has revealed that the order of efficacy against feline herpes virus is idoxuridine > virabadine > trifluridine. The least effective drug is aciclovir.

Formulations and dose rates

Aciclovir

Apply a small amount of ointment to the affected eye six times daily. It has been suggested that aciclovir therapy needs to be combined with interferon to be effective. Clinically, the author has found a much improved clinical response when aciclovir is used in combination with interferon given by subcutaneous injection.

It has also been suggested that oral aciclovir may be of benefit in the treatment of feline herpetic keratitis. However, even at a dose of 50 mg/kg, the resultant concentration of aciclovir achieved was inadequate to inhibit viral replication.

Trifluridine and idoxuridine

These drugs will usually need to be compounded by a manufacturing pharmacist as they are no longer commercially made.

One drop every 1–2 h until a clinical response (reduction in the size of the ulcer) is seen, then apply four times daily until the ulcer heals. Trifluridine and idoxuridine are only virostatic and therefore need to be applied frequently to achieve a clinical response. Clinically, the best results are seen when the drug is used hourly for the first 24 h, then 6–8 times daily until the corneal ulceration has resolved.

Both drugs can be irritating to the cornea, resulting in blepharospasm and conjunctival hyperemia. If this occurs, drug treatment may have to be discontinued.

ADDITIONAL THERAPIES FOR THE TREATMENT OF VIRAL KERATITIS

Lysine

Lysine has been demonstrated to substantially reduce replication and shedding of feline herpes virus when given orally at a dose of 250 mg q.12 h. Clinically its efficacy is unproven in controlled clinical trials but anecdotal reports suggest that it may be of some use.

Interferon

Interferons are produced by leukocytes during an immune response and induce an antiviral reaction in cells. Experimentally, interferons greatly increase the efficacy of aciclovir in in vitro testing against feline herpes virus.

Formulations and dose rates for the treatment of viral keratitis

TOPICAL THERAPIES

- Idoxuridine eye drops 0.1%: idoxuridine is the preferred drug for viral keratitis. Apply 1 drop to the affected eye(s) hourly for the first 24 h, then 6–8 times daily. This will need to be compounded by a pharmacist

Alternatively:

- Aciclovir (Zovirax, Glaxo SmithKline) ointment: apply to the affected eye(s) 6–8 times daily

Alternatively:

- Betadine eye drops 1% or poviodine solution diluted in 9 parts saline: one drop to the affected eye(s) 6–8 times daily. This inexpensive treatment may resolve some cases of viral keratitis

ORAL THERAPIES

- Lysine (Lysine, Musashi): 250 mg (1/8th of a teaspoon) PO q.12 h. Lysine may help reduce viral replication; its greatest benefit may be to reduce the risk of recurrence of viral activation
- Doxycycline (Vibravet, Pfizer) 5 mg/kg orally twice daily. Antimicrobial treatment can be beneficial as many cases of viral keratitis are complicated by secondary chlamydial infection

IMMUNE STIMULATION

- Interferon injections subcutaneously 10,000 IU twice weekly. Dilute Interferon (Interon A, Schering-Plough) in water for injection. This treatment is thought to stimulate the antiviral state of the immune system. In the author's experience concurrent interferon treatment enhances the efficacy of idoxuridine

Summary

Feline viral keratitis is a challenging condition to treat. Intensive treatment in the early stages is more likely to result in a clinical response. Some cases may require surgical intervention.

DRUGS AFFECTING PUPIL SIZE

MYDRIATICS

Mydriatics dilate the pupil and can be used diagnostically to allow fundus examination and therapeutically to treat uveitis.

Relevant pathophysiology

The pupil can be dilated by activation of the sympathetic dilator muscle by an adrenergic agonist or by paralyzing the parasympathetic iris sphincter constrictor muscle with a parasympatholytic drug.

Inflammation causes production of many inflammatory mediators, including prostaglandin iridin. This particular prostaglandin causes an intense pupillary constriction. This miosis can cause adhesions of the iris onto the lesion which can result in vision loss. Clinically, it is important to dilate the pupil with a mydriatic.

Tropicamide

Tropicamide is a short-acting parasympatholytic drug. Inhibition of the parasympathetic constrictor muscle in the iris results in dilation of the pupil because the action of sympathetic dilator muscles is unopposed.

Tropicamide is used at a 1% concentration to dilate the pupil for diagnostic purposes. The pupil is usually dilated within 15 min and remains dilated for 4–5 h. Tropicamide is bound by pigment so in heavily pigmented eyes, tropicamide takes longer to work and the pupil stays dilated longer. Tropicamide is not used clinically to treat miosis because of its short duration of action.

Phenylephrine

Phenylephrine is a sympathomimetic drug that causes pupillary dilation by activating the sympathetic dilator iris muscle. It is usually administered with tropicamide to maximally dilate the pupil. Maximal pupil dilation may be useful when attempting to examine the fundus when a cataract is present or during cataract removal. It is administered 15–30 min before maximal mydriasis is required.

Atropine

Atropine is a long-acting parasympatholytic mydriatic used in management of uveitis-induced miosis. As it can cause mydriasis for up to a week in a pigmented canine eye, it is not usually used for diagnostic purposes. Melanocytes take up excess atropine and then release it as the intraocular concentration of atropine falls, prolonging the duration of action of the drug in heavily pigmented eyes.

Formulations and dose rates

One drop is administered to the affected eye q.6–8 h until the pupil dilates. This usually takes 1–2 d and is dependent on how much intraocular inflammation is present. Once the pupil is dilated, atropine is used as required to maintain dilation. If the eye is inflamed, atropine may be required 2–3 times a day to maintain mydriasis. If inflammation is controlled, then atropine administration may only be required once every second day or twice a week.

The degree of pupillary dilation maintained or achieved by 1 drop of atropine can be used as a guide to how well inflammation is controlled; if the pupil stays dilated with 1 drop of atropine, uveitis is well controlled. Rapid onset of miosis after atropine administration suggests that inflammation is not well controlled.

In refractory cases subconjunctival atropine can be administered as an epibulbar injection. The dose is 0.05 mg (cats and small dogs) or 0.1 mg (larger dogs). In these cases it is important to increase anti-inflammatory therapy by using subconjunctival depot cortisone injections with the epibulbar atropine injection.

MIOTICS

Clinical applications

Miotics (drugs that cause the pupil to contract) improve the outflow of aqueous as part of the treatment of glaucoma and reduce the risk of a posteriorly luxated lens entering the anterior chamber.

The importance of miotics in veterinary ophthalmology has decreased substantially over the last few years. They have been replaced in glaucoma management by more effective drugs such as topical carbonic anhydrase inhibitors and topical prostaglandin agonists. The use of miotics in animals with loose or luxated lenses has also reduced as it is now recommended that posteriorly luxated or subluxated lenses should be removed surgically.

Relevant physiology

Pupillary constriction (miosis) results from stimulating the parasympathetic nerve which innervates the iris. This can be achieved with direct-acting drugs (parasympathomimetic) or indirect-acting drugs that block hydrolysis of acetylcholine by cholinesterases.

Miotics also cause contraction of the ciliary body and increased vascular permeability within the eye. They reduce intraocular pressure by opening the drainage angle to increase outflow of aqueous. In some cases, production of aqueous humor is also reduced.

Direct-acting miotics – pilocarpine

There are many brands of pilocarpine available in a wide range of concentrations. Pilocarpine has a direct effect on muscarinic receptors in the eye. It is used predominantly as a glaucoma prophylactic drug. It is no longer considered the drug of choice for treatment of glaucoma as there are more effective drugs available.

Pilocarpine is also used in the treatment of dry eye. Increased lacrimal production can be achieved by its parasympathomimetic effect. It can be administered topically or orally.

Formulations and dose rates

Glaucoma therapy

Drops 1–2%: 1 drop to the predisposed eye q.6–12 h

Pilocarpine gel 4%: apply to the predisposed eye q.12 h. This preparation is formulated as an extended-contact hydrophilic gel, which reduces pilocarpine-induced irritation

Pilocarpine drops can be extremely irritating, resulting in blepharospasm and conjunctival hyperemia. This irritation seems to reduce after 2–3 d. In some cases irritation is so severe that the drug must be discontinued.

Dry eye therapy

Topical: topical pilocarpine will only be effective for dry eye if there is some existing lacrimal activity (Schirmer tear test >5 mm wetting/min). Use a concentration of 0.25% q.8–12 h. In some cases even dilute formulations (0.25%) can cause severe conjunctival irritation

Oral: mix 1 drop of 2 % pilocarpine well into the food, initially q.12 h. Every couple of days add an extra drop until tearing results. In many cases signs of toxicity (salivation, vomiting and diarrhea, colic and anorexia) will develop before lacrimation is stimulated. This form of therapy is of greatest benefit when neurogenic dry eye is present. Neurogenic dry eye is suspected when an ipsilateral dry nose is present

Indirect-acting miotics

Indirect-acting miotics are rarely used because of their potential toxicity, especially if animals are concurrently treated with organophosphate flea preparations such as flea collars.

Formulations and dose rates

Phospholine iodide

- 0.125% concentration, 1 drop to the affected eye q.12 h. Once miosis is achieved this can often be reduced to q.24 h

Demecarium

- Demecarium seems to be well tolerated in dogs. Use 0.125–0.25% concentration q.12 h

GLAUCOMA TREATMENTS

Glaucoma is a complex disease in which elevated intraocular pressure (IOP) is incompatible with normal optic nerve function. In contrast to humans, glaucoma in small animals is most commonly acute, when intraocular pressure rapidly increases. Prompt treatment is essential if there is to be any chance of saving vision.

Relevant pathophysiology

Aqueous humor is produced at a fairly constant rate by the passive filtration of blood and active production via carbonic anhydrase, an enzyme located in the ciliary body epithelium. The aqueous exits through the iridocorneal (drainage) angle. Increased intraocular pressure is usually the result of decreased outflow of aqueous. The aim of any glaucoma treatment is to reduce intraocular pressure to under 20–25 mmHg.

Intraocular pressure can be reduced by:

- increasing the outflow of aqueous. Drugs such as miotics, adrenergics and prostaglandin agonists can increase aqueous outflow
- decreasing aqueous production. Carbonic anhydrase inhibitors can be used either topically or systemically to reduce aqueous production. Adrenergics, β-blockers and prostaglandin agonists also reduce aqueous production
- osmotic removal of intraocular fluid, using systemic osmotic diuretics.

TOPICAL GLAUCOMA TREATMENT

Miotics

This class of drug is rarely used. They have been replaced by newer drugs such as the topical carbonic anhydrase inhibitors and prostaglandin agonists. (See the previous section on miotics.)

Carbonic anhydrase inhibitors

Carbonic anhydrase inhibitors (CAIs) are extremely useful in reducing intraocular pressure by about

15 mmHg. They reduce aqueous production by inhibition of carbonic anhydrase. Dozolamide (Trusopt®, MSD) is the topical carbonic anhydrase inhibitor used most frequently in managing glaucoma in dogs and cats. Other topical CAIs are brinzolamide (Azopt®, Alcon) and dorzolamide/timolol (Cosopt®, MSD).

In veterinary ophthalmology this class of drug is most useful in treating glaucoma that is secondary to uveitis or hyphema and following luxated lens removal. They do not seem to be effective in treating acute, primary glaucoma.

Prostaglandin agonists

This is a new class of drugs that have made a huge impact on the treatment of glaucoma in dogs. The prostanoids act to reduce the IOP by reducing aqueous production and increasing aqueous outflow. Latanoprost is the prostaglandin agonist used most commonly to reduce IOP in dogs. Profound miosis is produced once intraocular pressure is reduced. It is administered once daily. In humans, long-term use can cause increased iris pigmentation and lengthening of the eyelashes. Such side effects have not been noted in the domestic species.

Latanoprost (Xalatan®, Pharmacia & Upjohn) is indicated to treat acute, primary glaucoma. This is seen clinically in breeds predisposed to glaucoma and is characteristically acute in onset with a rapid and dramatic increase in the IOP. Travaprost (Travatan®, Alcon) is another prostaglandin agonist that has been used to treat glaucoma in dogs. It appears to work in a very similar manner to latanoprost. In some cases travaprost may reduce IOP when latanoprost has failed.

Prostaglandin agonists do not seem to be effective in cats. It is believed this species lacks the necessary receptors for this class of drug to be effective.

SYSTEMIC GLAUCOMA TREATMENT

Carbonic anhydrase inhibitors

Systemic carbonic anhydrase inhibitors (CAIs) used clinically include acetazolamide, dichlorphenamide and methazolamide. In many countries these drugs are no longer available.

Adverse effects of carbonic anhydrase inhibitors include anorexia, vomiting, diarrhea, diuresis and increased respiratory effort, secondary to acidosis. They may also cause hypokalemia.

There are now a number of topical CAIs available. These drugs appear to be more effective in reducing the IOP compared to the systemic CAIs. Topical CAIs are also advantageous in that they do not have systemic side effects. Today there are very few indications for systemic CAI therapy.

Formulations and dose rates

Acetazolamide
- 10 mg/kg PO q.8–12 h

Dichlorphenamide
- 2.5 mg/kg PO q.8–12 h

Methazolamide
- 5 mg/kg PO q.8–12 h

Systemic osmotic therapy

Traditionally, osmotic diuretics such as intravenous mannitol or oral glycerin have been used to reduce IOP. Water needs to be withheld after administration. These drugs are only effective for 4–6 h and are not used for chronic therapy. Today these drugs are used much less commonly, as raised IOP can be more effectively lowered by using topical therapies such as dozolamide or latanoprost.

GLAUCOMA SUMMARY

EMERGENCY TREATMENT OF ACUTE, PRIMARY GLAUCOMA IN THE DOG

Lantanoprost: 1 drop q.12–24 h, to reduce the IOP
Amlodipine: 2.5–5 mg orally q.24 h for 4 d, to protect the optic nerve from reperfusion injury
Sodium prednisolone succinate: 10 mg/kg IV, to protect the optic nerve from reperfusion injury

SECONDARY GLAUCOMA IN THE DOG

Dorzolamide: 1 drop q.8 h
Treat the underlying cause of the glaucoma, e.g anti-inflammatory therapy for uveitis.

MISCELLANEOUS THERAPY FOR GLAUCOMA

Calcium channel blockers

When IOP is reduced by glaucoma treatment, blood flow to the optic nerve increases. This results in a sudden release of calcium from mitochondria, which can damage the optic nerve. Calcium channel blockers are believed to protect the optic nerve from damage. Clinical data regarding the efficacy of calcium channel blockers in this setting have not been published.

Drugs used for this purpose include amlodipine. Mechanism of action, relevant pharmacokinetics and adverse effects are discussed in Chapter 18.

Dose rate is 2.5–5 mg q.12 h PO for 2–4 d while IOP is being reduced.

TOPICAL ANESTHETICS

Topical anesthetics provide local anesthesia and allow minor procedures to be performed, e.g. eversion of the third eyelid or removal of a superficial corneal foreign body. Topical anesthetics may also facilitate eye examination when there is considerable ocular pain. In such cases it may also be necessary to use sedatives and/or systemic analgesics to facilitate eye examination.

Topical anesthetics are toxic to corneal epithelium and therefore can only be used once for diagnostic procedures. If their use is continued, e.g. to relieve ocular pain, corneal ulceration will develop. This is the result of reduced blinking producing exposure of the cornea and inhibition of the normal neurogenic function needed for normal corneal health.

Formulations and dose rates

Apply 1 drop to the eye q.30 s for 3–4 applications. Corneal anesthesia develops quickly but to maintain conjunctival anesthesia, repeated applications are required. If the eye is severely inflamed or painful, additional applications will be required.

Proparacaine

Proparacaine is the most commonly used topical ophthalmic anesthetic. It causes roughening of the corneal surface, which may make intraocular examination difficult. It may be necessary to use artificial tears to smooth the corneal surface to permit fundus examination after its use.

Proparacaine should be refrigerated to delay degeneration of the preparation, which results in brownish discoloration. If this occurs the preparation should be discarded.

Lidocaine (lignocaine)

Injectable preparations of lidocaine (lignocaine) can be used topically to achieve local anesthesia. Compared with other local anesthetics, they can be irritating when first applied and may result in conjunctival hyperemia.

CORNEAL DEHYDRATING AGENTS

The normal cornea is kept relatively dehydrated by the metabolic activity of corneal endothelial cells. Corneal edema can develop for a variety of reasons. In these cases corneal dehydrating agents (topical hyperosmotics) can be used to reduce corneal edema for diagnostic purposes to allow intraocular examination. Longer-term therapy can also be used.

Topical glycerin can be used to temporarily clear the cornea to allow intraocular examination. Because it can be quite irritating, pretreatment with topical anesthesia is recommended.

Sodium chloride (5%) has been used as either a drop or an ointment to treat corneal edema and corneal bullous keratopathy. It must be administered at least four times daily.

DRY EYE THERAPY

Keratoconjunctivitis sicca is a common condition in dogs but less common in cats. Diagnosis is made with a Schirmer tear test strip. The normal Schirmer tear test is 15 mm wetting/min or greater for the dog and 10 mm/min or greater for the cat.

Clinically dry eye in dogs can manifest as corneal and conjunctival disease and is characterized by a copious mucopurulent discharge. The aim of dry eye therapy is to improve the precorneal tear film.

Ciclosporin

In over 80% of early dry eye cases, tear production can be restored to normal with ciclosporin. Ciclosporin is primarily used in humans to prevent organ transplant rejection. It is believed that dry eye in the dog may be the result of an immune-mediated reaction against the lacrimal glands. Ciclosporin may have efficacy in dry eye because it reduces this reaction. It is also believed that ciclosporin may have a direct lacrimogenic effect, possibly via prolactin receptors.

Ciclosporin is considered the treatment of choice for dry eye. It has also been used to treat pannus in German shepherds, punctate keratitis, vascular keratitis and other inflammatory corneal and conjunctival disease. Usually, a minimum of 3 months' treatment is necessary to reduce corneal pigmentation and lipidosis in dogs.

Formulations and dose rates

A commercial preparation of 0.2% ciclosporin ointment (Optimmune®, Schering-Plough) is available in many countries. If this product is not available, systemic ciclosporin can be diluted to a 1% or 2% concentration in white mineral oil.

Apply a small amount of ointment or 1 drop of solution to the affected eye q.12 h for at least 3–4 weeks. In some cases maximal response is not seen for up to 8 weeks. Initially, when the eye is dry, it is important to also treat the eyes with ocular lubricants such as artificial tears and protective ointments. To maximize effectiveness the eye should be clear of all discharge before ciclosporin is applied.

If a good clinical response is seen, ciclosporin treatment can be reduced to q.24 h or once every second day. Even if the Schirmer tear test readings are not increased by ciclosporin therapy, clinical signs are often relieved as ciclosporin inhibits the mediators that cause clinical signs of dry eye.

Adverse effects

- Local irritation can be seen with the solution preparations of ciclosporin, particularly those derived from the commercial preparation Neoral®. Intense blepharospasm and conjunctival hyperemia may occur. In some cases, the reaction is sufficiently severe to necessitate discontinuation of therapy.
- Topical ciclosporin can also cause periocular and eyelid hyperemia and hair loss.

Contraindications and precautions

Because of the immunosuppressive effects of ciclosporin, feline herpetic keratitis can be exacerbated by topical ciclosporin, resulting in development of secondary complications such as eosinophilic keratitis and corneal sequestration.

In dogs, it is possible that blepharitis can develop due to the overgrowth of *Malassezia*.

Tacrolimus

Similarly to ciclosporin, tacrolimus is used in humans to prevent graft rejection. Like ciclosporin, tacrolimus seems to be very effective as a 0.2% ointment in treating dry eye in dogs. Tacrolimus is also effective in treating pannus and can be used to reduce corneal pigmentation.

Formulations and dose rates

Tacrolimus is applied to the affected eye q. 8 h for at least 4–6 weeks. Due to the expense of compounding tacrolimus, clinically the author uses tacrolimus to treat cases which have failed to respond to the various forms of ciclosporin.

Artificial tears

The precorneal tear film has aqueous, lipid and mucin components. It is a complex fluid that is difficult to replace artificially. A huge number of artificial tear preparations are available. The effectiveness of tear substitutes can be increased by using agents such as methylcellulose, polyvinyl alcohol and polyvinylpyrrolidone to prolong corneal contact time. Prolonged contact time is important to minimize the frequency with which the medications need to be applied.

Adverse effects

Local irritation resulting in blepharospasm and conjunctival hyperemia can occasionally occur. This is usually the result of sensitivity to preservatives in the preparation. This occurs much less commonly in cats and dogs than in humans.

OCULAR LUBRICANTS

When the eye is dry, during and after general anesthesia, ocular lubricants are used to form an occlusive film over the cornea to protect it against desiccation. Lubricants may cause local irritation. The occlusive nature of these preparations may affect vision.

Ocular lubricants may be useful in the management of dry eye, as they have superior contact times compared to artificial tear preparations. However, the occlusive nature of these preparations may reduce oxygen transfer to the cornea, resulting in clinical disease.

Clinically the author has found that Viscotears is much more soothing to dry eyes than is Lacrilube.

FURTHER READING

Blogg JR, Stanley RG 1991 Common eye diseases. Proceedings 158. University of Sydney Post Graduate Committee in Veterinary Science

Martin CL 2004 Ophthalmic disease in veterinary medicine. Blackwell, Oxford

Mathis G, Regnier A, Ward DA 1999 Clinical ophthalmic pharmacology and therapeutics. In: Gelatt KN (ed.) Veterinary ophthalmology, 3rd edn. Lippincott Williams and Wilkins, Philadelphia, PA

Moore CP 2001 Ocular pharmacology. In: Adams HR (ed.) Veterinary pharmacology and therapeutics, 8th edn. Iowa State University Press, Ames, IA

Severin GA 1996 Severin's veterinary ophthalmology notes, 3rd edn. Veterinary Ophthalmology Notes, Fort Collins, CO

Slatter DH 2001 Fundamentals of veterinary ophthalmology, 3rd edn. WB Saunders, Philadelphia, PA

Willis AM, Diehl K, Robbin TE 2002 Advances in topical glaucoma therapy. Vet Ophthalmol 5: 9-12

Index

A

α-adrenergic receptors 70, *71*
α_1-adrenergic receptors 73
α_2-adrenoceptors 73
α-adrenoceptor agonists 143
α_1-adrenoceptor agonists 96–97, **120–124**
  and ketamine combinations 105
α-adrenoceptor antagonists 73–74, 144
α_1-adrenoceptor antagonists 471
α_2-adrenoceptor antagonists 74, **124**, 471
Abortifacient 541
Abortion
  induction 534, 535, 537, 538, 541, 542
  prevention 536
Absorbants 488–489
Absorption
  dogs vs cats 47
  half-life 2–3
  physiological basis of 29–31
ACE inhibitors *see* Angiotensin-converting enzyme (ACE) inhibitors
Acemannan 279
Acepromazine 114–116
Acepromazine (ACP) 114–115, 116, 315
Acetaminophen *see* Paracetamol (Acetaminophen)
Acetazolamide 571
Acetonide 263
Acetyl salicylic acid *see* Aspirin
Acetylcholine (ACh) 60–65
  airway diameter regulation 458–459, 462
  behavior-modification 127
  inactivation 69
  nicotinic receptors 9, 66
  sedative action 114
  vascular action 65
  see also Muscarinic receptors; Nicotinic receptors
Acetylcholinesterase 67
Acetylcysteine 466–467
Acetylpromazine 130–131
N-Acetyltransferase (NAT) *53–54*
Aciclovir *9*, 568
Actinomycin D 333, *336*, **353–354**
Activated charcoal 489
Active transport 29
Adenosine *8*
Adenosine triphosphate *63*
S-adenosyl methionine (SAMe) 494
Adrenal cortex
  drugs acting on 520–524
  physiology 519
Adrenal dysfunction
  hyperadrenocorticism 517–524
  hypoadrenocorticism 524–527
Adrenaline *see* Epinephrine (Adrenaline)
Adrenergic agonists 459–461
  see also α-adrenoceptor agonists; α_2-adrenoceptor agonists; β_2-adrenoceptor agonists
Adrenergic receptors *8*, 69–70, *71*, 73
Adrenocorticotrophic hormone (ACTH) 519, 520, 521
Adrenoreceptor agonists 73, **78–81**
Adrenoreceptor antagonists 73–74, **81–82**
Adriamycin *see* Doxorubicin
Adverse drug reactions (ADRs) 41–58
  augmented (type A) 41, 47–*55*
  bizarre (Type B) 41
  chronic (Type C) 41
  classification 41–42
  delayed (Type D) 41
  diagnostic difficulties 43–44
  end of treatment (Type E) 42
  failure of treatment (Type F) 42
  hypersensitivity *55–56*
  identification 46–47
  incidence 42–46
  postmarketing surveillance (pharmacovigilance) 44–46
  prescribing principles *25*
  reporting 44–46, *56–57*
    Australia *56*
    Canada *57*
    New Zealand *57*
    South Africa *57*
    UK *57*
    USA *57*
  vs adverse events (AEs) 41
  see also specific drugs/drug classes
Aerosols, adrenergic agonists 459–460
Age
  adverse drug reaction (ADRs) *50*
  influence on pharmacokinetics 18, *19*
Aglepristone (RU534) 537–538
Agonists 6
Albaconazole 193–194, *238*
Albendazole *204*, 208, *238*
Albuterol (salbutamol) sulfate 460–461
Aldosterone antagonists 418–419
Alfacalcidol 508
Alfentanil *319*, 324–325
Alkylating agents 340–348
Allopurinol 236–240
  antiprotozoal dosages *239*
  caution in renal disease *53*
  drug interactions 240
    azathioprine 272
    cyclophosphamide 334
    theophylline 462
  receptors and ligands 9
  selective toxicity *201*
Allylamines 195
Aloe vera extracts 553–554
Alphaxalone (alphadolone) 96, **101–103**
Alprazolam 134–136, *135*
Aluminum hydroxide 482–483
Alveolar inhalational anesthesia 85–87
Alveolar ventilation 86
Amfetamines 133–134
Amikacin 173
Aminocridine *237*
Aminocyclitols 170–173
Aminoglycosides *9*, *77*, *151*, *155*, 170–173
  adverse effects *56*, **171–172**
  antiprotozoal *239*
  cats, sensitivity of 48
  caution/avoidance in renal and hepatic disease *53*
  interactions 17, 188, 392, 448, 454
  mechanism of action 9, 170–171
  mechanism of resistance 171
  ocular therapy *565*
  pharmacokinetics 171
  therapeutic drug monitoring (TDM) *37*
  see also Amikacin, Framycetin, Gentamicin, Kanamycin, Neomycin, Paromomycin, Streptomycin, Tobramycin
Aminopenicillins *155*, 162
Aminophylline 461–462
8-Aminoquinolone *237*
Amiodarone *384*, *427*, 438–439
Amitraz *204*, *222*, 224–225
Amitriptyline 136, 136–138, *137*
  in pruritis 267
Amlodipine *384*, *403*, 404–405
  emergency glaucoma treatment 571
Amorphous state 12

Amoxicillin 162–163
  Helicobacter species eradication 483
Amoxicillin-clavulanate 164, *564*
AMPA receptors 114
cAMP 7–8
  bronchoconstriction 458, 460
  NSAIDs 293
  second messenger system 121
Amphotericin B 186–188, *239*
  interactions
  lipid complex 188–189
  ocular therapy *567*
Ampicillin 162–163
Ampicillin-sulbactam 164
Amprolium *239*, 240–241
Amrinone 400–402
Anal sac inflammation, antibacterial drug choice *153*
Anaphylactoid reactions 56
Anaphylaxis 55, 149–150
Anesthesia/anesthetic agents **83–112**
  adverse drug reactions (ADRs) 45
  caution/avoidance in renal and hepatic disease *53*
  inhalational 83–95
  injectable 95–108
  local 108–111
  opioid induction 316
  topical ocular therapy 572
Angiotensin receptor blockers 422
Angiotensin-converting enzyme (ACE) inhibitors *9*, *53*, 411, **412–418**
  and potassium-sparing diuretic interactions 395
Anidulafungin 196
Antacids 482–483
Antagonists 6
Anthelmintics 200–221
  adverse drug reactions (ADRs) 45
  arsenicals 217–219
  avermectins 211–213
  benzimidazoles 200–208
  cestocides 214–217
  macrocyclic lactones 210–211
  milbemycins 213–214
  miscellaneous 219–221
  nicotinic 208–210
  spectrum of activity *206–207*
Anthracycline antibiotics 348–352
Anti-inflammatory therapy
  caution/avoidance in renal and hepatic disease *53*
  ocular *558*, *559–564*
  respiratory 462–463
  see also Corticosteroids; Glucocorticoids; NSAIDS; Steroids
Antiandrogenic drugs 539–540
Antibacterials **148–185**
  adjunctive treatments 156–157
  adverse effects 51–52, 148–149
    see also named drugs/drug classes
  aims of therapy 148
  assessment and duration of therapy 154
  β-lactam 159–163
  β-lactamase inhibitors *9*, *151*, 163–164
  bacterial protein synthesis inhibiting 170–173
  bacterial susceptibility 150
  carbapenems 168
  caution/avoidance in renal and hepatic disease *53*
  cell membrane inhibiting function 170
  cephalosporins and cephamycins *151*, *155*, 164–168
  choice of drug 152, *153*
  classification 157–158, *159*
  client compliance 151–152
  clofazimine 185
  combination therapy 154–156
  distribution to infection site (pharmacokinetic phase) 150, *151*
  dosage and frequency 154, *155–156*
  factors affecting success 150–152
  favorable environmental conditions 150–151
  fluoroquinolones *9*, *151*, *155*, 180–183, *565–566*
  history 148
  hypersensitivity 149–150
  lincosamides *151*, *156*, 176–178
  macrolides *9*, *151*, *156*, 176–178
  nitrofurans 184–185
  nosocomial infections 149
  nucleic acid synthesis inhibiting 178–185
  ocular therapy *558*, *564–566*, *567*
  oral administration and feeding *154*
  otitis externa *555*
  peptide antibiotics 169–170
  principles of therapy 148–157
  prophylactic treatment 157
  route of administration 152–154
  selection or promotion of resistance 149
  skin 152, **552–553**
  summary of activity/inactivity *185*
  treatment failure 42, *43*
  see also Metronidazole; Rifampicin (Rifampin)
Antibiotic responsive diarrhoea/ small intestinal bacterial overgrowth *153*, 154, 174, 178, 183
Anticholinergics
  antiemesis 475–476
  in bradycardia 451–452
  GIT motility-modifying 488
  in respiratory disease 462
  see also Atropine
Anticholinesterase parasiticides 232–234
Anticoagulants 453–456
Anticonvulsants 132, 367–379
  adverse effects 132
    see also named drugs
  clinical applications 132, 367–368
  formulations and dose rates 132, *368*
  physiology and pathophysiology 367
  status epilepticus *368*, 374
  therapeutic drug monitoring (TDM) *37*
Antidepressants 136–141
Antidiarrheal drugs 487–490
Antidotes, prescribing 26
Antiemetics 469–471
  cats vs dogs 48
  classes 471–477
Antiestrogens 541
Antifungals
  ocular therapy *567–568*
  otitis externa *555*
  systemic 186–197
  targets 186
Antihistamines 266–268
  adverse effects 129, 268, 477
  antiemesis 476–477
  antipruritic agents 267, *553–554*
  behavior-modification 129–130
  clinical applications 129, 267
  contraindications and precautions 129, 268
  drug interactions 130, 268, 477
  examples 266
  formulations and dose rates 129, 267
  H_1-receptor blockers 266
  H_2-receptor blockers 478–479
  ocular therapy 564
  pathophysiology 266
  pharmacokinetics 129, 268, 477
Antihypertensives 67
Antileukotrienes 467–468
Antimetabolites 358–361
Antimonials *202*, *203*, 241–242
  antiprotozoal *239*
Antiparasitic drugs 198–244, *245–260*
  adverse effects *see named drugs/drug classes*
  anticholinesterase 232–234
  antiprotozoal *199*, 236–244
  apparent inefficacy 198
  approved agents *199*
  cyclo-octadepsipeptides 214
  DEET 231–232
  external *199*, 221–244
    dosage forms *221–222*
  formamidines 224–225
  insect growth regulators/ development inhibitors (IGR/IDI) 225–226
  internal *199*, 200–221
  neonicotinoids 228
  otitis externa *556*
  phenyl pyrazoles 228–230
  public health considerations 198
  repellents 230–231
  selective toxicity 199–200, *200–204*
  semicarbazone 230
  synergists 232
  see also Pyrethrins

- Antiplatelet drugs 456–457
  - pimobendan 400
  - *see also* Aspirin
- Antiprogestins 537–538
- Antiprotozoal drugs *199*, 236–244
- Antipruritic agents *267*, *553–554*
- Antipseudomonal parenteral cephalosporins 167
- Antipseudomonal penicillins *155*, 163
- Antipsychotics (neuroleptics) 130–132
- Antisebborrheic agents *550–552*
- Antistaphylococcal penicillins *155*, 162
- Antithyroid drugs 501–503
- Antitussives *463–465*
  - nonopioid 464
  - opioid 464–465
- Antiulcer drugs 477–483
- Antiviral ocular therapy *568–569*
- Apomorphine 48, **497**
- Appetite stimulants 490–491
- Aquaretics 423
- Aqueous diffusion 28
- Area under the curve (AUC) 3, 38, 39
- Aromatase inhibitors 543
- Aromatic diamidines *204*, *237*
- Arsenicals 217–219
- Articular cartilage injury, NSAIDs 297
- Artificial tears 573
- L-asparaginase *336*, 361–362
- Aspirin 303–304
  - adverse reactions 50, 51, 56, **304**
    - cats vs dogs 47, *49*
    - articular cartilage injury 297
  - clinical applications 303
  - drug interactions 304
  - formulations and dose rates 303, *386*
  - mechanism of action 304
  - ocular therapy 563
  - pharmacokinetics 304
  - preoperative 287
  - special considerations 304
- Atenolol *384*, *386*, 419, 420, *427*, **436–437**
- Atipamezole 124
  - as antidote 74, *124*, 225
- Atovaquone *200*, *238*, 242
- Atracurium besylate 75–77
- Atropine *65*, 68, **75**
  - adverse effects 75, 452, 476
  - antiemesis 475–476
  - in bradycardia 451–452
  - carbamate poisoning 234
  - clinical applications 75
  - drug interactions 75
  - formulations and dose rates *427*, 452, 476
  - mechanism of action 75
  - mydriasis 569
  - organophosphate intoxication 234
  - pharmacokinetics 75
- Auranofin 276
- Aurothiomalate 276
- Australia, regulatory agency 56
- Autonomic nervous system (ANS) *59–82*
  - anatomical organization 59–60
  - digitalis toxicity 449
  - drugs and their clinical applications 74–82
  - parasympathetic nervous system 59–60, 61–69
  - physiological and pharmacological organization 60–61
  - sympathetic nervous system/ catecholamine synapses *59–61*, 69–74
- Avermectins 211–213
  - -milbemycin class (endectocides) 210–211
- Avoparcin 169–170
- Azaperone 116–117
- Azaspirodecanediones (azaspirones) 141–142
- Azathioprine 270–272
  - adverse effects *48*, 272
  - clinical applications 270–271
  - drug interactions 272
  - formulations and dose rates 271
  - *Helicobacter* species eradication 483
  - mechanism of action 271
  - ocular therapy 563
- Azithromycin 178, *240*
- Azlocillin 163
- Azo dye *237*
- Azocillin 163
- Azole *9*
  - antifungals 189–193
  - antiprotozoals *238*
  - selective toxicity *202*

B

- β-adrenoceptor antagonists *see* β-blockers
- β_2-adrenoceptor agonists 452–453, 459–460
- β-adrenoreceptors 70, *71*
- β_1-adrenoreceptors 73, 74, 459
- β_2-adrenoreceptors 73, 74, 459
- β-blockers *53*, 74, **419–422**
  - behavior modification 132–133
  - in canine heart disease *383*, 419–420
  - cardiac arrhythmias 426, *427*, 434–437
  - ventricular relaxation 423
- β-glucan synthase inhibitors 196
- β-lactam antibacterials 159–163
- β-lactamase inhibitors *9*, *151*, 163–164
- Bacitracin 170
  - adverse effects 45, 170
  - ocular therapy 565
- Bacterial endocarditis, drug choice *153*
- Bacterial pneumonia, drug choice *153*
- Bacterial protein synthesis inhibiting antibacterials 170–173
- Bacterial susceptibility 150
- Bactericidal drugs 158
- Bacteriostatic drugs 157
- Baquiloprim 178
- Barbiturates
  - anesthesia 96
  - in liver disease 52
- BCNU 333, *336*, **340–341**
- Behavior
  - between-species differences 18, 48
  - diagnosis 126
  - neurophysiology and neurochemistry 127–129
- Behavior-modifying drugs 126–147
  - applications 126
  - client consent and compliance 126
  - drug classes 127, 129–147
  - pretreatment screening 127
- Benazepril *384*, *403*, 417–418
- Benzene acetonitriles *239*
- Benzimidazoles 200–208
- Benznidazole *239*, 242
- Benzocaine *48*
- Benzodiazepines
  - adverse effects 119, 135–136, 375
  - antagonists 120
  - as anticonvulsant 373–375
  - behavior-modification 134–136
  - clinical applications 118, 134–135, 373–374
  - contraindications and precautions 119, 136
  - drug interactions 119, 375
  - formulations and dose rates 135, 374
  - and ketamine combinations 105
  - mechanism of action 118, 134, 374
  - pharmacokinetics 118–119, 135, 374–375
  - sedation 114, **118–120**
  - special considerations 119–120
  - therapeutic drug monitoring (TDM) *37*
- Benzoyl peroxide 552
- Benzyl benzoate 226–227
- Benzylpenicillin (penicillin G) 161
- Betamethasone (betametasone) 263
- Betamethasone (betametasone) dipropionate 561
- Betamethasone (betametasone) valerate 555
- Bethanechol 74–75
- Between-species differences 18–19, 47–48, *49*, 60
- Biguanides 513 514
- Bile acid activity 15, 30
- Biliary excretion 33
- Biliary tract obstruction 52
- Bioavailability (*F*) 3, 34, 35, 36, 39
- Bioequivalence 3
- Biophysical cellular mechanisms of drug action 4
- Biotransformation 32
- Bisacodyl 486
- Bismuth subsalicylate 489
  - *Helicobacter* species eradication 483
- Bisphosphonates 505–506
- Bite wounds, antibacterial drug choice *153*

Bleomycin *336*, 354
Blood flow, distribution by 32
Blood parasites *251*
Blood solubility of inhalational anesthesia 86–87
Blood tests, behavior-modifying drugs 127
Blood–brain barrier 67–68, 69, 292–293
Blood–eye barrier 557–559
Body fluids, modification of composition 4
Body size 49–50
Body surface area (BSA) 332
Bowel cleansers 485–486
Bradycardia 451–453
  opioid analgesics 314
Bretylium 439–440
Bromhexine hydrochloride 466
Bromide *368*, 372–373
Bromocriptine
  in adrenal dysfunction 518
  adverse effects 146, 518, 535
  mechanism of action 145–146, 518, 533
  pharmacokinetics 146, 518, 534–535
  reproductive system applications 534
  urine spraying in cats 145–146
  vascular effect 74
Bromosulphan 50
Bronchodilator drugs 459–462
Buccal administration 30
Budesonide 262–263
Bulk-forming laxatives 485
Bunamidine hydrochloride 215
Bupivacaine *9*
  adverse effects 111
  local anesthetic techniques 109–110
  pharmacokinetics 110–111
Buprenorphine *319*, 326
Buspirone 141–142
Busulfan 341
Butorphanol *319*, 326–327, *386*
  antitussive 465
Butylscopalamine 475–476
N-Butyl chloride 220
Butyrophenones
  adverse effects 117
  behavior modification 131
  clinical applications 116–117
  contraindications and precautions 117
  drug interactions 117
  formulations and dose rates 117
  mechanism of action 117
  sedation 116–117

C

Cabergoline
  adverse effects 535
  interaction with metoclopramide 473
  mechanism of action 533
  reproductive system applications 533, 534
  vascular effect 74
Calciferol 507
Calcitonin 506
Calcitriol 508
Calcium
  entry into cells 8
  homeostasis derangements 504–508
  L-type channels 9, 458–459
  N-type channels 172
  T-type channels 378
  Voltage gated calcium channels 216, 369
  preparations 507
Calcium carbonate 482–483
Calcium channel blockers
  drug efflux inhibition 211
  drug interactions
    cimetidine 479
    halothane 90
    see also named drugs
  in glaucoma 571
  in heart disease
    afterload reducers 382
    arrhythmias 422–423, 426–428, 442–445
    vasodilation 402, 404–408
Canada, reporting adverse drug reactions (ADRs) 57
Cancer chemotherapy 330–366
  alkylating agents 340–348
  antibiotics 352–354
    anthracycline 348–352
  antimetabolites 358–361
  caution/avoidance in renal and hepatic disease *53*
  common protocols 365–366
  compounding drugs 335
  drug handling 334
  formulations *336*
  general indications 330
  in liver disease 52
  miscellaneous drugs 361–364
  platinum analogs 354–358
  stability of injectable drugs 334–335
  treatment principles 331–334
    agent selection 332
    dosing 331–332
    drug resistance 332–333
    drug toxicity 333–334
  tubulin-binding agents 335–340
Cancer pathophysiology 330–331
  cell cycle 331
  growth fraction 331
Canine chronic degenerative AV valve disease (CVD) *383*, 387–388
  drugs used in treatment *382–385*, 420
Canine dilated cardiomyopathy (DCM) *383*, 387
  drugs used in treatment *382–385*, 419–420
Canine heart disease *383*, *384–385*, 387–388, 419–420
Captopril 412, 415, 416, **418**
  adverse effects 418
  formulations and dose rates 418
  pharmacokinetics 418
'Capture myopathy' 88
Carbamates 234
Carbamazepine *9*
  adverse effects 132, 376–377
  anticonvulsant action 376–377
  behavior modification 132
  clinical applications 376
  drug interactions 377
  formulations and dose rates 376
  mechanism of action 376
  pharmacokinetics 376
Carbapenems 168
Carbenicillin 163
Carbimazole 501–502, *508*
Carbonic anhydrase inhibitors (CAIs) *9*
  systemic 571
  topical 570–571
Carboplatin *336*, 357–358
Carboxypenicillins 163
Cardiac arrhythmias 424–453
  catecholamine-induced 88, 113
  combination therapy 451
  drugs *382*
    class I 425–426, 428–434
    class II (β-blockers) 426, 434–437
    class III 426, 438–442
    class IV 426–428, 442–445
  physiology and pathophysiology 424–425
Cardiac output 87
Cardiovascular collapse 56
Cardiovascular disease
  ACE inhibitors 413–414
    preclinical 414
Cardiovascular system
  altered function 52–53
  inhalational anesthetic effects 88
  morphine effects 321
  parasites *250–251*
Carprofen 293, **297–298**
  adverse effects 45, 297, **298**
  clinical applications 297
  formulations and dose rates 297
  mechanism of action 297
  ocular therapy *560*, 563, *564*
  pharmacokinetics 297–298
Cartilage injury, NSAIDs 297
Carvedilol *384*, 419, 420
  formulations and dose rates 421, *427*
Caspofungin 9, 196
Catecholamine-induced cardiac arrhythmias 88, 113
Catecholaminergic neurotransmission 61, 69–74
Catecholaminergic transmitters 72
Catecholamines and behavior 127–128
CCNU (lomustine) *336*, 341–342
Cefalonium 167
Cefalothin 167
Cefamandole 167
Cefoperazone 167
Cefotaxime 168
Cefovecin 167

Ceftazidime 168
Ceftiofur 166–167
Ceftriaxone 166
Cefuroxime 165, 168
Cell membrane inhibiting antibacterials 170
Cell membrane, modification of 4
Cellular mechanisms of drug action 4
Central nervous system (CNS)
- inhalational anesthesia effects 87–88
- neurotransmitters 113–114
- opioid analgesic effects 315, 320–321
- parasites *258*
- stimulants (amfetamines) 133–134

Cephalosporins *151*, *155*, 164–168
- adverse effects 167–168
- classification 165–167
- clinical applications 165–167
- mechanism of action 164–165
- mechanism of resistance 165
- pharmacokinetics 167
- spectrum of activity *165*, *166*

Cephamycins 164–168
Cerebral metabolic oxygen requirements ($CMRO_2$) 103
Cestocides 214–217
Charcoal, activated 489
Chemical Abstracts Registry number (CAS RN) 8
Chemical characterization, new chemical entities (NCEs) 21
Chemical name 8
Chemical reactions, non-cellular mechanisms of drug action 4
Chemoreceptor trigger zone (CTZ) 469, **470**
- antiemesis 469, 470, 471, 473, 496, 497
- emesis 496, 497

Chemotherapy *see* cancer chemotherapy
Chitin synthase inhibitors 196
Chlorambucil 9, *336*, 342–343
Chloramphenicol 9, *151*, 175–176
- adverse effects 47, *49*, *56*, **176**
- clinical applications 175
- dosage *156*
- and imipenem, interaction 168
- mechanism of action 175
- ocular therapy 565
- pharmacokinetics 175–176
- resistance 175
- spectrum of activity 175

Chlorhexidine 552
Chlorofluorocarbons (CFCs) 89
Chlorothiazide 393–394
Chlorphenamine 267
Chlorpromazine 114–116, 130–131
Chlorpyrifos *201*
Cholangitis, antibacterial drug choice *153*
Cholecystitis, antibacterial drug choice *153*
Cholinergic agonists (parasympathomimetics) 74–75
Cholinergic antagonists 75–78
Cholinergic neurotransmission 61, 65–69
Cholinesterase inhibitors 69, **78**
Chondroprotective agents 306–307
- approved 307–308

Chronic (Type C) adverse drug reactions (ADRs) 41
Ciclosporin
- immunosuppressive therapy 272–275
- ocular therapy 572–573

Cimetidine 478, 479
- adverse effects 51, 479
- drug interactions 195, 479

Ciprofloxacin 181–183
Cisapride 483–484
- drug interactions 191

Cisplatin 9, *336*, 354–357
- adverse effects *48*, 356
- clinical applications 354–355
- contraindications and precautions 356
- drug interactions 356–357
- formulations and dose rates 355
- mechanism of action 355
- mechanism of resistance 355
- pharmacokinetics 355–356
- special considerations 357

Citalopram 138–140, 139
Clarithromycin 178
- *Helicobacter* species eradication 483

Clavulanic acid 163–164
Clearance (*Cl*) 2, 3, 34, 35, 39–40
- liver 50

Clemastine 266, 267
Client issues
- prescribing principles 25
- veterinarian–client–patient relationship (VCPR) 24–25
- *see also* Compliance

Clindamycin 9, 177–178
- antiprotozoal dosages *240*
- interaction with theophylline 462
- ocular therapy 565

Clinical pharmacology, definition 1
Clofazimine *156*, 185
Clomifene acetate 541
Clomipramine 136–138, 137, 138
Clonazepam 135, 374
Clopidogrel *385*, *386*, 456–457
Cloprostenol 542–543
Clorazepate dipotassium 135
- in status epilepticus 374

Clorazepate dipotassium 134–136
Clotrimazole 189, **192–193**
Cloxacillin 162
Clozapine 131–132
Codeine 325–326
- adverse effects 326, 464
- antitussive 464
- clinical applications 325
- formulations and dose rates *319*, 325, 464
- mechanism of action 325, 464

Codeine phosphate 464
Colchicine 492–493
Collars, antiparasitic drugs 221–223
Communication with client 25
Compliance 13–14
- antibacterials 151–152
- behavior-modifying drugs 126

Concentration-dependent bactericidal drugs 158
Conjunctivitis, antibacterial drug choice *153*
Consent 25
- behavior-modifying drugs 126

Constipation
- laxatives, enemas and bowel cleansers 485–486
- opioid effects 314–315

Continuous infusion of opioids 316
Coombs' test 168
COP chemotherapy 365
Copper indomethacin 300–301
Copper storage hepatopathy 493
Corneal dehydrating agents 572
Corticosteroids
- adverse effects 50, *525*, *526*, *527*
- biosynthesis *520*
- hypoadrenocortism 524–527
- ocular therapy 263, *558*, **559–562**
  - systemic 561–562
  - topical 560–561
- respiratory disease 462–463
- structure *525*
- *see also* Glucocorticoids; Steroids

Cortisone acetate 525–526
Cough suppressants *see* Antitussives
COX *see* Cyclo-oxygenase (COX)
Cranial nerves 59
Creams
- emulsions and ointments 554
- tips for application 550

Curare 67
Cyclic adenosine monophosphate *see* cAMP
Cyclic guanosine monophosphate (cGMP) 65, 458
Cyclo-octadepsipeptides 214
Cyclo-oxygenase (COX) 9, 288, **289**, 294–295
- COX/LOX inhibitors 288, 292
- and non-COX-related mechanisms 292–293
- selectivity 289–292

Cyclophosphamide 9, *336*, 343–344
- adverse effects 51, **343–344**
- clinical applications 343
- formulations and dose rates 343
- pharmacokinetics 343

Cyclosporin *see* Ciclosporin
CYP enzymes/cytochrome P450 16, 32, 51, *52*, *53*
Cypermethrin *222*, 236
Cyproheptadine
- in adrenal dysfunction 517–518
- adverse effects 518
- appetite stimulation 490
- behavior-modification 129–130
- drug interactions 518
- formulations and dose rates 518
- mechanism of action 517–518

pharmacokinetics 518
in pruritis 267
Cyromazine *222*, 225
Cytochrome P450/CYP enzymes 16, 32, *51*, *52*, *53*
Cytokines
gene therapy 285
modulation 399
recombinant 282–284
Cytosine arabinoside *336*, 358–359
Cytotoxic drugs *see* cancer chemotherapy

D

D-MAC chemotherapy 366
Dacarbazine *see* DTIC chemotherapy
Danazol 275–276
Danofloxacin 181–183
Dantrolene 88
Decoquinate *201*, *238*, 242–243
Deet 231–232
Dehydration
corneal dehydrating agents 572
and prerenal azotemia 389
Delayed (Type D) adverse drug reactions (ADRs) 41
Deltamethrin *221*, 236
Demecarium 570
Deoxycortisosterone pivalate (DOCP) 526–527
Dependence, opioid analgesics 315
Depolarizing muscle relaxants 67, **77–78**
adverse effects 77
clinical applications 77
drug interactions 78
formulations and dose rates 77
mechanism of action 77
pharmacokinetics 77
'Depot' injections 30
Deracoxib 298
Desflurane 85, *89*, **92–93**
Desipramine 136–138
Deslorelin 530
Detomidine 120–124
Dexamethasone (dexametasone)
clinical applications 527, 541
drug interactions 287
ocular therapy 560, 561, *564*
structure *525*
topical 263
Dexamfetamine 133–134
Dexrazoxane 350
Dextromethorphan 464
Di-*N*-propylisocinchomeronate (MGK 326) 232
Diabetes mellitus 509–515
Diagnostic difficulties, adverse drug reactions (ADRs) 43–44
Diamino pyrimidine *239*
Diazepam
adverse effects 119, 135, 136
appetite stimulation 490, 491
behavior-modification 135
dosages 135, *368*, 374
pharmacokinetics 118–119, 135
premedication 315
special considerations 119–120
in status epilepticus *368*, 374
teratogenic effects 119
Diazinon 45, *221*, *222*
Dichlorophen *201*, *206*, 215
Dichlorphenamide 571
Dichlorvos *206*, 220, *222*
Diclofenac *558*
Dicloxacillin 162
Diethylcarbamazine citrate (DEC) *206*, 219–220
Diethylstilbestrol (DES) 540–541
Difloxacin 181–183
Digitalis glycosides *9*, *53*, 445–451
adverse effects 449–451
clinical applications 395–396, 445–446
dosing strategy 448
factors that alter dosage 447–448
formulations and dose rates 447
mechanism of action 446–447
pharmacokinetics 448–449
Digitalis toxicity 449–450
treatment 450–451
Digoxin *49*, *384*, *386*, 422, *427*
therapeutic drug monitoring (TDM) *37*
Dihydrocodeine tartrate 465
Dihydrotachysterol 507–508
Diltiazem *384*
cardiac arrhythmias *427*, 444–445
ventricular relaxation 422–423
Dimenhydrinate 476–477
Diminazene 45, 199, 237, 243, 251
Dinoprost tromethamine 542–543
Diphenhydramine 129–130
antiemesis 476–477
in systemic anaphylaxis 267
Diphenoxylate 487–488
Dips, antiparasitic drugs *222*, 223
Dipyrone 298–299
adverse effects 47, **299**
clinical applications 298
drug interactions 299
formulations and dose rates 298
and hyoscine 483
pharmacokinetics 298
Discospondylitis, antibacterial drug choice *153*
Disease and pharmacokinetics 18, 36–37, 50–52
Disophenol *201*
Disopyramide 432
Disposal of medicines
drug labeling 23
prescribing principles 26
Dissociative anesthetics 96–97
Distribution
dogs vs cats 47
physiological basis 31–32
Diuretics 388–395
adverse effects 55, **389–390**
caution/avoidance in renal and hepatic disease *53*
clinical applications 388
in glaucoma 571
loop 390–393
mechanism of action 388–389
potassium-sparing 394–395
thiazide 393–394
Dobutamine 80
in heart failure *384*, 396–397
Docusate sodium 485
Dog Appeasement Pheromone 144–145
Dolasetron 475
Domperidone 473–474
Dopamine *62*, *69*, *72*
agonists 533–535
antagonists 535
and behavior 127–128
cardiovascular applications 397
sedative action 114
Dopamine receptors *8*, 74
GIT 471
Doramectin 199, 210, 213, 245, 251, 253, 257
Dorzolamide 571
Dosage
choice 35
drug effects 11–19
form 12–13
individualized regimens 34–36
see also species differences
Dose–response curve 5, 6
Dose–response effect 46
Dosing frequency (*T*) 35–36, 39–40
Doxepin 129, 136, 136–138, 137
Doxorubicin *336*, 348–351
adverse effects *49*, 52, 333, **350–351**
clinical applications 348, *349*
drug interactions 351
formulations and dose rates 348–349
mechanism of action 348
mechanism of resistance 348
pharmacokinetics 349–350
Doxycycline *9*
antiprotozoal dosage *240*
ocular therapy *564*, *566*, *568*
toxicity 152
Dozolamide 571
Droperidol 116–117
Drug action 3–4
Drug choice 35
antibacterials 152, *153*
Drug classification 10
Drug concentration 33–34, 35–36, 37, 38–40
analyses 27
gradient 28–29
'steady-state' 36, 39–40
Drug and dosage form 12–13
Drug interactions 16–17, 54
classification 54
mechanisms 17
see also named drugs/drug classes
Drug labeling 22–23
and drug knowledge 25
extra-label uses 26, 45, 68
Drug nomenclature 8–10
Drug receptor binding 4–6

Drug receptors 4–8
Drug–drug hypersensitivity *55*
Drug–receptor interaction 5–6
effect 6–7
Drug-induced antibody production 150
Drugs compendia 11
Dry eye therapy *570*, **572–573**
DTIC chemotherapy *336*, 363

E

Ear *see* Topical ear medications
eCG (PMSG) *531*, *532*
Echinocandins 196
Econazole 189
Edrophonium chloride 78
EDTA 506
Efficacy studies, new chemical entities (NCEs) 21
Eflornithine *202*
Eicosanoid fatty acids 541–543
Electrolyte abnormalities
digitalis 450
diuretics 389
Elimination half-life 2–3, 34, 38–39
Emetic agents 496–497
Emodepside *204*, *206*, 214
Emollients 553
laxative 485
Emulsions 554
Enalapril 381, 412, 413–414, **416–417**
adverse effects 416
formulations and dose rates *384*, *386*, *403*, 416
pharmacokinetics 416–417
End of treatment (Type E) adverse drug reactions (ADRs) 42
Endectocides (avermectin-milbemycin class) 210–211
Endothelin receptor antagonists 424
Enrofloxacin 46, *49*, 181–183
antiprotozoal uses *240*
ocular therapy *564*
Enteric nervous system (ENS) 60
Enteric-coated tablets 16
Enterohepatic circulation 30, 33, 50
antibacterial drug recycling 149, 174
atovaquone recycling 238`
diazepam recycling 119
fipronil sulfone recycling *229*
leflunomide metabolite recycling 278
methotrexate recycling 361
NSAID recycling 292, *295*
Ursodeoxycholic acid recycling 491
warfarin recycling 456
Environmental issues
antibacterials 150–151
drug labeling 23
inhalational anesthesia 89
new chemical entities (NCEs) 21
shampoos 548–549
Enzyme induction 17, 32–33, 51
Enzyme inhibition 4, 17, 33, 51
Ephedrine 80–81, 143
Epidural 110
morphine effects 321
Epinephrine (adrenaline) 61, 69, 72, **78–79**
adverse effects 79
clinical applications 78–79
contraindications and precautions 79
convertion of noradrenaline to 128
drug interactions 79, **79**, 110, 111, 116
formulations and dose rates 79
pharmacokinetics 79
Epirubicin 352
Epsiprantel *203*, *206*, 217
Ergocalciferol 507
Ergot alkaloids 74
behavior modification 145–146
Ergotamine 74
Errors, medical and medication 14–15
Erythromycin 484–485
adverse effects 152, **484**
clinical applications 178
drug interactions 484–485
formulations and dose rates 484
mechanism of action 484
ocular therapy *565*
pharmacokinetics 484
prokinetic action 484–485
Esmolol 419, *427*, **437**
Esophageal parasites *245*
Estradiol and derivatives 540–541
Estrogen receptor *9*
Estrogens 540–541
Estrus cycle 528–529
Estrus induction *529*, *530*, 531–532, 534
Estrus postponement/suppression 536, 539
Ethanol 51
Ethanolamine derivatives 266
Ethylenediamine derivatives 266
Ethyl lactate 552
Etodolac 299
Etomidate 96, **103–104**
Etoposide *9*, 333, *336*, **338–339**
European Agency for the Evaluation of Medicinal Products (EMEA) 46–47
Excipients 13
Excretion, physiological basis of 33
Exocrine pancreatic enzyme replacements 516
Exocrine pancreatic insufficiency 515–516
Expectorants 467
Extra-label uses 26, 45, 68
Extradural administration of opioids 316–317
Eye
parasites *257–258*
see also Topical ophthalmic therapy

F

Facilitated diffusion 29
Failure of treatment (Type F) adverse drug reactions (ADRs) 42, *43*
Famotidine 478, 479
Helicobacter species eradication 483
Fat
anesthetic agent solubility 89, 91, 92, 93, 98
body composition and dose calculation 48–49
blood flow 32
body fat and pharmacokinetic effects 19
drug accumulation 31, 32, 48, 214, 232
high-fat meal and pharmacokinetic effects 15, 16
atovaquone 238, 242
benzimidazoles 205, 208
ciclosporin 274
griseofulvin 194
voriconazole 191
Febantel *204*, *206*, *207*, 208
adverse effects 48, 208
antiprotozoal action *238*
Felbamate *368*, 377–378
Feline cardiomyopathies *383*, *386*, 388
Feline infectious anemia *153*
Feliway 144–145
Female reproductive physiology 528–529
Fenbendazole *204*, *206*, 208
antiprotozoal action *238*
Fenoxycarb *225*
Fentanyl *319*, 323–324
patches 317–318
Fenthion *201*, *222*
Fever
antibacterials, adjunctive treatments 156
drug metabolism in *19*, *52*
nonimmunologically mediated 56
NSAIDs 288
Fick's law of diffusion 28
Finasteride 539–540
Fipronil *203*, *222*, 228–229
Firocoxib 287, **299–300**
First aid
drug labeling 23
prescribing principles 26
First-order process 34
First-pass effect 2, 30, 50–51
Florfenicol *156*, 176
Fluanisone 116–117
Flubendazole *206*, 207
Flucazole *567*
Flucloxacillin 162
Fluconazole 189, **192**
adverse effects 191
pharmacokinetics 190
Flucytosine 189
ocular therapy *567*
9α-fludrocortisone 526

Flumazenil 120
and propoxur *221*
Flumethasone (Flumetasone) *262*
Flumethrin 236
Flunixin meglumine 287, 300
ocular therapy 563
Fluocinolone acetonide *555*
5-fluorouracil *9*, *336*, 359–360
Fluoroquinolones *9*, *151*, *155*, 180–183
antiprotozoal *240*
ocular therapy 565–566
Fluoxetine 138–140
Flurazepam 134–136, 135
Flurbiprofen *558*
Flutamide 539–540
Fluticasone propionate 462–463
Fluvoxamine 138–140
Follicle-stimulating hormone (FSH) 528, 531, 532
Follow-up 25
Food–drug interactions 15–16
oral antibacterials and feeding *154*
Formamidines 224–225
Formestane 543
Formulation, food–drug interaction 16
Framycetin 172
FSH *see* Follicle-stimulating hormone
Fungal cell wall synthesis inhibitors 196
Furazolidone *156*, 185, *238*, **243**
Furosemide 9, 390–393
adverse effects *49*, 50, 55, **392–393**
clinical applications 390
drug interactions 168, **393**
formulations and dose rates *384*, *386*, 391–392
in hypercalcemia 505
mechanism of action 390–391
pharmacokinetics 392
special considerations 393
Fusidic acid *564*, *566*

G

G protein-coupled receptors (GPCR) *8*
adrenergic receptors 70, 121
amitraz action 224
cholinergic receptors 66
emodepside action 204, 214
neurotransmitter actions 62
opioid receptors 310
GABA (γ-aminobutyric acid)
and behavior 128–129
and benzodiazepines 134
mediated inhibition 98
receptors *9*, *63*, 96, 101–102, 118
sedative action 114, 118
Gabapentin *368*, 378
Ganglion blockers 67
Gastric acid 16, 30
Gastric adaptation, NSAIDs 295
Gastric dissolution, food–drug interactions 15
Gastric emptying 29–30
food–drug interactions 15
Gastric pH 15, 16
Gastric ulceration, NSAIDs 294–296
Gastrin releasing peptide (GRP) *63*
Gastrointestinal drugs 469–497
antidiarrheal 487–490
antiulcer 477–483
appetite stimulants 490–491
combinations 483
emetics 496–497
Helicobacter species eradication 483
laxatives, enemas and bowel cleansers 485–486
prokinetic 483–485
see also Antiemetics
Gastrointestinal tract (GIT)
absorption 29–30
cytotoxic agents 333
drug interaction mechanisms 17
muscarinic receptors 476
opioid effects 321
serotonin (5-hydroxytryptamine) receptors 470, 471
Gated ion channels 7
Gemcitabine 360
Genetics, influence on pharmacokinetics 19, 53–54
Gentamicin 172–173
adverse effects
combination therapy 45
nephrotoxicity 152
ocular therapy *564*, 565
therapeutic drug monitoring (TDM) *37*
Gingivitis, antibacterial drug choice *153*
Glaucoma therapy *558*, 570–571
Glucocorticoids 261–265
adjunctive treatments
antibacterials 156–157
antihistamines 267
adverse effects 264
anti-inflammatory effects 261–262
clinical applications 263
contraindications and precautions 265
examples 262–263
formulations and dose rate 263–264
immune system effects 262
known drug interactions 265
mechanism of action 263
metabolic effects 261
pathophysiology 261–262
pharmacokinetics 264
receptor *9*
treatment
hypercalcemia 505
otitis externa *555*
see also Corticosteroids; Steroids
α-glucosidase inhibitors 515
Glucuronidation 32, 47, 48, 51
Glutamate 114
Glutamate receptor *9*
Glycine 114
Glycopeptides 169–170
P-glycoprotein (P-gp) 54
drug transport 28, 29, 210, 211
gene mutation and pharmacogenomics 19, 54, 212, 337, 473, 475
resistance by drug efflux 212, 333
CGMP 65, 458
Gold 276–277
Gonadotropin-releasing hormone (GnRH) 528, **529–531**
Gonadotropins 531–532
Good Clinical Practice (GCP) code 21
Good Laboratory Practice (GLP) code 21
Good Manufacturing Practice (GMP) code 21
Granisetron 475
Granulocyte colony-stimulating factor (G-CSF) 282–283
Griseofulvin 194–195
adverse effects *49*, 50, **194**
clinical applications 194
contraindications and precautions 194
drug interactions 194–195
formulations and dose rates 194
mechanism of action 194
pharmacokinetics 194
Guaifenisin 467

H

H_1-receptor blockers 266
H_2-receptor blockers 478–479
Half-life 2–3, 34, 38–39
NSAIDs 295
Haloperidol 131
and fluoxetine, interaction 140
Halothane 89–90
adverse effects 51, 90
clinical applications 89
contraindications and precautions 90
drug interactions 90
pharmacokinetics 89–90
hCG 531
Heart failure 380–387
backward (WET) 381, 385–386
causes *381*
forward (COLD) 381–386
new/experimental drugs 423–424
preclinical 386–387
Helicobacter species eradication 483
Hematology
cytotoxic agents 333
NSAIDs 296–297
Hemoglobin 48
Henry's law 85
Heparin
caution/avoidance in renal and hepatic disease *53*
drug interactions 454
low molecular weight (LMWH) 455
unfractionated 453–455
Hepatic disease 36, 52, *53*
management 491–496
Hepatic enzymes *see* Cytochrome P450/CYP enzymes; Enzyme induction; Enzyme inhibition

Hepatic excretion 33
Hepatic extraction 50–51
Hepatic shunting 50–51
Hepatotoxicity 51–52
  inhalational anesthesia 88
  NSAIDs 296
Hetacillin 162–163
Hexachlorophene 47
Hexamethonium *65*, 67
Histamine
  release, opioid analgesics 315, 321
  sedative action 114
Histamine receptor antagonists *8*, 478–479
Hormones, behavior modification 142–143
5-HT *see* Serotonin
5-HT_{2A} antagonists 517
5-HT_3
  agonists 484
  antagonists 475
5-HT_4 agonists 484
Hyaluronic acid (HA) 306–307
Hydralazine *384*, *403*, 405–407
Hydrochlorothiazide *384*, *386*, 393–394
Hydrocodone 133
Hydrocodone tartrate 464–465
Hydrocortisone 263, *525*
  antipruritic therapy 553–554
  ocular therapy 561
Hydrocortisone sodium succinate (HSS) 524–525
5-hydroxytryptamine *see* Serotonin (5-HT)
Hydroxycarbamide (hydroxyurea) *336*, 363–364
Hydroxyl daunorubicin *see* Doxorubicin
Hydroxynaphthoquinone *238*
Hydroxyquinoline *238*
Hydroxyzine 129–130
Hyoscine 68
  and dipyrone 483
Hyperadrenocorticism 517–524
Hypercalcemia 504
  treatment 505–506
    diuretics 505
    glucocorticoids 505
    IV fluids 505
Hyperosmotic laxatives 486
Hypersensitivity
  antibacterials 149–150
  sulfonamides 149, 152
  Type B adverse drug reactions (ADRs) 41, **55–56**
Hypertension 67
Hyperthyroidism 499
Hypertrophic cardiomyopathy *383*
Hypnotics *see* Sedatives
Hypoadrenocorticism 524–527
Hypocalcemia 504–505
  treatment 507–508
Hypotension 407
Hypothalamic-pituitary axis, drugs acting on 517–519
Hypothyroidism 499

I

Ibuprofen 304
  adverse effects 297, 304
Idarubicin *336*
  and epirubicin 352
Idoxuridine, ocular therapy 568
Ifosfamide *336*, 344
Imidacloprid *203*, *206*, *222*, 228
Imidazole carboxamide *see* DTIC chemotherapy
Imidazoles 189
  adverse effects 51
  mechanism of action 190
  ocular therapy 567
Imidocarb dipropionate *237*
Imipenem 168
Imipenem-cilastin 168
Imipramine 136–138
Immune complex deposition 150
Immune complex formation 55
Immune response genes 54
Immune system effects of glucocorticoids 262
Immunoglobulins 466
  intravenous 277
Immunomodulatory therapy 270–286
  future 285
  pathophysiology 270
Immunoregulin 280
Immunostimulatory drugs 279–285
Immunosuppressive drugs 270–279
  ocular therapy 563
Indoleamines 128
Indometacin (indomethacin)
  articular cartilage injury 297
  and copper indometacin (indomethacine) 300–301
Infectious tracheobronchitis, antibacterial drug choice *153*
Infiltrative block 110
Information sources 10–11
Inhalational administration 30
Inhalational anesthetics
  adverse effects 87–88
    see also named drugs
  agents 89–95
  anesthetic potency: minimum alveolar concentration 87
  chemical structure 84
  clinical applications 83
  hazards 88–89
  metabolism and elimination 87
  physical properties 84–86
    solubility 85–86
    vapor pressure 84–85
  physiological principles 83–84
  rate of change of anesthetic depth 86–87
Injectable anesthetics 95
  administration guidelines 97
  adverse effects 97
    see also named drugss
  agents 97–108
  chemical structure 96
  mechanism of action 96–97
  pharmacokinetics 96
  physical properties 96
Inodilators **398–402**, 411
Inositol 1,4,5-triphosphate (ITP) 458–459
Inotropy, pimobendan 399
Insect growth regulators/development inhibitors (IGR/IDI) 225–226
Inspired concentration of inhalational anesthesia 86
Instructions to client, prescribing principles 25
Insulin 509–510
  classes 510–512
  deficiency 509–515
  glargine 512
  isophane 510–11
  neutral/soluble 510
  lente 511
  Lispro 510
  protamine zinc 511
  receptor 9
  ultralente 511–512
Interferon 568
Interferon-α 283
Interferon-ω 283–284
Interleukin-2 284
Intermittent intravenous bolus, opioids 316
Interpleural blockade 110
Intestinal mucosal enzyme activity 15
Intra-arterial administration 30–31
Intra-articular analgesia 110
Intra-articular morphine 317
Intra-ocular pressure (IOP) *see* Glaucoma
Intramuscular administration 30
Intraoperative uses of opioids 316
Intrathecal administration 30
  opioids 316–317
Intravenous administration 30
Intravenous immunoglobulins 277
Iodine 552–553
  stable 503
  see also Povidone-iodine
Ion channels 7, *9*
Ipecac syrup 496–497
Ipodate 503
Ipratropium 68–69
Irbesartan 422
Isoflurane *89*, 90–91
Isophane insulin 510–511
Isoprenaline (isoproterenol) 452
Isopropamide 68, **475–476**
Isosorbide mononitrate/dinitrate 409–410
ITP (inositol 1,4,5-triphosphate) 458–459
Itraconazole 189, **191–192**
  adverse effects 191, **192**
  ocular therapy 567
  pharmacokinetics 190
Ivermectin 211–212, 280
  adverse effects 45, 54, **211–212**, **280**
  clinical applications
    antiparasitic 211–212
    immunoregulatory 280

contraindications and precautions 280
formulations and dose rates 280
mechanism of action 211, 280
pharmacokinetics 211
selective toxicity *203*
spectrum of activity *206*, *207*

J

Jaffe reaction, cephalosporins 168
Journals 10
online 11

K

Kainate receptors 114
Kanamycin 172
Kaolin and pectin 488
Ketamine 96–97, **104–107**
adverse effects 106–107, 124
clinical applications 104–105
contraindications and precautions 107
formulations and dose rates 105
mechanism of action 105
pharmacokinetics 106
Ketoconazole
in adrenal dysfunction 521–522
adverse effects *49*, *50*, *51*, **191**, **522**
antiprotozoal action *238*
clinical applications 189, **191**
contraindications 191
drug interactions 522
formulations and dose rates 522
mechanism of action 521–522
ocular therapy 567
pharmacokinetics 190, 522
Ketoprofen 293, **301**
Ketorolac 305, *558*
Kidney *see entries beginning* Renal

L

L-deprenyl *see* Selegiline
L-thyroxine 499–500
L-tri-iodothyronine 499
L-type calcium channels *9*, 458–459
Lactation, adverse drug reactions (ADRs) 50
Lactulose 495–496
Large intestine parasites *248–249*
Latamoxef 167
Latanoprost 571
Laxatives, enemas and bowel cleansers 485–486
LD_{50} 6
Leflunomide 277–278
Lente insulin 511
Leukotrienes 467–468
Levamisole
as anthelmintic *203*, *206*, 209–210
as immunostimulant 280–281
Levetiracetam *368*, 379
Levothyroxine 499–500, *508*
LH *see* Luteinizing hormone
Lidocaine (lignocaine) *9*, *53*
adverse effects *49*, *51*, **428–429**
as antiarrhythmic 428–429
clinical applications 428
drug interactions 429
formulations and dose rates *427*, 428
local anesthetic techniques/dosages 109–110
mechanism of action 428
ocular therapy 572
special considerations 429
therapeutic drug monitoring (TDM) *37*
Ligand-gated ion channel receptors *9*
Ligands, receptors and *8–9*
Lime sulfur 227
D-limonene 227
Linalool oil 227
Lincomycin 177
Lincosamides *151*, *156*, 176–178
antiprotozoal dosages *240*
Lindane *203*
Lineweaver–Burke plot *5*
Liothyronine 499
Lipid diffusion 28–29
Lipid solubility
antibacterials 151
distribution 32
Lipid theory of anesthesia 83–84
Lipopeptides 196
Lipoxygenase (LOX) *9*, 288, 292
Liquid–gas interface, inhalational anesthesia 84–85
Lisinopril *384*, 412, 418
Lithium 146
therapeutic drug monitoring *37*
Liver
blood flow 50–51
drug metabolism 50–52
function tests 127
parasites *249*
see also entries beginning Hepatic
Loading dose (LD) 35, 40
Local anesthetics 108–111
adverse effects 111
clinical applications 108–109, *110*
comparative pharmacology *111*
formulations and dose rates 109
mechanism of action 109
ocular therapy *558*, 572
pharmacokinetics 110–111
techniques 109–110
Lomustine (CCNU) *336*, 341–342
Loop diuretics 390–393
Loperamide 487–488
Lorazepam 134–136
in status epilepticus 374
Losartan 422
Low molecular weight heparin (LMWH) 455
LOX (lipoxygenase) 288, 292
Lubricants
laxatives 486
ocular 573
Lufenuron
as antifungal 196
as antiparasitic *201*, *206*, *222*, 226
Lumbosacral epidural *see* Epidural
Luteinizing hormone (LH) 528, 529, 531, 532
Lymphatic parasites *252*
Lysine 568

M

Macrocyclic lactone 210–211
Macrolides *9*, *151*, *156*, 176–178
antiprotozoal *240*
Magnesium compounds 482–483
Malathion *201*
Male reproductive physiology 528
Malignant hyperthermia 88
Malnourishment, influence on pharmacokinetics 18–19, 52
Mannitol 571
Manufacturing process, new chemical entities (NCEs) 21
Marbofloxacin 51, 181–183
Maropitant 474–475
Mast cell stabilizers, ocular therapy 564
Mastitis, antibacterial drug choice *153*
Material Safety Data Sheet (MSDS) 23
Maximum effect 5
Maximum tolerated dose (MTD), cancer chemotherapy 332
Meal type and size, food–drug interactions 16
Mebendazole *206*, 207
Mechlorethamine 333, **345**
Meclofenamic acid 301
Medetomidine *71*, 120–124
atipamezol as antidote to 74
pharmacokinetics 121–122
as premedicant 315
Medical and medication errors 14–15
Medroxyprogesterone acetate 142–143, 535
Megestrol acetate 142–143, 278, 535
adverse effects *49*, 278
clinical applications 278
contraindications and precautions 278
mechanism of action 278
Meglumine antimonate *9*, *239*, 241–242
Melarsomine hydrochloride *206*, 218–219
Melatonin, and behavior 128
Meloxicam 287, **301–302**
adverse effects 297, 302
clinical applications 301
formulations and dose rates 301
mechanism of action 301–302
pharmacokinetics 302
Melphalan *336*, 345–346
Membrane permeation 32
Mepacrine *see* Quinacrine hydrochloride
Meperidine (pethidine) *319*, 322
Mepivacaine 109–110

Metabolism
- dogs vs cats 47
- and elimination of inhalational anesthesia 87
- physiological basis 32–33

Metabotropic receptors 114
Metaflumizone *204*, *222*, 230
Metered dose inhalers (MDI) and spacers 463
Metergoline *533*, *535*
Methadone *319*, 322–323
Methazolamide *571*
Methimazole *49*
Methicillin *see* Meticillin
S-methoprene *204*, *221*, *222*, *225*
Methotrexate *9*, *336*, 360–361
Methoxyflurane 93–94
- adverse effects 51, 93–94
- drug interactions 94
- pharmacokinetics *89*, 93

N-methyl-D-asparate (NMDA) *see* NMDA receptors
Methylergometrine *543*
Methylphenidate 133–134
Methylprednisolone 51
Methylxanthines *459*, **461–462**
Meticillin 162
- resistance (MRSA) *162*, *164*, *165*, 168, 169, *179*, *181*, *184*

Metoclopramide **472–473**, *535*
Metronidazole *151*, 183
- adverse effects *49*, 183
- antiprotozoal dosages *238*
- clinical applications 183
- dosage *156*
- *Helicobacter* species eradication 483
- mechanism of action and resistance 183
- pharmacokinetics 183
- selective toxicity *202*
- spectrum of activity 183

Metyrapone 523–524
Mexiletine *385*, *427*, 432–433
Mezlocillin 163
MGK 264 (*N*-Octyl bicycloheptene dicarboximide) *202*, 232
MGK 326 (Di-*N*-propylisocinchomeronate) *222*, 232
Mibolerone 538–539
Micafungin 196
Miconazole 189
- emollient *553*
- ocular therapy *567*

Midazolam 118–120
- drug interactions 191
- as premedicant 315
- in status epilepticus 374

Mifepristone 537–538
Milbemycin oxime *206*, 213
Milbemycins 213–214
Milrinone and amrinone 400–402
Miotics *558*, 569–570
Misoprostol 480–481
Mithramycin *see* Plicamycin
Mitotane 522–523
Mixoxantrone (mitozantrone) 351–352
Mobility, influence on pharmacokinetics 19
Moisturizing agents *553–554*
Monoamine oxidase inhibitors (MAOIs) *9*, 140–141
- drug interactions 141
  - amitraz *204*
  - antihistamines 129, 130
  - SSRIs 139–140
  - tricyclic antidepressants 138

Monoamine oxidase (MAO) 72
Monoclonal antibody therapy 285
Montelukast 467–468
Montmorillonite 488–489
MOPP chemotherapy 365
Morphine 318–322
- adverse effects 47, 48, *49*, 50, 51, **320–322**
- clinical applications 320
- contraindications and precautions 322
- drug interactions 322
- formulations and dose rates 320
- intra-articular 317
- mechanism of action 320
- pharmacokinetics 320

Motility-modifying drugs 487–490
Moxidectin *206*, 213–214, *222*
MRSA resistance *162*, *164*, *165*, 168, 169, *179*, *181*, *184*
Mucolytics 465–467
Multidrug resistance protein 1 (Mdr1) 54 (see also P-glycoprotein or P-gp)
Mupirocin 554
Muramyl tripeptide 282
Muscarinic acetylcholine (ACh) receptor 60–61, 65
Muscarinic agonists 67–68, 127
Muscarinic antagonists 68–69, 127
Muscarinic receptors *8*, 60–61, 65, *68*
- airways 462
- and behavior 127
- drugs affecting 67–69, 127
- GIT 476

Musculoskeletal system
- inhalational anesthesia effects 88
- morphine effects 321
- parasites *252*

Mydriatics *558*, *569*
Myocardial toxicity due to doxorubicin 350
Myocardial toxicity *see* Digitalis toxicity

N

Nalbuphine *319*, 328–329
Nalmefene *319*, 329
Nalorphine *319*, 328
Naloxone 133, *319*
Naltrexone 133
Naproxen 305
- adverse effects 30, 297
- clinical applications 305
- mechanism of action 305
- pharmacokinetics 305

Narrow-spectrum penicillins 161
Natamycin *567*
Natural remedies and hepatic enzymes 51
Nausea and vomiting, opioid analgesics 314, 321
Naxolone 133, **328**
Neomycin 172
- ocular therapy *565*

Neonates
- adverse drug reaction (ADRs) 50
- antibacterials in 152
- drug metabolism in *19*

Neonicotinoids 228
Neosporin ointment *564*
Neostigmine *65*, 78
Neuroendocrine modulation 412–418
Neuroleptanesthesia 113
Neurones, pre- and postganglionic 59–60, 61
Neurotransmission, ANS 61
Neurotransmitters
- ANS 61, *62–64*, 69–74
- CNS 113–114
- enteric 60

New drugs/new chemical entities (NCEs)
- chemical characterization 21
- development 20–22
- discovery 20–21
- efficacy studies 21
- environmental fate and toxicity 21
- heart failure 423–424
- manufacturing process 21
- pharmacovigilance/postmarketing experiences 22
- regulatory review 22
- research 21
- safety 21
- triazoles 193–194

New Zealand, reporting adverse drug reactions (ADRs) 57
Niacinamide 279
Nicergoline 144
Niclosamide *201*, *206*, *207*, 215–216
Nicotinic acetylcholine receptor nAChR 61, 65, 203
Nicotinic agonists 66–67
Nicotinic antagonists 67, 75–78
Nicotinic anthelmintics 208–210
Nicotinic receptors *9*, 61, 65, *66*
Nifurtimox *203*, *238*, 243
Nikkomycin Z 196
Nikkomycins 196
Nitenpyram *203*, 228
Nitrate tolerance 408
Nitrates 408–411
Nitric oxide (NO) 60–61, *64*, *65*
Nitrofurans 184–185, *238*
Nitrofurantoin *156*, 184–185
Nitroglycerin *385*, *403*, 408–409
- paste *386*

Nitroimidazole *238*
Nitroprusside *403*, 408, **410–411**
Nitroscanate *206*, 220–221

Nitrous oxide *89*, 94–95
Nizatidine 478, 479
NK_1 receptor antagonists 474–475
NMDA receptors 114
  antagonism 94–95, 96
Noise phobia 135, 145
Non-cellular mechanisms of drug action 4
Nonadrenergic and noncholinergic (NANC) transmitters 61
Nondepolarizing muscle relaxants 67, **75–77**
  adverse effects 76–77
  clinical applications 75–76
  drug interactions 77
  formulations and dose rates 76
  mechanism of action 76
  pharmacokinetics 76
Nonopioid antitussives 464
Nonproprietary (common or generic) name 8
Nonreceptor binding sites 31
Nonsteroidal antiinflammatory drugs *see* NSAIDs
Nonsystemic antacids 482–483
Noradrenaline *see* Norepinephrine (noradrenaline)
Noradrenergic transmission *71*, 72
Norepinephrine (noradrenaline) 61, *62*, 69, 70, 72
  and behavior 128
  sedative action 114
Norfloxacin 181–183
Nortriptyline 136–138
Nosocomial infections 149
NSAIDs 287–308
  adverse effects 45, **294–297**
  approved for small animal practice 297–303
  clinical applications 287–288
  known drug interactions 297
  in liver disease 52
  mechanism of action 288–293
  metabolism in cats vs dogs 47
  ocular therapy *558*, 562–563
  pharmacokinetics and pharmacodynamics 293–294
  prostaglandins and inflammation 288–289
  in renal disease 52
  unapproved agents for small animal practice 303–306
Nuclear receptors *9*
Nucleic acid synthesis inhibiting antibacterials 178–185
Nucleic acids *9*
Nystatin 555

O

Obesity, influence on pharmacokinetics 18–19
N-Octyl bicycloheptene dicarboximide (MGK 264) 232
Ocular therapy 557–573
  achieving adequate tissue concentrations 557–559
  anti-inflammatory *558*, 559–564
  antibacterial *558*, 564–566, 567
  antifungal 567–568
  antiviral 568–569
  corneal dehydrating agents 572
  drug characteristics 559
  dry eye 570, **572–573**
  glaucoma *558*, 570–571
  lesion location and routes of administration 557
  lubricants 573
  miotics *558*, 569–570
  mydriatics *558*, *569*
  parasites *257–258*
  special considerations 557–559
  topical anesthetics *558*, 572
Off-label (extra-label) uses 26, 45, 68
Ofloxacin *564*
Ointments 554, *564*
Omeprazole *9*, 481–482
  adverse effects 51, 482
Ondansetron 475
Online journals 11
Opioid agonists 133, **318–326**
  partial 326–328
Opioid analgesics 310–329
Opioid antagonists 133, *319*, **328–329**
Opioid antitussives 464–465
Opioid GIT motility-modifying drugs 487–488
Opioid receptors *8*, *63*
  adverse effects in relation to 313
  agonist and antagonist activities *318*
  classes 310–311, *313*
  drug interactions 311–313
  effector mechanisms 311
Opioids
  adverse effects 314–315
  chemical structure 310
  clinical applications 310
  dosages and duration of action *318–319*
  importance of pre-emptive analgesia 309–310
  indications and techniques 315–318
  pharmacodynamics *318*
  pharmacokinetics 313–314
  and sedatives, 'neuroleptanesthesia' 113
Oral administration 29–30
Oral antibacterials 152
Oral calcium preparations *507*
Oral cephalosporins 167
Oral glycerin 571
Oral hypoglycemic agents 55, **512–515**
Orbifloxacin 181–183
Organophosphates *9*, 68, **232–234**
  adverse effects *49*, 233
  drug interactions 234
  pharmacokinetics 232–233
  toxicity 233–234
  treatment of toxicity 233
Ormetoprim *156*, 178, *239*
Osteo-arthritis 297
Osteomyelitis, antibacterial drug choice *153*
Otitis externa, topical medications *153*, *554–556*
Otitis media/interna, antibacterial drug choice *153*
Ototoxicity 556
Ovulation induction 529, 530, 532
Oxacillin 162
Oxantel *203*, *207*, 209
Oxatomide 266, 267
Oxazepam 134–136, 135, 491
Oxibendazole 205, *206*, *207*
Oximes 233–234
Oxymorphone *319*, 323
Oxytocin 532–533

P

P-glycoprotein (P-gp) 54
Paclitaxel *336*, 339–340
Pain
  animals presenting in 315
  importance of pre-emptive analgesia 309–310
  recognition and management 309
Pancreatic enzyme activity 15
Pancreatic enzyme replacements 516
Pancreatic function disorders 509–516
Pancreatic insufficiency 515–516
Pancreatic parasites *249*
Pancuronium bromide 75–77
Paracetamol (acetaminophen) 305–306
  adverse effects 47, *48*, 51, **305–306**
  clinical applications 305
  CNS action 293
  toxicity 306
Paraffin 486
Parasites *245–260*
Parasympathetic nervous system 59–60, 61–69
Parasympatholytics 75–78
Parasympathomimetics (cholinergic agonists) 74–75
Parathyroid disease 503–508
Parathyroid hormone (PTH) replacement 508
Paregoric 487–488
Parenteral antibacterials 152–154
Parenteral calcium preparations *507*
Parenteral cephalosporins 167
Paromomycin *239*
Paroxetine 138–140
Partial agonists 6
  opioid 326–328
Partial coefficients, solubility of inhalational anesthesia 85–86
Particle size and drug absorption 13
Parturition induction 533, 538
Pathology and pharmacokinetics 18, 36–37, 50–52
Penicillamine 493
Penicillin G 161
Penicillin V 161
Penicillin-induced hypersensitivity 55
Penicillins *151*, *155*, 159–161
  classes 161–163
Pentamidine isetionate 234, *237*, 243, 250, 251

Pentazocine *319*, 327
Pentobarbital *96*
Pentosan polysulfate 307–308
Pentoxifylline 278–279
Peptide antibiotics 169–170
Peptide immunotherapy for autoimmune/allergic disease *285*
Periodontitis, antibacterial drug choice *153*
Peripheral muscle relaxants 67
Peripheral nerve blocks 110
Peripheral nervous system (PNS) *59*
Permethrin *221*, *222*, 235–236
  adverse drug reactions (ADRs) 45, 48, **236**
  toxicology 236
Pethidine (meperidine) *319*, 322
Pharmaceutical drug interactions 54
Pharmacodynamics
  between-species differences 18
  definition 3
  drug interactions 54
Pharmacogenetic differences 19, *53–54*
Pharmacokinetics 27–40
  between-species differences 18
  definition 2–3
  and disease 18, 36–37, *50–52*
  dose calculations 38–40
  drug interactions 54
  physiological basis 27–33
  and prescribing issues 33–37
  and therapeutic drug monitoring (TDM) 37
  within-species differences 18–19
Pharmacology, definition 1
Pharmacovigilance (postmarketing surveillance) 22, 44–46
Phenethicillin 161
Phenobarbital (phenobarbitone) 368–371
  adverse effects 51, **132**, **370**
  behavior modification 132
  clinical applications 368
  drug interactions 194–195, **370–371**
  formulations and dose rates *368*, 369
  mechanism of action 368–369
  pharmacokinetics 269–270
Phenobarbitone *see* Phenobarbital
Phenothiazines
  adverse effects 115–116, 471
  antiemetic action 471–472
  behavior modification 130–131
  clinical applications 114–115
  contraindications and precautions 116
  derivatives 266
  drug interactions 116, 471–472, 535
  formulations and dose rates 115, 471
  and ketamine combinations 105
  mechanism of action 115, 471
  pharmacokinetics 115, 471
  sedative action 114–116
Phenoxybenzamine *71*, 73–74, 81–82
Phenoxymethyl-penicillin (penicillin V) 161
Phentolamine *71*, 73–74, 81–82
Phenyl pyrazoles 228–230
Phenylbutazone 302
Phenylephrine *569*
Phenylpropanolamine **79–80**, 143
  adverse effects 80
  clinical applications 79–80, *543*
  contraindications and precautions 80
  drug interactions 80
Phenytoin *9*
  adverse effects 376, 429
  antiarrhythmic action 429
  anticonvulsant action 375–376
  clinical applications 375
  drug interactions 376, 429
  formulations and dose rates 375, *427*, 429
  mechanism of action 375, 429
  pharmacokinetics 375–376, 429
Pheromones 144–145
Phospholine iodide *570*
Physical effects of non-cellular mechanisms of drug action 4
Physical state, influence on pharmacokinetics 18–19
Physicochemical cellular mechanisms of drug action 4
Physicochemical non-cellular mechanisms of drug action 4
Physicochemical properties, food–drug interaction 16
Physiological effects 13
Pilocarpine *570*
  extra-label uses 68
Pimobendan *385*, 398–400, *403*
Pindolol 133
Pinocytosis (receptor-mediated endocytosis) 29
Piperacillin 163
Piperazine *53*, *203*, *206*, 219
  derivatives 266
Piperonyl butoxide (PBO) *202*, 232
Piroxicam 287, **306**
Placebo effects 19–20
Plasma membrane enzymes 7–8
Plasma membrane-bound protein kinases, stimulation of 8
Platinum analogs 354–358
Plicamycin
  cancer chemotherapy *336*, 352–353
  in hypercalcemia *506*
PMSG (eCH) *531*, 532
Pneumocandins 196
Poiseuille–Hagan formulation 458
Polyene antibacterials, ocular therapy *567*
Polyethylene glycol 3350 (PEG) 486
Polymorphous state 12
Polymyxin B, ocular therapy *566*
Polymyxins *56*, *151*, **170**
Polypeptide hormones 529–535
Polysulfated glycosaminoglycans (PSGAGs) 306–307, **308**
Ponazuril *239*
Posaconazole 193
Positive inotropic drugs *382*, *395–397*
Positive lusitropic agents (ventricular relaxation) *382*, 400, **422–423**
Postganglionic synapses 69, *70*
Postmarketing surveillance (pharmacovigilance) 22, 44–46
Potassium-sparing diuretics 394–395
Povidone-iodine *552–553*
  ocular therapy *567*
  see also Iodine
Praziquantel *203*, *206*, *207*, 216–217
Prazosin 74, *403*, **407–408**
Prednisolone 263, *525*, **527**
  and aurothiomalate 276
  and ciclosporin 272
Prednisolone acetate, ocular therapy *558*, *560*
Pregnancy
  adverse drug reaction (ADRs) 50
  and antibacterials 152
  influence on pharmacokinetics 18–19
  see also Abortion
Preoperative analgesia 315–316
Prerenal azotemia 389
Prescribing
  instructions 26
  pharmacokinetics 33–37
  principles 23–26
Prilocaine 111
Primaquine phosphate *237*, 243–244
Primidone 371–372
Procainamide *37*, *53*, *385*, *427*, 431–432
Procarbazine 346–347
Prochlorperazine 114–116
Progesterone *535–537*
Progesterone receptor *9*
Progestins *535–537*
  behavior modification 142–143
Prokinetic gastrointestinal drugs 483–485
Prolactin *533*, *534*, *535*
Promazine 114–116
Promethazine 114–116
Propanolol *71*, 419, *427*, **435–436**
  adverse effects *50*, 51, **133**, **436**
  behavior modification 132–133
  clinical applications 435
  drug interactions 436
  formulations and dose rates 436
  mechanism of action 435–436
  pharmacokinetics 436
  special considerations 436
Propantheline 475–476
Propantheline bromide 68
Proparacaine *572*
Propentofylline 146–147
Propofol 99–101
Proprietary names 10
Propylamine derivatives 266
Propylene glycol *56*
Propylthiouracil *9*, *48*
Prostacyclin analogs 424
Prostaglandin agonists *571*
Prostaglandin inhibition 294–295

Prostaglandins 288–289
 $F_{2\alpha}$ ($PGF_{2\alpha}$) and derivatives 541–543
Prostanoid receptors *8*
Prostatitis, antibacterial drug choice *153*
Protamine zinc insulin 511
Protectants, GIT 488–489
Protein binding
 age, effect on *50*
 atovaquone 200
 diazepam *375*
 drug distribution 31
 drug interactions 17, *54*
 in liver disease 36, 52
 local anesthetic agents 111
 macrolides 177
 niclosamide 201, 216
 NSAIDs 293
 phenytoin 376
 sulfonamides 180
 tricyclic antidepressants (TCAs) 137
 valproic acid 377
 warfarin 456
Protein synthesis 7
Protein theory of anesthesia 83, 84
Proton pump inhibitors 481–482
Pruritic skin diseases 267, 548, 553–554
Pseudoallergic drug reactions 56
Psyllium 485
Puberty, postponement of 529, 530
Pustular dermatitis, antibacterial drug choice *153*
Pyelonephritis, antibacterial drug choice *153*
Pyexia *see* Fever
Pyoderma, antibacterial drug choice *153*
Pyometra 534, 537–538
Pyrantel *203*, *206*, *207*, 209
Pyrethrins *222*, 231, **235**
 and synthetic pyrethroids *204*, 234–236
Pyrimethamine 178, *201*, *239*
Pyrimidine derivatives *567*
Pyriprole *203*, *222*, 229–230
Pyriproxyfen *204*, 221, 226
Pyrothorax, antibacterial drug choice *153*

Q

Quinacrine *204*
Quinacrine hydrochloride *237*, 244
Quinidine *37*, *53*, *427*, 429–431

R

Ramipril 398, 412
Ranitidine 478, 479
 Helicobacter species eradication 483
Reassessment, prescribing principles 25
Receptor sites, drug interactions mechanisms 17
Receptor-mediated effects 4
 endocytosis (pinocytosis) 29
Receptors
 cats vs dogs 48
 downregulation 7
 and ligands *8–9*
 occupancy 7
 regulation 7
 selectivity and specificity 6
 upregulation 7
Recombinant cytokines 282–284
Record keeping, prescribing principles 25
Rectal administration 30
Regressin-V 284
Regulatory agencies *56–57*
 Australia *56*
 Canada *57*
 New Zealand *57*
 South Africa *57*
 UK *57*
 USA *57*
Regulatory agency approval number 23
Regulatory review of new drugs 22
Remifentanil *319*, 324–*325*
Renal clearance 39
Renal disease 36–37, *52*, *53*
Renal excretion 33
 drug interactions mechanisms 17
Renal function tests 127
Renal toxicity
 cisplatin 356
 digitalis 450
 gentamicin 152
 inhalational anesthesia 88
 NSAIDs 296
Repellents 230–231
Reporting adverse drug reactions (ADRs) 44–46, *56–57*
Reproduction *528–545*
 physiology 528–*529*
 therapies
  eicosanoid fatty acids *541–543*
  miscellaneous *543*
  polypeptide hormones *529–535*
  steroids *535–541*
Research, new drugs/new chemical entities (NCEs) 21
Resistance
 antibacterials 149
  MRSA *162*, *164*, *165*, 168, 169, *179*, *181*, *184*
 antiparasitic drugs 223–224
 cancer chemotherapy 332–333
 diuretic 389–390
Resmethrin 235
Respiratory disease
 clinical signs 458–459
  pathological regulation of airway size 458–459
 management **458–468**
  anticholinergics 462
  antileukotrienes 467–468
  antitussives 463–*465*
  bronchodilator drugs 459–462
  expectorants 467
  methylxanthines 459, **461–462**
  mucolytics 465–467
  topical anti-inflammatory therapy 462–463
Respiratory system
 depression, opioid analgesics 314, 321
 inhalational anesthesia effects 88
 parasites *249–250*
Ribosomes *9*
Rifampicin *151*, 184
 dosage *155*
 and terbinafine interaction 195
Romifidine 120–124, 121–122
Ropivacaine 109
Rotenone *200*, 227–228
Routes of administration 29–31

S

S-adenosyl methionine (SAMe) 494
S-methoprene *204*, *221*, *222*, *225*
Safety issues
 antiparasitic drugs 198
 cancer chemotherapy 334
 drug labeling 23
 inhalational anesthesia 88–89
 Material Safety Data Sheet (MSDS) 23
 new drugs/new chemical entities (NCEs) 21
Salbutamol (albuterol) sulfate 460–461
Salicylic acid 551
Salt forms 13
Sarafloxacin 181–183
Seborrheic disorders 548
Second messengers 121
 accumulation of multiple intracellular 8
Sedatives 113–125
 agents 114–124
 clinical applications 113
 CNS physiology 113–114
 vs tranquilizers 113
Selamectin *206*, 212, *222*
Selective serotonin reuptake inhibitors (SSRIs) 138–140
Selectivity 6–7
 autonomic drug selectivity
 SSRI
 agonists
 antagonistis/inhibitors
 antibacterial drugs
 antiparasitic drugs 199–204
 antifungal drugs
 immunomodulation
 NSAIDs and COX selectivity
 opioids
 cancer chemotherapy
 cardiac drugs
 GIT drugs
Selegiline
 in adrenal dysfunction 518–519
 behavior modification 140–141
Selenium sulfide 551–552

Semicarbazone 230
Septic arthritis, antibacterial drug choice *153*
Septicemia, antibacterial drug choice *153*
Serotonin (5-hydroxytryptamine or 5-HT)
  agonists 484
  antagonists 475, *533–535*
  and behavior 128
  receptors *8*, *63*
    GIT 470, 471
  sedative action 114
Serotonin syndrome 138, 139–140
Serratia marcescens 284
Sertraline 138–140
Sevoflurane *89*, 91–92
Sex
  adverse drug reaction (ADRs) 50
  influence on pharmacokinetics 18
Sex hormones 50
Shampoos, moisturizers and conditioners *547*, 550–554
Signalling mechanisms and drug action 7–8
Sildenafil *385*, 411–412
Silver sulfadiazine 567–568
Silymarin 494–495
Skin
  diseases *153*, 548, 552–553
    pruritic 267, 548, 553–554
  parasites *252–257*
  reactions
    to antibacterials 150
    to cytotoxic agents 333–334
  see also Topical dermatological therapy
Sleep/wake cycle 128
Small intestine
  bacterial overgrowth/antibiotic-responsive diarrhea *153*, 174, 178, 183
  parasites *245–248*
Sodium chloride 572
Sodium cromoglycate 564
Sodium phosphate enemas *48*
Sodium stibogluconate *239*
Solubility of inhalational anesthesia 85–87
Solvated state 13
Sotalol *385*, *386*, *427*, 440–442
South Africa, reporting adverse drug reactions (ADRs) 57
Spacers 463
Species differences 18–19, 47–48, *49*, 60
Specificity 6–7
Spectinomycin *151*, 173
Spiramycin 178
Spironolactone *385*, *386*, **394–395**, 418–419
  and HCT *384*
Splanchnic blood flow 15
Spot-ons 549
  antiparasitic drugs *222*, 223
Sprays 549
  antiparasitic drugs *222*, 223
Staphage lysate 284
Staphoid AB 284–285
Status epilepticus *368*, 374
Sterculia 485
Steroids 535–541
Stimulant laxatives 486
Stomach parasites *245*
Storage of medicines
  instructions, drug labeling 23
  prescribing principles 25
Streptomycin 172
Streptozocin 347
Structural nonspecificity 3–4
Structure-dependent drug action 3
Subconjunctival corticosteroids 561
Subconjunctival ocular injections 557
Subcutaneous administration 30
Sublingual administration 30
Succinylcholine 47, **77–78**
Sucralfate 479–480
Sufentanil 324–325
Sulfadimethoxine *240*
Sulfasalazine 489–490
Sulfonamides *151*, *155*
  adverse effects 47, 48, 53–54, 55, **180**
  antiprotozoal dosages *240*
  clinical applications 179
  hypersensitivity 149, 152, 180
  mechanism of action 178–179
  mechanism of resistance 179
  ocular therapy 566
  pharmacokinetics 179–180
  and potentiators 178–180
  selective toxicity *201*
  spectrum of activity 179
Sulfonylureas *9*, 512–513
Sulfur 550–551
Supraventricular arrhythmias 426
Surgery, prophylactic antibacterial treatment 157
Suxamethonium *53*, *65*, 67
Sympathetic nervous system 59–61
  catecholamine synapses 69–74
Sympathomimetics 72–74
  in bradycardia 452–453
  in heart failure 396–397
  indirect *71*, 73
Synergists 232
Synthetic L-tri-iodothyronine 499
Synthetic levothyroxine 499–500
Systemic allergic reaction 55

T

Tachyarrhythmia
  reflexive 407
  therapy 425–451
Tacrolimus 554
  ocular therapy 573
Tamoxifen acetate 541
Tar shampoos 551
Tegaserod 484
Teicoplanin 169, 170
Tepoxalin 302
Terbinafine 195
Terbutaline *427*, 453
Terbutaline sulfate 460
Testosterone 528
  and deriviatives 538–539
Tetracyclines *151*, *156*, 173–175
  adverse effects *49*, 50, *56*, **174–175**
  antiprotozoal dosages *240*
  clinical applications 174
  mechanism of action 173
  mechanism of resistance 173
  and niacinamide 279
  ocular therapy 566
  pharmacokinetics 174
  spectrum of activity 173–174
Theophylline *8*, *37*
  and aminophylline 461–462
Therapeutic drug monitoring (TDM) 37
Thiabendazole *see* Tiabendazole
Thiacetarsamide sodium *206*, 217–218
Thiamazole 501–502, *508*
Thiamine 56
Thiamphenicol 176
Thiazide diuretics *9*, 393–394
Thiazolidinediones 514–515
Thienopyridines 456–457
Thiopental 96, **97–99**
Thiopeta 347–348
Thiopurine S-methyltransferase (TPMT) 54
Thioridazine 130–131
Thiourylene antithyroid drugs 501–502
Thyroid disease 498–499
  antithyroid drugs 501–503
Thyroid extract 499
Thyroid hormone
  receptor *9*
  replacement therapy 499–500
  secretion and transport 498–499
  synthesis 498
  therapeutic drug monitoring *37*
Thyroxine 499–500
Tiabendazole 205, *555*
Ticarcillin 163
Ticarcillin-clavulanate 164
Ticlopidine 457
Tiletamine 96–97
Tiletamine-zolazepam 107–108, 118–120
Time-dependent bactericidal drugs 158
Tissue binding 32
Tissue plasminogen activator (TPA) *563*
Tissue solubility
  distribution 32
  of inhalational anesthesia 87
Tobramycin 173
  ocular therapy *565*
Tocainide *427*, 433–434
Tolazoline 124
Tolerance and dependence, opioid analgesics 315
Tolfenamic acid 303
Toltrazuril *239*
Toluene 220
Topical administration 30

Topical anti-inflammatory therapy, respiratory disease 462–463
Topical dermatological therapy *546–556*
- antimicrobials 152, **552–553**
- creams, emulsions and ointments *554*
- glucocorticoids 263
- otitis externa *153*, *554–556*
- pathophysiology 546
- practical tips 546–550
- shampoos, moisturizers and conditioners *547*, 550–554

Topical ear medications 548
- application 549–550
- otitis externa *153*, *554–556*

Topical ophthalmic therapy 557–558, *558*
- anesthetics *558*, *572*
- corticosteroids 263, *558*, **560–561**
- glaucoma *558*, 570–571
- glycerin 572
- NSAIDs *558*, 563

Total intravenous anesthesia (TIVA) 95, 316
Toxicity 35
- antibacterials 152
- antiparasitics 199–200, *200–204*, 556
- cancer chemotherapy 333–334
- new drugs/new chemical entities (NCEs) 21
- organophosphates 233–234
- paracetamol (acetaminophen) 306
- *see also* Digitalis toxicity; Hepatotoxicity; Renal toxicity

Toxoplasmosis, antibacterial drug choice *153*
Tramadol 327–328
Tranquilizers
- vs sedatives 113
- *see also* Sedatives

Transdermal administration 30
- fentanyl patches 317–318
- thiamazole 502

Transfereases 32
Transmembrane carriers 29 (see also P-gp)
Transport across membranes 27–29
Transport proteins *9*
Travaprost 571
Tri-iodothyronine 499, *508*
Triamterene 394, **395**
Triazines *239*
Triazolam 135
Triazoles 189
- new 193–194
- pharmacokinetics 190

Tricin ointment *564*
Triclosan 553
Tricyclic antidepressants (TCAs) *9*, *71*, 136–138
- and SSRIs interaction 140

Trifluralin *204*
Trifluridine 568
Trilostane 520–521
Trimethoprim *151*, 179, 180, *201*
- antiprotozoal dosage *239*

Trimethoprim-sulfonamide 179, 180
- and imipenem interaction 168

Tropicamide 569
Tropisetron 475
Trypan blue *238*, 244
Tubulin-binding agents 335–340
'Two neurone' rule of ANS 59
Tylosin 178
Tyrosine kinase-associated receptors *9*

U

Ulcerative stomatitis, antibacterial drug choice *153*
Ultralente insulin 511–512
Unfractionated heparin 453–455
United Kingdom, reporting adverse drug reactions (ADRs) 57
United States of America, reporting adverse drug reactions (ADRs) 57
Ureidopenicillins 163
Urinary retention, opioid analgesics 315
Urinary tract infection, antibacterial drug choice *153*
Urine glucose test 168
Urine pH 33
- drug interactions mechanisms 17

Urine spraying in cats 145–146
Urogenital parasites *252*
Ursodeoxycholic acid (ursodiol) 491–492
University of Wisconsin-Madison chemotherapy protocol 365

V

Vaccines
- adverse drug reactions (ADRs) 46, 50, 54
- immune response genes 54

Valproic acid *9*, 377
Vancomycin 169
Vapour pressure, inhalational anesthesia 84–85
Vascular actions of acetylcholine (ACh) 65
Vasoactive intestinal peptide (VIP) *64*
Vasodilators 402–404
- with additional properties 411–412
- pimobendan 399
- pure 404–411

Vecuronium bromide *75–77*
Vedaprofen 293, **303**
Ventricular arrhythmias 426, *427*
Ventricular relaxation *see* Positive lusitropic agents
Verapamil 443–444
- adverse effects 50, 51, **444**
- clinical applications 427, 443
- drug efflux inhibition 211
- drug interactions 275, 322, 333, 444, 479
- formulations and dose rates *427*, 443–444
- inhibition of drug metabolising enzymes 17, 33
- mechanism of action 9, 443
- pharmacokinetics 11, 444

Veterinarian–client–patient relationship (VCPR) 24–25
Vinblastine *333*, *336*, **337–338**
Vincristine 333, *336*, **336–337**
Vinorelbine 338
Vitamin D 503–504
- oral preparations 507–508
- receptor *9*

Volume of distribution (*V*) 2, 3, 31, 32, 34, 35, 39–40
Vomit center 469
Vomiting
- cisplatin toxicity *356*
- opioid analgesics 314, 321

Voriconazole 189, **193**
- adverse effects 191
- pharmacokinetics 190

W

Warfarin 455–456
Websites 11
- regulatory agencies 11, *12*

White soft paraffin 486
Wolf–Chaikoff effect 503
Wounds, antibacterial drug choice *153*

X

Xanthine derivative glial cell modulators 146–147
Xylazine *71*, 120–124
- atipamezole as antidote to 74
- and nicergoline interaction 144

Y

Yohimbine 124
- adrenoceptor antagonist 71
- amitraz antidote 224

Z

Zafirlukast 467–468
Zero-order process 33–34
Zileuton 467–468
Zinc 494
Zolazepam 118–120
Zonisamide *368*, 378–379